A TEXT-BOOK

of

VETERINARY ANATOMY

BY

SEPTIMUS SISSON, S.B., V.S.

PROFESSOR OF COMPARATIVE ANATOMY IN OHIO STATE UNIVERSITY, COLUMBUS, OHIO

MEMBER OF THE AMERICAN ASSOCIATION OF ANATOMISTS

WITH 588 ILLUSTRATIONS

MANY IN COLORS

PHILADELPHIA AND LONDON

W. B. SAUNDERS COMPANY

1910

ILLUSTRATED &

PUBLISHED BY

E-KİTAP PROJESİ & CHEAPEST BOOKS

www.facebook.com/EKitapProjesi

www.cheapestboooks.com

Copyright, 2016

by

e-Kitap Projesi

Istanbul

ISBN:

978-625-6629-36-3

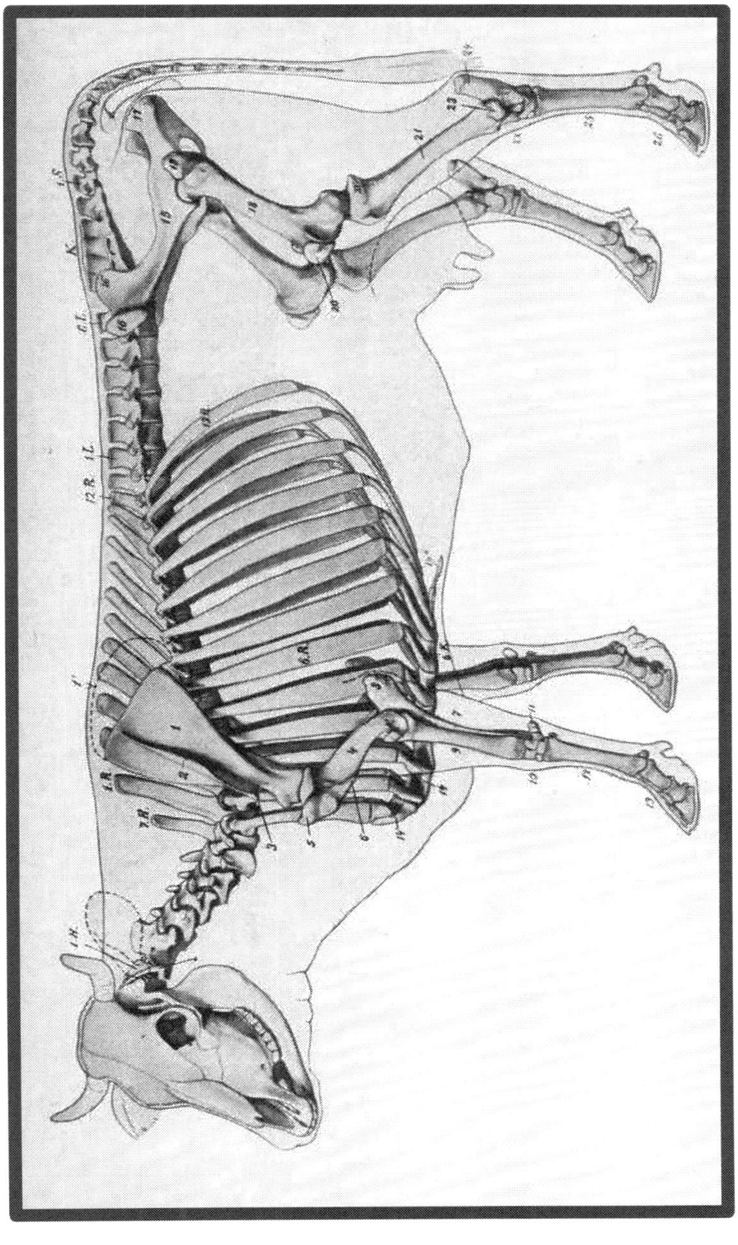

TO

KATHERINE OLDHAM SISSON

IN GRATEFUL RECOGNITION OF CONSTANT
INSPIRATION AND ENCOURAGEMENT
THIS BOOK IS DEDICATED

BY THE AUTHOR

PREFACE

THE lack of a modern and well-illustrated book on the structure of the principal domestic animals has been acutely felt for a long time by teachers, students, and practitioners of veterinary medicine. The work here offered is the expression of a desire to close this gap in our literature.

The study of frozen sections and of material which has been hardened by intravascular injection of formalin has profoundly modified our views concerning the natural shape of many of the viscera and has rendered possible much greater precision in topographic statements. The experience of the author during the last ten years, in which almost all of the material used for dissection and for frozen sections in the anatomical laboratory of this University has been hardened with formalin, has demonstrated that many of the current descriptions of the organs in animals contain the same sort of errors as those which prevailed in regard to similar structures in man previous to the adoption of modern methods of preparation.

While the method of treatment of the subject is essentially systematic, topography is not by any means neglected either in text or illustrations; it is hoped that this will render the book of value to the student in his clinical courses and to the practitioner. Embryological and histological data have been almost entirely excluded, since it was desired to offer a text-book of convenient size for the student and a work of ready reference for the practitioner. It is believed that the use of black type for the names of important structures and of small print for certain details or matter of secondary importance will prove useful in this respect.

Veterinary anatomical nomenclature is at present quite chaotic in English-speaking countries. In this work an attempt is made to eliminate some terms which do not appear to the author to fulfil any useful purpose, and others which are clearly erroneous or otherwise undesirable. In many cases the terms agreed upon by the Congresses at Baden and Stuttgart are adopted either in the original Latin or in anglicized form; otherwise these terms are added in parenthesis. The author favors the substantial adoption of this terminology, but considered it desirable to offer a sort of transitional stage at present.

The original illustrations are chiefly reproductions of photographs, many of which were taken by Mr. F. H. Haskett. The preparation of the pictures for reproduction was carried out by Messrs. J. V. Alteneder and W. J. Norris. The author takes pleasure in expressing his appreciation of the care and skill exercised by these gentlemen in this often difficult task.

The author is under great obligation to Professors Ellenberger and Baum in Dresden, to Professor Schmaltz in Berlin, and to their publishers for permission to use or to copy figures from their most excellent works. Their generosity in this matter has made it possible to supply this text with a larger number of high-class illustrations than is to be found in any other. A few figures have been taken from other sources, and proper credit has been given in each case.

For checking over certain data and for assistance in the correction of the proofs the author is much indebted to his associate, Dr. F. B. Hadley.

The author desires to express his high appreciation of the determination and constant effort of the publishers to do all in their power to render the book worthy of favorable reception by the profession for whom it is intended.

OHIO STATE UNIVERSITY, COLUMBUS, OHIO
September, 1910

SEPTIMUS SISSON.

CONTENTS

INTRODUCTION

OSTEOLOGY

ARTHROLOGY

THE MUSCULAR SYSTEM—MYOLOGY

SPLANCHNOLOGY—THE DIGESTIVE SYSTEM

THE RESPIRATORY SYSTEM

THE UROGENITAL SYSTEM

THE MALE GENITAL ORGANS

THE FEMALE GENITAL ORGANS

ANGIOLOGY

NEUROLOGY.—THE NERVOUS SYSTEM

THE RESPIRATORY SYSTEM

THE UROGENITAL SYSTEM

THE MALE GENITAL ORGANS

THE FEMALE GENITAL ORGANS

ANGIOLOGY

NEUROLOGY.—THE NERVOUS SYSTEM

ÆSTHESIOLOGY

VETERINARY ANATOMY

INTRODUCTION

Anatomy is the branch of biological science which deals with the form and structure of organisms, both animal and vegetal. It is therefore in close correlation with physiology, which treats of the functions of the body.

Etymologically the word "anatomy" signifies the cutting apart or disassociating of parts of the body. In the earlier phases of its development anatomy was necessarily a purely descriptive science, based on such observations as were possible with the unaided eye and simple dissecting instruments—the scalpel, forceps, and the like. At this time, therefore, the term adequately expressed the nature of the subject. But as the scope of the science extended and the body of anatomical knowledge grew, subdivisions became necessary and new terms were introduced to designate special fields and methods of work. With the introduction of the microscope and its accessories it became possible to study the finer details of structure and minute organisms hitherto unknown, and this field of inquiry rapidly developed into the science of **microscopic anatomy** or **histology** as conventionally distinguished from **gross** or **macroscopic anatomy**. In the same way the study of the changes which organisms undergo during their development soon attained sufficient importance to be regarded on practical grounds as a separate branch known as **embryology**.

This term is usually limited in its application to the earlier phases of development during which the tissues and organs are formed. The term **ontogeny** is used to designate the entire development of the individual. The ancestral history or **phylogeny** of the species is constituted by the evolutionary changes which it has undergone as disclosed by the geological record.

Comparative anatomy is the description and comparison of the structure of animals, and forms the basis for their classification. By this means—including extinct forms in the scope of inquiry—it has been possible to show the genetic relationship of various groups of animals and to elucidate the significance of many facts of structure which are otherwise quite obscure. The deductions concerning the general laws of form and structure derived from comparative anatomical studies constitute the science of **morphology** or **philosophical anatomy**. The morphologist, however, deals only with such anatomical details as are necessary to form a basis for his generalizations. The anatomical knowledge required in the practice of medicine and surgery is evidently of a different character and must include many details which are of no particular interest to the morphologist.

Special anatomy is the description of the structure of a single type or species, *e. g.*, anthropotomy, hippotomy.

Veterinary anatomy is the branch which deals with the form and structure of the principal domesticated animals. It is usually pursued with regard to professional requirements, and is therefore largely descriptive in character. As a matter of convenience the horse is generally selected as the type to be studied in detail and to form a basis for comparison of the more essential differential characters in the other animals.

Two chief methods of study are employed—the **systematic** and the **topographic**. In the former the body is regarded as consisting of systems of organs or apparatus which are similar in origin and structure and are associated in the performance of certain functions. The divisions of **systematic anatomy** are:

1. Osteology
2. Arthrology
3. Myology
4. Splanchnology
    (1) Digestive System
    (2) Respiratory System
    (3) Urogenital System
        (*a*) Urinary Organs
        (*b*) Genital Organs

. Angiology

. Neurology

5. Æsthesiology
    (1) Sense Organs
    (2) Common Integument.

The term **topographic anatomy** designates the methods by which the relative positions of the various parts of the body are accurately determined. It presupposes a fair working knowledge of systematic anatomy.

Descriptive Terms.—In order to indicate precisely the position and direction of parts of the body, certain descriptive terms are employed, and must be understood at the outset. In the explanation of these terms it is assumed here that they apply to a quadruped such as the horse in the ordinary standing position. The surface directed toward the plane of support (the ground) is termed **inferior** or **ventral,** and the opposite surface is **superior** or **dorsal**; the relations of parts in this direction are named accordingly. The longitudinal **median plane** divides the body into similar halves. A structure or surface which is nearer than another to the median plane is **internal** or **medial** to it, and an object or surface which is further than another from the median plane is **external** or **lateral** to it. Planes parallel to the median plane are **sagittal.** Transverse or **segmental** planes cut the long axis of the body perpendicular to the median plane, or an organ or limb at right angles to its long axis. A frontal plane is perpendicular to the median and transverse planes. The head end of the body is termed **anterior, cephalic,** or **cranial**; and the tail end **posterior** or **caudal**; relations of structures with regard to the longitudinal axis of the body are designated accordingly. Certain terms are used in a special sense as applied to the limbs. **Proximal** and **distal** express relative distances of parts from the axis of the body. The anterior face of the thoracic limb from the elbow downward is also termed dorsal, and the opposite face **volar.** In the corresponding part of the pelvic limb the terms are dorsal and **plantar** respectively. In the same regions radial and ulnar (thoracic limb), tibial and **fibular** (pelvic limb), may be used to designate that side of the extremity on which the corresponding bone is situated; they are therefore equivalent respectively to internal or medial and external or lateral in the animals with which we are concerned.

It is evidently advantageous to employ terms which are as far as possible independent of the position of the body in space and capable of general application, *e. g.*, dorsal, ventral, proximal, etc. It is also desirable that the terms internal and external be reserved to indicate relations of depth in cavities or organs, and medial and lateral to designate relations to the median plane. Such terms are coming into more extensive use in human and veterinary anatomy, but the older nomenclature is very firmly established and cannot well be discarded at once and entirely.

OSTEOLOGY

THE SKELETON

The term **skeleton** is applied to the framework of hard structures which supports and protects the soft tissues of animals. In the descriptive anatomy of the higher animals it is usually restricted to the bones and cartilages, although the ligaments which bind these together might well be included.

In zoölogy the term is used in a much more comprehensive sense, and includes all the harder supporting and protecting structures. When the latter are situated externally, they form an **exoskeleton,** derived from the ectoderm. Examples of this are the shells and chitinous coverings of many invertebrates, the scales of fishes, the shields of turtles, and the feathers, hair, and hoofs of the higher vertebrates. The **endoskeleton** (with which we have to deal at present) is embedded in the soft tissues. It is derived chiefly from the mesoderm, but includes the notochord or primitive axial skeleton, which is of entodermal origin.

The skeleton may be divided primarily into three parts: (1) axial; (2) appendicular; (3) splanchnic.

The **axial skeleton** comprises the vertebral column, ribs, sternum, and skull.

The **appendicular skeleton** includes the bones of the limbs.

The **splanchnic skeleton** consists of certain bones developed in the substance of some of the viscera or soft organs, *e. g.*, the os penis of the dog and the os cordis of the ox.

The **number** of the bones of the skeleton of an animal varies with age, owing to the fusion during growth of skeletal elements which are separate in the fœtus or the young subject. Even in adults of the same species numerical variations occur, *e. g.*, the tarsus of the horse may consist of six or seven bones, and the carpus of seven or eight; in all the domestic mammals the number of coccygeal vertebræ varies considerably.

The bones are commonly divided into four **classes** according to their shape and function.

(1) **Long bones** (Ossa longa) are typically of elongated cylindrical form with enlarged extremities. They occur in the limbs, where they act as supporting columns and as levers. The cylindrical part, termed the shaft or body (Corpus), is tubular, and incloses the **medullary cavity,** which contains the medulla or marrow.

(2) **Flat bones** (Ossa plana) are expanded in two directions. They furnish sufficient area for the attachment of muscles and afford protection to the organs which they cover.

(3) **Short bones** (Ossa brevia), such as those of the carpus and tarsus, present somewhat similar dimensions in length, breadth, and thickness. Their chief function appears to be that of diffusing concussion. Sesamoid bones, which are developed in the capsules of some joints or in tendons, may be included in this group. They diminish friction or change the direction of tendons.

(4) **Irregular bones.** This group would include bones of irregular shape, such as the vertebræ and the bones of the cranial base; they are median and unpaired. Their functions are various and not so clearly specialized as those of the preceding classes.

This classification is not entirely satisfactory; some bones, *e. g.*, the ribs, are not clearly provided for, and others might be variously placed.

STRUCTURE OF BONES[1]

Bones consist chiefly of bone tissue, but considered as organs they present also an enveloping membrane, termed the **periosteum**, the **medulla** or **marrow**, vessels, and nerves.

The architecture of bone can be studied best by means of longitudinal and cross-sections. These show that the bone consists of an external shell of dense **compact substance**, within which is the more loosely arranged **spongy substance.**

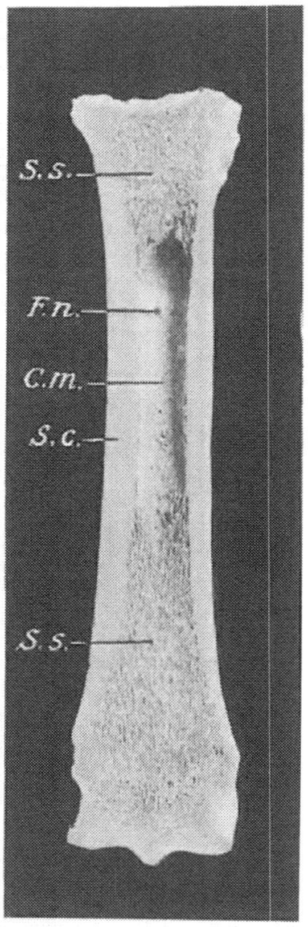

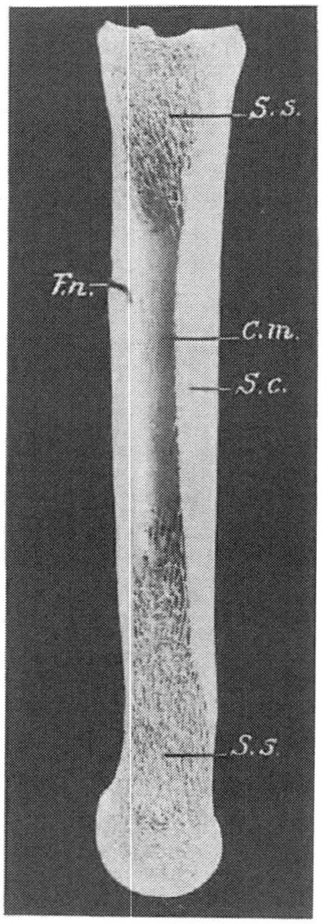

FIG. 1.—FRONTAL SECTION OF LARGE METATARSAL BONE OF HORSE, POSTERIOR PART.

FIG. 2.—SAGITTAL SECTION OF LARGE METATARSAL BONE OF HORSE.

S.c., Compact substance; *S.s.*, spongy substance; *C.m.*, medullary cavity; *F.n.*, nutrient foramen. Note the greater thickness of the compact substance of the inner and anterior parts of the shaft.

In typical long bones the shaft is hollowed to form the **medullary cavity** (Cavum medullare).

The **compact substance** (Substantia compacta) differs greatly in thickness in various situations, in conformity with the stresses and strains to which the bone is subjected. In the long bones it is thickest in the middle part of the shaft and thins out toward the extremities. On the latter the layer is very thin, and is especially dense and smooth on joint surfaces.

[1] Only the gross structure is discussed here. For the microscopic structure reference is to be made to histological works.

The **spongy substance** (Substantia spongiosa) consists of delicate bony plates and spicules which run in various directions and intercross. These plates are definitely arranged with regard to mechanical requirements, so that systems of pressure and tension plates can be recognized, in conformity with the lines of pressure and the pull of tendons and ligaments respectively. The intervals (marrow spaces) between the plates are occupied by marrow. The spongy substance forms the bulk of short bones and of the extremities of long bones; in the latter it is not confined to the ends, but extends a variable distance along the shaft also. Some bones (Ossa pneumatica) contain **air-spaces** or **sinuses** within the compact substance instead of spongy bone and marrow. In certain situations the two compact layers of flat bones are not separated by spongy bone, but fuse with each other; in some cases of this kind the bone is so thin as to be translucent, or may even undergo absorption, producing an actual deficiency.

The flat bones of the cranial vault and sides are composed of an outer layer of ordinary compact substance, an inner layer of very dense bone, the **tabula vitrea,** and between these a variable amount of spongy bone, here termed **diploë**.

The **periosteum** is the membrane which invests the outer surface of bone, except where it is covered with cartilage. It consists of an outer protective fibrous layer, and an inner cellular osteogenic layer. During active growth the osteogenic layer is well developed, but later it becomes much reduced. The fibrous layer varies much in thickness, being in general thickest in exposed situations. The adhesion of the periosteum to the bone also differs greatly in various places; it is usually very thin and easily detached where it is thickly covered with muscular tissue which has little or no attachment. The degree of vascularity conforms to the activity of the periosteum.

The **marrow** (Medulla ossium) occupies the interstices of the spongy bone and the medullary cavity of the long bones. There are two varieties in the adult—red and yellow. In the young subject there is only **red marrow** (Medulla ossium rubra), but later this is replaced in the medullary cavity by **yellow marrow** (Medulla ossium flava). The red marrow contains several types of characteristic cells and is a blood-forming substance, while the yellow is practically ordinary adipose tissue.

Since yellow marrow is formed by regressive changes in red marrow, including fatty infiltration and degeneration of the characteristic cells, we find transitional forms or stages in the process. In aged or badly nourished subjects the marrow may undergo gelatinous degeneration, resulting in the formation of gelatinous marrow.

Vessels and Nerves.—It is customary to recognize two sets of **arteries**—the **periosteal** and the **medullary.** The former ramify in the periosteum and give off innumerable small branches which enter minute openings (Volkmann's canals) on the surface and reach the Haversian canals of the compact substance. Other branches enter the extremities of the long bones and supply the spongy bone and marrow in them. In the case of the larger bones—and especially the long bones—the large **medullary** or **nutrient artery** enters at the so-called **nutrient foramen** (Foramen nutricium), passes in a canal (Canalis nutricius) through the compact substance, and ramifies in the marrow; its branches anastomose with the central branches of the periosteal set. The larger **veins** of the spongy bone do not, as a rule, accompany the arteries, but emerge chiefly near the articular surfaces. Within the bone they are destitute of valves.

The **lymph-vessels** form perivascular channels in the periosteum and the Haversian canals of the compact substance. Lymph-spaces exist at the periphery of the marrow.

The **nerves** appear to be distributed chiefly to the blood-vessels. Special nerve-endings (Vater-Pacini corpuscles) in the periosteum are to be regarded as sensory, and probably are concerned in mediating the muscle sense (Kopsch).

DEVELOPMENT AND GROWTH OF BONE[1]

The primitive embryonal skeleton consists of cartilage and fibrous tissue, in which the bones develop. The process is termed **ossification** or **osteogenesis**, and is effected essentially by bone-producing cells, called **osteoblasts**. It is customary, therefore, to designate as **membrane bones** those which are developed in fibrous tissue, and as **cartilage bones** those which are preformed in cartilage. The principal membrane bones are those of the roof and sides of the cranium and most of the bones of the face. The cartilage bones comprise, therefore, most of the skeleton. Correspondingly we distinguish **intramembranous** and **endochondral ossification.**

In intramembranous development the process begins at a definite **center of ossification** where the cells (osteoblasts) surround themselves with a deposit of bone. The process extends from this center to the periphery of the future bone, thus producing a network of bony trabeculæ. The trabeculæ rapidly thicken and coalesce, forming a bony plate which is separated from the adjacent bones by persistent fibrous tissue. The superficial part of the original tissue becomes periosteum, and on the deep face of this successive layers of periosteal bone are formed by osteoblasts until the bone attains its definitive thickness.

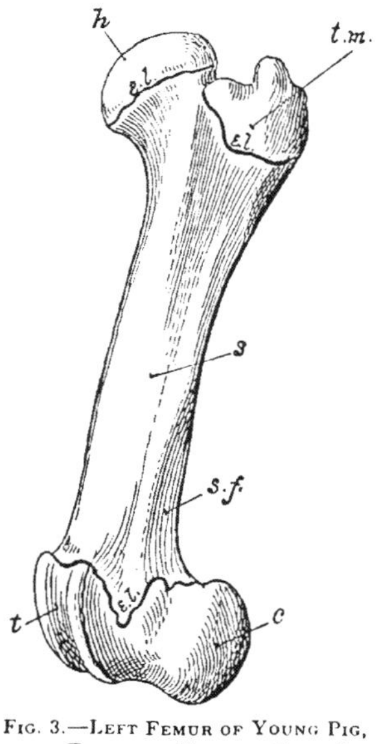

FIG. 3.—LEFT FEMUR OF YOUNG PIG, EXTERNAL VIEW, TO SHOW DIVISION OF A LONG BONE INTO SHAFT (*s*) AND EXTREMITIES.

Proximal extremity consists of two parts, head (*h*) and trochanter major (*t. m.*), which have separate centers of ossification. Distal extremity consists of trochlea (*t*) and condyles (*c*); *e.l.*, epiphyseal cartilages; *s.f.*, supracondyloid fossa.

In endochondral ossification the process is fundamentally the same, but not quite so simple. Osteoblasts emigrate from the deep face of the perichondrium or primitive periosteum into the cartilage and cause calcification of the matrix or ground-substance of the latter. Vessels extend into the calcifying area, the cartilage cells shrink and disappear, forming primary marrow cavities which are occupied by processes of the osteogenic tissue. There is thus formed a sort of scaffolding of calcareous trabeculæ on which the bone is constructed by the osteoblasts. At the same time perichondral bone is formed by the osteoblasts of the primitive periosteum. The calcified cartilage is broken down and absorbed through the agency of large cells called **osteoclasts,** and is replaced by bone deposited by the osteoblasts. The osteoclasts also cause absorption of the primitive bone, producing the marrow cavities; thus in the case of the long bones the primitive central spongy bone is largely absorbed to form the medullary cavity of the shaft, and persists chiefly in the extremities. Destruction of the central part and formation of subperiosteal bone continue until the shaft of the bone has completed its growth.

A typical long bone is developed from three primary centers of ossification, one for the diaphysis or shaft and one for each epiphysis or extremity. Many bones have secondary centers from which processes or apophyses develop.

The foregoing outline accounts for the growth of bones except in regard to length. Increase in length may be explained briefly as follows: Provision for continued ossification at either end of the diaphysis is made by a layer of actively growing cartilage—the **epiphyseal cartilage**—which intervenes between the diaph-

[1] Only a brief general statement of osteogenesis can be made here; details must be sought in embryological literature.

ysis and the epiphysis. It is evident that so long as this cartilage persists and grows, new bone may continue to be formed at its expense, and increase of length is possible. When the epiphyseal cartilage ceases to grow, it undergoes ossification, the bone is consolidated, and no further increase in length is possible. This fusion takes place at fairly definite periods in the various bones, and it is of value to know the usual times at which it occurs in the larger bones of the limbs at least.

After the bones have reached their full size, the periosteum becomes relatively reduced and inactive so far as its osteogenic layer is concerned; the bone-forming function may be stimulated by various causes, as is well seen in the healing of fractures and the occurrence of bony enlargements.

CHEMICAL COMPOSITION OF BONE

Dried bone consists of organic and inorganic matter in the ratio of 1 : 2 approximately. The animal matter gives toughness and elasticity, the mineral matter hardness, to the bone tissue. Removal of the organic matter by heat does not change the general form of a bone, but reduces the weight by about one-third, and makes it very fragile. Conversely, decalcification, while not affecting the form and size of the bone, renders it soft and pliable. The animal matter when boiled yields gelatin. The following table represents the composition in 100 parts of ox bone of average quality:

Gelatin	33.30
Phosphate of lime	57.35
Carbonate of lime	3.85
Phosphate of magnesia	2.05
Carbonate and chlorid of sodium	3.45
	100.00

PHYSICAL PROPERTIES OF BONE

Fresh dead bone has a yellowish-white color; when macerated or boiled and bleached, it is white. The specific gravity of fresh compact bone is a little over 1.93. It is very hard and resistant to pressure; a 5-millimeter cube of compact bone of the ox will resist pressure up to 852 pounds, if the pressure be applied in the line of the lamellæ (Rauber). Its tensile strength is estimated to be nearly twice that of oak.

DESCRIPTIVE TERMS

The surfaces of the bones present a great variety of eminences and depressions, as well as perforations. The prominences and cavities may be articular, or non-articular, furnishing attachment to muscles, tendons, ligaments or fascia. A number of descriptive terms are used to designate these features, and the following are some of those in general use:

Process (Processus) is a general term for a prominence.

A **tuberosity** (Tuber, Tuberositas) is a large, rounded projection; a **tubercle** (Tuberculum) is a smaller one.

The term **trochanter** is applied to a few prominences, *e. g.*, the trochanters of the femur.

A **spine** (Spina) or **spinous process** (Processus spinosus) is a pointed projection.

A **crest** (Crista) is a sharp ridge.

A **line** (Linea) is a very small ridge.

A **head** (Caput) is a rounded articular enlargement at the end of a bone; it may be joined to the shaft by a constricted part, the **neck** (Collum).

A **condyle** (Condylus) is an articular eminence which is somewhat cylindrical; a non-articular projection in connection with a condyle may be termed an **epicondyle**.

A trochlea is a pulley-like articular mass.

A glenoid cavity (Cavitas glenoidalis) is a shallow articular depression, and a cotyloid cavity or acetabulum is a deeper one.

The term facet is commonly applied to articular surfaces of small extent, especially when they are not strongly concave or convex.

The terms fossa, fovea, groove or sulcus, and impression are applied to various forms of depressions.

A foramen is a perforation for the transmission of vessels, nerves, etc.

A sinus or antrum is an air-cavity.

Other terms, such as canal, fissure, notch, etc., require no explanation.[1]

VERTEBRAL COLUMN

The vertebral column (Columna vertebralis) is the fundamental part of the skeleton. It consists of a chain of median, unpaired, irregular bones which extends from the skull to the end of the tail. In the adult certain vertebræ have become fused to form a single bony mass with which the pelvic girdle articulates. Vertebræ so fused are termed **fixed** or **"false" vertebræ** (Vertebræ immobiles), as distinguished from the **movable** or **"true" vertebræ** (Vertebræ mobiles).

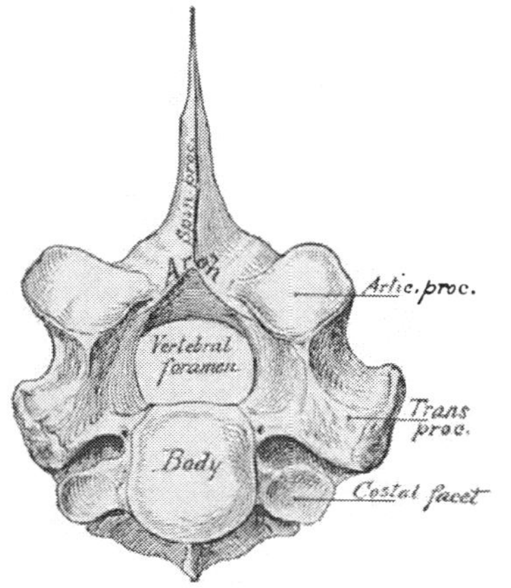

FIG. 4.—FIRST THORACIC VERTEBRÆ OF HORSE. To illustrate plan of structure of vertebræ.

The column is subdivided for description into **five regions,** which are named according to the part of the body in which they are placed. Thus the vertebræ are designated as **cervical, thoracic** (or dorsal), **lumbar, sacral,** and **coccygeal** or **caudal** (Vertebræ cervicales, thoracales, lumbales, sacrales, coccygeæ). The number of vertebræ in a given species is fairly constant in each region except the last, so that the **vertebral formula** may be expressed (for the horse, for example) as follows:

$$C_7T_{18}L_6S_5Cy_{15-21}.$$

The vertebræ in a given region have special characters by which they may be distinguished from those of other regions, and individual vertebræ have characters which are more or less clearly recognizable. All typical vertebræ have a common plan of structure, which must first be understood. The parts of which a vertebra consists are the body or **centrum,** the **arch,** and the **processes.**

The body (Corpus vertebræ) is the more or less cylindrical mass on which the other parts are constructed. The anterior and posterior extremities of the body are attached to the adjacent vertebræ by intervertebral fibro-cartilages, and are usually convex and concave respectively. The dorsal surface is flattened and enters into the formation of the vertebral canal, while the ventral aspect is rounded laterally, and is in relation to various muscles and viscera. In the thoracic region the body presents two pairs of demifacets (Foveæ costales) at the extremities for articulation with the heads of two pairs of ribs.

The arch (Arcus vertebræ) is constructed on the dorsal aspect of the body. It consists originally of two lateral halves, each of which is considered to consist of a pedicle and a lamina. The pedicles form the lateral parts of the arch, and are

[1] As might be expected from the history of anatomy, a good many of these terms are more or less interchangeable; furthermore, a given skeletal feature may differ greatly in various species.

cut into in front and behind by the **vertebral notches** (Incisura vertebralis cranialis, caudalis). The notches of two adjacent vertebræ form **intervertebral foramina** for the passage of the spinal nerves and vessels; in some vertebræ, however, these are complete foramina instead of notches. The laminæ are plates which complete the arch dorsally, uniting with each other medially at the root of the spinous process.

The body and the arch form a bony ring which incloses the **vertebral foramen** (Foramen vertebrale); the series of vertebral rings, together with the ligaments which unite them, inclose the **vertebral canal** (Canalis vertebralis), which contains the spinal cord and its coverings and vessels.

The **articular processes,** two **anterior** and two **posterior** (Processus articulares craniales, caudales), project from the borders of the arch on either side. They present joint surfaces adapted to those of adjacent vertebræ, and the remaining surface is roughened for muscular and ligamentous attachment.

The **spinous process** (Processus spinosus) is single, and projects dorsally from the middle of the arch. It varies greatly in form, size, and direction in different vertebræ. It furnishes attachment to muscles and ligaments.

The **transverse processes** (Processus transversi) are two in number and project laterally from the side of the arch, or from the junction of the arch and body. In the thoracic region each has a facet for articulation with the tubercle of a rib (Fovea costalis transversalis). They also give attachment to muscles and ligaments.

Some vertebræ have also a **ventral** or **hæmal spine.**

Mammillary processes (Processus mammillares) are found in most animals on the last thoracic and anterior lumbar vertebræ between the transverse and anterior articular processes or on the latter.

Accessory processes (Processus accessorii), when present, are situated between the transverse and posterior articular processes.

Development.—The vertebræ are developed by ossification in the cartilage which surrounds the notochord and forms the sides of the neural canal. There are **three primary centers of ossification,** one for the body and one for each side of the arch. **Secondary centers** appear later for the summit of the spinous process (except in the cervical region), the extremities of the transverse processes, and the thin epiphyseal plates at the extremities of the body.

Sometimes there are at first two centers for the body which soon fuse. The process of ossification extends from the lateral centers to form not only the corresponding part of the arch, but also the processes and a part of the body next to the root of the arch (Radix arcus). In the horse and ox the body and arch are usually fused at birth, but the epiphyses do not fuse till growth is complete. In the pig, sheep, and dog the body and arch are united at birth by cartilage (neurocentral synchondrosis), but fuse in the first few months.

THE RIBS

The **ribs** (Costæ) are elongated curved bones which form the skeleton of the lateral thoracic walls. They are arranged serially in pairs which usually correspond in number to the thoracic vertebræ. Each articulates dorsally with the spine and is continued ventrally by a **costal cartilage.** Those which articulate with the sternum by means of their cartilages are termed **sternal** or **"true"** ribs (Costæ sternales s. veræ); the remainder are **asternal** or **"false"** ribs (Costæ asternales s. spuriæ). Ribs at the end of the series which have their ventral ends free in the abdominal wall are named **floating ribs** (Costæ fluctuantes). The intervals between the ribs are termed **intercostal spaces** (Spatia intercostalia).

A typical rib[1] consists of a **shaft** and two **extremities.** The **shaft** (Corpus costæ)

[1] The term is employed here, as is usual in descriptive anatomy, to designate only the bony part of the rib (Os costale); morphologically it includes the cartilaginous part also.

is band-like and varies much in length, breadth, and curvature. In the case of some ribs the curvature is not uniform, but is most accentuated at a certain point, termed the **angle of** the rib (Angulus costæ); this occurs at a variable distance from the vertebral end, and is usually marked by a rough ridge. The direction also varies; the first rib is almost vertical, while the remainder slope backward in increasing degree. The **external** surface is convex, and the **internal** flattened from edge to edge; on the latter, close to the posterior border, is the **costal groove** (Sulcus costalis), which fades out ventrally. It contains the intercostal vein. The **anterior** and **posterior borders** are thin and sharp on some ribs, rounded on others.

The **vertebral extremity** (Extremitas vertebralis) consists of the **head, neck,** and **tubercle.** The head (Capitulum costæ) is the actual end of the rib, and is rounded and somewhat enlarged. It presents two facets (Facies articularis capituli costæ) for articulation with the bodies of two adjacent thoracic vertebræ; these surfaces are separated by a groove in which the conjugal ligament is attached. The **neck** (Collum costæ) joins the head to the shaft. It varies in length and diameter. Its outer surface is rough, its inner smooth. The **tubercle** (Tuberculum costæ) projects backward at the junction of the neck and shaft. It has a facet (Facies articularis tuberculi costæ) for articulation with the transverse process of the posterior vertebra of the two with which the head articulates. The tubercle gradually approaches the head in the posterior ribs, and eventually fuses with it.

The **sternal extremity** (Extremitas sternalis) is commonly slightly enlarged, and has a rough depression in which the costal cartilage is embedded.

Development.—The ribs are ossified in cartilage from three centers—one each for the shaft (and sternal end), head, and tubercle; the third center does not occur in the last two ribs.

THE COSTAL CARTILAGES

These (Cartilagines costales) are bars of hyaline cartilage which continue the ribs. Those of the sternal ribs articulate with the sternum, while the remainder overlap and are attached to each other to form the **costal arch** (Arcus costalis)

THE STERNUM

The **sternum** or breast-bone is a median segmental bone which completes the skeleton of the thorax ventrally, and articulates with the cartilages of the sternal ribs laterally. It consists of six to eight bony segments (Sternebræ) connected by intervening cartilage in the young subject. Its form varies with that of the thorax in general and with the development of the clavicles in animals in which they are present. Its anterior extremity, the **manubrium sterni** or **presternum,** is specially affected by the latter factor, being broad and strong when the clavicles are well developed and articulate with it (as in man), relatively small and laterally compressed when they are absent (as in the horse) or rudimentary (as in the dog). The cartilages of the first pair of ribs articulate with it. The body or **mesosternum** (Corpus sterni) presents laterally, at the junction of the segments, concave facets (Incisuræ costales) for articulation with the cartilages of the sternal ribs. The posterior extremity or **metasternum** presents the **xiphoid** (or ensiform) **cartilage** (Processus xiphoideus); this is thin and plate-like, as in the horse and ox, or narrow and short, as in the pig and dog.

Development.—The cartilaginous sternum is formed by the fusion medially of two lateral bars which unite the ventral ends of the first eight or nine costal cartilages, and is primitively unsegmented. The manubrium ossifies from a single center, but the centers for the other segments appear to be primitively paired. The sternum never becomes completely ossified; details in regard to persisting cartilage will be given in the special descriptions. The layer of compact tissue is for the greater part very thin and the spongy substance is open-meshed and very vascular.

THE THORAX

The skeleton of the thorax comprises the thoracic vertebræ dorsally, the ribs and their cartilages laterally, and the sternum ventrally. The **thoracic cavity** (Cavum thoracis) resembles in shape an irregular truncated cone; it is compressed laterally, especially in front, and the dorsal wall or roof is much longer than the ventral wall or floor. The **anterior aperture** (Apertura thoracis cranialis) is bounded by the first thoracic vertebra dorsally, the first pair of ribs and their cartilages laterally, and the manubrium sterni ventrally. The **posterior aperture** (Apertura thoracis caudalis) is bounded by the last thoracic vertebra, the last pair of ribs, the costal arches, and the anterior part of the xiphoid cartilage.

It may be noted here that the diaphragm (which forms the partition between the thoracic and abdominal cavities) does not follow the costal arches in its posterior attachment, so that the posterior ribs enter also into the formation of the abdominal wall.

THE SKULL

The term skull is usually understood to include all of the bones of the head. The head consists of the cranium and the face, and it is therefore convenient to divide the bones into cranial and facial groups.

The **cranial bones** (Ossa cranii) inclose the brain with its membranes and vessels and the essential organs of hearing. They concur with the facial bones in forming the orbital and nasal cavities, in which the peripheral organs of sight and of smell are situated.

The **facial bones** (Ossa faciei) form the skeleton of the oral and nasal cavities, and also support the larynx and the root of the tongue.

Most of the bones of the skull are flat bones, developed in membrane; those of the cranial base may be classed as irregular, and are cartilage bones. Only two form permanent movable joints with other parts of the skull. The mandible or lower jaw-bone forms diarthrodial joints with the temporal bones, and the hyoid bone is attached to the latter by bars of cartilage. The other bones form immovable joints, most of which disappear with age.

In order to study the separate bones, skulls of young subjects are necessary, since later most of the lines of demarcation become effaced. The relations of each bone to its surroundings should be specially noted, since the final object is to understand the skull as a whole. In the descriptions which follow the skull is considered with its long axis horizontal, and that of the horse will serve as a type.

THE BONES OF THE THORACIC LIMB

The thoracic limb consists of four chief segments, viz., the shoulder girdle, the arm, the forearm, and the forefoot or manus.

The **shoulder girdle** (Cingulum extremitatis thoracicæ), when fully developed, consists of three bones—the **scapula** or shoulder-blade, the **coracoid,** and the **clavicle** or collar-bone. In the domesticated mammals only the scapula, a large, flat bone, is well developed, and the small coracoid element has fused with it, while the clavicle is either absent or is a small rudiment embedded in the mastoido-humeralis muscle. There is therefore no articulation of the shoulder with the axial skeleton.

The shoulder girdle is fully developed in birds and the lower mammals (monotremata). In the higher mammals the coracoid is reduced to the coracoid process of the scapula, and the development of the clavicle is in conformity with the function of the limb. Thus in typical quadrupeds, such as the horse and ox, in which the forelimbs are used only for support and locomotion, the clavicle is absent. Other animals which use these limbs for grasping, burrowing, climbing, etc. (*e. g.*, man, apes, moles), have well-developed clavicles which connect the scapula with the sternum.

The **arm** (Brachium) contains a single long bone, the **humerus** or arm bone.

In the **forearm** (Antibrachium) are two long bones, the **radius** and **ulna**. These vary in relative size and mobility. In the horse and ox the two bones are fused, and the lower part of the limb is fixed in the position of pronation. The radius is placed in front and supports the weight. The ulna is well developed only in its upper part, which forms a lever for the extensor muscles of the elbow. In the pig the ulna is the larger and longer of the two bones, but is closely attached to the back of the radius. In the dog the ulna is also well developed and a small amount of movement is possible between the two bones.

The forefoot or **hand** (Manus) consists of three subdivisions, viz., the **carpus, metacarpus,** and **digit or digits.**

The **carpus,** popularly termed the "knee" in animals, and homologous with the wrist of man, contains a group of short bones (Ossa carpi). These are typically eight in number and are arranged in two transverse rows—a proximal or antibrachial, and a distal or metacarpal. The bones of the proximal row, named from the radial to the ulnar side (*i. e.*, from within outward), are the **radial, intermediate, ulnar,** and **accessory** carpal bones. The bones of the distal row are designated numerically, in the same direction, as **first, second, third,** and **fourth** carpal bones.

This nomenclature, introduced by Gegenbaur, and now used largely by comparative anatomists, seems decidedly preferable to the variety of terms borrowed from human anatomy and based on the form of the bones in man. The following table of synonyms in common use is appended for comparison. The Latin terms and abbreviated notations are given in parenthesis.

Radial (Os carpi radiale, Cr)	Scaphoid
Intermediate (Os carpi intermedium, Ci)	Semilunar
Ulnar (Os carpi ulnare, Cu)	Cuneiform
Accessory (Os carpi accessorium, Ca)	Pisiform
First carpal (Os carpale primum, C1)	Trapezium
Second carpal (Os carpale secundum, C2)	Trapezoid
Third carpal (Os carpale tertium, C3)	Os magnum
Fourth carpal (Os carpale quartum, C4)	Unciform

The central carpal bone (Os carpi centrale) is omitted, since it is not a separate element in the animals under consideration here.

The **metacarpus** contains typically five **metacarpal bones** (Ossa metacarpalia I–V), one for each digit; they are long bones and are designated numerically from within outward. This arrangement occurs in the dog, although the first metacarpal is much smaller than the others, and the second and fifth are somewhat reduced. Further reduction has taken place in the other animals, resulting in the perissodactyl and artiodactyl forms. In the horse the first and fifth metacarpals are absent, the third is the large supporting metacarpal bone and carries the single digit, while the second and fourth are much reduced. In artiodactyls (*e. g.*, ox, sheep, pig) the third and fourth are the chief metacarpals and carry the well developed digits; they are fused in the ox and sheep. The others are variously reduced or absent as noted in the special descriptions to follow.

The fossil remains of the ancestors of the existing Equidæ illustrate in a most complete manner the reduction which has occurred in this respect. The earliest known ancestor of the horse, Eohippus or Hyracotherium of the Lower Eocene, had four well developed metacarpal bones, each of which carried a digit; the first metacarpal bone was small. Eleven intermediate stages show the gradual evolution of the race from this primitive animal, which was about the size of the domestic cat. There is reason to believe that earlier forms had five digits.

The digits (Digiti manus) are homologous with the fingers of man, and are typically five in number. They are designated numerically from the radial to the ulnar side, in correspondence with the metacarpus. The full number is present in the dog. In the ox and pig the third and fourth are well developed and support the weight, while the second and fifth are reduced. The existing horse has a single digit, the third of his polydactyl ancestors. The skeleton of each fully developed digit consists of three **phalanges** and certain **sesamoid** bones. The **first** or **proximal phalanx** (Phalanx prima) articulates with the corresponding metacarpal bone above and with the **second** or **middle phalanx** (Phalanx secunda) below. The **third** or **distal phalanx** (Phalanx tertia) is inclosed in the hoof or claw, and is modified to conform to the latter. The **sesamoid bones** (Ossa sesamoidea) are developed along the course of the flexor tendons or in the joint capsules. Two **proximal sesamoids** (Ossa sesamoidea phalangis primæ) occur at the flexor side of the metacarpo-phalangeal joint and form a pulley for the flexor tendon. The **distal sesamoids** (Ossa sesamoidea phalangis tertiæ) are similarly placed between the deep flexor tendon and the joint between the second and third phalanx; they are absent in the dog, which has a small sesamoid on the extensor side of the metacarpo-phalangeal joints, and often at the proximal interphalangeal joint also.

Numerous cases are recorded of the occurrence of supernumerary digits (hyperdactylism) in the horse and other animals. In some pigs, on the other hand, the two chief digits are fused, and the condition appears to be inherited.

THE BONES OF THE PELVIC LIMB

The pelvic limb, like the thoracic, consists of four segments, viz., the pelvic girdle, thigh, leg, and the hind foot or pes; the last is subdivided into tarsus, metatarsus, and digits.

The **pelvic girdle** (Cingulum extremitatis pelvinæ) consists of the **os coxæ** or hip bone, which joins its fellow of the opposite side ventrally at the symphysis pelvis, and articulates very firmly with the sacrum dorsally. The two coxal bones, together with the sacrum and the first two or three coccygeal vertebræ, constitute the bony pelvis. The os coxæ consists originally of three flat bones, the **ilium, ischium,** and **pubis,** which meet at the acetabulum, a large cotyloid cavity that articulates with the head of the femur. These three parts are fused before growth is complete, but are considered separately for convenience of description. The **ilium** (Os ilium) is situated in the lateral wall of the pelvis, the **pubis** (Os pubis) in the anterior part, and the **ischium** (Os ischii) in the posterior part of the ventral wall.

The **thigh** (Femur), like the arm, contains a single large, long bone, the **femur** or thigh bone (Os femoris). This articulates with the acetabulum above and the tibia and patella below.

The skeleton of the **leg** (Crus) comprises three bones (Ossa cruris), viz., the **tibia, fibula,** and **patella.** The **tibia** is a large prismatic long bone which supports the weight, and articulates below with the tibial tarsal bone. The **fibula** is situated along the outer border of the tibia, from which it is separated by the **interosseous space** of the leg. It is much more slender than the tibia and does not articulate with the femur. In the pig and dog it has a complete shaft and two extremities, but in the horse and ox it is much reduced and otherwise modified. The **patella** or "knee-cap" is a short bone which articulates with the trochlea of the distal end of the femur; it is to be regarded as a large sesamoid bone intercalated in the tendon of the quadriceps femoris muscle.

The **tarsus** or "hock" consists of a group of short bones (Ossa tarsi) numbering five to seven in the different animals. The proximal or crural row consists of two bones, the **tibial** and **fibular tarsals;** the former is situated at the inner or tibial side, and has a trochlea for articulation with the distal end of the tibia; the latter, situated externally, has a process, the **tuber calcis,** which projects upward and backward and constitutes a lever for the muscles which extend the hock joint. The distal or metatarsal row consists of four bones when seven tarsal elements are present, as in the pig and dog. They are best designated numerically as **first tarsal, second tarsal,** etc. The **central tarsal** is interposed between the rows.

The preceding terms are anglicized abbreviations of those introduced by Gegenbaur into comparative anatomy. The Latin names and synonyms are given in the following table.

Tibial (Os tarsi tibiale, Tt.)	Astragalus or Talus
Fibular (Os tarsi fibulare, Tf.)	Calcaneus or Os calcis
Central (Os tarsi centrale, Tc.)	Scaphoid or Navicular
First Tarsal (Os tarsale primum, T1)	First or internal cuneiform
Second Tarsal (Os tarsale secundum, T2)	Second or middle cuneiform
Third Tarsal (Os tarsale tertium, T3)	Third or external cuneiform
Fourth Tarsal (Os tarsale quartum, T4)	Cuboid.

The **metatarsal** and **digital bones** resemble in general those of the corresponding regions of the thoracic limb; the differential features will be noted in the special descriptions.

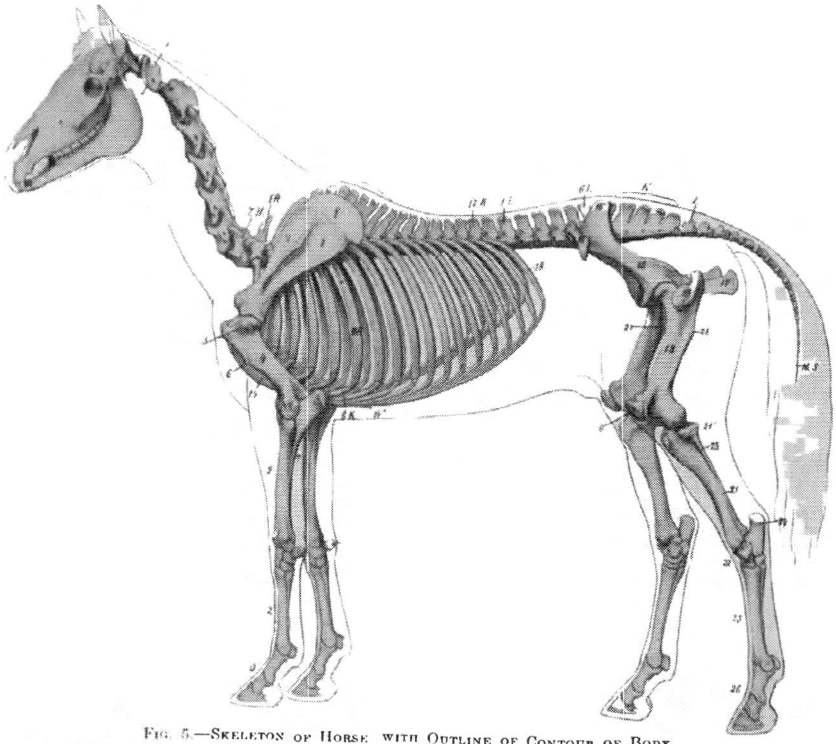

FIG. 5.—SKELETON OF HORSE WITH OUTLINE OF CONTOUR OF BODY.

1.H., Atlas; *7.H.*, seventh cervical Vertebra; *1.R.*, first thoracic vertebra; *17.R.*, seventeenth thoracic vertebra; *1.L.*, first lumbar vertebra; *6.L.*, sixth lumbar vertebra; *K*, sacrum; *1.S.*, first coccygeal vertebra; *16.S.*, sixteenth coccygeal vertebra; *6.R.*, sixth rib; *6.K.*, costal cartilage; *18.R.*, last rib; 1, scapula; 1', cartilage of scapula; 2, spine of scapula; 4, humerus; 4' external epicondyle of humerus; 5, external tuberosity of humerus; 6, deltoid tuberosity; 7, shaft of ulna; 8, olecranon; 9, radius; 10, carpus; 11, accessory carpal bone; 12, metacarpus; 13, digit; 14, sternum; 14", xiphoid cartilage; 15, ilium; 16, 16', external and internal angles of ilium; 17, ischium; 18, femur (shaft); 19, trochanter major; 27, trochanter minor; 28, trochanter tertius; 20, patella; 21, tibia (shaft); 21', external condyle of tibia; 23, fibula; 22, tarsus; 24, tuber calcis; 25, metatarsus; 26, digit. (After Ellenberger-Baum, Anat. für Künstler.)

THE SKELETON OF THE HORSE

The skeleton of the horse consists of 205 bones, as shown in the following table.

Vertebral column	54
Ribs	36
Sternum	1
Skull (including auditory ossicles)	34
Thoracic limbs	40
Pelvic limbs	40
	205

In this enumeration the average number of coccygeal vertebræ is taken to be 18, the temporal and os coxæ are not divided into parts, the usual number of carpal and tarsal elements is taken, and the sesamoids are included.

The Vertebral Column

The vertebral formula of the horse is $C_7T_{18}L_6S_5Cy_{15-21}$.

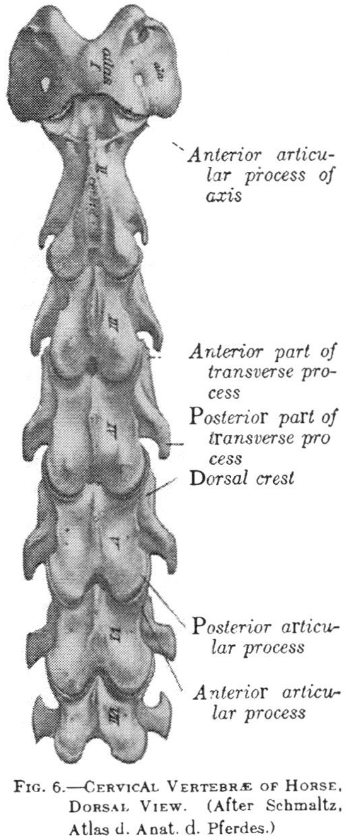

Fig. 6.—Cervical Vertebræ of Horse, Dorsal View. (After Schmaltz, Atlas d. Anat. d. Pferdes.)

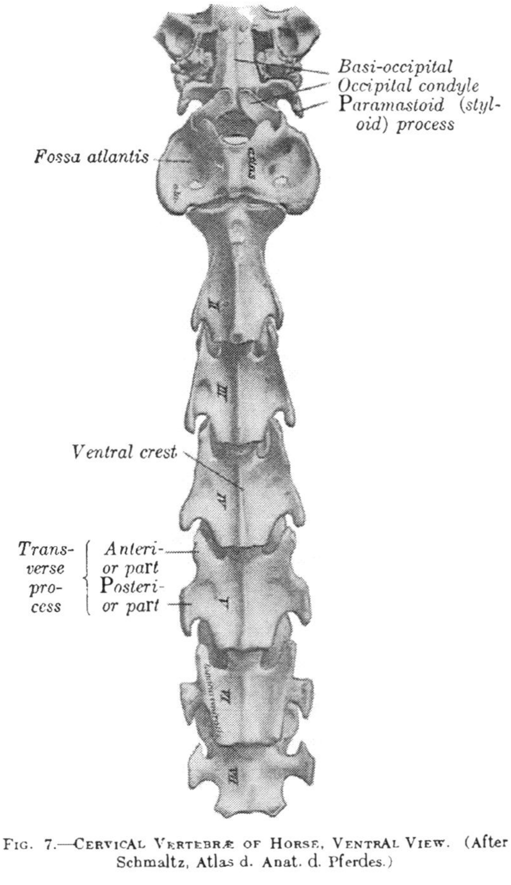

Fig. 7.—Cervical Vertebræ of Horse, Ventral View. (After Schmaltz, Atlas d. Anat. d. Pferdes.)

THE CERVICAL VERTEBRÆ

These are quadrangular, massive, and longer than the vertebræ of other regions; they decrease in length from the second to the last. The **third, fourth,** and **fifth** are typical, and have the following characters:

1. The **bodies** are long as compared with those of other vertebræ. Each presents a median **ventral spine** or **crest,** which becomes more prominent as it is traced backward, and is tuberculate at its posterior end. The **lateral aspect** is concave. The **dorsal surface** has a flat central area which is narrow in the middle of the vertebræ, and wide at either end; it gives attachment to the superior common ligament. On either side of this area is a groove which lodges the longitudinal spinal vein. These lateral grooves are connected at the middle of the surface by a transverse furrow, in which there are several foramina through which veins emerge from the spongy substance of the body. The **anterior extremity** presents a head which has an oval articular surface, strongly convex, and wider above than below. The **posterior extremity** is larger and has a nearly circular cotyloid cavity.

2. The **arches** are large and strong. They are perforated on either side by a

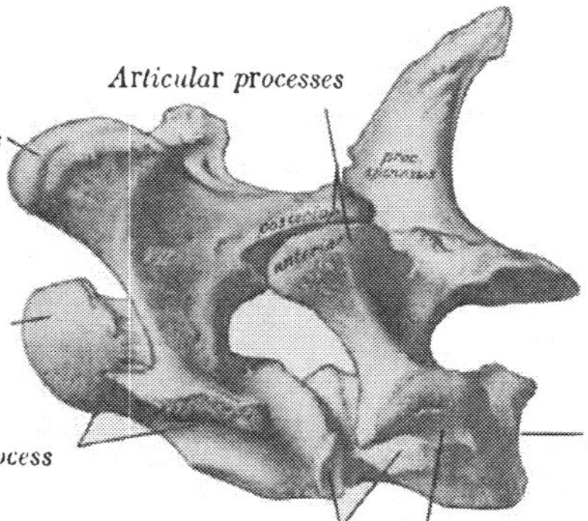

FIG. 8.—LAST CERVICAL AND FIRST THORACIC VERTEBRÆ OF HORSE, LATERAL VIEW. (After Schmaltz Atlas d. Anat. d. Pferdes.)

foramen which communicates with the foramen transversarium. The vertebral notches are large.

3. The **articular processes** are large. Their articular surfaces are extensive, oval in outline, and slightly concave; the anterior ones are directed upward and inward, the posterior downward and outward. The remaining surface is mainly roughened for ligamentous and muscular attachment. A crest connects the articular processes of the same side on the fourth and fifth; on the third it does not reach the anterior process.

4. The **transverse processes** are large and plate-like. Each arises by two roots, one from the arch and one from the body; between these is the **foramen transversarium,** through which the vertebral artery passes. The process divides externally into anterior and posterior branches, which are thickened and rough for muscular attachment.

5. The **spinous process** is represented by a crest (Crista spinosa), which widens behind, and is connected by ridges with the posterior articular processes.

The **sixth** cervical vertebra has the following distinctive features: It is shorter and wider than the fifth. The **arch** is large, especially posteriorly. The **posterior** articular processes are shorter, thicker and further apart; they are connected with the anterior ones by a thick ridge. The spinous process is less rudimentary; it is half an inch or more (ca. 1.5 cm.) in height. The transverse processes have three branches; the third part is a thick, almost sagittal plate, which forms with its fellow and the body a wide ventral groove on the posterior part of the vertebra; the other branches correspond to those of the typical vertebræ, but are short and thicker. The foramen transversarium is large; below its posterior end is a fossa. The ventral crest is small and is less prominent posteriorly.

The third branch of the transverse process and the fossa are sometimes absent on one side.

The seventh cervical vertebra is readily distinguished by the following characters: It is shorter and wider than the others. The body is flattened dorso-ventrally and wide, especially behind; here it has a demifacet on either side for articulation with part of the head of the first rib. The arch and its notches are large. The anterior articular processes are wider and longer than the posterior pair. The spinous process is an inch or more (ca. 3 cm.) in height. The transverse process is undivided, and has no foramen transversarium. The ventral crest is replaced by a pair of tubercles.

In some specimens a large foramen transversarium is present on one side or (rarely) on both.

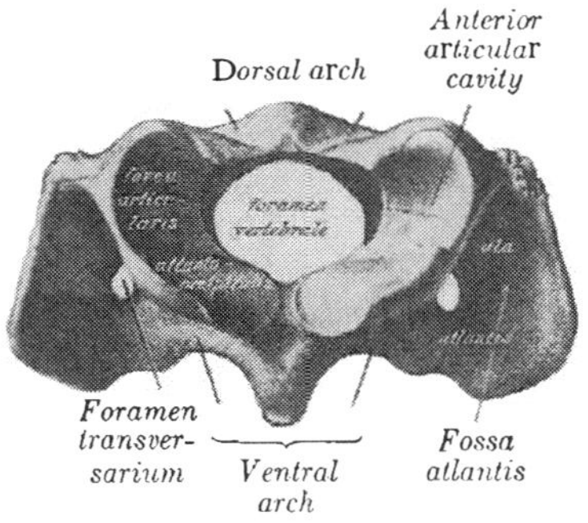

Fig. 9.—Atlas of Horse, Anterior View. (After Schmaltz, Atlas d. Anat. d. Pferdes.)

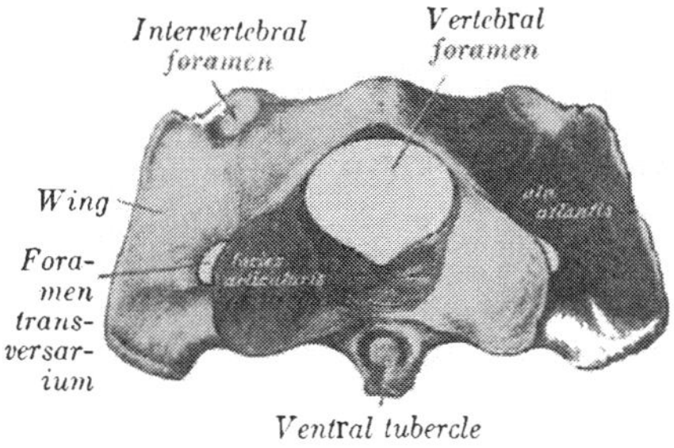

Fig. 10.—Atlas of Horse, Posterior View. (After Schmaltz, Atlas d. Anat. d. Pferdes.)

The Atlas

This vertebra is decidedly atypical in form and structure. The body and spinous process are absent. It has the form of a strong ring, from which two curved plates, the wings, project laterally. The ring incloses a very large vertebral foramen, and consists of two lateral masses connected by dorsal and ventral arches.

The lateral masses (Massæ laterales) present two deep oval anterior articular cavities (Foveæ articulares craniales) which receive the occipital condyles; they are separated by a wide notch above and a narrow one below. The outer margin is also notched, and a triangular non-articular depression cuts into the inner part of each cavity. The posterior articular surfaces (Facies articulares caudales) are somewhat saddle-shaped; they are confluent on the ventral arch below, but are widely separated above, and do not conform in shape to the corresponding surfaces of the axis.

The dorsal arch (Arcus dorsalis) presents a median dorsal tubercle (Tuberculum dorsale) and is concave below. It is perforated on either side near its anterior margin by the intervertebral foramen. The anterior border is deeply notched, and the posterior is thin and concave.

The ventral arch (Arcus ventralis) is thicker, narrower, and less curved than the dorsal. On its lower surface is the **ventral tubercle** (Tuberculum ventrale), into which the terminal tendon of the longus colli muscle is inserted. The upper face has posteriorly a transversely concave articular surface (Fovea dentis), on which the dens or odontoid process of the axis rests. In front of this is a transverse rough excavation for the attachment of the odontoid ligament.

The **wings** (Alæ) are modified transverse processes. They are extensive curved plates which project outward, downward, and backward from the lateral masses. The dorsal surface is concave. Between the ventral aspect of the wing and the lateral mass is a cavity, the **fossa atlantis**; in this there is a foramen which opens into the vertebral canal. The border is thick and rough. Two foramina perforate each wing. The anterior one, the **foramen alare**, is connected with the intervertebral foramen by a short groove. The posterior one is the **foramen transversarium.**

Development.—The atlas ossifies from three or four centers, one or two for the ventral arch, and one on either side for each lateral mass, wing, and half of the dorsal arch. At birth the bone consists of three pieces—the ventral arch and two lateral parts, which are separated by a layer of cartilage in the dorsal median line. These parts are usually fused at about six months.

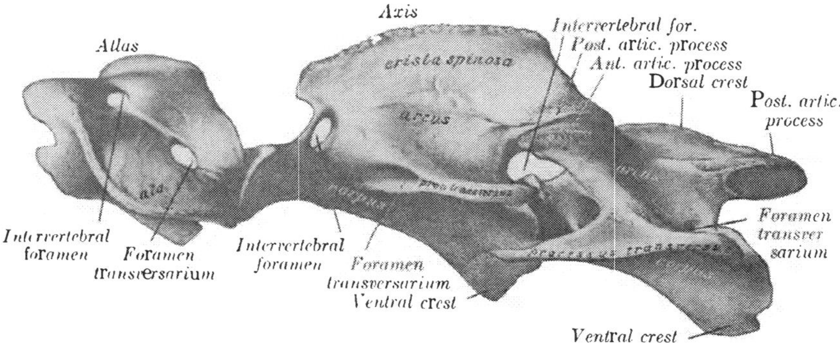

FIG. 11.—FIRST THREE CERVICAL VERTEBRÆ OF HORSE, LATERAL VIEW. (After Schmaltz, Atlas d. Anat. d. Pferdes.)

THE AXIS

The **axis** (Epistropheus) is the longest of the vertebræ, and is characterized by the presence of the odontoid process, which projects from the anterior part of the body.

The body has a median ventral crest which terminates in a tubercle behind. The anterior extremity presents centrally the **odontoid process** (Dens); this has a convex articular surface ventrally for articulation with the ventral arch of the atlas, and two rough depressions for the attachment of the odontoid ligament dorsally. Flanking this on either side are the modified **anterior articular processes,** which have saddle-shaped articular surfaces confluent below with that of the dens. The posterior extremity has the usual cavity.

The **arch** presents in the young subject a notch on each side of its anterior border; this is converted into a foramen by a ligament which usually ossifies later. The posterior border has the usual notches.

The **posterior articular processes** are typical.

The **transverse processes** are small, single, and project backward. The **foramen transversarium** is small.

The **spinous process** is very large and strong. Its free border is rough, thickens posteriorly, and is continued to the articular processes by two ridges. The lateral surfaces are concave and rough for muscular attachment.

Development.—The axis has **six or seven centers** of ossification. In addition to the usual five, one or two appear for the dens, which is regarded as the displaced body of the atlas. A nucleus behind the dens, which remains distinct to three or four years of age, is considered by Lesbre to be the head of the axis.

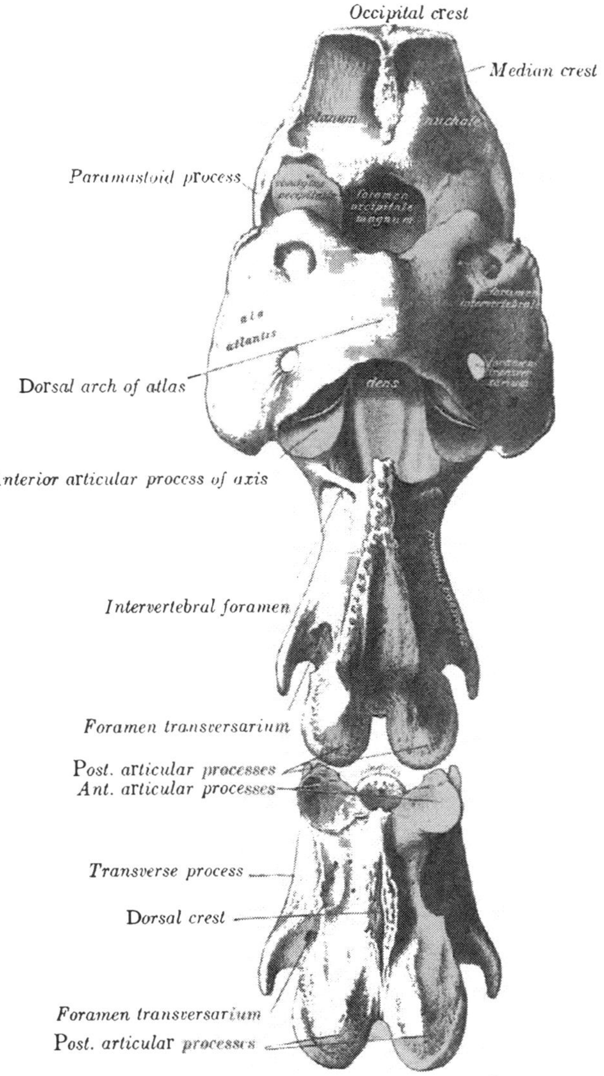

FIG. 12.—OCCIPITAL BONE AND FIRST THREE CERVICAL VERTEBRÆ OF HORSE, DORSAL VIEW. (After Schmaltz, Atlas d. Anat. d. Pferdes.)

THE THORACIC VERTEBRÆ

These (Vertebræ thoracales) are usually eighteen in number in the horse, but there are sometimes nineteen, rarely seventeen. As regional characters we note the surfaces for articulation with the ribs and the length and form of the spinous processes. Those in the middle of the series are the most typical and present the following features:

1. The **bodies** are short and constricted in the middle. The ends are expanded and have articular surfaces which are not strongly curved. On the upper part of each side are anterior and posterior **costal facets** (Fovea costalis cranialis, caudalis), which, with those of adjacent vertebræ, form sockets for the heads of the ribs.

2. The **arches** are small. Their posterior notches are relatively large and are often converted into foramina.

3. The **articular processes** are small. The anterior pair are in fact represented

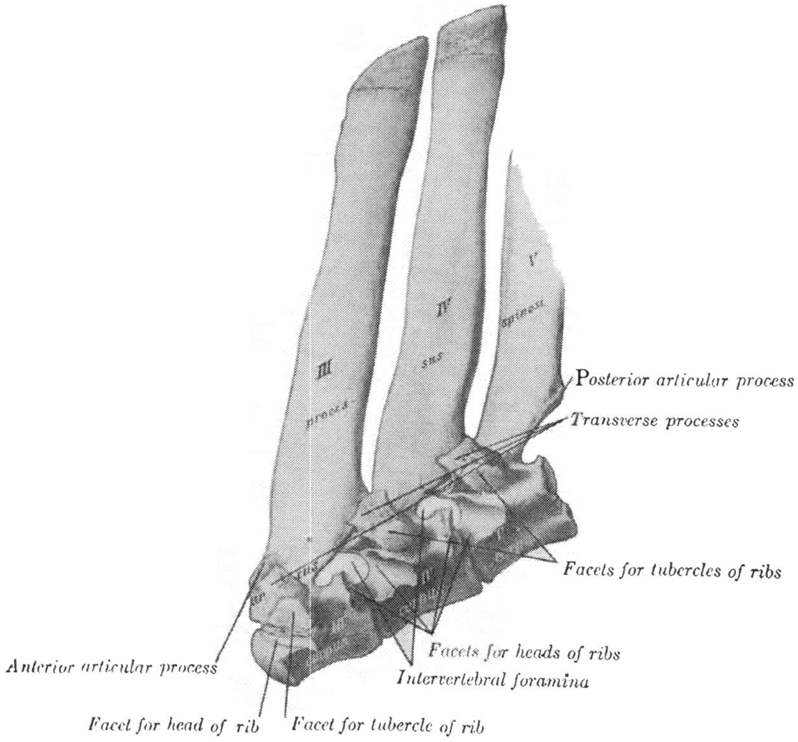

FIG. 13.—THIRD, FOURTH, AND FIFTH THORACIC VERTEBRÆ OF HORSE, LATERAL VIEW. (After Schmaltz Atlas d. Anat. d. Pferdes.)

only by two oval facets on the anterior part of the laminæ which face almost directly upward. The posterior pair spring from the base of the spinous process; their facets face almost directly downward.

4. The **transverse processes** are short, thick, and tuberous at the free end. Each has a facet (Fovea transversaria) for articulation with the tuberosity of the rib which has the same serial number

5. The **spinous process** is large, narrow, and slopes upward and backward. The anterior border is thin, the posterior wider and furrowed. The summit is expanded and rough.

The **first thoracic vertebra** is easily recognized by the following specific characters: The body is wide and flattened dorso-ventrally. In front it has a head like the cervical vertebræ, and behind a cavity somewhat deeper than any other thoracic vertebra. Two **costal facets** are found on either side, and a well-marked spine ventrally. The **arch** is large and strong, and has large notches. The **articular processes** are much larger than those of other thoracic vertebræ, and resemble a good deal those of the seventh cervical in form. The **transverse processes** are short and thick, and each has on its ventral aspect a large concave facet for articulation with the tubercle of the first rib. The spinous process is curved backward and tapers to a point. Its length is usually about three or four inches (ca. 8 to 10 cm.). It may be mistaken at first glance for the last cervical, but is promptly identified by the three costal facets on each side and the length of the spine.

The **last thoracic vertebra** is distinguished by the absence of the posterior pair of costal facets, and the confluence of the anterior pair with those on the transverse processes.

The serial position of others may be determined at least approximately by the following data: (1) The bodies gradually diminish in length and width to the middle of the region and then increase slightly. Their costal facets become smaller and less concave from first to last. The ventral crest is distinct on three or four vertebræ at either end of the region. (2) The transverse processes diminish in size and are placed lower down as they are traced backward. Their costal facets become smaller and lower in position; on the last (and sometimes on its predecessor also) it fuses with the costal facet of the body. The upper non-articular part of the process gradually becomes more sharply defined, and in the last four or five separates to form the **mammillary process.** (3) The spinous processes increase in length to the third and fourth, and then gradually diminish to the fifteenth, beyond which they have about the same length. The backward inclination is most pronounced in the second, the sixteenth is vertical, and the last two are directed a little forward. The longest spines (*i. e.*, those of the withers) are the thickest and have expanded summits which remain more or less cartilaginous; the others are more plate-like, and are surmounted by a thick lip. The second spine is more than twice as large as the first. The summits of the fourth and fifth usually form the highest point of the withers.

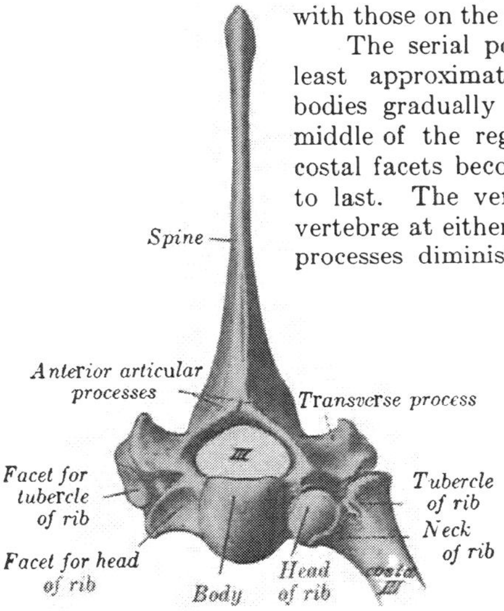

Fig. 14.—Third Thoracic Vertebræ and Upper Part of Rib of Horse, Anterior View. (After Schmaltz, Atlas d. Anat. d. Pferdes.)

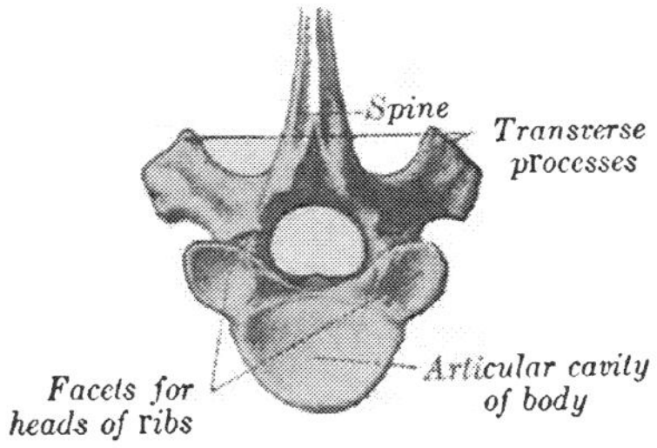

Fig. 15.—Lower Part of Ninth Thoracic Vertebra of Horse, Posterior View. (After Schmaltz, Atlas d. Anat. d. Pferdes.)

Development.—There are **six or seven centers,** three for the body, two for the arch, and one for the spinous process; some of the latter have an additional center for the summit.

THE LUMBAR VERTEBRÆ

The lumbar **vertebræ** (Vertebræ lumbales) are usually six in number in the horse. They are characterized by the size and form of their transverse processes.

The bodies of the first three are triangular on cross-section, and present a

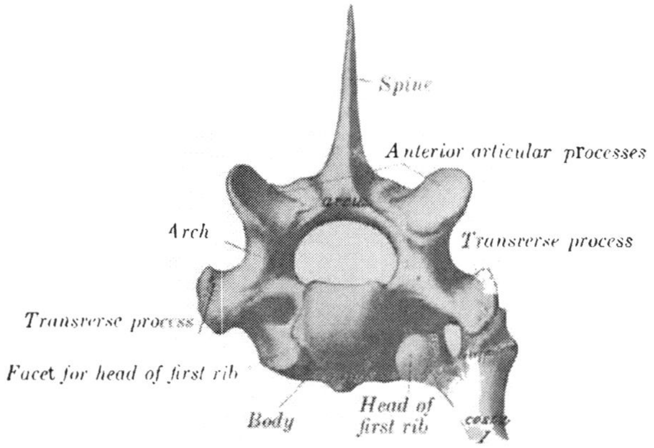

FIG. 16.—FIRST THORACIC VERTEBRA AND UPPER PART OF FIRST RIB OF HORSE, ANTERIOR VIEW. (After Schmaltz, Atlas d. Anat. d. Pferdes.)

distinct ventral crest. From the fourth backward they become wider and flatter and the ventral crest fades out.

The **arches** of the first two or three are about equal in size and similar to that of the last thoracic; from the fourth they decrease noticeably in breadth and height.

The **anterior articular processes** are fused with the mammillary processes, and

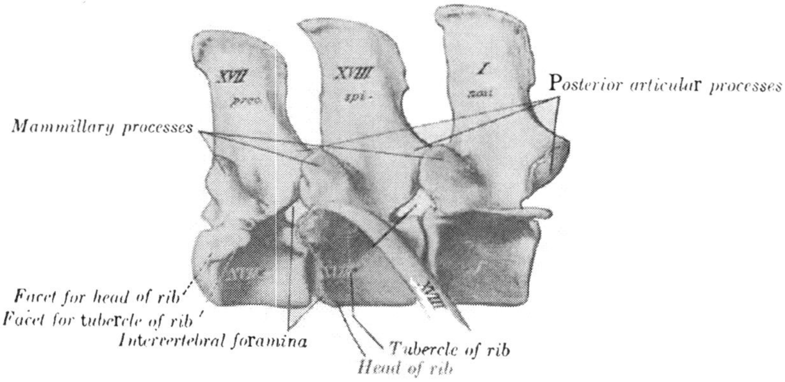

FIG. 17.—LAST TWO THORACIC AND FIRST LUMBAR VERTEBRÆ OF HORSE, LATERAL VIEW. (After Schmaltz Atlas d. Anat. d. Pferdes.)

present superiorly concave surfaces for articulation with the posterior pair of the preceding vertebra. The **posterior articular processes** project distinctly from the arch at the base of the spinous process, and have ventrally convex articular surfaces, which fit into the grooved surfaces of the anterior pair of the next vertebra.

The **transverse processes** are large plates, flattened dorso-ventrally, which project outward and usually curve slightly downward; their length increases to the third and fourth, and then diminishes to the last, which is the shortest. The first one or two usually curve somewhat backward, the last two decidedly forward. Those of the fifth have an oval concave facet on the inner part of the posterior border for articulation with the sixth process; the latter has a corresponding convex facet on the anterior border, and a larger concave surface on the posterior border for articulation with the wing of the sacrum. Sometimes the fifth process has a small surface for articulation with the fourth. The inner part of the sixth process is thick, the outer part thinner, narrower, and curved forward. The inner part of the fifth is also somewhat thickened.

The **spinous processes** resemble those of the last two thoracic vertebræ. They are usually about equal in height, but minor differences are common, and the width diminishes in the last three.

Development.—This is similar to that of the thoracic vertebræ. The extremities of the transverse processes remain cartilaginous for some time after ossification is otherwise complete.

The transverse processes of this region are considered equivalent to the proper transverse process + the costal element, and hence the distinctive term processus lateralis (s. costarius) has been proposed. The occurrence of a lumbar rib in connection with the transverse process of the first lumbar is not rare. Reduction of the number to five has been observed frequently, and

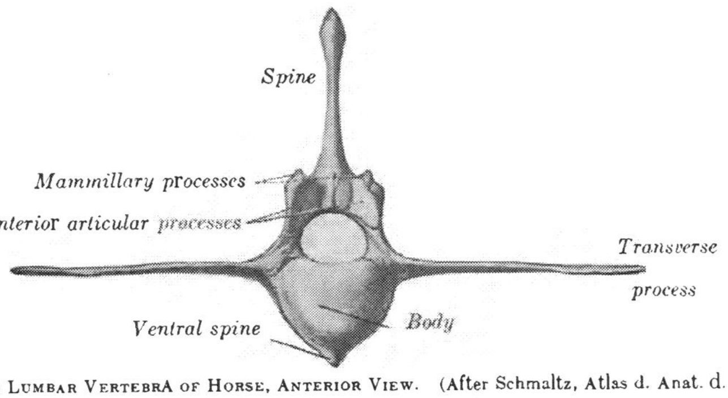

Fig. 18.—Second Lumbar Vertebra of Horse, Anterior View. (After Schmaltz, Atlas d. Anat. d. Pferdes.)

may or may not be compensated by an additional thoracic vertebra. This variation is not more common in certain races as Sanson and others have maintained. Very few cases are recorded of seven lumbar vertebræ—especially with the normal thoracic number. An anomalous vertebra with mixed thoracic and lumbar characters sometimes occurs at the junction of the two regions.

THE SACRUM

The **sacrum** (Os sacrum) is formed by the fusion of five vertebræ usually, and is conveniently described as a single bone. It is triangular in form and is wedged in between the ilia, with which it articulates very firmly on each side. Its long axis is gently curved, and slightly oblique, so that the posterior end is a little higher than the anterior. It presents two surfaces, two borders, a base, and an apex.

The **dorsal surface** presents centrally the five sacral spines, which are directed upward and backward, and have (with the exception of the first) tuberous summits which are sometimes bifid.

The first spine is relatively thin and narrow, and is not so high as the internal angle of the ilium. The second is the longest, and the height diminishes rapidly to the last. The bases of the spines are often fused in old subjects.

On either side of the spines is a groove, in which are the four dorsal sacral foramina (Foramina sacralia dorsalia); the dorsal branches of the sacral nerves emerge through them.

The ventral or pelvic surface (Facies pelvina) is concave in its length, wide in front, narrow behind. It is marked by four more or less distinct transverse lines (Lineæ transversæ), which indicate the demarcation of the bodies of the vertebræ. At the ends of these lines are the ventral sacral foramina (Foramina sacralia ventralia), which are larger than the dorsal series and diminish in size from first to last; they transmit the ventral divisions of the sacral nerves.

The dorsal and ventral foramina communicate with the sacral canal and are together equivalent to the usual intervertebral foramina.

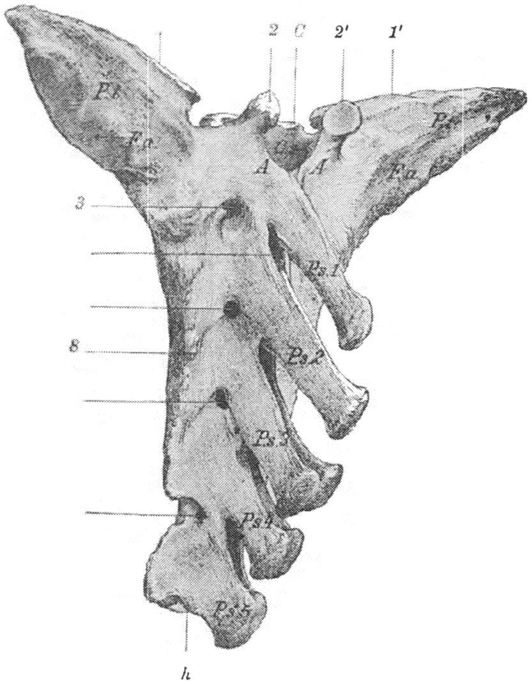

FIG. 19.—SACRUM OF HORSE, DORSO-LATERAL VIEW.

Body of first sacral vertebra; *A*, arch of first vertebra; *Cs*, sacral canal; *P.s.* 1–5, sacral spines; *P.t.*, wings of sacrum; 1, 1', surfaces for articulation with transverse processes of last lumbar vertebra; *F.a.*, auricular surface; 2, 2', articular processes; 3–6, dorsal sacral foramina; 7, interarcuate space; 8, lateral border; *h*, apex. (Struska, Anat. d. Haustiere.)

The lateral borders are rough, thick in front, thin behind.

The base (Basis ossis sacri) is directed forward, and is relatively very wide. It presents centrally the body of the first sacral segment, which is wide transversely, flattened dorso-ventrally, and has a rounded surface which articulates with the last lumbar vertebra through the medium of an intervertebral fibro-cartilage. The ventral margin projects slightly, forming the promontory (Promontorium). Above the body is the entrance to the sacral canal, flanked by a pair of articular processes, which project upward and forward from the arch, and have concave surfaces internally for articulation with those of the last lumbar vertebra. On each side of these is a smooth notch which is converted into a foramen by apposition with the last lumbar. The lateral parts of the base, the wings or alæ (Alæ sacrales), are strong prismatic masses with pointed ends, which result from the fusion of the first with part of the second transverse process. Each has in front a large, oval, slightly convex surface for articulation with the transverse process of the last lumbar. Posteriorly there is an elongated oval area which faces upward, backward, and outward. This is the **auricular surface** (Facies auricularis), which articulates with the ilium; it is slightly concave in its length, and somewhat rough and irregular. The rest of the dorsal surface of the wing is roughened for ligamentous attachment, while the ventral surface is smooth.

The **apex** (Apex ossis sacri) is the posterior aspect of the last sacral vertebra and is quite small. It presents the elliptical flattened surface of the body, above which is the triangular posterior opening of the sacral canal, surmounted by the last sacral spine. There is a pair of narrow notches between the arch and body, above which rudiments of articular processes may occur.

The name **sacral canal** (Canalis sacralis) is applied to that part of the vertebral canal which traverses the sacrum. Its anterior part is large and has the form of a triangle with the angles rounded off; its width is about twice its height. Traced backward it is seen to diminish in size rapidly, and the posterior opening is quite small and triangular.

The term **lateral part** (Pars lateralis) designates the portion external to the foramina, which results from the fusion of the transverse processes.

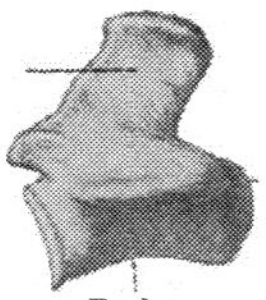

Fig. 20.—First Coccygeal Vertebra of Horse Left View. (After Schmaltz, Atlas d. Anat. d. Pferdes.)

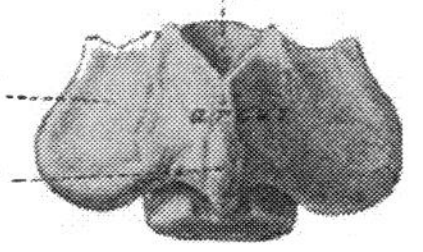

Fig. 21.—First Coccygeal Vertebra of Horse Dorsal View. (After Schmaltz, Atlas d. Anat. d. Pferdes.)

Development.—The several sacral vertebræ ossify in the typical manner. Separate centers for costal elements in the lateral parts have not yet been found in the domesticated animals. Fusion begins in front, and is usually not complete behind till near adult age. The lateral parts unite before the bodies. It is rather curious that the epiphyseal plates of adjacent segments unite with each other before they fuse with the main portion of the bodies.

THE COCCYGEAL VERTEBRÆ

These (Vertebræ coccygeæ) vary considerably in number, but eighteen may be taken as an average. From first to last they become reduced in size and, with the exception of a few at the beginning of the series, consist of bodies only. The first three have bodies which are somewhat flattened dorso-ventrally, constricted in the middle, and have at the ends slightly convex, elliptical, articular surfaces. The ventral surface has a median groove for the coccygeal artery. The arch is small and triangular; it is formed of two flat plates which are prolonged to form a short spinous process with a thickened and often double summit. The anterior notches are absent. Functional articular processes are not present, but small rudiments of the anterior pair commonly occur. The transverse processes are relatively large plates which project horizontally outward. Further back the arch becomes incomplete, open above, and soon disappears; the transverse processes gradually fade out, and the vertebræ are reduced to cylindrical rods of diminishing size. The last one has a pointed end.

Variations.—The number is said by good observers to vary between fourteen and twenty-one. In old age the first is often fused with the sacrum, and sometimes with the second. The arch of the third may be open.

THE VERTEBRAL COLUMN AS A WHOLE

In the mid-dorsal line is the series of **spinous processes**, which are low ridges in the cervical region with the exception of the second and seventh, reach their maximum height at the fourth and fifth thoracic vertebræ, and diminish to the fifteenth or sixteenth thoracic. Behind this they are about equal in height as far as the last lumbar and first sacral, which are somewhat lower. The second sacral spine is about as high as the middle lumbar; behind this they diminish rather rapidly in height and fade out about the third coccygeal. Their **inclination** backward is most decided at the second thoracic, diminishes from the sixth or seventh to the fifteenth or sixteenth, which is vertical and is termed the **anticlinal** or **diaphragmatic vertebra.** Behind this they are inclined a little forward until the sacrum is reached; here there is an abrupt change to the backward inclination, so that a considerable interspinous angle is formed.

On either side of the spinous processes is a vertebral groove which contains the deep muscles of the spine. The floor of the groove is formed by the laminæ and articular processes. It is wide in the neck and narrows progressively in the back.

Viewed from the side, the column presents a series of **curves.** When the head and neck are in the ordinary neutral position, the anterior part of the cervical spine forms a gentle curve, concave ventrally. The posterior cervical and first thoracic vertebræ form a more pronounced curve in the opposite direction. At the junction of the cervical and thoracic regions there is a marked change of direction, forming a ventral projection or angle. At the second thoracic vertebra a gentle curve, concave ventrally, begins. This is continued to the lumbo-sacral junction, where there is a change of direction, and hence a promontory. The sacrum has a variable, but never very pronounced, ventral concave curvature, which is continued in a much accentuated form in the coccygeal region. It may be remarked that a line through the summits of the spines does not correspond to these curves formed by the bodies.

The vertebral **canal,** of course, corresponds in curvature to the bodies. Its **caliber** varies greatly at different points. The greatest diameter (ca. 5 cm.) is in the atlas, where it contains the dens of the axis in addition to the spinal cord, and provision must be made for extensive movement. It is very much smaller in the axis (ca. 2.5 cm. wide, 3 cm. high). It widens considerably at the junction of the cervical and thoracic regions to accommodate the cervical enlargement of the spinal cord. Beyond this it diminishes, and is smaller in the middle of the back than at any preceding point; this is correlated with the small size of the spinal cord and the very limited movement of the spine. At the middle of the lumbar region it again widens considerably to contain the lumbar enlargement of the spinal cord. The caliber diminishes very rapidly from the second sacral segment backward, and the canal ceases to be complete at the fourth coccygeal vertebra.

The **articular processes** are very large and wide apart in the neck, greatly reduced and much closer together in the back, larger and interlocking in the lumbar region.

The **transverse processes** are large and outstanding in the neck, where they form the outer boundary of a ventral groove occupied by the longus colli muscle. In the back they are short and stout, and are characterized by the facets for the tubercles of the ribs. On the first thoracic vertebra this facet is large, deeply concave, and situated almost directly outward from the cavity for the head of the rib; traced backward it becomes smaller and flatter, and gradually comes to lie behind the cavity for the head of the rib, with which it is fused on the last and often also on the next to the last thoracic vertebra. The processes in the lumbar region have a characteristic elongated plate-like form. In the sacral region they are fused to form the wings and lateral parts of the sacrum. In the coccygeal region they are at first of considerable size relatively, but undergo rapid reduction, and disappear at the fifth or sixth vertebra.

The cavities for the heads of the ribs diminish progressively in size and depth from first to last.

The **mammillary processes** are usually distinct on the fourteenth to the seventeenth thoracic vertebræ. In front of these they blend with the transverse, behind with the anterior articular processes.

The length of the vertebral column (including the intervertebral fibro-cartilages) in a horse of medium size is about 260 to 265 cm. (ca. 8 feet 8 inches to 8 feet 10 inches). The relative lengths of the various regions appear to vary most in the neck and back.

The table below gives the measurements in centimeters in a trotting stallion of medium size and in an adult Percheron stallion. The percentages are in round numbers.

	Trotter		Percheron	
Cervical..	60.0	22.7%	74.0	25.4%
Thoracic.	98.0	37.2%	100.0	34.4%
Lumbar..........	31.5	12.0%	36.5	12.5%
Sacral....	20.0	7.6%	22.5	7.7%
Coccygeal............	54.0	20.5%	58.0	20.0%
	263.5	100.0	291.0	100.0

The Ribs

There are usually eighteen pairs of ribs in the horse, but a nineteenth rib on one side or both is not at all rare. Eight are **sternal** or "true" ribs, the remainder **asternal** or "false." Ribs from different parts of the series vary much in length, curvature, and other characters. We will therefore consider as a type a rib from the middle of the series first, and afterward note the chief serial differences A **typical rib** has the following characters:

The **shaft** or **body** (Corpus costæ) is elongated, relatively very narrow, and strongly curved; the curvature is most pronounced in the dorsal third, and the ventral part is twisted and inclined inward, so that when a rib is laid with its outer surface on the table, the ventral end is raised. The **external surface** is convex in its length and also transversely; its anterior part is, however, grooved longitudinally. A distinct angle, *i. e.*, a point at which the curve of the rib changes rather suddenly, as in man, can scarcely be said to exist in the horse. The term is often applied, however, to a corresponding rough elevation which gives attachment to the ilio-costalis muscle; it is most distinct on the fourth to the eighth inclusive. The **internal surface** is smooth, concave in its length, and rounded from side to side; the costal groove, situated posteriorly, is very distinct above and fades out about the middle. The **anterior border** is concave, the **posterior** convex.

The **vertebral extremity** (Extremitas vertebralis) consists of the head, neck, and tubercle. The **head** (Capitulum costæ) has an articular surface (Facies articularis capituli costæ), composed of two convex facets, anterior and posterior, separated by a groove for the attachment of the conjugal ligament. It articulates with the cavity formed by facets on the bodies of two adjacent thoracic vertebræ and the intervertebral fibro-cartilage. The **neck** (Collum costæ) is roughened above and in front. The tubercle (Tuberculum costæ) is placed above and behind the junction of neck and shaft; it has a small surface (Facies articularis tuberculi costæ) for articulation with the transverse process of the corresponding thoracic vertebra.

The **sternal extremity** (Extremitas sternalis) is somewhat expanded, and is continued by the costal cartilage.

The **first rib** is easily distinguished. It is the shortest and least curved. At the lower part of the anterior border there is a smooth impression where the brachial vein curves around it; above this is usually the scalene tubercle. The costal groove is absent. The head is large and has two facets of unequal extent which meet at an acute angle in front; the smaller one faces forward and articulates with the last cervical vertebra; the larger one is directed inward and articulates with the first thoracic vertebra. The neck is thick and very short. The tubercle is larger than that of any other rib and has an extensive articular surface which is convex in its length. The sternal end is larger than that of any other rib; it is thick and very wide, and is turned a little forward.

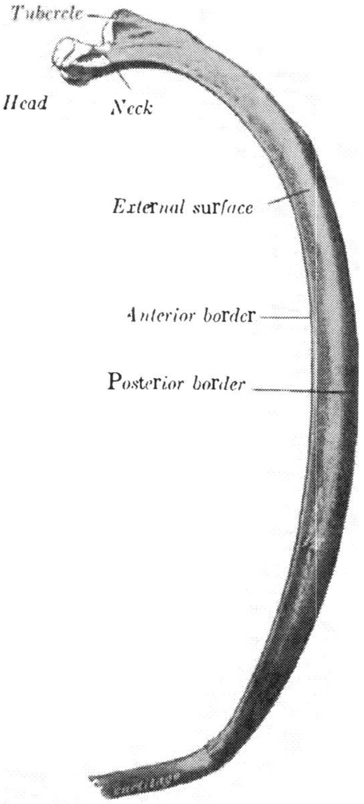

FIG. 22.—LEFT SEVENTH RIB OF HORSE, ANTERO-EXTERNAL VIEW. (After Schmaltz, Atlas d. Anat. d. Pferdes.)

The **last rib** is the most slender and regularly curved. It is usually but little longer than the second. The facet on the tubercle is confluent with that of the head. (This feature, however, is usual on the seventeenth also, and not rare on the sixteenth.)

The serial position of the other ribs may be determined approximately by the following considerations: The **length** increases from the first to the tenth and eleventh and then diminishes. The **width** increases somewhat to the sixth and then diminishes. The **anterior** border is thin and sharp from the second to the eighth, and behind this becomes thick and rounded. The **external** groove is distinct on the fourth to the eighth inclusive. The **curvature** increases in degree rapidly from the first to the seventh, remains about the same to the sixteenth, and then decreases very noticeably. In regard to dorso-ventral **direction**, the first rib inclines a little forward, the second is about vertical, while behind this they slope backward in increasing degree, so that a plane tangent to the ventral ends of the last pair cuts the third lumbar vertebra. The **head** and tubercle diminish in size from first to last. Their relative positions change in that the tubercle of the first rib lies almost directly outward from the head, while further back it gradually comes to lie behind it. The **neck** is longest on the longest ribs, and is absent on the last two or three. A costo-transverse foramen is formed between the neck and the transverse process.

Development.—The ribs ossify in cartilage from **three centers**, one each for the shaft, head, and tubercle; the third center is absent in some of the posterior ribs.

Variations.—A nineteenth rib on one side or both is not rare. It is usually imperfectly developed and quite variable. In some cases it is a mere strip of cartilage connected by ligament with the first lumbar transverse process; in other cases it is ossified, and may be fused with the process; in others again it is connected with an additional presacral vertebra which may be thoracic or lumbar or ambiguous in character. It is commonly floating, but may be attached to the eighteenth. Reduction in number is uncommon. Fusion of adjacent ribs sometimes occurs.

THE COSTAL CARTILAGES

The first costal cartilage is an inch or more (2.5 to 3 cm.) in length. The upper part is very wide and thick. The sternal end is small. The two articulate with each other as well as with the sternum. The cartilages of the other sternal ribs increase progressively in length and become more rounded. The sternal end is expanded and has an elliptical convex facet for articulation with the sternum. The cartilages of the asternal ribs are long, slender, and pointed. The ninth is the

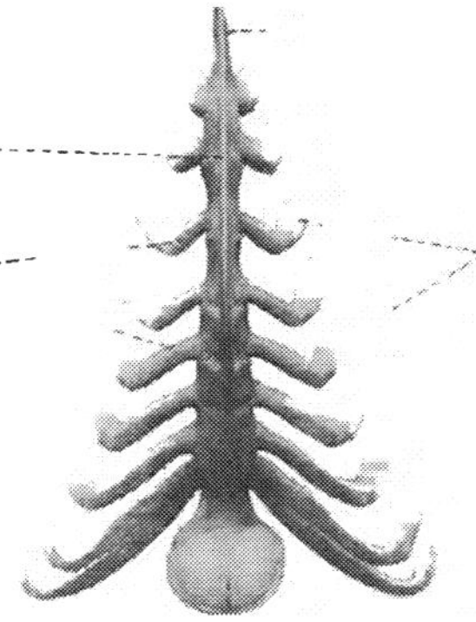

Fig. 23.—Sternum and Costal Cartilages of Horse, Ventral View. (After Ellenberger-Baum, Anat. f. Künstler.)

longest, and is very firmly attached to the eighth; behind this they diminish progressively in size, and are attached to each other by elastic tissue. Except in the case of the first, the cartilage does not continue the direction of the rib, but forms with the latter an angle which is open in front, and decreases in obtuseness from second to last.

More or less extensive ossification is to be regarded as a normal occurrence, especially in the cartilages of the sternal ribs.

The Sternum

The sternum of the horse is shaped somewhat like a canoe; it is compressed laterally, except in its posterior part, which is flattened dorso-ventrally. It is inclined obliquely so that the posterior end is about six to eight inches (15 to 20 cm.) lower than the anterior.

The **dorsal surface** has the form of a very narrow isosceles triangle with the apex in front. It is concave longitudinally, flattened transversely.

The **lateral surfaces** are convex above, slightly concave below, and diminish in extent behind. Each presents on its upper part seven **articular cavities** (Foveæ costales), which receive the sternal ends of the second to the eighth costal cartilages inclusive. These cavities are situated in series at the intersternebral junctions.

The first four are elliptical in outline with the long diameter vertical, and are separated by considerable regular intervals. The others are progressively smaller, more circular, and closer together. The area below these cavities gives attachment to the pectoral muscles.

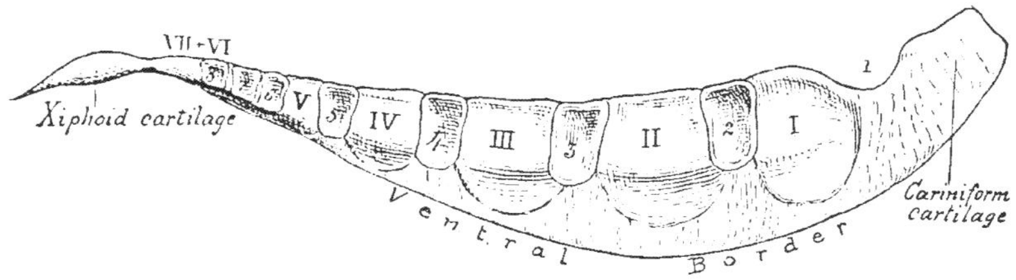

FIG. 24.—STERNUM OF HORSE, LATERAL VIEW.
The sternebræ are designated by Roman numerals and the costal facets by ordinary figures.

The dorso-lateral borders separate the dorsal and lateral surfaces. They give attachment to the lateral branches of the sternal ligament.

The ventral border forms the prominent keel-like crest of the sternum (Crista sterni) which may be felt in the living animal; it fades out behind.

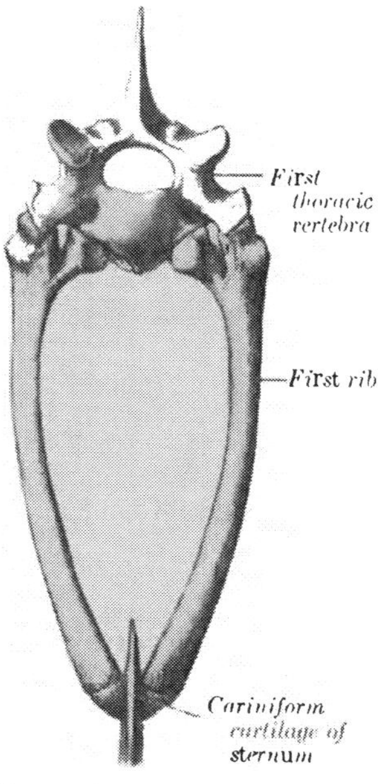

FIG. 25.—ANTERIOR APERTURE OF THORAX OF HORSE. (After Schmaltz, Atlas d. Anat. d. Pferdes.)

The **anterior extremity** or **manubrium sterni**[1] can be distinctly felt in the central furrow of the breast. It consists of a laterally compressed cartilaginous prolongation, commonly called the **cariniform cartilage.** Its lateral surfaces are flat and furnish attachment to muscles of the breast and neck. The ventral border is rounded, and is continued backward on the body of the bone. The dorsal border is concave and has an articular cavity for the first pair of costal cartilages.

The **posterior extremity** is formed by the **xiphoid** or **ensiform cartilage** (Processus xiphoideus). This is a thin plate, connected in front with the last bony segment by a relatively thick, narrow neck, and expanding in nearly circular form behind and laterally. Its dorsal surface is concave, and gives attachment to the diaphragm. The ventral surface is convex. The free margin is very thin.

Development.—At birth the sternum of the horse consists of seven bony segments or sternebræ united by intersternebral cartilages. The last two sternebræ fuse in the second month, but the others do not usually unite completely even in old age. The sternebræ consist of very vascular spongy bone covered by a very thin layer of compact substance. The adult sternum thus consists to a very considerable extent of persisting cartilage, viz., the intersternebral cartilages, the ventral keel, and the extremities; in old age these undergo partial ossification.

[1] The manubrium sterni of man is equivalent, strictly speaking, to the cariniform cartilage + the first osseous segment of the horse.

THE THORAX

The bony thorax of the horse is remarkably compressed laterally in its anterior part, but widens greatly behind. The **anterior aperture** is oval and very narrow below; in a horse of medium size its greatest width is about 4 inches (10 cm.), and its height 7 to 8 inches (ca. 18 to 20 cm.). The **ventral wall** or **floor** is about 16 inches (40 cm.) long, and the **dorsal wall** or **roof** about 38 to 40 inches (95 to 100 cm.) long. The height from the last segment of the sternum to the seventh or eighth thoracic vertebra is about twice that of the anterior aperture; this is due to the obliquity and divergence of the roof and floor. The greatest width of the posterior aperture is about 20 to 24 inches (50 to 60 cm.). The intercostal spaces increase in width from the first to the seventh or eighth, and then diminish. Their average width is about 1¼ to 1½ inches (3 to 3.5 cm.).

THE BONES OF THE SKULL

(A) BONES OF THE CRANIUM

The bones of the cranium (Ossa cranii) are the Occipital, Sphenoid, Ethmoid, Interparietal, Parietal, Frontal, and Temporal. The first four are single, the others paired.

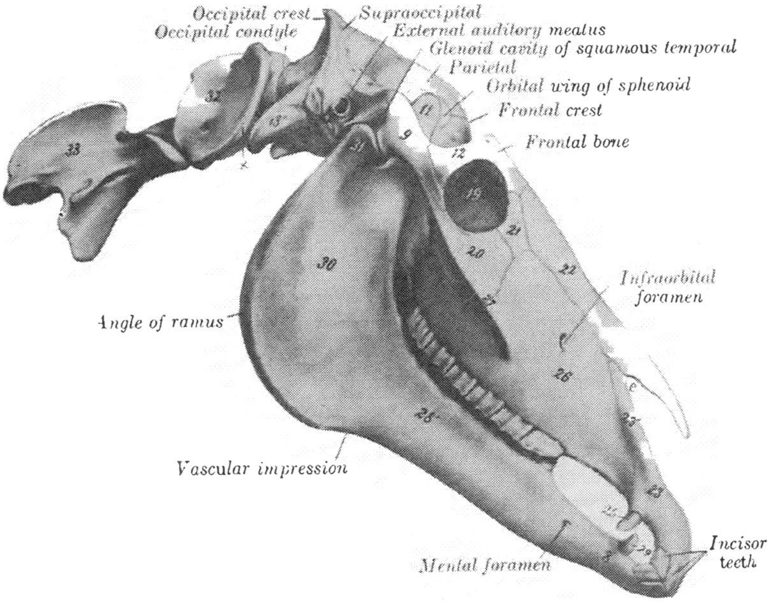

FIG. 26.—SKULL, ATLAS, AND AXIS OF HORSE, LATERAL VIEW.

8, Body of mandible; 28′, horizontal (molar) part of ramus; 30, vertical part of ramus; 9, zygomatic process of squamous temporal; 11, coronoid process of mandible; 12, supraorbital process; 13″, paramastoid (styloid) process of occipital; 19, orbit; 20, malar bone; 21, lacrimal bone; 22, nasal bone; 23, premaxilla; 23′, nasal process of premaxilla; 25, 29, canine teeth; 26, maxilla; 27, facial crest; 31, condyle of mandible; 32, atlas; 33, axis; x, wing of atlas; e, naso-maxillary notch. (After Ellenberger-Baum, Anat. für Künstler.)

THE OCCIPITAL BONE

The **occipital bone** (Os occipitale) is situated at the posterior part of the cranium, of which it forms the posterior wall and part of the ventral wall or base.[1]

[1] The long axis of the skull is considered to be horizontal in these descriptions.

Its lower part is perforated centrally by a large, almost circular opening, the **foramen magnum** (Foramen occipitale magnum), at which the brain and spinal cord join. The foramen is bounded laterally and dorsally by the **lateral parts** of the bone, and ventrally by the **basilar part** or **process**. Above the lateral parts—but not entering into the formation of the foramen magnum—is the **squamous part**.

The **lateral parts** (Partes laterales) bear the **occipital condyles** (Condyli occipitales), which articulate with the atlas. The condyles are obliquely placed, wide apart dorsally, and separated by a small interval ventrally. The articular surface is curved so sharply in the dorso-ventral direction as to form a blunt ridge

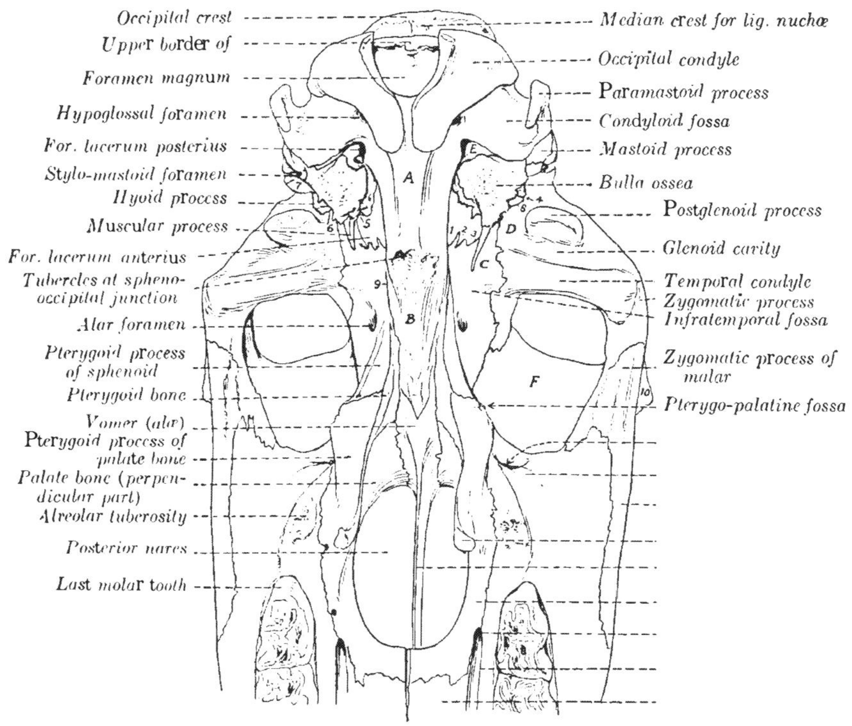

Fig. 27.—Line Drawing of Posterior Half of Base of Skull of Horse, Without Mandible. (Key to Fig. 28.)

1, Incisura carotica; 2, incisura ovalis; 3, incisura spinosa; 4, external orifice of parieto-temporal canal; 5, Eustachian canal; 6, petro-tympanic fissure; 7, external auditory canal; 8, hyoid process; 9, Vidian groove; 10, supraorbital process; *A*, basilar part of occipital; *B*, body of sphenoid; *C*, temporal wing of sphenoid; *D*, squamous temporal bone; *E*, petrous temporal bone; *F*, orbital part of frontal bone.

externally. The cranial surface is concave and smooth. External to the condyle is the **paramastoid** or **styloid process** (Processus jugularis), a strong flattened bar of bone which projects downward and backward; its external surface is convex and roughened for muscular attachment. Between the root of this process and the condyle is a smooth depression, the **condyloid fossa** (Fossa condyloidea inferior); in this is the **hypoglossal foramen** (Foramen hypoglossi), which transmits the nerve of like name.

The **basilar part** or **process** (Pars basilaris) is a strong, somewhat prismatic bar which extends forward from the ventral margin of the foramen magnum. It is much narrower in front than behind. The ventral surface is rounded. The cranial surface is concave and smooth; its posterior part supports the medulla, and its anterior part has a shallow cavity on which the pons rests. The lateral borders are thin and sharp, and form the inner margin of the **foramen lacerum** (Foramen lacerum et jugulare). The anterior end has, in the young subject, a

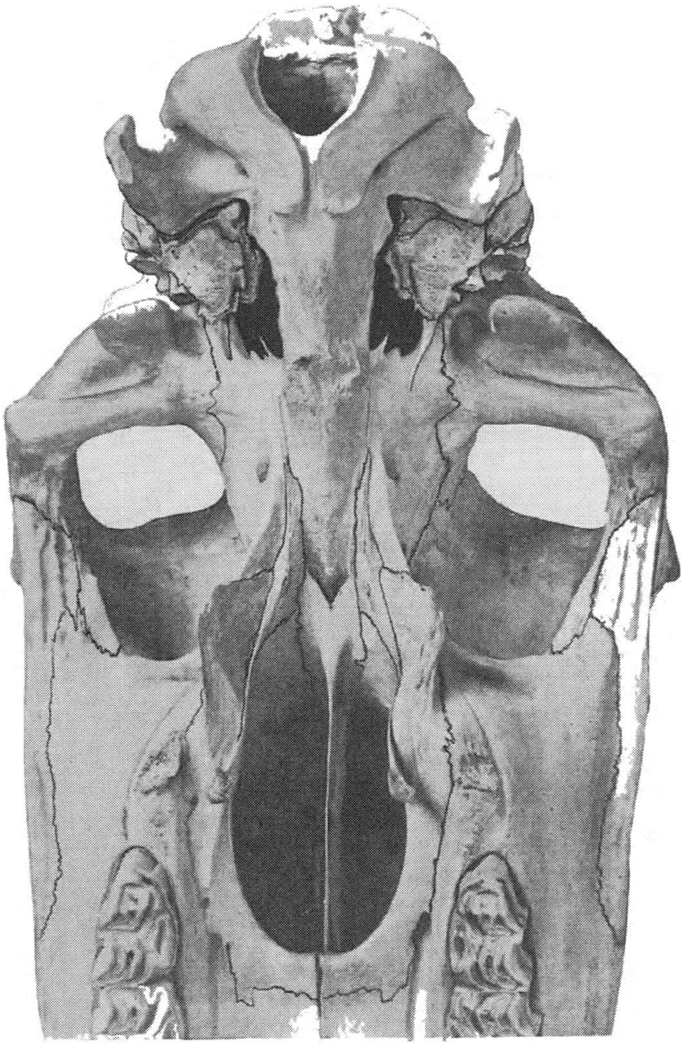

Fig. 28.—Ventral Surface of Skull of Horse, Posterior Half Without Mandible. The skull is inclined slightly. (Notation on key Fig. 27.)

semicircular, flat, pitted surface which is attached to the body of the sphenoid bone by a layer of cartilage; in the adult there is complete fusion. On the ventral aspect of the junction are tubercles for the attachment of the ventral straight muscles of the head.

The **squamous part** (Squama occipitalis) is the somewhat quadrilateral mass situated above the lateral portions, from which it remains distinct till the second year. The outer **surface** is crossed by a very prominent ridge, the **occipital crest**; the middle part of this is thick, transverse in direction, and forms the highest point of the skull when the head is in the ordinary position; laterally it becomes thinner and runs downward and forward to join the temporal crest.[1] The crest divides the surface into two very unequal parts; the small anterior area (Planum parietale) presents a median ridge which is the posterior part of the external sagittal crest; the large area below the crest (Planum nuchale) also has a central eminence, the **external occipital protuberance**, on the sides of which the funicular part of the ligamentum nuchæ is attached. The **internal surface** is concave and presents a deep central depression and two shallower lateral ones which adapt it to the surface of the cerebellum.

The occipital bone is connected by suture with the interparietal, two parietals, and two temporals, and by synchondrosis with the sphenoid; the condyles articulate with the atlas.

Development.—The occipital ossifies in cartilage from four **centers,** and consists at birth of four pieces as described above.[2] The lateral parts unite with the basilar at three to four months, and with the squama in the second year, when the bone is consolidated.

The parieto-occipital suture and the spheno-occipital synchondrosis are obliterated about the fifth year usually. The temporo-occipital suture partially ossifies in old subjects.

THE SPHENOID BONE

The **sphenoid bone** (Os sphenoidale) is situated in the base of the cranium, its central part lying in front of the basilar part of the occipital. It consists of a central part, the body, two pairs of wings, and two pterygoid processes.

The **body** (Corpus) is a cylindrical bar, flattened dorso-ventrally, and wider in front than behind. Its **ventral surface** (Facies externa) is convex in the transverse direction; and its anterior part is concealed to a large extent by the vomer and pterygoid bones. The **cerebral surface** (Facies cerebralis) presents the following features: (1) In front is a raised, flattened part which is subdivided by a median elevation into two slightly concave lateral areas; this part has a posterior, thin, free margin (Limbus sphenoidalis), which overlies the entrance to the optic foramina. (2) Just behind this and at a lower level is a smooth transverse depression, the **optic** groove (Sulcus chiasmatis), on which the optic chiasma rests. (3) From each end of this groove the **optic foramen** passes forward and outward to terminate in the posterior part of the orbital fossa.[3] (4) Near the posterior end is a central depression, the **hypophyseal** or **pituitary** fossa (Fossa hypophysea), which lodges the hypophysis cerebri or pituitary body. On each side of this is an ill-defined groove for the internal carotid artery and the cavernous sinus. The **anterior end** is expanded, and is excavated to form the **sphenoidal sinuses.** These cavities extend back as far as the optic groove, and are usually continuous in front with the cavities in the vertical parts of the palate bones; they are separated by a complete septum which is not always median.[4] The **posterior end** is flat and is

[1] The occipital crest of this description is equivalent to the external occipital protuberance and superior nuchal line of man. A curved line a little lower down, which is continued on the paramastoid process, represents the inferior nuchal line of man.

[2] Other terms for these parts are basioccipital (basilar part), exoccipitals (lateral parts), and supraoccipital (squamous part). It should be noted, however, that the lines between the basioccipital and exoccipitals pass through the lower part of the condyles.

[3] This foramen might well be called a canal, since it is an inch or more in length.

[4] The cavity so formed may be termed the sphenopalatine sinus. The sphenoidal sinus may be a separate cavity which communicates only with the ventral ethmoidal meatuses; this arrangement exists in about a third of the cases, according to Paulli.

joined to the basilar part of the occipital; at the line of junction there is dorsally a transverse elevation, the **spheno-occipital** crest (Crista spheno-occipitalis).

The **orbital wings** (Alæ orbitales) curve upward and somewhat outward from the sides of the body of the pre-sphenoid. Their **inner** or **cerebral surfaces** are concave, and are marked by **digital impressions** (Impressiones digitatæ) for the gyri of the cerebrum. The **external surface** is convex and is largely concealed by the overlapping temporal wing and the squamous temporal and frontal bones; a narrow part of it (Facies orbitalis) is uncovered on the inner wall of the orbital cavity at the sphenoidal notch of the frontal bone. The **dorsal border** unites with the frontal bone at the spheno-frontal suture. The **anterior border** joins the ethmoid at the spheno-ethmoidal suture; at its lower part it concurs with the frontal in the formation of the **ethmoidal** (or internal orbital) **foramen.** The **posterior border** is overlapped by the temporal wing and the squamous temporal. The root of the wing is perforated by the **optic foramen.** Immediately below and behind the latter (*i. e.*, beneath the root) is the **foramen lacerum orbitale** or **orbital fissure.** Below this, and separated from it usually by a thin plate, is a larger opening, the **foramen rotundum,** which is bounded externally by the root of the pterygoid process. Behind these foramina is the **pterygoid crest** (Crista pterygoidea), which is continued downward and forward on the pterygoid process; on its upper part may be found the small and inconstant **trochlear** (or pathetic) **foramen.** Just behind the crest is the **temporal foramen** (For. alare parvum), through which the anterior deep temporal artery emerges from the alar canal of the pterygoid process.

The **temporal wings** (Alæ temporales) extend outward and somewhat upward from the body of the post-sphenoid; they are irregularly quadrilateral in outline. The **external surface** (Facies temporalis) enters into the formation of the infratemporal fossa, and bears the pterygoid process on its anterior part; at the junction with the body there is a small groove for the pterygoid nerve. The **internal surface** (Facies cerebralis) presents, at the junction with the body, two longitudinal **grooves** (Sulci nervorum). The outer groove is the larger, and leads forward to the foramen rotundum; it contains the maxillary nerve. The inner groove conducts to the orbital fissure, and contains the third, sixth, and ophthalmic nerves. The outer groove is bounded externally by a thin overhanging crest, on which is a small groove for the fourth nerve. The remainder of the surface is concave and supports the pyriform lobe of the brain. The **dorsal border** joins the squamous temporal at the spheno-squamous suture. The **anterior border** joins the orbital wing. The **posterior border** forms the anterior boundary of the foramen lacerum; it presents **three notches,** which are (from within outward) the carotid, oval, and spinous (Incisura carotica, ovalis, spinosa). The angle of junction of the dorsal and posterior borders articulates with the parietal bone.

The **pterygoid processes** (Processus pterygoidei) arise from the temporal wings and the body. They project downward and forward, and curve outward at the lower part. The root is perforated by the **alar canal** (Canalis alaris),[1] which transmits the internal maxillary artery. From this canal a branch leads upward and forward to open at the temporal foramen. The **external surface** is concave, and is marked by lines for muscular attachment. The **internal surface** is largely concealed by the overlapping palate and pterygoid bones, with which it concurs in the formation of the **pterygoid** or **Vidian canal.**

Development.—The sphenoid is ossified in cartilage, and consists in early life of two distinct parts, the pre-sphenoid and post-sphenoid. The former develops from two centers, one in each wing; the latter has three centers, one for the body and one for each wing. The pterygoid processes ossify from the centers of the temporal wings.

[1] This is also called the subsphenoidal canal or pterygoid foramen.

Variation.—The dorsal border of the orbital wing may come to the surface through a defect in the frontal bone at the place where the horn process is situated in animals which have frontal horns.

The Ethmoid Bone

The **ethmoid** (Os ethmoidale) is situated in front of the body and orbital wings of the sphenoid. It projects forward between the orbital plates of the frontal bones and enters into the formation of the cranial, nasal, and paranasal cavities.[1] It consists of four parts—the cribriform plate, two lateral masses, and the perpendicular plate.

The **cribriform plate** (Lamina cribrosa) is a sieve-like partition between the cranial and nasal cavities. Its margin joins the orbital wings of the sphenoid laterally, and the cranial plate of the frontal bones dorsally. Its **cranial surface** is divided into two parts by a median ridge, the **crista galli,** which is the intracranial portion of the perpendicular plate. Each half forms a deep oval cavity, the **ethmoidal** or **olfactory fossa,** which lodges the olfactory bulb. The plate is perforated by numerous small foramina for the passage of the olfactory nerve filaments, and on either side is the much larger **ethmoidal foramen.** The **nasal surface** is convex, and has the lateral masses attached to it.

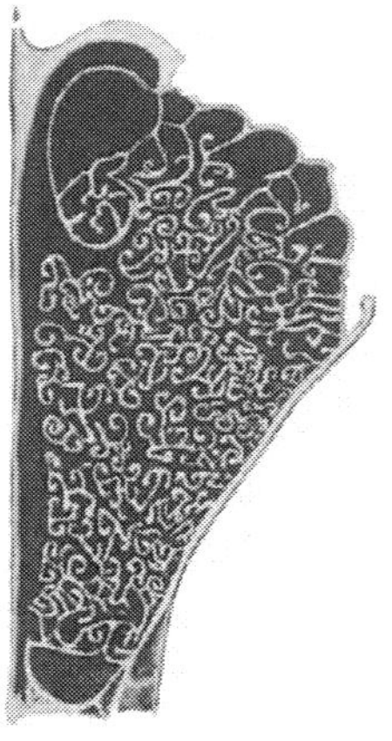

Fig. 29.—Cross-section of Lateral Mass of Ethmoid Bone of Horse.

The **lateral masses** or **labyrinth** project forward from the cribriform plate into the posterior part of the nasal cavity, which they nearly fill. Each mass is somewhat conical in shape, with the base attached to half of the cribriform plate. The **inner surface** is separated by a narrow space from the perpendicular plate. The outer **surface** is convex and faces chiefly into the frontal and maxillary sinuses, but is attached behind to the inner wall of the orbital cavity; it is covered by a very thin layer of bone, the **lamina papyracea.** The mass consists of a large number of delicate, scroll-like plates of bone, termed **ethmo-turbinals** or **ethmoidal cells.** These are attached to the lamina papyracea, and are separated by narrow intervals termed **ethmoidal meatuses,** which communicate with the nasal cavity. In the living animal the ethmo-turbinals are covered with mucous membrane.

The lateral mass is a very complex structure, the arrangement of which may be studied on cross-sections of decalcified specimens with the mucous membrane retained. Each mass consists of six turbinals which extend almost to the perpendicular plate and are termed **endoturbinals.** These diminish in size from above downward; the largest is attached to the nasal bone, and is hence usually called the naso-turbinal or superior turbinal; the second is much smaller, and is very commonly termed the great ethmoid cell. Between the endoturbinals are twenty-one small **ectoturbinals,** and all are beset with secondary and tertiary coiled lamellæ.

The **perpendicular plate** or **mesethmoid** (Lamina perpendicularis) is median, and forms the posterior part of the septum nasi. Its **lateral surfaces** are nearly plane, but are marked below by some grooves and ridges; they are covered by the nasal mucous membrane. The **anterior border** is irregular and is continuous with the septal cartilage. The **posterior border** projects into the cranial cavity as a ridge, the **crista galli.** The **dorsal border** joins the frontal bones at their line of junction—the frontal suture. The **ventral border** is received into the groove of the vomer.

Development.—The ethmoid develops in cartilage from five centers, two for

[1] On account of its deep situation, and the fact that it cannot be separated from its surroundings, the ethmoid must be studied by means of appropriate sagittal and transverse sections of the skull.

each lateral mass, and one for the perpendicular plate; from the latter ossification extends into the cribriform plate. At birth the perpendicular and cribriform plates are entirely cartilaginous. By the time ossification is complete the ethmoid has united with surrounding bones to such an extent that it cannot be separated intact for study.

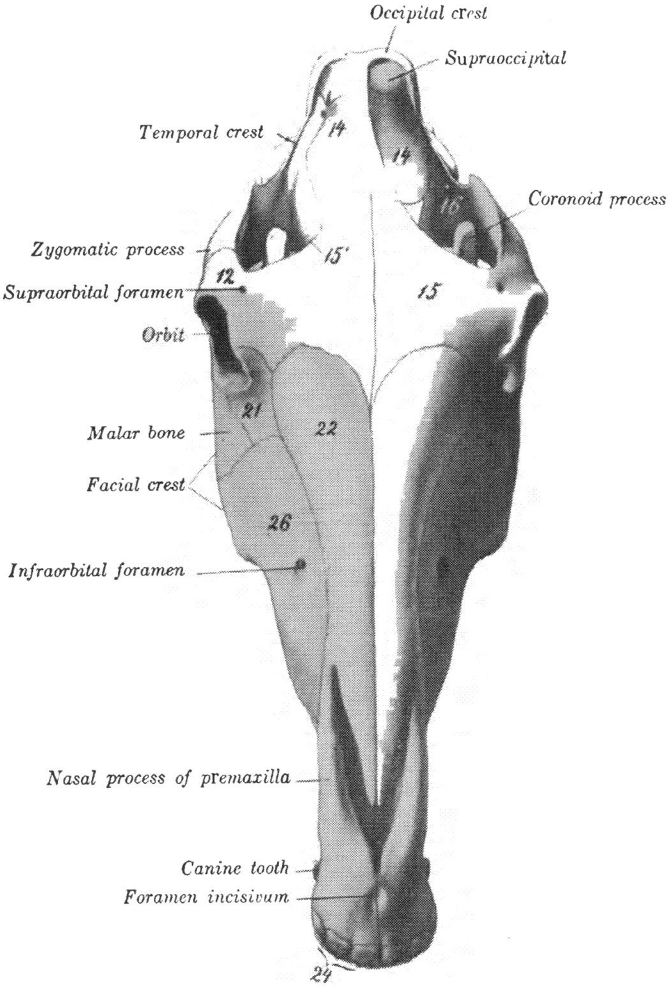

FIG. 30.—SKULL OF HORSE, DORSAL VIEW.

12, Supraorbital process; 14, parietal bone; 14', external sagittal crest; 15, frontal bone; 15', frontal crest; 21, lacrimal bone; 22, nasal bone; 26, maxilla; 24, incisor teeth. (After Ellenberger-Baum, Anat. für Künstler.)

THE INTERPARIETAL BONE

This bone (Os interparietale) is centrally placed between the squamous part of the occipital and the parietal bones. It is usually described as a single bone, although it ossifies from two chief lateral centers, and is sometimes distinctly paired in skulls of young foals.

The **external surface** (Facies externa) is quadrilateral and is flat and smooth in the very young foal; later it presents the median external sagittal crest.

The **internal surface** (Facies cerebralis) presents the **internal occipital protuberance,** a three-sided process which projects downward and forward into the cranial cavity between the cerebral hemispheres and the cerebellum; it has three concave surfaces and three sharp borders which form part of the tentorium osseum.

The **posterior** border is thick; it joins the squamous part of the occipital bone. The **lateral** and **anterior borders** are united by suture with the parietal bones.

Development.—The interparietal ossifies in membrane from two chief lateral centers.[1] It fuses first with the parietals, somewhat later with the occipital, but the period at which this union takes place is quite variable.

The Parietal Bones

The two **parietal bones** (Ossa parietalia) form the greater part of the roof of the cranium; they unite in the median line, forming the **sagittal suture.** Each is quadrilateral in outline and has two surfaces and four borders.

The **external surface** (Facies parietalis) is convex, and is marked by a more or less prominent curved line, the **external sagittal crest**; this is median in its posterior part, and is continuous with the crest of like name on the occipital bone; in front it curves outward and is continuous with the frontal crest. The surface external to the crest (Planum temporale) enters into the formation of the temporal fossa, and is roughened for the attachment of the temporal muscle.

The **internal** or **cerebral surface** (Facies cerebralis) is concave. It presents numerous **digital impressions** (Impressiones digitatæ) which correspond to the gyri of the cerebrum. There are also furrows (Sulci vasculosi) for the meningeal arteries. Along the inner border there is a **sagittal groove** (Sulcus sagittalis) for the superior longitudinal sinus.

The **anterior border** joins the frontal bone at the **parieto-frontal suture** (Sutura coronalis).

The **posterior** border meets the occipital bone at the **parieto-occipital suture** (Sutura lambdoidea). Below this junction it curves inward and concurs with the temporal bone in the formation of the **parieto-temporal canal** (Meatus temporalis). A **transverse groove** (Sulcus transversus) connects this canal with the sagittal sulcus.

The **internal** border is thick and serrated. It joins its fellow at the **sagittal suture,** and (in the young subject) meets the interparietal at the **interparietal suture.** The line of junction is marked internally by the **internal sagittal crest** (Crista sagittalis interna).

The **external** border is beveled and is overlapped by the squamous temporal bone, forming the parieto-temporal suture (Sutura parieto-squamosa). The angle of junction of the external and posterior borders articulates with the posterior angle of the temporal wing of the sphenoid.

Development.—Each parietal bone ossifies in membrane from a single center. In the young foal the central part of the bone is much more convex than in the adult and forms a prominence similar to the pronounced tuber parietale of the young child; the external sagittal crest is not present, and the external surface is smooth.

The sagittal suture is usually closed at four years, the parieto-occipital at five years, and the parieto-temporal at twelve to fifteen year

[1] According to Martin, there are originally four centers, two anterior and two posterior (smaller) ones, which fuse in a variable manner.

The Frontal Bones

The **frontal bones** (Ossa frontalia) are situated on the limits of the cranium and face, between the parietals behind and the nasal bones in front. Each is irregularly quadrilateral, and consists of frontal, orbital, and temporal parts.

The **frontal part** (Pars naso-frontalis) forms the basis of the forehead. Its **external surface** (Facies frontalis) is nearly flat, and is smooth and subcutaneous; it is separated from the temporal part by the external frontal crest (Crista frontalis externa). At the junction with the orbital part the **supraorbital** or **zygomatic process** (Proc. zygomaticus) curves outward and downward to join the zygomatic arch. The process partially separates the orbit from the temporal fossa; its root is perforated by the **supraorbital foramen,** or presents instead a notch on its anterior border; its upper surface is convex, while the lower or orbital surface is concave and smooth, forming a shallow fossa for the lacrimal gland (Fossa glandulæ lacrimalis). The **internal surface** enters into the formation of the cranial cavity and the frontal sinus. The cranial surface presents digital impressions for the cerebral gyri. The two plates of the bone separate and diverge in front, and thus inclose a large air-space which is part of the **frontal sinus.** The cranial plate curves downward and articulates with the cribriform plate of the ethmoid bone; the facial plate extends forward and joins the nasal and lacrimal bones.

The **orbital part** (Pars orbitalis) forms the major part of the inner wall of the orbital cavity. It is separated from the frontal part by a prominent ridge which is part of the orbital margin. Its **external** or **orbital surface** is concave and smooth, and presents superiorly a small depression (Fovea trochlearis), which is bridged by a small bar of cartilage, around which the superior oblique muscle of the eye is reflected. The lower border concurs with the orbital wing of the sphenoid in the formation of the ethmoidal or internal orbital foramen. The **internal surface** faces into the frontal sinus and gives attachment to the lateral mass of the ethmoid.

The **temporal part** is separated from the orbital part by the deep **sphenoidal notch** (Incisura sphenoidalis), which is occupied by the orbital wing of the sphenoid. Its **external surface** forms part of the inner wall of the temporal fossa. The **internal surface** is largely covered by the orbital wing of the sphenoid in the young subject, but later forms part of the wall of the frontal sinus.

The principal connections of the frontal bone are as follows: (1) The inner border joins its fellow at the **frontal suture.** (2) The anterior border meets the nasal and lacrimal at the **naso-frontal** and **fronto-lacrimal sutures.** (3) Laterally it forms the **spheno-frontal** suture with the orbital wing of the sphenoid, and also joins the palate bone and maxilla. (4) Posteriorly it meets the parietal at the **parieto-frontal** (or coronal) **suture,** and articulates below this with the squamous temporal. (5) The extremity of the supraorbital process unites with the zygomatic process of the temporal bone.

Development.—Each ossifies in membrane from one center which appears in the root of the supraorbital process. In the new-born foal there is a slit between the cranial plate and the orbital and temporal plates which receives the cartilaginous margin of the orbital wing of the sphenoid.

The Temporal Bones

The **temporal bone** (Os temporale) forms the greater part of the lateral wall of the cranium. It is situated between the occipital behind, the parietal above, the frontal in front, and the sphenoid below. It consists of two distinct parts, **squamous** and **petrous.**

1. The **squamous temporal** (Squama temporalis) is a shell-like plate which has two surfaces and four borders.

The **internal surface** (Facies cerebralis) is largely overlapped by the surrounding bones, but its central part is free and presents digital impressions and vascular grooves.

The **external surface** (Facies temporalis) is convex, and enters into the formation of the temporal fossa. From its lower part there springs the **zygomatic process** (Processus zygomaticus), which forms the external boundary of the temporal fossa. It is at first directed outward, and is wide and flattened dorso-ventrally. It then turns forward, becomes narrower, and is twisted so that its surfaces are internal and external. Its anterior end is pointed and joins the zygomatic process of the malar bone, with which it forms the **zygomatic arch** (Arcus zygomaticus). The narrow anterior part has a convex outer surface and a concave inner one. Its upper border has a rough area for articulation with the supraorbital process of the frontal. Its lower border is wide and rough. The wide posterior part presents on its ventral face a surface for articulation with the condyle of the mandible. This surface consists of a transversely elongated **condyle** (Tuberculum articulare), behind which is the **glenoid fossa** (Fossa mandibularis). The fossa is limited behind by the **post-glenoid process,** the anterior surface of which is articular. Behind this process is a fossa in which is the external opening of the parieto-temporal canal. The dorsal surface is concave and forms the outer boundary of the temporal fossa. The superior border is sinuous and is continuous behind with the temporal crest.

The **posterior process** (Processus posterior) springs from the posterior part of the squama. Its external surface is crossed by the temporal crest, which forms here the outer limit of the temporal fossa. The internal surface forms the outer boundary of the parieto-temporal canal, and is elsewhere applied to the petrous portion. It divides into two branches, upper and lower; the upper branch unites with the occipital bone, while the lower one curves downward behind the external auditory process and overlaps the mastoid process.

The **superior border** of the squamous temporal articulates with the parietal, forming the **parieto-temporal suture.** The **inferior border** joins the temporal wing of the sphenoid at the **spheno-squamous suture.** The **anterior border** unites with the frontal bone, and the **posterior** with the parietal.

2. The **petrous temporal** (Os petrosum) is placed between the occipital behind and the parietal in front, and is largely overlapped externally by the squamous temporal. It has the form of a four-sided pyramid, the base of which is ventral.

The **external surface** is mainly concealed by the squamous temporal, but two features are visible. A short tube of bone, the **external auditory process,** protrudes from the lowest part through the notch of the squamous temporal. The process is directed outward, upward, and a little forward. It gives attachment to the annular cartilage of the ear. Its lumen, the **external auditory meatus** (Meatus acusticus externus), conducts to the cavity of the middle ear (tympanum) in the dry skull, but is separated from it by the tympanic membrane in the natural state. The **mastoid process** projects ventrally in the interval between the posterior process of the squamous temporal and the root of the paramastoid (or styloid) process of the occipital bone; its outer surface is crossed by a curved groove which leads to the parieto-temporal canal.

The **internal surface** faces into the cerebellar fossa of the cranium. It is concave and smooth but irregular. In its lower part is the entrance to a short canal, the **internal auditory meatus,** which transmits the seventh and eighth cranial nerves.

The fundus of the meatus is divided by a crest into a superior and an inferior fossa. In the superior one is the origin of the **facial canal**, which curves through the bone and opens externally at the stylo-mastoid foramen; it transmits the facial (seventh cranial) nerve. The inferior fossa presents small foramina for the passage of fibers of the auditory (eighth cranial) nerve.

Behind the meatus and near the posterior margin of the surface is the slit-like opening of the aquæductus vestibuli, covered by a scale of bone. Below this is a narrow fissure, the orifice of the aquæductus cochleæ.

The **anterior surface** looks upward and forward. The outer part articulates with the parietal bone and the inner part faces into the cerebral fossa of the cranium. A sharp border, the **petrosal crest** (Crista petrosa), separates this surface from the inner one.

The **posterior surface** joins the lateral part of the occipital bone.

The **base** forms the outer boundary of the foramen lacerum basis cranii. It is very irregular and presents a number of important features. The hyoid **process** is a short rod which projects downward and forward below the base of the external auditory process, inclosed in a bony tube; it is connected by a bar of cartilage with the hyoid bone. The **stylo-mastoid foramen** is situated between the root of the hyoid process and the mastoid process; it is the external opening of the facial canal, through which the facial nerve emerges. The **bulla ossea** is a considerable eminence situated centrally; it is thin-walled and incloses a cavity which is part of the tympanum. The **muscular process**[1] is a sharp spine which projects downward and forward from the anterior part of the base; it gives origin to the tensor and levator palati muscles. External to the root of the preceding is the small **petro-tympanic** or **Glaserian** fissure (Fissura petro-tympanica) for the passage of the chorda tympani nerve. The osseous **Eustachian tube** is a semicanal at the inner side of the root of the muscular process; it leads to the tympanum. At the inner side of the preceding is the slit-like orifice of the petrosal canal, which communicates with the facial canal.

The **apex** projects upward and backward between the squamous temporal and the occipital bone.

Development.—The petrous temporal may be regarded as consisting of petro-mastoid and tympanic parts. The latter includes the external auditory process, the bulla ossea, and the muscular process; it is developed in membrane. The petro-mastoid is developed in the cartilaginous ear capsule. Its petrous part consists of very dense bone which contains the labyrinth or internal ear and forms the inner wall of the tympanum.

The **parieto-temporal canal** (Meatus temporalis) is a continuation of the transverse groove which extends outward from the base of the tentorium osseum. It is directed downward, forward, and somewhat outward, and opens externally in front of the root of the auditory process. It is bounded by the squamous temporal externally, the petrous behind, and the parietal in front and internally. Several foramina open from it into the temporal fossa. It contains a large vein (Vena cerebralis dorsalis), the continuation of the transverse sinus of the dura mater.

The **foramen lacerum basis cranii** (Foramen lacerum et jugulare) is a large irregular opening in the cranial base, bounded internally by the basilar part of the occipital bone, externally by the petrous temporal, and in front by the temporal wing of the sphenoid. It consists of a large anterior part (Foramen lacerum anterius), and a narrow posterior part (Foramen lacerum posterius s. jugulare). It transmits the internal carotid artery, the middle meningeal artery, the mandibular, ninth, tenth, and eleventh cranial nerves, and the inferior cerebral vein.

In the fresh state the foramen is occupied by a dense fibrous membrane which is perforated by apertures for the various structures transmitted. Thus there are three openings in front for the internal carotid artery, the mandibular nerve, and the middle meningeal artery; these are (from within outward) the foramen caroticum, ovale, spinosum.

(B) BONES OF THE FACE

The bones of the face (Ossa faciei) are the Maxilla, Premaxilla, Palatine, Pterygoid, Nasal, Lacrimal, Malar, Superior Turbinal, Inferior Turbinal, Vomer, Mandible, and Hyoid. The last three are single, the others paired.

[1] This is commonly termed the styloid process. It is not the homologue of the styloid process of man.

The Maxillae

The **maxillæ** are the principal bones of the upper jaw and carry the upper cheek teeth. They are situated on the lateral aspect of the face, and articulate with almost all of the facial bones and the frontal and temporal also. For description each may be divided into a body and two processes.

The body (Corpus maxillæ) presents two surfaces, two borders, and two extremities. The **external or facial surface** (Facies lateralis) is somewhat concave in front and convex behind. On its posterior part is a horizontal ridge, the **facial or zygomatic crest** (Crista facialis); in a skull of medium size its anterior end is about an inch and a half (3 to 4 cm.) above the third or fourth cheek tooth, and it is continued behind by a corresponding ridge on the malar bone. About two inches (5 cm.) above and a little in front of the anterior end of the crest is the **infraorbital foramen** (Foramen infraorbitale); this is the external opening of the infraorbital canal.

In the young horse the anterior part of the surface is convex over the embedded parts of the teeth. As the latter are extruded the surface flattens and becomes concave in old subjects.

The **internal or nasal surface** (Facies nasalis) is concave dorso-ventrally; it forms the greater part of the lateral wall of the nasal cavity. Its upper part is crossed obliquely forward and downward by the shallow **lacrimal groove** (Sulcus lacrimalis), which contains the naso-lacrimal duct; in the adult the posterior part of the groove is converted into a canal, which is continuous with that on the inner surface of the lacrimal bone. Below the groove is the **inferior turbinal crest** (Crista conchalis inferior), to which the inferior turbinal bone is attached. Lower down and parallel with the turbinal crest is the **palatine process,** which projects inward like a shelf. Behind this the surface is rough for articulation with the palate bone; this area is crossed by a groove which concurs with a furrow on the palate bone in the formation of the **palatine canal.** The posterior part of the bone is excavated to form part of the maxillary sinus.

The **superior border** is irregular and scaly. Its anterior part is grooved and its posterior part beveled for articulation with the nasal process of the premaxilla and the nasal and lacrimal bones.

The **inferior or alveolar border** (Processus alveolaris) is thick, and presents six large cavities, the **alveoli,** for the cheek teeth. The alveoli are separated by transverse **interalveolar septa.** There is often a small alveolus for the first premolar ("wolf tooth") close to the first large one. Further forward the border is narrow and forms part of the **interdental or interalveolar space** (Margo interalveolaris). Behind the last alveolus is a rough area, the **alveolar tuberosity.**

The **anterior extremity** is pointed. It joins the premaxilla, and forms with it the alveolus for the canine tooth.

The **posterior extremity** forms a rounded prominence, the **maxillary tuberosity** (Tuber maxillare). Internal to the tuberosity is a deep cavity, the maxillary hiatus, in which are three foramina. The upper one, the **maxillary foramen,** leads into the infraorbital canal. The lower one, the **posterior palatine foramen,** is the entrance to the palatine canal. The **spheno-palatine foramen** perforates the inner wall of the hiatus and opens into the nasal cavity.

The **zygomatic or temporal process** (Processus temporalis) projects backward above and external to the tuberosity; it is overlapped by the corresponding part of the malar and also articulates with the zygomatic process of the temporal. A small curved plate extends inward from it and joins the frontal and palate bones, forming part of the floor of the orbit.

The **palatine process** (Processus palatinus) is a plate which projects horizontally inward from the lower part of the inner surface of the body. It forms the greater part of the basis of the hard palate. Its **superior** or **nasal surface** is smooth and concave transversely; on its anterior part, close to the inner border, is a shallow groove in which the organ of Jacobson is situated. The **inferior** or **palatine surface** is slightly concave from side to side, and presents along its outer part the **palatine groove** (Sulcus palatinus). The groove is a continuation of the palatine canal, and contains the palatine artery and nerve. The **internal** border unites with its fellow to form the median palatine suture; its nasal aspect bears the nasal crest, which forms, with that of the opposite process, a groove for the vomer. The **posterior border** unites with the horizontal part of the palate bone at the transverse palatine suture.

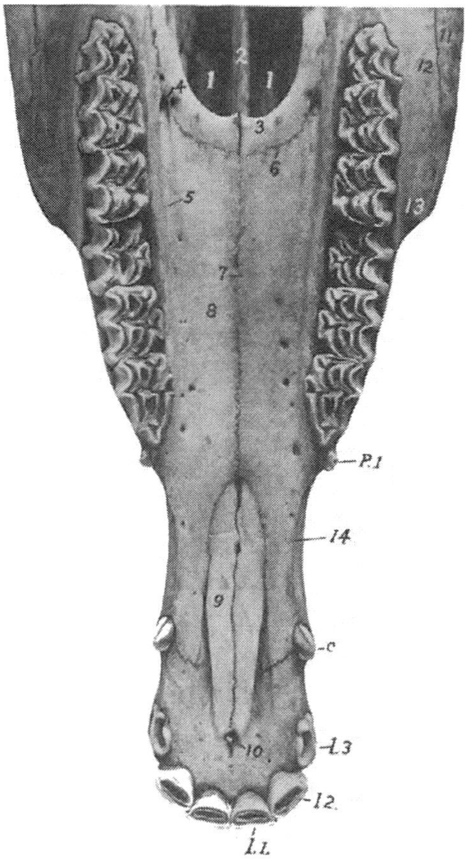

Fig. 31.—Upper Jaw of Horse About Four and a Half Years Old, Ventral View.

1, 1, Posterior nares; 2, vomer; 3, horizontal part of palate bone; 4, anterior palatine foramen; 5, palatine groove; 6, transverse palatine suture; 7, median palatine suture; 8, palate process of maxilla; 9, palate process of premaxilla; 10, foramen incisivum; 11, malar bone; 12, maxilla; 13, anterior end of facial crest; 14, interalveolar space; I. 1–3, incisor teeth; *C*, canine tooth; *P*1, first premolar or "wolf" tooth.

The **infraorbital** or **superior dental canal** extends almost horizontally from the maxillary foramen to the infraorbital foramen. It is placed at the upper edge of the inner plate of the maxilla, and traverses the maxillary sinus. Near the infraorbital foramen it gives off a small canal (Canalis alveolaris incisivus) which lies above the roots of the premolars and extends also into the premaxilla, carrying vessels and nerves to the teeth there.

Development.—The maxilla ossifies in membrane below and external to the cartilaginous nasal capsule. It has one chief center and a supplementary one in the region of the deciduous canine tooth (Martin).

The Premaxillae

The **premaxillæ** (Ossa incisiva) form the anterior part of the upper jaw and carry the incisor teeth. Each consists of a bodv and two processes, nasal and palatine.

The **body** is the thick anterior part which carries the incisor teeth. Its **labial** or **superior surface** is convex and smooth, and is related to the upper lip. The **palatine** or **inferior surface** is concave and presents a foramen a little behind its middle.[1] The **internal surface** is rough, and joins the opposite bone; it is marked by a curved groove, which forms with that on the opposed surface, the **incisive**

[1] This foramen is somewhat variable in position, but is commonly opposite the corner incisor. Smaller inconstant foramina are often present.

foramen (Foramen incisivum). The alveolar border (Limbus alveolaris) separates the palatine and labial surfaces; it is curved and thick, and presents three alveoli for the incisor teeth; behind the third alveolus it is rounded and free, forming part of the interalveolar space.

The nasal process (Processus nasalis) projects backward and upward from the body, forming here the lateral wall of the nasal cavity. The two surfaces, facial and nasal, are smooth and rounded. The superior border is free, thick, and smooth. The inferior border is dentated and joins the maxilla; at its anterior end it forms with the latter the alveolus for the permanent canine tooth.[1] The posterior extremity fits into the interval between the nasal bone and the maxilla.

The palatine process (Processus palatinus) is a thin plate which forms the anterior part of the basis of the hard palate. Its nasal or superior surface has a longitudinal ridge which forms with that of the other side a groove for the septal cartilage. The palatine or inferior surface is flat. The internal border is serrated and meets its fellow at the median palatine suture. The external border is separated from the maxilla and the nasal process by the palatine cleft (Fissura palatina). The posterior extremity fits into the interval between the vomer and the palatine process of the maxilla.

Development.—The premaxilla ossifies from a single center. Fusion of the two bones is complete at the end of the third or the beginning of the fourth year.

The Palatine Bones

The palatine bones (Ossa palatina) are situated on either side of the posterior nares, and form the posterior margin of the hard palate. Each is twisted so as to form a horizontal and a perpendicular part.

The horizontal part (Pars horizontalis) is a narrow plate which forms the posterior part of the hard palate. It presents smooth nasal and palatine surfaces. The internal border meets its fellow at the median palatine suture, on the nasal aspect of which is the nasal crest. The anterior border joins the palate process of the maxilla at the transverse palatine suture, and forms with it the anterior palatine foramen. The posterior border is concave and free; it gives attachment to the aponeurosis of the soft palate.

The perpendicular part (Pars perpendicularis) is more extensive and forms the outer boundary of the posterior nares. The nasal or internal surface is in the greater part of its extent concave and smooth; it is marked by a narrow rough area to which the pterygoid bone is attached. Below this the bone curves outward, forming the pterygoid process. The maxillary or external surface (Facies maxillaris) presents three areas for consideration. The largest articulates with the maxilla; it is rough and is crossed by a groove which enters into the formation of the palatine canal. Behind this is a smooth part which assists in forming the pterygo-palatine fossa. The rough area below this is overlapped by the pterygoid process of the sphenoid bone. The superior border is perforated by the spheno-palatine foramen. Behind the foramen the two plates of the bone separate to inclose part of the spheno-palatine sinus. The inner plate curves inward to articulate with the vomer. The outer plate joins the maxilla and frontal and the orbital wing of the sphenoid.

Development.—The palatine bone ossifies in membrane from a single center.

The Pterygoid Bones

The pterygoid bones (Ossa pterygoidea) are narrow, thin, bent plates, situated on either side of the posterior nares. Each has two surfaces and two extremities. The internal surface is smooth, and forms part of the boundary of the posterior nares. The external surface articulates with the palatine, vomer, and sphenoid,

[1] The alveolus for the temporary canine is commonly formed in the maxilla alone.

concurring with the last in the formation of the **pterygoid** or **Vidian canal.** The **anterior extremity** is free, turned slightly outward, and forms the **hamulus,** a pulley around which the tendon of the tensor palati muscle is reflected.

Development.—The pterygoid ossifies in membrane from a single center.

The Nasal Bones

The **nasal bones** (Ossa nasalia) are situated in front of the frontal bones and form the greater part of the roof of the nasal cavity. They have an elongated triangular outline, wide behind, pointed in front. Each presents two surfaces, two borders, a base, and an apex.

The **external** or **facial surface** is smooth and is convex transversely; the profile contour is usually slightly wavy, with a depression about its middle and a variably prominent area in front.

The **internal** or **nasal surface** is smooth and concave from side to side. About in its middle it presents the **superior turbinal crest** (Crista conchalis dorsalis), which is parallel with the inner border, and has the superior turbinal bone attached to it. Most of this surface faces into the nasal cavity, but its posterior part enters into the formation of the frontal sinus; the latter area is marked off by an oblique ridge.

The **internal border** is straight, and meets the opposite bone at the **nasal suture.**

The **external border** is irregular. Its anterior third is free and concurs with the nasal process in forming the **naso-maxillary notch** (Incisura naso-maxillaris). Behind this it is scaly for articulation with the end of the nasal process, the maxilla, and the lacrimal, forming the **naso-maxillary** and **naso-lacrimal sutures.**

The **base** or posterior end is beveled and overlaps the frontal bone, forming the **naso-frontal suture.**

The **apex** is pointed and thin.

Development.—Each nasal bone ossifies in membrane from a single center. The nasal suture does not close completely even in old age. In some cases the two plates separate to inclose a small air-space in the posterior part.

The Lacrimal Bones

The **lacrimal bones** (Ossa lacrimalia) are situated at the anterior part of the orbit, and extend forward on the face to the posterior border of the maxilla. Each presents three surfaces and a circumference.

The external aspect is clearly divided into orbital and facial parts by the orbital margin. The **orbital surface** (Facies orbitalis) is triangular in outline, smooth and concave; it forms part of the inner and front wall of the orbit. Near the orbital margin it presents a funnel-like **fossa** for the lacrimal sac (Fossa sacci lacrimalis), which is the entrance to the osseous lacrimal canal. Behind this is a depression in which the inferior oblique muscle of the eye takes origin. The **facial surface** (Facies facialis) is more extensive, and has the form of an irregular pentagon. It is slightly convex and smooth in the foal, flattened in the adult. It usually bears the small **lacrimal tubercle,** situated nearly an inch (ca. 2 cm.) from the orbital margin.

The **nasal** or **internal surface** (Facies nasalis) faces into the frontal and maxillary sinuses. It is concave and very irregular, and is crossed almost horizontally by the osseous **lacrimal canal** (Canalis lacrimalis osseus).

The **orbital margin** (Margo orbitalis) is concave, rough above, smooth below.

The **circumference** articulates above with the frontal and nasal bones, below with the malar and maxilla, in front with the maxilla, and behind with the frontal. The various sutures so formed are designated by combinations of the names of the bones.

Development.—Each ossifies in membrane from a single center.

The Malar Bones

The **malar** or **zygomatic bones** (Ossa zygomatica) are placed between the lacrimal above and the maxilla below and in front. Each is irregularly triangular in outline and presents three surfaces, three borders, a base, and an apex.

The **facial surface** is smooth, slightly convex, wide in front, and narrow behind. At its lower part it presents the **facial** or **zygomatic crest**, which is continuous in front with the similar ridge on the maxilla and behind with the zygomatic process of the temporal: the crest is rough below, where the masseter muscle is attached to it.

The **orbital surface** is separated from the facial surface by the concave **orbital margin**. It is concave and smooth, and forms part of the lower and front wall of the orbit.

The **nasal surface** is concave and faces into the maxillary sinus. In the young foal a considerable part of it articulates with the maxilla.

The **superior border** articulates with the lacrimal chiefly, but to a small extent behind with the maxilla also.

The **inferior border** and the **base** articulate with the maxilla.

The **apex** is beveled above and is overlapped by the zygomatic process of the temporal bone.

Development.—Each ossifies in membrane from one or two centers.

The Turbinal Bones

These (Ossa turbinata) are delicate, scroll-like bones, four in number, which are attached to the lateral walls of the nasal cavity. They project into the cavity and greatly diminish its extent. Each is composed of a very thin lamina, cribriform in many places, and covered on both sides with mucous membrane in the fresh state. They are arranged in two pairs, superior and inferior.

The **superior** or **naso-turbinal** (Concha dorsalis)[1] is somewhat cylindrical in form, small at its anterior part, and flattened transversely. It is attached to the turbinal crest of the nasal bone and the nasal plate of the frontal bone. The anterior part is rolled like a scroll one and a half times, thus inclosing a cavity which communicates with the middle meatus nasi. The arrangement is best seen on a cross-section (Fig. 37). The posterior part is not rolled, but its lower border is attached to the lateral nasal wall, thus helping to inclose a large space which is part of the frontal sinus. This cavity is separated from that of the scroll-like part by a transverse septum. The **internal surface** is flattened, and is separated from the septum nasi by a narrow interval, the **common meatus** (Meatus nasi communis). Another narrow passage, the **superior meatus** (Meatus nasi superior), separates the upper surface from the roof of the nasal cavity. The space between the lower surface and the inferior turbinal is the **middle meatus** (Meatus nasi medius). The anterior extremity is prolonged toward the nostril by two small bars of cartilage.

The **inferior** or **maxillo-turbinal bone** (Concha ventralis) is shorter and smaller posteriorly than the upper one. It is attached to the inferior turbinal crest, and consists, like the upper one, of an anterior coiled and a posterior uncoiled portion.

To express briefly the mode of coiling of the two bones of the same side we may say that they are rolled toward the septum and each other.

The inferior and posterior borders of the posterior part are attached to the maxilla, thus helping to inclose a cavity which is part of the maxillary sinus. The lower surface is separated from the floor of the nasal cavity by the **inferior meatus** (Meatus nasi inferior), which is much larger than the other nasal passages. The anterior extremity is prolonged to the nostril by a curved bar of cartilage.

Development.—Each ossifies in cartilage from a single center.

[1] This bone is really a greatly developed first ethmo-turbinal.

The Vomer

The vomer is a median unpaired bone, which assists in forming the lower part of the septum nasi. It is composed of a thin lamina which is bent (except in its posterior part) so as to form a narrow groove (Sulcus septi narium), in which the lower part of the perpendicular plate of the ethmoid bone and the septal cartilage are received. The **lateral surfaces,** right and left, are highest near the posterior end and diminish gradually to the anterior end; they are slightly convex dorso-ventrally, and are covered by the nasal mucous membrane during life. The **inferior border** is thin and free in its posterior third, and divides the posterior nares into right and left halves; in the remainder of its extent it is wider and is attached to the nasal crest. The **anterior extremity** lies above the ends of the palatine processes of the premaxillæ. The **posterior extremity** consists of two wings (Alæ vomeris) which extend outward below the body of the pre-sphenoid; posteriorly they form a notch (Incisura vomeris), and laterally join the palate and pterygoid bones.

Development.—The vomer is primitively double, and ossifies from a center on either side in the membrane covering the cartilaginous septum nasi; the two laminæ then fuse below and form a groove.

The Mandible

The **mandible** or **inferior maxilla** (Mandibula) is the largest and the only movable bone of the face. The two halves of which it consists at birth unite during the second or third month, and it is usually described as a single bone. It carries the lower teeth, and articulates by its condyles with the squamous temporal on either side. It consists of a body and two rami.[1]

The **body** (Corpus mandibulæ) is the thick anterior part which bears the incisor teeth. It presents two surfaces and a border. The **lingual** or **superior surface** (Facies lingualis) is smooth and slightly concave; during life it is covered by mucous membrane, and the tip of the tongue overlies it. The labial or **mental surface** (Facies mentalis) is convex and is related to the lower lip. It is marked by a median furrow which indicates the position of the primitive symphysis mandibulæ. The curved **alveolar border** (Limbus alveolaris) presents six alveoli for the incisor teeth, and a little further back two alveoli for the canine teeth in the male; in the mare the latter are usually absent or small.

The **rami** (Rami mandibulæ) extend backward from the body and diverge to inclose the **submaxillary space** (Spatium mandibulare). Each ramus is bent so as to consist of a horizontal part (Pars molaris) which bears the lower cheek teeth, and a vertical part (Ramus mandibulæ) which is expanded and furnishes attachment to powerful muscles; the term **angle** is applied to the most prominent part of the curve. The ramus presents two surfaces, two borders, and two extremities. The **external surface** is smooth and slightly convex from edge to edge on the horizontal part; at the junction with the body it presents the **mental foramen** (Foramen mentale), which is the external opening of the mandibular or inferior dental canal. On the vertical part it is somewhat concave and presents a number of rough lines for the attachment of the masseter muscle. The **internal surface** of the horizontal part is smooth, and presents a shallow longitudinal depression in its middle; above this there is often a faint mylo-hyoid line for the attachment of the muscle of like name. At the lower part of the junction with the body there is a small fossa for the attachment of the genio-hyoid and genio-glossus muscles. On the vertical part the surface is concave, and is marked in its lower and

[1] In the Stuttgart Nomenclator Anatomicus (S. N. A.) the body (Corpus) is the part which bears the teeth, and is divided into a pars incisiva and a pars molaris. The ramus is the rest of the bone.

posterior part by rough lines for the attachment of the internal pterygoid muscle. In front of its middle is the **mandibular** or **inferior maxillary foramen** (Foramen mandibulare), which is the posterior orifice of the **mandibular** or **inferior dental canal** (Canalis mandibulæ). The canal curves downward and passes forward below the cheek teeth, opening externally at the mental foramen; it is continued into the body of the bone as a small canal (Canalis alveolaris incisivus), which carries the vessels and nerves to the incisor teeth. The **superior** or **alveolar border** forms anteriorly part of the interalveolar space; here it is thin. Behind this it is thick and is excavated by six alveoli for the lower cheek teeth. Behind the last alveolus it curves sharply upward and is narrow and rough. In the young foal there is commonly a small alveolus for the vestige of the first premolar ("wolf tooth") close to the first large one. The **inferior border** of the horizontal part is nearly straight; it is thick and rounded in the young horse, becoming narrower and sharp in old subjects. At its posterior part there is a smooth impression (Incisura vasorum) where the facial vessels and parotid duct turn round the bone. Behind this point the border curves sharply upward, forming the **angle** (Angulus mandibulæ); this part is thick and has two roughened lips, internal and external, separated by a considerable intermediate space; near the condyle it becomes narrower. The **anterior extremity** joins the body. The **superior extremity** comprises the **coronoid process** in front and the **condyle** behind, the two being separated by the **sigmoid notch** (Incisura mandibulæ), through which the nerve to the masseter muscle passes. The **coronoid process** (Processus coronoideus) is thin transversely and curved slightly inward and backward. It projects upward in the temporal fossa, and furnishes insertion to the temporal muscle. The **condyle** (Capitulum mandibulæ) lies at a much lower level than the end of the coronoid process. It is elongated transversely and articulates with the squamous temporal through the medium of an articular disc. The part below the condyle is usually termed the **neck** (Collum mandibulæ); on its antero-internal part is a depression (Fovea pterygoidea) for the attachment of the external pterygoid muscle. The middle of the vertical part of the ramus consists to a large extent of a single plate of compact substance which may be so thin in places as to be translucent.

Development.—The mandible develops from two chief centers in the connective tissue which overlies the paired Meckel's cartilages. At birth it consists of two symmetrical halves which meet at a median symphysis. Fusion usually occurs in the second or third month.

Age changes.—These are associated largely with the growth and later with the reduction of the teeth. In the young horse, in which the teeth are large and are in great part embedded in the bone, the body is thick and strongly curved, and the horizontal part of the ramus is also thick. Later, as the teeth are extruded from the bone, the body becomes flattened and narrower, and the horizontal part of the ramus is thinner, especially in its lower part; the angle and the impression in front of it are more pronounced.

The Hyoid Bone

The hyoid bone (Os hyoideum) is situated chiefly between the vertical parts of the rami of the mandible, but its upper part extends somewhat further back. It is attached to the petrous temporal bones by rods of cartilage, and supports the root of the tongue, the pharynx, and larynx. It consists of a body, a lingual process, and three pairs of cornua.

The **body** or **basihyoid** (Basis ossis hyoidei) is a short transverse bar, compressed dorso-ventrally. The upper surface is concave and smooth in its middle, and presents at each end a convex facet or tubercle for articulation with the small cornu. The lower surface is slightly roughened for muscular attachment. The anterior border carries medially the lingual process. The posterior border is concave and smooth in its middle, and carries on either side the thyroid cornu. The body, the lingual process, and the thyroid processes are fused together, and may be compared to a spur or a fork with a very short handle.

The **lingual process** (Processus lingualis) projects forward medially from the body, and is embedded in the root of the tongue during life. It is compressed laterally and has a blunt-pointed free end. The lateral surfaces are slightly concave. The upper border is narrow, the lower thick and irregular.

The **thyroid cornua** or **thyrohyoids** (Cornua laryngea)[1] extend backward and upward from the lateral parts of the body. They are compressed laterally (except at their junction with the body), and their posterior ends are connected with the anterior cornua of the thyroid cartilage of the larynx.

The **small cornua** or **keratohyoids** (Cornua minora) are short rods which are directed upward and forward from either end of the upper surface of the body. Each is somewhat constricted in its middle part and has slightly enlarged ends. The lower end has a small concave facet which articulates with the body. The upper end articulates with the great cornu, or with the middle cornu when present.

The **great cornua** or **stylohyoids** are much the largest parts of the bone. They are directed upward and backward, and are connected above with the base of the petrous temporal bones. Each is a thin plate, seven or eight inches (ca. 18 to 20 cm.) long, which is slightly curved in its length, so that the external surface is concave and smooth. The internal surface is convex and smooth. The borders are thin. The upper extremity is large and forms two angles; the upper angle is connected by a rod of cartilage with the hyoid process of the petrous temporal bone; the lower angle is somewhat thickened and rough for muscular attachment. The lower extremity is small, and articulates with the small or the middle cornu.

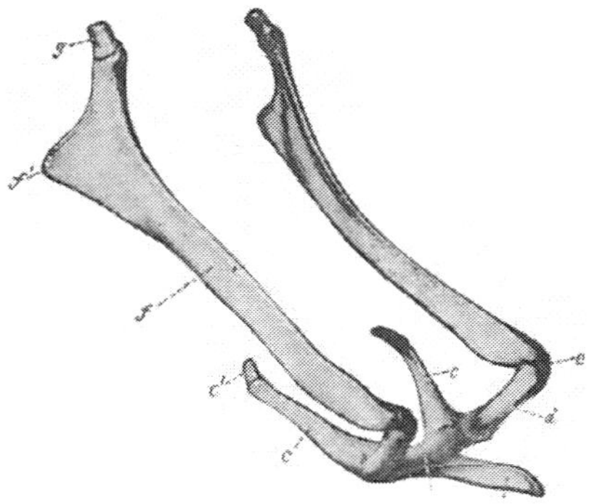

FIG. 32.—HYOID BONE OF HORSE, VIEWED FROM THE SIDE AND SOMEWHAT FROM IN FRONT.

a, Body; *b*, lingual process; *c*, thyroid cornu; *c'*, cartilage of *c*; *d*, small cornu; *e*, middle cornu; *f*, great cornu; *f'*, muscular angle of great cornu; *g*, cartilage of great cornu. (Ellenberger-Baum, Anat. d. Haustiere.)

The **middle cornua** or **epihyoids** are small wedge-shaped pieces or nodules interposed between the small and great cornua. They are usually transitory, and unite with the great cornua in the adult.

Development.—The hyoid ossifies in the cartilages of the second and third visceral arches. Each part has a separate center, except the lingual process, which ossifies by extension from the body. The latter has primarily two centers (Martin).

THE SKULL AS A WHOLE

The skull of the horse has the form of a long four-sided pyramid, the base of which is posterior. It is convenient to exclude the mandible and hyoid from present consideration. The division between the cranium (Cranium cerebrale) and the face (Cranium viscerale) may be indicated approximately by a transverse plane through the anterior margins of the orbits.

The **superior** or **frontal surface** (Norma frontalis) is formed by the upper part of the occipital, the interparietal, parietal, frontal, and nasal bones. It may be

[1] These correspond to the great cornua of man.

divided into parietal, frontal, nasal, and premaxillary regions. The **parietal region** extends from the occipital crest to the parieto-frontal or coronal suture. It is marked medially by the **external sagittal crest,** which bifurcates in front, the branches becoming continuous with the **frontal crests.** The latter curve outward to the root of the supraorbital process. The **frontal region** is the widest part of the surface, and is smooth and almost flat. It is bounded in front by the naso-frontal suture. On either side of it is the root of the **supraorbital process,** pierced

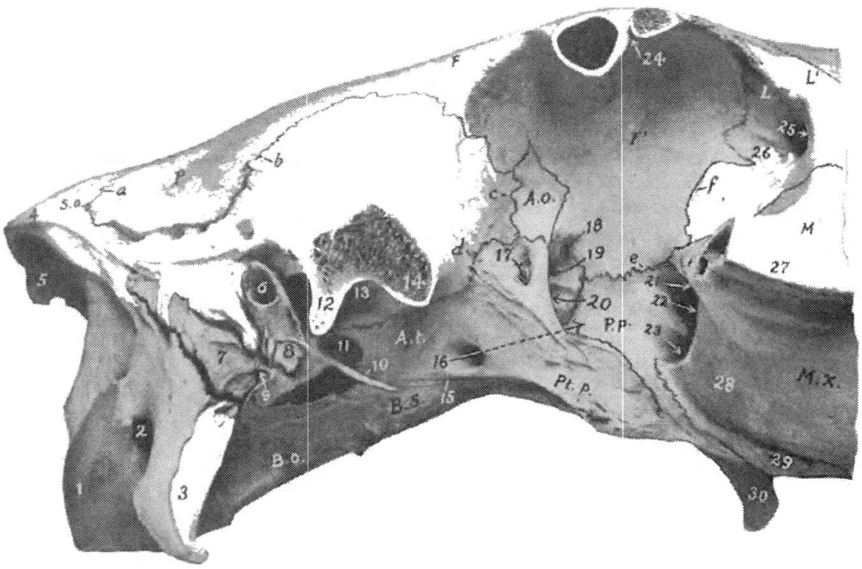

FIG. 33.—CRANIAL AND ORBITAL REGIONS OF SKULL OF HORSE, LATERAL VIEW. THE ZYGOMATIC ARCH AND SUPRAORBITAL PROCESSES HAVE BEEN SAWN OFF.

1, Occipital condyle; 2, condyloid fossa; 3, paramastoid or styloid process; 4, occipital crest; 5, external occipital protuberance; 6, external auditory meatus; 7, mastoid process; 8, hyoid process; 9, stylomastoid foramen; 10, muscular process; 11, foramen lacerum anterius; 12, postglenoid process; 13, glenoid cavity; 14, temporal condyle; 15, Vidian groove; 16, alar canal of pterygoid process indicated by arrow; 17, temporal foramen; 18, ethmoidal foramen; 19, optic foramen; 20, foramen lacerum orbitale; 21, maxillary foramen; 22, sphenopalatine foramen; 23, posterior palatine foramen; 24, supraorbital foramen (opened); 25, lacrimal fossa; 26, depression for origin of obliquus oculi inferior; 27, facial crest; 28, maxillary tuberosity; 29, alveolar tuberosity; 30, hamulus of pterygoid bone; *S.o.*, supraoccipital; *P*, parietal; *S*, squamous temporal; *B.o.*, basioccipital; *B.s.*, basisphenoid; *A.t.*, temporal wing of sphenoid; *A.o.*, orbital wing of sphenoid; *Pt.p.*, pterygoid process of sphenoid; *P.p.*, perpendicular part of palate bone; *F,F'*, facial and orbital parts of frontal bone; *L,L'*, orbital and facial parts of lacrimal bone; *M*, facial part of malar bone; *M.x.*, maxilla; *a*, parieto-occipital suture; *b*, parieto-temporal or squamous suture; *c, d*, spheno-squamous suture; *e*, palato-frontal suture; *f*, fronto-lacrimal suture.

by the **supraorbital foramen.** The **nasal region** is convex from side to side, wide behind, narrow in front. Its profile is in some cases nearly straight; in others it is undulating, with a variably marked depression about its middle and at the anterior end. The **premaxillary region** presents the **osseous nasal aperture** (Apertura nasalis ossea) and the **foramen incisivum.**

The **lateral surface** (Norma lateralis) may be divided into cranial, orbital, and maxillary or preorbital regions.

The **cranial region** presents the temporal fossa, the zygomatic arch, and the outer part of the petrous temporal bone.

The **temporal fossa** is bounded internally by the sagittal and frontal crests, externally by the temporal crest and the zygomatic arch, and behind by the occipital crest. Its upper and middle parts are rough for the attachment of the temporal muscle. In its lower posterior part are several **foramina** which communicate with the parieto-temporal canal. The fossa is continuous in front with the orbital cavity.

The **zygomatic arch** is formed by the zygomatic processes of the temporal, malar, and maxilla. Its ventral face presents the **condyle** and **glenoid cavity** for articulation with the lower jaw, through the medium of the articular disc. Behind the glenoid cavity is the **post-glenoid process.**

The **external auditory process** projects outward through a deep notch in the lower margin of the squamous temporal below the temporal crest. A little further back is the **mastoid process,** crossed in its upper part by a groove for the mastoid artery.

The **orbital region** comprises the orbit and the pterygo-palatine fossa.

The **orbit** is a cavity which incloses the eyeball, with the muscles, vessels, and nerves associated with it. It is not separated in the skeleton from the temporal fossa. The long **axis** of the cavity, taken from the optic foramen to the middle of the inlet, is directed forward, outward, and slightly upward. The **inner wall** (Paries medialis) is complete and extensive. It is concave and smooth, and is formed by the frontal and lacrimal and the orbital wing of the sphenoid. In its extreme anterior part is the fossa for the lacrimal sac. Behind this is a small depression in which the inferior oblique muscle of the eye arises; here the plate which separates the orbit from the maxillary sinus is very thin. The **upper wall** (Paries superior) is formed by the frontal and to a small extent by the lacrimal bone. It presents the supraorbital foramen, which perforates the root of the supraorbital process. The lower **wall** (Paries inferior) is very incomplete, and is formed by the malar, the zygomatic process of the temporal, and to a small extent by the maxilla. The **external boundary** (Paries lateralis) is the supraorbital process. At the extreme posterior part is the **orbital group** of **foramina.** Four are situated in front of the pterygoid crest. Of these, the uppermost is the **ethmoidal** or **internal orbital foramen,** which transmits the ethmoidal vessels and nerve. The **optic foramen** is situated a little lower and further back; it transmits the optic nerve. Immediately below the optic is the **foramen lacerum orbitale,** which transmits the ophthalmic, third, sixth, and sometimes the fourth nerve; commonly there is a very small **trochlear** or **pathetic foramen** in the crest for the last named nerve. The **foramen rotundum** is below the foramen lacerum, from which it is separated by a thin plate; it transmits the superior maxillary nerve. The **alar canal** opens in common with the foramen rotundum, and the anterior opening of the pterygoid or Vidian canal is also found here. The **temporal foramen** (For. alare parvum) is just behind the pterygoid crest and on a level with the foramen lacerum. It is the upper opening of a canal which leads from the alar canal, and through it the anterior deep temporal artery emerges. The **inlet** of the orbital cavity (Aditus orbitæ) is circumscribed by a complete bony ring, which is nearly circular. Its antero-inferior part (Margo infraorbitalis) is smooth and rounded; the remainder (Margo supraorbitalis) is rough and irregularly notched. During life the cavity is completed by the periorbita or ocular sheath, a conical fibrous membrane, the apex of which is attached around the optic foramen.

Below the orbital cavity is the **pterygo-palatine** fossa. Its wall is formed by the pterygoid process, the perpendicular part of the palate bone, and the tuber maxillare. Its deep anterior part (maxillary hiatus) contains three foramina. The upper one, the **maxillary foramen,** is the entrance to the infraorbital canal, which transmits the infraorbital nerve and vessels. The **spheno-palatine foramen** transmits vessels and nerves of like name to the nasal cavity. The lower foramen, the **posterior palatine**, transmits the palatine artery and nerve to the palatine canal. The upper part of the fossa is smooth, and is crossed by the internal maxillary artery and the maxillary nerve. The lower part is chiefly roughened for the attachment of the internal pterygoid muscle, but is crossed in front by a smooth groove in which the palatine vein lies.

The **maxillary** or **preorbital region** is formed chiefly by the maxilla, but also by the premaxilla, and the facial parts of the lacrimal and malar bones. Its contour is approximately triangular, the base being posterior. It offers two principal features. The **facial crest** extends forward from the lower margin of the orbit, and ends abruptly at a point about an inch and a half (3 to 4 cm.) above the third or fourth cheek tooth;[1] its inferior aspect is rough for the attachment of the masseter muscle. The **infraorbital foramen** is situated in a transverse plane about an inch (ca. 2 to 3 cm.) in front of the end of the crest and about two inches (5 cm.) above it. The foramen opens forward, and through it the infraorbital artery and nerve emerge. The surface over the premolar teeth varies greatly with age, in conformity with the size of the embedded parts of the teeth. In the young horse the surface here is strongly convex, the outer plate of bone is thin and even defective sometimes in places, and the form of the teeth is indicated by eminences (Juga alveolaria). In the old animal the surface is concave on account of the extrusion of the teeth from the bone. The downward curve of the premaxilla is pronounced in the young subject, very slight in the aged.

The **inferior** or **basal surface** (Norma basalis), exclusive of the mandible, consists of cranial, guttural, and palatine regions.

The **cranial region** (Basis cranii externa) extends forward to the vomer and pterygoid processes (Fig. 28). At its posterior end is the **foramen magnum**, flanked by the **occipital condyles**. External to the latter is the **condyloid fossa**, in which is the **hypoglossal foramen**, which transmits the hypoglossal nerve and the condyloid artery and vein. Further outward are the **paramastoid** or **styloid processes** (Processus jugulares) of the occipital bone. Extending forward centrally is a prismatic bar, formed by the basilar part of the occipital and the body of the sphenoid bone; at the junction of these parts are tubercles for the attachment of the ventral straight muscles of the head. On either side of the basilar part of the occipital is the **foramen lacerum basis cranii**, bounded externally by the base of the petrous temporal bone. In front of these the region becomes very wide on account of the lateral extension of the **zygomatic processes**, bearing on the ventral aspect the **condyle** and **glenoid cavity** for articulation with the mandible. Beyond this the process turns forward and joins the zygomatic process of the malar, completing the zygomatic arch and the surface for the attachment of the masseter muscle. On either side of the body of the sphenoid is the infratemporal fossa, formed by the temporal wing and the root of the pterygoid process of the sphenoid bone. It is bounded in front by the pterygoid crest, which separates it from the orbit and the pterygo-palatine fossa. In it is the **pterygoid** or **alar foramen**, which transmits the internal maxillary artery. A little lower is the entrance to the **pterygoid** (Vidian) **canal**.

The **guttural region** presents the pharyngeal orifice of the nasal cavity. This is elliptical and is divided in its depth medially by the vomer into two **posterior nares** or **choanæ**. It is bounded in front and laterally by the palate and pterygoid bones, behind by the vomer. It is flanked by the hamular process of the pterygoid bones. The plane of the opening is nearly horizontal, and the length is about twice the width.

The **palatine region** comprises a little more than half of the entire length

[1] This relation varies with age; in the young horse the third tooth, in the old subject the fourth, lies below the end of the crest.

of the base of the skull (Fig. 31). The hard **palate** (Palatum durum) is concave from side to side, and in its length also in the anterior part. It is formed by the palatine processes of the premaxillæ and maxillæ, and the horizontal parts of the palate bones. It is circumscribed in front and laterally by the **superior alveolar arch,** in which the upper teeth are implanted. The **interalveolar space** (Margo interalveolaris) is that part of the arch in which alveoli are not present. Behind the last alveolus is the **alveolar tuberosity,** and internal to this is a groove for the palatine vein. In the middle line is the **median palatine suture** (Sutura palatina mediana). In the line of the suture, a little behind the central incisors, is the **foramen incisivum,** through which the palato-labial artery passes. On either side, parallel with the alveolar part of the maxilla, is the **palatine groove** (Sulcus palatinus), which contains the palatine vessels and nerve. It is continuous at the anterior palatine foramen with the palatine canal, which is situated between the maxilla and the palate bone. The **palatine cleft** (Fissura palatina) is the narrow interval along the outer margin of the palatine process of the premaxilla; it is closed in the fresh state by cartilage. Scattered along each side of the palate are several vascular foramina. The **transverse palatine suture** (Sutura palatina transversa) is about half an inch from the posterior border. The latter is in a plane through the last molar teeth, and is concave and free.

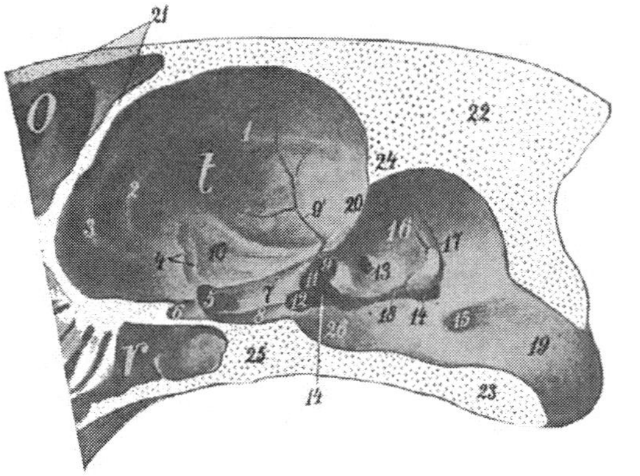

FIG. 34.—CRANIAL CAVITY OF HORSE AS SEEN ON SAGITTAL SECTION OF SKULL.

O, Frontal sinus; *r*, sphenoidal sinus; *t*, cerebral compartment of cranium; 1–3, ridges (juga) corresponding to fissures of lateral surface of cerebrum; 4, groove for middle cerebral artery; 5, entrance to for. lacerum orbitale; 6, entrance to optic foramen; 7, 8, grooves on sphenoid bone; 9, incisura spinosa; 9′, groove for middle meningeal artery; 10, fossa for pyriform lobe of cerebrum; 11, incisura ovalis; 12, incisura carotica; 13, internal auditory meatus; 14, foramen lacerum basis cranii; 15, hypoglossal foramen; 16, petrous temporal; 17, orifice of aquæductus vestibuli; 18, orifice of aquæductus cochleæ; 19, foramen magnum; 20, petrosal crest; 21, two plates of frontal bone; 22, supraoccipital; 23, basioccipital; 24, tentorium osseum; 25, body of sphenoid. (After Ellenberger-Baum, Top. Anat. d. Pferdes.)

The posterior or **nuchal surface** (Norma occipitalis) is formed by the occipital bone. It is trapezoidal in outline, wider below than above, concave dorso-ventrally, convex transversely. It is separated from the superior surface by the **occipital crest,** and from the lateral surfaces by the **superior curved lines** (Lineæ nuchæ superiores). Below the crest are two rough areas for the attachment of the complexus muscles. A little lower is a central eminence on the sides of which the ligamentum nuchæ is attached. At the lowest part centrally is the **foramen magnum,** at which the brain and spinal cord meet; this is bounded laterally by the **occipital condyles,** which are flanked by the **paramastoid** or **styloid processes** (Processus jugulares).

The **apex** of the skull is formed by the bodies of the premaxillæ and mandible, carrying the incisor teeth.

THE CRANIAL CAVITY

This cavity incloses the brain, with its membranes and vessels. It is relatively small and is ovoid in shape.

The superior wall or roof (Calvaria) is formed by the supraoccipital, interparietal, parietal, and frontal bones. In the middle line is the internal sagittal crest, which joins the crista galli in front, and furnishes attachment to the falx cerebri. Posteriorly the crest is continued by the sharp anterior margin of the tentorium osseum, which projects downward and forward into the cavity, and gives attachment to the tentorium cerebelli by its sharp lateral edges. Behind this the roof is grooved centrally for the middle lobe or vermis of the cerebellum. Transverse grooves pass from the base of the tentorium osseum to the parieto-temporal canals. The anterior part of the roof is hollowed by the frontal sinus. The occipital part is very thick and strong.

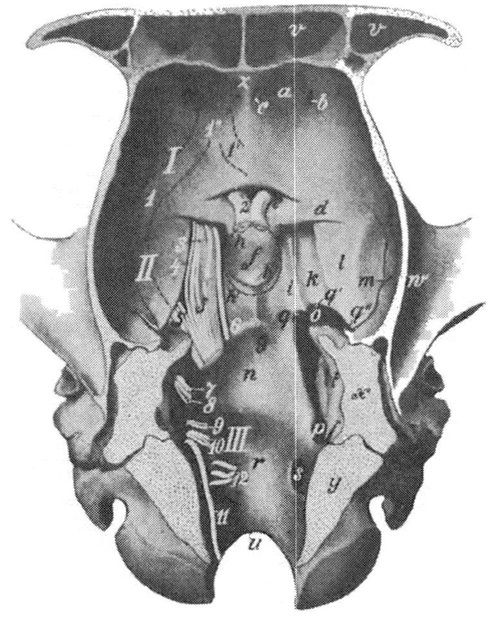

FIG. 35.—FLOOR OF CRANIAL CAVITY OF HORSE.

The roots of the cranial nerves are shown on the left side and are designated by number. *I*, Anterior cranial fossa; *II*, middle cranial fossa; *III*, posterior cranial fossa; *a*, ethmoidal fossa; *b*, ethmoidal foramen; *c*, foramen for nasal branch of ophthalmic artery; *d*, orbital wing of sphenoid bone; *e*, optic fossa; *f*, sella turcica; *g*, spheno-occipital crest; *h*, *h'*, dotted line indicating contour of pituitary body; *h''*, slight elevation representing dorsum sellæ; *i*, k, grooves for nerves and cavernous sinus; *l*, depression for pyriform lobe of cerebrum; *m*, groove for middle meningeal artery; *n*, depression for pons; *o*, foramen lacerum anterius; *p*, foramen lacerum posterius; *q*, incisura carotica; *q'*, incisura ovalis; *q''*, incisura spinosa; *r*, depression for medulla oblongata; *s*, hypoglossal foramen; *t*, internal auditory meatus; *u*, foramen magnum; *v*, frontal sinus; *w*, zygomatic process of temporal bone; *x*, section of petrous temporal; *y*, section of occipital bone; *z*, crista galli; 1, 1', 1'', dotted lines indicating position of olfactory tracts and peduncle. (After Ellenberger-Baum, Top. Anat. d. Pferdes.)

The **lateral walls** are formed by the occipital, parietal, temporal, and frontal bones, and in part by the orbital wings of the sphenoid. Each is crossed obliquely by the **petrosal crest**, which concurs with the projecting margin of the parietal bone and the tentorium osseum in dividing the cavity into cerebral and cerebellar compartments. Behind the crest is a depression for the lateral lobe (hemisphere) of the cerebellum. Below this are the internal auditory meatus and the openings of the aquæductus vestibuli and aquæductus cochleæ.

The roof and lateral walls are marked by digital impressions and vascular grooves.

The **inferior wall or floor** (Basis cranii interna) may be regarded as forming three fossæ. The **anterior fossa** (Fossa cranii anterior) supports the frontal and olfactory parts of the cerebrum. It is formed chiefly by the presphenoid, and lies at a higher level than the middle fossa. In front the fossa is divided medially by the **crista galli**, lateral to which are the deep **ethmoidal** or **olfactory fossæ** for the olfactory lobes. The **ethmoidal** or **internal** orbital **foramen** perforates the cranial wall at the outer side of these fossæ. Further back the central part of the surface is slightly elevated, and is flanked by shallow depressions which support the olfactory peduncles. Posteriorly is a bony shelf which covers the entrance to the **optic foramina**; the edge of this shelf and the posterior borders of the orbital wings of the sphenoid may be taken as the line of demarcation between the anterior and middle fossæ. The **middle fossa** (Fossa cranii media) is the widest part of the cavity. It extends backward to the internal spheno-occipital and petrosal crests, thus corresponding to the post-sphenoid. In its middle is a small fossa, the **sella turcica,** in which the pituitary body, or hypophysis cerebri, is situated. On either side are two grooves for nerves; the inner one transmits the ophthalmic, third, and sixth nerves to the foramen lacerum orbitale; the outer one leads to the foramen rotundum, and lodges the maxillary nerve. External to the grooves is a depression for the pyriform lobe of the cerebrum. The **posterior fossa** (Fossa cranii posterior) corresponds to the basilar part of the occipital bone. It contains the medulla, pons, and cerebellum. In front is a median depression (Fossa pontis) for the pons. The surface behind this is concave transversely and slopes gently downward to the foramen magnum; it supports the medulla. On either side are the **foramen lacerum basis cranii** and the **hypoglossal foramen.**

The **anterior** or **nasal wall** is formed by the cribriform plate of the ethmoid, which separates the cranium from the nasal cavity. It is perforated by numerous foramina for the passage of the olfactory nerve-bundles.

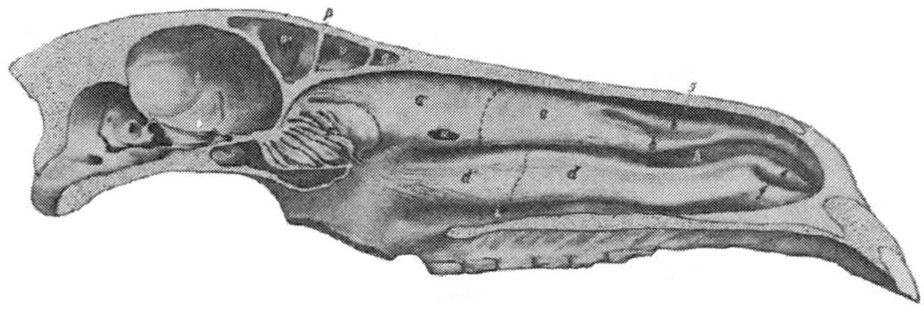

FIG. 36.—MEDIAN SECTION OF SKULL OF HORSE WITHOUT THE MANDIBLE.

The septum nasi is removed, but the mucous membrane on the turbinal bones is retained. *a, a'*, Superior turbinal bone, dotted line indicating limit between anterior coiled part and posterior uncoiled part; *b, b'*, superior turbinal folds, inclosing bars of cartilage; *c*, fold of mucous membrane formed by union of *b* and *b'*; *d, d'*, anterior coiled and posterior uncoiled part of inferior turbinal, dotted line indicating septum between them; *e, f*, inferior turbinal folds, former (alar fold) inclosing bar of cartilage; *g, h, i*, superior, middle, inferior meatus; *o, o'*, frontal sinus; partial septum between *o* and *o'*; *q*, nasal part of frontal sinus (nasal sinus); *r*, lateral mass of ethmoid bone; *s*, sphenoidal sinus; *t*, cranial cavity; *u*, opening made in superior turbinal bone at point where drainage of frontal sinus may be obtained. (After Ellenberger, in Leisering's Atlas.)

THE NASAL CAVITY

The **nasal cavity** (Cavum nasi) is a longitudinal passage which extends through the upper part of the face. It is divided into right and left halves by a median **septum nasi.** The **lateral walls** are formed by the maxilla, premaxilla, and the perpendicular part of the palate bones. Attached to them are the turbinal bones, which subdivide each nasal fossa into three **meatuses** (Meatus nasi). This wall is crossed obliquely by the **canal** and **groove** for the **naso-lacrimal duct,** and its posterior part is perforated by the **spheno-palatine foramen.** The superior wall or roof is formed by the frontal and nasal bones. It is concave from side to side, and nearly straight longitudinally, except in the posterior part, where it curves downward. It presents a median elevation, the **nasal crest.** The **inferior wall** or **floor** is formed by the palatine processes of the premaxillæ and maxillæ, and the horizontal parts of the palate bones. It is wider but considerably shorter than the roof. It is concave transversely, and nearly horizontal from before backward, except in the posterior third, where there is a slight declivity. The anterior part presents a median groove for the cartilaginous septum, and a furrow for the organ of Jacobson on either side. On either side of the palatine processes of the premaxillæ is the **palatine** cleft.

The **septum nasi** is incomplete in the macerated skull. It is formed by the perpendicular plate of the ethmoid behind, and the vomer below. In the fresh state it is completed by a plate of cartilage.

The **superior meatus** (Meatus nasi superior) is a narrow passage between the roof and the superior turbinal bone. It ends at the cribriform plate of the ethmoid. The **middle meatus** (Meatus nasi medius) is the space between the two turbinal bones. In its posterior part is the very narrow opening into the maxillary sinus. The **inferior meatus** (Meatus nasi inferior) is the channel along the floor which is overhung by the inferior turbinal bone. It is much the largest and is the direct path between the anterior and posterior nares.

The external aperture is bounded by the nasal bones and the premaxillæ.

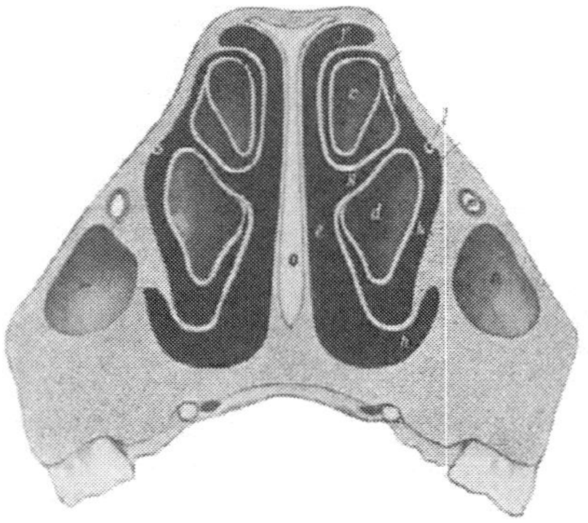

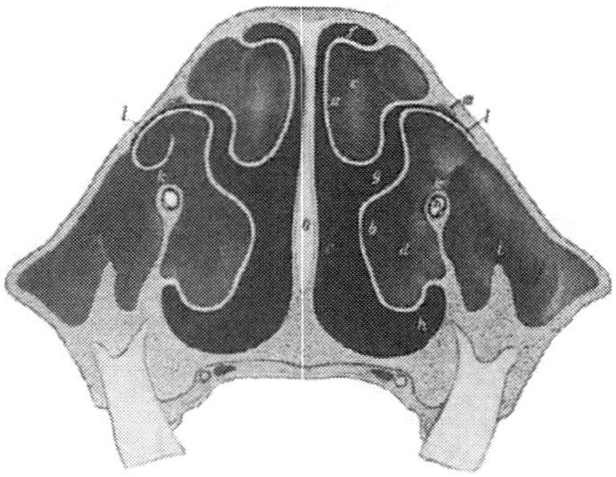

Fig. 37.—Cross-section of Nasal Region of Skull of Horse; the Section Passes Through the Anterior End of the Facial Crest, and Between the Third and Fourth Cheek Teeth.

a, Superior, *b*, inferior turbinal bone; *c*, *d*, cavities of *a* and *b*; *e*, common meatus; *f*, *g*, *h*, superior, middle, inferior meatus; *i*, k, passages to cavities of turbinal bones; *l*, naso-lacrimal duct; *m*, infraorbital canal; *n*, anterior end of maxillary sinus; *o*, septal cartilage. (After Ellenberger, in Leisering's Atlas.)

Fig.

The posterior extremity or fundus is separated from the cranial cavity by the cribriform plate of the ethmoid, and is largely occupied by the lateral masses of that bone.

THE PARANASAL SINUSES

Connected directly or indirectly with the nasal cavity, of which they are diverticula, are four pairs of air-sinuses (Sinus paranasales), viz., maxillary, frontal, spheno-palatine, and ethmoidal.

The **maxillary sinus** (Sinus maxillaris) is the largest. Its external wall is formed by the maxilla, the lacrimal, and the malar. It is bounded internally by the maxilla, the inferior turbinal, and the lateral mass of the ethmoid bone. It extends backward to a transverse plane in front of the root of the supraorbital process, and its anterior limit is indicated approximately by a line drawn from the anterior end of the facial crest to the infraorbital foramen. Its upper boundary corresponds to a line drawn backward from the supraorbital foramen parallel to the facial crest. The floor is formed by the alveolar part of the maxilla; it is very irregular and is crossed by bony plates running in various directions. The last three cheek teeth project up into the cavity to an extent which varies with age; they are covered by a thin plate of bone. The cavity is divided into anterior and posterior parts by an oblique **septum.** The outer margin of the septum is commonly about one and a half to two inches (ca. 3.5 to 5 cm.) from the anterior end of the facial crest; from here it is directed inward, backward, and upward. The upper part of the septum (formed by the posterior end of the inferior turbinal bone) is very delicate and usually cribriform.

The position of the septum is quite variable. It is not rare to find it further forward, and in some cases it is further back than is stated above. In the recent state, *i. e.*, when covered by the mucous membrane on both surfaces, it is nearly always complete, but in very exceptional cases there is an opening of variable size in the upper part.

The **anterior compartment,** often called the **inferior maxillary sinus,** is partially divided by the infraorbital canal into an external maxillary part and an internal smaller turbinal part. The latter communicates with the middle meatus by a very narrow slit situated at its highest part. The **posterior compartment,** often called the **superior maxillary sinus,** is also crossed by the infraorbital canal, internal to which it opens freely into the spheno-palatine sinus. It communicates dorsally

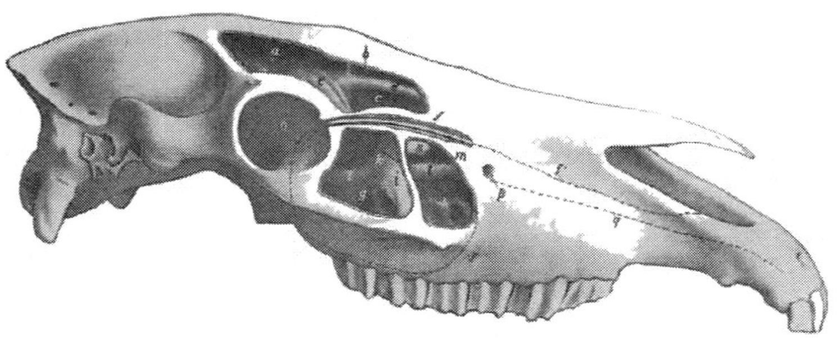

FIG. 39.—SKULL OF HORSE LATERAL VIEW WITHOUT MANDIBLE. THE SINUSES ARE OPENED UP.

a, Posterior part, *b* and *c*, anterior part of frontal sinus; *d*, roof of superior meatus; *e*, lateral mass of ethmoid bone; *f*, *f'*, naso-lacrimal duct, exposed in its posterior part; *g*, *h*, posterior and anterior compartments of maxillary sinus (also designated as superior and inferior maxillary sinuses); *i*, septum between *g* and *h*; *k*, lower limit of upper thin and partly membranous portion of septum; *l*, infraorbital canal; *m*, turbinal part of maxillary sinus; *n*, bullous prominence of inferior turbinal; *o*, orbit; *p*, infraorbital foramen; *q*, continuation of infraorbital canal to premaxilla; *r*, limit of maxillary sinus. (After Ellenberger, in Leisering's Atlas.)

with the frontal sinus through the large oval **fronto-maxillary opening,** situated at the level of the osseous lacrimal canal and the corresponding part of the inner wall of the orbit; the orifice is commonly about one and a half to two inches (ca. 4 to 5 cm.) long and an inch or more (2 to 3 cm.) wide. Just in front of this, and covered by a thin plate, is the narrow **naso-maxillary fissure** (Aditus naso-maxillaris), by which the sinus opens into the posterior part of the middle meatus.

The foregoing statements refer to the arrangement in the average adult animal. In the foal the cavity (with the exception of its turbinal part) is largely occupied by the developing teeth. In horses five to six years of age the maxillary part of the sinus is still filled up to a large degree by the embedded parts of the teeth. As the teeth are extruded to compensate the wear, more and more of the cavity becomes free, until in old age only the short roots project up in the floor, covered by a layer of bone. Other facts in this connection will be given in the description of the teeth. In exceptional cases the posterior part of the inferior turbinal is smaller than usual and leaves a considerable interval, through which the maxillary sinus communicates with the nasal cavity.

The **frontal sinus** (Sinus concho-frontalis) consists of frontal and turbinal parts. The frontal part is bounded chiefly by the two plates of the frontal bone, but its floor is formed in part by the lateral mass of the ethmoid. It extends forward to a plane through the anterior margins of the orbits, backward to one through the temporal condyles, and outward into the root of the supraorbital process. It is separated from the sinus of the opposite side by a complete **septum**. It is partially subdivided by a number of bony plates. The turbinal part is situated in the posterior part of the superior turbinal bone, roofed in by the nasal and lacrimal bones. It extends forward to a transverse plane about half-way between the anterior margin of the orbit and the end of the facial crest. Behind it is in free communication with the frontal part over the lateral mass of the ethmoid. It is separated from the nasal cavity by the thin turbinal plate. The frontal and maxillary sinuses communicate through the large opening described above.

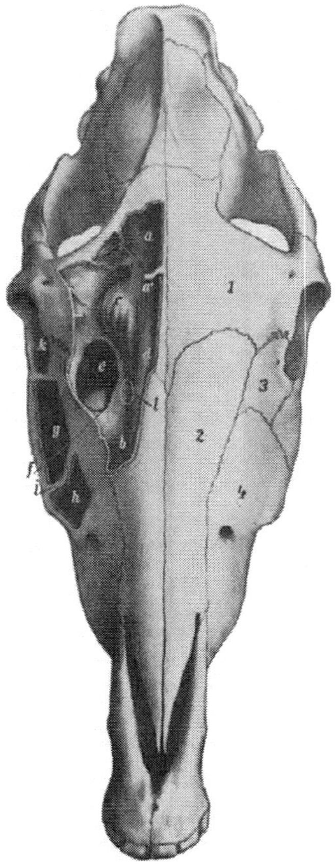

FIG. 40.—SKULL OF HORSE DORSAL VIEW WITH SINUSES EXPOSED BY REMOVAL OF THE OUTER PLATE OF BONE.

1, Frontal bone; *2*, nasal bone; *3*, lacrimal bone; *4*, maxilla; *a*, posterior part of frontal sinus; *a'*, middle part of frontal sinus; *b*, anterior (turbinal) part of frontal sinus; *c*, lateral mass of ethmoid bone; *d*, roof of superior meatus; *e*, fronto-maxillary opening; *f*, naso-maxillary opening below plate which forms the anterior margin of *e*; *g*, *h*, posterior and anterior compartments of maxillary sinus—often called the superior and inferior maxillary sinuses; *i*, septum between *g* and *h*; *k*, orbit; *l*, point at which superior turbinal bone may be perforated to obtain drainage into nasal cavity. (After Ellenberger, in Leisering's Atlas.)

The **spheno-palatine sinus** (Sinus sphenopalatinus) consists of two parts which communicate under the lateral mass of the ethmoid. The sphenoidal (posterior) part is excavated in the body of the pre-sphenoid. The palatine (anterior) part is between the two plates of the perpendicular part of the palate bone, under the lateral mass of the ethmoid; it communicates freely with the maxillary sinus. The septum between the right and left sinuses is not usually median in the sphenoidal part.

In about one-third of the cases (according to Paulli) the sphenoidal and palatine parts are separated by a transverse septum, and the sphenoidal part then communicates only with the lower ethmoidal meatuses.

The term **ethmoidal sinus** is often applied to the cavity of the largest ethmo-turbinal. It communicates with the maxillary sinus.

THE BONES OF THE THORACIC LIMB

THE SCAPULA

The **scapula** is a flat bone, situated on the anterior part of the lateral wall of the thorax, and extending obliquely from the vertebral end of the seventh or eighth rib to the sternal end of the first rib. It is curved slightly and slopes outward in adaptation to the form of the thoracic wall. It is triangular in outline, and has two surfaces, three borders, and three angles.

The **external surface** or **dorsum** (Facies lateralis s. dorsalis) is divided into two fossæ by the **spine** (Spina scapulæ), which extends from the vertebral border to the neck of the bone, where it gradually subsides. The free edge of the spine is thick, rough, and in great part subcutaneous. A little above its middle is a variable prominence, the **tubercle** of the spine (Tuber spinæ), to which the trapezius muscle is attached. The **supraspinous fossa** (Fossa supraspinata) is situated in front of the spine, and the **infraspinous** fossa (Fossa infraspinata) behind it. The former is much the smaller of the two; it is smooth and is occupied by the supraspinatus muscle. The infraspinous fossa lodges the infraspinatus muscle; it is wide and smooth in its upper part, narrower below, where it is marked by several rough lines for the attachment of the teres minor muscle; near the neck is the nutrient foramen, and a little lower is a vascular groove.

The **costal surface** or **venter** (Facies costalis) is hollowed in its length by the

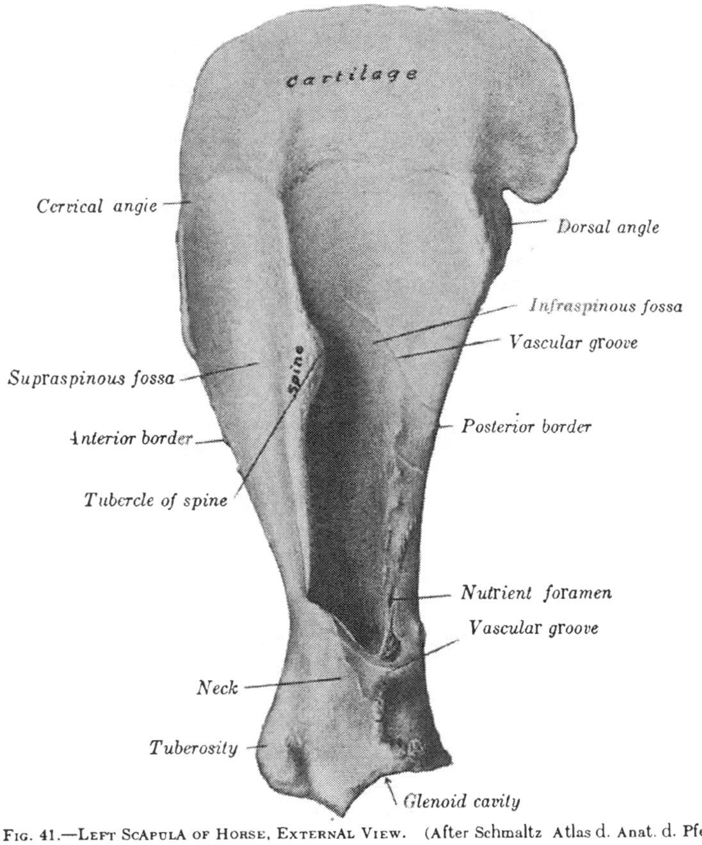

Fig. 41.—Left Scapula of Horse, External View. (After Schmaltz Atlas d. Anat. d. Pferdes.)

subscapular fossa (Fossa subscapularis); this occupies nearly the whole of the lower part of the surface, but is pointed above and separates two rough triangular areas (Facies serrata), to which the serratus magnus is attached. In the lower third there is a vascular furrow with several branches.

The **anterior** or **cervical border** (Margo cranialis) is convex and rough above, concave and smooth below.

The **posterior** or **dorsal** border (Margo caudalis) is slightly concave. It is thick and rough in its upper third, thin in its middle, and thickens again below.

The **superior** or vertebral border (Margo dorsalis s. basis) carries the **scapular cartilage** (Cartilago scapulæ). In the young subject the edge of the bone is thick, and is pitted by impressions into which the cartilage fits. The cartilage is the unossified part of the fœtal scapula. Its lower edge fits the depressions and elevations of the bone. It thins out toward the free edge, which is convex and lies alongside of the upper parts of the vertebral spines. In front it continues the line of the scapula, but behind it forms a rounded projection. The lower part of the cartilage undergoes more or less ossification, so that the vertebral border of the bone in old subjects is thin, irregular, and porous.

The **anterior** or **cervical angle** (Angulus cranialis) is at the Junction of the

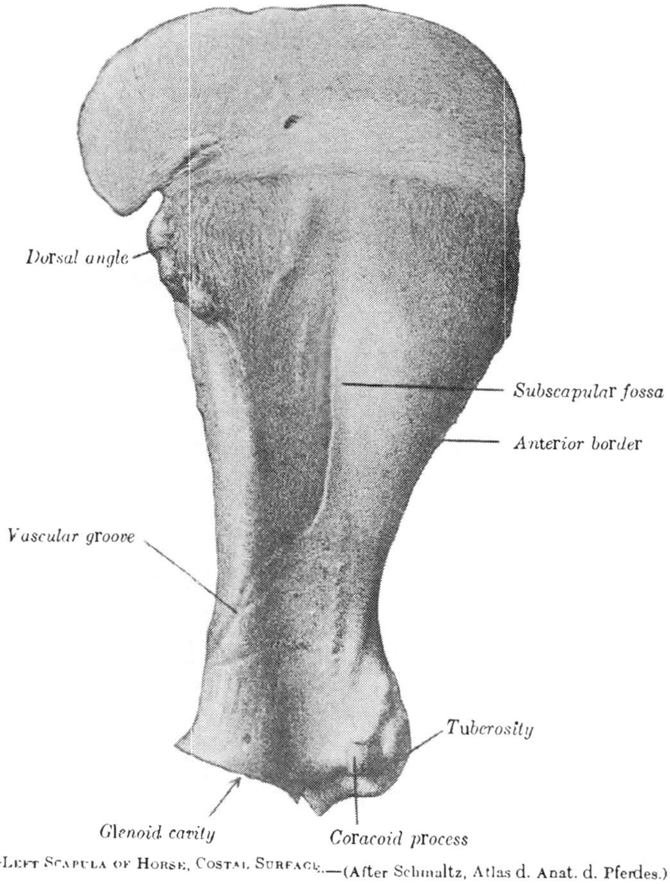

FIG. 42.—LEFT SCAPULA OF HORSE, COSTAL SURFACE.—(After Schmaltz, Atlas d. Anat. d. Pferdes.)

anterior and vertebral borders and lies opposite to the second thoracic spine. It is relatively thin and is about a right angle.

The **posterior** or **dorsal angle** (Angulus caudalis) is thick and rough; its position can be determined readily in the living animal.

The **inferior** or **articular angle** (Angulus glenoidalis) is joined to the body of the bone by the **neck** of the scapula (Collum scapulæ). It is enlarged, especially in the sagittal direction. It bears the glenoid cavity (Cavitas glenoidalis) for articulation with the head of the humerus. The cavity is oval in outline, and its margin is cut into in front by the **glenoid notch** (Incisura glenoidalis), and is rounded off externally; just above its postero-external part is a tubercle to which a tendon of the teres minor is attached. The **bicipital tuberosity** or **tuber scapulæ** is the large rough prominence in front, to which the tendon of origin of the biceps brachii is attached; projecting from its inner side is the small **coracoid process** (Processus coracoideus), from which the coraco-brachialis muscle arises.

Development.—The scapula has four centers of ossification, viz., one each for the body of the bone, the bicipital and coracoid processes, the anterior part of the glenoid cavity, and the tuber spinæ. The last ossifies after birth and fuses with the spine about the third year. The bicipital tuberosity and coracoid fuse with the body of the bone about the end of the first year.

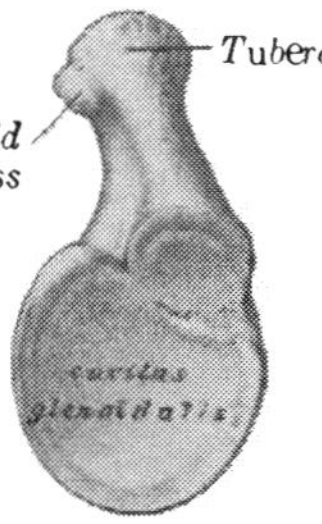

Fig. 43.—Distal End of Left Scapula of Horse, End View. (After Schmaltz, Atlas d. Anat. d. Pferdes.)

In old subjects the spongy substance disappears at the middle part of the fossæ, so that the bone consists here of a thin layer of compact substance. Considerable ossification of the cartilage is usual, the borders become much rougher, the muscular lines are more pronounced, and a medullary cavity may appear in the neck. Much variation occurs in dimensions and slope. The average ratio between the length and breadth (scapular index) is about 1 : 0.5, but in many cases the base is relatively wider. The inclination on a horizontal plane varies from 50 to 65 degrees. Exceptionally the coracoid process reaches a length of an inch or more (2½ to 3 cm.), and the chief nutrient foramen may be on the posterior border or in the subscapular fossa.

THE HUMERUS

The **humerus** is a long bone which extends from the shoulder above, where it articulates with the scapula, to the elbow below and behind, where it articulates with the radius and ulna. It is directed obliquely downward and backward, forming an angle of about 55 degrees with a horizontal plane. It may be divided into a shaft and two extremities.

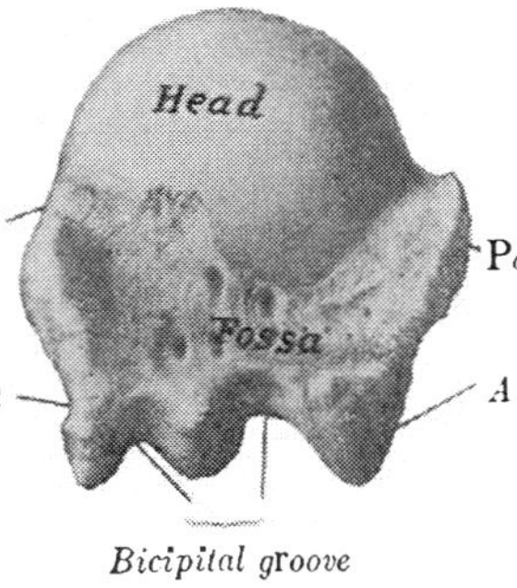

Fig. 44.—Proximal End of Left Humerus of Horse, End View. (After Schmaltz, Atlas d. Anat. d. Pferdes.)

The **shaft** or **body** (Corpus humeri) is irregularly cylindrical and has a twisted appearance. It may be regarded as having four surfaces. The **external surface** is smooth and is spirally curved, forming the **musculo-spiral groove** (Sulcus musculi brachialis), which contains the brachialis muscle; the groove is continuous with the posterior surface above and winds around toward the front below. The **internal surface** is nearly straight in its length, rounded from side to side, and blends with the anterior and posterior surfaces. Just above its middle is the **internal** or **teres** tubercle (Tuberositas teres), to which the tendon of the latissimus dorsi and teres major muscles is attached. The **nutrient foramen** is in the lower third of this surface. The **anterior surface** is triangular, wide and smooth above, narrow and roughened below. It is separated from the external surface by a distinct border, which bears on its upper part the **deltoid tuberosity** (Tuberositas deltoidea). From the latter a rough line curves upward and backward to the outer surface of the neck, and gives origin to the external head of the triceps muscle. Below the

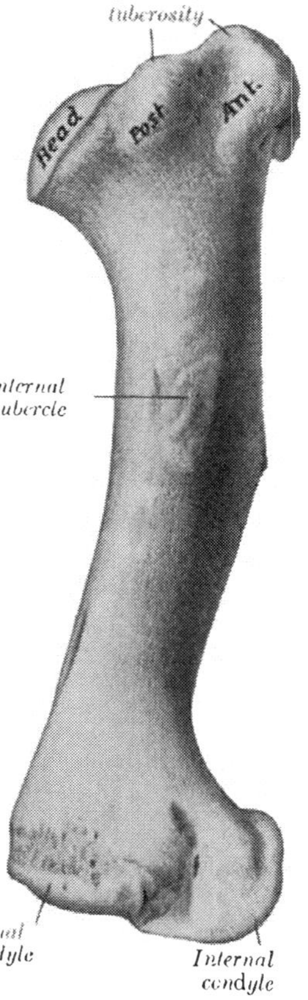

FIG. 45.—LEFT HUMERUS OF HORSE, INTERNAL SURFACE. (After Schmaltz, Atlas d. Anat. d. Pferdes.)

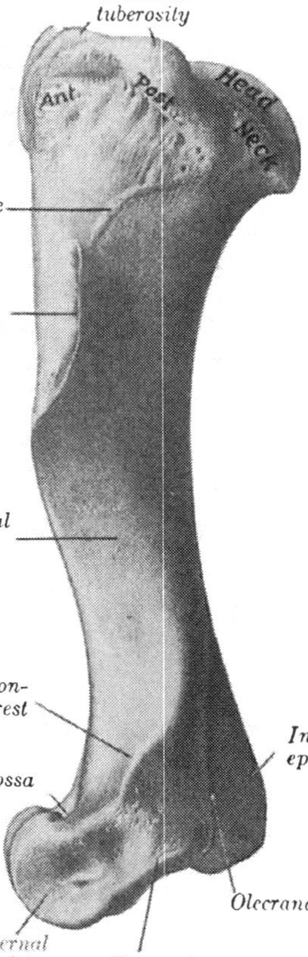

FIG. 46.—LEFT HUMERUS OF HORSE, EXTERNAL SURFACE. (After Schmaltz, Atlas d. Anat. d. Pferdes.)

tuberosity the border inclines forward, becomes less salient, and ends at the coronoid fossa. The **posterior surface** is rounded from side to side and smooth.

The **proximal extremity** consists of the head, neck, two tuberosities, and the bicipital groove. The **head** (Caput humeri) presents an almost circular convex articular surface, which is about twice as extensive as the glenoid cavity of the scapula, with which it articulates. In front of the head is a fossa, in which are several foramina. The **neck** (Collum humeri) is well defined behind, but is practically absent elsewhere. The **external tuberosity** (Tuberculum majus) is placed antero-externally, and consists of two parts; the anterior part forms the outer boundary of the bicipital groove and gives attachment to the external branch of the supraspinatus muscle; the posterior part gives attachment to the short insertion of the infraspinatus, while its outer surface is coated with cartilage, over which the chief tendon of the same muscle passes to be inserted into a triangular facet on the outer aspect of the anterior part. The **internal tuberosity** (Tuberculum minus) is less salient, and consists of anterior and posterior parts; the anterior part forms the inner boundary of the bicipital groove, and furnishes insertion to the inner branch of the supraspinatus above, and the posterior deep pectoral muscle below;

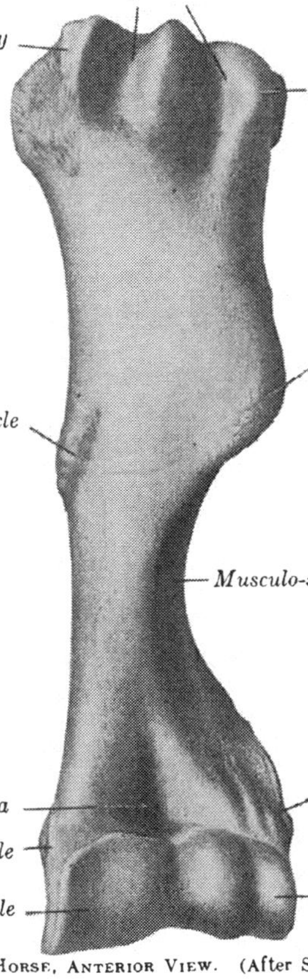

FIG. 47.—LEFT HUMERUS OF HORSE, ANTERIOR VIEW. (After Schmaltz Atlas d. Anat. d. Pferdes.)

the posterior part gives attachment to the subscapularis muscle. The **bicipital** or **intertubercular** groove (Sulcus intertubercularis) is situated in front; it is bounded by the anterior parts of the tuberosities, and is subdivided by an intermediate ridge. The groove is covered in the fresh state by cartilage, and lodges the tendon of origin of the biceps brachii muscle. Just below the intermediate ridge is a small fossa in which several foramina open.

The **distal extremity** has an oblique surface for articulation with the radius and ulna, which consists of two condyles of very unequal size, separated by a ridge. The **internal condyle** (Condylus medialis) is much the larger, and is crossed by a sagittal groove, on the anterior part of which there is usually a synovial fossa. Posteriorly the groove extends upward considerably above the rest of the articular surface and reaches the olecranon fossa, and this part articulates with the semilunar notch of the ulna. The **external condyle** (Condylus lateralis) is much smaller and is placed somewhat lower and further back, giving the extremity an oblique appearance; it is marked by a wide shallow groove. The **coronoid fossa** (Fossa coronoldea) is situated in front above the groove on the internal condyle; it furnishes origin to part of the extensor carpi, and external to it is a rough depression from which the anterior or common extensor of the digit arises. Behind and above the condyles are two thick ridges, the epicondyles. The **internal** or **flexor epicondyle** (Epicondylus medialis s. flexorius) is the more salient; it furnishes origin to flexor muscles of the carpus and digit, and presents internally a tubercle for the attachment of the internal lateral ligament of the elbow joint. The **external** or **extensor epicondyle** (Epicondylus lateralis s. extensorius) bears externally the **external supracondyloid crest** (Crista condyloidea lateralis), which forms here the outer boundary of the musculo-spiral groove, and gives origin to the extensor carpi. Below this is a rough excavation in which the external lateral ligament is attached. The lower border of the epicondyle gives attachment to the flexor carpi externus. Between the epicondyles is the deep **olecranon fossa** (Fossa olecrani).

Development.—The humerus ossifies from six centers, viz., three primary centers for the shaft and epiphyses, and three secondary centers for the external tuberosity, the deltoid tuberosity, and the internal condyle. The proximal end fuses with the shaft at about three and one-half years, the distal at about one and a half years of age.

THE RADIUS

The **radius** is much the larger of the two bones of the forearm in the horse. It extends in a vertical direction from the elbow, where it articulates with the humerus, to the carpus below. It is gently curved, the convexity being anterior. It consists of a shaft and two extremities.

The **shaft** (Corpus radii) is curved in its length, somewhat flattened from before backward, and expanded at its ends. It presents for description two surfaces and two borders. The **anterior surface** (Facies dorsalis) is smooth, slightly convex in its length, and rounded from side to side. The **posterior surface** (Facies volaris) is correspondingly concave in its length and is flattened in the transverse direction. At its upper part there is a smooth shallow groove, which concurs with the ulna in the formation of the **interosseous space** of the forearm; the nutrient foramen is in the lower part of this groove. Below this there is in the young subject a narrow, rough, triangular area to which the ulna is attached by an interosseous ligament; in the adult the two bones are fused here. A variable rough elevation below the middle of the surface and close to the internal border gives attachment to the superior check ligament. The **internal border** (Margo medialis) is slightly concave in its length and is largely subcutaneous; at its proximal end there is a smooth area on which the tendon of insertion of the brachialis muscle lies, and a small rough area just below gives attachment to that muscle and the long internal lateral ligament of the elbow-joint. The **external border** (Margo lateralis) is more strongly curved, but presents no special features.

The **proximal extremity** or **head** (Capitulum radii) is flattened from before backward and wide transversely. It presents an articular surface (Fovea capituli) which corresponds to that on the distal end of the humerus; it is crossed by a central sagittal ridge, which has a synovial fossa on its posterior part, and ends in front at a prominent lip, the **coronoid process** (Processus coronoideus). Just below the posterior border there are two concave facets for articulation with the ulna, and between these and the interosseous space is a quadrilateral rough area at which the two bones are united by an interosseous ligament. At the inner side of the anterior surface is the **bicipital tuberosity** (Tuberositas radii), into which the biceps tendon is inserted. The **internal tuberosity** is continuous with the preceding eminence, and furnishes attachment to the short part of the internal lateral

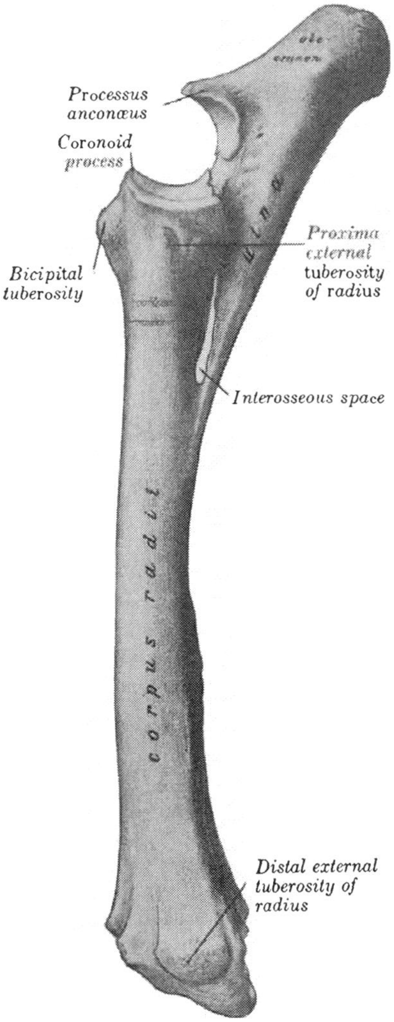

Fig. 48.—Left Radius and Ulna of Horse, External View. (After Schmaltz, Atlas d. Anat. d. Pferdes.)

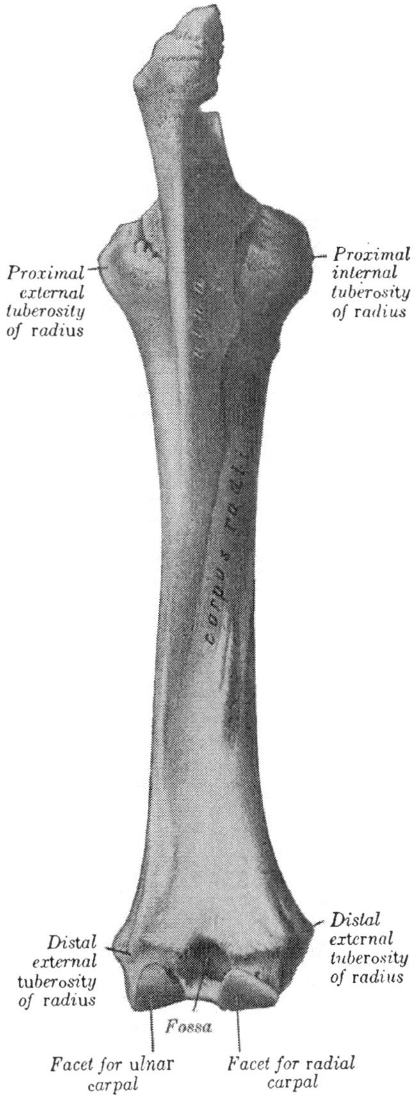

Fig. 49.—Left Radius and Ulna of Horse. Posterior View. (After Schmaltz, Atlas d. Anat. d. Pferdes.)

ligament. The **external tuberosity** is more salient; it gives attachment to the external lateral ligament and to the anterior and lateral extensor muscles of the digit.

The **distal extremity** is also compressed from before backward. It presents the carpal articular surface (Facies articularis carpea) which consists of three parts. The inner facet is the largest, is quadrilateral, concavo-convex from before backward, and articulates with the radial carpal bone (or scaphoid); the middle one is somewhat similar in form but smaller, and articulates with the intermediate carpal bone (or semilunar); the outer facet is smaller, is convex, and articulates below with the ulnar carpal (or cuneiform) and behind with the accessory carpal (or pisiform). The anterior surface presents three grooves, separated by ridges. The middle one is vertical and gives passage to the tendon of the extensor carpi radialis; the outer one is similar and contains the tendon of the anterior extensor of the digit; the inner one is small and oblique and lodges the tendon of the extensor carpi obliquus. The posterior aspect is crossed by a rough ridge, below which are three depressions. On either side is a tuberosity (Tuberculum ligamenti) to which the lateral ligament is attached. The outer one is marked by a small vertical groove for the passage of the lateral extensor tendon.

Development.—The radius ossifies from four centers, viz., one each for the shaft, the two extremities, and the outer part of the distal end; the last is morphologically the distal end of the ulna which has fused with the radius, and the line of fusion is often indicated by a distinct groove on the carpal articular surface. The proximal extremity unites with the shaft at about one and a half years, the distal end at about three and a half years.

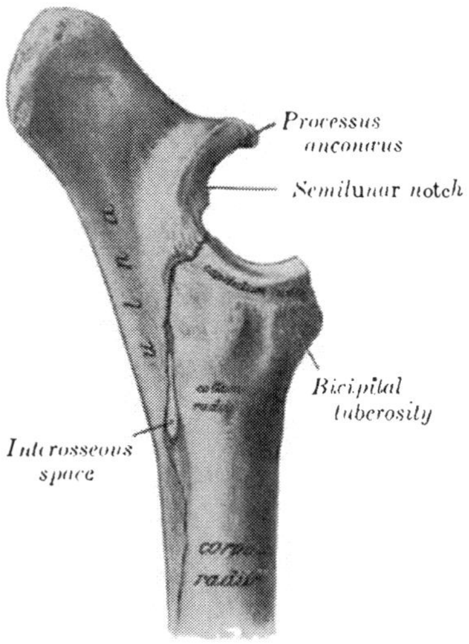

FIG. 50.—UPPER HALF OF RADIUS AND ULNA OF HORSE, INTERNAL VIEW. (After Schmaltz, Atlas d. Anat. d. Pferdes.)

THE ULNA

The ulna of the horse is a reduced long bone situated behind the radius, with which it is partially fused in the adult.

The shaft (Corpus ulnæ) is three-sided and tapers to a point below. The anterior surface (Facies dorsalis) is applied to the posterior surface of the radius, and below the interosseous space the two bones are fused in the adult. The surface which enters into the formation of the space is smooth and usually presents a small nutrient foramen, directed upward. Above the space it is rough and is attached to the radius by an interosseous ligament which is usually permanent. The internal surface (Facies medialis) is smooth and slightly concave. The external surface (Facies lateralis) is flattened. The internal and external borders are thin and sharp, except at the interosseous space. The posterior border is slightly concave in its length and is rounded. The lower end is pointed and is usually a little below the middle of the radius. It is commonly continued by a fibrous cord to the distal external tuberosity of the radius, but this band may be replaced in part or entirely by bone.

The proximal extremity is the major part of the bone. It projects upward and somewhat backward behind the lower end of the humerus, and forms a lever arm for the extensor muscles of the elbow. The internal surface is concave and smooth. The external surface is convex and is roughened above. The anterior border bears on its middle a pointed projection, the processus anconæus or "beak," which overhangs the semilunar notch or sigmoid cavity (Incisura semilunaris). The latter is triangular in outline, concave from above downward, and articulates with the humerus; in the middle of its lower part is an extensive synovial fossa. Just below the notch are two convex facets which articulate with those on the posterior aspect of the proximal end of the radius. The posterior border is nearly straight, and is thick and rounded. The free end or summit is a rough tuberosity, the olecranon, which gives attachment to the triceps brachii and other muscles.

The primitive distal extremity has, as previously stated, fused with the radius.

Development.—The ulna ossifies from three centers, of which one is for the main part of the bone, one for the olecranon, and one for the distal end. The cartilaginous embryonic ulna extends the entire length of the forearm. The lower part of the shaft is usually reduced to a small fibrous band or may disappear entirely; in some cases a variable remnant of it ossifies. The distal extremity fuses early with the radius. The olecranon unites with the rest of the bone at three to three and a half years. A medullary canal appears to occur constantly in the adult—contrary to the statements of some authors.

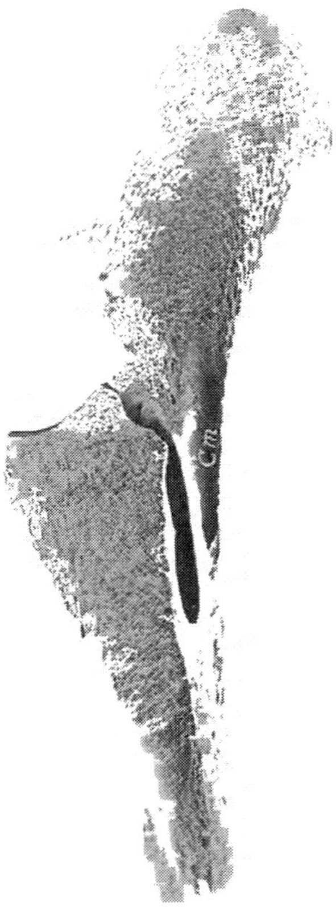

Fig. 51.—Sagittal Section of Upper Part of Radius and Ulna of Horse. *Cm*, Medullary cavity of ulna.

THE CARPUS

The carpus of the horse consists of seven or eight bones (Ossa carpi) arranged in two rows, proximal or antibrachial, and distal or metacarpal. The (abbreviated) names and relative positions of the bones of the left carpus as seen from in front are indicated below.

Proximal Row:

Radial	Intermediate	Ulnar	Accessory

Distal Row:

First	Second	Third	Fourth

The Radial Carpal Bone

The radial carpal bone (Os carpi radiale, scaphoid) is the largest bone of the upper row; it is somewhat compressed laterally, and is clearly six-sided. The superior or proximal surface is convex in front, concave behind, and articulates with the inner facet on the distal end of the radius. The inferior or distal surface is also convex in front and concave behind; it articulates with the second and third carpal bones. The external surface bears upper and lower facets on its anterior part for articulation with the intermediate; between and behind these it is excavated and rough. The anterior or dorsal surface is rough and slightly convex. The internal surface and the posterior or volar surface are rough and tuberculate.

The Intermediate Carpal Bone

The intermediate carpal bone (Os carpi intermedium, semilunar, lunar) is somewhat wedge-shaped, wider in front than behind. The superior or proximal surface is saddle-shaped, and articulates with the middle facet on the distal end of the radius. The inferior or distal surface is smaller, convex in front, concave behind, and articulates with the third and fourth carpal bones. The internal surface has upper and lower facets for articulation with the radial carpal, and between these it is excavated and rough. The external surface is similar to the preceding and articulates with the ulnar carpal. The anterior or dorsal surface is rough and slightly convex. The posterior or volar surface bears a tuberosity on its lower part.

The Ulnar Carpal Bone

The ulnar carpal bone (Os carpi ulnare, cuneiform) is the smallest and most irregular bone of the upper row. The superior or proximal surface is concave, and fits the lower part of the outer facet on the distal end of the radius. The inferior or distal surface is oblique and undulating for articulation with the fourth carpal bone. The internal surface has upper and lower facets for articulation with the intermediate. The anterior or dorsal and external surfaces are continuous, convex, and rough. The posterior or volar surface is oblique, and bears a concave facet for articulation with the accessory carpal bone; below this is a tubercle.

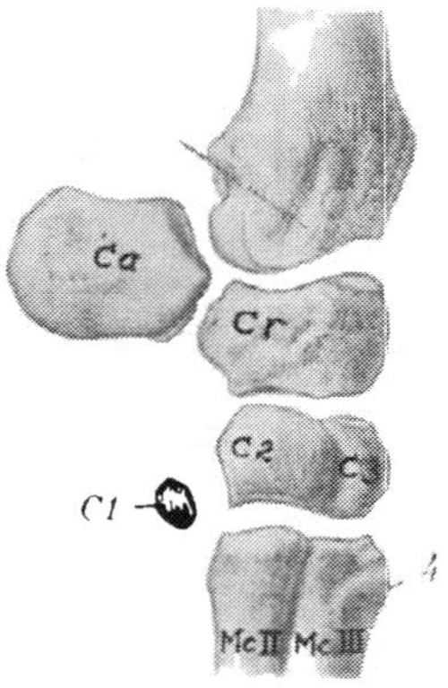

Fig. 52.—Left Carpal Bones of Horse, with Distal End of Radius and Proximal End of Metacarpus; Internal View.

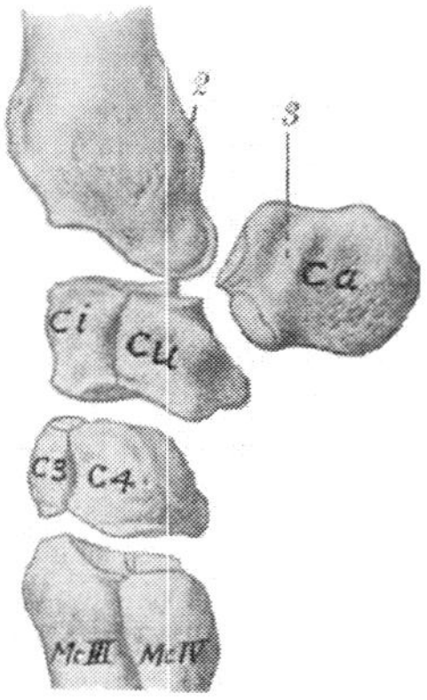

Fig. 53.—Left Carpal Bones of Horse with Adjacent Ends of Radius and Metacarpus; External View.

Ca, Accessory carpal bone; *Cr*, radial carpal; *Ci*, intermediate carpal; *Cu*, ulnar carpal; *C1–4*, first to fourth carpals; *Mc. II, III, IV*, metacarpal bones; *1*, groove for tendon of extensor carpi obliquus; *2*, groove for lateral extensor tendon; *3*, groove for tendon of flexor carpi externus; *4*. metacarpal tuberosity. (After Schmaltz, Atlas d. Anat. d. Pferdes.)

The Accessory Carpal Bone

The accessory carpal bone (Os carpi accessorium, pisiform) is situated behind the ulnar carpal bone and the outer part of the distal end of the ulna. It is discoid and presents for description two surfaces and a circumference. The internal surface is concave and forms the outer wall of the carpal groove. The external surface is convex and rough; a smooth groove for the outer tendon of the flexor carpi externus crosses its anterior part obliquely downward and slightly forward. The anterior border bears two facets; the upper one is concave and articulates with the back of the outer facet on the distal end of the radius; the lower one is convex and articulates with the ulnar carpal bone. The remainder of the circumference is rounded and rough.

The accessory does not directly bear weight, and may be regarded as a sesamoid bone interposed in the course of the tendons of the middle and external flexors of the carpus, which it enables to act at a mechanical advantage. The posterior border furnishes attachment to the transverse carpal ligament, which completes the carpal canal for the flexors of the digit.

The First Carpal Bone

The **first carpal** bone (Os carpale primum, trapezium) is a small inconstant bone, commonly about the size and shape of a pea, which is situated in the lower part of the internal lateral ligament behind the second carpal bone.

This bone appears to be absent on both sides in about half of the cases; in a good many subjects it is present on one side only. In size it varies from a minute nodule to a discoid mass 10 to 12 mm. in length. In exceptional cases it articulates with both the second carpal and the second (inner) metacarpal bone, in other cases with the former only, but in the majority of specimens no articular facet is present.

The Second Carpal Bone

The **second carpal** bone (Os carpale secundum, trapezoid) is the smallest constant bone of the lower row, and is irregularly hemispherical in shape. The **superior** or **proximal surface** is a convex facet which is continued upon the **posterior** or volar **surface** and articulates with the posterior part of the radial carpal. The **external surface** faces obliquely outward and forward, and bears three facets for articulation with the third carpal bone. The **anterior** or **dorsal** and the **internal surface** bear a tuberosity to which the lateral ligament is attached. The **inferior** or **distal**

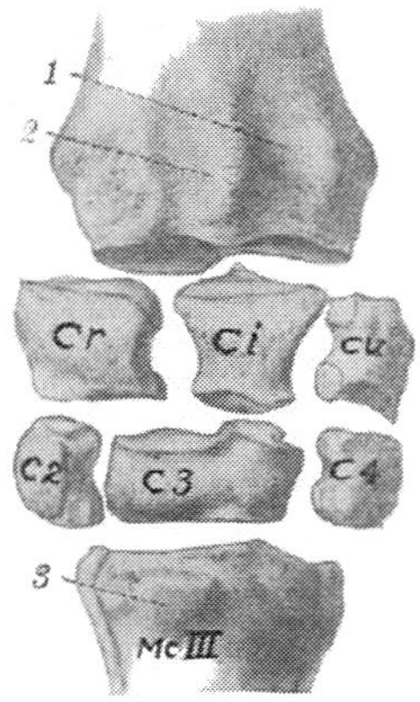

Fig. 54.—Carpal Bones of Horse, with Adjacent Ends of Radius and Metacarpus; Anterior View. The Accessory and First Carpal Bones are Not Shown.

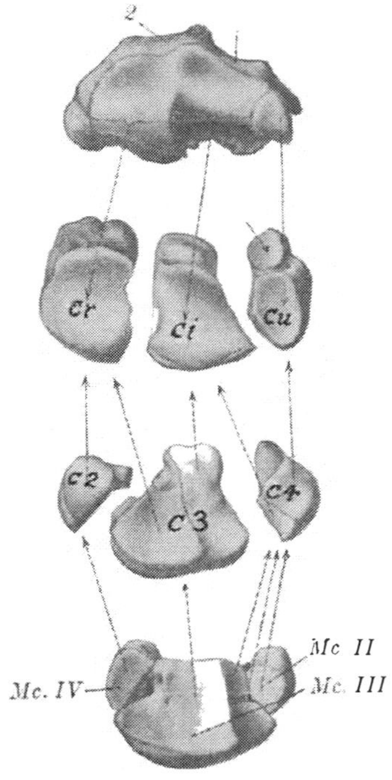

Fig. 55.—Carpal Articular Surface of Radius and Proximal Articular Surfaces of Carpal and Metacarpal Bones. Left Side. The Accessory and First Carpal Bones are not Shown.

Cr, Radial carpal; *Ci*, intermediate carpal; *Cu*, ulnar carpal; *C2*, *C3*, *C4*, second, third, and fourth carpals; *Mc.II*, second or inner small metacarpal bone; *Mc.III*, third or large metacarpal bone; *Mc.IV*, fourth or outer small metacarpal bone; *1*, *2*, grooves for tendons of anterior extensor and extensor carpi radialis; *3*, metacarpal tuberosity. Arrows indicate relations of facets. Short arrow points to facet on ulnar carpal for articulation with accessory carpal. (After Schmaltz, Atlas d. Anat. d. Pferdes.)

surface is articular and consists of a large flattened facet for the inner (second) metacarpal bone, and a small one for the large (third) metacarpal bone. Some specimens have a small facet on the lower part of the posterior surface which articulates with the first carpal bone.

THE THIRD CARPAL BONE

The third carpal bone (Os carpale tertium, os magnum) is much the largest bone of the lower row, forming more than two-thirds of the width of the latter. It is flattened from above downward, and is twice as wide in front as behind. The superior or proximal surface consists of two facets separated by an antero-posterior ridge; the inner facet is concave and articulates with the radial carpal; the outer facet—for the intermediate carpal—is concave in front and convex behind, where it encroaches on the posterior surface. The inferior or distal surface is slightly undulating, and articulates almost entirely with the large (third) metacarpal bone, but it usually bears a small oblique facet at its inner side for the inner (second) metacarpal, and there is commonly a non-articular depression externally. The internal surface faces backward and inward, and bears three facets for articulation with the second carpal, between which it is excavated and rough. The external surface has two facets for articulation with the fourth carpal, and is depressed and rough in its middle. The anterior or dorsal surface is convex and is crossed by a rough transverse ridge. The posterior or volar surface is relatively small, and is rounded; its upper part is encroached upon by the superior articular surface, below which it is rough.

THE FOURTH CARPAL BONE

The fourth carpal bone (Os carpale quartum, unciform) is somewhat wedge-shaped, and is readily distinguished from the second by its greater size and its posterior tubercle. The superior or proximal surface articulates with the intermediate and ulnar; it is convex and curves outward, backward, and downward, encroaching on the external and posterior surfaces. The inferior or distal surface bears two inner facets for the large (third) metacarpal and an outer one for the external (fourth) metacarpal bone. The internal surface has two or three facets for articulation with the third carpal, between which it is excavated and rough. The anterior or dorsal surface is convex and rough. The external surface is small, being encroached upon by the superior articular surface. The posterior or volar surface bears a tubercle on its lower part.[1]

THE CARPUS AS A WHOLE

The bones of the carpus, exclusive of the accessory, form an irregular quadrangular mass, the width of which is about twice the height or the antero-posterior diameter. The anterior or dorsal surface is convex from side to side, depressed along the line of junction of the two rows, and prominent below. The posterior or volar surface is in general slightly convex, but very irregular. It forms with the accessory the carpal groove (Sulcus carpi), which in the recent state is rendered smooth by the posterior ligament; it is converted into the carpal canal (Canalis carpi) for the flexor tendons by the transverse carpal ligament, which stretches across from the accessory bone to the inner side. The proximal surface is widest internally and is elevated in front, concave behind; it is entirely articular and adapted to the carpal articular surface of the radius. The distal surface is also articular and is irregularly faceted in adaptation to the surfaces of the metacarpal bones; each of the lower bones usually articulates with two metacarpal bones, but sometimes the third does not bear on the inner metacarpal bone. The lateral surfaces are both irregular and rough, the internal one being the wider. With the exception of the accessory, ulnar, and second, each bone articulates with two bones of the other row.

Development.—Each ossifies from a single center.

[1] This bone is probably equivalent to the fourth and fifth carpals of forms in which five carpal elements are present in the lower row.

THE METACARPUS

Three **metacarpal bones** (Ossa metacarpalia) are present in the horse. Of these, only one, the third or large metacarpal bone, is fully developed and carries a digit; the other two, the second and fourth, are much reduced, and are commonly called the internal and external small metacarpal or "splint" bones.

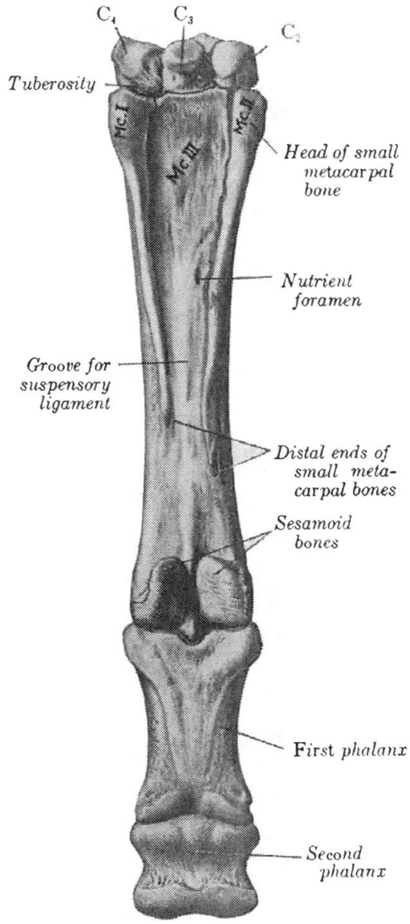

FIG. 56.—DISTAL ROW OF CARPAL BONES, METACARPUS, FIRST AND SECOND PHALANGES, AND PROXIMAL SESAMOID BONES OF HORSE; POSTERIOR VIEW, LEFT SIDE.

The fourth (external) metacarpal bone is wrongly numbered as I. (After Schmaltz, Atlas. d. Anat. d. Pferdes.)

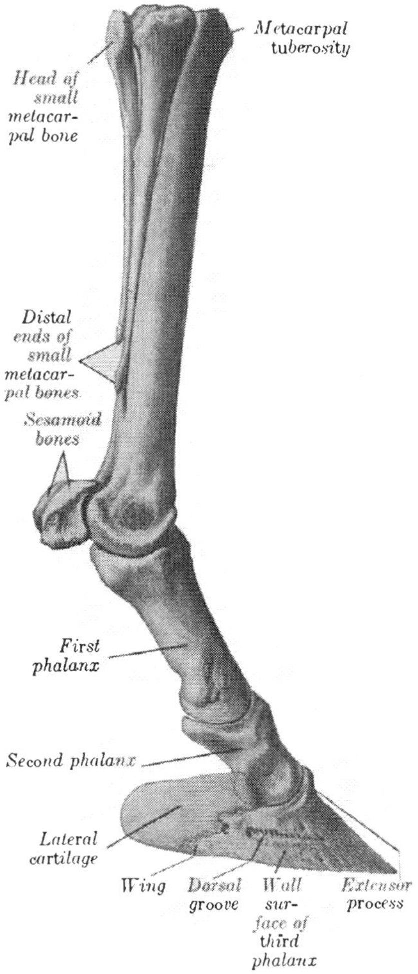

FIG. 57.—LEFT METACARPAL AND DIGITAL BONES OF HORSE, INTERNAL VIEW. (After Schmaltz Atlas d. Anat. d. Pferdes.)

THE LARGE METACARPAL BONE

This (Os metacarpale tertium) is a very strong long bone, placed vertically between the carpus above and the first phalanx below. It consists of a shaft and two extremities.

The shaft (Corpus) is semicylindrical, and presents two surfaces and two borders. The anterior or dorsal surface is smooth, convex from side to side, and nearly straight in its length. The posterior or volar surface is somewhat convex from side to side and, with the small bones, forms a wide groove which lodges the suspensory ligament. On either side of its upper two-thirds it is roughened for the attachment of the small metacarpal bones. The nutrient foramen occurs at the junction of the upper and middle thirds. The lower third is wider and flattened. The borders are rounded.

The proximal extremity (Basis) bears an undulating articular surface adapted to the lower row of carpal bones. The greater part supports the third carpal bone; the oblique outer part, separated from the preceding by a ridge, articulates with the fourth, and a small facet for the second is usually found at the postero-internal angle. On either side is a notch separating two small facets which articulate with the proximal ends of the small metacarpal bones. Toward the inner side of the anterior surface is the metacarpal tuberosity, into which the extensor carpi radialis is inserted. The posterior surface is roughened for the attachment of the suspensory ligament.

The distal extremity (Trochlea s. Capitulum) presents an articular surface for the first phalanx and the proximal sesamoid bones, which is composed of two condyles, separated by a sagittal ridge; the inner condyle is slightly the larger. On either side is a small fossa, surmounted by a tubercle, for the attachment of the lateral ligaments of the fetlock joint.

The large metacarpal is one of the strongest bones in the skeleton. The compact substance is specially thick in front and internally. The medullary canal extends further toward the ends than in most of the long bones of the horse and there is little spongy bone.

THE SMALL METACARPAL BONES

These are situated on either side of the posterior surface of the large metacarpal bone, and form the sides of the metacarpal groove. Each consists of a shaft and two extremities.

The shaft (Corpus) is three-sided and tapers to the distal end. It is variably curved, convex toward the middle line of the limb. The anterior surface is flattened and is rough, except in its lower part; it is attached to the large metacarpal bone by an interosseous ligament, except near the distal end. The abaxial surface is smooth and rounded from side to side above, grooved below. The axial surface is smooth and concave from edge to edge, except below, where it forms a rounded edge.

The proximal extremity or head (Basis) is relatively large. In the case of the inner bone it usually bears two facets above which support the second and third carpal bones, while the outer bone has here a single facet for articulation with the fourth carpal bone. Each has also two facets for articulation with the large metacarpal, and is elsewhere roughened for the attachment of ligaments and muscles. The inner bone may present a small facet behind for the first carpal bone.

The distal extremity (Capitulum) is usually a small nodule, which projects to a variable extent in different subjects, and is easily felt in the living animal. It is situated two-thirds to three-fourths of the way down the region.

The small metacarpal bones vary much in length, thickness, and curvature. In the majority of cases the inner bone is the longer; in other subjects the outer one is the longer or there no material difference. Sometimes the curvature is very pronounced, so that the distal end causes a decided projection. The distal end is very variable in size and may be a mere point.

Development.—The large metacarpal bone ossifies from three centers. The proximal extremity unites with the shaft before birth, the distal extremity toward the middle of the second year. The small metacarpal bones ossify from two centers, one of which is for the proximal extremity. Their distal ends are cartilaginous at birth. Fusion of the middle part of the shaft with the large metacarpal bone is common.

THE PHALANGES

The First Phalanx

The **first phalanx** (Phalanx prima)[1] is a long bone, situated between the large metacarpal bone above and the second phalanx below. It is directed obliquely downward and forward, forming an angle of 50 to 55 degrees with the horizontal plane in well-formed limbs. It consists of a shaft and two extremities.

The **shaft** (Corpus) is wider and much thicker above than below, and presents two surfaces and two borders. The anterior or dorsal surface is convex from side to side and smooth. The posterior or volar surface is flattened, and bears a triangular rough area, bounded laterally by ridges which begin at the tuberosities above and converge below; this area furnishes attachment to the inferior sesamoidean ligaments. The **borders, internal** and **external,** are rounded and have a rough area or a tubercle on their middle parts.

The **proximal extremity** (Basis) is relatively large. It bears an articular surface adapted to the distal end of the large metacarpal bone, consisting of two glenoid cavities separated by a sagittal groove; the inner cavity is a little larger than the outer one. The posterior angles are formed by buttress-like tuberosities for ligamentous attachment. The anterior surface has a slight elevation for the attachment of the lateral extensor tendon.

The **distal extremity** is smaller, especially in its antero-posterior diameter. It presents a trochlea for articulation with the second phalanx, consisting of a shallow central groove and two lateral convex areas or condyles; the inner area is a little the larger. On either side, just above the margin of the articular surface, is a depression surmounted by a tubercle, to both of which the lateral ligament is attached. Behind the tubercle is a distinct facet to which the superficial flexor tendon is attached.

Development.—The first phalanx ossifies from three centers. The distal end unites with the shaft before birth, the proximal end early in the first year.

The first phalanx contains a small medullary canal in the middle of the shaft. It may be remarked that the bone is twisted slightly; when placed volar surface down on the table, it touches the latter by three points only, the proximal tuberosities and the internal condyle.

The Second Phalanx

The **second phalanx** (Phalanx secunda)[2] is situated between the first and third phalanges, its direction corresponding to that of the first phalanx. It is flattened from before backward, and its width is greater than its height. It may be described as possessing four surfaces.

The **upper** or **proximal surface** presents two glenoid cavities separated by a low ridge, and articulates with the first phalanx. The middle of the anterior border is elevated and roughened in front for the attachment of the anterior or common extensor tendon. The posterior border is thick and overhanging; in the fresh state its middle part is covered with cartilage, over which the deep flexor tendon passes. On either side there is an eminence, to which the lateral ligament and the superficial flexor tendon are attached.

The **inferior** or **distal surface** is trochlear, and articulates with the third phalanx and third sesamoid bone. It resembles somewhat the trochlea of the first phalanx, but is more extensive and encroaches more on the anterior and posterior surfaces.

The **anterior** or **dorsal surface** is convex from side to side and smooth in its

[1] It is also called the large pastern bone or os suffraginis.
[2] This bone is also called the small pastern bone or os coronæ.

middle; on its lower part are lateral rough depressions, surmounted by tuberosities, to both of which ligaments are attached.

The posterior or volar surface is smooth, flattened, and slopes obliquely downward and forward. The borders which separate the anterior and posterior surfaces are concave from above downward, rounded from before backward.

Development.—The second phalanx ossifies like the first, but the proximal end unites with the shaft two or three months earlier.

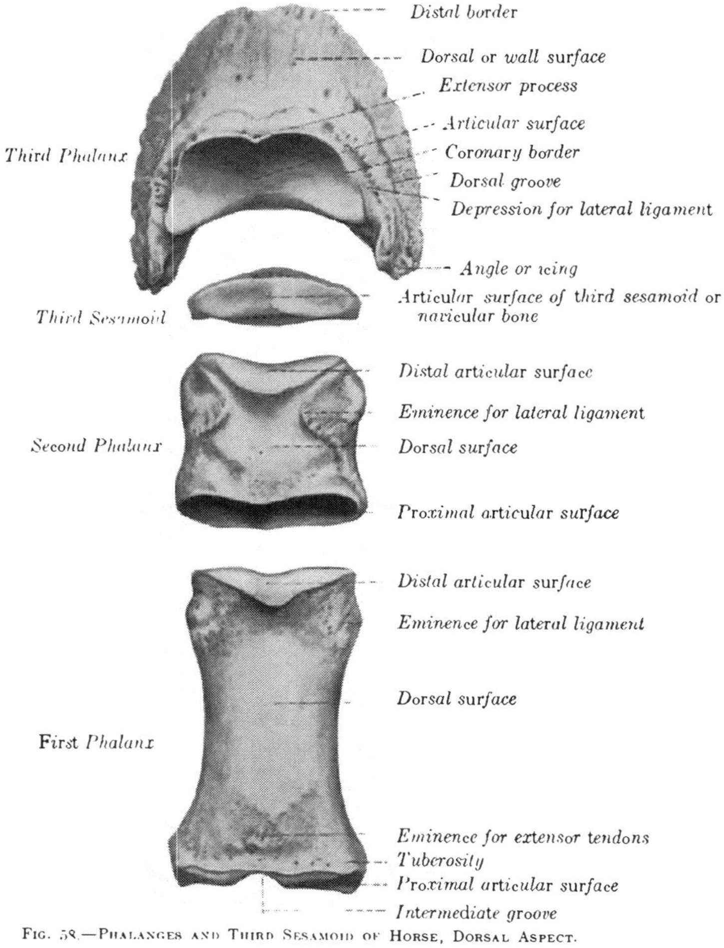

FIG. 58.—PHALANGES AND THIRD SESAMOID OF HORSE, DORSAL ASPECT.

THE THIRD PHALANX

The **third** or **ungual phalanx** (Phalanx tertia)[1] is entirely inclosed by the hoof, to which it conforms in a general way. It presents for examination three surfaces, three borders, and two angles or wings.

The articular **surface** (Facies articularis) faces upward and backward, and is chiefly adapted to the distal surface of the second phalanx, but a narrow flattened area along the posterior border articulates with the third sesamoid. The an-

[1] This bone is also called the os pedis or coffin bone.

terior or **coronary border** forms a central eminence, the **extensor** (or pyramidal) **process** (Processus extensorius), to the front of which the anterior extensor tendon is attached. On either side is a depression for the attachment of the lateral ligament.

The **dorsal** or **wall surface** (Facies dorsalis) slopes downward and forward. The angle of inclination on the ground plane is about 45 to 50 degrees in front. Laterally the height diminishes, and the slope becomes steeper, especially on the inner side. From side to side the curvature is almost semicircular. The surface is rough and porous, resembling pumice stone somewhat. It is perforated by numerous foramina of various sizes; a series of larger ones is situated on or near the lower border. On either side the **dorsal** (or preplantar) **groove** (Sulcus dorsalis) passes forward from the wing and ends at one of the larger foramina. In the fresh state this surface is covered by the matrix of the wall of the hoof. The **inferior** or **distal border** is thin, sharp, and irregularly notched; there is commonly a wider notch in front.

The **volar** or **inferior surface** (Facies volaris) is arched, and divided into two unequal parts by a curved rough line, the **semilunar crest** (Crista semilunaris). The larger anterior area is crescent-shaped, concave, and comparatively smooth; it corresponds to the sole of the hoof, and may be termed the **sole surface**. The posterior part is much smaller, and is semilunar; it is related to the deep flexor tendon, and is hence called the **flexor** or **tendon surface** (Facies flexoria). It presents a central prominent rough area, on either side of which is the **volar** (or plantar) **foramen** (Foramen volare), to which the **volar** (or plantar) **groove** (Sulcus volaris) conducts from the wing. The foramina lead into the **semilunar canal** within the bone, from which small canals lead to some of the foramina of the wall surface. The deep flexor tendon is inserted into the semilunar crest and the central rough area behind it.

The volar grooves and foramina transmit the terminations of the digital arteries into the semilunar canal, where they meet and form a terminal arch, from which branches pass through canals in the bone and emerge through the foramina on the wall surface.

The **angles** or **wings** (Anguli) are prismatic masses which project backward on either side; the inner one is usually the shorter. Each is divided into upper and lower parts by a notch, or is perforated by a foramen which leads to the vascular groove on the side of the wall surface.[1] The upper border carries the lateral cartilage.

The **lateral cartilages** (Cartilagines ungulæ) are rhomboid curved plates, which surmount the wings on either side. They are relatively large and extend above the margin of the hoof sufficiently to be distinctly palpable. The abaxial surface is convex, the axial concave. The upper border is convex and thin; the lower is thicker and is in part attached to the wing. The anterior end is attached by ligament to the side of the second phalanx. The posterior end curves toward its fellow at the heel, and is perforated by numerous foramina for the passage of veins. The central part is mainly hyaline, the periphery mainly fibrous.

It will be noted that the size and form of the wings vary much in different specimens. In the new-born foal the wing is a small, pointed projection. Later the process of ossification invades the lower part of the cartilage to a varying extent. In some cases the greater part of the cartilage is ossified—a condition commonly termed "sidebone."

Development.—The ossification of the terminal phalanx is peculiar. While the proximal articular part is still cartilaginous, a perichondrial cap of bone is formed in relation to the hoof. Later the process extends into the upper part.

Structure.—The interior of this bone is channeled by numerous canals for

[1] The upper and lower divisions of the wing are sometimes termed the basilar and retrossal processes respectively.

vessels, most of which radiate from the semilunar canal to the wall surface; these are not canals for nutrient vessels of the bone, but transmit arteries to the matrix of the hoof. Thick layers of compact substance are found at the articular and flexor surfaces and the extensor process, *i. e.*, at the points of greatest pressure and traction.

THE SESAMOID BONES

The two proximal or great sesamoids (Ossa sesamoidea phalangis primæ) are situated behind the distal end of the large metacarpal bone, and are closely attached to the first phalanx by strong ligaments. Each has the form of a three-sided pyramid. The anterior or articular surface conforms to the corresponding part of the distal end of the large metacarpal bone. The posterior or flexor surface is flattened and oblique; in the fresh state it is covered by a layer of cartilage which also fills the interval between the opposed borders of the two bones, and forms a smooth groove for the deep flexor tendon. The abaxial surface is concave, and gives attachment to part of the suspensory ligament; it is separated from the posterior surface by a rough everted border. The base faces downward, and furnishes attachment to the inferior sesamoidean ligaments. The apex is directed upward and is rounded.

The third sesamoid or navicular bone (Os sesamoideum phalangis tertiæ) is shuttle-shaped, and is situated behind the junction of the second and third phalanges. Its long axis is transverse, and it possesses two surfaces, two borders, and two extremities. The articular surface (Facies articularis) faces upward and forward; it consists of a central eminence, flanked by concave areas, and articulates with the distal end of the second phalanx. The flexor or tendon surface (Facies flexoria) is directed downward and backward. It resembles the articular surface in form, but is more extensive and not so smooth. In the fresh state it is coated with cartilage and the deep flexor tendon plays over it. The proximal border (Margo liber) is wide and grooved in its middle, narrower and rounded on either side. The distal border (Margo ligamenti) bears in front a narrow facet for articulation with the third phalanx. Behind this is a groove, which contains a number of relatively large foramina, and is bounded behind by a prominent edge. The extremities are blunt-pointed.

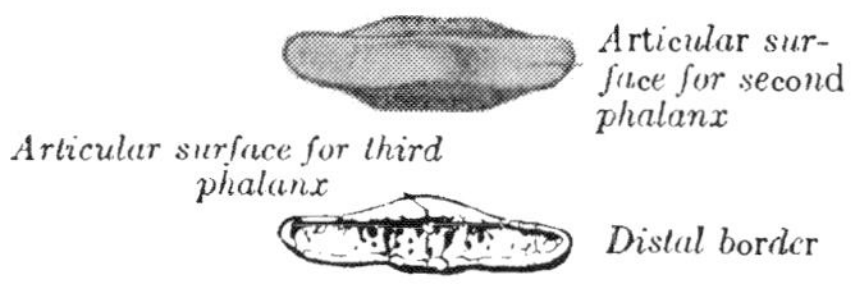

Fig. 59.—Third Sesamoid or Navicular Bone of Horse. (After Schmaltz, Atlas d. Anat. d. Pferdes.)

Development.—It ossifies from a single center.

THE BONES OF THE PELVIC LIMB

The pelvic girdle consists of the ossa coxæ, which unite ventrally at the symphysis pelvis, and articulate with the sacrum dorsally.

OS COXÆ

The os coxæ (or os innominatum) forms the skeleton of the hip or haunch, and is the largest of the flat bones. It consists primarily of three parts, the ilium, ischium, and pubis, which meet to form the acetabulum, a large cotyloid cavity for articulation with the head of the femur. These parts are fused at about one year of age, but it is convenient to describe them separately.

THE ILIUM

The **ilium** (Os ilium) is the largest of the three parts. It is irregularly triangular and presents two surfaces, three borders, and three angles.

The **gluteal surface** (Facies glutæa) faces upward, backward, and outward. It is wide and concave in front, narrower and convex behind. The wide part is crossed by the curved **gluteal line** (Linea glutæa), which extends from the middle of the inner border toward the external angle. This surface gives attachment to the middle and deep gluteal muscles.

The **pelvic surface** (Facies pelvina) faces in the opposite direction; it is convex,

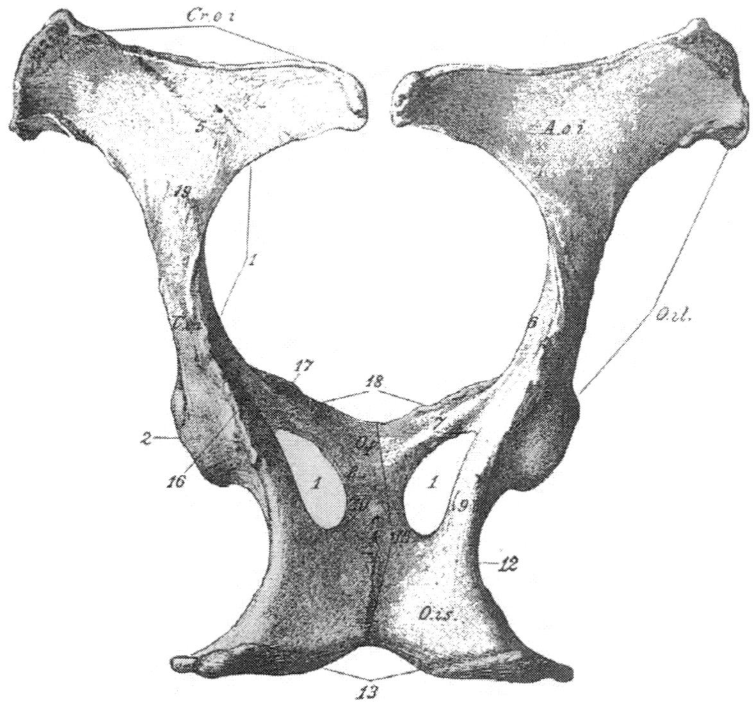

FIG. 60.—OSSA COXARUM OF MARE, DORSAL VIEW.

O. il., Ilium; *O.p.*, pubis; *O.is.*, ischium; *A.o.i.*, wing of ilium; *C.o.i.*, shaft of ilium; *Cr.o.i.*, anterior border (crest) of ilium; *1*, obturator foramen; *2*, acetabulum; *3*, internal angle of ilium; *4*, external angle of ilium; *5*, gluteal line; *6*, psoas tubercle; *7*, *8*, acetabular and symphyseal branches of pubis; *9*, *10*, acetabular and symphyseal branches of ischium; *12*, lesser sciatic notch; *13*, ischial arch; *14*, great sciatic notch; *15*, symphysis pelvis; *17*, ilio-pectineal eminence; *18*, anterior borders of pubic bones; *19*, posterior gluteal line. (Struska, Anat. d. Haustiere.)

and consists of two distinct parts. The inner triangular part (Pars articularis) is roughened for ligamentous attachment, and bears an irregular facet, the **auricular surface** (Facies auricularis), for articulation with the sacrum. The outer quadrilateral part (Pars iliaca) is in general smooth. It is crossed by the **ilio-pectineal line** (Crista iliopectinea), which begins below the auricular surface and is continued on the shaft of the bone to join the anterior border of the pubis. The line is interrupted by furrows for the iliaco-femoral vessels, and below these it bears the **psoas tubercle** (Tuberculum psoadicum), which gives attachment to the psoas minor muscle. The iliacus muscle is attached to the surface external to the ilio-pectineal line.

The **anterior border** or **crest** (Crista iliaca) is concave, thick, and rough.

The **internal border** is deeply concave; its middle part forms the lower boundary of the **great sciatic foramen**, and it is continuous behind with the **superior ischiatic spine**.

The **external border** is concave and in great part rough. Its fore part is crossed by grooves for the ilio-lumbar vessels, which are continued on the pelvic surface. The **nutrient foramen** is usually situated on or near the posterior part of this border.

The **internal** or **sacral angle** (Tuber sacrale) curves upward and a little back-

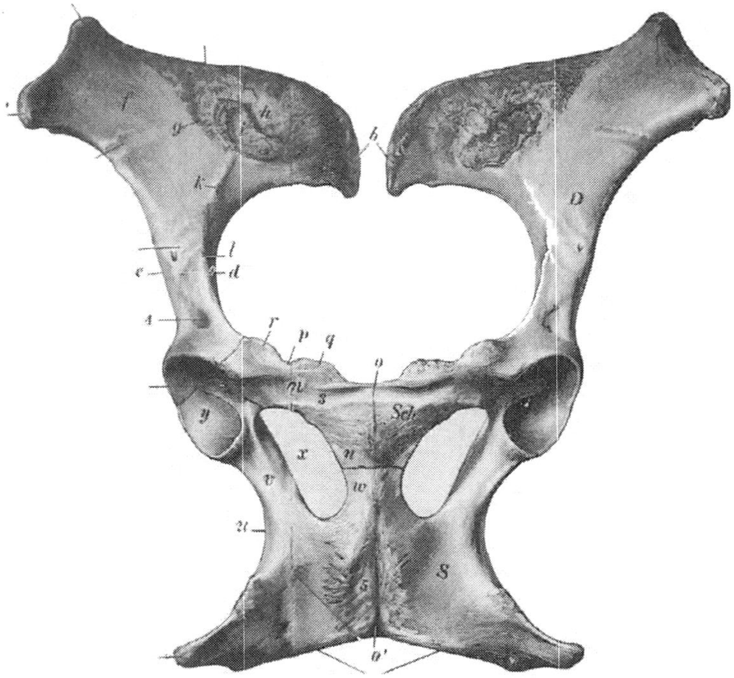

Fig. 61.—Ossa Coxarum of Mare, Ventral View.

D, ilium; *Sch.*, pubis; *S*, ischium; *a*, anterior border (crest) of ilium; *b*, internal angle of ilium; *c'*, external angle of ilium; *d*, great sciatic notch; *e*, external border of ilium; *f*, iliac surface; *g*, linea arcuata; *h*, rough ligamentous area; f, auricular surface; k, ilio-pectineal line; *l*, psoas tubercle; *m*, transverse branch, and *n*, symphyseal branch of pubis; *o*, *o'*, symphysis pelvis; *p*, anterior border of pubis (pecten); *q*, tuberculum pubicum; *r*, ilio-pectineal eminence; *s*, tuber ischii; *t*, ischial arch; *u*, lesser sciatic notch; *v*, acetabular branch, and *w*, symphyseal branch of ischium; *x*, obturator foramen; *y*, articular surface of acetabulum; *z* fossa acetabuli; *1*, groove for ilio-lumbar artery, *2*, groove for iliaco-femoral artery; *3*, subpubic groove; *4*, depression for inner tendon of origin of rectus femoris; *5*, rough area for attachment of adductor muscles. (Ellenberger-Baum, Anat. d. Haustiere.)

ward close to the first sacral spine, and forms here the highest point of the skeleton. It is somewhat thickened and rough.

The **external** or **coxal angle** (Tuber coxæ) forms the basis of the point of the hip. It is a large quadrangular mass, narrow in its middle, and enlarged at either end, where it bears a pair of tuberosities. It is roughened for muscular attachment.

The **posterior** or **acetabular angle** meets the other two bones at the acetabulum, of which it forms about two-fifths. Its prominent upper border forms part of the **superior ischiatic spine**, which is roughened externally, smooth internally. Two depressions above and in front of the acetabulum give attachment to the tendons of origin of the rectus femoris muscle. This angle is connected with the **ala** or wide part of the bone by a constricted part, often termed the shaft. The latter is of three-sided prismatic form. Its external surface is convex and rough, and gives attachment to the deep gluteus muscle. Its pelvic surface is smooth and is grooved for the obturator vessels and nerves. Its ventral surface is crossed by vascular grooves, below which is a rough area, bounded internally by the psoas tubercle.

THE ISCHIUM

The **ischium** (Os ischii) forms the posterior part of the ventral wall or floor of the bony pelvis. It slopes a little downward and inward, but is practically horizontal in the longitudinal direction. It is irregularly quadrilateral, and may be described as having two surfaces, four borders, and four angles.

The **superior** or **pelvic surface** (Facies pelvina) is smooth and slightly concave from side to side.

The **inferior surface** (Facies externa) is nearly flat, and is in great part roughened for the attachment of the adductor muscles.

The **anterior border** forms the posterior margin of the obturator foramen.

The **posterior border** is thick and rough. It slopes obliquely inward and forward to meet the border of the other side, forming with it the **ischial arch** (Arcus ischiadicus).

The **internal border** meets the opposite bone at the symphysis.

The **external border** is thick and rounded, but concave in its length; it forms the **lesser sciatic notch,** the lower boundary of the lesser sciatic foramen.

The **antero-internal angle** or **symphyseal branch** (Ramus symphyseos) meets the pubis, with which it forms the inner boundary of the obturator foramen.

The **antero-external angle** or **acetabular branch** joins the other two bones at the acetabulum, of which it forms more than half. Superiorly it bears part of the **superior ischiatic spine** (Spina ischiadica), and internally it is grooved for the obturator vessels.

The **postero-external angle** is a thick three-sided mass, the **tuber ischii** (Tuber ischiadicum); its lower border is the **inferior ischiatic spine,** to which the biceps femoris and semitendinosus muscles are attached.

THE PUBIS

The **pubis** (Os pubis) is the smallest of the three parts of the os coxæ. It forms the anterior part of the pelvic floor, and may be described as having two surfaces, three borders, and three angles.

The **superior** or **pelvic surface** (Facies pelvina) is convex in the young subject and the stallion, concave and smooth in the mare and usually in the gelding also. The urinary bladder rests on it.

The **inferior** or **ventral surface** (Facies externa) is convex, and in great part rough for muscular attachment. Near the anterior border it is crossed by the **subpubic groove,** the inner part of which is occupied by a large vein, the outer part by the pubo-femoral ligament.

The **anterior** border is thin in its inner part (except in the young subject and the stallion), forming the pecten ossis pubis. Externally it bears the rough **ilio-pectineal eminence** (Eminentia iliopectinea), beyond which it is continuous with the ilio-pectineal line.

The **internal border** joins the opposite bone at the symphysis pubis.

The **posterior** border forms the anterior margin of the obturator foramen, and is marked externally by the obturator groove.

The **internal angle** meets its fellow at the anterior end of the symphysis. This part is very thick in the young subject and the stallion, but in the mare, and usually in the gelding also, it becomes thin with advancing age.

The **external** or **acetabular angle** joins the ilium and ischium at the acetabulum.

The **posterior angle** joins the ischium, with which it forms the inner boundary of the obturator foramen.

The pubis may conveniently be regarded as consisting of two branches which meet at a right angle; these are termed the **transverse** or **acetabular branch** (Ramus acetabularis) and the **longitudinal** or **symphyseal branch** (Ramus symphyseos).

The **acetabulum** is a cotyloid cavity which lodges the head of the femur. It faces downward and outward, and consists of an articular and a non-articular part. The **articular part** (Facies lunata) is crescentic, and is cut into internally by the non-articular part, which lies at a lower level, and is termed the **acetabular fossa** (Fossa acetabuli). The inner part of the rim is correspondingly cut into by the **acetabular notch** (Incisura acetabuli), which is converted into a foramen by the transverse ligament in the fresh state, and transmits the pubo-femoral and round ligaments to the head of the femur.

The **obturator foramen** (Foramen obturatum) is situated between the pubis and ischium. It is oval in outline, the longer axis being directed forward and outward. Its margin is grooved antero-externally for the obturator nerve and vessels.

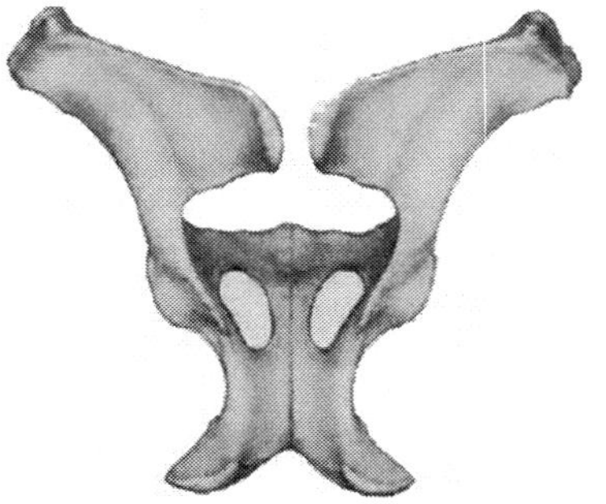

Fig. 62.—Ossa Coxarum of Stallion, Dorsal View. (After Ellenberger-Baum, Anat. für Künstler.)

Development.—Each division of the os coxæ ossifies from one chief center. The center for the ilium appears first near the acetabulum, followed quickly by one for the ischium, and a little later by the pubic center. Secondary centers appear for the crest and external angle of the ilium, the tuber and posterior border of the ischium, and the acetabular part of the pubis. The pubis and ischium are united at birth or soon after, but are not fused with the ilium until the second year. The epiphyseal parts fuse with the main mass at four and a half to five years of age.

The acetabular part of the pubis ossifies from a separate center. It is most distinct in the embryo at three months, and is often called the os acetabuli. Martin says that the ilium has a center for the acetabular part, one for the shaft and wing, and a third for the crest. He also states that there is a special center for the acetabular part of the ischium, and a transitory nucleus in the symphyseal part of the pubis.

THE PELVIS

The bony **pelvis** is composed of the ossa coxarum, the sacrum, and the first three coccygeal vertebræ. The **dorsal wall** or roof is formed by the sacrum and first three coccygeal vertebræ, and the **ventral wall** or floor by the pubic and ischial bones. The **lateral walls** are formed by the ilia and the acetabular part of the ischia. The defect in the skeleton here is supplied in the fresh state by the sacro-sciatic ligaments and semimembranosus muscles.

The **anterior aperture** or **inlet** (Apertura pelvis cranialis) is bounded by the **terminal line** (Linea terminalis) or brim, composed of the base of the sacrum dorsally, the ilio-pectineal lines laterally, and the anterior border of the pubis ventrally.

It is almost circular in the mare, semi-elliptical in the stallion, and faces obliquely downward and forward. It has two principal diameters. Of these, the **conjugate or sacro-pubic diameter** (Conjugata) is measured from the sacral promontory to the anterior end of the symphysis. The **transverse diameter** (Diameter transversa) is measured at the greatest width, *i. e.*, just above the psoas tubercle.

The **posterior aperture** or **outlet** (Apertura pelvis caudalis) is much smaller and is very incomplete in the skeleton. It is bounded above by the third coccygeal vertebra and below by the ischial arch; in the fresh state it is completed laterally by the sacro-sciatic ligament and the semimembranosus muscle.

The **axis** of the pelvis is an imaginary line drawn through the centers of the inlet, cavity, and outlet.

Sexual Differences.—Marked differences exist in the size and form of the pelvis in the two sexes. The average **conjugate diameter** is about 9½ inches (ca. 23 to 24 cm.) in the mare, 7½ inches (ca. 18 to 20 cm.) in the stallion. The **transverse diameter** of the inlet averages about 9 inches (ca. 22 to 23 cm.) in the mare, and 8 inches (ca. 20 cm.) in the stallion. The **obliquity** of the inlet is greater in the female; the difference is indicated by the fact that a vertical plane from the pecten cuts the fourth sacral segment in the female, the second in the male. The outlet is also larger in the mare, the **ischial arch** being about one-third wider than in the stallion. The **cavity** is much more roomy in the female; the transverse diameter between the middles of the superior ischiatic spines is about 8 inches (20 cm.) in the mare, 6 inches (15 cm.) in the stallion. The pubic part of the floor in the female is concave and lies considerably lower than the ischiatic part, which is wide and relatively flat. In the stallion the pubis is very thick centrally, and this part of the floor is convex, while the ischial part is relatively narrow, and is concave from side to side. The obturator **foramina** are correspondingly larger in the female. The **ilium** is shorter, and the greater sciatic notch deeper and narrower in the male. The pelvis of the gelding, when castration has been performed early, resembles that of the mare; otherwise the male characters appear to be retained to a large degree.

THE FEMUR

The **femur** or thigh bone (Os femoris) is the largest and most massive of the long bones. It extends obliquely downward and forward, articulating with the acetabulum above and the tibia and patella below. It presents for examination a shaft and two extremities.

The **shaft** or **body** (Corpus femoris) is in general cylindrical, but flattened behind, and larger above than below. The **anterior** and **lateral surfaces** are continuous and strongly convex from side to side; there is often a central vertical rough line on the proximal part, but otherwise these surfaces are smooth. They are covered by the quadriceps femoris muscle. The **posterior surface** is wide, flat, and smooth in its proximal fourth. Below this part there is a rough elevation externally for the attachment of the femoral tendon of the biceps femoris, and a rough line internally to which the quadratus femoris is attached. The middle third is narrower, and is rough for the attachment of the adductor muscle. Just below this area an oblique groove crosses the surface, indicating the position of the femoral vessels. The **internal border** bears on its proximal part the **internal trochanter** or **trochanter minor,** a thick rough ridge, to which the ilio-psoas muscle is attached. From this a rough line curves up to the front of the neck and indicates the limit of the attachment of the vastus internus muscle. A narrow rough area about the middle gives attachment to the pectineus muscle, and the **nutrient foramen** is usually found just in front of this mark. The **supracondyloid crest** is situated below the groove for the femoral vessels, and gives origin to the inner head

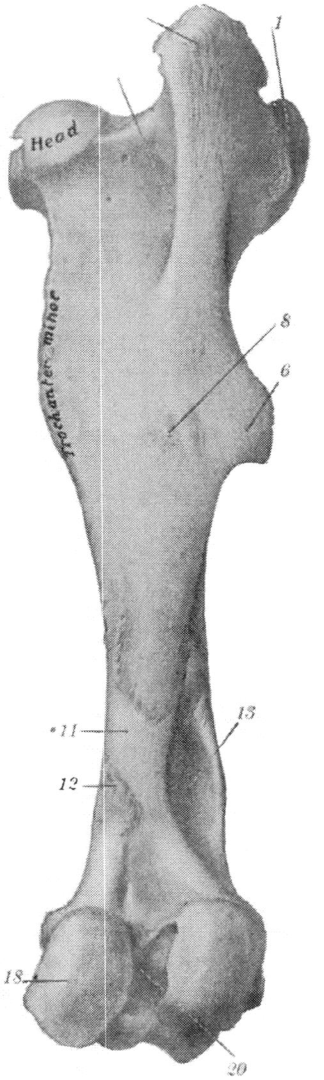

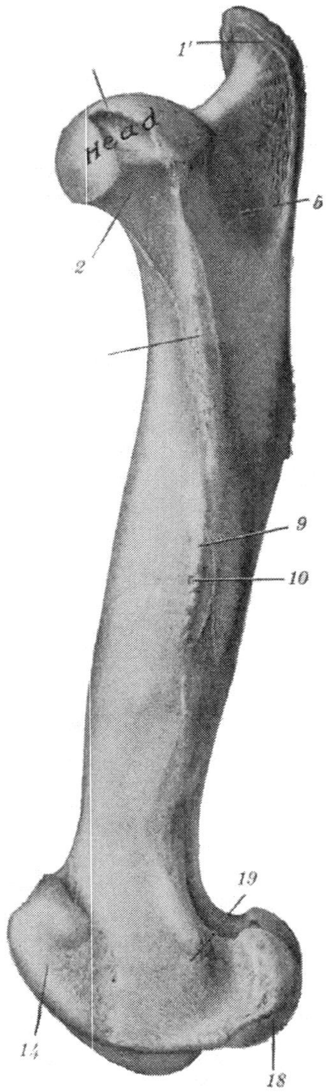

ɪɢʜᴛ Fᴇᴍᴜʀ ᴏғ Hᴏʀsᴇ
ᴇxᴛᴇʀɴᴀʟ Vɪᴇᴡ.

Fɪɢ. 64.—Rɪɢʜᴛ Fᴇᴍᴜʀ ᴏғ Hᴏʀsᴇ Pᴏsᴛᴇʀɪᴏʀ Vɪᴇᴡ.

Fɪɢ. 65.—Rɪɢʜᴛ Fᴇᴍᴜʀ ᴏғ Hᴏʀsᴇ, Iɴᴛᴇʀɴᴀʟ Vɪᴇᴡ.

terior part, *1'*, posterior part of trochanter major; *2*, neck; *3*, fovea capitis; *4*, crest; *5*, trochanteric fossa; *6*, ex-
rd trochanter; *7*, trochanter minor; *8*, eminence for attachment of biceps femoris; *9*, internal border; *10*, nutrient
, groove for femoral vessels; *12*, supracondyloid crest; *13*, supracondyloid fossa; *14*, trochlea; *15*, external epicon-
ternal condyle; *17*, extensor fossa; *18*, internal condyle; *19*, internal epicondyle; *20*, intercondyloid fossa. (After
tlas d. Anat. d. Pferdes.)

of the gastrocnemius. The **external** border is prominent in its upper part, and bears at the junction of its proximal and middle thirds the **external** or **third trochanter** (Trochanter tertius); this process is curved forward, and furnishes insertion to the tendon of the superficial gluteus muscle. At the lower part is found the **supracondyloid** or **plantar fossa** (Fossa plantaris), in which the superficial flexor arises; it is bounded externally by a thick rough margin, to which the outer head of the gastrocnemius muscle is attached.

The **proximal extremity** (Extremitas proximalis) is large and consists of the head, neck, and great trochanter. The **head** (Caput femoris) is placed at the inner side and is directed inward, upward, and somewhat forward. It is approximately hemispherical and articulates with the acetabulum. It is cut into internally by a deep notch, the fovea **capitis**, in which the pubo-femoral and round ligaments are attached. The articular surface is surrounded by a distinct margin. The **neck** (Collum femoris) is most distinct in front and internally. The **great trochanter** (Trochanter major) is situated externally; it presents three features. The **anterior part** or **convexity** is situated opposite to the head and rises little above the level of the latter; it gives attachment to the deep gluteus muscle, and in the fresh state its outer surface is coated with cartilage, over which a tendon of the middle gluteus passes, to be inserted into the **crest**, which is placed below and behind the convexity. The **posterior part** or **summit** is separated from the convexity by a notch; it is situated behind the plane of the head and rises to a much greater height. It furnishes insertion to part of the middle gluteus muscle. Its posterior border is continued downward as the **trochanteric ridge**, which forms the outer wall of the **trochanteric fossa**. A number of foramina are found in the concave area internal to the convexity.

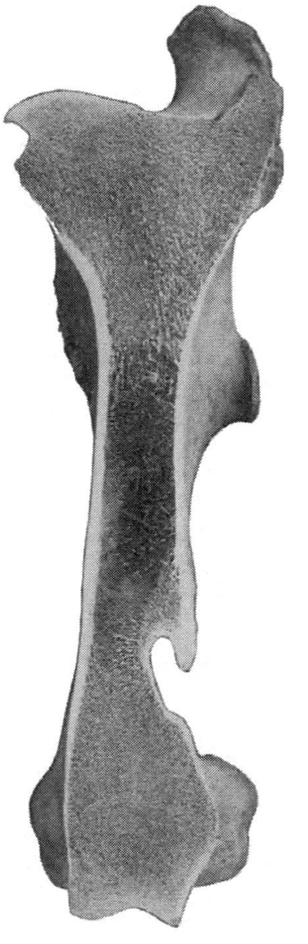

FIG. 66.—FRONTAL SECTION OF LEFT FEMUR OF HORSE, ANTERIOR VIEW.

The figure shows that the medullary cavity is traversed for the most part by fine bony trabeculæ.

The **distal extremity** (Extremitas distalis) is large in both directions and comprises the trochlea in front and two condyles behind. The **trochlea** consists of two ridges separated by a groove, and forms an extensive surface (Facies patellaris) for articulation with the patella. It is very unsymmetrical; the inner ridge or lip is much wider, more prominent, and extends up higher than the external one, and the two converge below. The **condyles, internal** and **external** (Condylus medialis, lateralis), are separated by the deep **intercondyloid fossa** (Fossa intercondyloidea), and articulate with the condyles of the tibia and the semilunar cartilages of the stifle joint. A ridge connects each condyle with the lower part of the corresponding lip of the trochlea. The intercondyloid fossa lodges the spine of the tibia and the crucial ligaments of the stifle joint, which are attached here.

The condyles are obliquely placed, with their long axes directed downward, forward, and inward. The articular surface of the external condyle is more strongly convex from side to side than that of the inner one, and the ridge which connects it with the trochlea is much narrower.

The **internal epicondyle** (Epicondylus medialis) is a rounded prominence on the internal surface of the internal condyle, to which the internal lateral ligament and the adductor muscle are attached. The corresponding **external epicondyle** (Epicondylus lateralis) is less distinct; it presents a mark where the lateral ligament is attached, below and behind which there is a depression (Fossa musculi poplitei) in which the popliteus muscle arises. Between the external condyle and trochlea is the **extensor fossa** (Fossa extensoria), in which the tendon of origin of the anterior extensor and peroneus tertius is attached.

Development.—The shaft and the distal end each ossify from one center, but the proximal end has two centers, one of which is for the great trochanter. The edge of the external trochanter also has a separate center. The proximal end fuses with the shaft at three to three and a half years, the distal at about three and a half years.

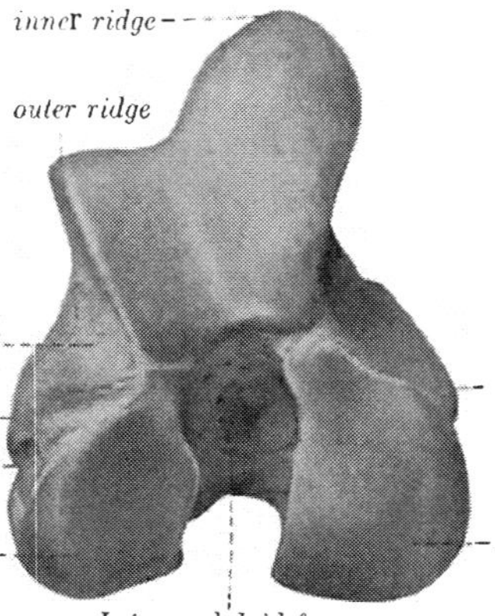

Fig 67.—Distal Extremity of Right Femur of Horse, End View.

THE TIBIA

The tibia is a long bone which extends obliquely downward and backward from the stifle to the hock. It articulates above with the femur, below with the tarsus, and externally with the fibula. It possesses a shaft and two extremities.

The **shaft** or body (Corpus tibiæ), large and three-sided above, becomes smaller and flattened in the sagittal direction below, but widens a little at the distal end. It presents for notice three surfaces and three borders. The **internal surface** (Facies medialis) is broad above, where it furnishes insertion to the internal lateral ligament and the sartorius and gracilis muscles; below this it is convex and subcutaneous. The **external surface** (Facies lateralis) is smooth and somewhat spiral. It is wide and concave in its upper part, below which it becomes narrower and slightly convex, and winds gradually to the front of the bone; near the distal end it widens a little, becomes flat, and faces forward. The **posterior surface** (Facies posterior) is flattened, and is divided into two parts by the rough **popliteal line,** which runs obliquely from the upper part of the external border to the middle of the internal border. The triangular area above the line is occupied by the popliteus muscle, while the area below is marked by rough lines (Lineæ musculares) to which the deep flexor muscle of the digit is attached; the lines fade out below, where the surface is smooth and flat. The **nutrient foramen** is situated on or near the popliteal line. The **anterior** border is very prominent in its upper third, forming the **tibial crest** (Crista tibiæ); below it is reduced to a rough line, which ends at a small elevation near the distal end of the bone. The **internal** border (Margo medialis) is rounded in its upper half, to which the popliteus muscle is attached, and a tubercle is found on this part. The lower part is a rough line on well-marked bones. The **external border** (Crista interossea) is concave in its upper part and concurs with the fibula in the formation of the interosseous space of the leg; a smooth impression indicates the course of the anterior tibial vessels through the space to the

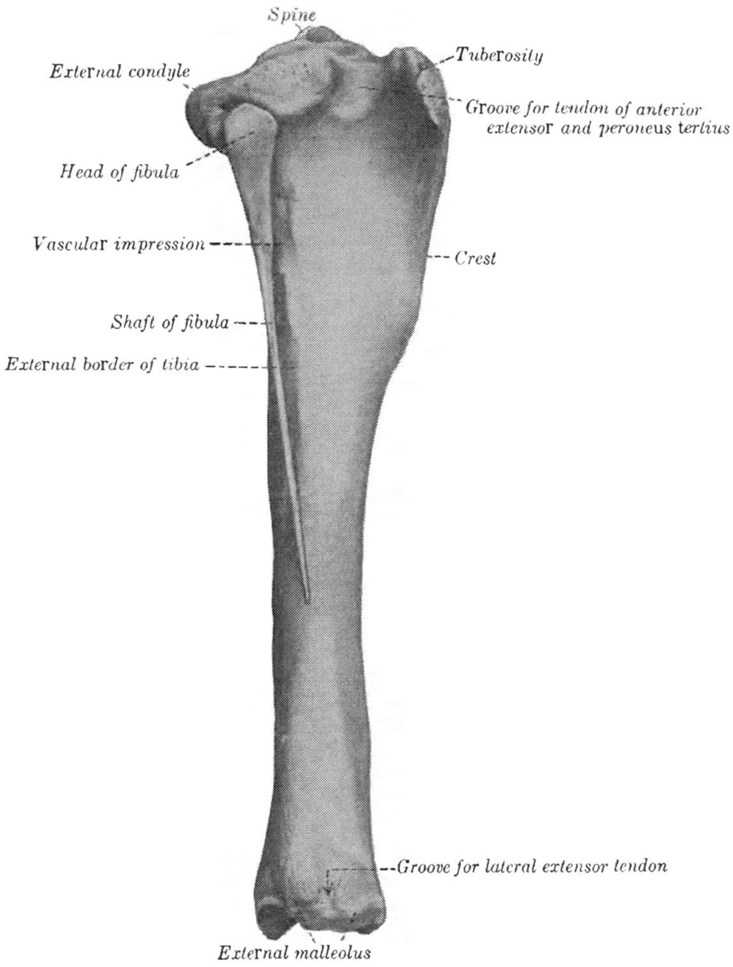

FIG. 68.—RIGHT TIBIA AND FIBULA OF HORSE, EXTERNAL VIEW.

front of the leg. Lower down the border divides and incloses a narrow triangular surface.

The **proximal extremity** (Extremitas proximalis) is large and three-sided. It bears two lateral eminences, the **internal** and **external condyles** (Condylus medialis, lateralis). Each presents a somewhat saddle-shaped surface for articulation with the condyle of the femur and the semilunar cartilage. The **spine** or **intercondyloid eminence** (Eminentia intercondyloidea) is the central prominence, upon which the articular surfaces are continued; it consists of a high inner part and a lower outer part (Tuberculum intercondyloideum mediale, laterale). On, before, and behind the spine are the **anterior** and **posterior intercondyloid fossæ,** in which the anterior crucial ligament and the semilunar cartilages are attached. The condyles are separated behind by the deep **popliteal notch** (Incisura poplitea), on the inner side of which is a tubercle for the attachment of the posterior crucial ligament. The external condyle has an overhanging outer margin, below which is

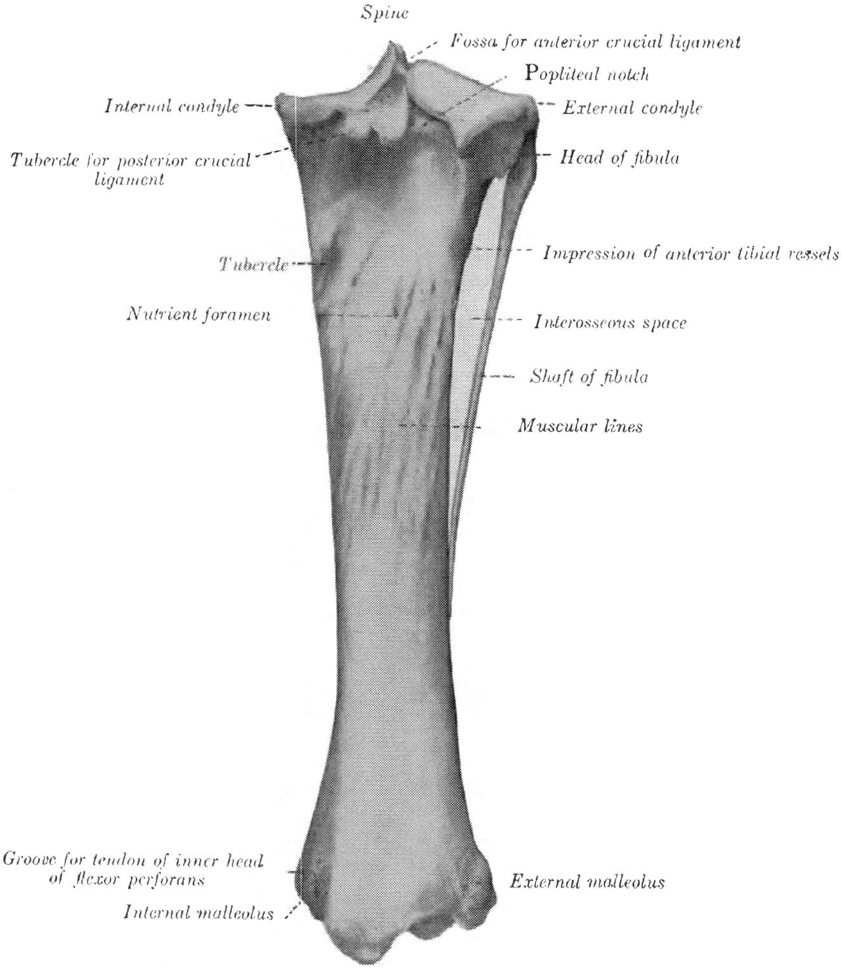

Fig. 69.—Right Tibia and Fibula of Horse, Posterior View.

a facet for articulation with the fibula. The large anterior eminence is the **tuberosity** of the tibia (Tuberositas tibiæ). It is marked in front by a **groove,** the lower part of which gives attachment to the middle patellar ligament, and the groove is flanked by rough areas for the attachment of the internal and external patellar ligaments. A semicircular smooth **notch** (Sulcus muscularis) separates the tuberosity from the external condyle, and gives passage to the tendon of origin of the anterior extensor and the peroneus tertius.

The **distal extremity** (Extremitas distalis) is much smaller than the proximal; it is quadrangular in form and larger internally than externally. It presents an **articular surface** (Cochlea tibiæ), which is adapted to the trochlea of the tibial tarsal bone (astragalus), and consists of two grooves separated by a ridge. The ridge and grooves are directed obliquely forward and outward, and are bounded laterally by the **malleoli,** to which the lateral ligaments of the hock joint are at

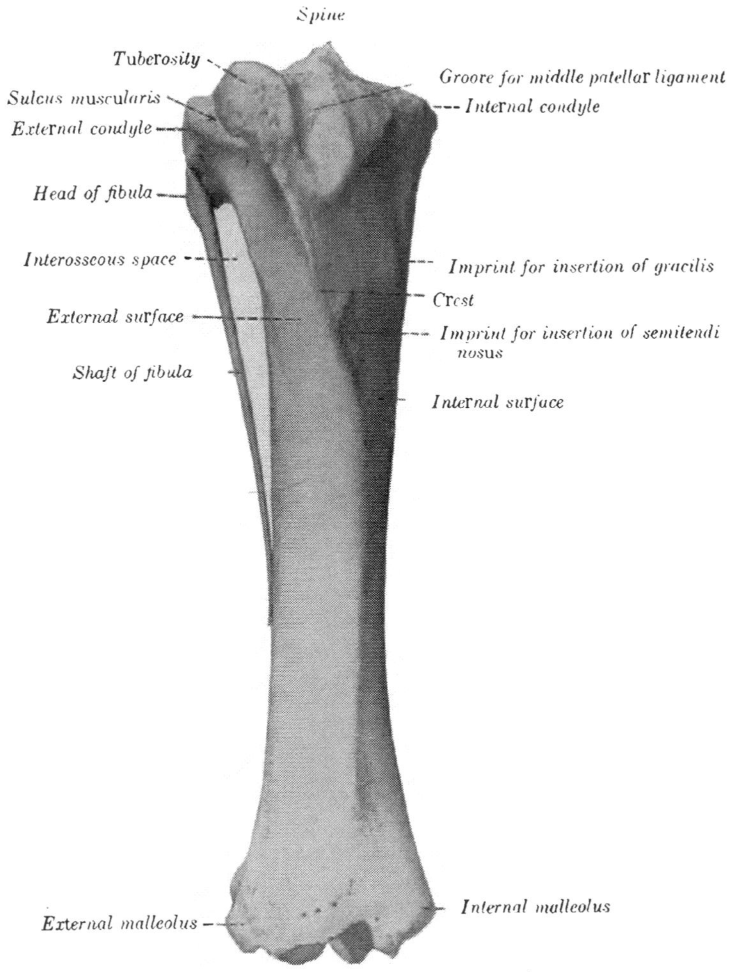

Fig. 70 — Right Tibia and Fibula of Horse, Anterior View

tached. The **internal malleolus** (Malleolus tibialis) is the more prominent of the two, and forms the anterior boundary of a groove for the tendon of the inner head of the flexor perforans. The **external malleolus** (Malleolus fibularis) is broader, and is marked by a vertical groove for the passage of the lateral extensor tendon.

Development.—The tibia has the usual three chief centers of ossification and supplementary ones for the tuberosity and the external malleolus. The latter is really the distal end of the fibula; it is a separate piece at birth, and the line of union is commonly quite evident in the adult in the external articular groove. The proximal end unites with the shaft at about three and a half years, and the distal end at about two years of age.

THE FIBULA

The fibula of the horse is a much reduced long bone, situated along the outer side of the tibia.

The **shaft** or **body** (Corpus fibulæ) is a slender rod which forms the outer boundary of the interosseous space; it usually terminates below in a pointed end about one-half to two-thirds of the way down the external border of the tibia.

The **proximal extremity** or **head** (Capitulum fibulæ) is relatively large, and is flattened transversely. Its internal surface presents a narrow area along the upper border for articulation with the tibia. The external surface is rough and gives attachment to the external lateral ligament of the stifle joint. It has rounded anterior and posterior borders.

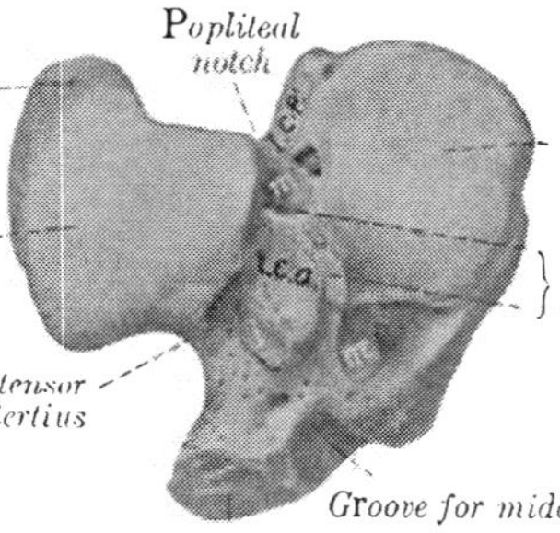

FIG. 71.—PROXIMAL EXTREMITY OF RIGHT TIBIA OF HORSE, END VIEW.
l.c.a., *l.c.p.*, Depressions for attachment of anterior and posterior crucial ligaments; *l*, *m*, *m*, depressions for attachment of semilunar cartilages.

The **distal extremity** is fused with the tibia, constituting the external malleolus.

Development.—This resembles that of the ulna. The embryonic cartilaginous fibula extends the entire length of the leg, but does not articulate with the femur. The lower part of the shaft is usually reduced to a fibrous band. Three centers of ossification appear, one each for the shaft and the extremities. The distal end unites early with the tibia, forming the external malleolus.

It is interesting to note that in some cases the entire shaft of the fibula develops, a reversion to the condition in the Miocene ancestors of the present horse.

THE PATELLA

The **patella** is a large sesamoid bone which articulates with the trochlea of the femur. It presents for description two surfaces, two borders, a base, and an apex.

The **anterior** or **free surface** (Facies libera) is irregularly quadrilateral, convex, and rough for muscular and ligamentous attachment.

The **posterior** or **articular surface** is smaller and is triangular in outline. It presents a vertical rounded ridge, which corresponds to the groove on the trochlea of the femur, and separates two concave areas. Of the latter, the inner cavity is much the larger, and is not very well adapted to the inner lip of the trochlea; in the fresh state, however, it is completed and rendered more congruent by the curved **accessory fibro-cartilage.**

The **lateral borders** converge to the apex below, and each forms a prominence or angle at the base. The inner angle and the adjacent part of the border give attachment to the fibro-cartilage of the patella, which increases the articular surface. The external border is rounded and its angle is less prominent.

The **base** (Basis patellæ) faces upward and backward, and is convex transversely, concave from before backward.

The **apex** forms a blunt point directed downward.

Development.—The patella develops as a sesamoid bone from a single center in a cartilaginous deposit in the tendon of the quadriceps femoris muscle.

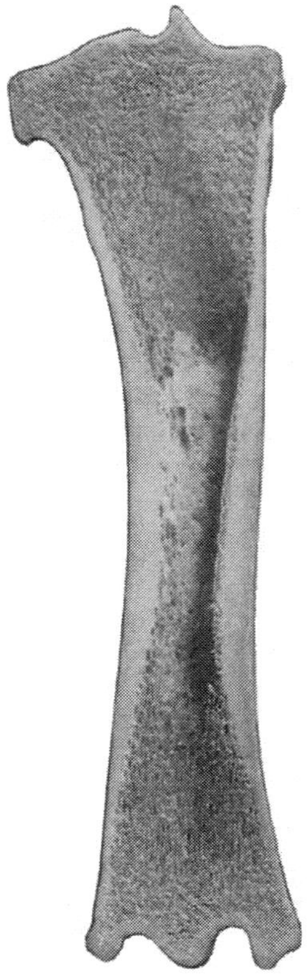

FIG. 72.—FRONTAL SECTION OF RIGHT TIBIA OF HORSE, ANTERIOR VIEW.

THE TARSUS

The **tarsus** or hock of the horse usually comprises six short bones (Ossa tarsi), but exceptionally seven are present.

THE TIBIAL TARSAL BONE

The **tibial tarsal** bone (Os tarsi tibiale, astragalus, or talus) is the inner bone of the proximal row. It is extremely irregular in form, but may be considered as offering six surfaces for description.

The **superior** and the **anterior** or **dorsal surface** are continuous, and form a **trochlea** for articulation with the distal end of the tibia. The trochlea consists of two oblique ridges with a deep groove between them, which curve spirally forward, downward, and outward. There is usually a shallow **synovial fossa** in the groove. The **inferior surface** is convex from before backward, and most of it articulates with the central tarsal; externally it has an oblique facet for the fourth tarsal, and a non-articular groove cuts into the surface to its middle. The **posterior** or **plantar surface** is oblique and extremely irregular; it presents four facets for articulation with the fibular tarsal bone; the facets are separated by rough excavated areas, and the largest fossa (Sulcus tali) forms with a corresponding one on the fibular

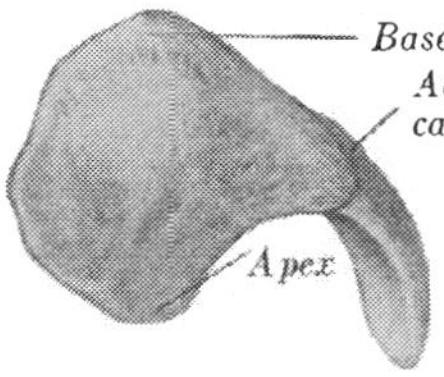

FIG. 73.—RIGHT PATELLA OF HORSE, ANTERIOR VIEW.

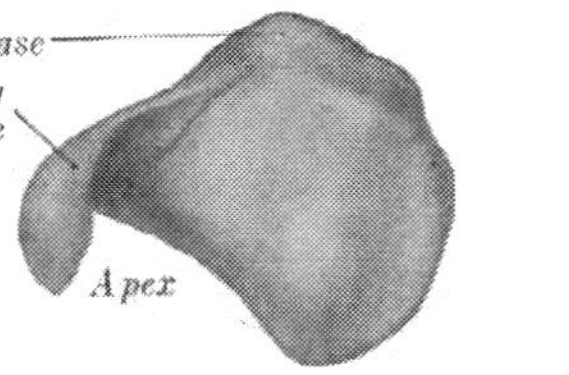

FIG. 74.—RIGHT PATELLA OF HORSE, POSTERIOR VIEW.

tarsal a cavity termed the **sinus tarsi.** The **internal surface** bears on its lower part a large tuberosity, and on its upper part a small one for the attachment of the internal lateral ligament. The external surface is smaller than the internal, and is marked by a wide rough fossa in which the external ligament is attached.

The Fibular Tarsal Bone

The fibular tarsal bone (Os tarsi fibulare, calcaneum, os calcis) is the largest bone of the hock. It is elongated, flattened from side to side, and forms a lever

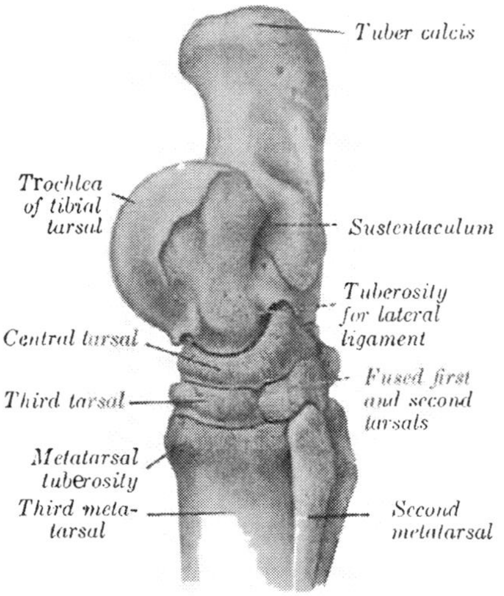

Fig. 75.—Right Tarsus and Upper Part of Metatarsus of Horse, Internal View. (After Schmaltz, Atlas d. Anat. d. Pferdes.)

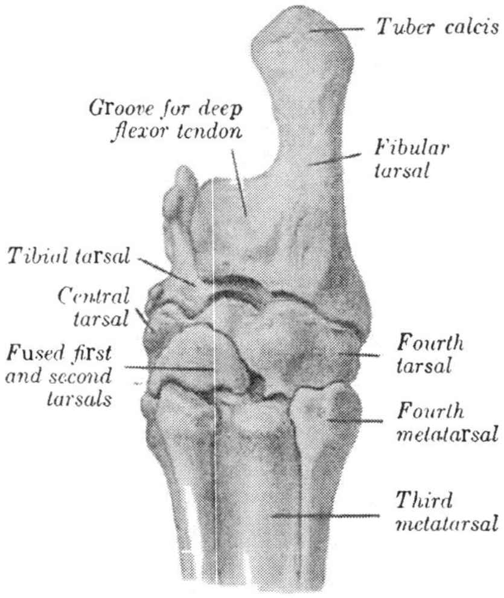

Fig. 76.—Right Tarsus and Upper Part of Metatarsus of Horse, Posterior (Plantar) View. (After Schmaltz, Atlas d. Anat. d. Pferdes.)

for the muscles which extend the hock joint. It consists of a body and an inner process, the sustentaculum tali.

The body (Corpus calcanei) is enlarged at its proximal end to form the tuber

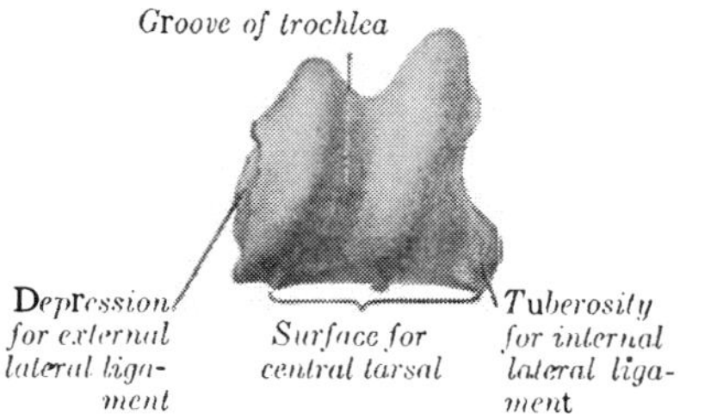

Fig. 77.—Right Tibial Tarsal Bone of Horse. Anterior View. (After Schmaltz, Atlas d. Anat. d. Pferdes.)

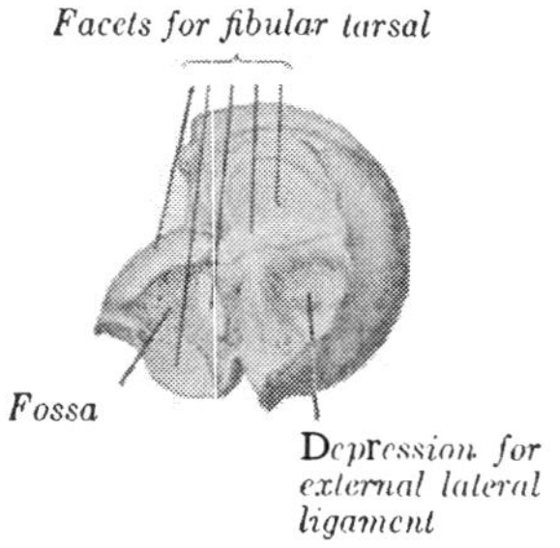

Fig. 78.—Right Tibial Tarsal Bone of Horse External View. (After Schmaltz, Atlas d. Anat. d. Pferdes.)

calcis or "point of the hock." The posterior part of this eminence gives attachment to the tendon of the gastrocnemius, while in front and laterally it furnishes insertion to tendons of the flexor perforatus, biceps, and semitendinosus muscles. The inferior extremity bears a concave facet for articulation with the fourth tarsal bone. The internal surface has on its lower part a strong process, the sustentaculum tali, which projects inward. The process has a large, oval, slightly concave facet in front for articulation with the tibial tarsal, and sometimes a small articular surface below for the central tarsal bone. Its plantar surface forms with the smooth inner surface of the body a groove for the deep flexor tendon (Sulcus musculi flexoris hallucis longi). Its inner surface has a prominence on the lower part for the attachment of the lateral ligament. The **external surface** of the body is flattened, except below, where there is a rough prominence for the attachment of the lateral

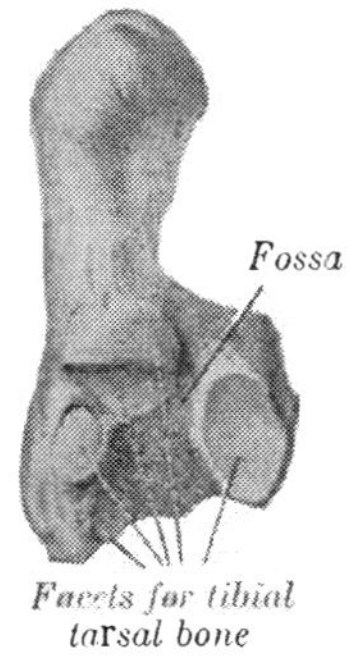

FIG 79.—RIGHT FIBULAR TARSAL BONE OF HORSE, ANTERIOR VIEW. (After Schmaltz, Atlas d. Anat. d. Pferdes.)

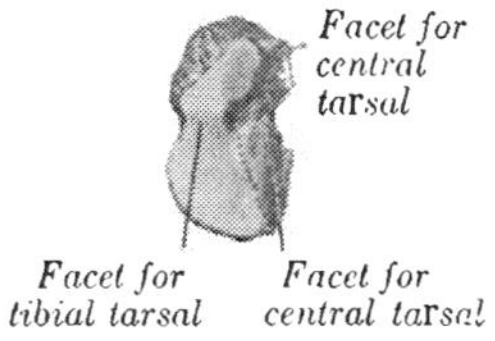

FIG. 80.—RIGHT FOURTH TARSAL BONE OF HORSE UPPER SURFACE. (After Schmaltz, Atlas d. Anat. d. Pferdes.)

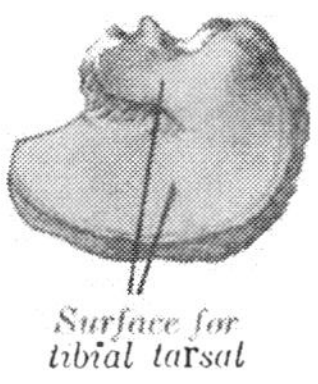

FIG. 81.—RIGHT CENTRAL TARSAL BONE OF HORSE UPPER SURFACE. (After Schmaltz, Atlas d. Anat. d. Pferdes.)

ligament. The **anterior** or **dorsal border** is concave in its length, smooth and rounded in its upper part. About its middle is a blunt-pointed projection (Processus cochlearis) which bears facets on its inner and lower surfaces for articulation with the tibial tarsal bone, and is roughened outwardly for ligamentous attachment. Below this are two facets for the tibial tarsal, and an extensive rough fossa which concurs in the formation of the sinus tarsi. The **posterior** or **plantar border** is

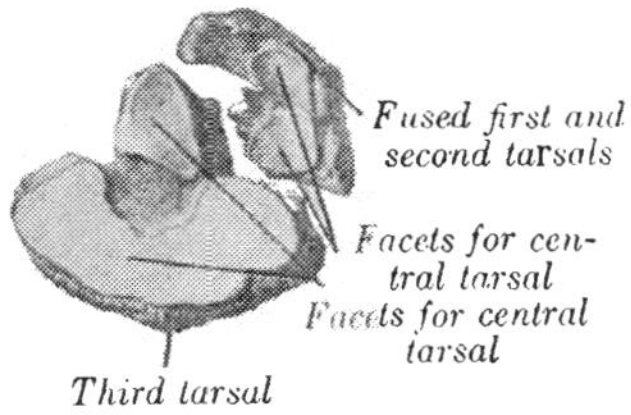

FIG. 82.—RIGHT FIRST, SECOND, AND THIRD TARSAL BONES OF HORSE, UPPER SURFACE. (After Schmaltz, Atlas d. Anat. d. Pferdes.)

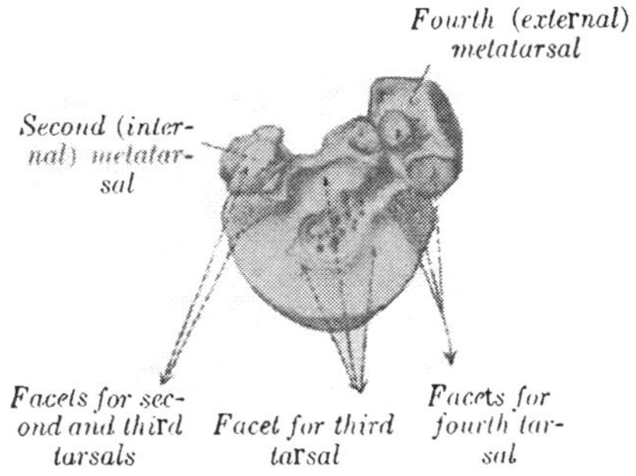

FIG. 83.—PROXIMAL ARTICULAR SURFACES OF LEFT METATARSAL BOXES OF HORSE. (After Schmaltz, Atlas d. Anat. d. Pferdes.)

straight and thick, and widens a little at either end; it is rough, and gives attachment to the long plantar ligament.

THE CENTRAL TARSAL BONE

The **central tarsal** bone (Os tarsi centrale, scaphoid, or navicular) is irregularly quadrilateral, and is situated between the tibial tarsal above and the third tarsal below. It is flattened from above downward, and may be described as having two surfaces and four borders. The superior surface is concave from before backward, and almost all of it articulates with the tibial tarsal; a non-articular depression cuts into its outer part, and sometimes there is a facet for the fibular tarsal bone on the posterior angle. The inferior surface is convex, and is crossed by a non-articular groove, which separates facets for articulation with the third and the first and

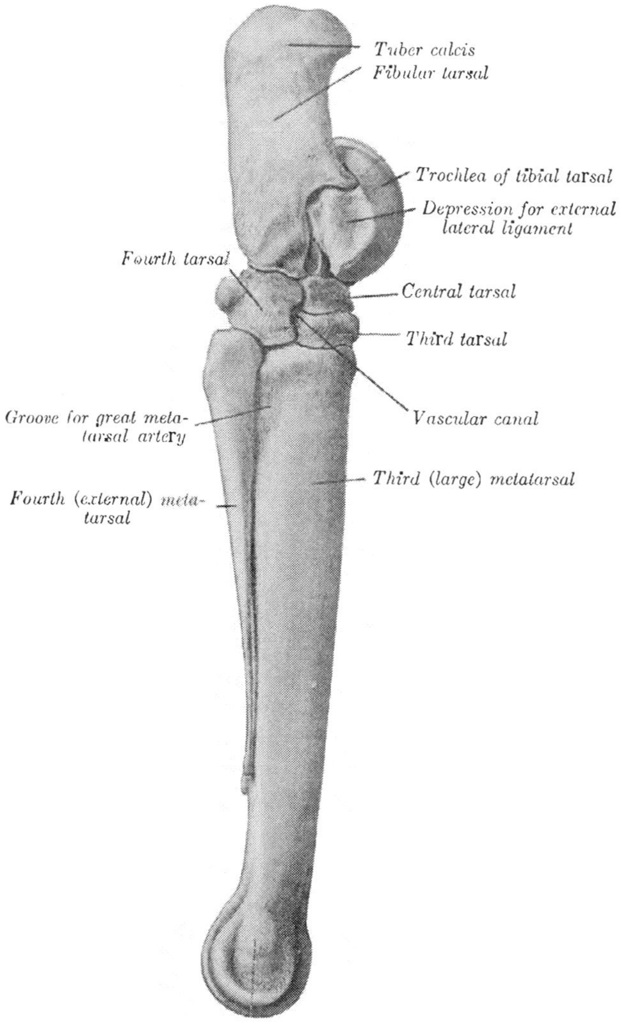

FIG. 84.—RIGHT TARSAL AND METATARSAL BONES OF HORSE, EXTERNAL VIEW. (After Schmaltz, Atlas d. Anat. d. Pferdes.)

second (fused) tarsals. The anterior or dorsal border and the internal border are continuous, convex, and rough. The posterior or plantar border bears two prominences, separated by a notch. The external border is oblique, and bears anterior and posterior facets for articulation with the fourth tarsal, between which it is excavated and rough.

First and Second Tarsal Bones

The **first** and **second tarsal** bones (Os tarsale primum et secundum, cuneiform parvum) are usually fused in the horse, forming a bone of very irregular shape, situated in the inner and posterior part of the lower row, below the central and behind the third tarsal. It is the smallest of the tarsal bones, and may be described as having two surfaces, two borders, and two extremities. The **internal surface** faces backward and inward, and is convex. Its anterior part is ridged, and gives attachment to the internal lateral ligament, and its posterior part bears an imprint where the inner tendon of the tibialis anterior is inserted. The **external surface** is marked by a deep notch which indicates the division between the first and second tarsal elements; it bears on its anterior part a large concave facet for the central tarsal. The **superior border** is convex. The **inferior border** is broad in front, where it articulates with the large and inner small metatarsal bones. The **anterior extremity** has a small facet for articulation with the third tarsal, and bears internally a ridge or tubercle. The **posterior extremity** is a blunt point.

In some cases the first and second tarsal bones remain separate—a remarkable reversion to the condition in the early ancestors of the horse. In such specimens the first tarsal is a discoid bone, articulating above with the central, below with the small metacarpal bone. The second tarsal is quadrangular, equivalent to the thick anterior part of the bone as described above, and overlapped by the anterior part of the first tarsal.

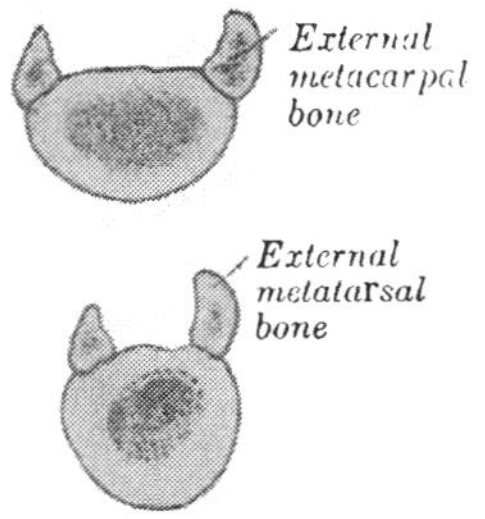

Fig. 85.—Cross-sections of Metacarpal and Metatarsal Bones of Horse. (After Schmaltz, Atlas d. Anat. d. Pferdes.)

The Third Tarsal Bone

The **third tarsal** bone (Os tarsale tertium, third or great cuneiform) resembles the central, but is smaller and triangular in outline. It is situated between the central above and the large metatarsal bone below. It possesses two surfaces and three borders.

The **superior surface** is concave, and is crossed by a non-articular depression which divides it into two unequal facets; it articulates with the central tarsal. The **inferior surface** is slightly convex, and rests on the large metatarsal bone; it has an extensive central rough excavation. The **anterior** or **dorsal border** is convex and bears a rounded ridge on its inner part. The **internal border** is deeply notched and has a small facet for the second tarsal on its anterior part. The **external border** is also divided by a notch into two parts, and bears two diagonally opposite facets for articulation with the fourth tarsal. In some cases there is a facet for the inner small metatarsal bone.

The Fourth Tarsal Bone

The **fourth tarsal** bone (Os tarsale quartum, cuboid) is the outer bone of the lower row, and is equal in height to the central and third together. It is cuboid in shape and presents six surfaces.

The **superior surface** is convex from side to side, and articulates chiefly with the fibular tarsal, but to a small extent with the tibial tarsal also. The **inferior surface** rests on the large and external small metatarsal bones. The **internal surface** bears four facets for articulation with the central and third tarsal bones. It is crossed from before backward by a smooth groove, which by apposition with the adjacent bones forms the **canal of the tarsus** (Canalis tarsi) for the passage of the perforating tarsal vessels. The **anterior** or **dorsal, external,** and **posterior** or **plantar surfaces** are continuous and rough. A tuberosity behind gives attachment to the plantar ligament.

Development.—The fibular tarsal bone has two centers of ossification, one for the main mass and the other for the tuber calcis; the latter fuses with the rest of the bone at about three years of age. The first and second tarsals have separate centers, but fusion usually occurs before birth. Each of the other bones ossifies from a single center.

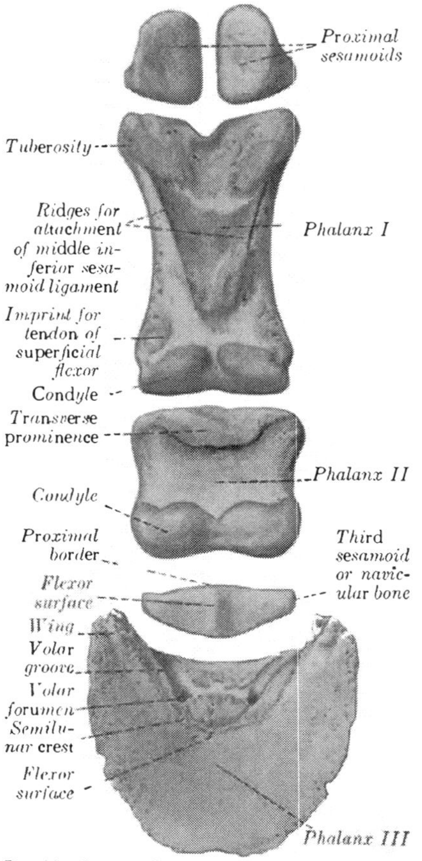

FIG. 86.—DIGITAL BONES OF FORE LIMB OF HORSE, VOLAR ASPECT.

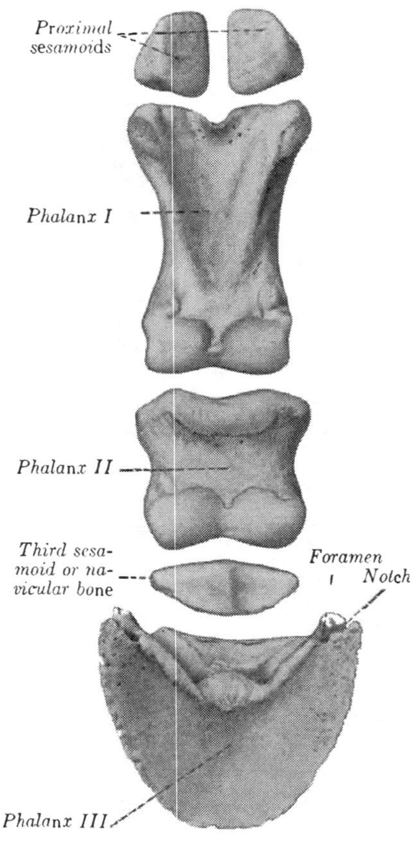

FIG. 87.—DIGITAL BONES OF HIND LIMB OF HORSE VOLAR ASPECT.

THE METATARSUS

The metatarsal bones (Ossa metatarsalia), three in number, have the same general arrangement as the metacarpal bones, but present some important differences. Their direction is slightly oblique, downward and a little forward

The large or third metatarsal bone is about one-sixth longer than the corresponding metacarpal; in an animal of medium size the difference is about two inches. The shaft is more cylindrical, and is almost circular on cross-section, except in its lower part. At the upper part of its external surface there is a groove, which is directed obliquely downward and backward, and is continued by the furrow formed by the apposition of the external metatarsal bone; it indicates the course of the great metatarsal artery. A faint impression in a similar place on the inner side marks the position of the corresponding vein. The nutrient foramen is relatively higher than on the metacarpal bone. The proximal extremity is much wider from before backward than that of the metacarpal bone. Its articular surface is slightly concave, and is marked by a large central non-articular depression, continued outward by a deep notch. The greater part of the surface articulates with the third tarsal, but there is an outer facet for the fourth, and usually a small facet postero-internally for the second tarsal bone. Posteriorly there are two pairs of facets for articulation with the small metatarsal bones. The front is crossed by a rough ridge for insertion, which becomes larger and turns downward on the outer side behind the vascular groove. The distal extremity closely resembles that of the corresponding metacarpal bone.

In some cases the lower part of the shaft is bent backward somewhat. The articular surface extends a little higher behind than in the case of the metacarpal bone. The large metatarsal bone is even more strongly constructed than the metacarpal. The shell of compact substance is very thick in the middle of the shaft, especially in front and internally.

The small metatarsal bones are a little longer than the corresponding metacarpals. The external (fourth) metatarsal is relatively massive, especially in its upper part. The head is large and outstanding, and bears two facets above for the fourth tarsal, and two in front and internally for articulation with the large metatarsal; elsewhere it is roughened for attachment. The internal (second) metatarsal is much more slender than the outer one, especially in its upper part. The head bears two facets above for the first and second tarsals, and sometimes one for the third tarsal.

THE PHALANGES AND SESAMOIDS

The axis of the phalanges of the hind limb is about five degrees less oblique than that of the fore limb, and the chief differences in the form and size of the bones are as follows:

The first phalanx is a little shorter, wider above, and narrower below.

The second phalanx is narrower and slightly longer.

The third phalanx is narrower, the angle of inclination of the wall surface is a little (ca. 5 degrees) greater, the sole surface is more concave, and the wings are less prominent and closer together.

The proximal sesamoids are a little smaller, except in thickness. The third sesamoid or navicular bone is narrower and shorter.

SKELETON OF THE OX

VERTEBRAL COLUMN

The vertebral formula is $C_7T_{13}L_6S_5Cy_{18-20}$.

The cervical vertebræ are much shorter than those of the horse and are smaller in their other dimensions. The articular processes are smaller than in the horse, and a plate of bone connects each two of the same side. The transverse processes of the third, fourth, and fifth are double; the upper part projects backward, and is short and stout; the lower part is directed downward and forward, and is longer and more plate-like. The lower part of the sixth transverse process is a large, thick, quadrilateral and almost sagittal plate, directed downward. The seventh transverse process is single, short, and thick, and presents no foramen transversarium; it is in series with the upper part of the preceding processes. The spinous processes are well developed, and increase in height from before backward. They are directed upward and forward, with the exception of the last, which is nearly vertical and is about four or five inches (ca. 10 to 12 cm.) in height. The summit of that of the third bone is usually bifid. The ventral spines are prominent and thick in their posterior part; they are absent on the last two.

The atlas has a large rough tuberosity on its dorsal arch. The ventral arch is very thick. The wings are less curved than in the horse, and the foramen transversarium (posterior foramen) is absent. The cavities for the occipital condyles are divided into upper and lower parts by a non-articular area, and are separated by a narrow interval below. The posterior articular surfaces are flattened behind and are continued into the vertebral canal, forming an extensive area for the odontoid process of the axis.

The axis is short. The spine projects a little in front, and increases in height and thickness behind; its posterior border descends abruptly. The odontoid process (dens) is wide, and its upper surface is deeply concave from side to side. The intervertebral foramen is circular and not so close to the anterior border of the arch as in the horse. The posterior notches are not so deep. The transverse processes are stouter, but the foramen transversarium is small and sometimes absent.

The thoracic vertebræ, thirteen in number, are larger than those of the horse. The bodies are longer and are distinctly constricted in the middle. They bear a thin-edged ventral crest. The arches—in addition to the usual notches, which are shallow—are perforated in the posterior part by a foramen. The transverse processes are thick and strong, and bear rounded mammillary processes (except at the posterior end of the series); the last two, although prominent, do not always articulate with the ribs. The spinous processes are long. The first is much higher than in the horse, the next two are usually the most prominent, and behind this there is a very gradual diminution in height. The backward slope, slight at first, increases to the tenth; the last is vertical and lumbar in character. The summit is usually pointed on the first, and the thickening on those further back is less than in the horse. The width diminishes from the fifth to the eleventh usually. Both borders of the spines are in general thin and sharp, but the last three or four sometimes have thick posterior margins.

The lumbar vertebræ, six in number, are much longer than in the horse. The bodies are much constricted in the middle, expanded at either end, and bear rudimentary ventral crests. The fourth and fifth are usually the longest. The intervertebral foramina are often double in the anterior part of the series, and are

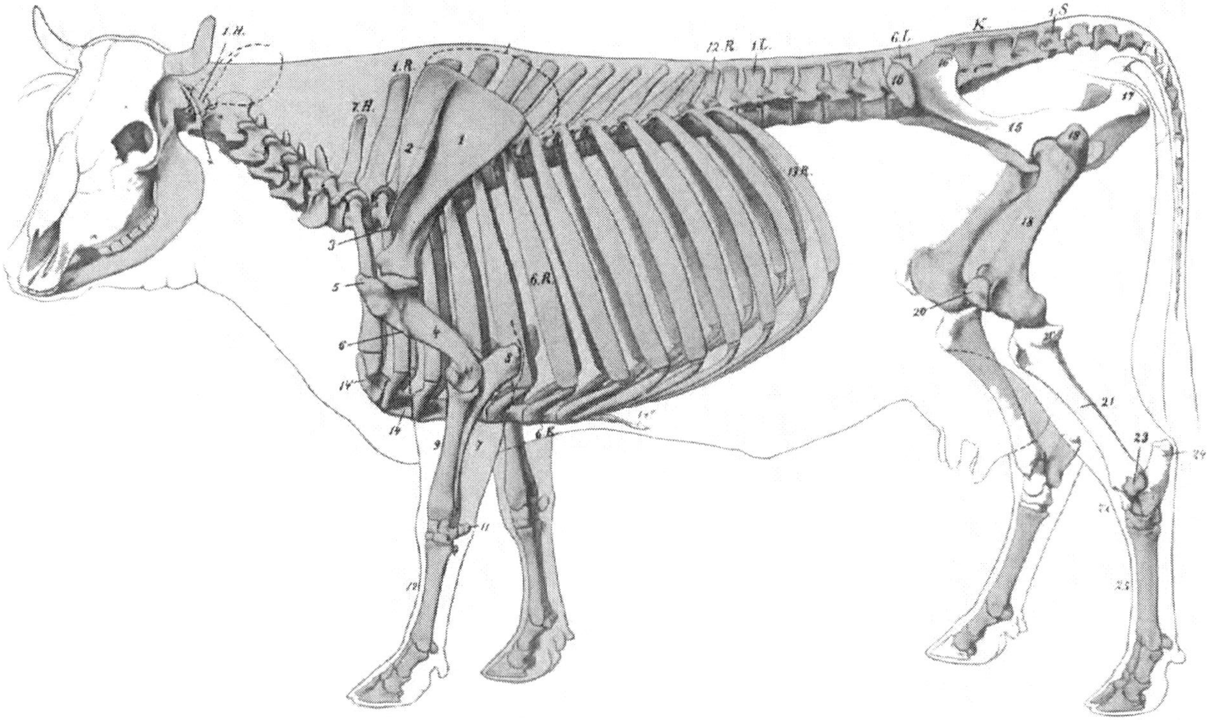

FI 88.—SKELETON OF CO

1.H., Atlas; *7.H.*, seventh cervi ; ., re ; ., sixth rib; *12.R.*, ; ; *L.*, rst, *6.L.*, last lu dr vertebra
K, sacrum; *1.S.*, first coccygeal vertebra; .*K.*, ; wi ; *1*, scapula; *1'*, ; ; a mion; *4*, humerus; *4'*, externa
condyle of humerus; *5*, external tuberosi ; , *8* olecranon; *9*, ; *10*, ; n ; *12*, ps; *13*, pha anges
14, sternum; *14'*, manubrium; *14''*, xiph ; *1* , ili ; m; *16'*, internal of iliu ; ii; ; trochanter major; *20*, atella
21, tibia; *21'*, external condyle of tibia; *22*, , distal ; *25*, metatarsus; t. für Künstler.)

very large further back. The articular processes are large, and their facets are more strongly curved than in the horse. The transverse processes all curve forward. They are separated by considerable intervals, and form no articulations with each other or with the sacrum. Their borders are thin and irregular, and often bear projections of variable size and form. The first is the shortest and the length increases to the fifth, the last being considerably shorter. The spinous processes are relatively low and wide, the last being the smallest; their summits are moderately thickened.

The sacrum is longer than that of the horse. It consists originally of five segments, but fusion is more complete and involves the spinous processes, which are united to form a median sacral crest, with a convex thick and rough margin. A lateral crest is formed by the fusion of the articular processes. The pelvic surface is concave in both directions, and is marked by a central groove, which indicates the course of the middle sacral artery. The inferior sacral foramina are large. The wings are quadrangular, short, compressed from before backward, and high dorso-ventrally. They have an extensive anterior surface, which is concave from side to side, and non-articular. The posterior surface is rough, and bears a triangular area below for articulation with the ilium. The body of the first segment is very wide, and the entrance to the sacral canal correspondingly wide and low. The anterior articular processes are large, and are concave and semi-cylindrical in curvature internally. The lateral borders are thin, sharp, and irregular. The apex is wider than in the horse, and the posterior end of the crest forms a pointed projection over the opening of the sacral canal.

The coccygeal vertebræ are longer and better developed than in the horse. The first five or six have complete arches and spinous processes. The transverse processes are relatively large in the anterior part of the series, in which there are also anterior articular processes (which do not articulate), and a pair of ventral spines which form a hæmal groove for the middle coccygeal artery.

Vertebral curves: The cervical curve is very slight and is concave dorsally. The thoracic and lumbar regions form a gentle curve, concave ventrally. The promontory is more pronounced than in the horse, especially in subjects in which the sacrum is inclined upward behind. Another promontory occurs at the junction of the sacrum and first coccygeal vertebræ.

Length: The following table gives the lengths of the regions of a shorthorn cow of medium size:

Cervical	47 cm.
Thoracic	75 cm.
Lumbar	40 cm.
Sacral	24 cm.
Coccygeal	75 cm.
	261 cm.

Variations: Sometimes fourteen thoracic vertebræ and fourteen pairs of ribs are present; reduction to twelve with the normal number of lumbar vertebræ is very rare. According to Franck, there are sometimes seven lumbar vertebræ with the normal number in the thoracic region. The number of coccygeal vertebræ may vary from sixteen to twenty-one.

THE RIBS

Thirteen pairs of ribs are normally present, of which eight are sternal and five asternal. They are in general longer, wider, flatter, less curved, and less regular in form than in the horse. The eighth, ninth, and tenth are the longest and widest. The width of most of the ribs increases considerably in the middle, and the breadth of the intercostal spaces is correspondingly diminished. The neck is long, and forms (except in the posterior part of the series) a smaller angle with the shaft than in the horse. The articular surface of the tubercle is concave transversely, except on the last two or three, where the facet is small and flat or absent. The lower ends of the second to the tenth or eleventh inclusive form diarthrodial joints with the costal cartilages. The first costal cartilages are very short; they articulate by their internal surfaces with the sternum, but not with each other.

The presence of a fourteenth rib is not very rare. It is usually floating and may correspond to an additional thoracic vertebra or to the first lumbar. Reduction of the thirteenth is more common. The eighth cartilage often does not reach the sternum, but articulates with the seventh.

The sternum consists of seven sternebræ, most of which are developed from two lateral centers. It is wider, flatter, and relatively longer than in the horse, and the ventral crest or "keel" is absent. The manubrium is somewhat wedge-shaped and laterally compressed. Its base forms a diarthrodial joint with the body of the bone, and laterally it bears extensive facets for articulation with the first pair of costal cartilages. The body widens from before backward, but behind the last pair of costal facets it becomes much narrower. The ventral surface is prominent on the second and third segments, concave further back. The lateral borders are notched for the passage of vessels. The cariniform cartilage is absent. The xiphoid cartilage is like that of the horse but is smaller.

THE THORAX

The bony thorax is shorter than in the horse. The inlet is higher. The roof is short, and the floor wider and relatively longer. The transverse diameter is wider in the posterior part. The summits of the spinous processes are almost in a straight line from the second thoracic to the middle of the lumbar region.

BONES OF THE SKULL

BONES OF THE CRANIUM

The occipital bone is situated in the lower part only of the posterior surface of the skull, and is separated from the highest part (the frontal eminence) by the parietal and interparietal bones. The supraoccipital, interparietals, and parietals fuse before birth or soon after, and the mass so formed is separated from the lateral parts of the occipital bone by a transverse suture in the skull of the calf. Above this suture is a central tuberosity, to which the ligamentum nuchæ is attached, and the surface on either side is depressed and rough for muscular attachment. Below the suture the bone is much wider than that of the horse. The foramen magnum is wide, so that the condyles are further apart except below. The paramastoid processes are short and wide and are bent inward. Two constant foramina are found in the condyloid fossa; the anterior one is the hypoglossal, the other (sometimes double) conducts a vein from the condyloid canal. The latter passes upward from a foramen on the inner side of the condyle and opens into the parieto-temporal canal. The cranial surface of the supraoccipital presents a central depression, and above this is a variable but never very pronounced eminence, which corresponds to the tentorium osseum of the horse. On either side is a groove leading to the parieto-temporal canal. The basilar process is short and wide; its cranial surface is deeply concave, and the internal spheno-occipital crest is prominent. Two large tubercles below mark the junction with the sphenoid. The foramen lacerum is short and very narrow. In the adult animal the bone is excavated to contain an air-cavity which is regarded as a part of the frontal sinus.

The sphenoid bone is short. The cranial surface of the body presents a deep sella turcica, in front of which it rises abruptly. The high anterior part bears a central ridge (Rostrum sphenoidale), which joins the crista galli of the ethmoid. Two foramina occur on either side. Of these, the large anterior one is equivalent to the foramen rotundum, lacerum orbitale, and patheticum of the horse. The posterior one is the foramen ovale, which transmits the inferior maxillary nerve.

The orbital wing is thick and is overlapped by the frontal in such manner as to appear externally to divide into two branches; the anterior part joins the ethmoid close to the sphenopalatine foramen, and contains a small sinus which communicates with an ethmoidal meatus. The temporal wing is small, but forms a prominent thick pterygoid crest. The pterygoid process is wide, and the pterygoid or alar foramen is absent. The sphenoidal sinus is absent in the calf and small in

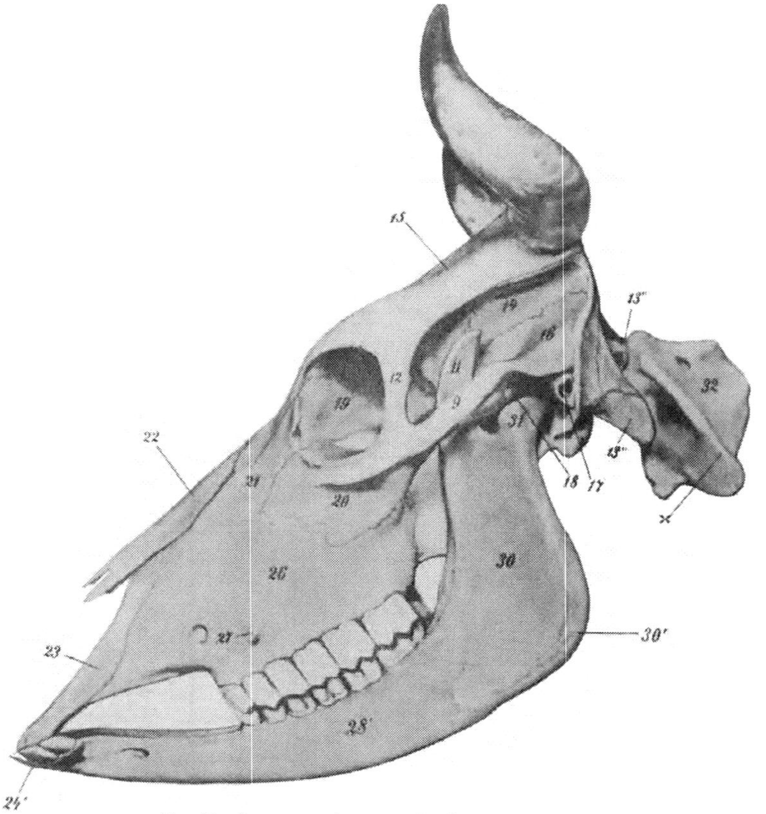

Fig. 89.—Skull and Atlas of Ox, Lateral View.

9, Zygomatic arch; *11*, coronoid process; *12*, supraorbital process; *13''*, paramastoid or styloid process; *13'''*, occipital condyle; *14*, parietal bone; *15*, frontal bone; *16*, squamous temporal bone; *17*, external auditory meatus; *18*, temporal condyle; *19*, orbital surface of lacrimal bone; *20*, malar bone; *21*, facial surface of lacrimal bone; *22*, nasal bone; *23*, nasal process of premaxilla; 24', incisor teeth; 26, maxilla; *27*, facial tuberosity; infraorbital foramen in front of *27*; *28'*, molar part of ramus of mandible; *30*, broad vertical part of ramus; *30'*, angle of jaw; *31*, condyle of mandible; *32*, atlas; *x*, wing of atlas. (After Ellenberger-Baum, Anat. für Künstler.)

the adult; it communicates by one or two small openings with an ethmoidal meatus, and so with the nasal cavity.

The ethmoid bone has an extensive perpendicular plate. The lateral mass consists of five endoturbinals and eighteen ectoturbinals (Paulli). The largest ethmoturbinal is so extensive as to be termed a third or middle turbinal bone; it projects forward between the upper and lower turbinals. The lamina papyracea appears to a small extent externally in the pterygo-palatine fossa, forming part of the upper margin of the sphenopalatine foramen.

The **interparietals** are primitively paired, but unite before birth. As already mentioned, fusion occurs before or shortly after birth with the parietals and supra-occipital. No distinct tentorium osseum is present.

The **parietal bones** do not enter into the formation of the roof of the cranium. They constitute the upper part of the posterior wall, and bend sharply forward

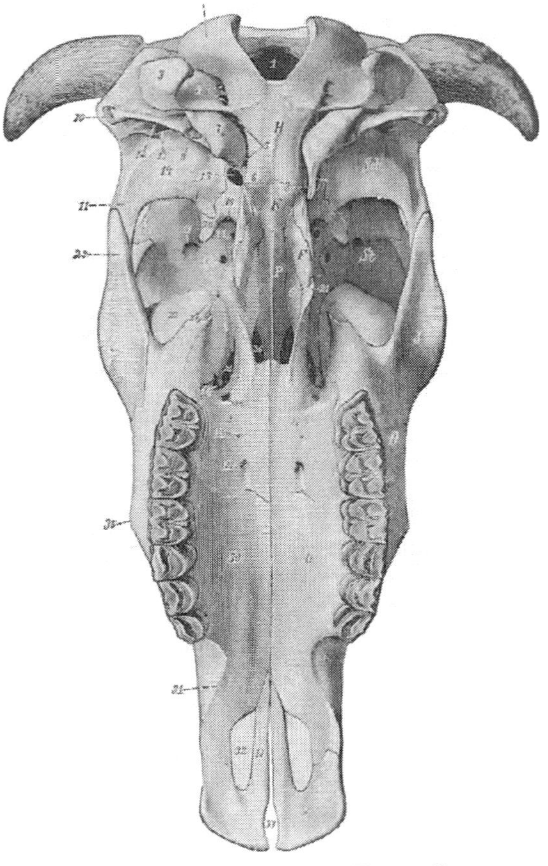

FIG. 90.—SKULL OF OX, BASAL VIEW, WITHOUT MANDIBLE.

F, Pterygoid bone; *G*, horizontal and *G'*, perpendicular part of palate bone; *H*, occipital bone; J, malar bone; *K*, sphenoid bone; *O*, maxilla; *P*, vomer; *Sch.*, squamous temporal; *St.*, frontal bone; *Z*, premaxilla; *1*, for. magnum; *2*, occipital condyle; *3*, paramastoid (styloid) process of occipital; *4*, hypoglossal and condyloid foramina; *5*, for. lacerum; *6*, pharyngeal tubercles; *7*, bulla ossea; *8*, muscular process (left one is removed to expose for. ovale); *9*, hyoid process; *10*, ext. auditory meatus; *11*, zygomatic process; *12*, external opening of parieto-temporal canal; *13*, postglenoid process; *14*, temporal condyle; *15*, for. ovale; *16*, for. lac. orbitale + for. rotundum; *17*, optic foramen; *18*, ethmoidal foramen; *19*, orbital opening of supraorbital canal; *20*, pterygoid crest; *21*, hamulus of pterygoid bone; *22*, lacrimal bulla; *23*, temporal process of malar; *24*, pterygoid process of maxilla; *25*, sphenopalatine foramen; *26*, maxillary foramen; *27*, posterior palatine foramen; *28*, anterior palatine foramen; *29*, accessory palatine foramina; *30*, palate process of maxilla; *31*, interalveolar border; *32*, palatine cleft; *33*, palate process of premaxilla; *34*, fissura incisiva; *35*, facial tuberosity; *36*, posterior nares. (Ellenberger-Baum, Anat. d. Haustiere.)

along the lateral wall, forming part of the wall of the temporal fossa. The line of inflection is marked by the prominent **parietal crest**, which is continuous with the temporal crest below. The parietals are excavated to form part of the frontal sinuses in the adult animal.

The condition in the young subject is as follows: The two parietals are united with each other and also with the interparietal and supraoccipital. The resulting mass is somewhat horseshoe-shaped. Its occipital part (Planum occipitale) forms the greater part of the posterior wall of the cranium and bears about its center the tuberosity for the attachment of the ligamentum nuchæ. From either side of this a line curves outward, and divides the surface into an upper smooth area and a lower area which is rough for muscular attachment. The upper border joins the frontal bone and concurs in the formation of the frontal eminence. The temporal parts (Plana temporalia) are much smaller and are concave externally; they join the frontal above and the squamous temporal below.

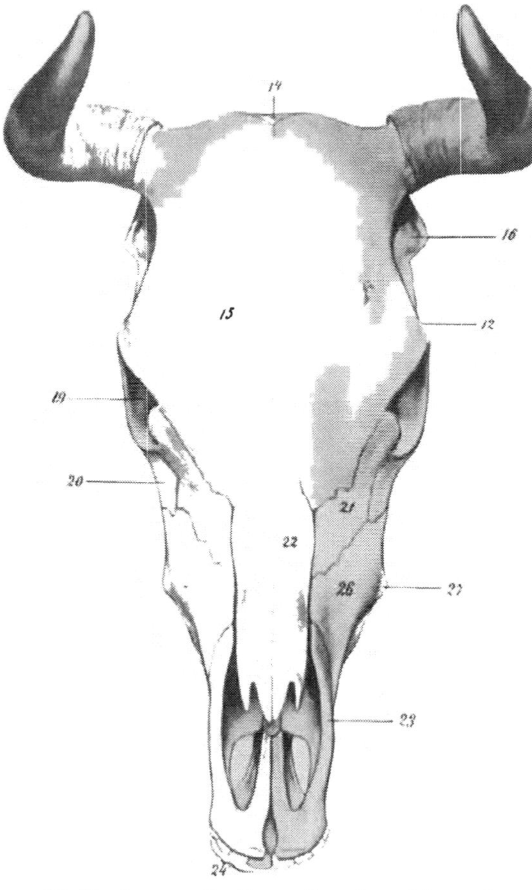

Fig. 91.—Skull of Ox, Dorsal View (with Mandible).

12, Supraorbital process; *14*, parietal bone; *15*, frontal bone; *16*, squamous temporal bone; *19*, orbit; *20*, malar bone; *21*, lacrimal bone; *22*, nasal bone; *23*, premaxilla; *26*, maxilla; *27*, facial tuberosity; *24*, incisor teeth. (After Ellenberger-Baum, Anat. f. Künstler.)

The frontal bones are very extensive, forming about one-half of the entire length of the skull, and all of the roof of the cranium. The posterior borders form with the parietals a large central frontal **eminence** (Torus frontalis), the highest point of the skull. At the junction of the posterior and the lateral borders are the **processus cornu** or "horn-cores," for the support of the horns. These processes are of elongated conical form, and vary greatly in size, length, curvature, and direction. The external surface is rough and porous, marked by numerous grooves and foramina; in the fresh state they are covered by the matrix of the horns. The base has a constriction, the neck. The interior is excavated to form a number of irregular intercommunicating spaces, divided by bony septa, and communicating with the frontal sinus. In the polled breeds these processes are absent, the skull is narrower in this region, and the frontal eminence more pronounced. The supraorbital process is situated about half-way between the anterior and posterior margins; it is short and joins the frontal process of the malar bone. The supra orbital foramen (often double) is situated about an inch inward from the root of the process; it is the external orifice of the **supraorbital canal** (Canalis supraorbi-

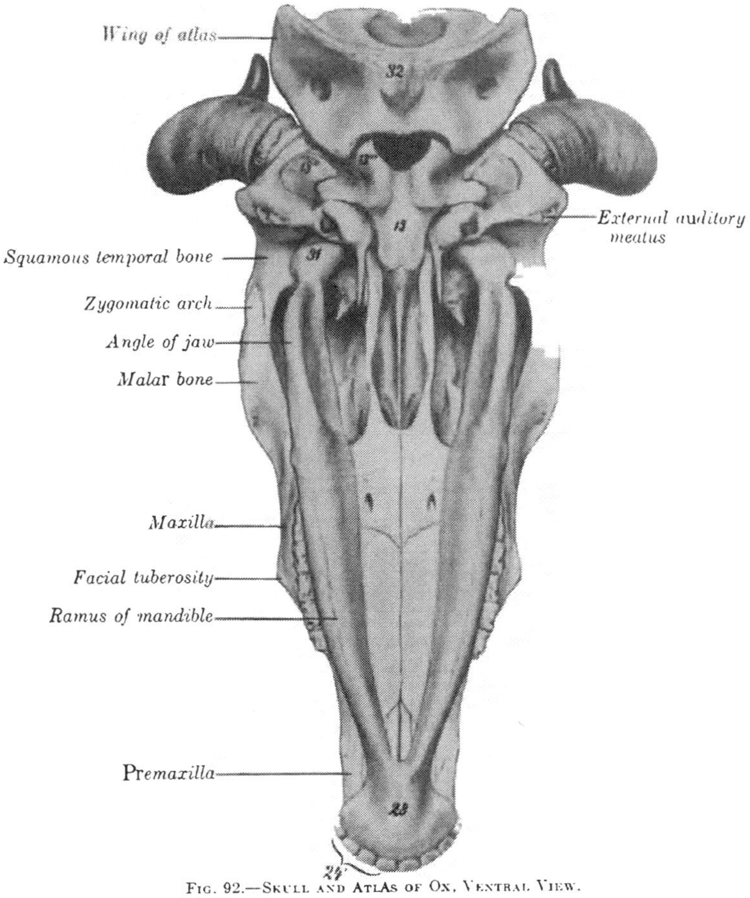

FIG. 92.—SKULL AND ATLAS OF OX, VENTRAL VIEW.

13, Basi-occipital; *13''*, paramastoid or styloid process; *13'''*, occipital condyle; *24'*, incisor teeth; *28*, body of mandible; *31*, condyle of mandible; *32*, ventral tubercle of atlas. (After Ellenberger-Baum, Anat. für Künstler.)

talis), which passes downward and forward into the orbit. The foramen is in the course of the **supraorbital groove** (Sulcus supraorbitalis), which marks the course of the frontal vein. The anterior ends of the naso-frontal parts form a notch which receives the nasal bones, and sutural or Wormian bones are often found at this junction (naso-frontal suture). The orbital part is extensive; it is perforated behind by the orbital opening of the supraorbital canal, and below by the ethmoidal or internal orbital foramen. It does not articulate with the palatine, from which it is separated by the orbital wing of the sphenoid. The temporal part is also more extensive than in the horse. The frontal sinus is very extensive, being continued into the parietals and occipital, and the horn processes when present.

The **squamous** and **petrous parts** of the temporal **bone** fuse early—in fact, union is nearly complete at birth. The squamous part is relatively small. Its external surface is divided into two parts by the prominent temporal crest, which is continuous with the parietal crest above and turns forward below, ending at a tubercle above the external auditory meatus. The part behind the crest faces backward, and is partly free, partly united with the occipital. The area in front of the crest is concave and enters into the formation of the temporal fossa; it is perforated by foramina which communicate with the parieto-temporal canal. The zygomatic process is much shorter and weaker than in the horse, and articulates with the malar only. The condyle is convex in both directions. The postglenoid process is less prominent, and behind it is the chief external opening of the parieto-temporal canal. The internal surface is almost completely overlapped by the parietal and sphenoid. The petrous part proper is small, but the tympanic part is extensive. The external auditory meatus is smaller than in the horse and is directed outward. From it a plate projects downward and helps to inclose the deep depression in which the hyoid process is placed. Behind this plate is the stylomastoid foramen. The muscular process is large and often bifid at its free end. The bulla ossea is large and laterally compressed. It is separated from the occipital bone by a narrow opening which is equivalent to part of the foramen lacerum basis cranii of the horse. The parieto-temporal canal is formed entirely in the temporal bone. The facial canal, on the other hand, is bounded partly by the occipital bone.

Bones of the Face

The **maxilla** is shorter but broader and relatively higher than in the horse. Its external surface bears instead of the facial crest a rough **facial tuberosity** (Tuber malare), placed above the third cheek tooth; a rough curved line often extends from it to the upper part of the malar bone. The infraorbital foramen—often double—is situated above the first cheek tooth. The tuber maxillare is small, laterally compressed, and usually bears a small pointed process (Processus pterygoideus). The zygomatic process is very small. The interalveolar border is concave, and there is no alveolus for a canine tooth. The palatine process is wider, but somewhat shorter than in the horse. It incloses a large air-space, which is continuous behind with a like cavity in the horizontal part of the palate bone, forming the **palatine sinus.** This communicates externally (over the infraorbital canal) with the maxillary sinus; in the macerated skull it communicates with the nasal cavity by a large oval opening, which is closed by mucous membrane in the fresh state. A median septum separates the two palatine sinuses. The alveoli for the cheek teeth increase in size from before backward. The maxillary sinus proper is small and is undivided. The maxillary foramen is a narrow fissure, deeply placed at the inner side of the lacrimal bulla. The maxilla takes no part in the formation of the palatine canal. Sutural (or Wormian) bones may be found at its junction with the lacrimal and malar bones.

The body of the **premaxilla** is thin and flattened, and has no alveoli, since the canine and upper incisor teeth are absent. A deep notch takes the place of the foramen incisivum. The nasal process is short, convex externally, and is not closely attached to the nasal bone; the space between the two processes is greater than in the horse. The palatine process is narrow and is grooved on its nasal surface for the septal cartilage and the vomer. The palatine cleft is very wide.

The **palatine bone** is very extensive. The horizontal **part** forms one-fourth or more of the hard palate. The anterior palatine foramen opens near the junction with the maxilla, about half an inch from the median palatine suture and crest.

Accessory palatine foramina are also present. The palatine groove is usually not very distinct. The palatine canal is formed entirely in this part, and there is no articulation with the vomer. A rounded ridge occurs on the nasal side of the median suture. The interior is hollow, forming part of the palatine sinus. The **perpendicular part** is an extensive, quadrilateral, thin plate, which forms the posterior part of the lateral wall of the nasal cavity and in part bounds the narrow posterior nares. Its internal surface is nearly flat, and is smooth and free, except behind, where it is overlapped by the pterygoid bone. The external surface is attached to a small extent to the pterygoid process behind, and is free elsewhere. The spheno-palatine foramen is a long elliptical opening, formed by a deep notch in the upper edge of the palate bone and completed by the ethmoid and sphenoid. The edge behind this foramen articulates with the orbital wing of the sphenoid, not the frontal as in the horse.

The **pterygoid bone** is wider than in the horse, and forms the greater part of the lateral boundary of the posterior nares. Its outer surface is almost entirely united

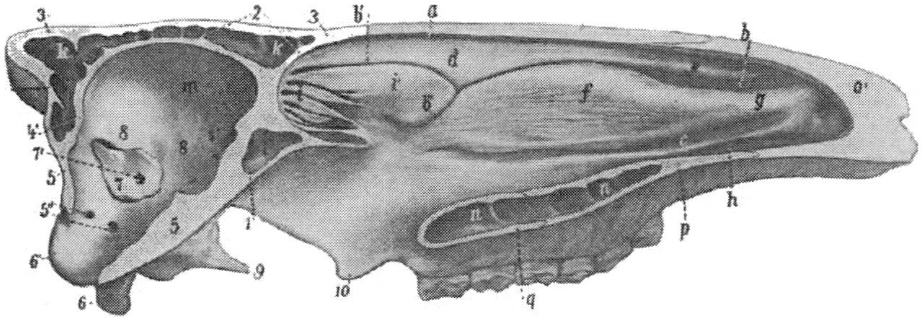

FIG. 93.—MEDIAN SECTION OF SKULL OF OX, WITHOUT THE MANDIBLE.

The mucous membrane is retained. The septum nasi is removed. *a*, Superior meatus; *b*, middle meatus, with *b'* and *b''*, its upper and lower divisions; *c*, inferior meatus; *d*, superior turbinal; *e*, superior turbinal fold; *f*, inferior turbinal; *g*, alar fold; *h*, inferior turbinal fold; *i*, lateral mass of ethmoid (ethmoturbinals); *i'*, large ethmoturbinal or middle turbinal; *k*, frontal sinus; *l*, sphenoidal sinus; *m*, cranial cavity; *n*, palatine sinus; *o*, nasal bone; *o'*, parietal cartilage; *p*, palate process of maxilla; *q*, palate bone (horizontal part); *1*, sphenoid bone; *2*, *3*, inner and outer plates of frontal bone; *4*, *4'*, outer and inner plates of parietal bone; *5*, *5'*, occipital bone; *5''*, condyloid and hypoglossal foramina; *6*, paramastoid or styloid process; *6'*, occipital condyle; *7*, petrous temporal bone; *7'*, internal auditory meatus; *8*, squamous temporal bone; *9*, muscular process; *10*, pterygoid bone (hamulus). (After Ellenberger, in Leisering's Atlas.)

to the palate bone and the pterygoid process, but a small part is free in the pterygopalatine fossa. The hamulus is distinctly hook-like, thin, and sharp.

The **nasal bone** is little more than half the length of that of the horse. It is straight in its length, but strongly curved from side to side. It does not fuse laterally with the adjacent bones, even in old age. The posterior extremity is pointed and fits into the notch between the frontal bones. The anterior end is broader, and is divided into two parts by a deep notch. In old animals there is a small extension of the frontal sinus into this bone.

The **lacrimal bone** is very large. The extensive facial part is concave in its length, and bears no lacrimal tubercle. The orbital margin is marked by several notches. The orbital part forms below the remarkable **lacrimal bulla**; this is a large and very thin-walled protuberance, which bulges backward into the lower part of the orbit, and contains an extension of the maxillary sinus. The lacrimal fossa is small, and is just behind the orbital margin.

The **malar bone** is relatively long. The facial surface is extensive; it bears a curved crest (Crista facialis) just below the orbital margin, and below this it is concave from above downward. The zygomatic process divides into two branches;

of these, the frontal process turns upward and backward and joins the supraorbital process of the frontal bone; the temporal process continues backward, and is overlapped by the zygomatic process of the temporal bone, completing the zygomatic arch.

The superior turbinal bone is less cribriform and fragile than in the horse, and is thickest in its middle, small at either end. It is attached to the turbinal crest of the nasal bone, and curves downward, outward, and upward to be applied outwardly to the frontal and lacrimal bones. It thus incloses a cavity which communicates with the middle meatus nasi. (In the macerated skull it opens into the frontal sinus, but this communication is closed by mucous membrane in the fresh state.)

The inferior turbinal bone is shorter but much broader than in the horse. It is attached to the maxilla by a basal lamella about an inch (ca. 2 to 3 cm.) wide, which slopes downward and inward. At the inner edge of this it splits into two plates which are rolled in opposite directions, and inclose two separate cavities, subdivided by several septa. The upper one opens into the middle meatus, the lower one into the inferior meatus nasi

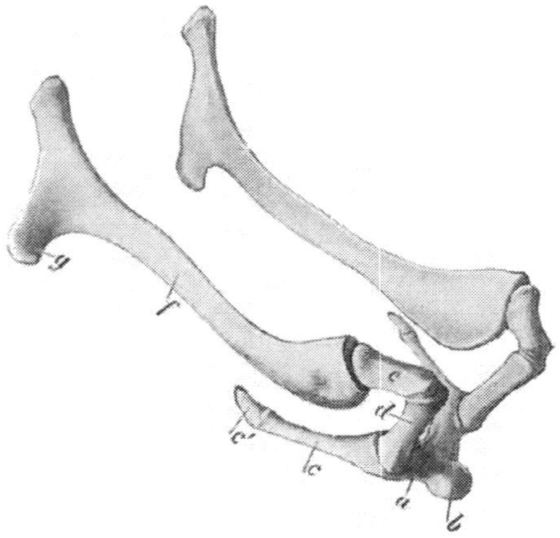

Fig. 94.—Hyoid Bone of Ox.
a, Body; b, lingual process; c, thyroid cornu and cartilage, c'; d, small cornu; e, middle cornu; f, great cornu; g, muscular angle of f. (Ellenberger-Baum, Anat. d. Haustiere.)

The two halves of the mandible do not fuse completely even in advanced age. The symphyseal surfaces are extremely rough and are marked by reciprocal projections and cavities. The body is shorter, wider, and flatter than in the horse, and has eight round and relatively shallow alveoli for the lower incisors. The interalveolar border is long, curved, thin and sharp. There are no alveoli for the canine teeth, which are absent. The anterior part of the ramus constitutes a long narrow neck. The mental foramen is further forward than in the horse, and is in the posterior end of a fossa. The rami diverge more, so that the submaxillary space is wider than in the horse. They are also more strongly curved, and the angle is more pronounced. The molar part is not so high, especially in its anterior part. Its lower border is convex in its length. Its upper border bears six alveoli for the lower cheek teeth; the first is quite small, and they increase in size from before backward. The vertical part is much smaller than in the horse and its posterior border is relatively thin below, concave and wider above. The mandibular foramen is about in the middle of its inner surface, and a groove for the lingual nerve curves downward and forward from it. The condyle projects inward further than in the horse, and is concave from side to side. The coronoid process is extensive and curves backward.

The hyoid bone has a short tuberous lingual process. The middle cornua are almost as large as the small cornua. The great cornua are narrow, except at the ends. The upper end divides into two branches, which correspond to the two angles of that of the horse. The thyroid cornua do not fuse with the body.

SKULL OF THE OX AS A WHOLE

The skull of the ox is more clearly pyramidal than that of the horse, and is shorter and relatively wider. The cranium is quadrangular and larger externally than in the horse; its large size is due mainly to the great extent of the frontal sinus, and does not affect the cranial cavity, which is smaller than in the horse.

The **superior** or **frontal surface** is formed by the frontals, nasals, and premaxillæ. The frontal part is quadrilateral and very extensive, the greatest width being at the orbits. It presents a central depression on its anterior part, and on either side are the supraorbital grooves and foramina. Behind is the median frontal eminence, and at the lateral angles the "horn-cores" project in horned cattle. The nasal part is very short. The osseous nasal aperture is wide. The premaxillæ do not bend downward as in the horse; they are relatively thin and weak, and are separated by an interval which has a wide anterior part in place of the foramen incisivum.

The **lateral surface** is more triangular than in the horse. The temporal fossa is confined to this surface. It is deep and narrow, and its boundaries are more complete. It is limited above by a crest which extends from the postero-external angle of the frontal to the supraorbital process, and is analogous to the sagittal crest of the horse. Behind it is bounded by the temporal crest. It is clearly marked off from the orbit by the rounded posterior orbital ridge and the pterygoid crest. The zygomatic process is short, weak, and flattened, and is formed by the temporal and malar only. Its condyle is convex and is wide from before backward. The glenoid cavity and postglenoid process are small. The orbit is encroached upon below by the lacrimal bulla, and presents the orifice of the supraorbital canal behind. The margin is completed behind by the frontal process of the malar; its lower part is prominent and rough, not smooth and rounded as in the horse. The pterygo-palatine fossa is much larger, deeper, and more clearly defined. It has a long narrow forward extension (maxillary hiatus) between the vertical plate of the palate bone internally and the maxilla and lacrimal bulla externally; thus the sphenopalatine and maxillary foramina are deeply placed. The preorbital region is short but relatively high. A tuberosity and curved line take the place of the facial crest. The infraorbital foramen is situated above the first cheek tooth and is often double.

The **basal surface** is short and wide, especially in its cranial part. The occipital condyles are limited in front by transverse ridges. The tubercles at the junction of the occipital and sphenoid are large. The condyloid fossæ contain two foramina, the hypoglossal below and in front, and the condyloid above and behind; other inconstant ones occur. The paramastoid processes are short and convergent. The foramen lacerum is slit-like. The bulla ossea is a large, laterally compressed prominence. The muscular processes are usually long and narrow triangular plates, with one or two sharp points. The external auditory process is directed almost straight outward. A curved plate extends downward from it and joins the bulla ossea internally, completing the deep cavity which receives the articular angle of the hyoid bone. The chief external opening of the temporal canal is in front of this plate, and an accessory one lies behind it. The infratemporal fossa is small, and presents the foramen ovale. The posterior nares are very narrow, and the vomer does not reach to the level of their margin. The hard palate is wide, and forms about three-fifths of the entire length of the skull. A small central part only of its posterior border enters into the formation of the posterior nares; the lateral parts are notched and just above them are the posterior palatine foramina.

The anterior palatine foramina are an inch or more from the posterior margin, and about the same distance apart. The palatine grooves are distinct for a short distance only. Just beyond the cheek teeth the palate narrows and becomes concave; beyond this it widens and flattens.

The **posterior or nuchal surface** is extensive and somewhat pentagonal in outline in the adult. About its center is the eminence for the attachment of the ligamentum nuchæ. From this a median crest extends toward the foramen magnum, and laterally two lines (Lineæ nuchæ superiores) curve outward, marking the upper limit of the area which is roughened for muscular attachment. The surface above the lines is relatively smooth, and is covered only by the skin and the thin auricular muscles in the living animal. It is separated from the cranial roof by a thick border, which forms centrally the frontal eminence, and bears at its extremi-

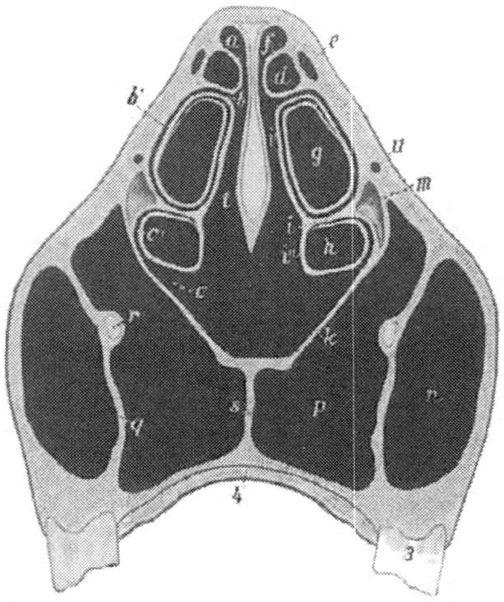

FIG. 95.—CROSS-SECTION OF SKULL OF OX. SECTION PASSES THROUGH FIFTH CHEEK TOOTH.

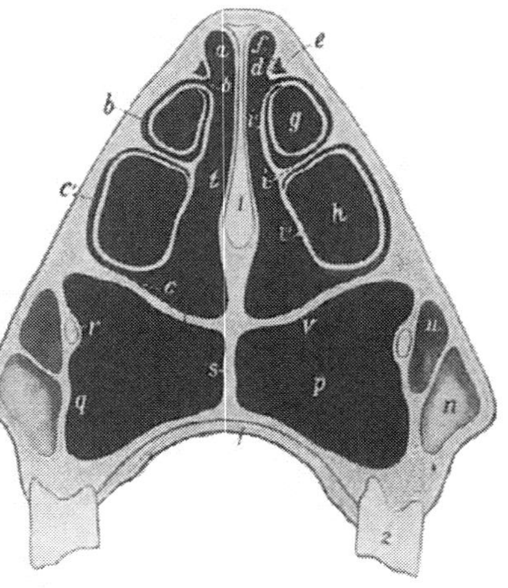

FIG. 96.—CROSS-SECTION OF SKULL OF OX. SECTION PASSES THROUGH SECOND CHEEK TOOTH.

a, b, c, Superior, middle, inferior meatus; *b'*, communication between middle meatus and cavity of upper part of inferior turbinal; *c'*, communication between inferior meatus and lower part of inferior turbinal; *d*, cavity of superior turbinal; *e, f*, outer and inner walls of *d*; *g, h*, upper and lower cavities of inferior turbinal bone; *i*, basal lamella of inferior turbinal; *i', i''*, upper and lower divisions of inferior turbinal bone; *k*, floor of nasal cavity; *m*, lacrimal sinus; *n*, maxillary sinus; *p*, palatine sinus; *q*, septum between maxillary and palatine sinuses; *r*, infraorbital canal; *s*, septum between palatine sinuses; *t*, common meatus; *u*, naso-lacrimal canal; *v*, floor of nasal cavity and roof of palatine sinus; *1*, septum nasi; *2*, posterior part of second cheek tooth; *3*, posterior part of fifth cheek tooth; *4*, hard palate. (After Ellenberger, in Leisering's Atlas.)

ties the processus cornu—except in the polled breeds. The condyles are further apart, and the articular surfaces are more clearly divided into upper and lower parts than in the horse.

The **cranial cavity** is shorter and its long axis is more oblique than in the horse, but it is relatively high and wide. The anterior fossa lies at a much higher level than the rest of the floor. The olfactory fossæ are smaller, and the sella turcica is much deeper than in the horse. A deep groove leads from the petrous temporal forward over the foramen ovale to the foramen rotundum. Behind the sella there is often a distinct prominence (Dorsum sellæ). The internal sagittal crest is prominent anteriorly, but absent further back. A faintly marked elevation takes the place of the tentorium osseum. The small petrous temporal bone projects into the cavity laterally. The ridges and digital impressions are very pronounced. The parieto-temporal canal is formed entirely in the temporal bone, and opens at the apex of the petrous, where it is joined by the condyloid canal. The foramen lacerum is divided into two parts (For. lacerum anterius et posterius).

The **nasal cavity** is incompletely divided by the septum, which does not reach the floor posteriorly. The floor is relatively long, and is more concave from side to side than in the horse. In the dry skull it has a large oval opening into the palatine sinus, which is closed during life by mucous membrane. The middle meatus is divided behind into upper and lower branches by the great ethmoturbinal. The posterior nares are narrow and oblique.

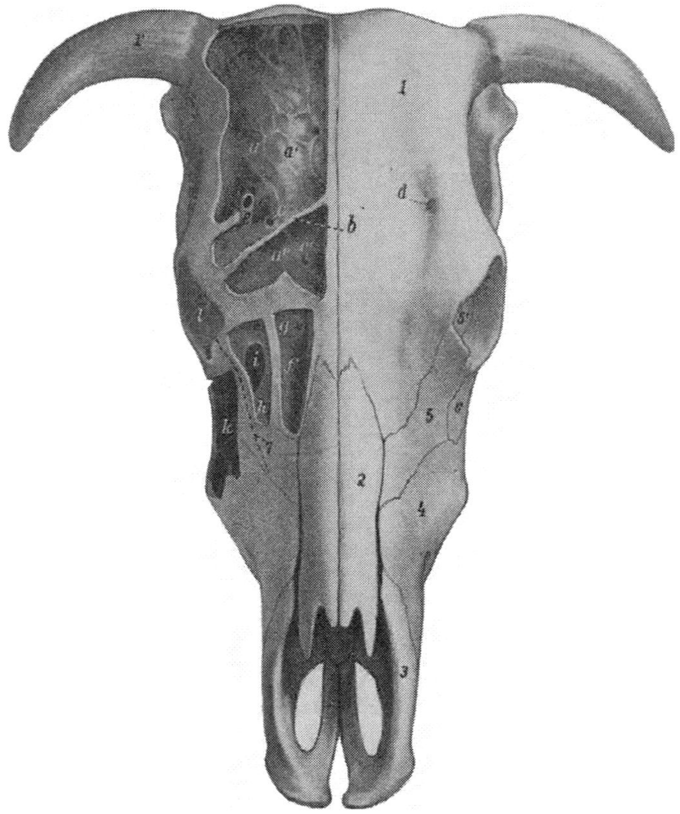

FIG. 97.—SKULL OF OX, DORSAL VIEW.

The outer plate of bone has been removed to show the sinuses. *a*, Frontal sinus; *a'*, cranial plate of frontal bone; *a''*, anterior part of frontal sinus, which is separated from remainder by a septum (*b*); *c*, *c'*, communications between frontal sinus and nasal cavity; *d*, supraorbital foramen; *e*, supraorbital canal; *f*, cavity of superior turbinal bone, and *g*, its opening into the nasal cavity; *h*, lacrimal sinus, *i*, its communication with the maxillary sinus; *k*, maxillary sinus; *l*, orbit; *1*, frontal bone; *1'*, processus cornu; *2*, nasal bone; *3*, premaxilla (nasal process); *4*, maxilla; *5*, lacrimal bone; *6*, malar bone; *7*, dotted line indicating course of naso-lacrimal duct. (After Ellenberger, in Leisering's Atlas.)

The **frontal sinus** is very large. It involves almost all of the frontal bone and a large part of the posterior wall of the cranium. It also extends for a variable distance into the horn processes when these are present. A complete median septum separates the right and left sinuses. The anterior limit is indicated by a transverse plane through the middle of the orbits. It extends externally to the crest which limits the temporal fossa above, and into the root of the supraorbital process. At the highest part of the cranial cavity and at the tuberosity on the posterior surface the two plates of the bone come together. The cavity is very irregular and is subdivided into numerous spaces by ridges and partial septa. This multilocular character is most marked in the anterior part, and here several small spaces appear to be cut off from the main cavity (Baum). The supraorbital canal passes through the sinus. Several small openings lead from the sinus to the ethmoidal meatuses, and thus indirectly to the upper division of the middle meatus nasi. The communications with the cavity of the superior turbinal and with the lacrimal part of the maxillary sinus which are seen in the macerated skull are closed in the fresh state by mucous membrane.

The **maxillary sinus** is excavated chiefly in the maxilla, lacrimal, and malar, and is not divided by a septum as in the horse. It extends forward as far as the facial tuberosity, or a little further in old animals. Its upper limit is indicated approximately by a line drawn from the infraorbital foramen to the upper margin of the orbit. It is continued directly backward into the lacrimal bulla to a point nearly opposite to the bifurcation of the zygomatic process of the malar. It also extends upward and backward through a large opening into a cavity formed by the

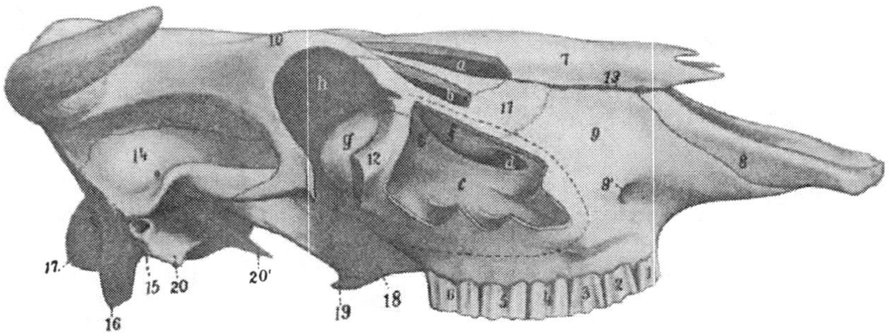

Fig. 98.—Skull of Ox, Lateral View without Mandible.

The maxillary, lacrimal, and turbinal sinuses have been opened, and a portion of the orbit removed. *a*, Cavity of superior turbinal bone; *b*, lacrimal sinus; *c*, maxillary sinus; *d*, communication between maxillary and palatine sinuses; *e*, opening between maxillary and lacrimal sinuses; *f*, thin osseous bulla; *g*, lacrimal bulla; *h*, orbit; *1–6*, cheek teeth; *7*, nasal bone; *8*, premaxilla (nasal process); *9*, maxilla; *9'*, infraorbital foramen; *10*, frontal bone; *11*, lacrimal bone; *12*, malar bone; *13*, fissure between nasal bone and maxilla; *14*, temporal bone (squamous); *15*, external auditory meatus; *16*, styloid or paramastoid process; *17*, occipital condyle; *18*, palate bone (perpendicular part); *19*, pterygoid bone (hamulus); *20*, tympanic part of temporal; *20'*, muscular process of petrous temporal. (After Ellenberger, in Leisering's Atlas.)

lacrimal, frontal, ethmoid, and turbinal bones, at the inner side of the orbit.[1] The floor of the cavity is irregular and the roots of the last three or four cheek teeth project up into it, covered by a plate of bone. The sinus communicates with the palatine sinus freely over the infraorbital canal through an oval opening about two to three inches (ca. 5 to 7.5 cm.) long. Above this it communicates by a shorter and much narrower opening with the middle meatus nasi.

The **palatine sinus** is excavated in the hard palate, and is separated from that of the opposite side by a median septum. It extends from the posterior border of the palate to a plane an inch or more (2.5 to 3 cm.) in front of the first cheek tooth. As mentioned above, there is a large communication with the maxillary sinus over the infraorbital canal, so that the cavity is sometimes regarded as a part of that sinus. The large defect in the bony roof of the sinus is closed by two layers of mucous membrane in the fresh state. The palatine canal passes obliquely through the posterior part of the sinus.

[1] This is termed the lacrimal sinus by some authors. It is similar in location and in the position of its orifice to the turbinal part of the frontal sinus of the horse, with the important difference that it does not communicate with the frontal sinuses in the ox.

The **sphenoidal sinus** is almost entirely in the sphenoid bone and does not communicate with the palatine and maxillary sinus. It has one or two openings into the ventral ethmoidal meatuses. There is no cavity in the perpendicular part of the palate bone.

There are several small air-cavities between the lateral mass of the ethmoid and the anterior part of the frontal sinus, which communicate separately with ethmoidal meatuses.

BONES OF THE THORACIC LIMB

The **scapula** is more regularly triangular than in the horse, relatively wider at the vertebral end and narrower at the lower end. The scapular index is about 1 : 0.6. The spine is more prominent and is placed further forward, so that the supraspinous fossa is narrow and does not extend to the lower part of the bone. The spine is sinuous, bent backward in its middle, forward below. Its free border is somewhat thickened in its middle, but bears no distinct tubercle. Instead of subsiding below as in the horse the spine becomes a little more prominent, and is prolonged by a pointed projection, the **acromion,** from which part of the deltoid muscle arises. The subscapular fossa is shallow. The areas for the attachment of the serratus muscle are not very distinct. The nutrient foramen is usually in the lower third of the posterior border. The glenoid cavity is almost circular and without any distinct notch. The tuberosity is small and close to the glenoid cavity. The coracoid process is short and rounded. The cartilage resembles that of the horse.

The **humerus** has a shallow musculo-spiral groove. The deltoid tuberosity is less prominent than in the horse, and the curved line running from it to the neck bears a well-marked tubercle on its upper part. The nutrient foramen is usually in the lower third of the posterior surface. The external tuberosity is very large, and rises an inch or more (ca. 3 cm.) above the level of the head. Its anterior part curves inward over the bicipital groove, and below it externally there is a prominent circular rough area for the insertion of the tendon of the supraspinatus. The anterior part of the internal tuberosity has a small projection which curves over the groove. The groove is undivided. The distal articular surface is decidedly oblique, and the grooves and ridge are very well marked. The coronoid and olecranon fossæ are deep and wide. The external condyloid crest is represented by a rough raised area. The proximal end unites with the shaft at three and one-half to four years, and the distal at about one and one-half years.

The **radius** is short and relatively broad. It is somewhat oblique, the lower end being nearer the median plane than the upper. The curvature is more pronounced below than above. The shaft is prismatic in its middle part and has anterior, external, and posterior faces. There is a marked increase in width and thickness below. The proximal articular surface presents a synovial fossa which extends inward from the deep groove between the two glenoid cavities. The bicipital tuberosity is represented by a slightly elevated rough area. The posterior facets for the ulna are larger than in the horse. The two bones commonly fuse above the proximal interosseous space and always fuse below it, except near the distal end, where there is a small distal interosseous space. A groove connects the two spaces externally. The distal extremity is large, and is thickest internally. Its articular surface is oblique in two directions, *i. e.*, from within upward and backward. The grooves for the extensor tendons are shallow. The proximal end unites with the shaft at one to one and one-half years, and the distal at three and one-half to four years.

The approximation of the lower ends of the forearms and the carpi gives the "knock-kneed" appearance in cattle. The obliquity of the joint surfaces produces lateral deviation of the lower part of the limb in flexion. The facets for the radial and intermediate carpals are narrower than in the horse and run obliquely forward and outward. The surface for the ulnar carpal is extensive and saddle-shaped; its outer part is furnished by the ulna.

The **ulna** is more fully developed than in the horse. The shaft is complete,

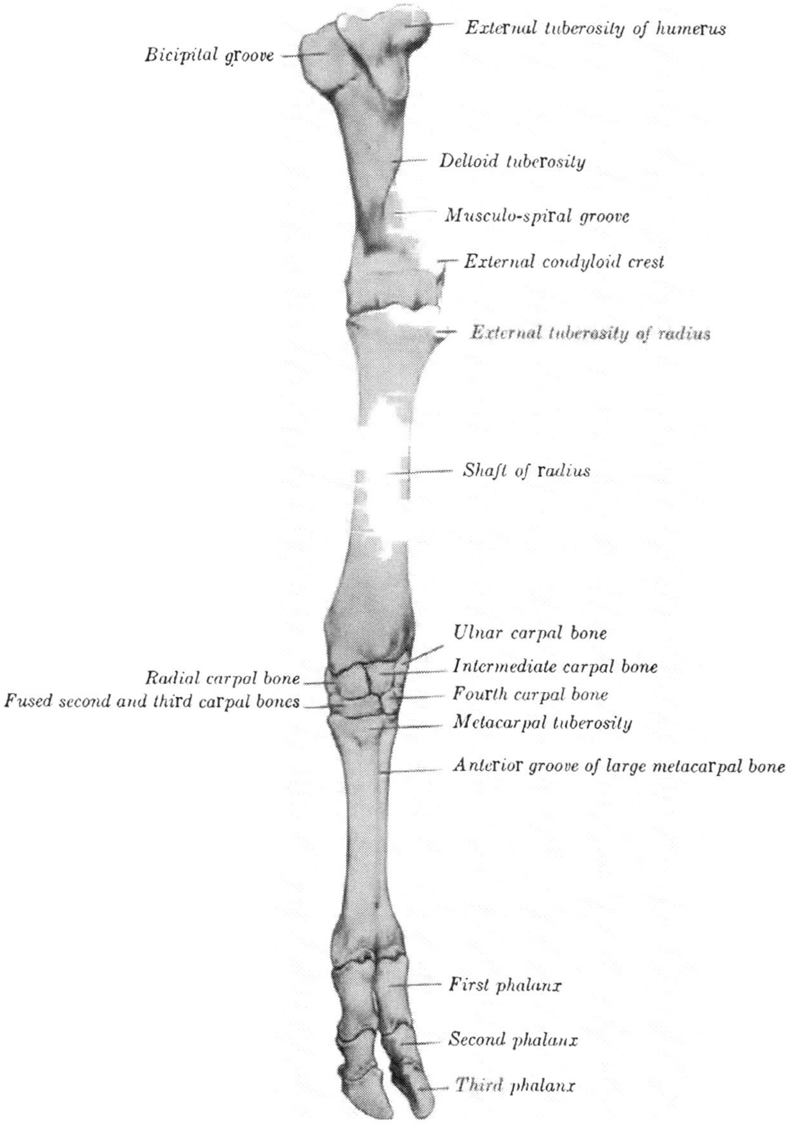

Fig. 99.—Skeleton of Left Fore Limb of Ox, from Shoulder Downward, Anterior View. (After Ellenberger-Baum, Anat. für Künstler.)

three-sided, and strongly curved. It is fused with the radius in the adult, except at the two interosseous spaces mentioned above. Its upper part contains a medullary canal which extends somewhat into the proximal end. The olecranon is large and bears a rounded tuberosity above. The distal end is fused with the radius; it projects below the level of the latter, forming the **styloid process** (Processus styloideus ulnæ), which furnishes part of the facet for the ulnar carpal. The proximal and distal ends unite with the shaft at three and one-half to four years.

The **carpus** consists of six bones, four in the upper row, and two in the lower. The upper row is oblique in conformity with the carpal articular surface of the radius. The radial and intermediate resemble in general those of the horse, but

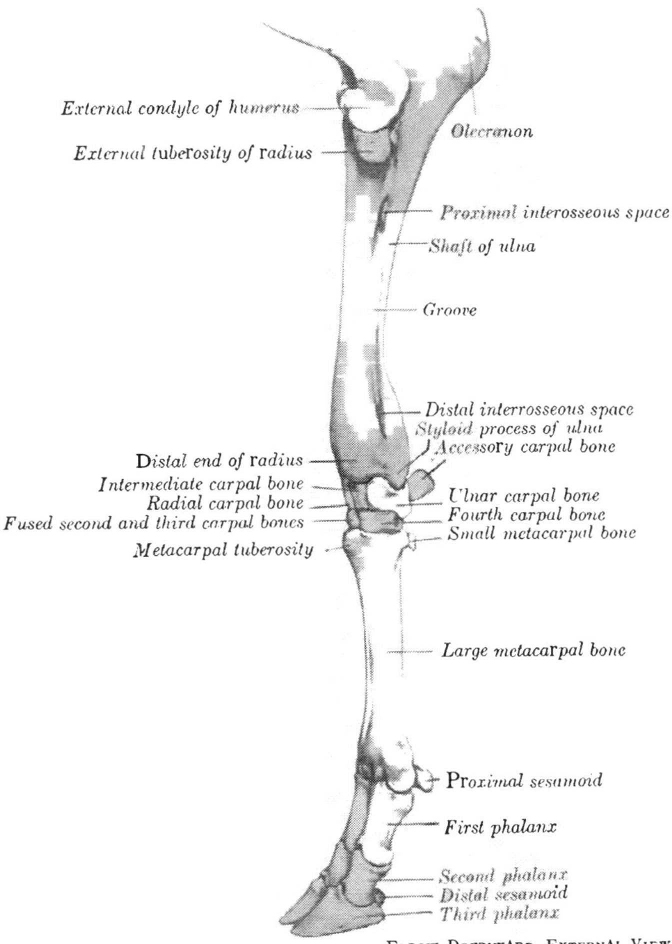

FIG. 100.—SKELETON OF LEFT FORE LIMB OF OX, FROM ELBOW DOWNWARD, EXTERNAL VIEW. (After Ellenberger-Baum, Anat. für Künstler.)

are less regular in shape, and their long axes are directed obliquely backward and inward. The radial is narrower than in the horse and curves upward behind. The intermediate is constricted in its middle, and wider behind than in front. The ulnar is large and very irregular. Its proximal surface is extensive and sinuous and articulates with both radius and ulna. Behind is a large oval facet for articulation with the accessory carpal. The accessory is short, thick, and rounded; it articulates with the ulnar carpal only. The first carpal is absent. The second and third carpals are fused to form a large quadrilateral bone. The fourth carpal is a smaller quadrilateral bone.

The **metacarpus** consists of a large metacarpal and an external small metacarpal bone. The large metacarpal bone (Mc. 3 + 4) results from the fusion of the third and fourth bones of the fœtus, and bears evidences of its double origin even in the adult state. The shaft is shorter than in the horse, and is relatively wider and flatter. The anterior surface is rounded, and is marked by a vertical vascular groove connecting two canals which traverse the ends of the shaft from before backward. The posterior surface is flat and presents a similar but much fainter groove. The borders are rough in the upper third. The proximal end bears two slightly concave facets for articulation with the bones of the lower row of the carpus; the inner area is the larger, and they are separated by a ridge in front and a notch behind. The outer angle has a facet behind for the small metacarpal bone. The inner part of the extremity has anterior and posterior tuberosities. The distal end is divided into two parts by a sagittal notch. Each division bears an articular surface similar to that in the horse, but much smaller. The **medullary canal** is divided into two parts by a **vertical septum** which is usually incomplete in the adult.

The **small metacarpal** bone (Mc. 5) is a rounded rod about an inch and a half (ca. 3.5 to 4 cm.) in length, which lies against the upper part of the outer border of the large bone. Its upper end articulates with the latter, but not with the carpus. The lower end is pointed.

Four cartilaginous metacarpals are present in the early fœtal state, viz., the second, third, fourth, and fifth. The second commonly either disappears or unites with the third; sometimes it develops as a small rod of bone. The third and fourth gradually unite, but can be cut apart at birth. Each has three centers of ossification; the proximal epiphysis fuses with the shaft before birth, the distal at two to two and one-half years

Four digits are present in the ox. Of these, two—the third and fourth—are fully developed and have three phalanges and three sesamoids each. The second and fifth are vestiges and are placed behind the fetlock; each contains one or two small bones which do not articulate with the rest of the skeleton.

The **first phalanges** are shorter and narrower than in the horse and are three-sided. The interdigital surface is flattened and its posterior part bears a prominence for the attachment of the interdigital ligaments. The proximal extremity is relatively large, and is somewhat compressed from side to side. The articular surface is concave from before backward and is divided by a sagittal groove into two areas, of which the abaxial one is the larger and higher. Behind these are two facets for articulation with the sesamoid bones. The posterior surface bears two tuberosities separated by a deep depression. The distal extremity is smaller than the proximal, especially in the antero-posterior direction. Its articular surface is divided by a sagittal groove into two convex facets, of which the abaxial one is decidedly the larger. There are depressions on either side for ligamentous attachment. The bone consists at birth of two pieces—the distal end and the fused shaft and upper extremity. Union occurs at one and one-half to two years.

The **second phalanges** are about two-thirds of the length of the first and are distinctly three-sided. The proximal articular surface is divided by a sagittal ridge into two glenoid cavities, of which the abaxial one is much the larger. There is a central prominence in front and two lateral tubercles behind. The distal extremity is smaller than the proximal. Its articular surface encroaches considerably on the anterior and posterior surfaces, and is divided into two lateral parts by a groove. There is a deep depression for ligamentous attachment on the interdigital side. The bone contains a small medullary canal. The distal end unites with the rest of the bone about the middle of the second year.

The **third phalanges** resemble in a general way one-half of the bone of the horse.

Each has four surfaces. The dorsal or wall surface is marked in its lower part by a shallow groove, along which there are several foramina of considerable size; the posterior one of the series is the largest, and conducts to a canal in the interior of the bone. Below the groove the surface is prominent, rough, and porous. Near and on the extensor process are several relatively large foramina. The slope of the surface is very steep posteriorly, but in front it forms an angle of 25 to 30 degrees with the ground plane. The articular surface is narrow from side to side, and slopes downward and backward. It is also oblique transversely, the interdigital side being the lower. It is adapted to the distal surface of the second phalanx, with the exception of a facet behind for the distal sesamoid. The extensor process is very rough. The volar or sole surface is narrow and slightly concave, and presents two or three foramina of considerable size. It is separated from the wall surface by a border which is sharp in front, rounded behind. There is no semilunar crest, since the deep flexor tendon is attached to the thick posterior border of the sole surface. The interdigital surface is smooth and grooved below, rough and porous above. At the upper angle it is perforated by a large foramen, which is equivalent to the volar foramen of the horse and leads to a cavity in the middle of the bone. The surface is separated by a rounded border from the wall surface, and by a sharp edge from the sole surface. The wing or angle is very short and blunt, and there is no lateral cartilage.

Four **proximal sesamoids** are present, two for each digit. They are much smaller than in the horse. The bones of each pair articulate with the corresponding part of the distal end of the large metacarpal bone by their anterior surfaces, with each other and with the first phalanx by small facets.

The two **distal sesamoids** are short and their ends are but little narrower than the middle.

BONES OF THE PELVIC LIMB

The **ilia** are almost parallel to each other and are also less oblique with regard to the horizontal plane than in the horse. They are relatively small. The gluteal line is prominent and is nearly parallel to the external border; it joins the superior ischiatic spine. A rounded ridge separates the two parts of the ventral surface. The surface for articulation with the sacrum is triangular. The internal angle is truncated, does not extend as high as the vertebral spines, and is separated from the opposite angle by a wider interval than in the horse. The external angle is relatively large and prominent; it is not so oblique as in the horse, and is wide in the middle, smaller at either end. The shaft is short and compressed from side to side.

The **ischium** is large. Its long axis is directed obliquely upward and backward, forming an angle of about 45 to 50 degrees with the horizontal plane. The transverse axis is oblique downward and inward at a similar angle, so that this part of the pelvic floor is deeply concave from side to side. The middle of the ventral surface bears a rough ridge or imprint for muscular attachment. The superior ischiatic spine is high and thin, and bears a series of almost vertical rough lines externally. The tuber ischii is large and three-sided, bearing upper, lower, and external tuberosities. The ischial arch is narrow and deep. The symphysis bears a ventral ridge, which fades out near the ischial arch.

The acetabular branch of the **pubis** is narrow, and is directed outward and a little forward. The anterior border is marked by a transverse groove which ends below the rough ilio-pectineal eminence. The longitudinal branch is wide and thin.

The **acetabulum** is smaller than in the horse. The rim is rounded and is usually marked by two notches. One of these is postero-internal and is narrow and deep; it leads to the deep acetabular fossa and is commonly almost converted into a foramen by a bar of bone. The other notch is antero-internal, small, and sometimes replaced by a foramen or absent.

The obturator foramen is large and elliptical. Its inner border is thin and sharp.

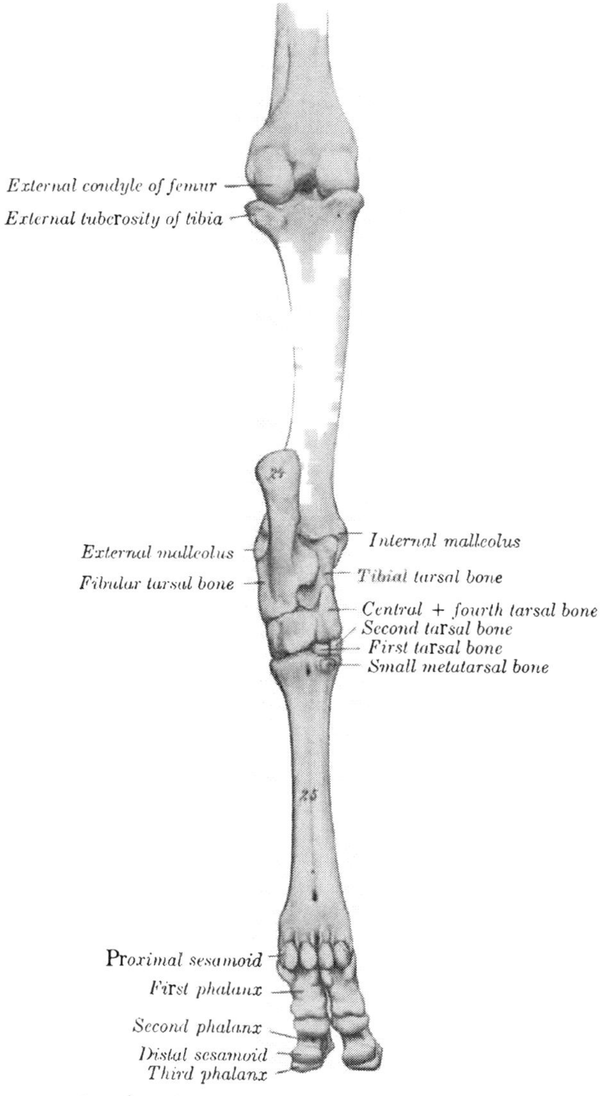

Fig. 101.—Skeleton of Left Hind Limb of Ox, from Middle of Thigh Downward Posterior View. 21, Tibia; 24, tuber calcis; 25, large metatarsal bone. (After Ellenberger-Baum, Anat. für Künstler.)

The pelvic inlet is elliptical and is more oblique than in the horse. In a cow of medium size the conjugate diameter is about nine and a half inches (ca. 23 to 24 cm.), and the transverse about seven inches (ca. 18 cm.). The anterior end of the symphysis lies in a transverse plane through the junction of the third and fourth sacral segments. The roof is concave in both directions. The floor is deeply concave, particularly in the transverse direction. The cavity is narrower and its axis is inclined strongly upward in the posterior part. The distance between the acetabulum and the external angle of the ilium is only a little (ca. 3 to 4 cm.) more than the distance between the former and the tuber ischii.

The femur has a relatively small shaft, which is cylindrical in its middle, prismatic below. The trochanter minor has the form of a rough tuberosity, and is situated higher up than in the horse and encroaches on the posterior surface. The trochanteric ridge (Crista intertrochanterica posterior) connects it with the tro-

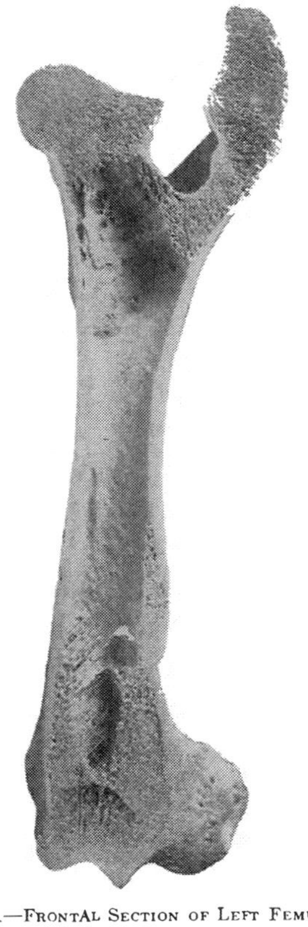

FIG. 102.—FRONTAL SECTION OF LEFT FEMUR OF OX, FRONT VIEW.

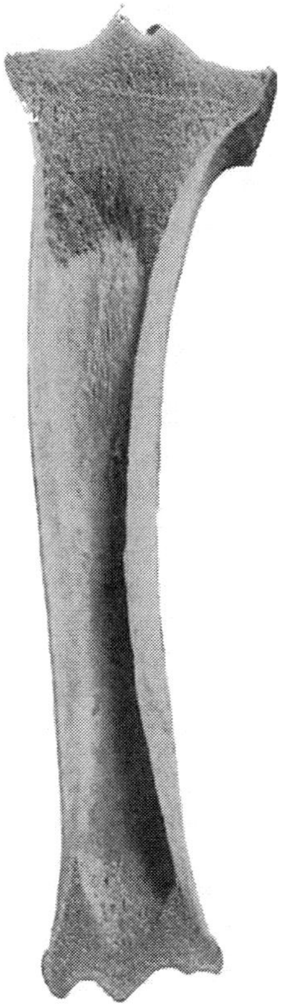

FIG. 103.—FRONTAL SECTION OF LEFT TIBIA OF OX, ANTERIOR VIEW.

These figures show the internal architecture of these bones, and especially the great extent of the medullary cavity as compared with those of the horse (Figs. 67 and 72).

chanter major. The third trochanter is absent. The supracondyloid (plantar) fossa is shallow. The proximal extremity is very wide. The head is smaller than in the horse and the articular surface extends considerably on the upper surface of the neck. Instead of the notch there is a small depression on the middle of the head for the attachment of the round ligament. The neck is well defined except above. The trochanter major is very massive and is undivided; its external surface is very rough. The trochanteric fossa is deep, but does not extend so far downward as in the horse. The distal end presents no very striking differential features, but the lips of the trochlea are less oblique than in the horse, and converge very slightly below. The proximal extremity unites with the shaft at about three and one-half years, the distal at three and one-half to four years.

The **tibia** resembles that of the horse rather closely, but is somewhat shorter. The shaft is distinctly curved, so that the inner side is convex. The posterior surface is not divided into two areas, and the lineæ musculares are fewer and extend up higher than in the horse. The articular grooves and ridge of the distal end are almost sagittal in direction, and present an extensive but shallow synovial fossa. The external groove is separated by a sharp ridge from an outer area which is for articulation with the external malleolus. The anterior part of the internal malleolus is prolonged downward and has a pointed end. The groove behind it is broad and well defined. Externally there is a deep narrow groove which separates two prominences. The proximal extremity fuses with the shaft at three and one-half to four years, the distal at two to two and one-half years.

The **fibula** usually consists of the two extremities only. The head is fused with the external condyle of the tibia and bears a small blunt-pointed prolongation below. The distal end remains separate and forms the external malleolus (sometimes called the os malleolare). It is quadrilateral in outline and compressed from side to side. The proximal surface articulates with the distal end of the tibia, and bears a small spine which fits into the groove on that bone. The distal surface rests on the fibular tarsal, and the inner articulates with the external ridge of the tibial tarsal bone. The outer surface is rough and irregular.

The early cartilaginous fibula is complete, but later the shaft is reduced and is usually represented by a fibrous cord which connects the two ends. In some cases, however, the upper part undergoes partial ossification, forming a slender rod which is usually united with the outer border of the tibia and is joined to the head by fibrous tissue.

The **patella** is long, narrow, and very thick. The anterior surface is strongly convex and very rough and irregular. The articular surface is convex from side to side and nearly straight in the vertical direction. The large prominence on the inner side for the attachment of the accessory cartilage allows prompt determination of the side to which the bone belongs. The apex is more pointed than in the horse.

The **tarsus** consists of five pieces; the central and fourth, and the second and third tarsal bones are fused.

The **tibial tarsal** bone is relatively long and narrow, and is somewhat flattened from before backward. It bears a trochlea at either end. The groove and ridges of the proximal trochlea are not spiral, but almost sagittal; the outer ridge is the wider, and articulates with both tibia and fibula. The distal trochlea consists of two condyles divided by a groove, and articulates with the combined central and fourth tarsals. The posterior surface bears a large oval facet for articulation with the fibular tarsal; this occupies most of the surface, and is convex and grooved from above downward. The outer surface presents two facets for articulation with the fibular tarsal, and is excavated and rough elsewhere. The inner surface bears a tuberosity at its upper part, and is flattened below.

The **fibular tarsal** bone is longer and more slender than in the horse. The distal part of the body is compressed laterally, and bears a projection in front which articulates with the external malleolus. The tuber calcis is marked posteriorly by a wide shallow groove, which is coated with cartilage in the fresh state.

The **central and fourth tarsals** are fused to form a large bone (Os centrotarsale quartum, scapho-cuboid), which extends across the entire width of the tarsus and articulates with all of the other bones. The greater part of the upper surface is molded on the distal trochlea of the tibial tarsal, and its inner part rises high above the rest posteriorly. Externally there is a narrow undulating surface for articulation with the distal end of the fibular tarsal bone. The posterior surface bears two tuberosities, of which the outer one is rounded, the inner more prominent and narrower.

The **first tarsal** bone is quadrilateral and small. It articulates with the central above, the metatarsus below, and the second tarsal in front.

The **second** and **third tarsals** are fused to form a rhomboid piece. The proximal surface is concavo-convex, and articulates with the central component. The distal surface is undulating and rests on the metatarsus. The external surface bears a small facet in front for the fourth tarsal component, and the posterior surface a very small one for the first tarsal bone.

The **large metatarsal** bone is about one-seventh (ca. 3 cm.) longer than the corresponding metacarpal. Its shaft is compressed laterally and is distinctly

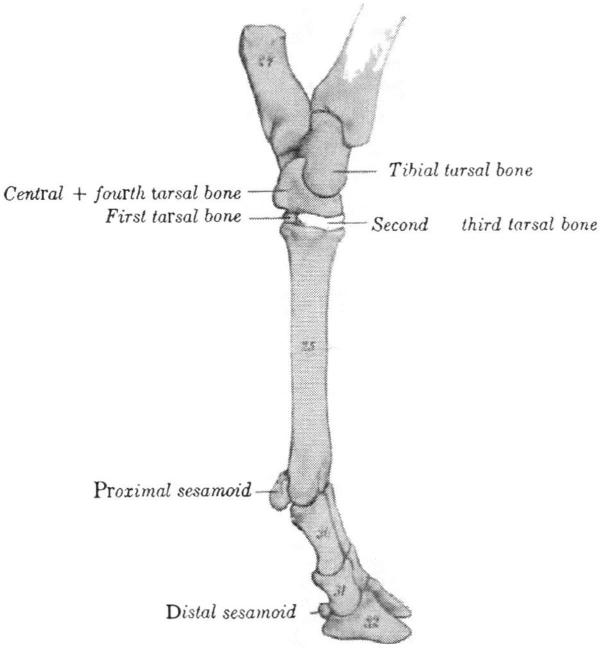

FIG. 104.—SKELETON OF DISTAL PART OF LEFT HIND LIMB OF OX, INTERNAL VIEW.
24, Tuber calcis; *25*, large metatarsal bone; *30*, first phalanx; *31*, second phalanx; *32*, third phalanx. (After Ellenberger-Baum, Anat. für Künstler.)

four-sided. The groove on the anterior surface is deep and wide. The posterior surface is marked by variable grooves. The upper foramen on this surface does not perforate the shaft, but passes obliquely through the extremity, opening on the posterior part of its proximal surface. The postero-internal angle of the proximal end bears a facet for articulation with the small metatarsal bone.

The **small metatarsal** bone is a quadrilateral disc a little less than an inch in width and height. Its anterior face bears a facet for articulation with the large metatarsal bone.

The large metatarsal bone is usually regarded as consisting of the fused third and fourth metatarsal bones. The medullary cavity is subdivided like that of the large metacarpal bone. Some anatomists, however, consider that the ridges at the upper end of each border represent the second and fifth metatarsals (Rosenberg and Retterer). On this basis the small bone would be the first metatarsal.

The **phalanges** and **sesamoids** resemble those of the thoracic limb so closely as to render separate description unnecessary.

SKELETON OF THE PIG

VERTEBRAL COLUMN

The vertebral formula is $C_7T_{14-15}L_{6-7}S_4Cy_{20-23}$.

The **cervical vertebræ** are short and wide. The bodies are elliptical in cross-section, the long diameter being transverse. The anterior articular surfaces are slightly convex from side to side and concave dorso-ventrally; the posterior ones are slightly concave. A ventral crest is not present. The arches are wide from side to side, but the laminæ are narrow, so that a considerable interval (Spatium interarcuale) separates adjacent arches dorsally. The pedicles are perforated by a foramen on either side in addition to the usual intervertebral foramina. The

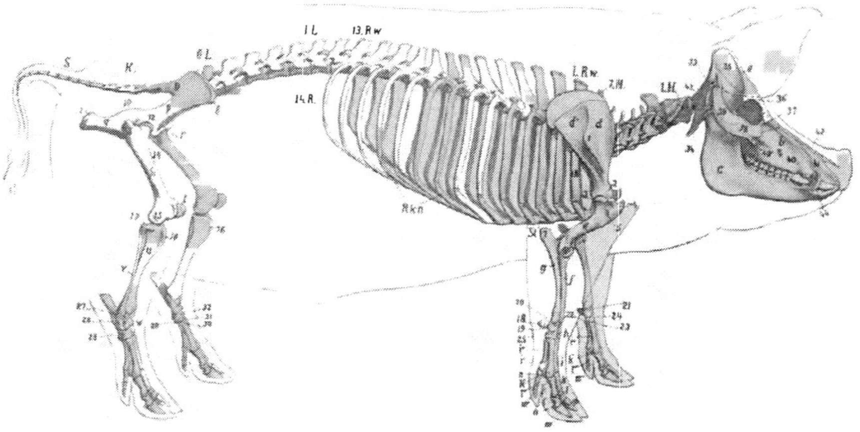

FIG. 105.—SKELETON OF PIG LATERAL VIEW.

a, Cranium; *b*, upper jaw; *c*, lower jaw; *1H.–7H.*, cervical vertebræ; *1R.w.*, first thoracic vertebra; *13 R.w.*, thirteenth thoracic vertebra (next to last); *1L.*, first lumbar vertebra; *6L.*, sixth lumbar vertebra (next to last usually); *K.*, sacrum; *S.*, coccygeal vertebra; *1R.*, first rib; *14R.*, last rib; *R.kn.*, costal cartilages; *St.*, sternum; *d*, supraspinous fossa of scapula; *d′*, infraspinous fossa; *1*, spine of scapula; *2*, neck of scapula; *e*, humerus; *3*, head of humerus; *4*, tuberosities of humerus; *5*, deltoid tuberosity; *6*, external epicondyle of humerus; *f*, radius; *g*, ulna; *7*, olecranon; *h*, carpus; *18–25*, carpal bones; *i–i′′′′*, metacarpus; *k–k′′′′*, proximal phalanges; *l–l′′′′*, middle phalanges; *m–m′′′′*, distal phalanges; *n*, *o*, sesamoids; *p*, ilium; *8*, external angle of ilium (tuber coxæ); *9*, internal angle of ilium (tuber sacrale); *10*, superior ischiatic spine; *q*, ischium; *11*, tuber ischii; *r*, pubis; *12*, acetabulum; *s*, femur; *13*, trochanter major; *14*, trochanter minor; *15*, external epicondyle; *t*, patella; *u*, tibia; *16*, crest of tibia; *17*, external condyle of tibia; *v*, fibula; *w*, tarsus; *26–31*, tarsal bones; *26′*, tuber calcis. (After Ellenberger, in Leisering's Atlas.)

transverse processes divide into two branches, both of which increase in size from the third to the sixth. The upper branch projects outward and backward; it is short and is thickened at its free end. The lower branch is a quadrilateral plate directed ventrally; each overlaps the succeeding one to a small extent, and the series forms the lateral boundary of a deep and wide groove beneath the bodies. The spines increase in height from the third to the last; the anterior ones are inclined backward, the posterior ones forward. The last cervical is recognized by the great length of its spine (ca. 10 cm. in the adult), the absence of the ventral plate of the transverse process, and the flatness of the body, which bears a pair of small facets on its posterior margin for the heads of the first ribs. It has foramina transversaria, and usually two foramina in either side of the arch.

The dorsal arch of the **atlas** bears a large tuberosity. The ventral tubercle is long, compressed laterally, and projects back under the axis. The wing is flattened and bears a posterior tuberosity. The foramen transversarium passes through the posterior border of the wing to the fossa under the latter, and is not visible dorsally; it is sometimes very small or absent. The sides of the vertebral foramen bear two lateral projections which partially divide it into a ventral narrow part, which receives the odontoid process, and a dorsal larger part for the spinal cord. In the fresh state the division is completed by the transverse ligament, which is attached to the projections.

The **axis** has a large spinous process, which is directed upward and backward. The odontoid process is a thick cylindrical rod. The transverse process is very small and the foramen transversarium is often incomplete.

The **thoracic vertebræ** are often fifteen in number. Their bodies are relatively long, constricted in the middle, and without ventral crests. Their extremities are

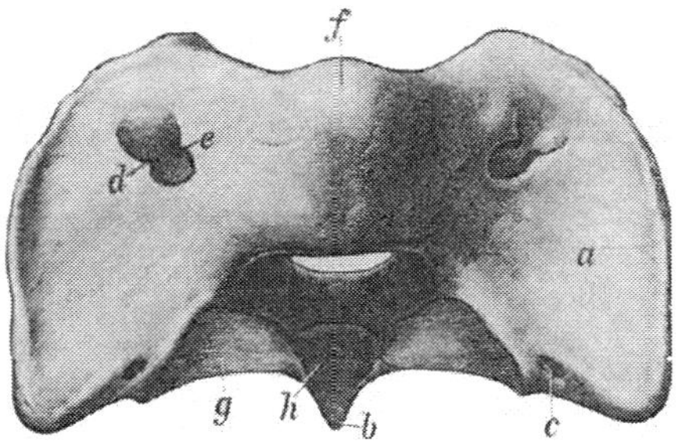

FIG. 106.—ATLAS OF PIG, DORSAL VIEW.

a, Wing; *b*, ventral tubercle; *c*, foramen transversarium; *d*, alar foramen; *e*, intervertebral foramen; *f*, dorsal tuberosity; *g*, articular surface corresponding to that of posterior articular process of typical vertebra; *h*, facet on ventral arch for odontoid process. (Ellenberger-Baum, Anat. d. Haustiere.)

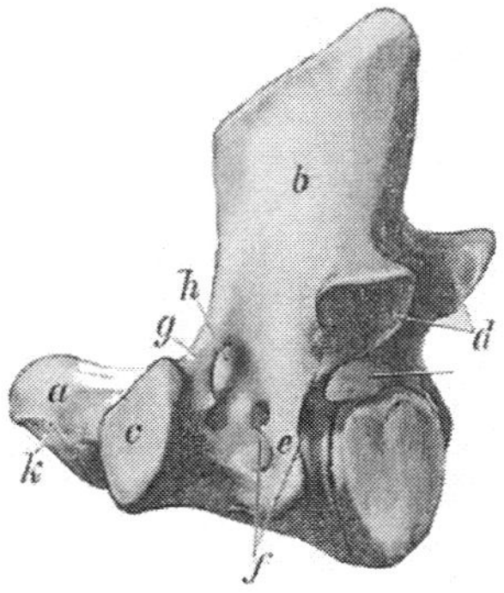

FIG. 107.—AXIS OF PIG, LEFT LATERAL VIEW.

a, Odontoid process (dens); *b*, spinous process; *c*, anterior articular process; *d*, posterior articular processes; *e*, transverse process; *f*, foramen transversarium; *g*, bar of bone which bounds *h*, intervertebral foramen; *i*, vertebral foramen. (Ellenberger-Baum, Anat. d. Haustiere.)

elliptical, depressed in the middle and prominent at the periphery. The arch is perforated by a foramen on either side, and in most of the series there is also a foramen in the posterior part of the root of the transverse process which communicates with the former or with the posterior intervertebral foramen. Sometimes there is a foramen in the anterior part of the process also. There are mammillary processes except on the first two; in the posterior five or six vertebræ they project from the anterior articular processes. The facet for the tubercle of the rib is absent or fused with that for the head in the last five or six. The last transverse process is lumbar in character, plate-like, and about an inch (2 cm.) long. Small accessory processes occur in the posterior part of the region. The first spinous process is broad, very high, and inclined a little forward. The others diminish very gradually in length to the tenth, beyond which they are about equal. The second to the ninth are inclined backward, the tenth is vertical (anticlinal), and the rest incline forward. The width decreases decidedly from the fourth to the tenth, beyond which there is a gradual increase. The summits are slightly enlarged and lie almost in a straight line.

The occurrence of fifteen thoracic vertebræ appears to be quite common, and some observers have recorded the existence of sixteen and even seventeen; a reduction to thirteen is rare.

The lumbar vertebræ are six or seven in number. The bodies are longer than in the thoracic region and bear a ventral crest. They become wider and flatter in the posterior part of the series. The arches are deeply notched, and are separated by an increasing space dorsally. The mammillary processes project outward and backward. The transverse processes are bent downward and incline a little forward. Their length increases to the fifth and is much diminished in the last. They form no articulation with each other or with the sacrum. The posterior edge of the root of the process is marked by a notch in the anterior part of the series, a foramen in the posterior part. The spines are broad and incline forward, with the exception of the last, which is narrow and vertical.

Lesbre states that six and seven lumbar vertebræ occur with almost equal frequency. The number may be reduced to five, and the number of presacral vertebræ varies from twenty-six to twenty-nine.

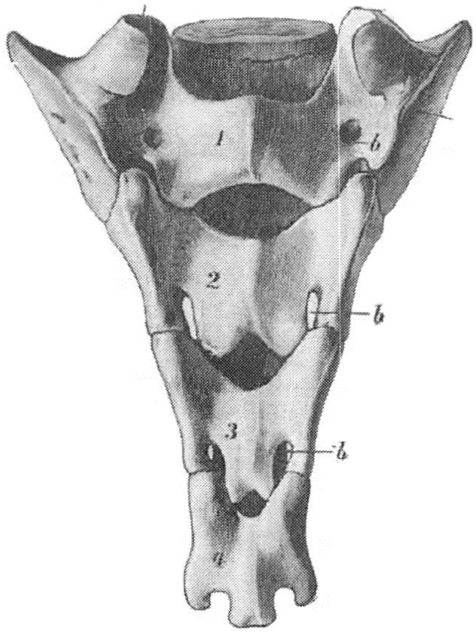

FIG. 108.—SACRUM OF PIG, DORSAL VIEW.
a, Wing; b, dorsal sacral foramina; c, articular process; 1–4, segments or sacral vertebræ. (Ellenberger-Baum, Anat. d. Haustiere.)

The sacrum consists usually of four vertebræ, which fuse later and less completely than in the other domesticated animals. It is less curved than in the ox. The spines are absent, excepting small rudiments on the last two segments. The middle of the dorsal surface is flattened and smooth, and presents openings into the sacral canal between adjacent arches (Spatia interarcualia). On either side are the superior sacral foramina, and tubercles which indicate the fused articular processes. The wings resemble those of the ox. The anterior articular processes are very large. The pelvic surface resembles that of the ox, but is not so strongly curved, and the transverse lines are very distinct.

The coccygeal vertebræ are specially characterized by the presence of functional articular processes on the first four or five, beyond which these processes become non-articular and smaller. The arches of the first five or six are complete. The transverse processes are broad and plate-like in the anterior part of the series and diminish very gradually.

The numerical variation here is twenty to twenty-six according to the observation of several anatomists. Lesbre states that he has found twenty-three most frequently.

Curves.—The cervical region is practically straight. The thoracic and lumbar regions form a gentle curve, concave ventrally, the highest point of which is at the junction of the two regions. The sacral promontory is not so pronounced as in the ox, and the sacral curve is flatter.

THE RIBS

The ribs number fourteen or fifteen pairs, of which seven are sternal and seven or eight asternal usually. They are in general strongly curved in the improved breeds, so that there is a fairly distinct angle, except toward the end of the series. The backward slope of the posterior ribs is slight. The first rib is prismatic, has a large sternal end, and a very short cartilage. The width is greatest in the third to the sixth, and the length in the sixth and seventh usually. The tuberosity fuses with the head on the last five or six. The second to the fifth form diarthrodial joints with their cartilages, which are wide and plate-like.

THE STERNUM

The **sternum** consists of six segments and resembles that of the ox in general form. The first segment (Manubrium) is long, flattened laterally, and bears a blunt-pointed cartilage on its anterior end; its posterior end forms a diarthrodial joint with the body. The latter is flattened, wide in its middle, narrow at either end. The widest segments are formed of two lateral parts, which are not completely fused in the adult. The last segment has a long narrow part which bears the xiphoid cartilage.

The **thorax** is long and is more barrel-shaped than in the horse or ox, since the ribs are more strongly curved and differ less in relative length.

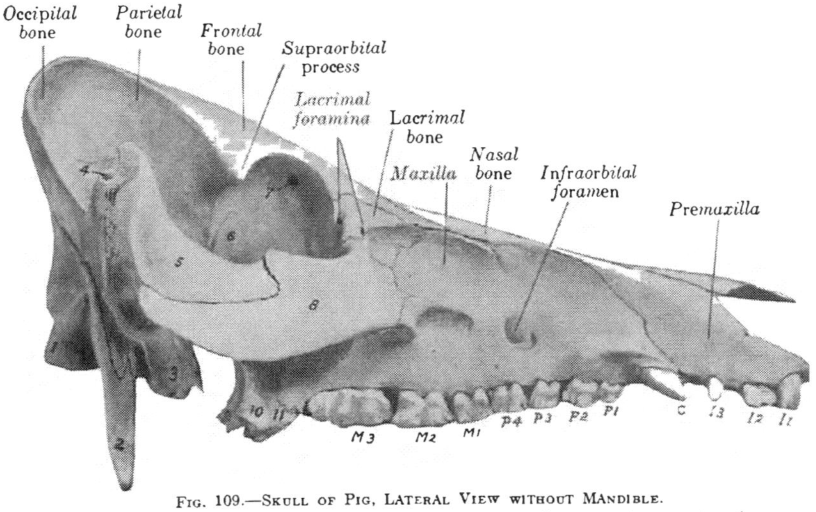

Fig. 109.—Skull of Pig, Lateral View without Mandible.

1, Occipital condyle; *2*, paramastoid or styloid process; *3*, bulla ossea; *4*, external auditory meatus, *5*, zygomatic process of temporal bone; *6*, sphenoid bone; *7*, orbital opening of supraorbital canal; *8*, malar bone; *9*, pterygoid bone; *10*, pterygoid process of sphenoid; *11*, pterygoid process of palate bone; *I1–3*, incisor teeth; *C*, canine tooth; *P1–4*, premolars; *M1–3*, molars.

BONES OF THE SKULL

Cranium

The **occipital bone** has an extensive squamous part or supraoccipital, which forms a very broad and prominent crest. The latter is concave, and is thick and rough above, where it forms the highest part of the skull; laterally it becomes thinner, turns downward, and is continuous with the temporal crest. Two divergent ridges pass upward from the foramen magnum, and the surface between them is concave and smooth. The greater part of the inner (or anterior) surface of the supraoccipital is united with the parietal bones, but a lower concave area faces into the cranial cavity. The foramen magnum is almost triangular, and is narrow above, where it is flanked by two small tuberosities. The paramastoid processes are extremely long and project almost straight downward. The hypoglossal foramen is at the inner side of the root of the process. The basilar part is short and wide; its lower surface bears a thin median ridge and two lateral imprints or tubercles which converge at the junction with the sphenoid bone.

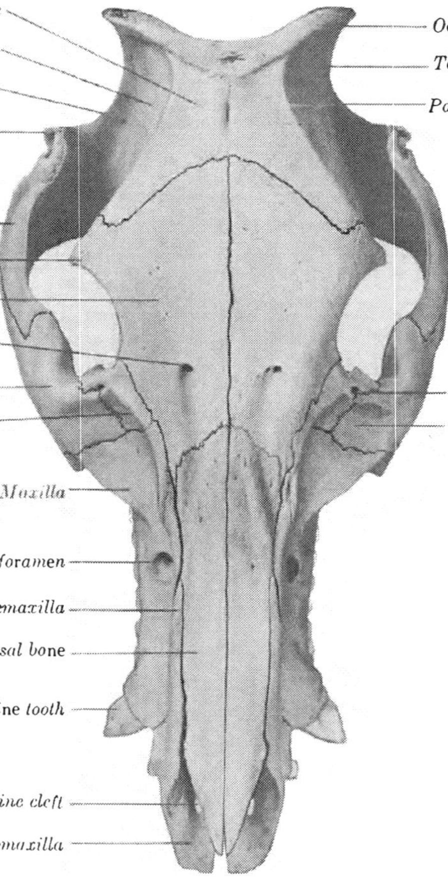

FIG. 110.—SKULL OF PIG, DORSAL VIEW.

The interparietal fuses before birth with the occipital. The tentorium osseum is absent.

The parietal is overlapped by the occipital bone behind and concurs in the formation of the occipital crest. Its external surface is divided by the parietal crest into two parts. The inner part (Planum parietale) faces upward and forward, and is flattened and smooth. Its inner border is short and straight and unites early with the opposite bone. Its anterior border is concave and joins the frontal bone. The outer part (Planum temporale) faces outward and is more extensive; it is concave, forms a large part of the temporal fossa, and is overlapped below by the squamous temporal. The parietal crest extends in a curve from the occipital crest forward and outward to the supraorbital process. The internal surface is concave and is marked by digital impressions. The lower border projects into the cranial cavity and forms a crest which separates the cerebral and cerebellar compartments laterally. The interior forms part of the frontal sinus in the adult. There is no parieto-temporal canal.

The frontal bone is long. The frontal surface slopes downward and forward, the inclination varying in different subjects. The anterior part is concave and is marked by the supraorbital foramen and the groove leading forward from the foramen to the nasal bone. The supraorbital canal opens into the orbit at the upper part of the inner wall of the latter. The supraorbital process is short and blunt-pointed, and is not connected with the zygomatic arch. The gap in the orbital margin is closed by the orbital ligament in the fresh state. The orbital part is extensive and forms the greater part of the inner wall of the orbit. Its upper part is perforated by the orbital orifice of the supraorbital canal, in front of which is the distinct fovea trochlearis. The ethmoidal or internal orbital foramen is situated in the lower part near the junction with the orbital wing of the sphenoid. The temporal part is very narrow and is separated from the orbital plate by a ridge which joins the pterygoid crest below. The interior of the bone is excavated by the frontal sinus in practically its entire extent in the adult. In the young subject the cavity is confined to the anterior part and the rest of the bone is thick.

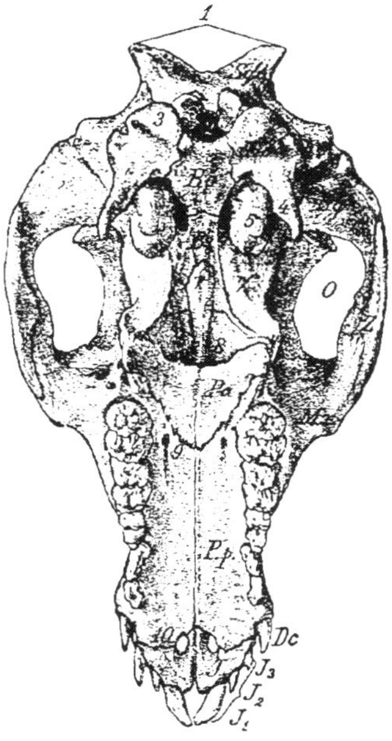

FIG. 111.—BASAL SURFACE OF SKULL OF YOUNG PIG, WITHOUT THE MANDIBLE.

Sq.o., Supraoccipital; *E.o.*, exoccipital; *B.o.*, basioccipital; *B.s.*, body of sphenoid; *Sq.*, squamous temporal bone; *V*, vomer; *Mx.*, maxilla; *Pa.*, horizontal part of palate bone; *P.p.*, palate process of maxilla; *Z.*, malar bone; *J*, premaxilla; *D.c.*, canine tooth; *J1–3*, incisor teeth; *O*, temporal fossa; *1*, occipital crest; *2*, for. magnum; *3*, occipital condyle; *4*, paramastoid (styloid) process; *5*, bulla ossea; *6*, for. lacerum basis cranii; *7*, pterygoid process of sphenoid; *8*, posterior nares; *9*, anterior palatine foramen; *10*, palatine cleft. (Struska, Anat. d. Haustiere.)

The temporal bone has a general resemblance to that of the ox. The zygomatic process is short and stout and is bent at a right angle. The upper border of the process is thin; traced from before backward it curves sharply upward and forms a high prominence in front of the external auditory meatus; beyond this it drops rather abruptly and is then continued upward to the occipital crest. The anterior part of the lower border joins the zygomatic process of the malar, which is deeply notched. The condyle is concave in the transverse direction. The postglenoid process is absent, but the articular surface is bounded behind and internally by a crest. There is no parieto-temporal canal. The external auditory canal is very long and is directed upward and outward. The bulla ossea is large, compressed laterally, and bears a pointed muscular process in front. A narrow space intervenes between the bulla and the basilar part of the occipital bone, so that the foramen lacerum resembles that of the horse. The small hyoid process is situated in a deep depression in front of the root of the paramastoid process, and the stylo-mastoid foramen is immediately external to it. The petrous part presents no important differential features. The squamous part (including the root of the zygomatic process) contains an air-cavity, which is continuous with the sphenoidal sinus.

The sphenoid bone is short and resembles that of the ox in general. The body is narrow. The pituitary fossa is very deep, and is limited behind by a prominent dorsum sellæ; the dorsum bears lateral projections, the **posterior clinoid processes.** The foramen ovale is absent, being included in the foramen lacerum anterius. The other foramina are like those of the ox. The pterygoid process is broad and twisted. Its base is not perforated and its free edge is thin and sharp. It concurs with the pterygoid and palate bones in the formation of the pterygoid fossa, which opens backward and is not present in the horse or ox. The sphenoidal sinus is very large and occupies the body, the temporal wings, and a great part of the pterygoid processes in the adult; it is continued into the temporal bone as mentioned above.

The **ethmoid bone** has a relatively long perpendicular plate, which is marked by ridges corresponding to the ethmoidal meatuses. The cribriform plate is extensive and very oblique, so that it and the crista galli are almost in line with the basi-cranial axis. A linear series of relatively large foramina is found on either side of the crista. The lateral mass consists of five endoturbinals and eighteen ectoturbinals (Paulli). The lamina papyracea concurs in the formation of the pterygo-palatine fossa.

Face

The **maxilla** is extensive. Its external surface forms a longitudinal groove, which is continued upon the premaxilla in front and the facial parts of the lacrimal and malar behind. The infraorbital foramen—sometimes double—is large and is situated above the third or fourth cheek tooth. The alveolus for the canine tooth produces a ridge at the anterior end which is very pronounced in the boar. The facial crest extends forward from the root of the zygomatic process and fades out behind the infraorbital foramen; in some specimens it is prominent and thin-edged, in others it is rounded and projects little. The zygomatic process is short but stout and buttress-like; it is overlapped externally by the malar. The maxillary tuberosity forms in the young subject a long bulla, which occupies most of the pterygo-palatine fossa and contains the developing permanent molars; after the eruption of the teeth the tuberosity flattens and joins the vertical part of the palate bone. The palatine process is very long and is marked in its anterior part by transverse ridges corresponding with those of the mucous membrane of the palate. The anterior palatine foramen is near the junction with the palate bone; from it the palatine groove can be traced distinctly along the entire length of the process. The alveolar border presents a large alveolus for the canine tooth at its anterior end; behind this are seven alveoli for the cheek teeth, which increase in size from first to last. The maxillary foramen and infraorbital canal are very large. The maxillary sinus is small.

The body of the **premaxilla** is narrow and prismatic. It presents three alveoli for the incisor teeth, which are separated by short intervals and diminish in size from before backward. As in the ox, a narrow space separates the right and left bones and takes the place of the foramen incisivum. The palatine process is long and narrow. The nasal process is very extensive and is somewhat rhomboid in outline. Its upper border forms a very long suture with the nasal bone, and the lower articulates tc about the same extent with the maxilla. The palatine fissure is relatively wide.

The horizontal part of the **palate bone** forms a fourth to a fifth of the length of the palate; its palatine surface is triangular, the apex being anterior; its nasal surface is deeply grooved and smooth. A pterygoid process (processus pyramidalis of man) projects backward and downward, and its thick rounded end is received between the pterygoid process of the sphenoid and the pterygoid bone. The perpendicular part is largely overlapped externally by the maxilla and concurs in forming part of the palatine canal. Superiorly the two plates separate and inclose an air-cavity which opens into an ethmoidal meatus. The inner plate curves inward and unites with the vomer and ethmoid to form a horizontal plate (Lamina transversalis), which divides the posterior part of the nasal cavity into an upper olfactory part and a lower respiratory part.

The **pterygoid bone** is nearly vertical in direction, and is narrow in its middle, wide at each end. The external surface is free below and forms the inner wall of the pterygoid fossa. The lower end is notched and forms a distinct hamulus.

The **nasal bone** is very long and its width is almost uniform, except at the anterior end, which is pointed and reaches almost as far forward as the premaxilla. The facial surface is flattened from side to side. In profile it is nearly straight in some subjects, variably concave in others. The external border is free to a small extent in front only; otherwise it is firmly connected with the premaxilla and maxilla. In the adult the frontal sinus extends into the posterior part of the bone.

The **lacrimal bone** is very sharply bent. Its facial surface presents a deep depression, surmounted by a ridge or tubercle. On or close to the orbital margin are two lacrimal foramina which lead to the lacrimal canals. The orbital surface presents a fossa in which the inferior oblique muscle of the eyeball arises, and its lower part bears a crest, which is crossed obliquely by a vascular furrow. The upper border articulates with the frontal only. The bone concurs in the formation of the maxillary sinus.

The **malar bone** is strongly compressed from side to side. Its facial surface is small and presents a fossa which is continuous with the depressions of the maxilla and lacrimal. The orbital surface is still smaller and is smooth and deeply grooved. The zygomatic process is very extensive, especially in the vertical direction. Its external surface is convex and free, and bears a rough eminence in its middle. Its internal surface is concave; it is overlapped in front by the maxilla, and in the remainder of its extent is free and smooth. The upper border is thick and rounded in front, where it forms the lower part of the orbital margin; behind this it forms an extensive notch which receives the zygomatic process of the temporal. (It might be regarded as dividing into frontal and temporal branches.) The lower border is convex and becomes thinner behind.

The **turbinal bones** resemble those of the ox. The superior turbinal is, however, relatively longer, less fragile, and more firmly attached to the nasal bone. There is no middle turbinal.

The **vomer** is very long. The anterior extremity reaches to the body of the premaxilla or very close to it. The lower border is received into a groove formed by the nasal crest of the maxillæ and palate bones and in front by the palatine processes of the premaxillæ. The posterior border is concave, thin, and sharp.

The **os rostri** (or prenasal bone) is situated in the snout between the nostrils. It has the form of a short three-sided prism. The upper surface is convex and is notched at each end. The lateral surfaces are concave, smooth, and converge below, forming a grooved lower border. The posterior surface is triangular, notched centrally, and rough laterally. The anterior surface is deeply pitted and is surrounded by an irregular sharp border.

The **mandible** is very strong, and differs very much from that of the horse or ox. The body narrows decidedly in front; the lingual surface is deeply concave; the mental surface is strongly convex, slopes downward and backward, and forms a distinct prominence at the point of divergence of the rami. Above this prominence is a pair of foramina. The alveolar border presents six alveoli for the incisor teeth, and a little further back two large cavities for the canine teeth. There are two pairs of mental foramina of considerable size and a variable number of smaller ones. The rami diverge more than in the horse or ox, and the upper part is somewhat incurved. The horizontal part is very thick and strong. Its outer surface is strongly convex from above downward. The inner surface is prominent over the roots of the molar teeth and overhangs the concave lower part. The alveolar border is thin in front and widens behind; it does not follow the axis of the ramus, but runs nearly straight and produces the marked overhang noted above. There are seven alveoli for the lower cheek teeth, which increase in size from before backward. The first is small, not always present in the adult, and is separated by short spaces from the second and the canine alveolus. The vertical part is relatively wide above. The condyle is convex in both directions, wide in front, narrow and declivitous behind. The very small and thin-edged coronoid process is not quite so high as the condyle, from which it is separated by a very wide notch. The mandibular foramen is large. The two halves of the bone unite soon after birth in the improved breeds.

The body of the **hyoid bone** is broad from before backward, short transversely, and bears on its ventral aspect a very short pointed lingual process. The thyroid cornua are wide and curved, concave and grooved dorsally; their ends are attached to the thyroid cartilage of the larynx by rather long bars of cartilage. The small cornua are short, wide, and flattened dorso-ventrally; they are attached to short bars which project from the junction of the body and thyroid cornua. The middle cornu is a little longer than the small cornu, but is relatively slender; it is largely cartilaginous in the young subject and does not ossify at either end. The great cornu is a very slender rod, slightly enlarged at either end; the upper extremity is attached to the hyoid process of the temporal by a rather long and wide bar of cartilage.

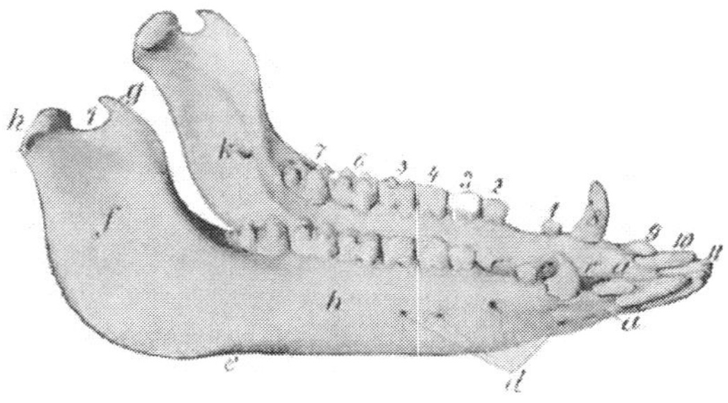

FIG. 112.—MANDIBLE OF PIG.

a, Body of mandible; *b*, horizontal part of ramus; *f*, vertical part of ramus; *c*, interalveolar border; *c'*, interval between canine and corner incisor; *c''*, interval between first and second premolars; *d*, mental foramina; *e*, vascular impression; *g*, coronoid process; *h*, condyle; *i*, sigmoid notch; k, mandibular foramen; *1–7*, cheek teeth, *8*, canine tooth; *9*, *10*, *11*, incisors. (Ellenberger-Baum, Anat d. Haustiere.)

THE SKULL AS A WHOLE

The **length** and the **profile** contour vary greatly in different subjects. Primitively the skull is long—especially in its facial part—and the frontal profile is almost straight. The condition is very pronounced in wild or semi-feral pigs, and exists also in the improved breeds during extreme youth. Most of the latter are decidedly brachycephalic when fully developed; the face is "dished" in a pronounced fashion. The frontal region slopes sharply upward, and the nasal region is shortened, and in some specimens even distinctly concave in profile. The supraorbital foramina are about midway between the orbital margin and the frontal suture. The supraorbital grooves extend forward from the foramina to the nasal region and turn outward and downward toward the infraorbital foramina over the ridges which separate the nasal and lateral regions.

The **lateral surface** is triangular when the mandible is included. The temporal fossa is entirely lateral and its long axis is almost vertical. It is bounded above by the occipital crest, behind by the temporal crest, in front by the parietal crest, and is marked off from the orbital cavity by the supraorbital process and a curved crest which extends from it to the root of the pterygoid process. The zygomatic arch is strong, high, and flattened from side to side. Its root is notched above and bears a projection below. It curves sharply upward behind and forms a pointed recurved projection above and in front of the external auditory meatus.

The orbit is small. Its margin is deficient behind in the dry skull, thick and rounded in front and below. The cavity is limited below by a ridge on the frontal and lacrimal bones, and is separated by a crest from the temporal fossa. The inner wall is perforated above by the orbital opening of the supraorbital canal, and below by the optic and ethmoidal foramina; on its antero-inferior part is the fossa in which the inferior oblique muscle of the eye takes origin. Two lacrimal foramina are found on or close to the anterior margin. The pterygo-palatine fossa is well defined; its upper part forms a deep groove which leads from the large foramen in the sphenoid (like that of the ox) to the very large maxillary foramen. The pre-orbital region is deeply grooved in its length and is clearly marked off by a ridge from the nasal and frontal regions. The facial crest is short, usually thin-edged, and lies above the fifth and sixth cheek teeth. A little (ca. 2 cm.) in front of it is the infraorbital foramen. There is a ridged prominence over the canine alveolus. In some skulls the anterior part of the upper jaw is inclined upward.

The most striking features of the **basal surface** are as follows: The paramastoid processes are extremely long, less flattened than in the horse and ox, and nearly vertical. At the inner side of the root of each is the hypoglossal foramen, and in front of it are the stylo-mastoid foramen and a deep cavity in which the hyoid process is concealed. The bulla ossea is long, compressed laterally, and bears a sharp, short, muscular process. The basioccipital is wide and flattened; it bears a median crest and two lateral tubercles. The posterior nares are small and are wider below than above. On either side of them is the tuberosity of the palate bone, and above this is the pterygoid fossa. The palate is remarkably long and is relatively narrow. It constitutes about two-thirds of the entire length of the skull. It is widest between the canines and premolars and narrow at each end. It is marked by a crest medially and by the palatine foramen and groove laterally. The anterior part bears transverse ridges. It is moderately arched from side to side. In some specimens it is nearly straight or slightly concave in its length; in others it curves upward to a variable degree in front. The posterior end always slopes upward more or less.

The **posterior** or **nuchal surface** is remarkable for its height and the breadth of the occipital crest. The central part above the foramen magnum is smooth and concave from side to side, and is bounded laterally by ridges, which converge below and end on two tubercles at the upper margin of the foramen magnum. The surface is separated from the temporal fossæ by the temporal crests, which curve downward and outward and blend with the external auditory canals. The mastoid process has the form of a plate which overlaps the root of the paramastoid process and bears a crest on its anterior part.

The **cranial cavity** is small, in spite of the great size of the cranium; the discrepancy is due to the enormous development of the frontal sinuses in the adult. It is relatively longer, but much lower than that of the ox. Its width is greatly diminished between the orbits. The olfactory fossæ are extensive and very oblique. The floor resembles that of the ox, but the foramen ovale is absent, the dorsum sellæ is more developed, and the foramen lacerum basis cranii is like that of the horse. Two oblique lateral crests clearly mark the limit between the cerebral and cerebellar compartments. The tentorium osseum and the parieto-temporal canals are absent.

The **nasal cavity** is very long. Its posterior part is divided by a horizontal plate into olfactory and respiratory parts. The olfactory part or fundus is above, and contains the ethmoturbinals and ethmoidal meatuses. The lower part is continuous with the inferior meatus and leads to the pharyngeal orifice; hence it is sometimes called the naso-pharyngeal meatus. The bony roof is almost complete in front on account of the great length of the nasal bones.

The **frontal sinus** is a vast excavation in the adult animal. It involves all of the roof and almost all of the sides of the cranium, and extends forward into the roof of the nasal cavity a variable distance—sometimes as far as a transverse plane through the infraorbital foramina. The septum between the right and left sinuses is usually deflected in an irregular manner in its middle part, but is practically median at either end. Each sinus is subdivided by numerous septa, some of which are complete. Thus the sinus is divided into compartments, each of which communicates with an ethmoidal meatus.

In the young pig the sinus is small and is confined to the anterior part of the frontal bone. Later it extends backward, outward, and to a less extent forward. In the old subject it penetrates laterally into the supraorbital process and the root of the zygomatic process of the temporal bone, and behind almost down to the foramen magnum and the occipital condyles. It then consists of six to eight compartments usually.

The **maxillary sinus** is relatively small. Its anterior end is a little less than an inch (ca. 2 cm.) behind the infraorbital foramen, and it extends upward into the lacrimal and backward into the malar bone. The infraorbital canal passes along its floor, and the roots of the molar teeth do not project up into it. It does not communicate with the frontal and sphenoidal sinuses, but with the posterior part of the middle meatus by means of a considerable orifice.

The **sphenoidal sinus** is very large. It involves the body, pterygoid processes, and temporal wings of the sphenoid bone, and extends into the squamous temporal. It communicates with the ventral ethmoidal meatus.

There is a small sinus in the perpendicular part of the palate bone which communicates with an ethmoidal meatus.

BONES OF THE THORACIC LIMB

The **scapula** is very wide, the index being about 1 : 0.7. The spine is triangular and is very wide in its middle, which curves backward over the infra spinous fossa and bears a large tuberosity. Its lower part bears a small projection (rudimentary acromion). The anterior border is strongly convex in profile, sinuous when viewed from the front, and thick and rough in its middle. The posterior border is wide, slightly concave, and bears an outer rough lip. The vertebral border is convex, and the cartilage is not so extensive as in the horse and ox. The cervical angle is thin and bent inward a little. The dorsal angle is thick and is about a right angle. The neck is well defined. The rim of the glenoid cavity is rounded and not notched. The tuberosity is just above the antero-internal part of the glenoid cavity and bears no distinct coracoid process.

The **humerus** has an appearance in profile somewhat like an italic *f* minus the cross-bar; this is due to the marked backward and forward inclination of the proximal and distal ends respectively. The shaft is decidedly compressed from side to side. The internal surface is extensive and flattened; it is separated from the anterior surface by a distinct border, and bears no teres tubercle. The musculo-spiral groove is shallow. The deltoid tuberosity is small, and there is a larger rounded eminence midway between it and the external tuberosity. The nutrient foramen is on the posterior surface below its middle. The head is more strongly curved and the neck better marked than in the horse or ox. The external tuberosity is very large and extends upon the front of the extremity. It is divided into two high prominences by a wide deep groove. There is a third eminence below and externally for the attachment of the supraspinatus muscle. The bicipital groove is at the front of the inner side; it is undivided and is almost converted into a canal. The outer groove on the distal articular surface is so shallow as to give the appearance of two condyles of similar size. The olecranon fossa is very deep, and the plate of bone which separates it from the coronoid fossa is thin and sometimes perforated. The proximal end unites with the shaft at three and a half years, the distal at one year.

The **radius** is short and narrow, but thick. The shaft increases in size from above downward. The greater part of the posterior surface is in apposition with the ulna; this part is marked by a vascular furrow which runs downward from the upper interosseous space, and has the nutrient foramen at its proximal end. The bicipital tuberosity is represented by a rough area. The distal end is relatively large. Its carpal surface consists of concavo-convex facets for the radial and intermediate carpal bones. There is a wide shallow groove on the middle of the front. The proximal end fuses with the shaft at one year, the distal at three and a half years.

The **ulna** is massive. It is much longer and considerably heavier than the radius. The shaft is curved. The anterior surface is convex and most of it is rough and attached to the radius by the interosseous ligament. There is a smooth area on the upper third, which concurs with the radius in forming the upper interosseous space, and is marked in its upper part by the nutrient foramen. From this space a vascular furrow passes downward to the lower part of the shaft, where there is often a distal interosseous space for the passage of vessels. The internal surface is extensive, concave, and smooth. The external surface is slightly convex, and its upper part is marked by an oblique rough line or ridge. The proximal extremity is large and is bent inward somewhat; its length is more than one-third of that of the entire bone. The distal extremity is relatively small; it articulates with the ulnar and accessory carpal bones, and is notched in front to accommodate the ridge on the radius. The bone contains a considerable medullary canal. The bone is consolidated at three to three and a half years.

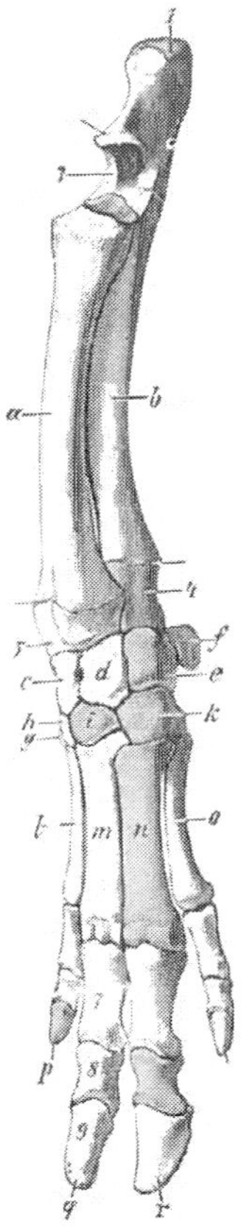

Fig. 113. — Skeleton of Forearm and Manus of Pig, Antero-external View.

a, Radius; *b*, ulna; *c*, radial carpal; *d*, intermediate carpal; *e*, ulnar carpal; *f*, accessory carpal; *g*, first carpal; *h*, second carpal; *i*, third carpal; *k*, fourth carpal; *l–o*, second to fifth metacarpal bones; *p–s*, second to fifth digits; *1*, olecranon; *2*, beak of ulna (proc. anconeus); *3*, semilunar notch; *4*, styloid process of ulna; *5*, styloid process of radius; *6*, distal epiphyseal lines; *7*, first phalanx; *8*, second phalanx; *9*, third phalanx. (Ellenberger-Baum, Anat. d. Haustiere.)

The **carpus** comprises eight bones, four in each row. The bones of the proximal row resemble those of the ox, with the exception of the accessory, which is more like that of the horse, but has no external groove. The first carpal is small, elongated from before backward, rounded, and articulates in front with the second carpal. The latter is high and narrow, and articulates with the second and third metacarpal bones below. The third carpal articulates with the radial and intermediate above, the third metacarpal bone below. The fourth is the largest bone of the row; it articulates with the intermediate and ulnar above, the fourth and fifth metacarpals below, and bears a tuberosity on its volar aspect.

Four **metacarpal bones** are present. The first is absent, the third and fourth are large and carry the chief digits, while the second and fifth are much smaller and bear the accessory digits. Their proximal ends articulate with each other and with the carpus as indicated above. The bones are consolidated at about two years of age.

The third and fourth metacarpals are flattened from before backward, three-sided, and placed close together. The distal end of each bears a trochlea for articulation with the first phalanx and the sesamoids. The third is the wider of the two, and articulates with all of the lower row of the carpus except the first. The fourth articulates with the fourth carpal chiefly, but has a small facet for the third. The second and fifth metacarpals are placed further back than the chief bones. The fifth is considerably the thicker of the two. The proximal ends are small and articulate with the corresponding carpal and metacarpal bones. The distal end is relatively large; its articular surface is condyloid in front, trochlear behind.

Each chief digit comprises three **phalanges** and three **sesamoids.** The bones of the chief digits resemble those of the ox in form, but there is no foramen on the interdigital side of the extensor process and the proximal sesamoids are narrow and ridged behind. The phalanges of the accessory digits (which do not reach the ground ordinarily) are similar in form but much smaller.

BONES OF THE PELVIC LIMB

The **os coxæ** is long and narrow. The ilium and ischium are almost in line with each other and sagittal in direction. The wing of the **ilium** bends outward much less than in the horse or ox. The gluteal surface is divided into two fossæ by a ridge, which is continuous with the superior ischiatic spine behind. The inner surface presents an extensive rough area behind, which is in apposition with the wing of the sacrum. The smooth iliac area is narrow, and is bounded above by a ridge. The crest or anterior border is convex, and is thick, rough, and prominent in its middle, which forms the highest point of the bone. The internal angle is lower than the crest, is directed backward, and articulates internally with the sacrum. The external angle is lower still and is very little thickened. The **ischia** in the female are somewhat divergent and flattened behind. The tubera are everted and bear three prominences. There is a crest or tuberosity on the ventral surface. The superior ischiatic spine is like that of the cow, but is slightly incurved and the muscular ridges on its outer face are more pronounced. The symphyseal part of the **pubis** is thick and the two bones are almost in a horizontal plane. The ilio-pectineal eminence is prominent and the psoas tubercle is well marked.

The **acetabulum** is placed a little further back than in the ox. The rim is thick and is cut into posteriorly by a narrow fissure, which leads into the deep fossa acetabuli. The three pieces of the os coxæ are fused by the end of the first year, but the crest and the ischial tubera are partially separate till the sixth or seventh year. The symphysis does not usually undergo complete anchylosis. Interischial bones are present.

The **inlet** of the **pelvis** is elliptical and very oblique. In a sow of full size the conjugate diameter is about five to six inches (10 to 12 cm.) and the transverse about three and a half to four inches (ca. 8.75 to 10 cm.). In the female the floor is relatively wide and flattened, especially at the outlet, where the tubera are everted; it also has a decided downward inclination behind. The pelvic axis is therefore correspondingly oblique. The ischial arch is wide. In the boar the pubis is much thicker and the ischia are not everted posteriorly. The inlet is smaller. The floor is concave from side to side and slopes decidedly less than in the sow. The superior ischiatic spines are more incurved, and the ischial arch is much narrower and deeper.

The **femur** has a relatively wide and massive shaft, on which four surfaces might be recognized. The principal nutrient foramen is situated in the proximal third of the anterior surface. The posterior surface is wide, and is limited outwardly by a ridge which extends from the trochanter major to the large external supracondyloid crest. There is no supracondyloid (plantar) fossa. The head is strongly curved, and is marked toward the inner side by a rather large depression for the attachment of the round ligament. The neck is distinct. The trochanter major, although massive, does not extend up as high as the head. The trochanteric ridge and fossa resemble those of the ox. The external (third) trochanter is absent. The ridges of the trochlea are similar and almost sagittal.

The shaft of the **tibia** is slightly curved, convex internally. The tuberosity is grooved in front, and a narrow sulcus separates it from the external condyle. The facet for the fibula is on the posterior border of the latter, and is bounded internally by an eminence. The upper part of the crest is very prominent and curves outward. The distal end resembles in general that of the ox, but is relatively narrower transversely and thicker from before backward.

The **fibula** extends the entire length of the region, and is separated from the tibia by a wide interosseous space. The shaft is flattened from side to side; the proximal part is wide and deeply grooved externally; the lower part is narrower and thicker. The proximal end is flattened, grooved externally, and articulates internally with the external condyle of the tibia. The distal end forms the external malleolus. It is grooved externally, and articulates with the tibia and tibial tarsal internally, with the fibular tarsal bone distally.

The **patella** is very much compressed laterally and presents three surfaces.

The **tarsus** comprises seven bones. The tibial and the fibular tarsal resemble in general those of the ox. The axis of the tibial is, however, slightly oblique downward and inward, and its distal end bears a double trochlea for articulation with the central and fourth tarsals. The tuber calcis is deeply grooved posteriorly. The central tarsal is narrow transversely and thick. Its proximal surface is deeply concave, and the posterior bears a large tubercle. The first tarsal is high and narrow; it articulates with the central and second tarsals and the second metatarsal bone. The second tarsal is small and somewhat prismatic; it articulates with the central above, the third in front, the first behind, and the second and third metatarsals below. The third tarsal is much larger, and is compressed from above downward, wide in front, narrow behind. It articulates with the central tarsal above, the third metatarsal below, the second tarsal internally, and the fourth tarsal externally. The fourth tarsal is large. Its external face is crossed by an oblique groove for the tendon of the peroneus longus. The internal surface articulates with the central and third tarsals. The proximal surface supports the tibial and fibular tarsal bones, and the distal surface rests on the fourth and fifth metatarsals. It ossifies from two centers.

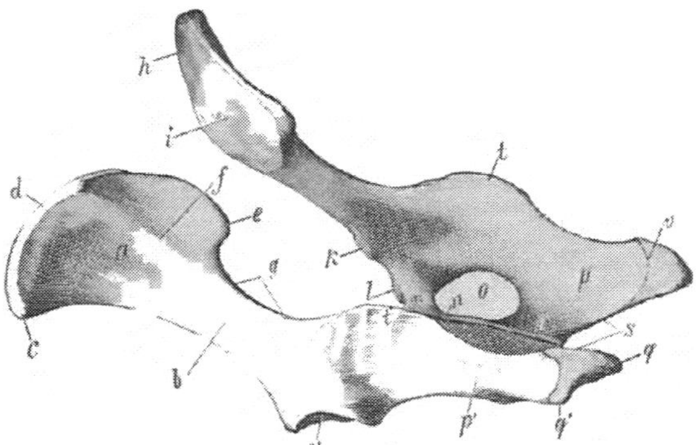

FIG. 114.—COXAL BONES OF PIG, LEFT POSTERIOR VIEW.

a, Wing, *b*, shaft, *c*, external angle, *d*, anterior border, *e*, internal angle, *f*, gluteal line of ilium; *g*, great sciatic notch; *h*, smooth, *i*, rough part of ventral surface of ilium; k, psoas tubercle; *l*, ilio-pectineal eminence; *m*, acetabular branch, *n*, symphyseal branch of pubis; *o*, obturator foramen; *p*, *p′*, ischium; *q*, *q′*, tuber ischii; *r*, symphysis; *s*, ischial arch; *t*, *t′*, superior ischiatic spine; *n*, acetabulum; *v*, epiphyseal line. (Ellenberger-Baum, Anat. d. Haustiere.)

The four **metatarsal bones** resemble the corresponding bones of the fore limb, but are somewhat longer. The proximal ends of the third and fourth each have a considerable projection behind; the process on the third has a facet for articulation with a discoid sesamoid bone. The second and fifth are placed more on the posterior aspect of the large bones than is the case in the fore limb.

The first and second **phalanges** are a little longer and narrower than those of the fore limb.

SKELETON OF THE DOG

VERTEBRAL COLUMN

The vertebral formula is $C_7T_{13}L_{7(6)}S_3Cy_{20-23}$.

The **cervical vertebræ** are relatively longer than in the ox and the pig. The bodies of the typical vertebræ diminish in length from first to last and are compressed dorso-ventrally. The anterior extremity is moderately convex and the posterior slightly concave; both are oblique. The median ridge and lateral grooves on the upper surface of the body are very well marked. The second, third, and fourth have distinct ventral spines. The spinous process of the third has the form of a long low crest; in the remainder it is higher, blunt-pointed, and inclined forward. The transverse processes of the third, fourth, and fifth project downward and backward, and divide into two branches; of these, the anterior one is thin, and the posterior is thick and tuberculate at its free end. The process of the sixth has two parts; one of these is an extensive quadrilateral plate directed downward and outward and ridged on its inner surface; the other part is short and blunt, and is directed outward and a little backward and upward. The seventh is readily distinguished by its shortness, the length of its spine, and the single transverse process. The posterior articular processes bear tubercles which are large on the third, fourth, and fifth.

The ventral arch of the **atlas** is narrow from before backward, and bears a small tubercle posteriorly. The upper surface of the dorsal arch is strongly convex and rough centrally. The wings are wide, flattened, and almost horizontal. The upper surface is rough. There is an alar notch (Incisura alaris) on the anterior border instead of the anterior foramen. The foramen transversarium is present.

The body of the **axis** is flattened dorso-ventrally, especially in front. The odontoid process is rounded and relatively long, reaching almost to the occipital bone; it is inclined upward a little. The articular surfaces which flank it are condyloid in form and very oblique. The inferior surface is wide, and is divided by a median crest into two fossæ. The transverse processes are single, pointed, directed backward and outward, and perforated by relatively large foramina transversaria. The spinous process is thin and of moderate height, but very long; it is prolonged forward so as to overhang the dorsal arch of the atlas, and is terminated behind by a tuberosity which is connected by two crests with the posterior articular processes. The anterior notches are large and are never converted into foramina.

The bodies of the **thoracic vertebræ** are wide and compressed dorso-ventrally, especially at each end of the region. Their convex anterior surfaces are depressed in the middle. The posterior facets for the heads of the ribs are absent on the last three or four. The transverse processes resemble those of the horse. They bear mammillary processes except at the anterior end of the region. The facets for the tubercles of the ribs are large and concave in the anterior part of the series, and become smaller and slightly convex further back. The last three have accessory processes also. The first three or four spinous processes are about equal in length. Behind this they become gradually shorter to the tenth, and then remain equal. The backward slope is most marked in the ninth and tenth. The eleventh is practically vertical (anticlinal vertebra) and the last two incline slightly forward.

The bodies of the **lumbar vertebræ** are decidedly flattened dorso-ventrally, and increase in width from first to last. The length increases to the sixth. The transverse processes are plate-like and are directed forward and downward. Their length increases to the fifth and sixth. They form no joints with each other or with the sacrum. Their extremities are enlarged, with the exception of the last. The accessory processes project backward over the posterior notches of the first five. The anterior articular processes are large, compressed laterally, and bear

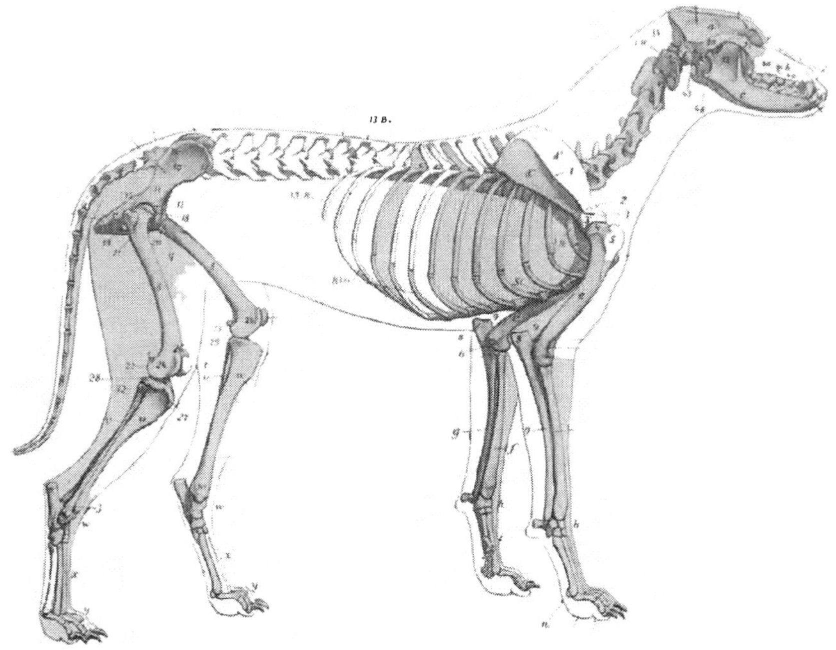

FIG. 115.—SKELETON OF DOG, LATERAL VIEW.

a, Cranium; *b*, face; *c*, mandible; *1H–7H*, cervical vertebræ; *13B*, last thoracic vertebra; *1L–7L*, lumbar vertebræ; *K*, sacrum; *S*, coccygeal vertebræ; *1R–13R*, ribs; *R.kn.*, costal cartilages; *St.*, sternum; *d*, scapula; *d'*, supraspinous fossa; *d''*, infraspinous fossa; *1*, spine of scapula; *2*, acromion; *3*, tuberosity of scapula; 3', articular end of scapula; *e*, humerus; *4*, head of humerus; *5*, external tuberosity of humerus; 5', deltoid ridge; 6, 6', epicondyles of humerus; *7*, external condyloid crest; *7'*, coronoid fossa; *f*, radius; *g*, ulna; *8*, olecranon; *9*, "beak" of ulna; *h*, carpus; *i*, metacarpus; k, proximal phalanges; *l*, middle phalanges; *m*, distal phalanges; *n*, sesamoid; *p*, ilium; *10*, wing of ilium; *11*, shaft of ilium; *12*, crest of ilium; *13*, external angle of ilium (tuber coxæ); *14*, internal angle of ilium (tuber sacrale); *15*, superior ischiatic spine; *q*, pubis; *r*, ischium; *16*, tuber ischii; *17*, acetabulum; *S*, femur; *18*, head of femur; *19*, trochanter major; *20*, trochanter minor; *21*, trochanter tertius; *22*, *23*, condyles; *24*, *25*, epicondyles; *26*, trochlea; *t*, patella; *u*, tibia; *27*, tuberosity of tibia; *28*, *29*, condyles of tibia; *30*, internal malleolus; *v*, fibula; *31*, external malleolus; *32*, head of fibula; *w*, tarsus; *x*, metatarsus; *y*, phalanges; *33*, occipital bone; *34*, paramastoid (styloid) process; *35*, parietal bone; *36*, frontal bone; *37*, lacrimal bone; *38*, malar bone; *39*, squamous temporal; *40*, maxilla; *40'*, infraorbital foramen; *41*, premaxilla; *42*, nasal bone; *43*, external auditory meatus; *44*, canine tooth; *45*, masseteric fossa; *46*, angular process of mandible. (After Ellenberger, in Leisering's Atlas.)

mammillary processes. The spinous processes are broad below, narrower above, and with the exception of the last, incline a little forward. Their height diminishes behind the fourth.

The **sacrum** results from the early fusion of three vertebræ. It is short, wide, and quadrangular. The spines are fused to form a median crest, which is notched, however, between the summits of the spines. On either side are two tubercles, vestiges of the fused articular processes. The pelvic surface is deeply concave and presents two pairs of foramina. The wings are prismatic and very high. Their lateral surfaces are extensive, face almost directly outward, and bear an auricular surface on the lower part. The anterior surface of the body of the first vertebra is extensive, depressed in its middle, and bears a prominent lip below The anterior articular processes are large and have extensive, slightly concave

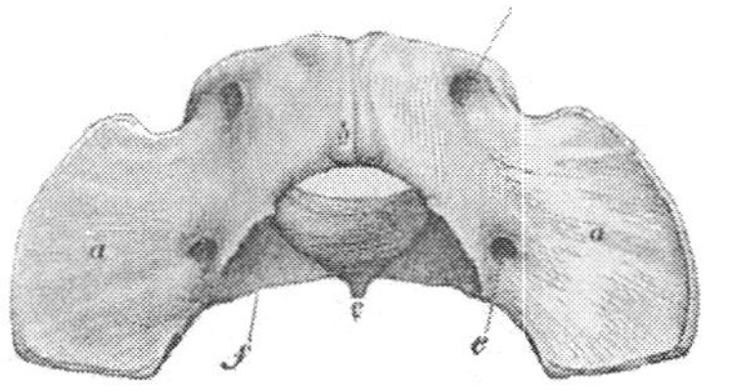

FIG. 116.—ATLAS OF DOG, VIEWED FROM ABOVE AND BEHIND.

a, Wing; *b*, dorsal arch and tubercle; *c*, ventral tubercle; *d*, intervertebral foramen; *e*, foramen transversarium; *f*, articular surface for axis. (Ellenberger-Baum, Anat. d. Hundes.)

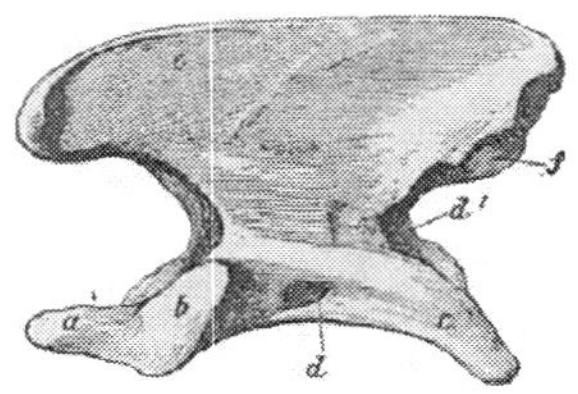

FIG. 117.—AXIS OF DOG, LEFT LATERAL VIEW.

a, Odontoid process; *b*, articular surface for atlas; *c*, transverse process; *d*; foramen transversarium; *d'*, posterior opening of *d*; *e*, spine; *f*, posterior articular process. (Ellenberger-Baum, Anat. d. Hundes.)

facets which face upward and inward. The posterior articular processes are small. The transverse processes of the last vertebra project backward and may articulate or fuse with those of the first coccygeal. The sacral canal is strongly compressed dorso-ventrally.

The **coccygeal vertebræ** are fully developed in the anterior part of the region. The arch is complete in the first six usually. The first three or four have well developed articular processes at each end. Behind this the posterior pair quickly disappears, and the anterior ones become non-articular and gradually reduced in size. The transverse processes of the first five or six

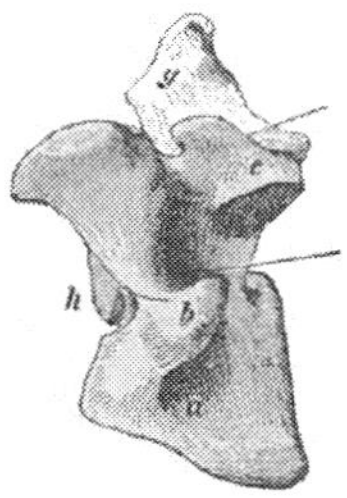

FIG. 118.—SIXTH CERVICAL VERTEBRA OF DOG, LEFT VIEW.

a, Ventral plate, *b*, lateral part of transverse process; *c*, foramen transversarium; *d*, anterior articular process; *f*, accessory process; *g*, spinous process; *h*, articular head of body. (Ellenberger-Baum, Anat. d. Hundes.)

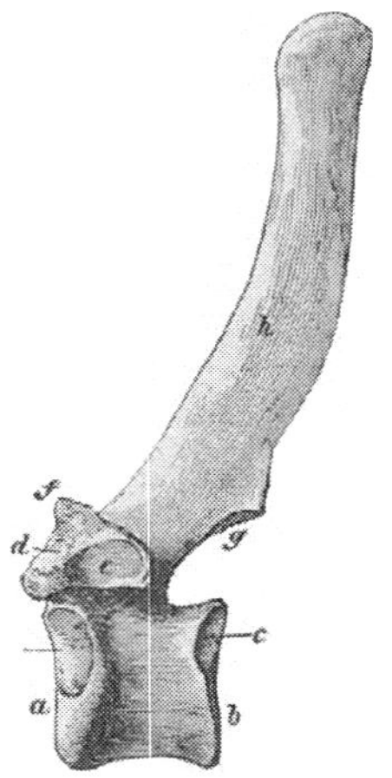

FIG. 119.—FOURTH THORACIC VERTEBRA OF DOG, LEFT VIEW.

a, Head; *b*, glenoid cavity; *c*, facet for head of rib; *d*, transverse process; *e*, facet for tubercle of rib; *f*, mammillary process; *g*, posterior articular process; *h*, spinous process. (Ellenberger-Baum, Anat. d. Hundes.)

are relatively large; behind this they quickly disappear. **Hæmal arches** (or chevron bones) in the form of a V or Y occur ventrally at the intercentral junctions of the third, fourth, and fifth usually. They transmit the middle coccygeal artery, which passes between pairs of ventral tubercles further back.

Curves.—A gentle curve, convex ventrally, is formed by the cervical and the anterior part of the thoracic region. The posterior thoracic and the lumbar vertebræ form a second curve, concave ventrally. The sacral promontory is well marked. The sacrum and the anterior part of the coccygeal region constitute a third and more pronounced curve, concave ventrally. In long-tailed dogs the sacro-coccygeal region is somewhat **S**-shaped.

Variations.—Numerical variations are not common except in the coccygeal region. The number of thoracic vertebræ may be twelve or fourteen, with or without compensatory change in the lumbar region. Girard recorded a case with eight lumbar and the usual number of thoracic vertebræ. Six lumbar with fourteen thoracic vertebræ have been met with. The first coccygeal sometimes unites with the sacrum.

THE RIBS

Thirteen pairs of ribs are present, of which nine are sternal and four asternal. They are strongly curved, narrow, and thick. Those in the middle of the series are the longest. The first eight or nine increase in width in their lower part. The last rib is usually floating.

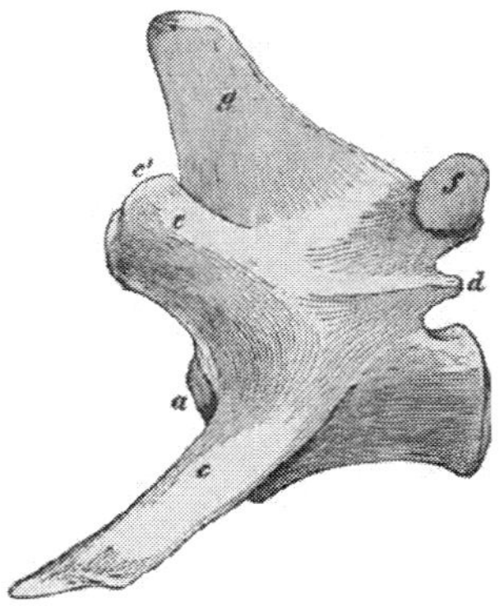

FIG. 120.—FOURTH LUMBAR VERTEBRA OF DOG, LEFT VIEW.

a, *b*, Articular surfaces of body; *c*, transverse process; *d*, accessory process; *e*, anterior articular process; *e'*, mammillary process; *f*, posterior articular process; *g*, spinous process. (Ellenberger-Baum, Anat. d. Hundes.)

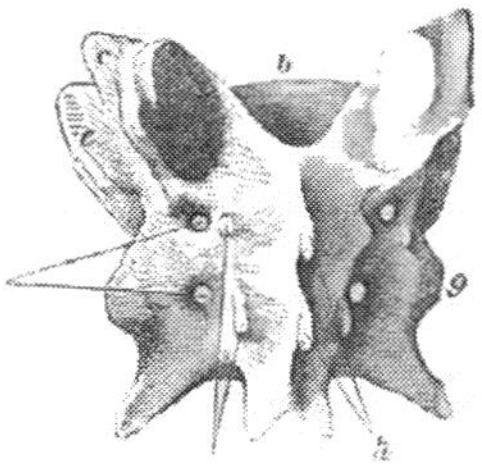

FIG. 121.—SACRUM OF DOG, DORSAL VIEW.

a, Dorsal sacral foramina; *b*, articular surface of body of first segment; *c*, *d*, anterior articular processes; *e*, wing; *f*, rudiments of articular processes; *g*, lateral part; *h*, spinous processes. (Ellenberger Baum, Anat. d. Hundes.)

The costal cartilages are long and curve forward; the length and curvature of the first pair is a striking special feature.

THE STERNUM

This is long, laterally compressed, and consists of eight sternebræ, which fuse only in exceptional cases and in extreme old age. The first segment is the longest; its anterior end is blunt-pointed and bears a short conical cartilage. It widens at the point of articulation of the first pair of cartilages. The last segment is also long, thinner than its predecessors, wide in front, and narrow behind, where it bears a narrow xiphoid cartilage.

The **thorax** is distinctly barrel-like and is not decidedly compressed anteriorly like that of the horse and ox. The inlet is oval and is relatively wide on account of the marked curvature of the first pair of ribs and cartilages.

BONES OF THE SKULL

In the following descriptions of the separate bones an intermediate type—*e. g.*, a fox terrier—is selected, and the most striking differences in the brachycephalic and dolichocephalic breeds will be considered in the section on the skull as a whole.

Cranium

The **occipital bone** is similar in position to that of the horse. The crest is prominent, angular, and directed backward. Just below the crest are two rough

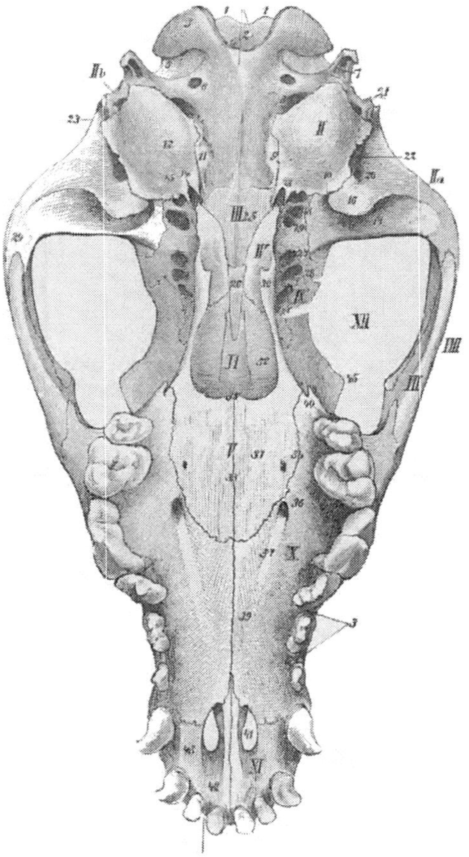

Fig. 122.—Base of Skull of Dog, without Mandible.

I, Occipital; *II*, tympanic part of temporal; *IIa*, squamous part of temporal; *IIb*, mastoid part of temporal; *III*, sphenoid; *IV*, pterygoid; *V*, palate bone; *VI*, vomer; *VII*, malar; *VIII*, zygomatic arch; *IX*, inner wall of orbit; *X*, palatine process of maxilla; *XI*, premaxilla; *XII*, orbital cavity; *1, 1*, tubercles above foramen magnum; *2*, foramen magnum; *3*, occipital condyle; *4*, notch between occipital condyles; *5*, condyloid fossa; *6*, hypoglossal foramen; *7*, paramastoid (styloid, jugular) process; *8*, for. lacerum and posterior opening of carotid canal; *9*, petro-occipital synchondrosis; *10*, petro-tympanic fissure; *11*, tubercle; *12*, bulla ossea; *13*, muscular process of petrous; *14*, carotid foramen; *15*, osseous Eustachian tube; *16*, postglenoid process; *17*, glenoid cavity; *18*, for. ovale; *19*, posterior opening of alar canal; *20*, external opening of parieto-temporal canal; *21*, stylomastoid foramen; *22*, external auditory meatus; *23*, temporal crest; *24*, zygomatic process of temporal bone; *25*, body of postsphenoid; *26*, body of presphenoid; *27*, anterior opening of alar canal; *28*, for. lacerum orbitale; *29*, optic foramen; *30*, hamulus of pterygoid; *31*, horizontal part of palate bone; *32*, perpendicular part of palate bone; *33*, median palatine suture; *34*, palato-maxillary suture; *35*, posterior nasal spine; *36*, anterior palatine foramen; *37*, palatine groove; *38*, alveolar border of maxilla; *39*, palatine process of maxilla; *40*, pterygoid process of maxilla; *41*, palatine fissure; *42*, body of premaxilla; *43*, palatine process of premaxilla; *44*, alveolar border of premaxilla; *45*, supraorbital process of frontal bone. (Ellenberger-Baum, Anat. d. Hundes.)

imprints or tubercles for muscular attachment. The surface below these is convex from side to side and concave from above downward. On either side, at the junction with the squamous, there is a foramen which communicates with the parieto-temporal canal. The condyles are somewhat flattened and are widely separated above; at the inner side of each is a short condyloid canal, which opens into the parieto-temporal canal. The paramastoid processes are very short. The basilar part is wide and joins the bulla ossea on either side; its lower surface is flattened and the tubercles are at the junction with the bulla. The hypoglossal foramen is small and is close to the foramen lacerum posterius; the latter is bounded in front by the bulla ossea, behind and internally by the occipital bone.

The **interparietal bone** fuses with the occipital before birth. It forms the high posterior part of the sagittal crest, and is wedged in between the two parietal bones. The tentorium osseum is thin and curved, concave ventrally. Its base concurs with the occipital and parietal bones in the formation of a transverse canal which is continuous with the parieto-temporal canals.

The **parietal bone** is rhomboid in outline and is strongly curved. It is extensive and forms the greater part of the roof of the cranial cavity. At the junction of the right and left bones there is a prominent sagittal crest which is continued upon the frontal bones. The lower border articulates with the temporal wing of the sphenoid by its anterior part and with the squamous temporal in the remainder of its extent. The external surface enters into the formation of the temporal fossa. The internal surface is marked by digital impressions, and by grooves for the middle meningeal artery and its branches.

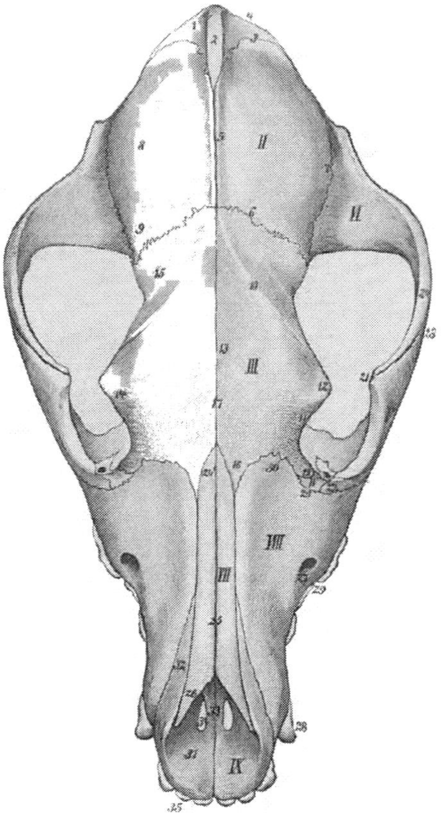

FIG. 123.—SKULL OF DOG, DORSAL VIEW.

I, Occipital; *II*, parietal; *III*, frontal; *IV*, lacrimal; *V*, malar; *VI*, squamous temporal; *VII*, nasal; *VIII*, maxilla; *IX*, premaxilla; *1*, supraoccipital; *2*, interparietal; *3*, parieto-occipital suture; *4*, occipital crest; *5*, sagittal crest; *6*, parieto-frontal suture; *7*, squamous suture; *8*, parietal eminence; *9*, antero-external angle of parietal bone; *10*, frontal crest; *11*, *14*, orbital margin; *12*, supraorbital process; *13*, frontal fossa; *15*, temporal part of frontal bone; *16*, nasal process of frontal bone; *17*, frontal suture; *18*, lacrimal foramen; *19*, maxillary process of frontal bone; *20*, lacrimo-maxillary suture; *21*, frontal process of malar bone; *22*, lacrimal process of malar; *23*, zygomatic process of malar; *24*, zygomatic process of squamous temporal; *24'*, posterior end of nasal bone; *25*, nasal suture; *26*, anterior end of nasal bone; *27*, infraorbital foramen; *28*, canine tooth; *29*, cheek tooth; *30*, frontal process of maxilla; *31*, body, *32*, nasal process, *33*, palatine process of premaxilla; *34*, palatine fissure; *35*, incisor teeth. (Ellenberger-Baum, Anat. d. Hundes.)

The external surface of the **frontal bone** is crossed by a frontal crest, which extends in a curve from the sagittal crest to the supraorbital process, and separates the frontal and temporal parts. The frontal parts of the two bones form a central depression and slope downward and forward. The supraorbital process is very short, so that the orbital margin is incomplete as in the pig. The supraorbital foramen is absent. In front there is a narrow pointed nasal part which fits in between the nasal bone and the maxilla. The orbital and temporal parts are relatively extensive. Two ethmoidal foramina are commonly present. The frontal sinus is confined to the frontal bone.

The parts of the **temporal bone** fuse early. The zygomatic process curves widely outward and forward. Its anterior part is beveled below and articulates extensively with the corresponding process of the malar. The articular surface for the condyle of the mandible consists of a transverse groove which is continued upon the front of the large postglenoid process. Behind the latter is the lower opening of the parieto-temporal canal. There is no condyle. The mastoid part is small, but bears a distinct mastoid process. The external auditory meatus is large and the canal very short, so that one can see into the tympanum in the dry skull. The bulla ossea is very large and is rounded and smooth; the inner side is united to the basioccipital. Above this junction and roofed in by the union of the petrous part and the basioccipital is the **petro-basilar canal** (Canalis petrobasilaris); this transmits a vein from the floor of the cranium to the foramen lacerum posterius. The latter is in reality a depression and is situated behind the bulla ossea. In its posterior part is a foramen which transmits the ninth, tenth, and eleventh cranial nerves. The **carotid canal** branches off from the petrobasilar, passes forward external to it through the inner part of the bulla ossea, and opens in front at the **carotid foramen**; it transmits the internal carotid artery. The Eustachian opening is immediately external to the carotid foramen. The muscular and hyoid processes are extremely rudimentary. The petrous part projects into the cranial cavity and forms a sharp prominent petrosal crest. The inner surface presents a deep **floccular fossa** above the internal auditory meatus. The anterior surface is also free. The anterior angle is perforated by a **canal** for the fifth cranial nerve (Canalis nervi trigemini).

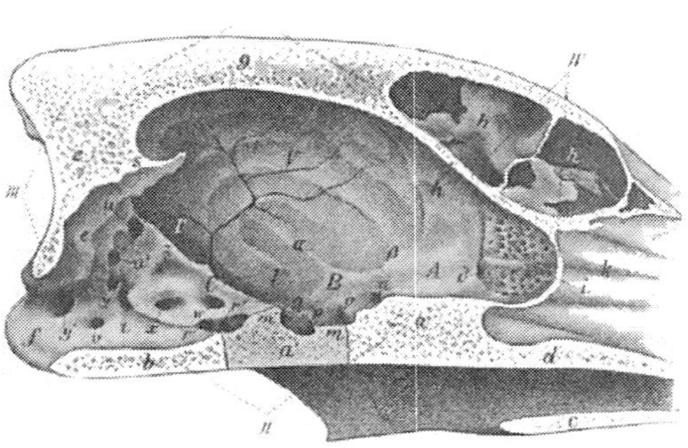

FIG. 124.—CRANIAL CAVITY OF DOG, AS SEEN ON SAGITTAL SECTION OF SKULL.

I, Roof of cranium; *II*, base of cranium; *III*, posterior wall of cranium; *IV*, anterior wall of cranium; *A*, anterior cranial fossa; *B*, middle cranial fossa; *C*, posterior cranial fossa; *a*, body of presphenoid; *a'*, body of postsphenoid; *c*, palate bone; *d*, vomer; *e*, occipital; *f*, occipital condyle; *g*, sagittal crest; *h*, frontal sinus; *h'*, cranial plate of frontal bone; *i*, cribriform plate of ethmoid bone; *i'*, ethmoidal foramen; *k*, ethmoturbinals; *l*, parietal bone; *l'*, *l''*, squamous temporal bone; *l'''*, temporal wing of sphenoid bone; *m*, sella turcica; *m'*, dorsum sellæ; *n*, optic foramen; *o*, foramen lacerum orbitale; *p*, foramen rotundum; *q*, foramen ovale; *r*, *r'*, carotid foramina; *s*, tentorium osseum; *t*, foramen lacerum; *u*, *u'*, orifices of parieto-temporal canal; *v*, condyloid canal; *w*, canal for trigeminal nerve; *x*, internal auditory meatus; *y*, *y'*, orifices of canal for inferior occipital sinus; *z*, floccular fossa. (After Ellenberger, in Leisering's Atlas.)

The body of the **sphenoid bone** is flattened dorso-ventrally. The sella turcica is shallow, but the dorsum sellæ is well developed and bears **posterior clinoid processes**. A pair of **anterior clinoid processes** project back from the roots of the orbital wings. The latter are relatively small and are crossed externally by a crest, which is continued forward upon the palate bone. The temporal wings are extensive and articulate above with the parietals. Perforating the roots of the wings are the following foramina, named from before backward: The optic passes through the orbital wing. The foramen lacerum orbitale is a little lower and is at the junction of the wings. The foramen rotundum opens into the alar canal, which passes through the root of the short but wide pterygoid process. The foramen ovale is near the posterior border of the temporal wing. There is no sphenoidal sinus.

The **ethmoid bone** is highly developed. The cribriform plate is extensive, and the olfactory fossæ are very deep. The crista galli is little developed, and often incomplete. The perpendicular plate is long. The lateral masses are greatly developed and bulge upward into the frontal sinus. There are four large endo-turbinals and six ectoturbinals. The lamina papyracea is extensive and forms the inner wall of the maxillary sinus. Its lower border joins the palatine process of the maxilla and the horizontal part of the palate bone. A shelf-like plate extends inward from its lower part and concurs with the similarly incurved part of the palate bone in forming the **transverse lamina** (Lamina transversalis), which divides the olfactory fundus of the nasal cavity from the naso-pharyngeal meatus.

Face

The **maxilla** is short, but very high posteriorly. The facial crest is absent. The infraorbital foramen is over the alveolus for the third premolar. The **frontal process** fits into a deep notch between the nasal and orbital parts of the frontal bone, and the middle part of the posterior border lies along the orbital margin. There are more or less pronounced ridges, juga alveolaria, over the canine and molar teeth. The zygomatic process is short and thin; it is completely overlapped outwardly by the malar, and is perforated by a number of foramina (Foramina alveolaria). A maxillary tuberosity is not present in the adult, but there is a pointed projection, the pterygoid process, behind the last alveolus. The internal surface bears a short turbinal crest on its anterior part, behind which it is deeply concave and forms the outer wall of the maxillary sinus. The palatine process is short, wide behind, and moderately arched from side to side. The anterior palatine foramen is situated at or close to the transverse palatine suture about midway between the median suture and the alveolar border. The palatine groove is distinct. The large alveolus for the canine tooth is completed by the premaxilla. The small alveolus for the first premolar is separated from the preceding one by a small interval. The next two consist of anterior and posterior parts for the roots of the teeth. The fourth and fifth are much larger and are divided into three parts. The last is small and consists of three divisions. The infraorbital canal is short.

The body of the **premaxilla** is compressed dorso-ventrally, and contains three alveoli for the incisor teeth, which increase in size from first to third; it also completes the inner wall of the large alveolus for the canine tooth. The foramen incisivum is very small except in large skulls. The interalveolar border is wide and very short. The nasal process is wide at its origin and tapers to a sharp point behind; the anterior part curves upward, backward, and a little inward, and forms the lateral margin of the osseous nasal aperture; the posterior part extends backward a long distance between the nasal bone and the maxilla. The palatine process turns upward and outward, forming with its fellow a wide groove for the septal cartilage; the posterior end is pointed and fits into a notch between the palatine processes of the maxillæ, and supports the end of the vomer. The palatine fissure is short but wide.

The horizontal part of the **palate bones** is extensive, forming about one-third of the hard palate. It presents a variable number of lesser palatine foramina. There is usually a pointed posterior nasal spine at the end of the median suture. The palatine canal is sometimes formed entirely in this bone. The perpendicular part is even more extensive. Its external surface is chiefly free and forms most of the inner wall of the large pterygo-palatine fossa. The maxillary foramen is situated in a deep recess between this bone and the zygomatic process of the maxilla. Just above it there is commonly another foramen which opens into the nasal cavity. The posterior palatine and spheno-palatine foramina are situated further back and a little lower; the former is immediately below the latter. A horizontal plate extends from the inner surface, meets that of the opposite bone and completes the lamina transversalis spoken of in the description of the ethmoid bone. There is no palatine sinus.

The **pterygoid bones** are very wide and short. They form a considerable part of the lateral boundaries of the posterior nares. The lower and posterior borders are free and at their angle of junction there is a variable hamulus.

The **nasal bones** are (in most breeds) long and wider in front than behind. The external surface is variably concave in its length and is inclined toward the median suture so as to form a central groove. The inner borders turn downward and form an internal nasal crest which becomes very prominent behind. The posterior parts fit into a notch formed by the frontal bones. The anterior ends form an almost semicircular nasal notch.

The **lacrimal bone** is very small. The facial part extends very little or not at all beyond the orbital margin. The orbital surface is small and triangular, and presents the entrance to the lacrimal canal.

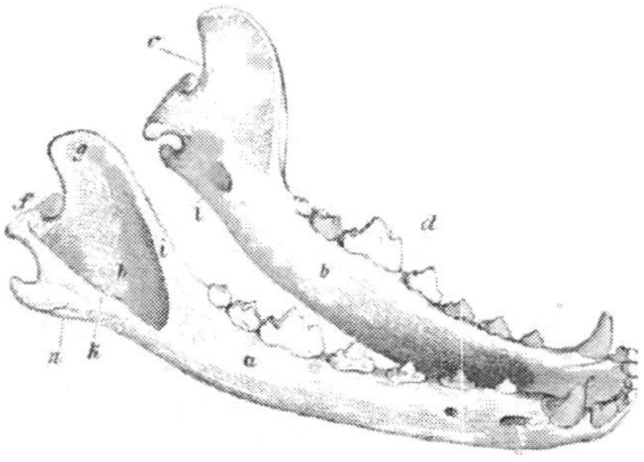

Fig. 125.—Mandible of Dog, Right Anterior View.

a, Right ramus; *b*, left ramus; *c*, body; *d*, alveolar border; *e*, processus angularis; *f*, condyle; *g*, coronoid process; *h*, masseteric fossa; *i*, k, crests which form the upper and lower boundaries of fossa; *l*, mandibular foramen; *m*, mental foramina; *n*, masseteric line; *o*, sigmoid notch. (Ellenberger-Baum, Anat. d. Hundes.)

The large zygomatic process constitutes the bulk of the **malar bone.** It is very long and is strongly curved. The upper border is convex, free in front, where it forms part of the orbital margin, beveled behind for articulation with the similar process of the temporal bone. Between these it bears an eminence, the processus frontalis, to which the orbital ligament is attached. The body of the bone may be considered to consist of a **lacrimal process** directed upward and fitting in between the lacrimal and maxilla, and a **maxillary process** directed downward. The facial surface is convex.

The **superior turbinal bone** is in its anterior part a simple plate, attached by one edge to the nasal bone; it curves downward and inward, and its free border is thickened and everted. The posterior part is wider and resembles the ethmo-turbinals, with which it is connected.

The **inferior turbinal bone** is short and very complex. It is attached to the nasal surface of the maxilla by a basal lamina, which divides into two secondary lamellæ. The latter detach numerous tertiary lamellæ, which are coiled and have thick free edges (Fig. 373).

The **vomer** is not in contact with the posterior part of the floor of the nasal cavity, and does not divide the posterior nares. The posterior end is narrow and deeply notched. Near the posterior nares the two plates curve outward and join the palate bones and assist in forming the lamina transversalis.

The two halves of the **mandible** do not fuse completely even in old age. The body presents six alveoli for the incisor teeth and two for the canines. The incisor alveoli increase in size from first to third. The canine alveoli extend deeply downward and backward. There are usually two or more foramina on the mental surface. The rami diverge less than in the pig. The inferior border of the horizontal part is convex in its length and is thick and rounded. The alveolar border is slightly concave in its length and is a little everted, especially in its middle;

it presents seven alveoli for the lower cheek teeth, which resemble those of the upper jaw except that the fourth and sixth are much smaller and the fifth is like the fourth of the upper series. The interalveolar space is very short or even absent. There are two or three mental foramina on either side. The vertical part is relatively small. Its external surface presents a deep **masseteric fossa** which encroaches on the coronoid process and is limited by ridges in front and below. The internal surface is convex and is marked by the usual foramen. At about the same level as the latter is the rough **angular process** (Processus angularis), which projects backward from the posterior border, and is equivalent to the angle of the other animals. The condyle is placed very low—not much higher than the apex of the canine tooth when the bone is resting on a flat surface. It is long transversely and the inner part of the articular surface is much the wider and extends over the posterior surface. Its long axis is a little oblique, the inner end being inclined somewhat downward and forward. The coronoid process is very extensive and is bent slightly outward and backward.

The body of the hyoid **bone** is a slightly curved transverse rod; it is compressed from before backward, and bears no lingual process. The thyroid cornua are permanently attached to the body by cartilage; they diverge widely, curve inward, and are compressed laterally. The small cornua are short, prismatic, and strong. The middle cornua are commonly a little longer than the great cornua; they are compressed laterally, and are slightly enlarged at the ends, which are joined by cartilage to the adjacent cornua. The great cornua are bent outward and are somewhat twisted.

THE SKULL AS A WHOLE

The different breeds of dog display great variations in the form and size of the skull. Those which have a long narrow skull (*e. g.*, greyhound, collie) are designated **dolichocephalic.** Other dogs (*e. g.*, bulldog, small spaniels, pugs) have very broad, short skulls and are termed **brachycephalic.** Intermediate forms (*e. g.*, fox terrier, dachshund) are **mesaticephalic.**

The length is usually measured from the occipital crest to the anterior end of the premaxillary suture, and the breadth between the summits of the zygomatic arches. The cephalic index is the relation of the breadth to the length, assuming the latter equal 100; the formula is: $\frac{\text{breadth} \times 100}{\text{length}}$ = cephalic index. The index of extreme dolichocephalic breeds is about 50 or even less, as in the greyhound, and that of brachycephalic specimens may be as high as 90, as in the bulldog and pugs. Among the mesaticephalic types are the fox terrier, with an index of about 70, and the white Pomeranian, with one about 72 to 75. The cranio-facial index is the relation of the distance from the occipital crest to the fronto-nasal suture to that between the latter and the nasal notch. It varies from 10 : 3 in extreme brachycephalic breeds to 10 : 7 in extreme dolichocephalic subjects.

The **superior surface** shows the wide outward curve of the zygomatic arches, and the great extent of the temporal fossæ. The latter are separated by the sagittal crest, which in the larger breeds is very strong and prominent, and is continued by the diverging frontal ridges to the supraorbital processes. The frontal and nasal regions are centrally depressed, and are more or less concave in profile. The nasal region is narrow and is terminated in front by a nasal notch. In the extreme brachycephalic breeds the differences are very striking. The cranium is strongly convex in both directions and is considerably longer than the face. The sagittal crest is more or less effaced and is formed by the interparietal only. The parieto-frontal crests are separated by an interval behind and diverge to the supraorbital processes, so that the temporal fossæ are widely separated. The frontal region is wide, strongly convex, and has a shallow central depression. The nasal region is very short, relatively wide, and centrally depressed. In profile there is a marked depression at the fronto-nasal junction, producing what is termed by fanciers the "stop" of the face.

On the **lateral surface** the great extent of the temporal fossa is seen. The orbit communicates freely with the fossa, the posterior part of the orbital margin being absent in the dry skull. The axis of the orbital cavity forms a much smaller angle with the median plane than in the horse and ox. A distinct crest marks the limit between the orbital cavity proper and the extensive pterygo-palatine fossa. The preorbital region is somewhat triangular, concave in its length, and convex from above downward. The infraorbital foramen is on its lower part above the third cheek tooth. In extreme brachycephalic breeds the orbit is relatively very large and the preorbital region extremely short but high. In the bulldog the lower jaw protrudes beyond the upper—a condition known as prognathism. The opposite condition, brachygnathism, is seen in the dachshund.

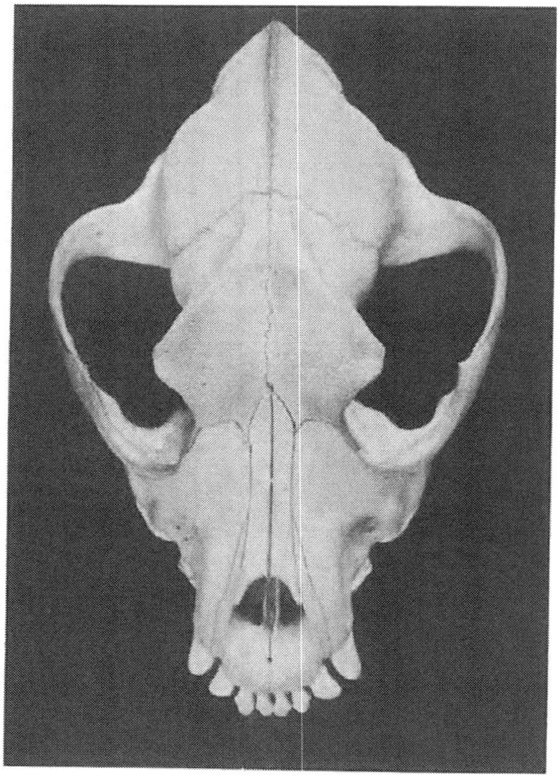

FIG. 126.—SKULL OF BRACHYCEPHALIC DOG, DORSAL VIEW WITHOUT MANDIBLE.

Striking features on the **basal surface** of the cranium are the width and flatness of the basioccipital, the small size of the paramastoid processes, the large size and rounded shape of the bulla ossea, and the grooved form of the articular surfaces for the mandible. The posterior nares are long and narrow and are not divided by the vomer. The hard palate is usually about half the length of the skull. It is commonly marked by a median crest or rough line, and on each side are the anterior and accessory palatine foramina and the palatine grooves. The width is greatest between the fourth pair of cheek teeth, and here there is in most skulls a pronounced depression on either side. The length, width, and contour vary greatly in different breeds.

The angle of divergence of the rami of the mandible varies from 25 to 30 degrees; it is smallest in the greyhound, largest in extreme brachycephalic types, *e. g.*, bulldog, pug.

The **posterior** or **nuchal surface** is somewhat triangular, with the base below. The summit is formed by the occipital crest, which projects very strongly backward in the large breeds. Below it there are two very distinct rough imprints for muscular attachment. In some skulls there is a thin median crest, in others a rounded elevation. Laterally are the temporal crests and the mastoid processes.

There is usually a foramen in the temporo-occipital suture above the root of the paramastoid process. The foramen magnum varies greatly in form; most often the transverse diameter is the greater, but in some skulls it is equaled or exceeded by the vertical diameter.

The **cranial cavity** (Fig. 124) corresponds in form and size with the cranium, specially in those breeds in which the various crests are more or less effaced and the frontal sinuses are small. The basi-cranial axis is almost parallel with the palate, and the floor is flattened. The anterior fossa is narrow and is only slightly higher than the middle one. The olfactory fossæ are very deep and the crista galli is little developed. The sella turcica is variable in depth, and the dorsum sellæ is relatively high and bears clinoid processes laterally. The cerebral and cerebellar compartments are well marked off laterally by the petrosal crests and above by the tentorium osseum. The base of the latter is traversed by a canal which connects the two parieto-temporal canals. The anterior angle of the petrous temporal is perforated by a canal for the fifth cranial nerve.

The **nasal cavity** (Fig. 373) conforms to the shape of the face. Its anterior

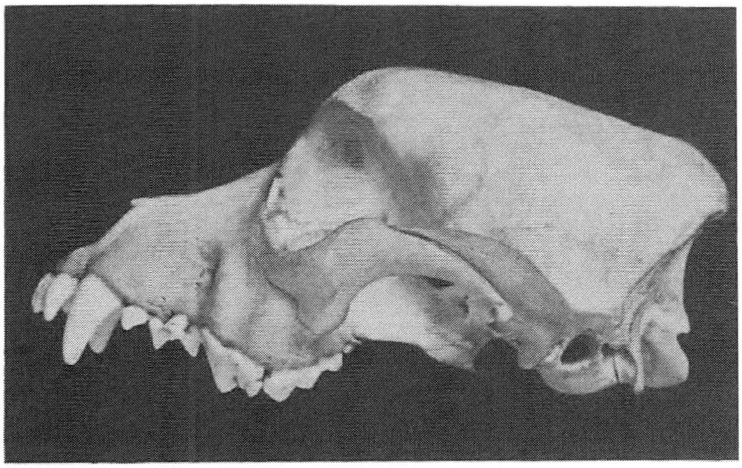

Fig. 127.—Skull of Brachycephalic Dog, Lateral View without Mandible.

aperture is large and nearly circular in most dogs. The complex inferior turbinals occupy the anterior part of the cavity to a large extent, except near the aperture. Behind the inferior turbinals is the large opening of the maxillary sinus. Behind this the cavity is divided by a horizontal plate (Lamina transversalis) into a large upper olfactory region or fundus nasi and a lower naso-pharyngeal canal. The fundus is occupied largely by the ethmoturbinals. The posterior nares are undivided and are in general long and narrow, but vary with the shape of the skull.

The **frontal sinus** is of considerable size in the large breeds, but is confined to the frontal bone. It is usually divided into a small anterior and a much larger posterior compartment, each of which opens into the superior ethmoidal meatus. The sinus is very small in extreme brachycephalic types.

The **maxillary sinus** is small, and is in such free communication with the nasal cavity as to make it rather a recess than a true sinus. It is bounded internally by the lamina papyracea of the ethmoid, and its outer wall is crossed obliquely by the lacrimal canal. The roots of the molar teeth do not project up into it.

BONES OF THORACIC LIMB

The **clavicle** is a small, thin, irregularly-triangular bony or cartilaginous plate. It is embedded in the mastoido-humeralis muscle in front of the shoulder-joint and forms no articulation with the rest of the skeleton. (It is nearly an inch long in a large cat and is a slender curved rod.)

The **scapula** is relatively long and narrow. The spine increases gradually in height from above downward and divides the external surface into two nearly equal fossæ. Its free edge is thick and rough above, and at the lower part is thin and bent backward. The **acromion** is short and blunt and is opposite the rim of the glenoid cavity. The subscapular fossa is very shallow and is marked by rough lines. The rough area above it for the attachment of the serratus magnus is large and quadrilateral in front, narrow and marginal behind. The anterior border is thin, strongly convex, and sinuous. The posterior border is straight and thick. The vertebral border is convex and thick and bears a band of cartilage. The cervical angle is rounded. The dorsal angle is thick and square. The neck is well defined and bears a rough eminence posteriorly. The glenoid cavity is continued

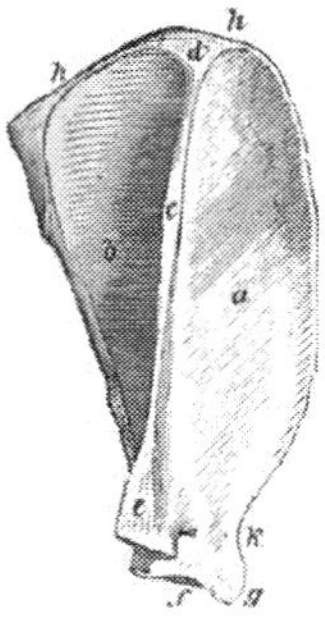

FIG. 128.—RIGHT SCAPULA OF DOG, EXTERNAL VIEW.
a, Supraspinous fossa; *b*, infraspinous fossa; *c*, spine; *d*, upper broad end of spine; *e*, acromion; *f*, glenoid cavity; *g*, tuberosity; *h*, vertebral border; *i*, posterior angle; k, scapular notch. (Ellenberger-Baum, Anat. d. Hundes.)

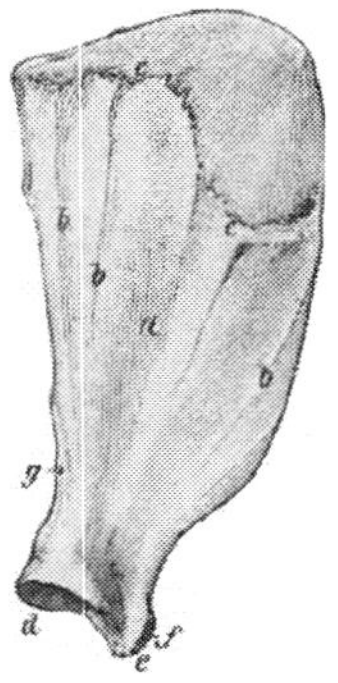

FIG. 129.—LEFT SCAPULA OF DOG, COSTAL SURFACE.
a, Subscapular fossa; *b*, *b*, *b*, muscular lines; *c*, *c*, limiting line between subscapular fossa and serratus area; *d*, glenoid cavity; *e*, *f*, tuberosity; *g*, nutrient foramen. (Ellenberger-Baum, Anat. d. Hundes.)

forward upon the lower face of the scapular tuberosity, which is blunt and bears no distinct coracoid process. There is a rough eminence on the posterior surface of the neck, from which the long head of the triceps arises. The cervical angle is opposite the first thoracic spine, the dorsal angle lies above the vertebral end of the fourth rib, and the articular angle at a point just in front of the sternal end of the first rib in the ordinary standing position. The shoulder has a great range of movement on the chest wall.

The **humerus** is relatively very long, rather slender, and has a slight spiral twist. The shaft is somewhat compressed laterally, especially in its upper two-thirds; this part is curved in varying degree, convex in front. The deltoid tuberosity has the form of a low ridge, and it is continued by a crest which runs upward and backward and bears a tubercle on its upper part. Another line runs from it down the anterior aspect and forms the inner boundary of the very shallow musculo-spiral groove. The nutrient foramen is about in the middle of the posterior surface. A slight elevation on the proximal third of the inner surface represents the teres tubercle. The head is long and strongly curved from before backward.

The neck is better marked than in the horse. The undivided external tuberosity is placed well forward and extends little above the level of the head. The internal tuberosity is small. The bicipital groove is undivided and is displaced to the inner side by the extension forward of the external tuberosity. The distal end bears an oblique trochlear articular surface for articulation with the radius and ulna, the outer part of which is the more extensive and is faintly grooved. The epicondyles are prominent. The coronoid and olecranon fossæ often communicate through a large **supratrochlear foramen.**

The two bones of the forearm are relatively long and articulate with each other at either end in such a manner as to allow of slight movement. A narrow interosseous space separates their shafts. The **radius** is flattened from before backward and increases in size from above downward. The shaft forms two curves; one of these, an anterior convexity, involves the whole shaft; the other,

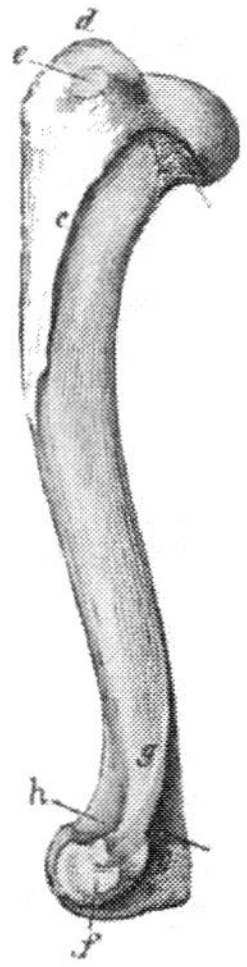

FIG. 130.—LEFT HUMERUS OF DOG EXTERNAL VIEW.

a, Head; *b*, neck; *c*, crest; *d*, external tuberosity; *e*, mark for insertion of infraspinatus tendon; *f*, external condyle; *g*, external condyloid crest; *h*, coronoid fossa; *i*, olecranon fossa. (Ellenberger-Baum, Anat. d. Hundes.)

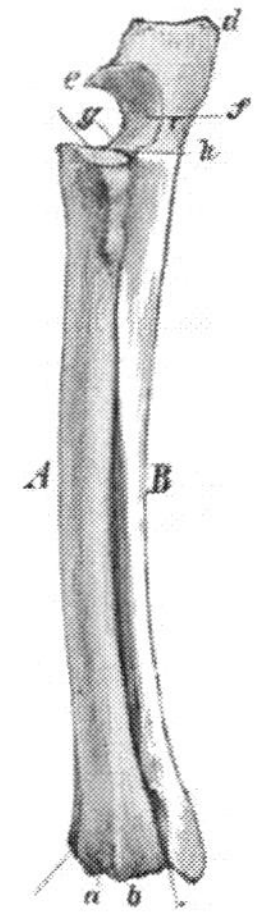

FIG. 131.—LEFT RADIUS AND ULNA OF DOG ANTERO-EXTERNAL VIEW.

A, Radius; *B*, ulna; *a*, groove for tendon of extensor carpi radialis; *b*, groove for common extensor tendon; *c*, proximal articular surface of radius; *d*, olecranon; *e*, beak (proc. anconeus) of ulna; *f*, semilunar notch; *g*, coronoid process; *h*, facet for radius; *i*, groove for lateral extensor tendon; k, groove for tendon of extensor carpi obliquus. (Ellenberger-Baum, Anat. d. Hundes.)

an inner convexity, affects the upper part. The anterior surface is convex in both directions and is marked by a groove for the oblique extensor of the carpus. The posterior surface presents the nutrient foramen in its upper third, and bears a rough line (Crista interossea) externally for the attachment of the interosseous ligament. The proximal end (Capitulum radii) is relatively small and is supported by a distinct neck (Collum radii). It bears a concave surface (Fovea capituli) above for articulation with the humerus, and a convex marginal area (Circumferentia articularis) behind for the ulna. The bicipital tuberosity is small. There is a large external tuberosity and below this a rough eminence. The distal extremity is much wider. It has an extensive concave carpal articular surface. Its inner border projects downward, forming the **styloid process** of the radius. Externally there is a concave facet (Incisura ulnaris radii) for the ulna. In front are three distinct grooves for the extensor tendons. The **ulna** is well developed, but diminishes in size from above downward. It crosses the posterior surface of the radius from within outward. The shaft is large and three-sided in its upper two-thirds, smaller and more rounded below. Its anterior surface is in general rough. The nutrient foramen is near the proximal end. A vascular groove descends from it and indicates the course of the interosseous artery. The proximal end is relatively short. It is concave and smooth internally, convex and rough externally. The olecranon is grooved and bears three prominences, of which the posterior one is large and rounded. The semilunar notch is wide below and completes the surface for articulation with the trochlea of the humerus. Below it is a concave surface (Incisura radialis) which articulates with the back of the head of the radius, and below this is a fossa, which receives a tuberosity of the radius. The distal end (Capitulum ulnæ) is small and is produced to a blunt point (Processus styloideus ulnæ). It articulates with the ulnar carpal below, and has a convex facet on its antero-internal aspect for the radius.

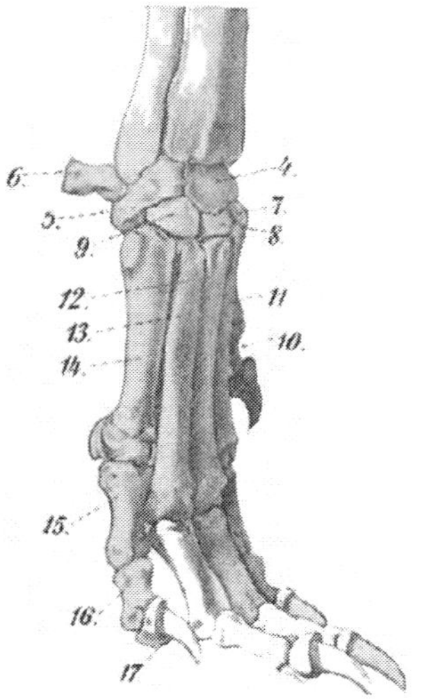

FIG. 132.—SKELETON OF DISTAL PART OF THORACIC LIMB OF DOG, EXTERNAL VIEW.

4, Radial + intermediate carpal bone; *5*, ulnar carpal; *6*, accessory carpal; *7*, second carpal; *8*, third carpal; *9*, fourth carpal; *10–14*, first to fifth metacarpals; *15*, first phalanx; *16*, second phalanx; *17*, third phalanx. (After Leisering's Atlas.)

The **carpus** comprises seven bones, three in the proximal row and four in the distal. The numerical reduction in the upper row is apparently due to the fusion of the radial and intermediate, constituting a large bone which articulates with almost all of the distal surface of the radius and with the bones of the lower row. It projects prominently on the posterior surface of the carpus. The ulnar carpal is long; it articulates with the radius and ulna above and the accessory behind; below it rests on the fourth carpal and is prolonged downward to articulate with the fifth metacarpal also. The accessory is cylindrical, constricted in its middle and enlarged at each end; the anterior extremity articulates with the ulna and ulnar carpal bone. The first carpal is the smallest bone of the lower row; it articulates with the second carpal externally and the first metacarpal distally. The second carpal is wedge-shaped, the base being posterior; its upper surface is convex, and its lower is concave and rests on the second metacarpal. The third carpal is somewhat like the second; its lower surface is concave and articulates chiefly with the third metacarpal. The fourth carpal is the largest of the row; it articulates with the fourth and fifth metacarpals below. Two small bones or cartilages may be found at the junction of the two rows behind, and a third small bone articulates with the inner side of the radio-intermediate.[1]

Five **metacarpal** bones are present. The first is much the shortest; the third and fourth are the longest, and are about one-fifth longer than the second and fifth. The fifth is the widest at the proximal end and is slightly shorter than the second. They are close together above, but diverge somewhat below; the first is separated from the second by a considerable interosseous space. They are so arranged as to form a convex dorsal surface, and a concave volar surface, which corresponds to the hollow of the palm of the hand in man. Each consists of a shaft and two extremities. The shaft is compressed from before backward. In the third and fourth it

[1] This third bone was termed the phacoid in the cat by Strauss-Durckeim, and is regarded by some authors as the vestige of an additional digit, the prepollex.

is almost four-sided, in the second and fifth three-sided, in the first rounded. The proximal ends (Bases) articulate with each other and with the corresponding carpal bones. The carpal articular surface formed by them is concave from side to side, convex from before backward. The distal ends (Capitula) have articular surfaces of the nature of a head, but bear a sagittal ridge behind, except the first, which is grooved.

The five **digits** have three phalanges each, except the first, which has two. The third and fourth digits are the longest; the first is very short and does not come in contact with the ground in walking. The first **phalanges** of the chief digits have four-sided shafts, which are slightly curved forward. The proximal end of each has a concave surface for articulation with the metacarpal bone and is deeply notched behind. The distal end has a trochlea for articulation with the second phalanx, and lateral depressions for ligamentous attachment. The **second phalanges** are about two-thirds of the length of the first phalanges. The proximal articular surface consists of two cavities separated by a sagittal ridge. The distal extremity is wider and flatter than that of the first. The **third phalanges** correspond in general to the form of the claws. The base has an articular surface adapted to the second phalanx and is encircled by a collar of bone. The volar surface bears a wing or tuberosity, and on either side of this is a foramen. The ungual part is a curved rod with a blunt-pointed free end. It is rough and porous. Its base forms with the collar previously mentioned a deep groove, into which the proximal border of the claw is received. The two phalanges of the first digit resemble in arrangement the first and third phalanges of the other digits.

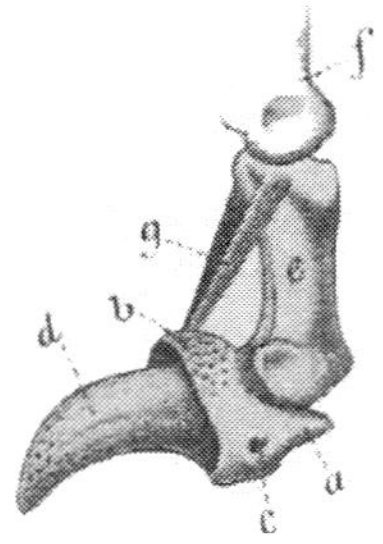

FIG. 133.—SECOND AND THIRD PHALANGES OF DOG.

a, Wing of third phalanx; *b*, coronary ridge; *c*, foramen for digital artery; *d*, ungual surface of third phalanx; *e*, second phalanx; *f*, first phalanx; *g*, elastic dorsal ligaments. (From Leisering's Atlas.)

Nine volar **sesamoids** are usually present. Two are found at each metacarpo-phalangeal joint of the chief digits. They are high and narrow, articulate with the distal end of the metacarpal bone in front, and have a small facet on the base for the first phalanx. On this joint of the first digit there is usually a single flattened sesamoid, but exceptionally two are present. The distal volar sesamoids remain cartilaginous. A nodular dorsal **sesamoid** occurs in the anterior part of the capsule of the metacarpo-phalangeal joints, and cartilaginous nodules are found in a similar position in connection with the joints between the first and second phalanges.

BONES OF THE PELVIC LIMB

The **ilium** is nearly parallel with the median plane and its axis is only slightly oblique with regard to the horizontal plane. The gluteal surface is concave. The iliac surface is almost flat. The auricular surface faces almost directly inward, and in front of it there is an extensive rough area. The ilio-pectineal line is very distinct and is uninterrupted. The anterior border or crest is strongly convex, thick, and rough. The internal angle is represented by a thickened part which bears two eminences, homologous with the posterior superior and posterior inferior iliac spines of man. The external angle also has two prominences, which are equivalent to the two anterior spines present in man. The shaft is almost sagittal and is compressed laterally. Above it is smooth and rounded, and below it bears a crest externally which terminates at a tuberosity in front of the acetabulum.

The **ischium** has a twisted appearance owing to the fact that its acetabular part is nearly sagittal while the posterior part is almost horizontal. The two bones also diverge behind and the tubera are flattened and everted. The superior ischiatic spine is low and thick; its posterior part is marked by transverse grooves

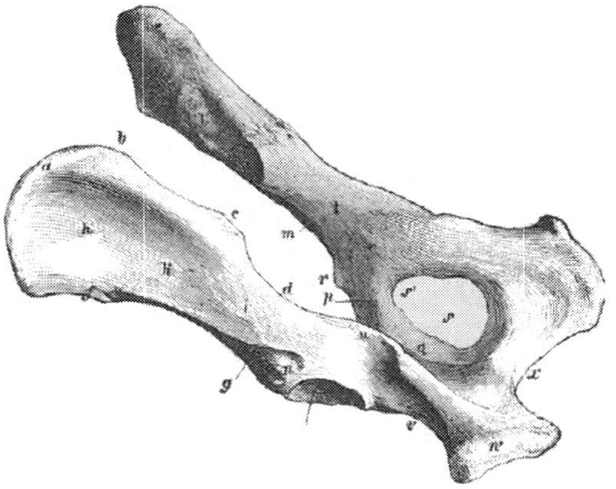

FIG. 134.—OSSA COXARUM OF DOG, LEFT POSTERIOR VIEW.

a, Crest; *b*, *c*, internal angle; *d*, great sciatic notch; *e*, *f*, external angle; *g*, posterior gluteal line; *h*, gluteal fossa of wing; *i*, shaft of ilium; k, anterior gluteal line; *l*, auricular surface; *m*, ilio-pectineal line; *n*, depression for origin of rectus femoris; *o*, acetabulum; *p*, acetabular, and *q*, symphyseal branch of pubis; *r*, psoas tubercle; *s*, obturator foramen; *s'*, obturator notch; *t*, line for origin of coccygeus; *u*, superior ischiatic spine; *v*, external border of ischium; *w*, tuber ischii; *x*, ischial arch. (Ellenberger-Baum, Anat. d. Hundes.)

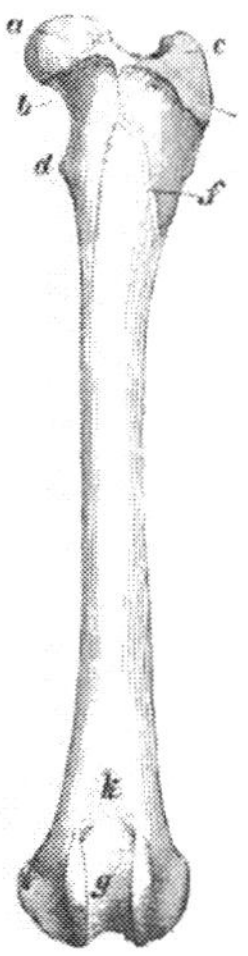

FIG. 135.—LEFT FEMUR OF DOG, ANTERIOR VIEW.

a, Head; *b*, neck; *c*, trochanter major; *d*, trochanter minor; *e*, rudimentary trochanter tertius; *f*, rough line; *g*, trochlea; *h*, *i*, condyles; k, suprapatellar fossa. (Ellenberger-Baum, Anat. d. Hundes.)

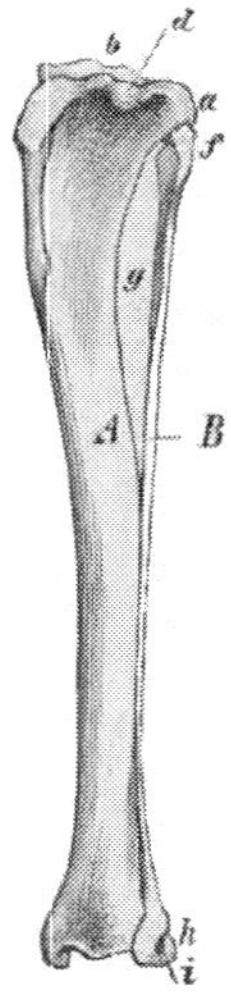

FIG. 136.—LEFT TIBIA AND FIBULA OF DOG, ANTERO-EXTERNAL VIEW.

A, Tibia; *B*, fibula; *a*, external condyle of tibia; *b*, spine; *c*, crest of tibia; *d*, muscular notch; *e*, internal malleolus; *f*, head of fibula; *g*, interosseous space; *h*, external malleolus (distal end of fibula); *i*, groove for tendon. (Ellenberger-Baum, Anat. d. Hundes.)

and has a prominent outer lip. There is no lesser sciatic notch. The ischial arch is relatively small and is semi-elliptical.

The symphyseal part of the **pubis** is thick and fuses late with the opposite bone. There is no subpubic groove.

The **acetabulum** is about twice as far from the external angle of the ilium as from the tuber ischii. The fossa acetabuli is deep, and is bounded internally by a flat plate of bone; its floor is so thin as to be translucent. There is a small notch behind.

The **obturator foramen** resembles in outline an equilateral triangle with the angles rounded off.

The inlet of the **pelvis** is very oblique. It is almost circular in the female, but in the male it is elliptical and the conjugate diameter is the longer. The cavity is narrowest between the acetabula, and very wide behind. The floor is concave and relatively narrow in front, wide and flat behind.

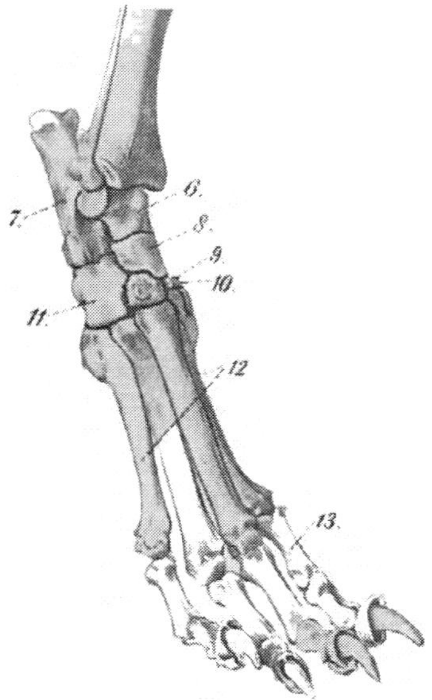

FIG. 137.—SKELETON OF DISTAL PART OF PELVIC LIMB OF DOG, EXTERNAL VIEW.

6, Tibial tarsal bone; *7*, fibular tarsal; *8*, central tarsal; *9*, second tarsal; *10*, third tarsal; *11*, fourth tarsal; *12*, metatarsal bones; *13*, first phalanx. The first tarsal bone is not visible in the figure. (After Leisering's Atlas.)

The **femur** is relatively much longer than in the horse or ox. The shaft is regularly cylindrical, except near the extremities, where it is wider and compressed from before backward. It is strongly curved in its lower two-thirds, convex in front. The posterior surface is flattened transversely, narrow in the middle, and widens toward each end. It is bounded by two rough lines (Labium laterale, mediale) which diverge toward the extremities. The third trochanter and the plantar (supracondyloid) fossa are absent. There are two supracondyloid crests, the inner one being small. The nutrient foramen is in the upper third of the posterior surface. The head is a little more than a hemisphere and has a shallow depression behind and external to its center. The neck is well defined. The trochanter major does not extend as high as the head; a thick ridge runs from its anterior surface to the neck. The internal trochanter has the form of a blunt tuberosity. The trochanteric fossa is round and deep. The ridges of the trochlea are practically sagittal in direction and are almost similar. The intercondyloid fossa is wide. Just above each condyle posteriorly there is a facet for articulation with the sesamoid (of Vesal), which is developed in the origin of the gastrocnemius muscle.

The **tibia** is about the same length as the femur. The shaft forms a double curve; the upper part is convex internally, the lower part externally. The proximal third is prismatic, but is compressed laterally and is long from before backward. The remainder is almost regularly cylindrical. The crest is short but very prominent. The nutrient foramen is usually in the upper third of the external border. The tuberosity is not grooved, but bears a distinct mark where the ligamentum patellæ is attached. There is a small facet for the fibula on the postero-external part of the external condyle, and a small sesamoid bone in the tendon of origin of the popliteus is in contact with the posterior angle of the latter. The distal end is quadrangular and relatively small. The articular grooves and ridge are almost sagittal. There is a facet externally for articulation with the fibula. There is a vertical groove internally and a shallower one behind—both for tendons.

The **fibula** extends the entire length of the region. It is slender, somewhat twisted, and enlarged at either end. The upper part of the shaft is separated from the tibia by a considerable interosseous space, but the lower part is flattened and closely applied to the tibia. The proximal end is flattened and articulates with the external condyle of the tibia. The distal end is somewhat thicker and forms the external malleolus. It articulates internally with the tibia and the tibial tarsal bone. Externally it bears two tubercles.

The **patella** is long and narrow. The anterior surface is convex in both directions. The articular surface is convex from side to side and slightly concave from above downward.

The **tarsus** comprises seven bones. The tibial tarsal consists of a body, neck, and head, like the bone in man. The body presents a trochlea above for articulation with the tibia and fibula. The posterior surface has three facets for articulation with the fibular tarsal bone. The head is directed a little inward and articulates with the central. The fibular tarsal has a long anterior process or "beak," but the inner process (sustentaculum) is short. The tuber calcis is grooved from before backward. The central has a concave proximal surface adapted to the head of the tibial tarsal. Its distal surface articulates with the first, second, and third tarsals. It bears two tubercles posteriorly. The first tarsal is flattened and irregularly quadrangular; it articulates above with the central and below with the first metatarsal. The second tarsal is the smallest and is wedge-shaped; it articulates below with the second metatarsal bone. The third tarsal is also wedge-shaped, the base being in front; it articulates with the third metatarsal below. The fourth tarsal is remarkably high, and resembles a quadrangular prism; it articulates with the fibular tarsal above, the fourth and fifth metatarsal below, and the central and third tarsal bones internally. A groove for the tendon of the peroneus longus crosses its outer and posterior surface, and above it are one or two tubercles.

Five **metatarsal bones** are present. The first is commonly very small and has the form of a blunt cone, somewhat compressed laterally. It articulates with the first tarsal and furnishes insertion to the tibialis anterior muscle. In some cases it fuses with the first tarsal; when the first digit is well developed, its metatarsal may resemble the others (except in size) or be reduced in its proximal part to a fibrous band. The other metatarsals are a little longer than the corresponding metacarpals. Their proximal ends are elongated from before backward and have posterior projections, which in the case of the third and fourth usually bear facets for articulation with two small rounded sesamoid bones. In other respects they resemble the metacarpals.

The first digit is often absent. When present, its development varies and it contains one or two phalanges. In other cases the digit is double. The phalanges of the other digits resemble those of the fore limb.

ARTHROLOGY

THE ARTICULATIONS OR JOINTS

An **articulation** or joint is formed by the union of two or more bones or cartilages by other tissue. Bone is the fundamental part of most joints; in some cases a bone and a cartilage, or two cartilages, form a joint. The uniting medium is chiefly fibrous tissue or cartilage, or a mixture of these. Union of parts of the skeleton by muscles (Synsarcosis), as in the attachment of the thoracic limb in the horse, will not be considered in this section.

Joints may be classified—(*a*) anatomically, according to their mode of development, the nature of the uniting media, and the form of the joint surfaces; (*b*) physiologically, with regard to the amount and kind of movement or the absence of mobility in them; (*c*) by a combination of the foregoing considerations.

The classification of joints is still in a very unsatisfactory state, and, unfortunately, the same term is used in various senses by different authors. The two main subdivisions proposed by Hepburn are: (1) Those in which the uniting medium is coextensive with the opposed joint surfaces, and in which a direct union of these surfaces is thereby effected. (2) Those in which the uniting medium has undergone interruption in its structural continuity, and in which a cavity of greater or less extent is thus formed in the interior of the joint. This distinction is of considerable importance clinically.

Three chief subdivisions of joints are usually recognized—viz., **synarthroses, diarthroses,** and **amphiarthroses.**

SYNARTHROSES

In this group the segments are united by fibrous tissue or cartilage, or a mixture of the two in such a manner as practically to preclude movement; hence they are often termed fixed or immovable joints. There is no joint cavity. Many of these joints are temporary, the uniting medium being invaded by the process of ossification, with a resulting ankylosis or synostosis. The chief classes in this group of joints are as follows:

(1) **Suture.**—This term (Sutura) is applied to those joints in the skull in which the adjacent bones are closely united by fibrous tissue—the sutural ligament. In many cases the edges of the bones have irregular interlocking margins, forming the **sutura serrata,** *e. g.*, the frontal suture. In others the edges are beveled and overlap, forming the **sutura squamosa,** *e. g.*, the parieto-temporal suture. If the edges are plane or slightly roughened, the term **sutura harmonia** is applied to the joint, *e. g.*, the nasal suture.

(2) **Synchondrosis.**—In these the two bones are united by cartilage, *e. g.*, the joint between the basioccipital and the sphenoid bone. Very few of these joints are permanent.

(3) **Symphysis.**—This term is usually limited to a few median joints which connect symmetrical parts of the skeleton, *e. g.*, symphysis pelvis, symphysis mandibulæ. The uniting media are cartilage and fibrous tissue. In some cases a cleft-like rudimentary joint cavity occurs.

(4) **Gomphosis.**—This term is applied to the implantation of the teeth in the alveoli.

DIARTHROSES

These joints are characterized by the presence of a joint cavity and by their mobility. They are often called movable or true joints. The structures which enter into their formation are:

1. The **joint surfaces** (Facies articulares), which are usually more or less expanded. They are in most cases smooth, and vary much in form. They are formed of specially dense bone, which differs histologically from ordinary compact substance. In certain cases (*vide* Osteology) the surface is interrupted by non-articular cavities known as **synovial fossæ.**

2. The **articular cartilages** (Cartilagines articulares), usually hyaline in type, form a covering over the articular surfaces of the bones. They vary in thickness in different joints; they are thickest on the areas of the greatest pressure, and usually tend to accentuate the curvature of the bone, *i. e.*, on a concave surface the peripheral part is the thickest, while on a convex surface the central part is the thickest. The articular cartilages are non-vascular, very smooth, and have a bluish tinge in the fresh state. They diminish the effects of concussion and greatly reduce friction.

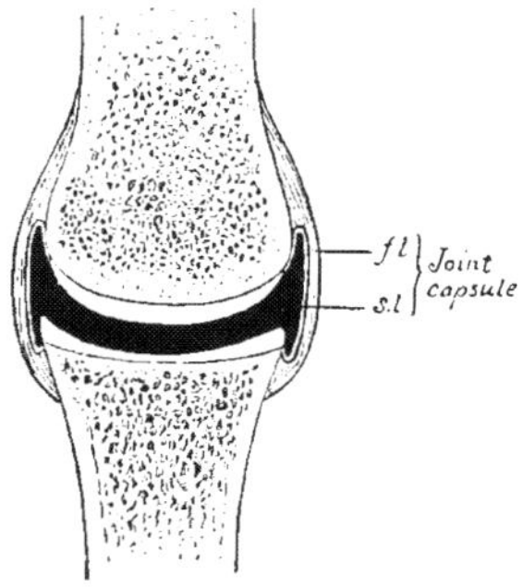

Fig. 138.—Diagram of Section of Diarthrosis.

f.l., Fibrous layer, *s.l.*, synovial layer of joint capsule. The articular cartilages are white, bones dotted, and the joint cavity black in the figure.

3. The **joint capsule** (Capsula articularis) is, in its simplest form, a sac, the margins of which are attached around the articulating surfaces. It consists of two layers—an external one, composed of fibrous tissue (Stratum fibrosum), and an internal one, the synovial layer or membrane (Stratum synoviale). The **fibrous layer,** sometimes termed the capsular ligament, is attached either close to the margins of the articular surfaces or at a variable distance from them. Its thickness varies greatly in different situations: in certain places it is extremely thick, and sometimes cartilage or bone develops in it; in other places it is practically absent, the capsule then consisting only of the synovial membrane. Parts of the capsule may undergo thickening and so form ligaments, which are not separable, except artificially, from the rest of the capsule. The **synovial layer** lines the joint cavity except where this is bounded by the articular cartilages; it stops normally at the margin of the latter. It is a thin membrane, and is richly supplied by close networks of vessels and nerves. It frequently forms **folds** (Plicæ synoviales) and **villi** (Villi synoviales), which project into the cavity of the joint. The folds commonly contain pads of fat which fill up interstices and vary in form and position in various phases of movement. The synovial membrane secretes a fluid, the **synovia,** which resembles white-of-egg and lubricates the joint.[1] In many places the membrane forms extra-articular pouches, which facilitate the play of muscles and tendons.

The **joint cavity** (Cavum articulare) is inclosed by the synovial membrane and the articular cartilages. Normally, it is, strictly speaking, only a potential cavity, which contains nothing but a small amount of synovia.

The student must guard against a false conception of the joint cavity which may result from dissections and diagrams, in which an actual cavity of considerable extent appears to exist. A correct idea of the intimate apposition of the parts is best obtained from the study of frozen sections. It is also instructive to examine joints which have been injected so as to distend the capsule fully. It is then seen that the cavity is often of much greater potential extent than

[1] It is doubtful whether the synovia is a true secretion or a transudate containing products of friction. The view given above is that which is more commonly accepted.

one might suppose, and that the capsule is often very irregular in form, *i. e.*, forms a variety of sacculations.

The foregoing are constant and necessary features in all diarthroses. Other structures which enter into the formation of these joints are ligaments, articular discs or menisci, and marginal cartilages.

4. **Ligaments.**—These are strong bands or membranes, usually composed of white, fibrous tissue, which bind the bones together. They are pliable, but practically inelastic. In a few cases, however, *e. g.*, ligamenta flava, ligamentum nuchæ, they are composed of elastic tissue. They may be subdivided, according to position, into **periarticular** and **intraarticular.** Periarticular ligaments are frequently blended with or form part of the fibrous capsule; in other cases they are quite distinct. Strictly speaking, intraarticular ligaments, though within the fibrous capsule, are not in the joint cavity; the synovial membrane is reflected over them. The term seems justifiable, however, on practical grounds. Ligaments which connect directly opposed surfaces of bones are termed interosseous. The special names are based usually on their position, form, and attachments, *e. g.*, lateral or collateral, cruciate, sacro-iliac, etc. In many places muscles, tendons, and thickenings of the fasciæ function as ligaments and increase the security of the joint. Atmospheric pressure and cohesion play a considerable part in keeping the joint surfaces in apposition.

5. **Articular discs** or **menisci** are plates of fibro-cartilage or dense fibrous tissue placed between the articular cartilages, and divide the joint cavity partially or completely into two compartments. They render certain surfaces congruent, *e. g.*, femoro-tibial joint, allow greater range or variety of movement, and diminish concussion.

6. A **marginal cartilage** (Labrum glenoidale) is a ring of fibro-cartilage which encircles the rim of an articular cavity. It enlarges the cavity and tends to prevent fracture of the margin.

Vessels and Nerves.—The **arteries** form anastomoses around the larger joints, and give off branches to the extremities of the bones and to the joint capsule. The synovial membrane has a close-meshed network of capillaries; the latter form loops around the margins of the articular cartilages, but do not usually enter them. The **veins** form plexuses. The synovial membrane is also well supplied with lymphatics. Nerve-fibers are especially numerous in and around the synovial membrane and there are special nerve-endings, *e. g.*, Pacinian bodies and the articular end-bulbs described by Krause.

Movements.—The movements of a joint are determined chiefly by the form and extent of the joint surfaces and the arrangement of the ligaments. They are usually classified as follows:

1. **Gliding.**—This refers to the sliding of one practically plane surface on another, as in the joints between the articular processes of the cervical vertebræ.

2. **Angular Movements.**—In these cases there is movement around one or more axes. Motion which diminishes the angle included by the segments forming the joint is termed **flexion,** while that which tends to bring the segments into line with each other is called **extension.**

With reference to the joints of the lower parts of the limbs, it seems advisable to employ the terms **dorsal** and **volar** or **plantar flexion,** since these joints can be "overextended." Similarly, the terms **dorsal** and **ventral flexion** should be applied to the corresponding movements of the spinal column. The meaning of the term **lateral flexion** is evident. These movements are all rotations around axes which are approximately either transverse or vertical. Depression, elevation, and lateral movement of the lower jaw fall in this category.

3. **Circumduction.**—This designates movements in which the distal part of the limb describes a circle or a segment of one. In man such movement is easily

performed, but in quadrupeds it is possible to a limited degree only, and is to be regarded usually as an indication of disease.

4. **Rotation.**—As a matter of convenience, this term is reserved to indicate rotation of one segment around the longitudinal axis of the other segment forming the joint. It is seen typically in the atlanto-axial joint.

5. **Adduction** and **abduction** designate respectively movement of a limb toward and away from the median plane, or of a digit toward and away from the axis of the limb.

Classification.—This is based on the form of the joint surfaces and the movements which occur. The following chief classes may be recognized

1. **Arthrodia,** or gliding joint. In these the surfaces are practically flat, admitting of gliding movement. Examples: carpo-metacarpal joints; joints between the articular processes of the cervical and thoracic vertebræ.

2. **Ginglymus,** or hinge-joint. In this class the joint surfaces consist usually of two condyles, or of a segment of a cylinder or cone, which are received by corresponding cavities. In typical cases the movements are flexion and extension, *i. e.,* around a single transverse axis. Examples: occipito-atlantal and elbow-joints.

3. **Trochoid,** or pivot joint. In these the movement is limited to rotation of one segment around the longitudinal axis of the other. Example: atlanto-axial joint.

4. **Enarthrosis,** or ball-and-socket joint. These are formed by a surface of approximately spherical curvature, received into a corresponding cavity. They are multiaxial, and allow of the greatest variety of movement, *e. g.,* flexion, extension, rotation, abduction, adduction, circumduction. Examples: hip and shoulder joints.[1]

AMPHIARTHROSES

These joints, as the name indicates, share some characters with both of the preceding groups. In them the segments are directly united by a plate of fibrocartilage, and usually by ligaments also. The amount and kind of movement are determined by the shape of the joint surfaces and the amount and pliability of the uniting medium.[2] These joints are all medial in position, and are best illustrated by the joints between the bodies of the vertebræ. There is usually no joint cavity, but in certain situations a rudimentary one exists.

THE ARTICULATIONS OF THE HORSE

JOINTS AND LIGAMENTS OF THE VERTEBRAE

The movable vertebræ form two sets of articulations, viz., those formed by the bodies, and those formed by the articular processes of adjacent vertebræ; the former are termed **intercentral,** and the latter, **interneural.** Associated with these are ligaments uniting the arches and processes; some of these are **special,** *i. e.,* confined to a single joint, while others are **common,** *i. e.,* extend along the entire

[1] This classification makes no claims to scientific accuracy, but is simply a statement of the terms in general use. A grouping based on mechanical principles seems desirable, but appears to be almost impossible on account of the great variety and irregularity of form of the articular surfaces.

[2] The movements in some of these joints are more extensive and varied than in some diarthroses. To illustrate this we may compare the movements of the cervical or coccygeal vertebræ with those possible in the carpo-metacarpal or the sacro-iliac joints.

vertebral column or a considerable part of it. The joints between the atlas and axis and between the former and the skull require separate consideration.

INTERCENTRAL ARTICULATIONS

These are **amphiarthroses,** formed by the junction of the extremities of the bodies of adjacent vertebræ. The **articular surfaces** in the cervical region consist of a cavity on the posterior end of the body of the anterior vertebra, and a corresponding convexity or head of the succeeding vertebra. In the other regions the surfaces are much flattened. The uniting media are:

1. The **intervertebral fibro-cartilages** (Fibrocartilagines intervertebrales). Each of these is a disc which fits into the space between the bodies of two adjacent vertebræ, to which it is intimately attached. The discs are thinnest in the middle of the thoracic region, thicker in the cervical and lumbar regions, and thickest in the coccygeal region. Each consists of a dense fibrous peripheral part (Annulus fibrosus), and a soft pulpy central part (Nucleus pulposus).

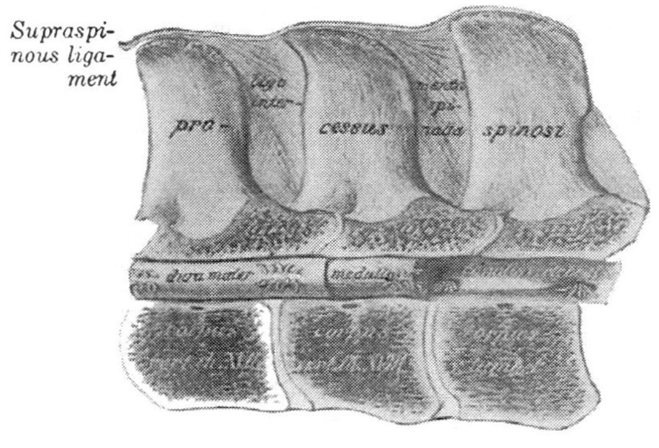

FIG. 139.—SAGITTAL SECTION OF LAST TWO THORACIC AND FIRST LUMBAR VERTEBRÆ, SHOWING LIGAMENTS AND SPINAL CORD (MEDULLA). (After Schmaltz, Atlas d. Anat. d. Pferdes.)

The fibrous ring consists of laminæ of fibrous tissue and fibro-cartilage, which pass obliquely between the two vertebræ and alternate in direction, forming an X-shaped arrangement. The central part of the ring is largely cartilaginous, and gradually assumes the character of the pulpy center. The latter is very elastic and is compressed, so that it bulges considerably from the surface of sections; it consists of white and elastic fibers, connective-tissue cells, and peculiar clear, transparent cells of various sizes. It is a remnant of the notochord. There are joint cavities in the cervical intercentral joints, and in those between the last cervical and the first thoracic, and between the last lumbar and the sacrum. In the latter the cavity is coextensive with the extremities of the bodies; in the former, it is usually not so extensive.

2. The **inferior common ligament** (Ligamentum longitudinale ventrale) lies on the ventral surface of the bodies of the vertebræ and the intervertebral fibro-cartilages, to which it is firmly attached. It begins about the fourteenth or fifteenth thoracic vertebra, and is at first a narrow, thin band. Further back it becomes gradually thicker and wider, and terminates on the pelvic surface of the sacrum by spreading out and blending with the periosteum. It is strongest in the lumbar region, where the tendons of the crura of the diaphragm fuse with it.

3. The superior common ligament (Ligamentum longitudinale dorsale) lies on the floor of the vertebral canal from the dens or odontoid process to the sacrum. It is narrow over the middles of the vertebral bodies, and widens over the intervertebral fibro-cartilages, to which it is very firmly attached.

This ligament is in relation with the spinal veins on either side, and in the middle of each vertebra a transverse anastomotic branch passes under the ligament.

INTERNEURAL ARTICULATIONS

Each typical vertebra presents two pairs of articular processes, which form diarthroses with the two adjacent vertebræ. The **articular surfaces** are extensive, flat, and oval in the cervical region, small and flat in the thoracic region, while in the lumbar region the anterior ones are concave and the posterior convex. The **joint capsule** is strong and ample in the cervical region, in conformity with the large size and greater mobility of these joints in the neck. In the thoracic and lumbar regions the capsule is small and close. These joints are arthrodia.

Associated with these joints are the **ligamenta flava,** which connect the arches of adjacent vertebræ. They are membranous and consist largely of elastic tissue.

The **supraspinous ligament** extends medially from the occipital bone to the sacrum. From the withers backward it consists of a strong cord of fibrous tissue, attached to the summits of the vertebral spines. In the neck and withers it is

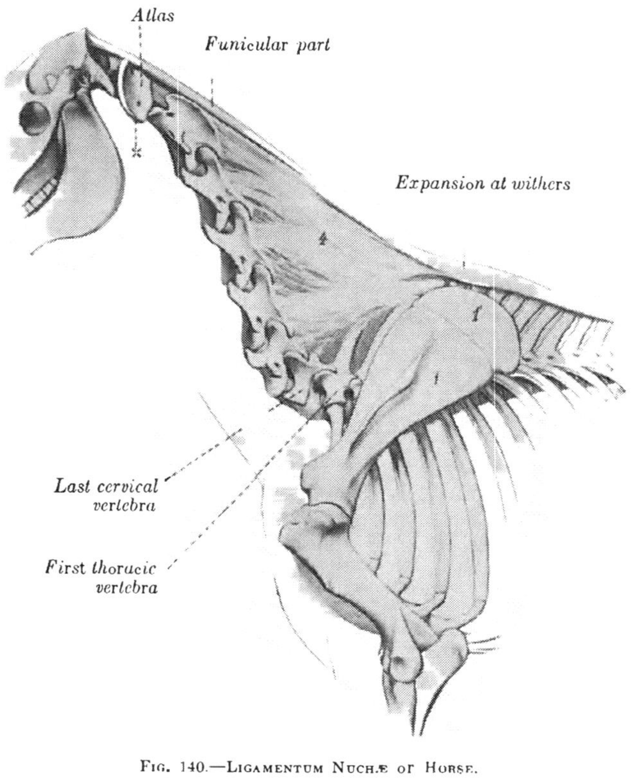

FIG. 140.—LIGAMENTUM NUCHÆ OF HORSE.
1, Scapula; *1'*, cartilage of scapula; *4*, lamellar part of ligamentum nuchæ; *x*, wing of atlas. (After Ellenberger-Baum, Anat. für Künstler.)

remarkably modified to form the ligamentum nuchæ, which requires more extended notice.

The **ligamentum nuchæ** is a powerful elastic apparatus, the principal function of which is to assist the extensor muscles of the head and neck. It extends from the occipital bone to the withers, where it is directly continuous with the supraspinous ligament. It consists of two parts—funicular and lamellar. The **funicular part** (Pars occipitalis) arises from the external occipital protuberance and the fossa below it, and is inserted into the summits of the vertebral spines at the withers. Two bursæ are usually found under it in the adult. The **supra-atloid bursa** lies between the ligament and the dorsal arch of the atlas. The **supra-**

spinous bursa occurs usually over the fourth thoracic spine, but may be over the third and may extend to the fifth.[1] In the neck the funicular part consists for the greater part of two bands closely applied and attached to each other. Near and at the withers it broadens greatly, forming an expansion three to five inches (ca. 8 to 12.5 cm.) in width, the lateral margins of which are thin and overlie the trapezius and rhomboideus muscles. Behind the higher spines it becomes narrower and thinner, and is continued by the white fibrous lumbo-dorsal ligament.[2] A mass of fat and elastic tissue lies upon the ligament as far back as the withers. It varies greatly in amount in different subjects, and is most developed in stallions of draft breeds, in which it forms the basis of the "crest." The **lamellar portion** (Pars cervicalis) consists of two laminæ separated medially by a layer of loose connective tissue. Each lamina is formed of digitations which arise from the second and third thoracic spines and from the funicular portion, are directed downward and forward, and end on the spines of the cervical vertebræ, except the first and last. The digitation which is attached to the spine of the axis is very thick and strong. Behind this they diminish in size and strength; that to the sixth cervical is quite thin and feeble, or may be absent.

The **interspinous ligaments** (Ligamenta interspinalia) extend between the spines of contiguous vertebræ. In the cervical region they are narrow elastic bands, and in the thoracic and lumbar regions they consist of white fibers directed obliquely downward and forward.

The **intertransverse ligaments** (Ligamenta intertransversaria) are membranes which connect adjacent transverse processes in the lumbar region.

INTERTRANSVERSE ARTICULATIONS

These joints (peculiar to equidæ) are diarthroses formed by the transverse processes of the last two lumbar vertebræ and the alæ of the sacrum. A similar joint between the fourth and fifth lumbar processes is frequently present. The **articular surfaces** have an elongated oval form, the anterior one being concave and the posterior one convex. The capsule is tight, and is reinforced ventrally.

SACRAL AND COCCYGEAL ARTICULATIONS

In the foal the bodies of the five sacral vertebræ form joints which resemble somewhat those in the posterior part of the lumbar region. These joints are invaded by the process of ossification early, so that the consolidation of the sacrum is usually complete, or nearly so, at three years.

The coccygeal vertebræ are united by relatively thick intervertebral fibrocartilages, which have the form of biconcave discs. Special ligaments are not present, but there is a continuous sheath of fibrous tissue. The movement in this region is extensive and varied. In old horses the first coccygeal vertebra is often fused with the sacrum.

MOVEMENTS OF THE VERTEBRAL COLUMN

The movements of the spine, exclusive of those at the atlanto-axial joint, are dorsal, ventral, and lateral flexion, and rotation. The range of movement at a single joint is very small, but the sum of the movements is considerable. The

[1] In dissecting-room subjects these bursæ and the adjacent structures are commonly the seat of pathological changes. They appear to be the starting-point of "poll evil" and "fistulous withers."

[2] No natural line of demarcation exists between the ligamentum nuchæ and the lumbo-dorsal continuation of the supraspinous ligament, since the change from the purely elastic to the white fibrous structure is gradual.

movements are freest in the cervical and coccygeal regions. Rotation is extremely limited in the thoracic and lumbar regions.

ATLANTO-AXIAL ARTICULATION

This is a trochoid or pivot joint, of a rather peculiar character. The articular surfaces are: (1) On the lateral masses of the atlas, two somewhat saddle-shaped facets, which are usually confluent ventrally; (2) on the axis, reciprocal saddle-shaped surfaces which extend upon the odontoid process and are confluent on its ventral aspect. It will be observed that the joint surfaces are not at all accurately adapted to each other, so that only limited areas are in contact at any time.

The joint capsule is attached around the margins of the articular surfaces. It is loose and ample enough laterally to allow extensive movement.

The superior atlanto-axial ligament (Ligamentum interarcuale) is membranous and reinforces the capsule dorsally.

The interspinous ligament (Ligamentum interspinale) consists of two elastic bands which extend from the dorsal arch of the atlas to the spine of the axis

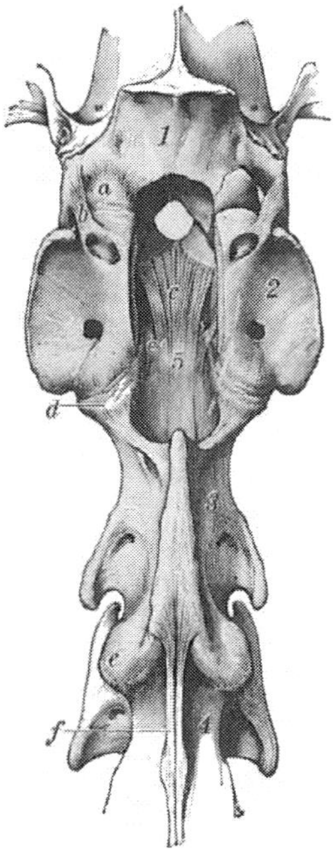

Fig. 141.—Atlanto-occipital and Atlanto-axial Joints of Horse, Dorsal View after Removal of Dorsal Arch of Atlas.

a, Joint capsule of left part of atlanto-occipital joint; *b*, lateral ligament of same; *c*, *c'*, odontoid ligament; *d*, atlanto-occipital joint capsule; *e*, joint capsule of articulation between axis and third cervical vertebra; *f*, interspinous ligament; *1*, occipital bone; *2*, atlas; *3*, axis; *4*, third cervical vetrebra. (Ellenberger-Baum, Anat. d. Haustiere.)

THE ATLANTO-OCCIPITAL ARTICULATION

This joint may be classed as a ginglymus. The articular surfaces of this joint are: (1) On the atlas, two deep oval cavities; (2) the corresponding condyles of the occipital bone.

The joint surfaces are oblique, coming very close to the median line ventrally, but separated by a considerable interval dorsally. Posteriorly, a triangular rough area cuts into the middle of each articular surface on the atlas.

There are two roomy joint capsules, which sometimes communicate ventrally, especially in old subjects.

The superior atlanto-occipital membrane extends from the dorsal arch of the atlas to the upper margin of the foramen magnum. It is blended with the capsules and contains many elastic fibers.

The inferior atlanto-occipital membrane extends from the ventral arch of the atlas to the lower margin of the foramen magnum. It is narrower and thinner than the superior membrane, and also fuses with the joint capsules.

The lateral **ligaments** are two short bands which are partially blended with the capsules. Each is attached to the border of the wing of the atlas near the intervertebral foramen, and to the outer surface of the paramastoid or styloid process of the occipital bone.

Movements.—These are chiefly flexion and extension. A small amount of lateral oblique movement is also possible.

ARTICULATIONS OF THE THORAX

COSTO-VERTEBRAL ARTICULATIONS

Each typical rib forms two joints with the vertebral column, one by its head, and one by its tubercle. They are termed respectively costo-central and costo-transverse joints.

I. The **costo-central articulations** (Articulationes capitulorum) are trochoid or rotatory joints, formed by the junction of the head of the rib with the bodies of two adjacent vertebræ and the intervertebral fibro-cartilage. The two facets on the head of the rib are separated by a non-articular groove, and correspond to the two concave facets (Foveæ costales) on the vertebral bodies. The capsules are rather tight, and are covered by the accessory ligaments, which are as follows: **1.** The **radiate ligament** (Ligamentum capituli costæ radiatum) extends ventrally from the neck of the rib to spread out on the vertebral bodies and the intervertebral fibro-cartilage. 2. The **conjugal ligament** (Ligamentum conjugale)—absent from the first joint—is attached to the groove on the head of the rib, passes transversely into the vertebral canal, and divides under the superior common ligament into two branches; one of these is attached to the body of the anterior vertebra; the other is continued across to the head of the opposite rib, and is attached to the intervertebral fibro-cartilage. The joint cavity is divided into two compartments by the conjugal ligament. 3. The **ligament of the neck** of the rib (Ligamentum colli costæ) is a strong band which crosses the joint dorsally. It is attached on the vertebra above the costal facet and on the neck of the rib.

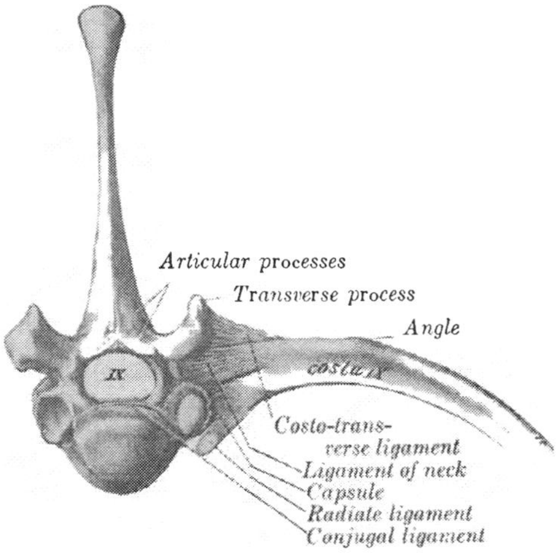

FIG. 142.—COSTO-VERTEBRAL ARTICULATION, ANTERIOR VIEW. (After Schmaltz, Atlas d. Anat. d. Pferdes.)

II. The **costo-transverse** articulations. These occur between the facets on the tubercles of the ribs and those on the transverse processes of the vertebræ. They are gliding joints. The **capsule** is reinforced by the superior costo-transverse **ligament** (Ligamentum costo-transversarium dorsale), a distinct strong band which arises on the transverse process and ends on the non-articular part of the tubercle. It is covered by the levatór costæ muscle, and begins to be quite distinct at the fifth joint.

The cavity for the head of the first rib is formed by concave facets on the bodies of the last cervical and first thoracic vertebræ. The conjugal ligament is absent, but the ligament of the neck is short and strong. The radiate ligament is very strong, and consists of two bands. In the case of the last two or three ribs the costo-central and costo-transverse joints are confluent, and the various structures are correspondingly modified.

Movements.—The chief movement is rotation around an axis which connects the centers of the head and tubercle of the rib. The movement is very limited in the anterior part of the series of joints, but very considerable in the posterior part.

In the case of the first rib, the movement is evidently extremely limited. The facet for the tubercle of the rib is deeply concave, and the axis of rotation is almost transverse. Further back the facets on the transverse processes become flat, and the axis of rotation gradually approaches a longitudinal direction. This, in connection with the mobility of the ventral ends of the asternal ribs and their elasticity, allows a great increase here in the range of movement, the effect of which is to enlarge (chiefly) the transverse diameter of the thorax.

COSTO-CHONDRAL ARTICULATIONS

The costo-chondral junctions are synarthroses. The rib has a concave surface which receives the convex end of the cartilage. They are united by the continuity of the strong periosteum and perichondrium.

CHONDRO-STERNAL ARTICULATIONS

These joints (Articulationes sternocostales) are diarthroses formed by the junction of the cartilages of the sternal ribs with the sternum. The articular ends of the cartilages (except the first) are somewhat enlarged, and present surfaces of cylindrical curvature. The articular surfaces on the sternum for the first pair of cartilages are placed close together on the dorsal border of the cariniform cartilage (Manubrium sterni); the other seven are placed laterally at the junction of the segments. The capsules are strong and tight; the first pair of joints has a common capsule, and the cartilages articulate with each other medially. The lower ends of the first pair of ribs are firmly attached to each other by dense fibrous tissue, which is prolonged forward along the upper margin of the cariniform cartilage and is continuous behind with the sternal ligament. Each of the other capsules is reinforced dorsally by the **superior costo-sternal ligament** (Ligamentum sternocostale radiatum), composed of radiating fibers which blend with the sternal ligament. The movement is rotation around a nearly vertical axis, except in the case of the first pair of joints.

INTERCHONDRAL LIGAMENTS

The eighth and ninth costal cartilages are firmly united by fibrous tissue. The chondro-xiphoid ligament attaches the ninth costal cartilage to the xiphoid cartilage. The remaining cartilages are rather loosely attached to each other by elastic tissue.

STERNAL ARTICULATIONS

In the new-born foal the sternum has seven bony segments (Sternebræ), united by persisting cartilage. The last two segments coalesce within a few weeks after birth. In old subjects there is more or less ossification of the intersegmental cartilage, which may lead to partial fusion of adjacent segments, especially posteriorly. The **sternal ligament** (Ligamentum sterni proprium internum) lies on the thoracic surface of the sternum. It arises on the first segment, and divides opposite the second chondro-sternal joint into three bands. The median band passes backward and spreads out on the last segment and the xiphoid cartilage. The lateral branches—thicker and wider—lie along the lateral borders above the chondro-sternal joints, and end at the cartilage of the eighth rib;. they are covered by the transversus thoracis muscle.

The Articulations of the Skull

TEMPORO-MANDIBULAR ARTICULATION

This joint (Articulatio mandibularis) is the only diarthrosis formed between bones of the skull.

The **articular surfaces** are dissimilar in form and size. That on the squamous temporal bone is concavo-convex, and the long axis is directed outward and somewhat forward; it consists of a glenoid cavity, which is continued upon the postglenoid process behind, and a condyle in front. The mandible presents a transversely elongated condyle.

The **articular disc** is placed between the joint surfaces, which it renders congruent. Its upper and lower surfaces are molded upon the temporal and mandibular surfaces respectively, and its circumference is attached to the joint capsule; thus it divides the joint cavity into upper and lower compartments, the former being the more roomy.

The **joint capsule** is strong and tight. It is reinforced by two ligaments. The **external ligament** (Ligamentum laterale) extends obliquely across the anterior part of the outer surface of the capsule, from which it is not distinctly separable. The **posterior ligament** (Ligamentum posterius) is an elastic band which is attached above to the postglenoid process, and below to a line on the posterior face of the neck of the mandible.

Movements.—The chief movements take place around a transverse axis passing through both joints. Associated with this hinge-like action is slight gliding movement, as in opening and shutting the mouth. When the mouth is shut, the condyle lies under the glenoid cavity. When the mandible is depressed, the condyle moves forward under the articular eminence of the temporal bone, carrying the disc with it. In protrusion and retraction of the lower jaw the gliding movement just described occurs without the hinge-like rotation of the condyle. These movements are similar in both joints. In the lateral movements (as usually performed in mastication) the action consists of rotation of the condyles around a vertical axis, while the disc glides forward on one side and backward on the other.

THE SYNARTHROSES OF THE SKULL

Most of the bones of the skull are united with the adjacent bones by **sutures**; a few are united by cartilage. The difference in the uniting medium depends on the fact that most of these bones are developed in membrane, but some are preformed in cartilage. Most of these joints are temporary, and are obliterated at various periods during development and growth. Their importance rests on the fact that so long as they persist, continuous growth is possible. They are usually designated according to the bones which enter into their formation, *e. g.*, spheno-squamous, naso-frontal, internasal, etc. Special names (borrowed from human anatomy) are sometimes used; thus the interparietal, the parieto-occipital, and the parieto-frontal sutures are often called the sagittal, lambdoid, and coronal respectively.

Detailed description of the sutures has not sufficient clinical value to justify much addition to the statements made in the osteology in this connection. The obliteration or closure of the sutures is, however, worthy of brief mention. The cranial sutures are usually all closed at seven years, but the apex only of the petrous temporal is fused with the occipital and squamous temporal. Most of the facial sutures are practically closed at ten years, although complete synostosis may in some be delayed for years or may not occur at all; the nasal suture, for example, often persists even in advanced age, so far as its anterior part is concerned.

The principal **synchondroses** are: (1) That between the basioccipital and the body of the sphenoid (Synchondrosis sphenooccipitalis); (2) that between the presphenoid and postsphenoid (Synchondrosis intersphenoidalis); (3) those between the parts of the occipital bone (Synchondroses intraoccipitales). The first is usually ossified at four years, the second at three years, and the occipital bone is consolidated at two years.

The **symphysis** of the lower jaw (Symphysis mandibulæ) ossifies at one to six months.

THE HYOIDEAN ARTICULATIONS

The **temporo-hyoid articulation** is an amphiarthrosis, in which the dorsal angle of the proximal end of the great cornu (Stylo-hyal) is attached by a short bar of cartilage to the hyoid process of the petrous temporal bone. The cartilage (Arthro-hyal) is about half an inch (ca. 1 to 1.5 cm.) in length. The chief movement is hinge like, the axis of motion passing transversely through both joints.

The **intercornual articulation** is an amphiarthrosis formed by the junction of the distal extremity of the great cornu with the proximal end of the small cornu (kerato-hyal). They are united by a very short piece of cartilage, in which there is usually a small nodule of bone in the young subject. This nodule, the epihyal or middle cornu, is usually fused with the great cornu in the adult. The chief movement here is also hinge-like, the angle between the cornua being increased or diminished.

The **basi-cornual articulation** is a diarthrosis formed by the junction of each small cornu (kerato-hyal) with the body (basi-hyal). The small cornu has a concave facet which articulates with the convex facet on either end of the dorsal surface of the body. The capsule is ample enough to allow considerable movement, which is chiefly hinge-like. The movements of the hyoid bone are concerned chiefly in the acts of mastication and swallowing. In the latter the distal parts of the hyoid bone are moved forward and upward, carrying the root of the tongue and the larynx with them, and then return to their former position.

THE ARTICULATIONS OF THE THORACIC LIMB

In the absence of the clavicle the thoracic limb forms no articulation with the trunk, unless we regard as such the union by muscles. The movement of the shoulder on the chest-wall is chiefly rotation around a transverse axis passing through the scapula behind the upper part of the spine.

THE SHOULDER JOINT

The shoulder or scapulo-humeral joint (Articulatio scapulo-humeralis) is formed by the junction of the distal end of the scapula with the proximal end of the humerus. The **articular surfaces** are: (1) On the scapula, the glenoid cavity; (2) on the humerus, the head. Both surfaces are approximately spherical and similar in curvature, but the humeral surface is much more extensive than that of the scapula.

The **joint capsule** is ample enough to allow the bones to be drawn apart about an inch (ca. 2 to 3 cm.); but this requires a very considerable amount of force unless air is admitted into the joint cavity. The fibrous layer (or capsular ligament) is not attached to the margin of the joint surfaces, but at a distance of one to two centimeters from it. It is strengthened in front by two diverging elastic bands, which arise on the scapular tuberosity and end on the lips of the bicipital groove. A pad of fat is interposed between the capsule and the tendon of the biceps.

Ligaments are absent from this joint, but the muscles and tendons around it afford remarkable security, so that dislocation seldom or never occurs. The large extent of the head of the humerus is also of importance in this regard.

The principal muscles which are attached around the joint and act as ligaments are: externally, the supraspinatus, infraspinatus, and teres minor; internally, the subscapularis; in front, the biceps and supraspinatus; behind, the triceps.

Movements.—While it is a typical enarthrosis in structure, and capable of the various movements of the ball-and-socket joint, the chief normal movements are flexion and extension. In the position of rest the angle formed between the scapula and humerus posteriorly is about 110° to 120°; in flexion it is reduced to about 80°, and in extension it is increased to about 145°. Adduction and abduction are very restricted, the former being limited chiefly by the infraspinatus, the latter by the subscapularis and the low insertion of the superficial pectoral muscles. Rotation is somewhat freer, but does not exceed 33°, when all the muscles are removed (Franck).

THE ELBOW JOINT

This, the cubital articulation (Articulatio cubiti), is a ginglymus formed between the distal extremity of the humerus and the proximal ends of the bones of the forearm.

The **articular surfaces** are: (1) A trochlear surface formed by the condyles of the humerus and the groove between them; (2) the corresponding glenoid cavities and ridge on the proximal extremity of the radius, together with the semilunar notch of the ulna.

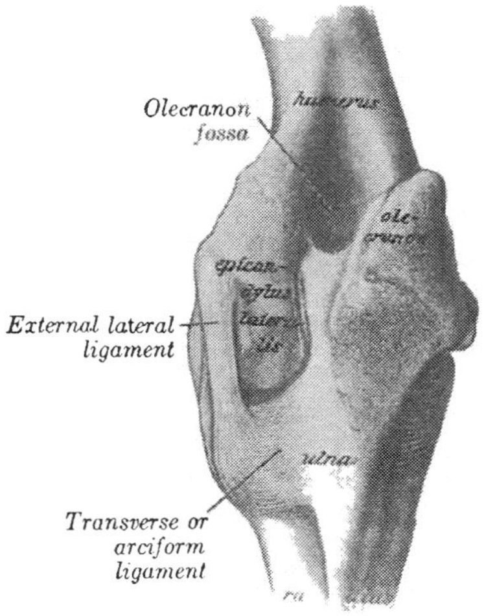

FIG. 143.—LEFT ELBOW JOINT OF HORSE, POSTERIOR VIEW. THE CAPSULE IS REMOVED. (After Schmaltz, Atlas d. Anat. d. Pferdes.)

The articular surface of the condyles does not extend upon the back of the extremity, but the groove which receives the semilunar notch of the ulna extends up into the olecranon fossa. In the fore part of the groove there is a synovial fossa. The surface on the outer condyle is smaller than that of the inner one, and is subdivided into two unequal parts by a shallow furrow. On e lower part of the semilunar notch and the adjacent part of the ridge on the radius are synovial fossæ.

The **joint capsule** is extremely thin behind, where it forms a pouch in the olecranon fossa under the anconeus muscle and a pad of fat. In front it is strengthened by oblique fibers (Ligamentum obliquum or anterior ligament), and laterally it fuses with the lateral ligaments. Small pouches of the synovial membrane lubricate the origins of the flexors of the carpus and digit and the small radio-ulnar joints. There are two lateral ligaments.

The **internal lateral ligament** (Ligamentum collaterale radiale) is attached above to an eminence on the internal epicondyle of the humerus, and divides into two parts: the long, superficial part ends on the inner border of the radius, just below the level of the interosseous space; the deep, short part is inserted into the internal tuberosity of the radius. (The superficial part represents the pronator teres muscle, which is only exceptionally present in the horse.)

The **external lateral ligament** (Ligamentum collaterale ulnare) is short and strong. It is attached above to a depression on the external epicondyle of the humerus, and below to the external tuberosity of the radius, just below the margin of the articular surface.

Movements.—This joint is a typical ginglymus, the only movements being flexion and extension around an axis which passes through the upper attachments of the lateral ligaments. In the standing position the articular angle (in front) is about 140° to 150°. The range of movement is about 55° to 60°. Complete extension is prevented chiefly by the tension of the lateral ligaments and the biceps muscle. (The axis of movement is slightly oblique, so that in flexion the forearm is carried somewhat outward.)

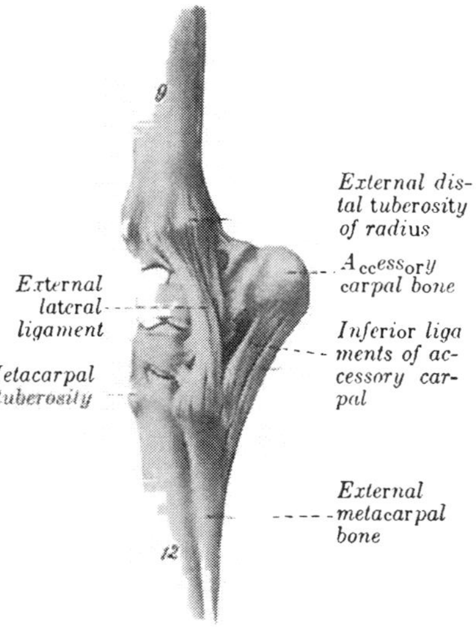

Fig. 144.—Left Carpal Joints of Horse, External View

The capsule has been removed. 9, Radius; 12, large metacarpal bone. (After Ellenberger-Baum, Anat. f. Künstler.)

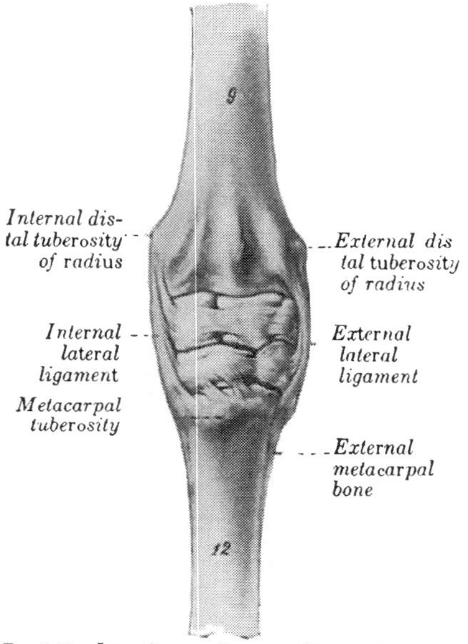

Fig. 145.—Left Carpal Joints of Horse, Anterior View.

The capsule has been removed. The smaller ligaments are shown. (After Ellenberger-Baum, Anat. f. Künstler.)

THE RADIO-ULNAR ARTICULATION

In the foal the shaft of the ulna is attached to the radius above and below the interosseous space by the **interosseous ligament**. Below the space the two bones become fused before adult age is reached.* Above the space the ligament usually persists, but may undergo more or less ossification in extreme old age. The **transverse** or **arciform ligaments** (Ligamentum transversum ulnare et radiale ulnæ et radii) consist of fibers which pass above the interosseous space from either border of the shaft of the ulna to the posterior surface of the radius. The proximal radio-ulnar articulation, formed by two small convex facets on the ulna and the corresponding facets on the posterior surface of the proximal extremity of the radius, is inclosed in the capsule of the elbow-joint and does not require separate consideration. The distal extremity of the ulna fuses early with the radius, and is, therefore, regarded usually as a part of the latter.

Movement.—This is inappreciable, the forearm being fixed in the position of pronation.

THE CARPAL JOINTS

These joints taken together constitute the composite **articulatio carpi,** or what is popularly termed the "knee-joint" in animals.[1] This consists of three chief joints, viz., (1) The **radio-carpal joint,** formed by the distal end of the radius and the proximal row of the carpus; (2) the **intercarpal joint,** formed between the two rows of the carpus; (3) the **carpo-metacarpal joint,** formed between the distal row of the carpus and the proximal ends of the metacarpal bones. The proximal and middle joints may be regarded as ginglymi, although they are not typical or pure examples of hinge-joints. The distal joint is arthrodial. In addition there are arthrodial joints formed between adjacent bones of the same row (Articulationes interosseæ). All these constitute a very composite joint, with numerous ligaments. The articular surfaces have been described in the Osteology.

The joint **capsule** may be regarded, so far as the fibrous part is concerned, as being common to all three joints. It is attached close to the margin of the articular surface of the radius above and the metacarpus below; its deep face is also attached to a considerable extent to the carpal bones and to the small ligaments. Its anterior part, the **dorsal** or **anterior common ligament,** is rather loose, and assists in forming the fibrous canals for the extensor tendons. Its posterior part, the **volar** or **posterior common ligament,** is very thick and dense, and is closely attached to the carpal bones. It levels up the irregularities of the skeleton here, and forms the smooth anterior wall of the carpal canal. It is continued downward to form the **subcarpal** or **inferior check ligament,** which blends with the tendon of the flexor perforans about the middle of the metacarpus.

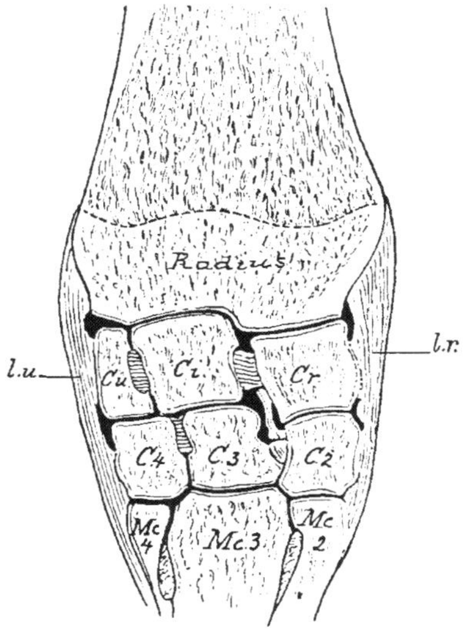

FIG. 146.—FRONTAL SECTION OF CARPAL JOINTS OF HORSE (RIGHT SIDE).

l.u., External, *l.r.*, internal, lateral ligament; *Cr*, radial carpal; *Ci*, intermediate carpal; *Cu*, ulnar carpal; *C2*, second carpal; *C3*, third carpal; *C4*, fourth carpal; *Mc2*, second (internal) metacarpal; *Mc3*, third (large) metacarpal; *Mc4*, fourth (external) metacarpal.

The **synovial membrane** forms three sacs corresponding to the three joints. The **radio-carpal sac** is the most voluminous; it includes the joints formed by the accessory carpal bone, and also those between the proximal carpal bones as far as the interosseous ligaments. The **intercarpal sac** sends extensions upward and downward between the bones of the two rows as far as the interosseous ligaments; it communicates between the third and fourth carpal bones with the **carpo-metacarpal sac.** The latter is very limited in extent, and is closely applied to the bones; it incloses the carpometacarpal joint, and lubricates also the lower parts of the joints between the distal carpal bones and the intermetacarpal joints.

The **external lateral ligament** (Ligamentum carpi collaterale ulnare) is attached above to the external tuberosity of the distal end of the radius. Its long superficial part is attached below to the proximal end of the external small metacarpal chiefly,

[1] The term is a very unfortunate one, since it is a distinct misapplication of the name as it is used in regard to man. It is, however, very firmly established, and appears likely to persist indefinitely in the absence of a convenient popular equivalent.

but some fibers end on the large metacarpal bone. A canal for the lateral extensor tendon separates a short deep band which ends on the ulnar carpal bone. Other deep fibers connect the latter with the fourth carpal bone, and the fourth carpal with the metacarpus.

The **internal lateral ligament** (Ligamentum carpi collaterale radiale) resembles the preceding in general, but is stronger and wider distally. It is attached above to the internal tuberosity of the distal end of the radius and ends below on the proximal ends of the large and inner small metacarpal bones. Deep fasciculi are detached to the radial and second carpal bones. The first carpal bone, when present, is usually embedded in the posterior part of the distal end of the ligament. The posterior part of the ligament is fused with the posterior annular ligament (Ligamentum carpi transversum), and concurs in the formation of a canal for the tendon of the flexor carpi internus.

A number of special short ligaments connect two or more adjacent bones; only the most distinct of these will be described here.

The accessory carpal bone is connected with adjacent bones by three ligaments (Fig. 444). The proximal one is a short band which extends from the accessory carpal in front of the groove on its outer face and is inserted into the distal end of the radius behind the groove for the lateral extensor tendon. A middle band connects the accessory with the ulnar carpal. The distal ligament consists of two strong bands which pass from the lower margin of the accessory to the fourth carpal and the proximal end of the outer metacarpal bone; these bands transmit the action of the muscles, which are inserted into the accessory carpal bone. The other bones of the proximal row are connected by two anterior or dorsal ligaments, which are transverse in direction, and two interosseous ligaments. An oblique ligament passes from an eminence on the posterior surface of the radial carpal bone to a small depression on the radius internal to the facet for the accessory carpal bone.

Two ligaments connect the proximal and distal rows posteriorly. The inner one joins the radial to the second and third carpal, and the outer one attaches the ulnar to the third and fourth carpals.

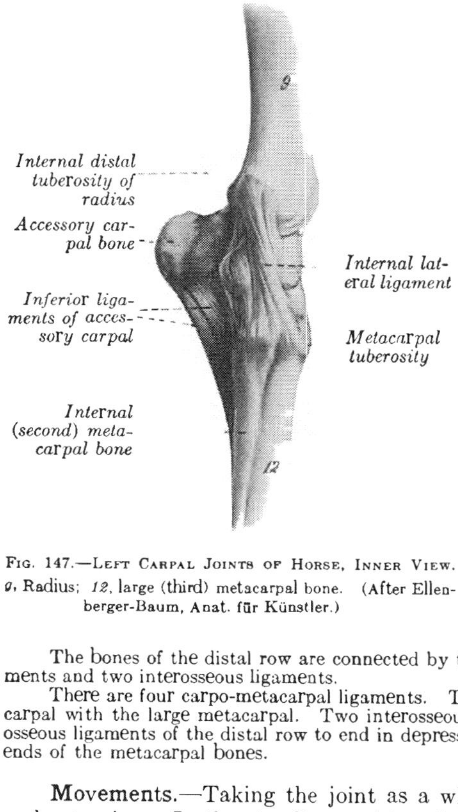

FIG. 147.—LEFT CARPAL JOINTS OF HORSE, INNER VIEW. *9*, Radius; *12*, large (third) metacarpal bone. (After Ellenberger-Baum, Anat. für Künstler.)

The bones of the distal row are connected by two strong transverse anterior or dorsal ligaments and two interosseous ligaments.

There are four carpo-metacarpal ligaments. Two oblique anterior bands connect the third carpal with the large metacarpal. Two interosseous ligaments pass downward from the interosseous ligaments of the distal row to end in depressions in the interstices between the proximal ends of the metacarpal bones.

Movements.—Taking the joint as a whole, the chief movements are flexion and extension. In the standing position the joint is extended. When the joint is flexed, slight lateral movement and rotation can be produced by manipulation. The anterior part of the capsule is, of course, tense during flexion, the posterior part in extension.

The movement practically all occurs at the radio-carpal and intercarpal joints, the articular surfaces of which are widely separated in front during flexion, but remain in contact behind. The distal row remains in contact with the metacarpus. The intermediate and ulnar carpals move together as one piece, but the radial does not move so far as the intermediate, so that the anterior and interosseous ligaments connecting these bones become tense and oblique in direction.

THE FETLOCK JOINT

This, the **metacarpo-phalangeal articulation** (Articulatio metacarpo-phalangea), is a ginglymus formed by the junction of the distal end of the large (third) metacarpal bone, the proximal end of the first phalanx, and the proximal sesamoid bones.

Articular Surfaces.—The surface on the large metacarpal bone is approximately cylindrical in curvature, but is divided into two slightly unequal parts by a sagittal ridge. This is received into a sort of socket formed by the first phalanx below and the two sesamoids together with the intersesamoid ligament behind. The latter is a mass of fibrocartilage in which the sesamoid bones are largely embedded. It extends above the level of the sesamoids, and is grooved to receive the ridge on the metacarpal bone; its posterior surface forms a smooth groove for the deep flexor tendon.

The joint **capsule** is attached around the margin of the articular surfaces. It is thick and ample in front; here a bursa is interposed between it and the extensor tendons, but the tendons are also attached to the capsule. Posteriorly it forms a thin-walled pouch which extends upward between the metacarpal bone and the suspensory ligament about as high as the point of bifurcation of the latter. The capsule is reinforced by two lateral ligaments.

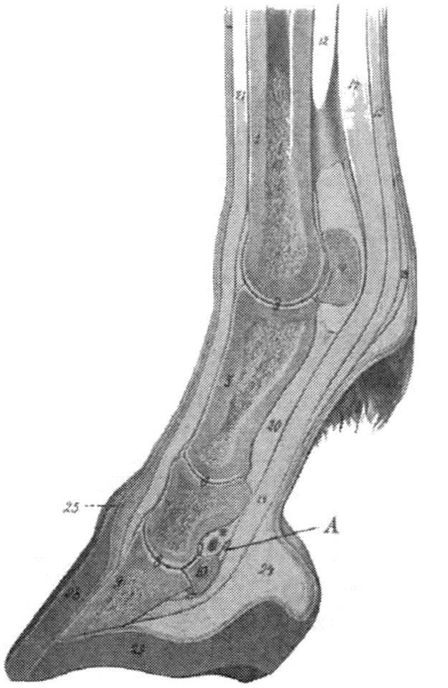

FIG. 148.—SAGITTAL SECTION OF DISTAL PART OF LIMB OF HORSE.

1, Large metacarpal bone; *3*, fetlock joint; *4*, proximal sesamoid bone; *5*, first phalanx; *6*, pastern joint; *7*, second phalanx; *8*, coffin joint; *9*, third phalanx; *10*, distal sesamoid (navicular bone); *12*, suspensory ligament; *14*, deep flexor tendon; *15*, superficial flexor tendon; *16*, posterior annular ligament of fetlock; *20*, inferior sesamoidean ligaments; *21*, extensor tendon; *24*, plantar cushion; *25*, periople; *28*, wall of hoof; *29*, sole of hoof; *A*, navicular bursa, proximal part. (After Ellenberger-Baum, Anat. für Künstler.)

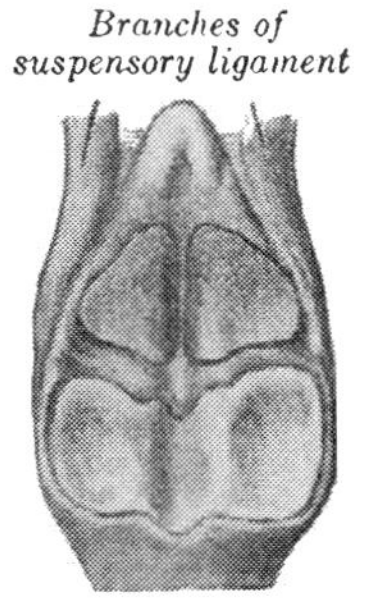

FIG. 149.—ARTICULAR SURFACES OF FIRST PHALANX AND SESAMOIDS AT FETLOCK, WITH INTERSESAMOID AND SUSPENSORY LIGAMENTS. (After Schmaltz, Atlas d. Anat. d. Pferdes.)

The **lateral ligaments, external** and **internal** (Ligamentum collaterale ulnare, radiale) are partially divided into two layers: the **superficial layer** arises from the eminence on the side of the distal end of the large metacarpal bone, and passes straight to the rough lateral area below the margin of the articular surface of the first phalanx; the **deep layer**, shorter and much stronger, arises in the lateral depression on the distal end of the metacarpal bone, and passes obliquely downward and backward to be inserted into the outer surface of the sesamoid and the proximal end of the first phalanx.

The capsule is further strengthened by a layer of oblique fibers which pass over the lateral ligament on either side and end on the extensor tendon and the proximal extremity of the first phalanx. It may properly be regarded as fascia rather than ligament.

Movements.—These are of the nature of flexion and extension, the axis of motion passing through the upper attachments of the lateral ligaments. In the ordinary standing position the joint is in a state of partial **dorsal flexion,** the articular angle (in front) being about 140° to 150°. (In the hind limb it is about 5° greater.) Diminution of this angle (sometimes termed "overextension") is nor-

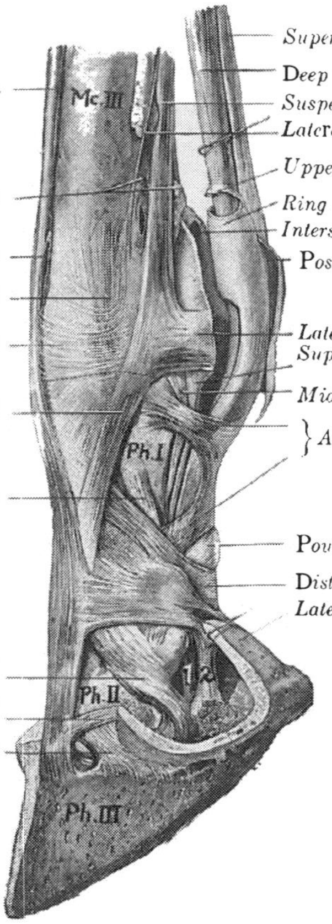

Fig. 150.—Ligaments and Tendons of Distal Part of Limb of Horse.
Mc.III, Large metacarpal bone; Ph.I, first phalanx; Ph.II, second phalanx; Ph.III, third phalanx; 1, deep flexor tendon; 2, band from first phalanx to plantar cushion. (After Schmaltz, Atlas d. Anat. d. Pferdes.)

mally very limited on account of the resistance offered by the sesamoidean apparatus, but it varies considerably in amount in different subjects. **Volar flexion** is limited only by contact of the heels with the metacarpus. During volar flexion a small amount of lateral flexion is possible.

THE SESAMOIDEAN LIGAMENTS

Under this head will be described a number of important ligaments which are connected with the sesamoid bones and form a sort of stay apparatus or brace.

The **intersesamoidean ligament** (Ligamentum intersesamoideum) not only fills the space between and unites the sesamoid bones, but also extends above them, entering into the formation of the articular surface of the fetlock joint. Other facts in regard to it have been given above.

The lateral **sesamoidean ligaments,** outer and inner (Ligamenta sesamoidea ulnare et radiale), arise on the abaxial surface of each sesamoid bone, pass forward, and divide into two branches, one of which ends in the depression on the distal end of the large metacarpal bone, the other on the eminence on the proximal end of the

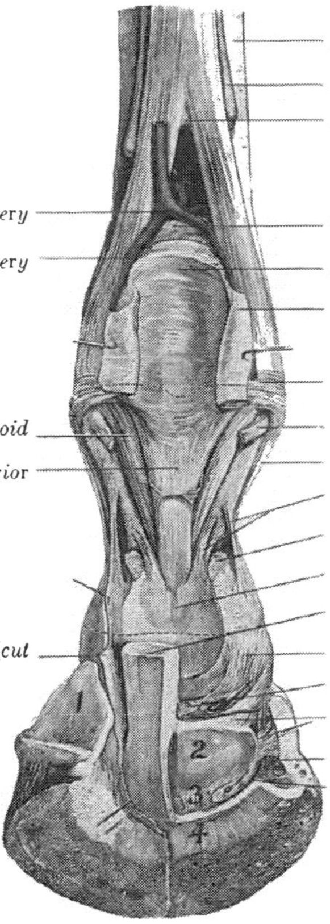

Fig. 151.—Deep Dissection of Distal Part of Right Fore Limb of Horse, Showing Joints and Ligaments, Posterior View.

1, Lateral cartilage; 2, tendon surface of navicular bone; 3, inferior navicular or interosseous ligament; 4, insertion of deep flexor tendon. Small arrows point to openings made in capsules of pastern and coffin joints. (After Schmaltz, Atlas d. Anat. d. Pferdes.)

first phalanx. They are partly covered by the branches of the suspensory or superior sesamoidean ligament.

The **suspensory** or **superior sesamoidean ligament** (Musculus interosseus medius) lies for the greater part in the metacarpal groove, where it has the form of a wide, thick band. It is attached above to the upper part of the posterior surface of the large metacarpal bone and to the distal row of carpal bones. At the lower fourth of the metacarpus it divides into two diverging branches. Each branch passes to the abaxial face of the corresponding sesamoid, on which a considerable part is attached. The remainder passes obliquely downward and forward to the anterior surface of the first phalanx, where it joins the extensor tendon. This ligament possesses considerable elasticity, and is the highly modified interosseous medius muscle. It consists mainly of tendinous tissue, but contains a variable amount of striped muscular tissue, especially in its deep part and in young subjects. Its principal function is to support the fetlock, *i. e.*, to prevent excessive dorsal flexion of the joint when the weight is put on the limb. The branches which join the common extensor tendon limit volar flexion of the interphalangeal joints in certain phases of movement.

The **inferior sesamoidean ligaments** are three in number—superficial, middle, and deep. The superficial or **straight ligament** (Ligamentum sesamoideum rectum) is a flat band and is somewhat wider above than below.[1] It is attached above to the bases of the sesamoid bones and the intersesamoid ligament, below to the complementary fibro-cartilage of the proximal end of the second phalanx. The **middle ligament** is triangular, with thick, rounded margins (Ligamenta obliqua) and a thin central portion.[2] Its base is attached to the sesamoid bones and intersesamoid ligament, and its deep face to the triangular rough area on the posterior surface of the first phalanx. The **deep or cruciate ligament** (Ligamenta sesamoidea cruciata) consists of two thin layers of fibers which arise on the base of the sesamoid bones, cross each other, and end on the opposite eminence on the proximal end of the first phalanx.

The short **sesamoidean ligaments** (Ligamenta sesamoidea brevia) are best seen by opening the joint in front and pushing the sesamoid bones backward; they are covered by the synovial membrane. Each is a short band which extends from the anterior part of the base of the sesamoid bone outward to the posterior margin of the articular surface of the first phalanx.

The inferior sesamoidean ligaments may be regarded as digital continuations of the suspensory ligament, the sesamoid bones being intercalated in this remarkable stay apparatus by which the fetlock is supported and concussion diminished.

THE PASTERN JOINT

This, the **proximal interphalangeal articulation** (Articulatio phalangis secundæ), is a ginglymus formed by the junction of the distal end of the first phalanx and the proximal end of the second phalanx.

The **articular surfaces** are: (1) On the first phalanx, two slightly unequal convex areas with an intermediate shallow groove; (2) on the second phalanx, a corresponding surface, completed behind by a plate of fibro-cartilage.

The joint capsule is close-fitting in front and laterally, where it blends with the extensor tendon and the lateral ligaments respectively. Behind it pouches upward a little and is reinforced by the straight sesamoidean ligament and the branches of the superficial flexor tendon.

There are two lateral and four volar ligaments.

The **lateral ligaments,** internal and external (Ligamentum collaterale radiale, ulnare) are very short and strong bands which are attached above on the eminence and depression on each side of the distal end of the first phalanx, and below on the eminence on either side of the proximal end of the second phalanx. The direction of the ligaments is about vertical and, therefore, does not correspond to the digital axis.

The volar or **posterior ligaments** consist of central and lateral pairs of bands which are attached below to the posterior margin of the proximal end of the second

[1] This is often called the Y-shaped ligament—a rather undesirable name, since it is not bifurcate.

[2] It is also called the V-shaped ligament.

phalanx and its complementary fibro-cartilage. The lateral pair is attached above to the middle of the borders of the first phalanx, the central pair lower down and on the margin of the triangular rough area.

These ligaments are very commonly thickened as a result of chronic inflammation, and then are not well defined. The central ones blend below with the branches of the superficial flexor tendon and with the straight sesamoidean ligament.

Movements.—These are very limited, and consist of flexion and extension. The axis of motion passes transversely through the distal end of the first phalanx. In the standing position the joint is extended. A small amount of volar flexion is possible, and in this position slight lateral flexion and rotation can be produced by manipulation. Dorsal flexion is prevented by the lateral, volar, and straight sesamoidean ligaments.

THE COFFIN JOINT

This joint, technically termed the distal interphalangeal articulation (Articulatio phalangis tertiæ), is a ginglymus formed by the junction of the second and third phalanges and the third sesamoid bone.

Articular Surfaces.—The surface on the distal end of the second phalanx is convex from before backward, concave transversely. The articular surface of the third phalanx slopes sharply upward and forward; its central part is prominent, and is flanked by two glenoid cavities. It is completed behind by the articular surface of the third sesmoid or navicular bone.

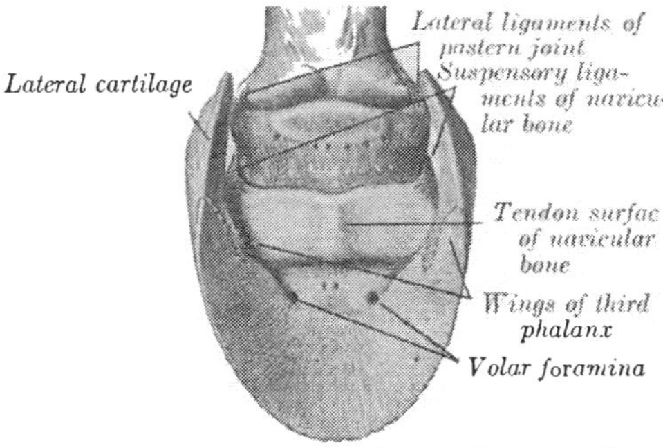

FIG. 152.—LATERAL LIGAMENTS OF PASTERN JOINT AND SUSPENSORY LIGAMENTS OF NAVICULAR BONE. (After Schmaltz, Atlas d. Anat. d. Pferdes.)

Joint Capsule.—This is attached around the margins of the articular surfaces. In front and laterally it is tight, and is blended with the extensor tendon and the lateral ligaments respectively. Posteriorly, it forms a considerable pouch which extends upward to about the middle of the second phalanx, where it is separated by a fibrous membrane from the digital synovial sheath. Laterally small pouches project outward (especially during volar flexion) against the lateral cartilages, just behind the lateral ligaments.[1]

Ligaments.—The lateral ligaments, external and internal (Ligamentum collaterale ulnare, radiale), are short strong bands which are attached above in the depressions on either side of the lower part of the second phalanx, under cover of the lateral cartilage. They widen below and end in the depressions on either side of the extensor process and on the anterior end of the lateral cartilages.

The suspensory navicular ligaments, external and internal (Ligamentum sesamoideum collaterale ulnare, radiale),[2] are strong, somewhat elastic bands, which form a sort of suspensory apparatus for the third sesamoid. They are attached superiorly in and above the depressions on either side of the distal end of the first

[1] This should be noted in regard to resection of the lateral cartilage or other operations in this vicinity.

[2] These are termed the postero-lateral ligaments by M'Fadyean. They may well be called, as by German authors, the suspensory ligaments of the navicular bone.

phalanx and are here partly blended with the lateral ligaments of the pastern joint. They are directed obliquely downward and backward, and end chiefly on the ends and proximal border of the third sesamoid, but detach a branch to the inner surface of each lateral cartilage and wing of the third phalanx.

The **inferior navicular ligament** (Ligamentum phalangeo-sesamoideum) reinforces the capsule inferiorly. It is a strong layer of fibers which extend from the distal border of the third sesamoid to the tendon surface of the third phalanx, near the posterior margin of the articular surface.

Movements.—The chief movements are flexion and extension. In the standing position the joint is extended. During volar flexion a very small amount of lateral movement and rotation can be produced by manipulation. Dorsal flexion is very limited.

Dorsal flexion appears to be checked mainly by the deep flexor tendon, since in cases of rupture of the latter the toe turns up. The slight mobility of the posterior part of the socket for the second phalanx (formed by the third sesamoid) diminishes concussion when the weight comes on the foot.

LIGAMENTS OF THE LATERAL CARTILAGES

In addition to the bands mentioned above, which attach the lateral cartilages to the extremities of the navicular bone, there are three ligaments on either side which attach the cartilages to the phalanges.

An ill-defined elastic band passes from the middle part of the border of the first phalanx to the upper part of the cartilage, detaching a branch to the plantar cushion.

A short strong band connects the anterior extremity of the cartilage with the rough eminence on the second phalanx in front of the attachment of the lateral ligament of the coffin joint.

The lower border of the cartilage is covered externally by fibers which attach it to the wing of the third phalanx.

THE ARTICULATIONS OF THE PELVIC LIMB

THE SACRO-ILIAC ARTICULATION

This joint (Articulatio sacro-iliaca) is a diarthrosis formed between the auricular surfaces of the sacrum and ilium. These surfaces are not smooth in the adult, but are marked by eminences and depressions, and are covered by a thin layer of cartilage. The joint cavity is a mere cleft, and is often crossed by fibrous bands.

The capsule is very close fitting, and is attached around the margins of the articular surfaces. It is reinforced by the **ventral sacro-iliac ligament** (Ligamentum sacro-iliacum ventrale), which surrounds the joint, and is exceedingly strong above.

The **movements** are inappreciable in the adult—stability, not mobility, being the chief desideratum.

The following ligaments may be regarded as accessory to the joint, although not directly connected with it.

The **dorsal sacro-iliac ligament** (Ligamentum sacro-iliacum dorsale breve) is a strong band which is attached to the internal angle (Tuber sacrale) of the ilium and the summits of the sacral spines.

The **lateral sacro-iliac ligament** (Ligamentum sacro-iliacum dorsale longum) is a triangular, thick sheet which is attached in front to the internal angle and border of the ilium above the great sciatic notch, and below to the lateral border of the sacrum. It blends above with the dorsal sacro-iliac ligament, below with the sacro-sciatic ligament, and behind with the coccygeal fascia.

The **sacro-sciatic ligament** (Ligamentum sacrospinosum et tuberosum) is a quadrilateral sheet which completes the lateral pelvic wall. Its upper border is attached to the border of the sacrum and the transverse processes of the first and second coccygeal vertebræ. Its lower border is attached to the superior ischiatic spine and tuber ischii. Between these it bridges over the external border of the ischium and completes the lesser sciatic foramen. The anterior border is concave, and completes the greater sciatic foramen. The posterior border is fused with the vertebral head of the semimembranosus muscle.

The **ilio-lumbar ligament** (Ligamentum ilio-lumbale) is a triangular sheet which attaches the ends of the lumbar transverse processes to the ventral surface of the ilium below the attachment of the longissimus muscle (Fig. 184).

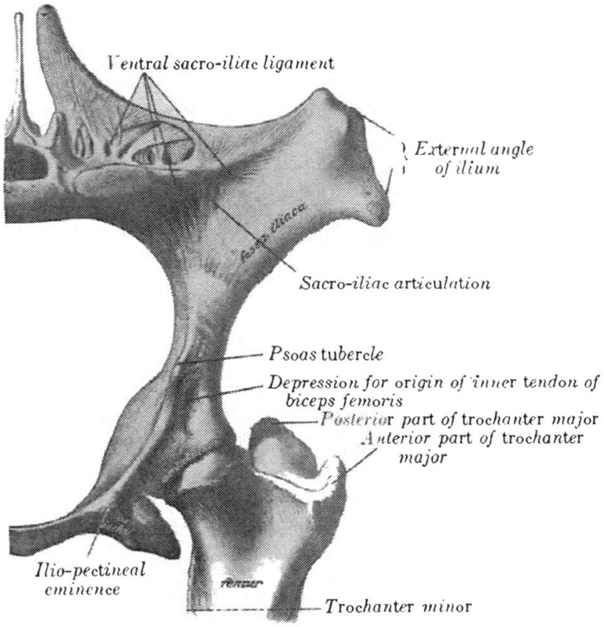

FIG. 153.—LEFT OS COXÆ AND ADJACENT PARTS OF SACRUM AND FEMUR OF HORSE. (After Schmaltz Atlas d. Anat. d. Pferdes.)

SYMPHYSIS PELVIS

The **symphysis pelvis** is formed by the junction of the two ossa coxarum at the ventral median line. In the young subject the bones are united by a layer of cartilage; in the adult the latter is gradually replaced by bone, the process beginning in the pubic portion and extending backward. The union is strengthened by white fibrous tissue above and below, and a transverse band also covers the anterior border of the pubis (pecten). No appreciable movement occurs even before synostosis takes place.

OBTURATOR MEMBRANE

This (Membrana obturatoria) is a thin layer of fibrous tissue which covers the obturator foramen, leaving, however, a passage (Canalis obturatorius) for the obturator vessels and nerve.

THE HIP JOINT

This joint (Articulatio coxæ) is an enarthrosis formed by the proximal end of the femur and the acetabulum.

Articular Surfaces.—The head of the femur presents an almost hemispherical articular surface, which is continued a short distance on the upper surface of the neck. It is more extensive than the socket which receives it. Internally it is cut into by a deep notch for the attachment of the round and pubo-femoral ligaments. The acetabulum is a typical cotyloid cavity. Its articular surface is somewhat crescentic, being deeply cut into internally by the acetabular notch and

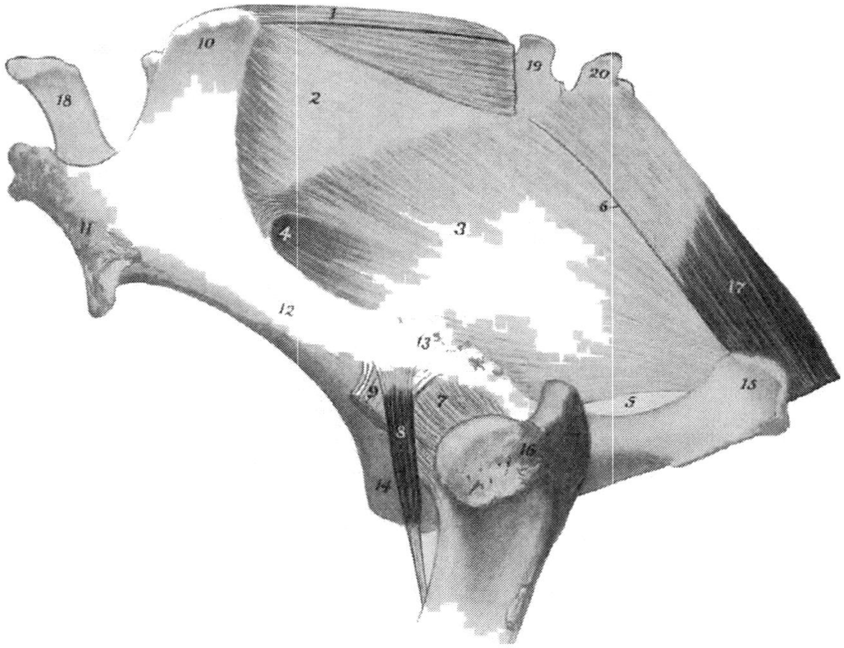

Fig. 154.—Pelvic Ligaments and Hip Joint.

1 Dorsal sacro-iliac ligament; *2*, lateral sacro-iliac ligament; *3*, sacro-sciatic ligament; *4*, greater sciatic foramen; *5*, lesser sciatic foramen; *6*, line of attachment of intermuscular septum between biceps femoris and semitendinosus; *7*, capsule of hip joint; *8*, rectus parvus or capsularis muscle; *9*, outer tendon of origin of biceps femoris; *10*, internal, *11*, external, angle of ilium; *12*, shaft of ilium; *13*, superior ischiatic spine; *14*, pubis; *15*, tuber ischii; *16*, trochanter major; *17*, semimembranosus; *18*, fifth lumbar spine; *19*, *20*, first and second coccygeal vertebræ.

fossa. It is increased and deepened by a ring of fibro-cartilage, the cotyloid ligament (Labrum glenoidale), which is attached to the bony margin; that part of the ligament which crosses the notch is called the transverse ligament (Fig. 456).

The joint capsule is roomy. It is attached around the margin of the acetabulum and the neck of the femur. It is thickest externally.

The attachment on the femur is about 1 cm. from the margin of the articular surface, except above, where 2 to 3 cm. of the neck is intracapsular. A thin oblique band corresponding in direction with the rectus parvus muscle reinforces the antero-external part of the capsule; this appears to be the feeble homologue of the very strong ilio-femoral ligament of man. The capsule is very thin under the ilio-psoas, and is adherent to the muscle. Internally, its fibrous part is perforated by the pubo-femoral and round ligaments and the articular vessels.

The **round ligament** (Ligamentum teres) is a strong band which is attached in the subpubic groove close to the acetabular notch, passes outward, and ends in the notch on the head of the femur (Fig. 456).

The **pubo-femoral ligament** (Ligamentum accessorium) does not occur in the domestic animals other than the equidæ. It is a strong band detached from the prepubic tendon of the abdominal muscles (Fig. 456). It is directed outward, backward, and upward, passes through the acetabular notch above the transverse ligament, and ends behind the round ligament in the notch on the head of the femur. The origin of the pectineus muscle is perforated by the ligament, which furnishes attachment to the greater part of the fibers of the muscle.

The **synovial membrane** is reflected over the intracapsular parts of these

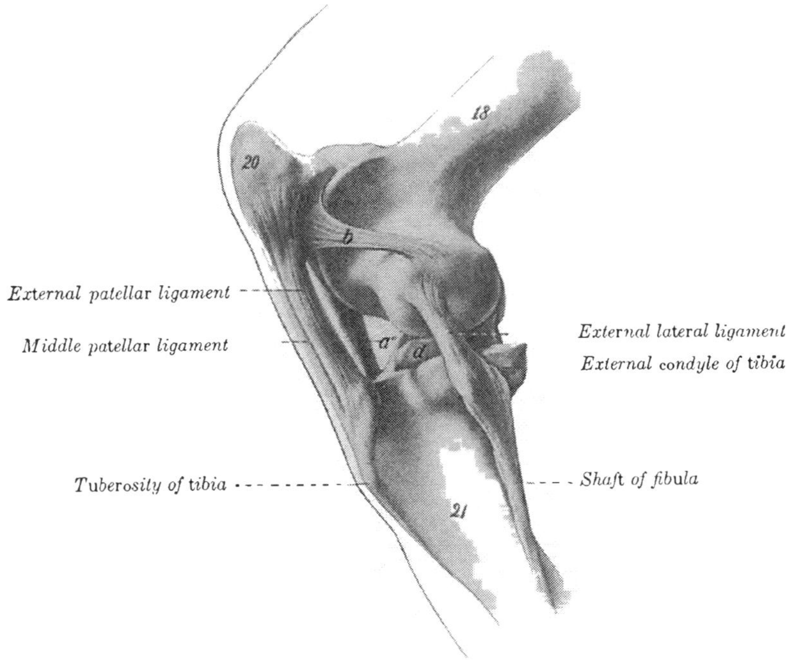

FIG. 155.—LEFT STIFLE JOINT OF HORSE, EXTERNAL VIEW, IN PARTIAL FLEXION.
The capsules have been removed. *18*, Femur; *20*, patella; *21*, tibia; *a''*, internal patellar ligament; *b*, external femoro-patellar ligament; *d*, external semilunar cartilage. (After Ellenberger-Baum, Anat. für Künstler.)

ligaments and covers the fossa acetabuli. A pouch also extends from the acetabular notch for a variable distance along the subpubic groove above the pubo-femoral ligament.

Movements.—This joint is capable of all the movements of a ball-and-socket joint, viz., flexion, extension, abduction, adduction, rotation, and circumduction. The greatest range of movement is displayed in flexion and extension. When standing at rest, the joint is partially flexed, the articular angle (in front) being about 100° to 115°. The other movements occur to a very limited extent in normal action.

Abduction appears to be checked by tension of the round ligament. The pubo-femoral ligament is tensed most promptly by inward rotation of the thigh.

THE STIFLE JOINT

This joint (Articulatio genu), which corresponds to the knee-joint of man, is the largest and most elaborate of all the articulations. Taken as a whole, it may be classed as a ginglymus, although it is not a typical example of the group. In reality it consists of two joints—the femoro-patellar and the **femoro-tibial.**

The **femoro-patellar articulation** (Articulatio femoro-patellaris) is formed between the trochlea of the femur and the articular surface of the patella.

Articular Surfaces.—The trochlea consists of two slightly oblique ridges, with a wide and deep groove between them. The inner ridge is much the larger of the two, especially at its upper part, which is wide and rounded. The outer

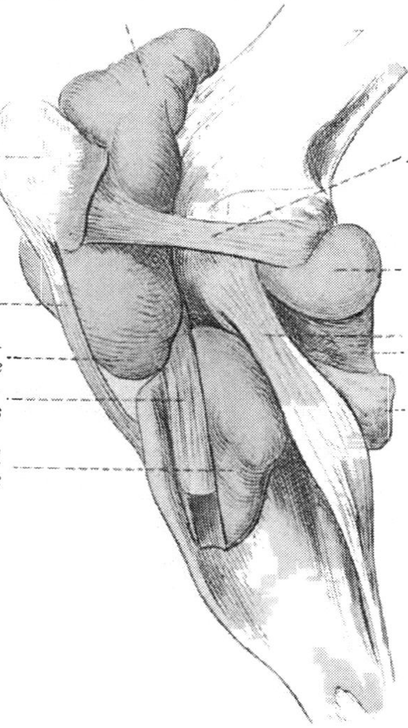

Fig. 156.—Left Stifle Joint of Horse, Lateral View.
The capsules are distended and the external patellar ligament is removed.

ridge is much narrower, and is more regularly curved; its upper part lies about an inch behind a frontal plane tangent to the inner ridge. The articular surface of the patella is much smaller than that of the trochlea. It is completed internally by a supplementary plate of fibro-cartilage (Fibrocartilago patellæ), which curves over the internal surface of the inner lip of the trochlea. A narrow strip of cartilage is found along the outer border also. The articular cartilage on the trochlea completely covers both surfaces of the inner ridge, but only a narrow marginal area on the external surface of the outer ridge.

Joint Capsule.—This is thin and is very capacious. On the patella it is attached around the margin of the articular surface, but on the femur the line of attachment is at a varying distance from the articular surface. On the inner side it is an inch or more from the articular cartilage; on the outer side and above, about half an inch. It pouches upward under the quadriceps femoris for a distance of two or three inches, a pad of fat separating the capsule from the muscle. Below the patella it is separated from the straight ligaments by a thick pad of fat, but inferiorly it is in contact with the femoro-patellar capsules. The joint cavity is the most extensive in the body. It usually communicates with the inner femoro-tibial joint cavity by a slit-like opening situated at the lowest part of the inner ridge of the trochlea. A similar, but smaller, communication with the outer femoro-patellar capsule is often found at the lowest part of the outer ridge.

The inner communication appears to be constant in adult horses, but is liable to be overlooked on account of the fact that it is covered by a valvular fold of the synovial membrane. It is about half an inch wide, and lies under the narrow articular area which connects the trochlea and internal condyle. The outer communication occurs in 18 to 25 per cent. of cases, according to Baum. It is instructive to distend this capsule and thus obtain an idea of its potential capacity and relations (Fig. 156).

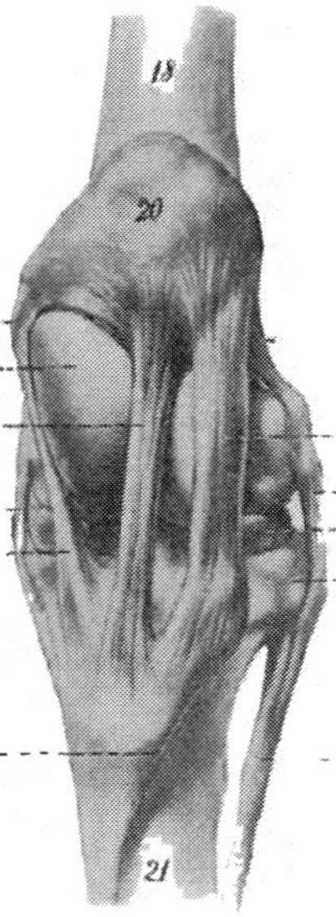

Fig. 157.—Left Stifle Joint of Horse, Front View, in Extension.

The capsules are removed. *18*, Femur; *20*, patella; *21*, tibia. (After Ellenberger-Baum, Anat. für Künstler.)

Ligaments.—The lateral **femoro-patellar ligaments**, external and internal (Ligamentum femoro-patellare fibulare, tibiale), are two thin bands which reinforce the capsule on either side. The external ligament is fairly distinct; it arises from the external epicondyle of the femur just above the lateral femoro-tibial ligament, and ends on the external border of the patella. The internal ligament is thinner and is not distinct from the capsule; it arises above the internal epicondyle, and ends on the patellar fibro-cartilage.

The **patellar ligaments** (Ligamenta patellæ), also called the straight ligaments of the patella, are three very strong bands which attach the patella to the tuberosity of the tibia. The **external** patellar **ligament** is attached above to the outer part of the anterior surface of the patella, and below to the outer part of the tuberosity. It receives a strong tendon from the biceps femoris muscle. The middle patellar **ligament** extends from the front of the apex of the patella to the lower part of the groove on the tuberosity of the tibia, a bursa being interposed between the ligament and the upper part of the groove. The **internal patellar ligament** is attached above to the patellar fibro-cartilage, and ends on the tuberosity of the tibia, internally to the groove. It is joined by the common aponeurosis of the gracilis and sartorius. These so-called ligaments are, in reality, the tendons of insertion of the quadriceps femoris muscle, and transmit the action of the latter to the tibia; they also function similarly for the other muscles attached to them as noted above.

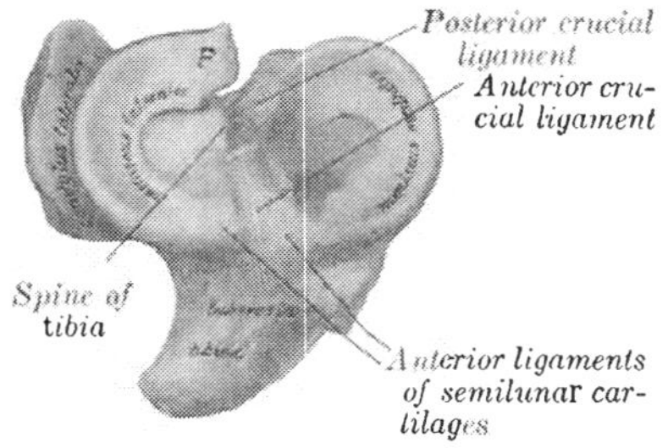

FIG. 158.—SEMILUNAR CARTILAGES AND CRUCIAL LIGAMENTS OF RIGHT STIFLE OF HORSE.

F, Femoral ligament of external cartilage. (After Schmaltz, Atlas d. Anat. d. Pferdes.)

It will be noticed that the upper attachments are further apart than the lower ones, so that the ligaments converge below. The inner ligament is especially oblique. The middle ligament is more deeply placed than the others, and therefore cannot usually be felt distinctly in the living animal.

The **femoro-tibial articulation** (Articulatio femorotibialis) is formed between the condyles of the femur, the proximal end of the tibia, and the interposed semilunar cartilages.

Articular Surfaces.—The condyles of the femur are slightly oblique in direction. The articular surface of the outer one is more strongly curved than that of the inner one; the latter is confluent below with the inner ridge of the trochlea, while the narrow ridge which connects the external condyle with the trochlea is usually non-articular. The saddle-shaped surfaces of the condyles of the tibia are not adapted to the femoral condyles, and are in contact with only a small part of them.

The **semilunar cartilages** (Meniscus lateralis, medialis) are two C-shaped or crescentic discs of fibro-cartilage which produce congruence in the articular surfaces. Each has an upper concave surface adapted to the condyle of the femur, and a lower surface which fits the corresponding condyle of the tibia. The external cartilage does not cover the outer and posterior part of the condyle, over which the tendon of origin of the popliteus muscle plays. The peripheral border is thick and convex, the central one very thin and concave. The fibrous ends or cornua are attached to the tibia in front of and behind the spine. The external cartilage has a third attachment by means of an oblique band (Ligamentum femorale menisci lateralis) which passes from the posterior cornu to the posterior part of the intercondyloid fossa of the femur.

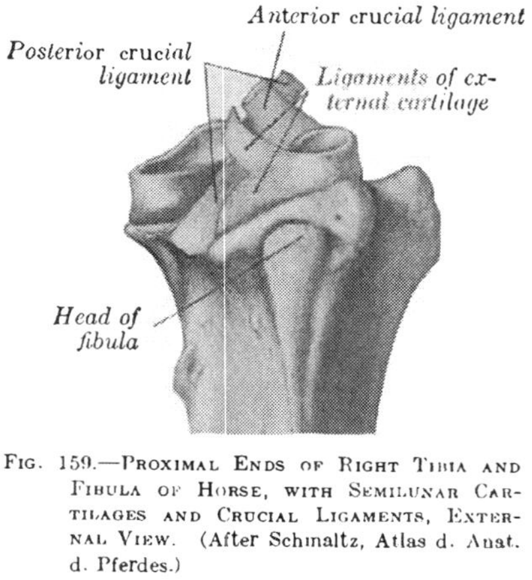

FIG. 159.—PROXIMAL ENDS OF RIGHT TIBIA AND FIBULA OF HORSE, WITH SEMILUNAR CARTILAGES AND CRUCIAL LIGAMENTS, EXTERNAL VIEW. (After Schmaltz, Atlas d. Anat. d. Pferdes.)

The cornua of the internal cartilage (Ligamenta tibiæ anterius et posterius menisci medialis) are attached in front of and behind the inner eminence of the spine. The anterior cornu of the external cartilage (Ligamentum tibiæ anterius menisci lateralis) is attached in front of the outer eminence of the spine. The posterior cornu bifurcates; the lower branch (Ligamentum tibiæ posterius menisci lateralis) is inserted at the popliteal notch, the upper (Ligamentum femorale menisci lateralis) in a small fossa in the extreme posterior part of the intercondyloid fossa.

The **joint capsule** is attached to the margin of the tibial articular surface, but on the femur the line of attachment is for the greater part about half an inch from the articular margin. It is also attached to the convex borders of the semilunar cartilages and to the crucial ligaments. It is strong posteriorly, but in front it practically consists only of the synovial layer. There are two synovial sacs, corresponding to the double nature of the articular surfaces; they do not usually communicate, and each is partially divided into an upper and a lower compartment by the semilunar cartilage. The inner sac pouches upward about half an inch over the condyle of the femur. The external sac invests the tendon of origin of the popliteus muscle, and also pouches downward about three or four inches (ca. 8 to 10 cm.) beneath the peroneus tertius and long extensor muscles (Fig. 156).

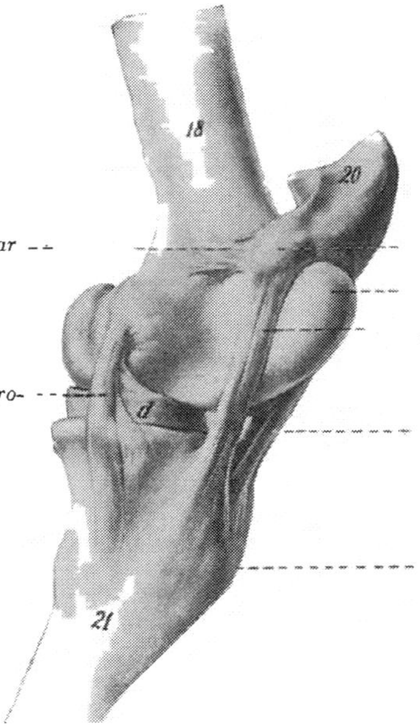

FIG. 160.—LEFT STIFLE JOINT OF HORSE, INTERNAL VIEW IN EXTREME EXTENSION.[1]
18, Femur; *20*, patella (base); *21*, tibia; *d*, internal semilunar cartilage. (After Ellenberger-Baum, Anat. für Künstler.)

As stated above, the outer sac sometimes communicates with the femoro-patellar joint cavity, and the inner sac usually, if not always, does so in the adult.

Ligaments.—There are four of these—two lateral and two crucial.

The **internal lateral ligament** (Ligamentum collaterale tibiale) is attached above to the prominent internal epicondyle of the femur, and below to a rough area below the margin of the internal condyle of the tibia.

The **external lateral ligament** (Ligamentum collaterale fibulare) is somewhat thicker; it arises from the upper depression on the external epicondyle, and ends on the head of the fibula. It covers the tendon of the origin of the popliteus muscle, and a bursa is interposed between the lower part of the ligament and the margin of the external condyle of the tibia.

[1] In this figure the patella is pushed up above the trochlea—a position which it does not occupy normally.

The **crucial ligaments** are two strong rounded bands situated mainly in the intercondyloid fossa of the femur, between the two synovial sacs. They cross each other somewhat in the form of an X, and are named according to their tibial attachments. The **anterior crucial ligament** (Ligamentum cruciatum anterius) arises in the central fossa on the tibial spine, extends upward and backward, and ends on the upper part of the inner surface of the external condyle of the femur. The **posterior crucial ligament** (Ligamentum cruciatum posterius) is internal to the preceding, and is somewhat larger. It is attached to an eminence at the popliteal notch of the tibia, is directed upward and forward, and ends in the anterior part of the intercondyloid fossa of the femur.

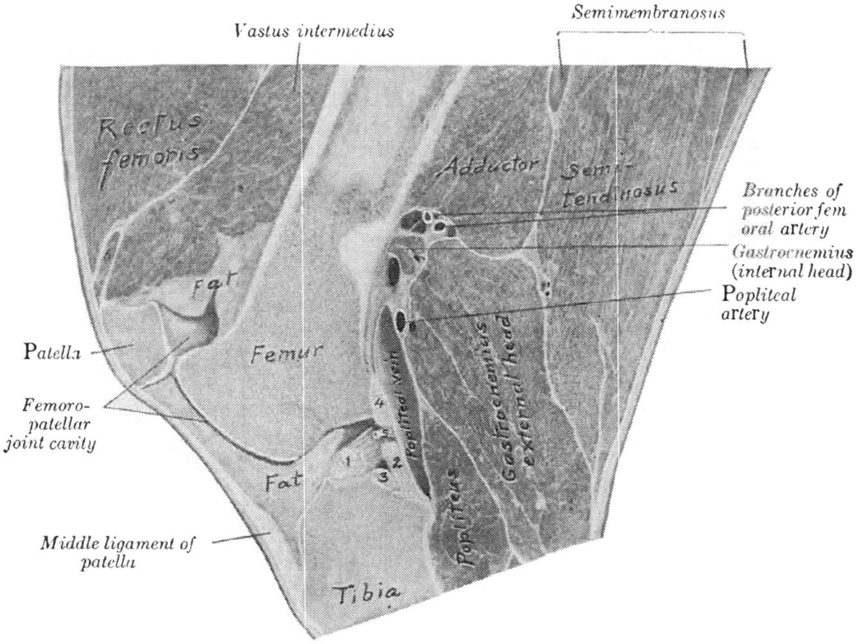

FIG. 161.—RIGHT STIFLE JOINT OF HORSE; SAGITTAL SECTION PASSING THROUGH OUTER PART OF INNER RIDGE OF TROCHLEA AND INTERCONDYLOID FOSSA.
1, Anterior crucial ligament; *2*, posterior crucial ligament; *3*, posterior cornu of internal semilunar cartilage; *4*, femoral ligament of external semilunar cartilage; *5*, articular artery; *6*, part of vastus internus.

It may be added that these ligaments do not lie in a sagittal plane, but are somewhat twisted across each other; outward rotation of the leg untwists and slackens them.

Movements.—The principal movements of the stifle joint as a whole are flexion and extension. In the ordinary standing position the articular angle (behind) is about 140° to 150°. Flexion is limited only by contact of the leg with the thigh if the hock is also flexed. Extension is incomplete, *i. e.*, the femur and tibia cannot be brought into the same straight line. Rotation is limited, and is freest during semiflexion. The patella glides on the femoral trochlea upward in extension, downward in flexion.

Extension is checked mainly by tension of the crucial and lateral ligaments. In extreme extension, which is accompanied by slight outward rotation of the leg, the patella can be pushed upward and inward so that its fibro-cartilage hooks over the upper end of the inner ridge of the trochlea, but it will not remain there unless held in position. When pressure is removed, the base of the patella tips forward and the cartilage lies upon the most prominent part of the trochlear ridge. During flexion, which is accompanied by slight inward rotation of the leg, the condyles of the femur and the semilunar cartilages glide backward on the tibia; the movement of the external condyle and cartilage is greater than that of the inner one. In extreme flexion the patellar and posterior crucial ligaments are tense; the other ligaments are relaxed. The movement of the patella is gliding with coaptation, *i. e.*, different parts of the opposing articular surfaces come into contact successively. Only a narrow transverse strip (ca. 1.5 to 2 cm. wide) of the patella is in contact with the trochlea at a time.

TIBIO-FIBULAR ARTICULATION

The head of the fibula articulates with a crescentic facet just below the outer margin of the external condyle of the tibia. The joint **capsule** is strong and close. The shaft of the fibula is attached to the external border of the tibia by the **interosseous membrane** of the leg (Membrana interossea cruris); this is perforated about an inch from its proximal end by an opening which transmits the anterior tibial vessels to the front of the tibia. A fibrous cord usually extends from the distal end of the shaft of the fibula to the external malleolus. The latter is the distal end of the fibula which has fused with the tibia. No appreciable movement occurs in this joint.

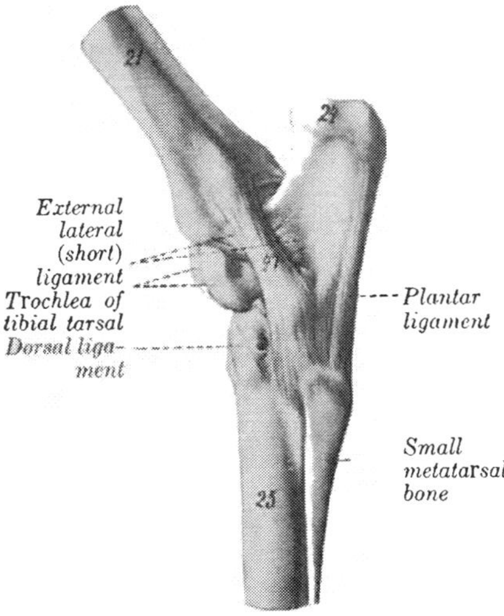

FIG. 162.—LEFT HOCK JOINT OF HORSE, EXTERNAL VIEW.

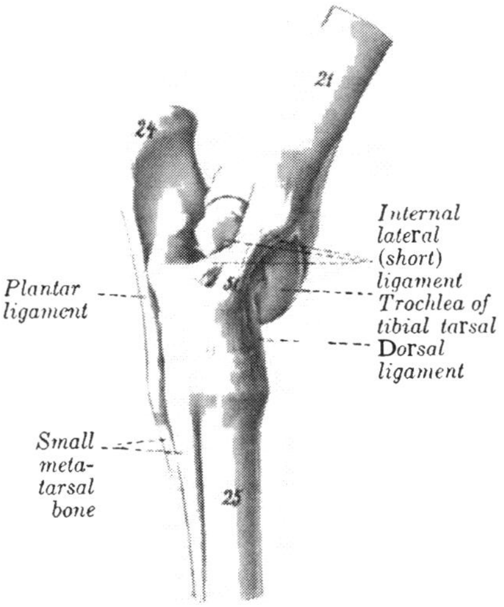

FIG. 163.—LEFT HOCK JOINT OF HORSE, INTERNAL VIEW.

21, Tibia; *24*, tuber calcis; *25*, large metatarsal bone; *47*, long external lateral ligament; *51*, long internal lateral ligament. (After Ellenberger-Baum, Anat. für Künstler.)

THE HOCK JOINT

This is a composite joint made up of a number of articulations (Articulationes tarsi). These are: (1) The tibio-tarsal articulation; (2) the intertarsal articulations; (3) the tarso-metatarsal articulation.

The **tibio-tarsal articulation** (Articulatio talo-cruralis) is a typical ginglymus formed by the trochlea of the tibial tarsal bone (astragalus or talus) and the corresponding surface of the distal end of the tibia. The ridges and grooves of these surfaces are directed obliquely forward and outward at an angle of about 12° to 15°, with a sagittal plane. The trochlear surface is about twice as extensive as that on the tibia, and its ridges have a spiral curvature. The other articulations are arthrodia, which have joint surfaces and ligaments of such a nature as to allow only a minimal amount of gliding motion.

As in the case of the carpal joints, it is convenient to describe first the common capsule and ligaments, which are the more important practically, and then to consider very briefly the special ligaments.

The fibrous part of the joint **capsule** is attached around the margin of the tibial articular surface above and the metatarsal surfaces below; it is also attached in part to the free surface of the bones which it covers, and blends with the lateral ligaments. Its anterior part (anterior ligament) is rather thin; in distention of the capsule, as in "bog-spavin," its antero-internal part, which is not bound down by the tendons passing over the joint, forms a fluctuating swelling over the inner ridge of the trochlea. The posterior part (posterior and tarso-metatarsal ligaments) is very thick, and is intimately attached to the tarsal bones. Its superficial face is in part cartilaginous, and forms a smooth surface for the perforans tendon. Superiorly, it pouches upward behind the distal end of the tibia for a distance of about

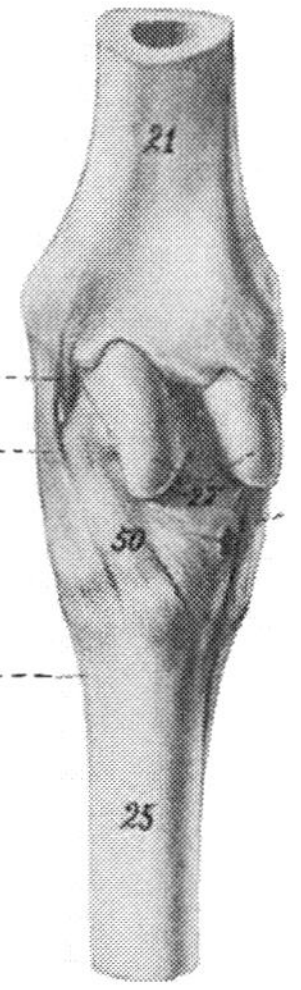

FIG. 164.—LEFT HOCK JOINT OF HORSE, ANTERIOR VIEW.
21 Tibia; *22*, trochlea of tibial tarsal bone; *25*, large metatarsal bone; *50*, dorsal or oblique ligament. (After Ellenberger-Baum, Anat. für Künstler.)

two inches (ca. 5 cm.). Inferiorly, it is continued downward, forming the **subtarsal** or **check ligament,** which unites with the perforans tendon about the middle of the metatarsus.

There are four **synovial sacs:** 1. The **tibio-tarsal sac** lubricates the proximal joint, and is much the largest and most important. It is chiefly involved in the swelling produced by excess of fluid in the joint cavity, when the capsule bulges antero-internally and postero-superiorly. 2. The first **intertarsal sac** lines the joints formed by the tibial and fibular tarsal bones above, and the central and fourth tarsals below; it communicates in front with the proximal synovial capsule. 3. The **second intertarsal sac** lubricates the joints formed between the central tarsal and the bones below and on either side. 4. The **tarso-metatarsal sac** lubricates the joints formed between the tarsal and metatarsal bones, those between the proximal ends of the metatarsal bones, and those formed by the third tarsal with the bones on either side.

Common Ligaments.—The **external lateral ligament** (Ligamentum collaterale fibulare longum et breve) consists of two distinct bands which cross each other. The **long** (superficial) **ligament** arises on the posterior part of the external malleolus, is directed almost straight downward, and is attached to the fibular and fourth tarsal bones and the large and external small metatarsal bones. It forms a canal for the lateral extensor tendon. The **short** (deep) **ligament** arises on the anterior part of the external malleolus, is directed chiefly backward, and ends on the rough excavation on the external surface of the tibial tarsal and the adjacent surface of the fibular tarsal bone.

The **internal lateral ligament** (Ligamentum collaterale tibiale longum et breve) also consists of two parts which cross each other. The **long ligament** arises on the posterior part of the internal malleolus, becomes wider below, and is attached on the lower tuberosity of the tibial tarsal, the large and outer small metatarsal bones, and the inner surface of the lower tarsal bones which it covers. The **short ligament** lies largely under cover of the long one. It extends from the anterior part of the internal malleolus runs backward and somewhat downward, and divides into two

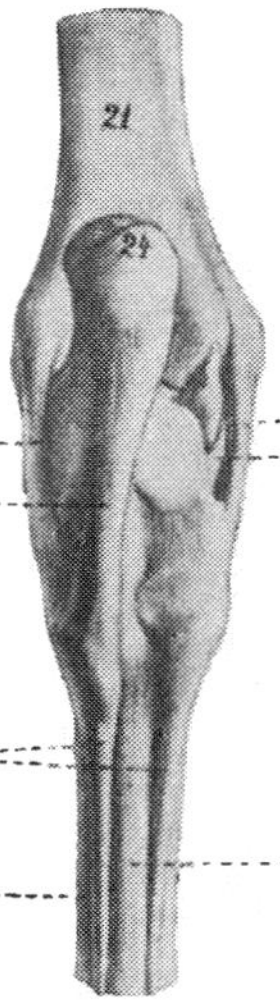

FIG. 165.—LEFT HOCK JOINT OF HORSE, POSTERIOR VIEW.
21, Tibia; *24*, tuber calcis. (After Ellenberger-Baum, Anat. für Künstler.)

branches; one of these ends on the upper tuberosity on the inner surface of the tibial tarsal bone, the other on the sustentaculum tali.

The **plantar** or **calcaneo-metatarsal ligament** (Ligamentum tarsi plantare) is a very strong flat band which covers the outer part of the posterior surface of the tarsus. It is attached to the posterior surface of the fibular and fourth tarsal bones and the proximal end of the external metatarsal bone.

The **dorsal** or **oblique ligament** (Ligamentum tarsi dorsale) is a triangular sheet which is attached above to the lower tuberosity on the inner face of the tibial tarsal bone, and spreads out below on the central and third tarsal bones, and the proximal ends of the large and inner small metatarsal bones, to all of which it is attached.

Special Ligaments.—A considerable number of short bands which connect adjacent bones of the tarsus and metatarsus are described by various authors; some of these are quite distinct; others are difficult to isolate. Most of them are not of sufficient importance to justify detailed description.

(1) The tibial and fibular tarsal bones are united by four bands (astragalo-calcaneal ligaments). The internal ligament extends from the sustentaculum tali to the adjacent part of the tibia tarsal, blending with the short lateral ligament. The external ligament extends from the anterior process of the fibular tarsal to the adjacent part of the external ridge of the trochlea. The superior ligament extends from the posterior margin of the trochlea to the fibular tarsal. The interosseous ligament is deeply placed in the sinus tarsi between the two bones, and is attached in the rough areas of the opposed surfaces.

(2) The smaller bones are attached to each other as follows: The central and third tarsal are united by an interosseous and an oblique anterior ligament (scaphoido-cunean ligaments). The central and fourth tarsal are united by an interosseous and a transverse external ligament (cuboido-scaphoid ligament). The third and fourth tarsals are similarly connected (cuboido-cunean ligaments). The third tarsal is joined by an interosseous (intercunean) ligament to the

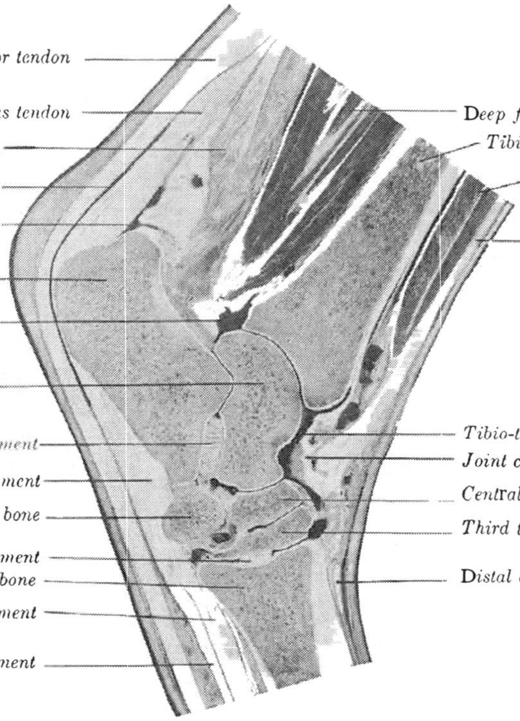

FIG. 166.—SAGITTAL SECTION OF HOCK OF HORSE.

(fused) first and second tarsals; the latter are connected with the fourth tarsal by a transverse posterior ligament.

(3) The smaller bones are connected with the upper row as follows: The central is attached to the tibial tarsal by posterior and interosseous (astragalo-scaphoid) ligaments, and to the fibular tarsal by a short oblique (calcaneo-scaphoid) band. The fourth is attached to the fibular tarsal by interosseous and posterior (calcaneo-cuboid) ligaments. The (fused) first and second tarsals are connected with the fibular tarsal by a posterior (calcaneo-cunean) ligament.

(4) The lower tarsal bones are connected with the metatarsus by tarso-metatarsal ligaments, which are not distinct from the common ligaments, except in the case of the interosseous ligament between the third tarsal and metatarsal bones.

Movements.—These are flexion and extension, which take place at the tibio-tarsal joint. The movements between the tarsal bones, and between the latter and the metatarsus, are so limited as to be negligible so far as the action of the joint as a whole is concerned. In the standing position the articular angle (in front) is about 150° to 160°. Complete extension is prevented by tension of the lateral ligaments. Flexion is checked only by contact of the metatarsus with the leg, provided the stifle joint is also flexed. Owing to the fact that the axis of motion is slightly oblique, the lower part of the limb deviates somewhat outward during flexion.

The movements of the hock joint must correspond with those of the stifle on account of the tendinous bands in front and behind (peroneus tertius and flexor perforatus), which extend from the lower part of the femur to the tarsus and metatarsus.

The remaining joints differ in no material respect from those of the thoracic limb.

COMPARATIVE ARTHROLOGY[1]

JOINTS AND LIGAMENTS OF THE VERTEBRÆ

Ox.—The ligamentum nuchæ is better developed than in the horse. The funicular part is clearly divided into two lateral halves, which are round at their occipital attachment, but from the axis backward become rapidly wider and flat. This wide portion is almost sagittal, lies on either side of the vertebral spines, and is covered by the trapezius and rhomboideus muscles. From the highest part of

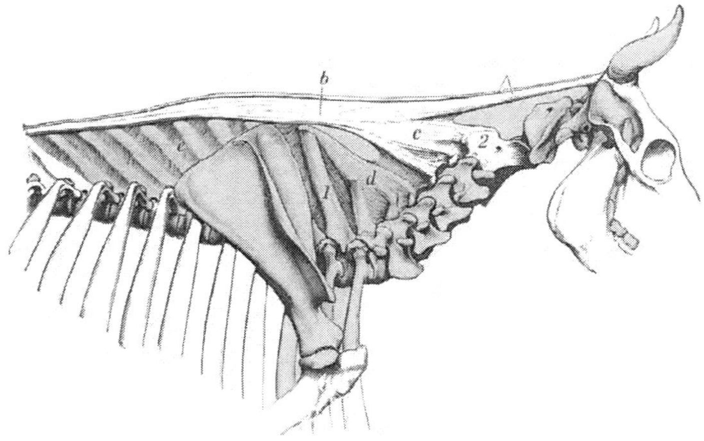

Fig. 167.—Ligamentum Nuchæ of Ox.

a, Funicular part; *b*, wide portion; *c*, *d*, lamellar part; *e*, interspinous ligaments; *1*, spinous process of first thoracic vertebra; *2*, axis. (Ellenberger-Baum, Anat. d. Haustiere.)

the withers (third thoracic spine) it gradually diminishes in size and fades out in the lumbar region. The lamellar part is thick, and consists of anterior and posterior parts. The anterior part is double; its fibers proceed from the funicular part to the second, third, and fourth cervical spines. The posterior part is single; its fibers extend from the first thoracic spine to the fifth, sixth, and seventh cervical spines.

The inferior common ligament is very strong in the lumbar region.

The intervertebral fibro-cartilages are thicker than in the horse.

The interspinous ligaments of the back and loins consist largely of elastic tissue.

[1]This section consists necessarily only of a brief statement of the most important differences in the joints of the other animals.

There are no intertransverse joints in the lumbar region.

Pig.—The ligamentum nuchæ is represented by a fibrous raphé and thin layers of elastic tissue which extend between the cervical spines.

The atlanto-occipital and atlanto-axial joints resemble those of the dog.

The interspinous ligaments of the neck are elastic.

Dog.—The ligamentum nuchæ consists of a small fibrous band which extends from the spine of the axis to the anterior thoracic spines; it may be regarded as a mere fibrous raphé between the right and left muscles.

There are interspinous muscles instead of ligaments in the neck.

There are three ligaments in connection with the odontoid process. The two alar ligaments (Ligamenta alaria) arise on either side of the odontoid process, diverge, and end on either side of the foramen magnum. The transverse ligament of the atlas (Ligamentum transversum atlantis) stretches across the dorsal surface of the odontoid process and binds it down on the ventral arch of the atlas, a bursa being interposed. It is attached on either side to the lateral masses of the atlas.

The two capsules of the atlanto-occipital joint communicate with each other, and usually with the capsule of the atlanto-axial joint also.

ARTICULATIONS OF THE THORAX

Ox.—The second to the eleventh costo-chondral joints inclusive are diarthroses with close capsules, reinforced externally. (They are synchondroses in the sheep.) The upper parts of the cartilages are attached to each other by distinct elastic ligaments (Ligamenta intercostalia).

The first pair of chondro-sternal joints are separate from each other; intercrossing fibers unite the costo-chondral junctions above the joints.

The first segment of the sternum forms a diarthrosis with the body. The anterior joint surface is concave, the posterior convex. The joint (Articulatio intersternalis) is surrounded by a close capsule, and the joint surfaces are attached to each by a small intra-articular ligament. Limited lateral movement is possible. (In the sheep the joint is a synchondrosis.)

Both surfaces of the sternum are covered by a layer of fibrous tissue.

Pig.—The second to the fifth or sixth costo-chondral joints are diarthroses. The intersternal articulation and the sternal ligaments resemble those of the ox.

Dog.—The first chondro-sternal joints do not coalesce.

The internal sternal ligament divides into three bands.

TEMPORO-MANDIBULAR ARTICULATION

Ox.—The articular surfaces are of such a character as to permit more extensive lateral movement than in the horse.

The condyle of the mandible is relatively small and is concave transversely. The temporal articular surface is extensive and is convex in both directions. The postglenoid process is small.

Pig.—The considerable longitudinal diameter of the temporal articular surfaces and the very small size of the postglenoid process allow great freedom of protraction and retraction of the lower jaw. Lateral movement is limited. The posterior ligament is absent.

Dog.—The articular surfaces allow extremely little lateral or gliding movement. They are cylindrical in curvature, and the interarticular disc is very thin. The posterior ligament is absent.

The other articulations of the skull are sufficiently described in the Osteology.

ARTICULATIONS OF THE THORACIC LIMB

SHOULDER JOINT

Ox.—The articular angle is about 100°.

Pig and Dog.—The joint capsule communicates freely with the bicipital bursa. There is a rudimentary marginal cartilage around the rim of the glenoid cavity. In the dog there is usually a strong band extending from the acromion to the outer part of the capsule; another band (Ligamentum coraco-acromiale) often stretches between the scapular tuberosity and the acromion.

ELBOW JOINT

Ox.—No important differences exist. The upper part of the interosseous radio-ulnar ligament is commonly ossified in the adult.

Pig.—There are no important differences. The radius and ulna are so firmly united by the interosseous ligament as to prevent any appreciable movement between them.

Dog.—The joint capsule is reinforced in front by an oblique ligament which arises on the front of the external condyle of the humerus above the joint surface, and joins the terminal part of the biceps and brachialis below. The external lateral ligament is thick and divides into two parts; the anterior part is attached to the radius and blends with the annular ligament; the posterior part widens below, forming a sort of cap, and is attached to the ulna. The internal lateral ligament also divides into two branches; the anterior branch ends on the inner surface of the neck of the radius; the posterior enters the interosseous space and is attached to both bones. An elastic band (Ligamentum olecrani) extends from the outer surface of the internal epicondyle to the anterior border of the ulna.

There are two radio-ulnar joints. The proximal radio-ulnar joint is included in the capsule of the elbow, but is provided with an annular ligament which extends from the lower part of the external ligament across the front of the proximal end of the radius to the ulna, blending with the biceps and brachialis tendons. The distal joint is formed by a concave facet on the radius and a convex one on the radius, and is surrounded by a tight capsule. The interosseous membrane unites the shafts of the two bones. The movements consist of limited rotation of the radius (ca. 20°), carrying the paw with it. The ordinary position is termed pronation; outward rotation is supination.[1]

THE CARPAL JOINTS

These have the same general arrangement as in the horse. Numerous minor differences naturally exist, but must be excluded from this brief account, which contains only important special features.

The lateral movements are freer, especially in the dog, but flexion is not so complete: the anatomical explanation of these facts lies in the nature of the articular surfaces and certain ligamentous differences. The lateral ligaments are much weaker, the long external one being especially small in the ox. Two oblique, somewhat elastic, bands cross the front of the radio-carpal and intercarpal joints. The proximal one is attached to the distal end of the radius and passes downward and outward to the ulnar carpal bone; the other one connects the radial and fourth carpal bones in a similar fashion.

In the ox the short lateral ligaments are well defined, a ligament connects

[1] These movements are best seen in man, in whom the back of the hand may be turned forward (pronation) or backward (supination).

the accessory carpal with the distal end of the ulna, and strong bands connect the distal bones with the metacarpus.

The interosseous and interordinal ligaments vary with the number of carpal bones present in the different species.

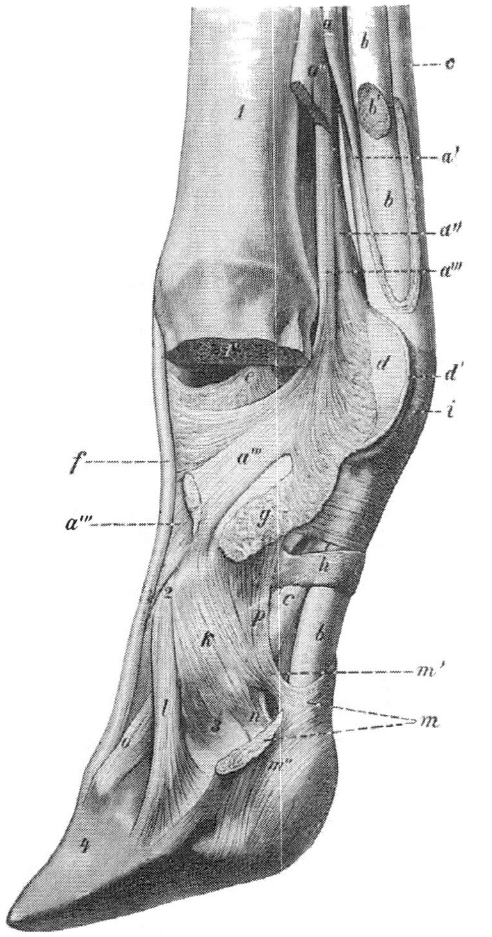

Fig. 168.—Distal Part of Limb of Ox, Showing Ligaments and Tendons. One Digit and Corresponding Articular Part of Metacarpal Bone are Removed.

a, Suspensory ligament; *a'*, branch of *a* to superficial flexor tendon; *a''*, *a'''*, lateral and central branches of *a*; *b*, deep flexor tendon; *b'*, branch of *b* to digit removed; *c*, *c*, superficial flexor tendon; *d*, *d'*, intersesamoid ligament (cut); *e*, interdigital lateral ligament of fetlock joint; *f*, tendon of common extensor; *g*, proximal interdigital ligament; *h*, digital annular ligament; *i*, posterior annular ligament of fetlock; k, lateral ligament of pastern joint; *l*, distal interdigital ligament; *m*, crucial interdigital ligament (cut); *m'*, *m''*, attachments of *m* to second phalanx and distal sesamoid bone; *n*, suspensory ligament of distal sesamoid; *o*, anterior elastic ligament; *p*, lateral volar ligament of pastern joint; *1*, metacarpus, sawn off at *1'*; *2*, first phalanx; *3*, second phalanx; *4*, third phalanx. (Ellenberger-Baum, Anat. d. Haustiere.)

METACARPO-PHALANGEAL JOINTS

Ox.—There are two joints, one for each digit. The two capsules communicate posteriorly. The two interdigital lateral ligaments (Ligamenta collateralia interdigitalia) result from the bifurcation of a band which arises in the furrow between the divisions of the distal end of the large metacarpal bone; they spread out and end on the proximal ends of the first phalanges. A strong superior **interdigital ligament** (Ligamentum interdigitale), consisting of short intercrossing fibers, unites the middles of the interdigital surfaces of the first phalanges.

Crucial ligaments (Ligamenta phalango-sesamoideæ) connect the sesamoids with the proximal end of the opposite first phalanx.

The intersesamoid ligament connects all four sesamoids, and extends upward much less than in the horse.

The lateral sesamoidean ligaments end almost entirely on the first phalanges.

The superficial inferior sesamoidean ligament is absent. The middle inferior sesamoidean ligaments of each digit are two short strong bands which extend from the distal margins of the sesamoids to the proximal ends of the first phalanges. The deep inferior sesamoidean ligaments are strong and distinctly crucial.

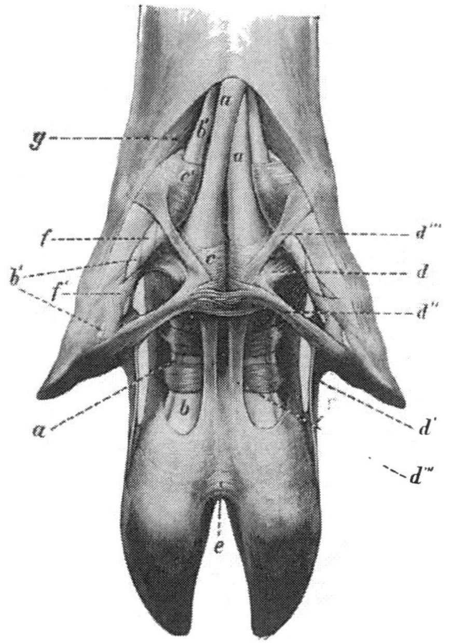

Fig. 169.—Ligaments and Tendons of Digits of Pig, Volar View.

a, Superficial flexor tendon; *b*, deep flexor tendon; *b'*, branches of *b* to accessory digits; *c*, *c'*, annular ligaments; *d–d'''*, ligaments of accessory digits; *e*, cruciate interdigital ligaments; *f*, *f'*, spiral band around the flexor tendons of the accessory digits; *g*, abductor of accessory digit. (Ellenberger-Baum, Anat. d. Haustiere.)

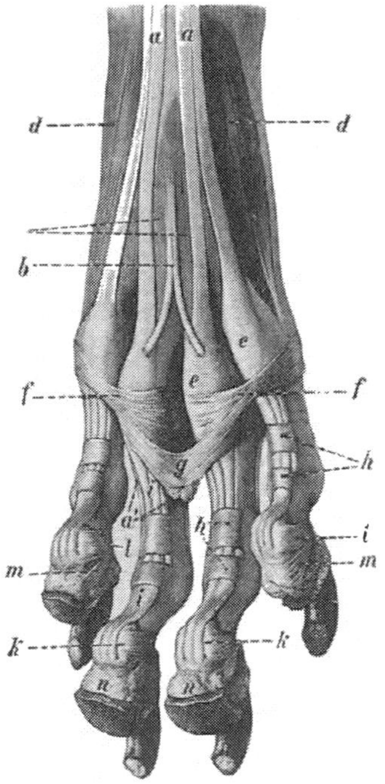

Fig. 170.—Ligaments and Tendons of Paw of Dog, Hind Limb, Volar View.

a, *a'*, Superficial flexor tendon; *b*, tendon to large pad; *c*, lumbricales muscles; *d*, interossei muscles; *e*, *f*, annular ligaments at metatarso-phalangeal joints; *g*, suspensory ligament of large pad; *h*, digital annular ligaments; *i*, deep flexor tendon; k, distal sesamoid; *l*, suspensory ligament of k; *m*, suspensory ligament of digital pad; *n*, digital pads. (Ellenberger-Baum, Anat. d. Haustiere.)

The suspensory or superior sesamoidean ligament is more distinctly muscular than in the horse—indeed in the young animal it consists almost entirely of muscular tissue. At the distal third of the metacarpus it divides into three branches. These give rise to five subdivisions, either by bifurcation of the lateral branches or trifurcation of the middle branch. The four lateral bands end on the sesamoid bones and the distal end of the large metacarpal bone, and detach slips to the extensor tendons. The middle band passes through the groove between the two divisions of the distal end of the metacarpus, and divides into two branches which join the tendons of the proper extensors of the digits; it sends fibers also to the interdigital lateral ligaments and to the central sesamoids. About the middle of the metacarpus the suspensory ligament detaches a band which unites lower down with the superficial flexor tendon, thus inclosing the tendon of the deep flexor of the digit; it also blends with the thick fascia of the region. The latter gives off a band on either side to the accessory digits, and a tendinous band descends from each accessory digit to the third phalanx and sesamoid bone, blending with the tendon of the corresponding proper extensor.

Pig.—There are four metacarpo-phalangeal joints, each of which has a capsule, lateral, intersesamoidean, and crucial sesamoidean ligaments. Since distinct interosseous muscles are present, there are, of course, no suspensory ligaments.

Dog.—There are five metacarpo-phalangeal joints, each having its own capsule and indistinct lateral ligaments. A small sesamoid bone occurs in the anterior part of each capsule, over which the corresponding extensor tendon plays. The intersesamoidean ligaments do not extend above the sesamoids. The cruciate ligaments are present, as well as a fibrous layer which attaches the distal margins of the sesamoids to the posterior surface of the proximal end of the first phalanx.

INTERPHALANGEAL JOINTS

Ox.—The two proximal joints have separate capsules, and broad, but rather indistinct, lateral ligaments. Each joint has also two central and two lateral volar ligaments. The central ligaments are largely fused to form a strong band. The lateral ones extend from the borders of the first phalanx to the proximal end of the second phalanx.

The distal interphalangeal joints have, in addition to the capsules and lateral ligaments, bands which reinforce them on either side. The central or interdigital pair arise in the depressions on the distal ends of the first phalanges, receive fibers from the second phalanges, and end on the interdigital surfaces of the third phalanges at the margin of the articular surface. The lateral pair have a similar course, but are thinner, and end on the corresponding third sesamoid. An elastic band crosses the front of the second phalanx obliquely, from the distal end of the first phalanx to the extensor process of the third phalanx.

The **crucial or inferior interdigital ligaments** (Ligamenta cruciata interdigitalia) are two strong bands which limit the separation of the digits. They are attached above to the lateral (or abaxial) eminences on the proximal ends of the second phalanges (blending with the lateral ligaments), cross the deep flexor tendon obliquely, and reach the interdigital space, where they intercross and blend. Most of the fibers end on the third sesamoid of the opposite side, but some are attached to the interdigital aspect of the second phalanx and the third sesamoid of the same side. In the sheep there is, instead of the foregoing, a transverse ligament which is attached on either side to the interdigital surfaces of the second and third phalanges and the third sesamoid bone. It is related below to the skin, above to a pad of fat.

Pig.—The interphalangeal joints of the chief digits resemble in general those of the ox. The inferior interdigital ligament resembles, however, that of the sheep, and is intimately adherent to the skin. There is, besides, a remarkable arrangement of ligaments which connect the small digits with each other and with the chief digits.

This apparatus is somewhat complex, but its chief features are as follows: A superior interdigital ligament is attached on either side to the third phalanges of the small digits, while centrally it blends with the annular ligaments of the flexor tendons behind the metacarpo-phalangeal joints of the chief digits. Two bands (central longitudinal interdigital ligaments) arise on the bases of the small digits, cross the flexor tendons obliquely downward and inward, pass through the superior interdigital ligament, and blend below with the inferior interdigital ligament. Two lateral bands (lateral longitudinal interdigital ligaments) are attached in common with the superior interdigital ligaments to the third phalanges of the small digits, and blend below with the outer part of the inferior interdigital ligament.

Dog.—Each joint has a capsule and two lateral ligaments. The distal joints have also two elastic **dorsal ligaments** (Ligamenta dorsalia), which extend from the proximal end of the second phalanx to the ridge at the base of the third phalanx (Fig. 133). They produce dorsal flexion of the joint, and thus raise or retract the claws when the flexor muscles relax. The distal sesamoids are represented by complementary cartilages attached to the volar margins of the articular surfaces of the third phalanges.

Three interdigital ligaments restrict the spreading apart of the digits. Two of these cross the volar surface of the proximal parts of the chief digits, *i. e.*, one for the second and third, the other for the fourth and fifth; they blend with the annular ligaments on either side. The third ligament is attached on either side to the foregoing ligaments and the annular ligaments of the third and fourth digits, and curves downward centrally, ending in the large pad on the paw.

ARTICULATIONS OF THE PELVIC LIMB

SACRO-ILIAC JOINT

This joint and the pelvic ligaments present no very striking differences in the other animals. The sacro-sciatic ligament in the dog is a narrow but strong band which extends from the posterior part of the lateral margin of the sacrum to the tuber ischii; it is the homologue of the ligamentum sacro-tuberosum of man.

HIP JOINT

Ox.—The shallowness of the acetabulum is compensated by the greater size of the marginal cartilage. The head of the femur has a smaller radius of curvature than that of the horse, and the articular surface extends a considerable distance outward on the upper surface of the neck. The round ligament is entirely intra-articular; it is small, and sometimes absent. The pubo-femoral or accessory ligament is absent.

There are no important differences in the other animals.

STIFLE JOINT

Ox.—There is a considerable communication between the femoro-patellar and inner femoro-tibial joint cavities; this is situated as in the horse, but is wider. A small communication with the external femoro-tibial capsule sometimes occurs. The two femoro-tibial capsules usually communicate. The middle patellar ligament is not sunken, as there is no groove on the tuberosity of the tibia where it is attached. The external patellar ligament fuses completely with the tendon of insertion of the biceps femoris, and a synovial bursa is interposed between them and the external condyle of the femur.

In the other animals there is a single ligamentum patellæ, and the synovial sacs communicate so freely as to constitute a common joint cavity. In the dog the semilunar cartilages are united anteriorly by a transverse ligament, and the posterior part of the capsule contains the two Vesalian sesamoids, which articulate with the condyles of the femur.

TIBIO-FIBULAR JOINTS

Ox.—The proximal end of the fibula fuses with the external condyle of the tibia. The distal end remains separate, and forms an arthrosis with the distal end of the tibia; the movement here is imperceptible, as the two bones are closely united by strong peripheral fibers.

Pig.—The superior joint is provided with a capsule which is reinforced in front and behind by fibrous tissue.

The interosseous ligament attaches the shaft of the fibula to the outer border of the tibia.

The inferior joint is included in the capsule of the hock joint, and is strength ened by oblique anterior and posterior ligaments. There is also an interosseus ligament.

Dog.—The arrangement is essentially the same as in the pig, but there is no interosseous ligament in the inferior joint.

HOCK JOINT

Ox.—There is very considerable mobility at the first intertarsal joint, the capsule of which is correspondingly roomy. The short external lateral ligament is attached below on the tibial tarsal only. A strong transverse ligament attaches the external malleolus (distal end of the fibula) to the back of the tibial tarsal bone. The dorsal or oblique ligament is narrow and thin.

Pig.—The arrangement in general resembles that of the ox.

Dog.—The long lateral ligaments are very small, and the short ones double. The plantar ligament is weak, and ends on the fourth metacarpal bone. No distinct dorsal (or oblique) ligament is present. Movement occurs almost exelusively at the tibio-tarsal joint.

The remaining joints resemble those of the thoracic limb.

THE MUSCULAR SYSTEM

MYOLOGY

The **muscles** (Musculi) are the active organs of motion. They are characterized by their property of contracting when stimulated. Muscular tissue is of three kinds: (*a*) **Striated** or striped; (*b*) **non-striated,** unstriped, or smooth; and (*c*) **cardiac.** Only the first of these varieties will be considered in this section. The striped muscles, being for the most part directly or indirectly connected with the skeleton, are often termed **skeletal** or somatic, while unstriped muscle may be spoken of as **visceral** or splanchnic. The former cover the greater part of the skeleton, and thus in a large measure determine the form of the animal. They are red in color, the shade varying in different muscles and under various conditions.

Muscles vary greatly in **form,** and may be classified as—(*a*) **Long**; (*b*) short; (*c*) **flat**; (*d*) **ring-like** or or**bicular**. Long muscles are found chiefly in the limbs, while the flat or broad muscles occur principally in the trunk, where they assist in forming the walls of the body cavities. The ring-like or orbicular muscles circumscribe orifices which they close, and are hence termed **sphincters.**

Attachments.—The muscles are attached to **bones, cartilages, ligaments, fasciæ,** or the **skin.** In all cases the attachment is by means of fibrous tissue, the muscle-fibers not coming into direct relation with the bone or cartilage. The perimysium of the muscle may fuse directly with the periosteum or perichondrium (fleshy attachment), or the union may be by means of intermediary fibrous strutures called **tendons** or **aponeuroses** (tendinous attachment). Tendons may be funicular, ribbon-like, or in the form of membranous sheets; to the latter the term aponeurosis is commonly applied.

In certain positions, especially where tendons play over joints or are subjected to great pressure, **sesamoid bones** develop in the original tendon tissue. Some of these are large and constant, as the patella and the great sesamoids of the fetlock.

The accessory structures connected with the muscles are the **synovial membranes** and the **fasciæ.**

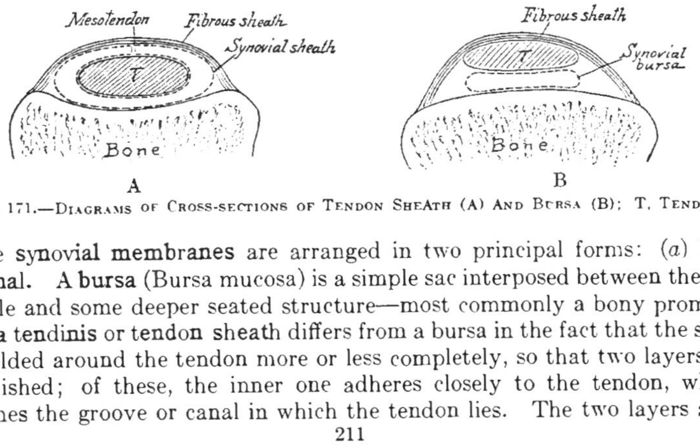

FIG. 171.—DIAGRAMS OF CROSS-SECTIONS OF TENDON SHEATH (A) AND BURSA (B); T, TENDON.

The **synovial membranes** are arranged in two principal forms: (*a*) **Bursal**; (*b*) **vaginal.** A **bursa** (Bursa mucosa) is a simple sac interposed between the tendon or muscle and some deeper seated structure—most commonly a bony prominence. A **vagina tendinis** or **tendon sheath** differs from a bursa in the fact that the synovial sac is folded around the tendon more or less completely, so that two layers can be distinguished; of these, the inner one adheres closely to the tendon, while the outer lines the groove or canal in which the tendon lies. The two layers are continuous along a fold termed the **mesotendon.** The arrangement is shown in Fig. 171.[1] The articular synovial membranes in some places form extra-articular pouches, which facilitate the play of tendons.

The **fasciæ** are sheets of connective tissue, mainly of the white fibrous variety, with a greater or less admixture of elastic fibers in certain cases. Two layers may usually be recognized. Of these, the **superficial fascia** (Fascia subcutanea) is composed of loose connective tissue which may contain more or less fat and is subcutaneous. The **deep fascia** is composed of one or more layers of dense fibrous tissue spread over the surface of the muscles chiefly. Its deep face may be very loosely attached to the underlying structures or may fuse with the epimysium, tendons, bones, or ligaments. In some parts, especially the limbs, septal plates pass between the muscles and are attached to the bones or ligaments; these are termed **intermuscular septa.** In this way many muscles are inclosed in fibrous sheaths which hold them in position. Not uncommonly special bands stretch across the grooves in which tendons play, converting these into canals. Such bands are termed **vaginal** or **annular ligaments.** The deep fascia is often so distinctly tendinous in structure, furnishing attachment to special tensor muscles, as to render the distinction between fascia and aponeurosis quite arbitrary. Bursæ occur in certain situations between the fascia and underlying structures (subfascial bursæ), or between the fascia and the skin (subcutaneous bursæ).

It is convenient to divide the description of a muscle into seven heads, viz.: (1) Name, followed by important synonyms; (2) position and form; (3) attachments; (4) action; (5) structure; (6) relations; (7) blood and nerve supply.

1. The **name** is determined by various factors, viz.: (*a*) The action, *e. g.*, extensor, adductor, etc.; (*b*) the shape, *e. g.*, quadratus, triangularis; (*c*) the direction, *e. g.*, rectus, obliquus; (*d*) the position, *e. g.*, the subscapularis, iliacus; (*e*) the division (into heads, etc.), *e. g.*, biceps, triceps, etc.; (*f*) the size, *e. g.*, major, minor, etc.; (*g*) the attachments, *e. g.*, sterno-cephalicus, mastoido-humeralis; (*h*) the structure, *e. g.*, semitendinosus. In most cases two or more of these factors have combined to produce the name, *e. g.*, adductor magnus, longus colli, obliquus externus abdominis.

2. The **shape** is, in many cases, sufficiently definite to allow the use of such terms as triangular, quadrilateral, fan-shaped, long, flat, fusiform, ring-like, etc.

3. The **attachments** are in most cases to bone, but many muscles are attached to cartilage, ligaments, fascia, the skin, etc. It is usual to apply the term **origin** to the attachment which always or more commonly remains fixed when the muscle contracts. The term **insertion** designates the movable attachment. Such a distinction cannot always be made, as the action may be reversible, or both attachments may be freely movable.

4. The **action** belongs rather to physiological study, but is briefly indicated in anatomical descriptions.

5. The **structure** includes the direction of the muscle-fibers, the arrangement of the tendons, the synovial membranes, and any other accessory structures, *e. g.*, annular ligaments and reinforcing sheaths and bands. The relation of the muscle-fibers to the tendon varies, and this fact has given rise to special terms. Thus a muscle in which the fibers converge to either side of the tendon is termed **bipennate**; while one in which this arrangement exists only on one side of the tendon is called **unipennate.** The terms fleshy and tendinous are used to indicate the relative amounts of muscular and tendinous tissue. The muscular tissue is often spoken of as the belly (Venter) of the muscle. In the case of the long muscles, the origin is

[1] The student will note in dissection that transition forms occur; also that the same sheath may belong to two or more tendons in common, *e. g.*, the sheath of the two flexors on the back of the carpus. In such cases the synovial membrane is reflected from one tendon to the other, and may form a secondary mesotenon.

often termed the **head** (Caput). Muscles having two or more heads are called biceps, triceps, etc. **Digastric** muscles are those which have two bellies joined by an intermediate tendon. Ring-like muscles which circumscribe openings are termed **sphincters,** on account of their action.

6. The **relations** are, of course, important on surgical grounds.

7. The **nerve-supply** is of clinical interest, and is important for the determination of homologies.

FASCIÆ AND MUSCLES OF THE HORSE

PANNICULUS CARNOSUS

The **panniculus carnosus** (Musculus cutaneus) is a thin muscular layer developed in the superficial fascia. It is intimately adherent in great part to the skin, but has very little attachment to the skeleton. It does not cover the entire body, and may be conveniently divided into facial, cervical, thoracic, and abdominal portions, each of which will be described with the muscles of the corresponding region.

THE FASCIÆ AND MUSCLES OF THE HEAD

The muscles of the head may be divided into three groups, viz.: (1) Superficial muscles, including the panniculus and those of the lips, cheeks, nostrils, eyelids, and external ear; (2) the orbital muscles; (3) the muscles of mastication.

The **superficial fascia** forms an almost continuous layer, but is very scanty around the natural orifices. It contains a number of the thin superficial muscles, so that care must be exercised in removing the skin. Over the frontal and nasal bones the fascia blends with the periosteum.

The **deep fascia** is of special interest in three regions. The **temporal fascia** covers the temporalis muscle, and is attached to the parietal and frontal crests internally, and to the zygomatic arch externally. The **buccal fascia** covers the buccinator muscle and the free part of the outer surface of the ramus of the jaw. Superiorly it is attached to the facial crest, and posteriorly it forms a band (Ligamentum pterygomandibulare) which stretches from the hamulus of the pterygoid bone to the mandible behind the last molar tooth. It is directly continuous with the **pharyngeal fascia,** which is attached to the great and thyroid cornua of the hyoid bone, covers the lateral walls of the pharynx, and blends dorsally with the median raphé of the constrictor muscles of the latter.

SUPERFICIAL MUSCLES

1. **Panniculus carnosus.**—The facial panniculus (M. cutaneus faciei) consists of a thin and usually incomplete muscular stratum, which covers the submaxillary space and the masseter muscle. A branch from it passes forward to the angle of the mouth and blends with the orbicularis oris; this part (M. cutaneus labiorum) retracts the angle of the mouth. (A number of the superficial muscles of the face may be considered modified parts of the panniculus, *e. g.*, the corrugator supercilii, malaris, zygomaticus, etc.)

MUSCLES OF THE LIPS AND CHEEKS

1. **Orbicularis oris.**—This is the sphincter muscle of the mouth; it is continuous with the other muscles which converge to the lips. It lies between the skin and the mucous membrane of the lips, and is intimately adherent to the

former. Most of the fibers run parallel to the free edges of the lips and have no direct attachment to the skeleton.

Action.—It closes the lips.

Blood-supply.—Palato-labial, facial, and mental arteries.

Nerve-supply.—Facial nerve.

2. **Levator nasolabialis** (Levator labii superioris alæque nasi).—This thin

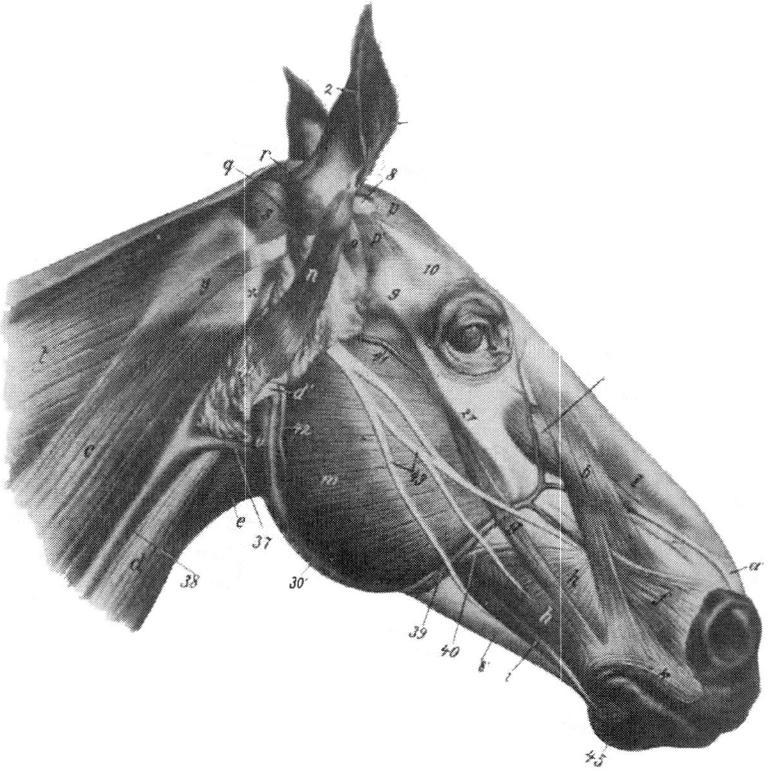

FIG. 172.—MUSCLES OF HEAD OF HORSE LATERAL VIEW. THE PANNICULUS IS REMOVED.

a, Levator labii superioris proprius; *b*, levator nasolabialis; *c*, mastoido-humeralis; *d*, sterno-cephalicus; *d'*, tendon of *d*; *e*, omo-hyoideus; *f*, dilatator naris lateralis; *g*, zygomaticus; *h*, buccinator; *i*, depressor labii inferioris; k, orbicularis oris; *l*, dilatator naris superior; *m*, masseter; *n*, parotido-auricularis; *o*, zygomatico-auricularis; *p*, interscutularis; *p'*, fronto-scutularis, pars temporalis; *q*, cervico-auricularis profundus major; *r*, cervico-auricularis superficialis; *s*, obliquus capitis anterior; *t*, splenius; *v*, stylo-maxillaris; *y*, mastoid tendon of mastoido-humeralis; *2*, posterior, *3*, anterior, border of external ear; *8*, scutiform cartilage; *9*, zygomatic arch; *10*, depression behind supraorbital process; *18*, temporo-mandibular articulation; *27*, facial crest; *30'*, angle of jaw; *37*, external maxillary vein; *38*, jugular vein; *39*, facial vein; *40*, parotid duct; *41*, transverse facial vein; *42*, masseteric vein; *43*, facial nerve; *44*, parotid gland; *45*, chin; *x*, wing of atlas. (After Ellenberger-Baum, Anat. für Künstler.)

muscle lies directly under the skin, and chiefly on the lateral surface of the nasal region.

Origin.—The frontal and nasal bones.

Insertion.—(1) The upper lip and the outer wing of the nostril; (2) the commissure of the lips.

Action.—(1) To elevate the upper lip and the commissure; (2) to dilate the nostril.

Structure.—The muscle arises by a thin aponeurosis. The belly is also thin, and divides into two branches, between which the lateral dilator of the nostril passes. The dorsal branch reaches the nostril and upper lip, blending with the lateral dilator; the ventral one is much smaller, and blends at the labial commissure with the orbicularis and buccinator.

Relations.—Superficially, the skin, fascia, and lateral dilator (in part); deeply, the levator labii superioris proprius, lateral dilator (in part), buccinator, branches of the facial vessels and nerve, and the infraorbital artery and nerve.

Blood-supply.—Facial and palato-labial arteries.

Nerve-supply.—Facial nerve.

3. Levator **labii** superioris **proprius.**—This lies on the dorso-lateral aspect of the face, partly covered by the preceding muscle.

Origin.—The lacrimal, malar, and maxillary bones at their junction.

Insertion.—The upper lip, by a common tendon, with its fellow.

Action.—Acting with its fellow, to elevate the upper lip. This action, if carried to the fullest extent, results in eversion. In unilateral action the lip is drawn upward and to the side of the muscle acting.

Structure.—The muscle has a short, thin tendon of origin. The belly is at first flattened, but becomes narrower and thicker, then tapers over the false nostril, to terminate in a tendon. The tendons of the two muscles unite over the alar cartilages of the nostrils, forming an expansion which spreads out in the substance of the upper lip.

Relations.—Superficially, the skin, the levator nasolabialis, and the angular vessels of the eye; deeply, the superior and transverse dilators of the nostril and the infraorbital artery and nerve.

Blood-supply.—Facial artery.

Nerve-supply.—Facial nerve.

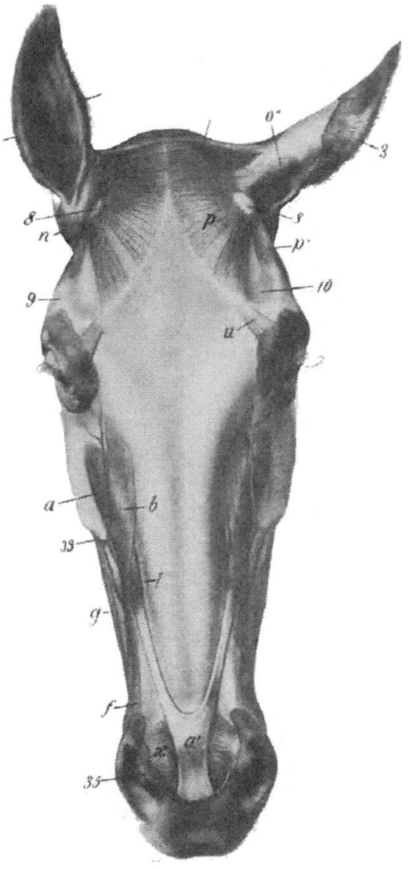

FIG. 173.—MUSCLES OF HEAD OF HORSE, DORSAL VIEW. THE PANNICULUS IS REMOVED.

a, Levator labii superioris proprius; *a′*, common tendon of *a* with opposite muscle; *b*, levator nasolabialis; *f*, dilatator naris lateralis; *g*, zygomaticus; *l*, dilatator naris superior; *n*, parotido-auricularis; *o″*, scutulo-auricularis superficialis superior; *p*, interscutularis; p′, fronto-scutularis, pars temporalis; r, cervico-auricularis superficialis; *u*, corrugator supercilii; *x*, transversus nasi; *2*, posterior, *3*, anterior, border of external ear; *8*, scutiform cartilage; *9*, zygomatic arch; *10*, supraorbital depression; *35*, inner wing of nostril, containing lamina of alar cartilage; *39*, facial vein. (After Ellenberger-Baum, Anat. für Künstler.)

4. **Zygomaticus.**—This very thin muscle lies immediately under the skin of the cheek.

Origin.—The fascia covering the masseter muscle below the facial crest.

Insertion.—The commissure of the lips, blending with the buccinator.

Action.—To retract and raise the angle of the mouth.

Structure.—Fleshy, with a thin aponeurotic origin.

Relations.—Superficially, the skin; deeply, the buccinator.

Blood-supply.—Facial artery.

Nerve-supply.—Facial nerve.

5. **Incisivus superior** (Depressor labii superioris).—This lies under the mucous membrane of the upper lip.

Origin.—The alveolar border of the premaxilla from the second incisor to the first cheek tooth.

Insertion.—The upper lip.

Action.—To depress the upper lip.

6. **Incisivus inferior.**—This is arranged in the lower lip like the preceding muscle in the upper one.

Origin.—The alveolar border of the mandible from the second incisor to a point near the first cheek tooth.

Insertion.—The skin of the lower lip and the prominence of the chin.

Action.—To raise the lower lip.

7. **Mentalis** (Levator menti).—This is situated in the prominence of the chin. Its fibers arise from each side of the body of the mandible and are inserted into the skin of the chin. It is mingled with fat and strands of connective tissue, in which the roots of the tactile hairs are embedded. It raises and corrugates the skin to which it is attached.

8. **Depressor labii inferioris.**—This muscle lies on the outer surface of the ramus of the mandible, along the ventral border of the buccinator.

Origin.—The alveolar border of the mandible near the coronoid process and the maxillary tuberosity, in common with the buccinator.

Insertion.—The lower lip.

Action.—To depress and retract the lower lip.

Structure.—The tendon of origin and the belly are fused with the buccinator as far forward as the first cheek tooth. From this point forward the belly is distinct and rounded, terminating in a tendon which spreads out in the lower lip, blending with the orbicularis and the muscle of the opposite side.

Relations.—Superficially, the skin, masseter, facial vessels, and parotid duct; deeply, the mandible and inferior labial artery.

Blood-supply.—Facial artery.

Nerve-supply.—Facial nerve.

9. **Buccinator.**—This muscle lies in the lateral wall of the mouth, extending from the angle of the mouth to the maxillary tuberosity

Origin.—The external surface of the maxilla above the interdental space and the molar teeth; the alveolar border of the mandible at the interdental space and also posteriorly where it turns upward to the coronoid process; the pterygo-mandibular ligament.

Insertion.—The angle of the mouth, blending with the orbicularis oris.

Action.—To flatten the cheeks, thus pressing the food between the teeth; also to retract the angle of the mouth.

Structure.—Two layers may be recognized. The superficial layer (Pars buccalis) extends from the angle of the mouth to the masseter. It is incompletely pennate, having a longitudinal raphé on which most of the muscle-fibers converge. The upper fibers are directed chiefly downward and backward, the lower ones upward and backward. The deep layer (Pars molaris) consists mainly of longitudinal fibers. It blends in part with the superficial layer of the orbicularis; it has a small tendinous attachment to the coronoid process behind, and is united below with the depressor labii inferioris.

Relations.—Superficially, the skin and fascia, the zygomaticus, levator nasolabialis, lateral dilator of the nostril, the superior buccal glands, the parotid duct, the facial vessels, and branches of the facial nerve; deeply, the mucous membrane of the mouth and the inferior buccal glands.

Blood-supply.—Facial and buccinator arteries.

Nerve-supply.—Facial nerve.

MUSCLES OF THE NOSTRILS

1. Levator **nasolabialis.**—This has been described (p. 214).

2. Dilatator **naris lateralis** (M. caninus).—This thin, triangular muscle lies on the lateral nasal region, and passes between the two branches of the levator nasolabialis.

Origin.—The maxilla, close to the anterior extremity of the facial crest.

Insertion.—The outer wing of the nostril.

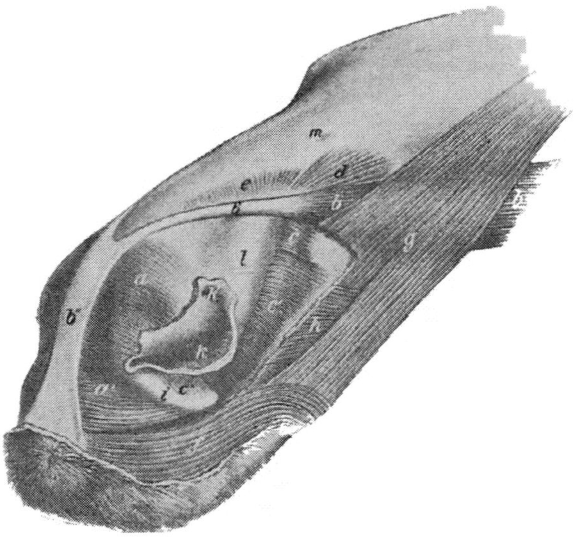

FIG. 174.—NASAL AND SUPERIOR LABIAL MUSCLES OF HORSE.

a, a', Dilatator naris transversus; *b*, levator labii superioris proprius; *b'*, tendon of *b*; *b''*, common tendon of two levatores labii superioris proprii; c, c', dilatator naris inferior; d, *e*, dilatator naris superior; *f*, orbicularis oris; *g*, levator nasolabialis, a portion of which is removed; *h*, dilatator naris lateralis (cut); *i*, cornu of alar cartilage; *k*, nostril; *k'*, false nostril; *l*, nasal diverticulum; *m*, nasal bone. (After Ellenberger-Baum, Top. Anat. d. Pferdes.)

Action.—To dilate the nostril.

Structure.—The muscle has a flat tendon of origin, passes between the two branches of the levator nasolabialis, and spreads out in the external wing of the nostril. The lower fibers blend with the orbicularis oris.

Relations.—Superficially, the skin, fascia, and the labial branch of the levator nasolabialis; deeply, the maxilla and the nasal branch of the levator nasolabialis.

Blood-supply.—Facial artery.

Nerve-supply.—Facial nerve.

3. Dilatator **naris** transversus (M. transversus nasi).—This is an unpaired, quadrilateral muscle, which lies between the nostrils. It consists of two layers.

Attachments.—Superficial layer, the superficial faces of the laminæ of the alar cartilages; deep layer, the convex edges of the cornua of the same.

Action.—To dilate the nostrils.

Structure.—It is composed of transverse fleshy fibers, which blend below with the orbicularis.

Relations.—Superficially, the skin, fascia, and tendinous expansion of the levator labii superioris proprius; deeply, the alar cartilages, the extremity of the septum nasi, and the palato-labial artery.

Blood-supply.—Palato-labial artery.

Nerve-supply.—Facial nerve.

4. **Dilatator naris superior** (Pars dorsalis m. lateralis nasi).—This very thin muscle occupies the angle between the nasal process of the premaxilla and the nasal bone.

Origin.—The lateral border of the nasal bone.

Insertion.—The inner wall of the false nostril and the parietal lamina of the septal cartilage.

Action.—To dilate the vestibule of the nasal cavity.

Structure.—Fleshy.

Relations.—Superficially, the skin, fascia, and levator labii superioris proprius; deeply, the parietal cartilage and false nostril.

Blood-supply.—Facial artery.

Nerve-supply.—Facial nerve.

5. **Dilatator naris inferior** (Pars ventralis m. lateralis nasi).—This is a similar but thicker muscle, which lies on the nasal process of the premaxilla.

Origin.—The maxilla and the nasal process of the premaxilla.

Insertion.—The cartilaginous prolongations of the turbinal bones and the inner wall of the false nostril.

Action.—To rotate the turbinal outward and dilate the nostril and the vestibule of the nasal cavity.

Structure.—Fleshy. A division into two or more parts may be recognized. A small part posteriorly is inserted into the cartilage of the dorsal turbinal bone, while the bulk of the muscle is inserted into the cartilage of the ventral turbinal bone. A few fibers also pass between the cornu of the alar cartilage and the outer wing of the nostril.

Relations.—Superficially, the levator labii superioris proprius, the levator nasolabialis, and the lateral nasal artery; deeply, the maxilla, the premaxilla, and the anterior nasal branch of the infraorbital nerve.

Blood-supply.—Facial artery.

Nerve-supply.—Facial nerve.

MUSCLES OF THE EYELIDS

1. **Orbicularis oculi.**—This is a flat, elliptical, sphincter muscle, situated in and around the eyelids, the portion in the upper lid being much broader than that in the lower. The chief attachment is to the skin of the lids, but some bundles are attached to the palpebral ligament at the inner canthus and to the lacrimal bone. Its action is to close the lids.

2. **Corrugator supercilii.**—This is a very thin, small muscle, which arises over the root of the supraorbital process and spreads out in the upper eyelid, blending with the orbicularis. Its action is to assist in raising the upper lid or, especially in pathological conditions, to wrinkle the skin.

3. **Malaris.**—This is a very thin muscle, which varies much in different subjects. It extends from the fascia in front of the orbit to the lower lid. Its action is to depress the lower lid.

The foregoing muscles receive their blood-supply from the facial, transverse facial, supraorbital, and infraorbital arteries; the nerve-supply is derived from the facial nerve.

4. **Levator palpebræ superioris.**—This slender, flat muscle is almost entirely within the orbital cavity. It arises on the pterygoid crest, passes forward above the rectus oculi superior and below the lacrimal gland, and terminates in a thin tendon in the upper lid.

Action.—To elevate the upper lid.

Blood-supply.—Ophthalmic artery.

Nerve-supply.—Oculomotor nerve.

MUSCLES OF MASTICATION

The muscles of this group are six in number in the horse. They arise chiefly from the upper jaw and the base of the cranium, and are all inserted into the mandible.

1. **Masseter.**—This muscle extends from the zygomatic arch and facial crest over the broad part of the mandibular ramus. It is semi-elliptical in outline.

Origin.—By a strong tendon from the zygomatic arch and the facial crest.

Insertion.—The outer surface of the broad part of the ramus of the mandible.

Action.—Its action is to bring the jaws together. Acting singly, it also carries the lower jaw toward the side of the contracting muscle.

Structure.—The superficial face of the muscle in its upper part is covered by a strong, glistening aponeurosis, and several tendinous intersections partially divide the muscle into layers. The fibers of the superficial layer take origin from the malar and maxilla only, and diverge somewhat to their insertion close to the thick ventral border of the lower jaw. The fibers of the deep layer arise from the entire area of origin, and pass straight to the border of the mandible; it will be noted that a small part, near the temporo-maxillary joint, is not covered by the superficial layer. The two layers are separable only above and behind; elsewhere they are fused.

Relations.—Superficially, the skin and panniculus, the parotid gland, the transverse facial and masseteric vessels, and the facial nerve; deeply, the ramus of the mandible, the buccinator, depressor labii inferioris, and mylo-hyoideus muscles, the superior buccal glands, the buccinator nerve, and two large varicose veins which join the facial vein at the anterior edge of the muscle. The facial vessels and parotid duct run along the anterior edge of the muscle; the duct, however, bends forward about the middle of the border and leaves the muscle.

Blood-supply.—Transverse facial and masseteric arteries.

Nerve-supply.—Mandibular nerve.

2. **Temporalis.**—This muscle occupies the temporal fossa.

Origin.—The rough part of the temporal fossa and the crests which surround it.

Insertion.—The coronoid process of the mandible, which it envelops.

Action.—Chiefly to raise the lower jaw, acting with the masseter and internal pterygoid muscles.

Structure.—The surface of the muscle is covered with a glistening aponeurosis, and strong tendinous intersections are found in its substance. The inner edge of the muscle is quite thin, but as the fibers converge toward the much smaller area of insertion, the muscle becomes nearly an inch thick. It fuses somewhat with the masseter.

Relations.—Superficially, the scutiform cartilage and anterior muscles of the external ear and the orbital fat; deeply, the temporal fossa and the deep temporal vessels and nerves.

Blood-supply.—Superficial and deep temporal, and mastoid arteries.

Nerve-supply.—Mandibular nerve.

3. **Pterygoideus internus** (s. medialis).—This muscle occupies a position on the inner surface of the ramus of the mandible similar to that of the masseter on the outside.

Origin.—The crest formed by the pterygoid process of the sphenoid and the palate bone.

Insertion.—The concave inner surface of the broad portion of the ramus of the mandible, and the inner lip of the lower border.

Action.—Acting together, to raise the lower jaw; acting singly, to produce also lateral movement of the jaw.

Structure.—The muscle is capable of division into two parts. The principal part is superficial (internal), and its fibers are, for the most part, vertical in direction. It contains much tendinous tissue (septa). The smaller portion is external to the foregoing, and its fibers are directed downward and backward.

Relations.—Externally, the ramus of the mandible, the external pterygoid muscle, the inferior alveolar vessels and nerve, and the lingual and mylo-hyoid nerves; internally, the great cornu of the hyoid bone, the tensor palati, pterygo-

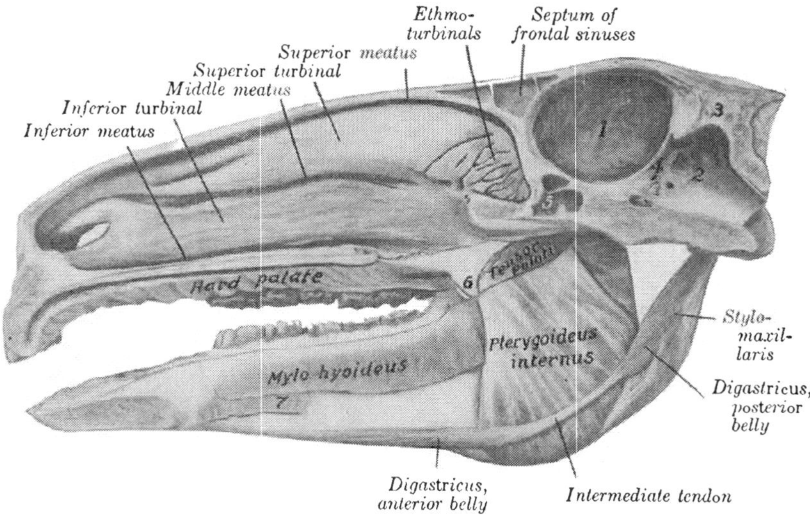

Fig. 175.—Sagittal Section of Head of Horse, Showing Deep Pterygo-maxillary Region, and Nasal and Cranial Cavities.

1, Cerebral compartment of cranial cavity; *2*, cerebellar compartment of same; *3*, tentorium osseum; *4*, tentorium cerebelli; *5*, sphenoidal sinus; *6*, hamulus of pterygoid bone-tendon of tensor palati cut off short at anterior border of hamulus; *7*, mylo-glossus. The olfactory mucous membrane is shaded.

pharyngeus, palato-pharyngeus, mylo-hyoideus, digastricus, and stylo-hyoideus muscles, the guttural pouch, the external maxillary vessels, the ninth and twelfth nerves, the submaxillary salivary gland, the submaxillary and parotid ducts, and the submaxillary and pharyngeal lymph-glands.

Blood-supply.—Internal maxillary, masseteric, and inferior alveolar arteries.

Nerve-supply.—Mandibular nerve.

4. **Pterygoideus externus (s. lateralis).**—This muscle is considerably smaller than the preceding one, and is situated external to its upper part.

Origin.—The external surface of the pterygoid process of the sphenoid bone.

Insertion.—The inner surface of the neck and the inner part of the anterior border of the condyle of the mandible.

Action.—Acting together, to draw the lower jaw forward; acting singly, to move the jaw laterally, *i. e.*, toward the side opposite to the muscle acting. The latter action is due to the fact that the origin is nearer to the median plane than the insertion.

Structure.—The muscle is almost entirely fleshy, and the fibers are almost

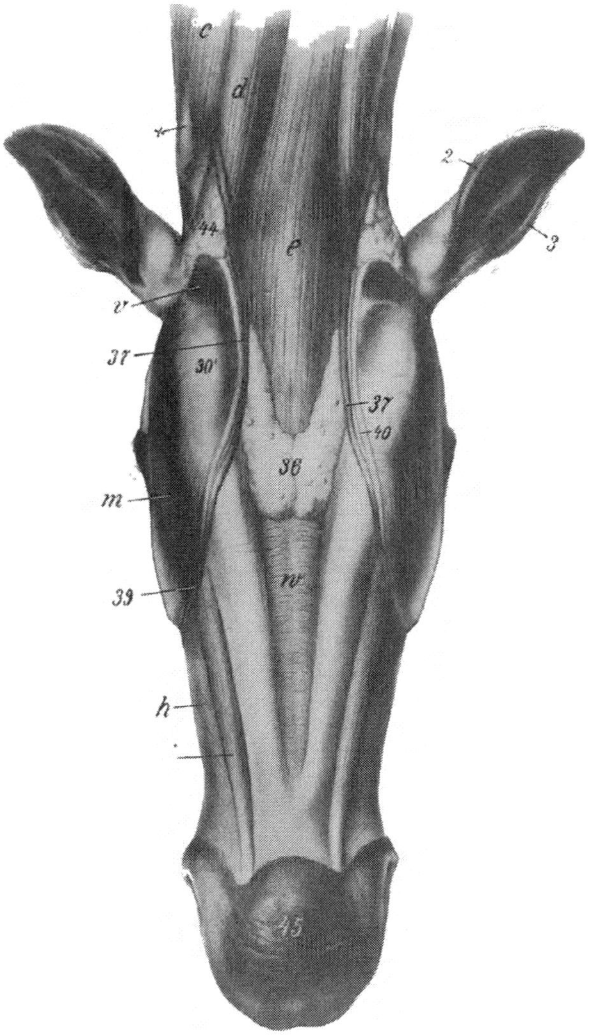

FIG. 176.—SUBMAXILLARY AND LARYNGEAL REGIONS OF HORSE, AFTER REMOVAL OF SKIN AND PANNICULUS.

c, Mastoido-humeralis; d, sterno-cephalicus; *e*, omo-hyoideus and sterno-hyoideus; *h*, buccinator; *i*, depressor labii inferioris; *m*, masseter; *v*, stylo-maxillaris; *w*, mylo-hyoideus; *2*, posterior, *3*, anterior, border of external ear; *30'*, angle of jaw; *36*, submaxillary lymph-glands; *37*, external maxillary vein; *39*, facial continuation of *37*; *40*, parotid duct; *44*, parotid gland; *45*, prominence of chin; *x*, wing of atlas. (After Ellenberger-Baum, Anat. für Künstler.)

longitudinal in direction. Some of them are inserted into the edge of the interarticular meniscus.

Relations.—Externally, the temporo-maxillary articulation and the temporalis muscle; internally, the internal pterygoid and tensor palati muscles. The internal maxillary artery crosses the lower face of the muscle and dips in between it and the tensor palati. The mandibular nerve lies on the ventral surface, and the buccinator nerve perforates the origin of the muscle.

Blood-supply.—Internal maxillary and inferior alveolar arteries.

Nerve-supply.—Mandibular nerve.

5. **Stylo-maxillaris** (s.-mandibularis) (M. jugulomandibularis).—This is a short muscle extending from the paramastoid or styloid process of the occipital bone to the posterior border of the lower jaw; it is covered by the parotid gland.

Origin.—The paramastoid or styloid process of the occipital bone, in common with the posterior belly of the digastricus.

Insertion.—The posterior border of the ramus of the mandible.

Action.—To depress the lower jaw and open the mouth.

Structure.—The muscle contains a good deal of tendinous tissue. It blends with the posterior belly of the digastricus.

Relations.—Superficially, the parotid gland, the tendon of the sterno-cephalicus, and the fibrous expansion which connects it with the tendon of the mastoido-humeralis; deeply, the guttural pouch, the external carotid artery, the ninth and twelfth nerves, the pharynx, and the submaxillary gland.

Blood-supply.—External carotid artery.

Nerve-supply.—Facial nerve.

6. **Digastricus.**—This muscle is composed of two fusiform, flattened bellies, united by a round tendon.

Origin.—The paramastoid or styloid process of the occipital bone, in common with the preceding muscle.

Insertion.—The inner surface of the lower border of the mandible behind the symphysis.

Action.—It assists in depressing the lower jaw and opening the mouth. If the mandible be fixed and both bellies contract, the hyoid bone and the base of the tongue are raised, as in the first phase of deglutition.

Structure.—The posterior belly has the appearance of a branch detached from the inner surface of the stylo-maxillaris. It passes downward and forward, and is succeeded by a small rounded tendon. The latter perforates the tendon of insertion of the stylo-hyoideus, and is provided with a **synovial sheath.** The anterior belly is larger and terminates by thin tendinous bundles.

Relations.—The posterior belly has practically the same relations as the stylo-maxillaris. The intermediate tendon is in contact externally with the internal pterygoid muscle, the submaxillary gland and duct, and the external maxillary artery. The anterior belly lies in the submaxillary space between the ramus of the jaw and the mylo-hyoideus muscle; the sublingual vessels run along its upper border.

Blood-supply.—External carotid and sublingual arteries.

Nerve-supply.—Facial and mandibular nerves.

THE HYOID MUSCLES

This group consists of eight muscles, one of which, the hyoideus transversus, is unpaired.

1. **Mylo-hyoideus.**—This muscle, together with its fellow, forms a sort of sling between the two rami of the lower jaw, in which the tongue is supported.

Origin.—The inner surface of the alveolar border of the mandible.

Insertion.—(1) A median fibrous raphé extending from the symphysis to the hyoid bone; (2) the lingual process and body of the hyoid bone.

Action.—It raises the floor of the mouth, the tongue, and the hyoid bone.

Structure.—Each muscle consists of a thin curved sheet, the fibers passing downward from their origin and then curving toward the median raphé. It is chiefly fleshy, and is thickest behind. The anterior superficial part of the muscle is termed the mylo-glossus.

Relations.—On the superficial surface of the muscles are the ramus, the internal pterygoid and digastricus muscles, and the submaxillary lymph-glands. The deep surface is in contact with the mucous membrane of the mouth, the stylo-glossus, hyo-glossus, and genio-hyoideus muscles, the sublingual gland and vessels, the submaxillary duct, and the lingual and hypo-glossal nerves.

Blood-supply.—Sublingual artery.

Nerve-supply.—Mylo-hyoid branch of the mandibular nerve.

2. **Stylo-hyoideus.**—This is a slender, fusiform muscle, having a direction nearly parallel to that of the great cornu of the hyoid bone (Fig. 436).

Origin.—The heel-like prominence on the proximal extremity of the great cornu of the hyoid bone.

Insertion.—The anterior part of the thyroid cornu of the hyoid bone.

Action.—It draws the base of the tongue and the larynx upward and backward.

Structure.—It arises by a thin, short tendon, and has a fusiform belly. The tendon of insertion is perforated for the passage of the intermediate tendon of the digastricus, and at this point there is a small synovial sheath.

Relations.—Superficially, the internal pterygoid muscle and the parotid gland; deeply, the guttural pouch, the pharynx, the external carotid and maxillary arteries, and the hypoglossal nerve.

Blood-supply.—External carotid artery.

Nerve-supply.—Facial nerve (stylo-hyoid branch).

3. **Occipito-hyoideus** (M. jugulo-hyoideus; occipito-styloideus).—This is a small triangular muscle, which lies in the space between the paramastoid process and the great cornu of the hyoid bone.

Origin.—The paramastoid (styloid) process of the occipital bone.

Insertion.—The proximal extremity and ventral edge of the great cornu of the hyoid bone.

Action.—It carries the distal extremity of the great cornu backward and upward. Acting with the genio-hyoideus and digastricus, it raises the hyoid bone and the larynx.

Structure.—The muscle is somewhat triangular, its fibers being longer as the ventral border is approached. It blends with the posterior belly of the digastricus.

Relations.—Superficially, the parotid gland; deeply, the guttural pouch.

Blood-supply.—Occipital artery.

Nerve-supply.—Facial nerve.

4. **Genio-hyoideus.**—This is a long, spindle-shaped muscle, which lies under the tongue in contact with its fellow of the opposite side (Fig. 243)

Origin.—The angle of union of the rami of the mandible.

Insertion.—The extremity of the lingual process of the hyoid bone.

Action.—It draws the hyoid bone and tongue forward.

Structure.—The muscle arises by a short tendon, which is succeeded by the belly, composed of long bundles of parallel fibers.

Relations.—Below, the mylo-hyoideus; above, the hyo-glossus, stylo-glossus, genio-glossus, the sublingual gland, submaxillary duct, and the lingual nerve.

Blood-supply.—Sublingual artery.

Nerve-supply.—Hypoglossal nerve.

5. **Kerato-hyoideus.**—This small triangular muscle lies in the space between the thyroid and small cornu, under cover of the hyo-glossus (Fig. 243).

Origin.—The posterior edge of the small cornu and the adjacent part of the ventral border of the great cornu.

Insertion.—The dorsal edge of the thyroid cornu.

Action.—It raises the thyroid cornu and the larynx.

Relations.—The muscle is crossed outwardly by the lingual artery.

Blood-supply.—Lingual artery.

Nerve-supply.—Glosso-pharyngeal nerve.

6. **Hyoideus Transversus.**—This is a thin, unpaired muscle, which extends transversely between the two small cornua of the hyoid bone.

Attachments.—The small cornua close to the junction with the great cornua.

Action.—When relaxed, its upper surface is concave; when it contracts, it elevates the root of the tongue.

Structure.—Fleshy, composed of parallel transverse bundles.

Blood-supply.—Lingual artery.

Nerve-supply.—Glosso-pharyngeal nerve.

7. **Sterno-thyro-hyoideus,** and

8. **Omo-hyoideus.**—These are described with the muscles on the ventral surface of the neck.

The Fasciæ and Muscles of the Neck

It is convenient to divide the muscles of the neck into ventral and lateral groups, the two lateral groups being separated from each other by the ligamentum nuchæ.

THE FASCIÆ OF THE NECK

The superficial fascia is in part two-layered, and contains the cervical portion of the panniculus. The fasciæ of the right and left sides are attached along the dorsal line of the neck to the ligamentum nuchæ, while along the ventral line they meet in a fibrous raphé. A deep layer is detached which passes underneath the panniculus, bridges over the jugular furrow, and crosses over the deep face of the mastoido-humeralis and omo-hyoideus to join the superficial layer. It again separates to pass under the cervical trapezius, and become attached to the ligamentum nuchæ. Along the ventral line a septum is detached which separates the sterno-cephalici. Two other layers in front of the shoulder inclose the prescapular lymph-glands.

The deep fascia also forms two layers. The superficial layer is attached to the wing of the atlas and the lower edge of the trachelo-mastoideus and scalenus. Passing downward, it incloses the trachea, and, together with the deep layer, furnishes sheaths for the vagus and sympathetic nerves and the carotid artery. Passing upward it detaches septa between the extensor muscles of the spine. Anteriorly it covers the thyroid gland, the guttural pouch, the adjacent vessels and nerves and the larynx, and is attached to the mastoid process of the temporal bone and the thyroid cornu of the hyoid bone. Posteriorly, it is attached to the first rib and the cariniform cartilage of the sternum. The deep layer (prevertebral fascia) covers the ventral surface of the longus colli, and incloses the trachea and œsophagus. Anteriorly, it forms, with the corresponding layer of the opposite side, a septum between the guttural pouches; posteriorly, it becomes continuous with the endothoracic fascia. A fascia propria forms a tubular sheath around the trachea, inclosing also the recurrent nerves.

VENTRAL MUSCLES

This group consists of eleven pairs of muscles which lie almost entirely ventral to the vertebræ.

1. **Panniculus carnosus.**—The cervical panniculus (platysma myoides of man) has a fleshy origin on the cariniform cartilage (manubrium) of the sternum.

It passes forward, outward, and upward, crossing over the sterno-cephalicus and jugular furrow obliquely. On reaching the surface of the mastoido-humeralis it adheres closely to this muscle, and soon thins out, to be continued over the splenius and trapezius by an aponeurosis which is difficult to remove from the latter muscle. Scattered bundles may be traced on the ventral surface of the neck to

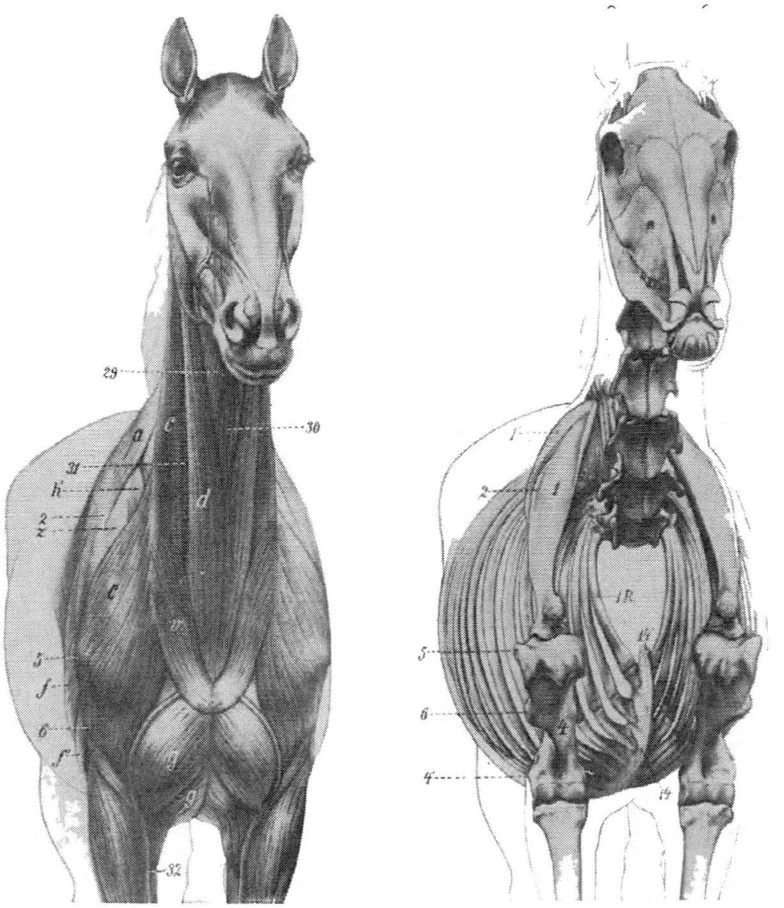

FIG. 177.—ANTERO-LATERAL VIEW OF MUSCLES AND SKELETON OF HORSE.

a, Trapezius; c, mastoido-humeralis; d, sterno-cephalicus; *f*, long head of triceps; *f'*, external head of triceps; *g*, anterior superficial pectoral muscle; *g'*, posterior superficial pectoral; *h'*, anterior deep pectoral; r, cervical panniculus; *z*, supraspinatus; *29*, omo-hyoideus; *30*, sterno-thyro-hyoideus; *31*, jugular vein; *32*, cephalic vein; *1*, scapula; *1'*, cartilage of scapula; *2*, spine of scapula; *4*, shaft of humerus; *4'*, external epicondyle; *5*, external tuberosity of humerus; *6*, deltoid tuberosity; *14*, ventral border ("keel") of sternum; *14'*, cariniform cartilage; *1.R.*, first rib. (After Ellenberger-Baum, Anat. für Künstler.)

the facial portion. The right and left muscles meet at a ventral median raphé in pennate fashion.

2. **Mastoido-humeralis.**—This is described on p. 252.

3. Sterno-cephalicus (Sterno-maxillaris s.-mandibularis).[1]—This is a long, nar-

[1] This muscle is probably the homologue of the sternal portion of the sterno-cleido-mastoid of man. On account of the differences in its insertion in the various animals, it seems desirable to adopt the name sterno-cephalicus.

row muscle, extending along the ventral and lateral aspects of the trachea from the sternum to the angle of the jaw. It forms the ventral boundary of the jugular furrow.

Origin.—The cariniform cartilage of the sternum.

Insertion.—The posterior border of the lower jaw.

Action.—Acting together, to flex the head and neck; acting singly, to incline the head and neck to the side of the muscle contracting.

Structure.—The two muscles are fused at their origin, which is fleshy. Near the middle of the neck they separate, and, becoming thinner, each muscle passes under the parotid gland and terminates in a flat tendon.

Relations.—Superficially, the cervical panniculus; deeply, the sterno-thyro-hyoideus and omo-hyoideus muscles. The upper edge of the muscle is related to the jugular vein, which lies in the jugular furrow. The carotid artery, the vagus, sympathetic, and recurrent nerves also lie along the upper edge at the root of the neck. The tendon passes under the submaxillary vein and the parotid gland, having the submaxillary gland and stylo-maxillaris muscle on its inner side.

Blood-supply.—Carotid artery.

Nerve-supply.—Ventral branches of the spinal accessory and first cervical nerves.

4. **Sterno-thyro-hyoideus** (Sterno-thyroideus et sterno-hyoideus).—This is a long, slender, digastric muscle, applied to the ventral surface of the trachea and its fellow of the opposite side.

Origin.—The cariniform cartilage of the sternum.

Insertion.—(1) The external surface of the thyroid cartilage of the larynx; (2) the body of the hyoid bone.

Action.—To depress and retract the hyoid bone, the base of the tongue, and the larynx, as in deglutition. It may also fix the hyoid bone when the depressors of the tongue are acting, as in suction.

Structure.—The origin of the muscle is fleshy, and as far as the middle of the neck it blends with its fellow. The common belly is then interrupted by a tendon, or sometimes two tendons, from which arise three or four fleshy bands. The lateral bands diverge to reach their insertion into the thyroid cartilage; while the inner bands, closely applied to each other and blending with the omo-hyoideus, pass straight forward to reach the ventral surface of the hyoid bone.

Relations.—At the root of the neck the common belly has the sterno-cephalicus below, and the carotid arteries and recurrent nerves above. Further forward the trachea becomes the upper relation, and near the head the skin and fascia, the lower one.

Blood-supply.—Carotid artery.

Nerve-supply.—Ventral branch of the first cervical nerve.

5. **Omo-hyoideus** (Subscapulo-hyoideus). — This is a thin, ribbon-like muscle, almost entirely fleshy, which crosses the trachea very obliquely under cover of the mastoido-humeralis.

Origin.—The subscapular fascia close to the shoulder joint.

Insertion.—The body of the hyoid bone, in common with the hyoid branch of the preceding muscle.

Action.—To depress the hyoid bone.

Structure.—The muscle is composed of parallel fleshy fibers, except at its origin, where it has a thin tendon.

Relations.—In the first part of its course the muscle passes forward between the supraspinatus, anterior deep pectoral, mastoido-humeralis (outwardly), and the scalenus (inwardly). It is intimately adherent to the mastoido-humeralis. In the middle of the neck it is related superficially to the mastoido-humeralis, sterno-cephalicus, and the jugular vein; deeply, to the rectus capitis anterior major, the carotid artery, the vagus, sympathetic, and recurrent nerves, the trachea, and, on the left side, the œsophagus. In its anterior part the muscle blends with the hyoid part of the sterno-thyro-hyoideus, the two covering the thyroid portion of the latter muscle, the thyroid gland, and the ventral face of the larynx.

Blood-supply.—Carotid and inferior cervical arteries.

Nerve-supply.—Ventral branches of the cervical nerves.

6. **Scalenus** (M. scalenus primæ costæ).—This muscle is deeply situated on the side of the posterior half of the neck. It is composed of two parts, between which the roots of the brachial plexus of nerves emerge.

Origin.—The anterior border and outer surface of the first rib.

Insertion.—(1) The dorsal (smaller) portion is attached to the transverse process of the seventh cervical vertebra; (2) the ventral portion is attached to the transverse processes of the sixth, fifth, and fourth cervical vertebræ.

Action.—The neck is flexed or inclined laterally, according as the muscles act together or singly. If the neck be the fixed point, the muscle may have a respiratory action by pulling forward or fixing the first rib.

Structure.—The dorsal portion is composed of three or four fleshy bundles.[1] The ventral portion, which is much larger, is almost entirely fleshy, and not so divided.

Relations.—Superficially, the anterior deep pectoral, mastoido-humeralis, and omo-hyoideus muscles, the phrenic nerve, and the other branches of the brachial plexus; deeply, the vertebræ, the longus colli and intertransversales muscles, the œsophagus (on the left side), the trachea (on the right side), the vertebral vessels, the vagus, sympathetic, and recurrent nerves. The roots of the brachial plexus form a flat anastomosis, which lies between the two portions of the muscle. The brachial vessels cross the ventral edge close to the first rib.

Blood-supply.—Carotid, vertebral, and inferior cervical arteries.

Nerve-supply.—Ventral branches of the cervical nerves.

7. **Rectus capitis anterior** major (M. longus capitis).—This is the largest of the three special flexors of the head, and lies along the ventro-lateral surface of the anterior cervical vertebræ and the base of the cranium.

Origin.—The transverse processes of the fifth, fourth, and third cervical vertebræ.

Insertion.—The tubercles at the junction of the basilar process of the occipital bone with the body of the sphenoid.

Action.—Acting together, to flex the head; acting singly, to incline it to the same side also.

Structure.—The origin of the muscle is by fleshy digitations. The belly increases in size by the union of these digitations, reaching its maximum at the axis. It then diminishes, passes toward the median plane, and terminates on a rounded tendon.

Relations.—Superficially, the mastoido-humeralis, omo-hyoideus, and rectus capitis anticus minor, the submaxillary gland, the carotid artery (which lies along the lower border), the occipital and internal carotid arteries, and the tenth, eleventh, and sympathetic nerves; deeply, the vertebræ, the longus colli, intertransversales, and the small straight muscle. The terminal part of the muscle lies in contact with its fellow above the pharynx and between the guttural pouches.

Blood-supply.—Carotid, vertebral, and occipital arteries.

Nerve-supply.—Ventral branches of the cervical nerves.

8. **Rectus capitis anterior** minor (M. rectus capitis ventralis).—This is a small muscle which lies under cover of the preceding one.

Origin.—The ventral arch of the atlas.

[1] The upper part of this may be separated from the scalenus proper, and is then termed the cervicalis ascendens or ilio-costalis cervicis—a continuation in the neck of the transversalis costarum.

Insertion.—The basilar process, close to the preceding muscle.

Action.—To flex the occipito-atlantal articulation.

Structure.—Fleshy.

Relations.—Below, to the preceding muscle; above, to the atlas, occipito-atlantal articulation, and the basilar process; externally, to the rectus capitis lateralis and the guttural pouch.

Blood-supply.—Occipital artery.

Nerve-supply.—Ventral branch of the first cervical nerve.

9. **Rectus** capitis lateralis.—This is a still smaller, entirely fleshy muscle, which lies for the most part under the small oblique muscle.

Origin.—The atlas, external to the preceding muscle.

Insertion.—The paramastoid or styloid process of the occipital bone.

Action.—The same as the preceding muscle.

Structure.—Fleshy.

Relations.—Superficially, the small oblique muscle, the occipital vessels, and the ventral branch of the first cervical nerve.

Blood-supply.—Occipital artery.

Nerve-supply.—Ventral branch of the first cervical nerve.

10. **Longus** colli.—This muscle covers the ventral surface of the vertebræ, from the sixth thoracic to the atlas, and is united with its fellow. It consists of two portions, thoracic and cervical.

Origin.—(1) Thoracic portion, the bodies of the first six thoracic vertebræ; (2) cervical portion, the transverse processes of the cervical vertebræ.

Insertion.—(1) Thoracic portion, the bodies and transverse processes of the last two cervical vertebræ; (2) cervical portion, the bodies of the cervical vertebræ and the tubercle on the ventral surface of the atlas.

Action.—To flex the neck.

Structure.—The muscle is composed of a succession of bundles. The largest of these constitute the thoracic part of the muscle, which has a strong tendon inserted into the last two cervical vertebræ. A bursa is interposed between the tendon and the spine at the first costo-vertebral articulation. The cervical portion consists of a number of smaller bundles, each of which passes from its origin on the transverse process of one vertebra forward and inward to its insertion into a vertebra further forward. The most anterior bundle is inserted by a strong tendon into the ventral tubercle of the atlas.

Relations.—The principal relations of the two muscles in the thorax are: ventrally, the pleura, and, further forward, the trachea and œsophagus; dorsally, the vertebræ and the costo-vertebral joints; laterally, the dorsal, superior cervical, and vertebral vessels, the sympathetic nerve, and the thoracic roots of the brachial plexus. In the neck, important relations are: ventrally, the trachea and œsophagus, the carotid artery, the vagus, sympathetic and recurrent nerves; dorsally, the vertebræ and, in the middle third of the neck, the intertransversales muscles; laterally, the scalenus, the rectus capitis anticus major, and the intertransversales (in the anterior third). The terminal part of the muscle is separated from the trachea by the œsophagus, which is here median in position.

Blood-supply.—Subcostal and vertebral arteries.

Nerve-supply.—Ventral branches of the spinal nerves.

11. **Intertransversales** colli (Mm. intertransversarii cervicis).—These are six fasciculi which occupy the spaces between the lateral aspects of the vertebræ and the transverse and articular processes. There is thus a bundle for each intervertebral articulation except the first. Each bundle consists of a dorsal and ventral portion.

Attachments.—The dorsal bundles pass from transverse process to articular process; the ventral bundles extend between adjacent transverse processes.

Action.—To bend the neck laterally.

Structure.—They contain strong tendinous intersections.

Relations.—Superficially, the mastoido-humeralis, rectus capitis anterior major, complexus, trachelo-mastoideus, splenius, scalenus, and longissimus muscles; deeply, the vertebræ, the longus colli muscle, and the vertebral vessels. The muscles are perforated by branches of these vessels and by the primary branches of the cervical nerves.

Blood-supply.—Vertebral artery.

Nerve-supply.—The cervical nerves.

LATERAL MUSCLES

This group consists of twelve pairs of muscles arranged in layers.

First Layer

1. **Trapezius cervicalis.**—Described on p. 250.

Second Layer

2. **Rhomboideus cervicalis.**—Described on p. 251.

3. **Serratus magnus** (M. serratus cervicis).—Described with the thoracic part on p. 254.

Third Layer

4. **Splenius.**—This is an extensive, flat, triangular muscle, partly covered by the preceding three muscles.

Origin.—The second, third, and fourth thoracic spines by means of the dorso-scapular ligament, and the funicular portion of the ligamentum nuchæ.

Insertion.—The occipital crest, the mastoid process, the wing of the atlas, and the transverse processes of the third, fourth, and fifth cervical vertebræ.

Action.—Acting together, to elevate the head and neck; acting singly, to incline the head and neck to the side of the muscle acting.

Structure.—The muscle arises in the withers from the anterior part of the dorso-scapular ligament, which also affords attachment to the rhomboideus, serratus anticus, and complexus muscles. The fibers pass upward and forward toward the head and the first cervical vertebra. The insertion on the occipital bone and the mastoid process is by means of a thin aponeurosis common to the splenius, trachelo-mastoideus, and mastoido-humeralis. The atlantal insertion is by a strong, flat tendon, also in common with these muscles. The remaining insertions are fleshy digitations.

Relations.—Superficially, the skin and fascia, the trapezius rhomboideus, cervicalis, serratus magnus, and posterior auricular muscles; deeply, the complexus, trachelo-mastoideus, and longissimus muscles.

Blood-supply.—Deep cervical and dorsal arteries.

Nerve-supply.—Dorsal branches of the last six cervical nerves.

Fourth Layer

5. **Trachelo-mastoideus** (M. longissimus capitis et atlantis).—This muscle consists of two parallel, fusiform portions. It lies between the deep face of the splenius and the ventral part of the complexus.

Origin.—(1) The transverse processes of the first two thoracic vertebræ; (2) the articular processes of the cervical vertebræ.

Insertion.—(1) The mastoid process; (2) the wing of the atlas.

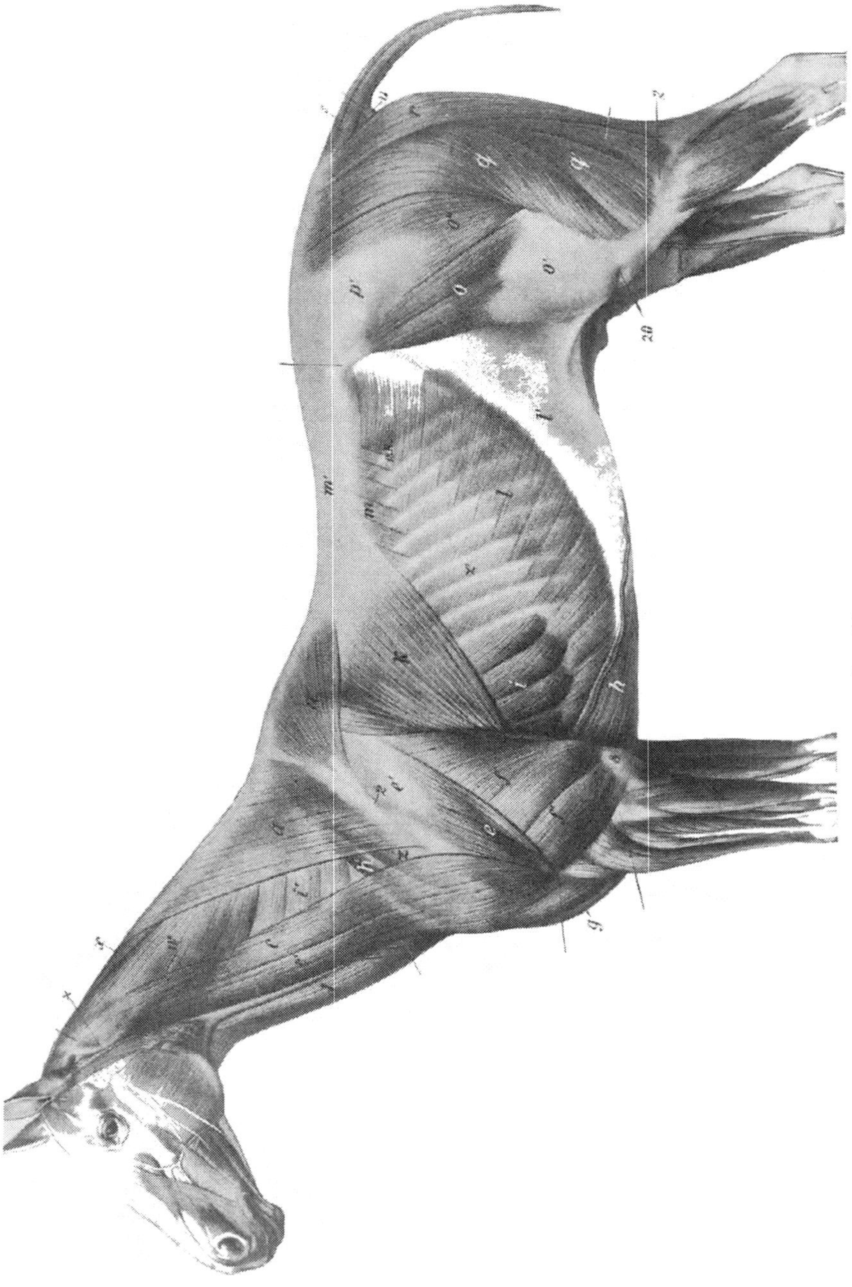

Fi 178.

Action.—Acting together, to extend the head and neck; acting singly, to flex the head and neck laterally or to rotate the atlas.

Structure.—The origin from the thoracic vertebræ is by aponeurotic slips which blend with the complexus. The succeeding fleshy portion, in passing along the neck, receives fasciculi from each of the cervical vertebræ except the first two. The dorsal division of the muscle is inserted into the mastoid process by a flat tendon which fuses with that of the splenius; the ventral division is inserted into the wing of the atlas by a ribbon-like tendon in common with the splenius and mastoido-humeralis.

Relations.—Superficially, the splenius muscle and dorsal branches of the cervical nerves; deeply, the complexus, the spinalis colli, and the oblique muscles of the head. The superior cervical vessels cross the deep face of the muscle obliquely at the level of the sixth and seventh cervical vertebræ.

Blood-supply.—Vertebral and superior cervical arteries.

Nerve-supply.—Dorsal branches of the last six cervical nerves.

6. **Complexus** (M. semispinalis capitis). — This is a large triangular muscle which lies chiefly on the ligamentum nuchæ, under cover of the splenius and trachelo-mastoideus muscles.

Origin.—(1) The second, third, and fourth thoracic spines, in common with the splenius and serratus anticus; (2) the transverse processes of the first six or seven thoracic vertebræ; (3) the articular processes of the cervical vertebræ.

Insertion.—The posterior surface of the occipital bone, external to the funicular portion of the ligamentum nuchæ.

Action.—It is the chief extensor of the head and neck. Acting singly, the muscle inclines the head to the same side.

Structure.—The origin of the muscle at the withers is aponeurotic. In the neck the bundles arising from the articular processes run obliquely upward and forward, giving the lower part of the muscle a distinct pennate character. The upper part of the belly is crossed obliquely by four or five tendinous intersections. The insertion is by a strong tendon.

Relations.—Superficially, the rhomboideus, serratus magnus, splenius, and trachelo-mastoideus muscles; deeply, the ligamentum nuchæ, the multifidus cervicis, longissimus, and the oblique and posterior straight muscles of the head, the deep or superior cervical vessels, and the dorsal cutaneous branches of the cervical nerves.

Blood-supply.—Deep cervical, vertebral, and occipital arteries.

Nerve-supply.—Dorsal branches of the last six cervical nerves.

7. **Multifidus** cervicis (M. semispinalis colli; transverse spinous muscle of neck).—This muscle lies on the arches of the last five cervical vertebræ. It consists of five or six segments.

Origin.—The articular processes of the last five (or four) cervical and the first thoracic vertebræ.

Insertion.—The spinous processes of the cervical vertebræ.

FIG. 8. —SUPERFICIAL MUSCLES OF HORSE.

The pand cu us, except the cervica pat , has ben remove . a, Trapez us cervica s; a', rapez us horacalis; c, c', mastoido-humeralis; d, sterno-cepl a cus; e, deltoid; f, ong head of triceps; f', externa hea dof r ceps; g, anter or superfic a pet bra ; h, pos er or pectoral; h', anter or deep pectoral; i, serra us cervic s; i', serra us horac s; k, a ts mus orsi; l, ob quus ab dom n s externus; l', aponeur s s of l; m, serra us pos icus; m', lum o- orsal fasc a; o, extensor asc æ a ae o', fasc a lata; o'', g u eus superficialis; q, q', q'', biceps femoris; r, sem ten nosus; s, sacro-coccygeus super or; , sacro-coccygeus a eral s; u, coccygeus; v, cervica pan cu us w, sp en us; x, rhomb o eus; y, ext dn of tricle o-mastoideus and mastoido-humeralis; z, supraspinatus; X, w ng of a as; 2, sp ne of scapu a; 4', externa epicondy e o humerus; 6, et al uberosity; 8, o ecranon 8, externa ang e of ilium; 9, patella; 9' external condyle of tibia. (A ter Elleb erger-Baum, Ana . für Kuns er.

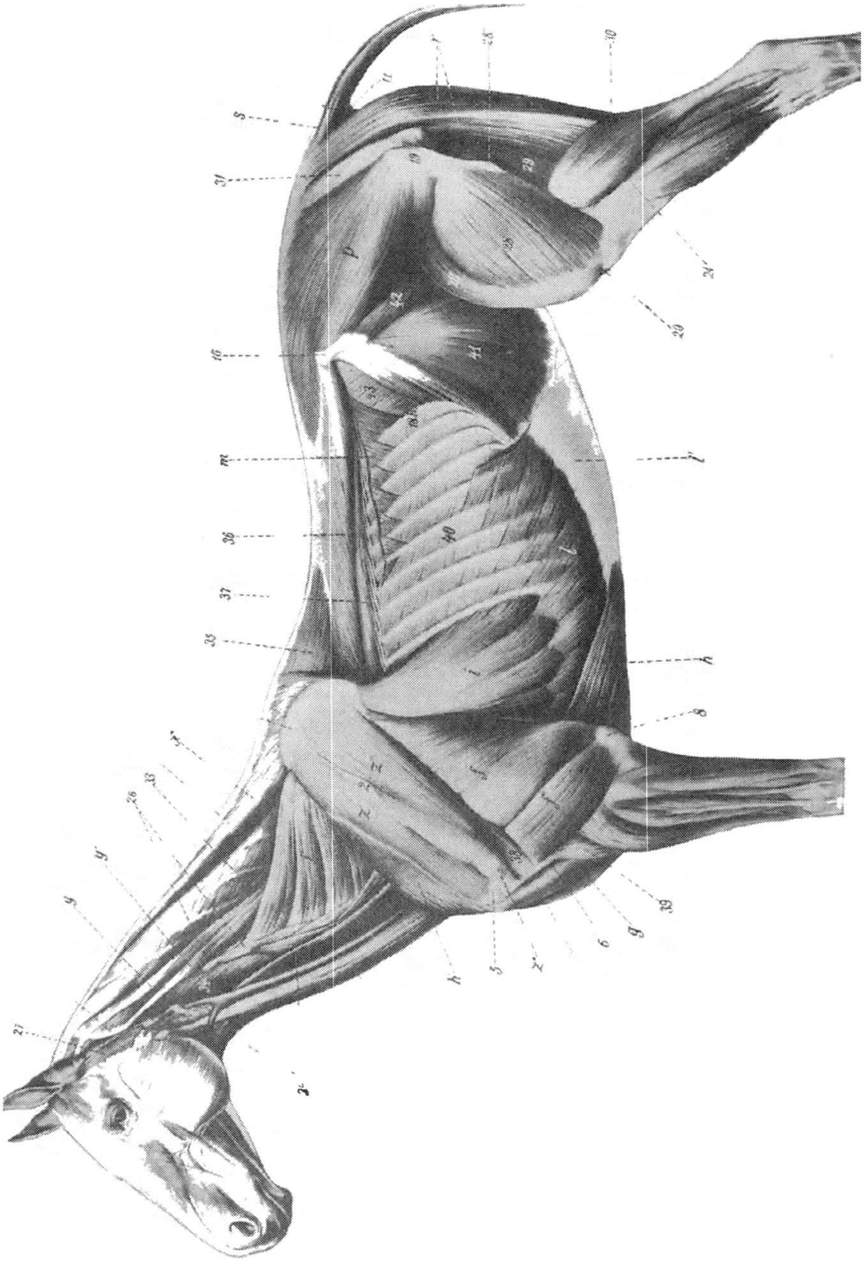

Fig. 179

Fig. 19. Deeper Muscles of Horse.

f, Long head of triceps; *f'*, external head of triceps; *g*, anterior or superficial pectoral; *h*, posterior deep pectoral; *h'*, anterior deep pectoral; *i*, serratus thoracis; serratus cervicis; , obliquus abdominis externus, and *l'*, its aponeurosis, the posterior part of which has been removed; *m*, serratus posticus; *p*, gluteus medius; *r*, semitendinosus; *s*, sacrococcygeus superior; , sacro-coccygeus lateralis; *u*, coccygeus; *v'*, deltoid; *x*, rhomboideus; *y*, *y'*, trachelo-mastoideus; *z*, supraspinatus; *z'*, infraspinatus; *1*, cartilage of scapula; *2*, spine of scapula; *6*, external tuberosity of humerus; *6*, external tuberosity; *8*, olecranon; *16*, external angle of ilium; *19*, trochanter major; *20*, patella; *21'*, external condyle of tibia; *26*, articular processes of cervical vertebræ; *2*, parotido-auricularis; *8*, vastus externus; *28'*, rectus femoris; *23''*, trochanter tertius; *9*, semimembranosus; *0*, gastrocnemius; *3*, sacro-sciatic ligament; *3*, omo-hyoideus; *3*, complexus; *34*, rectus capitis anterior major; *3*, spinalis dorsi; *36*, longissimus dorsi; *3*, transversalis costarum; *8*, teres minor; *39*, rhomboideus; *4*, external intercostal; *41*, obliquus abdominis internus; *2*, iliacus; *43*, transversus abdominis. (After Ellenberger-Baum, Anat. für Künstler.)

Action.—Acting together, to extend the neck; acting singly, to flex and rotate the neck to the opposite side.

Structure.—The muscle is composed of two sets of bundles. The superficial bundles are directed obliquely forward and inward, each passing from an articular process to the spine of the preceding vertebra. The deep bundles are shorter and run straight from an articular process to that of the preceding vertebra.

Relations.—Superficially, the complexus, longissimus, trachelo-mastoideus, and great oblique muscles; deeply, the spinalis muscle, the ligamentum nuchæ, and the arches of the vertebræ.

Blood-supply.—Deep cervical and vertebral arteries.

Nerve-supply.—Dorsal branches of the last six cervical nerves.

8. **Spinalis.**—Described with the longissimus on p. 237.

9. **Obliquus capitis posterior** (s. caudalis) (great oblique muscle of the head).—This is a strong, quadrilateral muscle, which covers the dorso-lateral aspect of the atlas and axis.

Origin.—The side of the spine and the posterior articular process of the axis.

Insertion.—The dorsal surface of the wing of the atlas.

Action.—Chiefly to rotate the atlas, and with it the head, to the same side; also to assist in extending and fixing the atlanto-axial joint.

Structure.—The muscle is composed almost entirely of parallel fleshy fibers directed obliquely forward and outward.

Relations.—Superficially, the skin, the splenius, complexus, trachelo-mastoideus, and mastoido-humeralis muscles; deeply, the arch and spine of the axis, the wing of the atlas, the atlanto-axial joint, the multifidus cervicis, the posterior straight muscles, the occipital and vertebral vessels, and the first and second cervical nerves. The terminal part of the vertebral artery joins the posterior branch of the occipital artery under cover of the muscle.

Blood-supply.—Occipital and vertebral arteries.

Nerve-supply.—Dorsal branch of the second cervical nerve.

10. **Obliquus capitis anterior** (s. cranialis) (small oblique muscle of the head).—A short, thick, quadrilateral muscle which lies on the side of the occipito-atlantal articulation.

Origin.—The anterior edge of the wing of the atlas and the fossa atlantis.

Insertion.—The styloid process and crest of the occipital bone, and the mastoid process.

Action.—Acting together, to extend the head on the atlas; acting singly, to flex the head laterally.

Structure.—The muscle contains a good deal of tendinous tissue. The direction of its fibers is forward, upward, and inward.

Relations.—Superficially, the posterior auricular muscles, artery, and nerve, the aponeurosis of the splenius, trachelo-mastoideus and mastoido-humeralis, and the parotid gland; deeply, the straight muscles, the complexus, the occipito-hyoideus, the occipito-atlantal articulation, branches of the occipital artery, and a branch of the occipital nerve.

Blood-supply.—Occipital artery.

Nerve-supply.—Dorsal branch of the first cervical nerve.

11. **Rectus capitis posterior major** (s. dorsalis major) (great posterior straight muscle of the head).—This muscle extends from the axis to the occipital bone, in contact with the ligamentum nuchæ.

Origin.—The edge of the spinous process of the axis.

Insertion.—The occipital bone, below and external to the complexus and ligamentum nuchæ.

Action.—To extend the head.

Structure.—The muscle is fleshy and may be divided into two parallel portions,

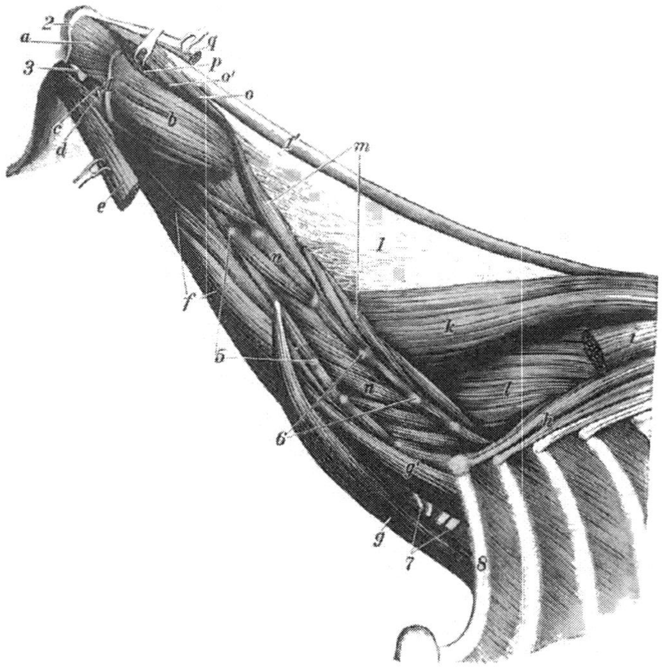

Fig. 180.—Deepest Layer of Muscles of Neck of Horse.

a Obliquus capitis anterior; *b*, obliquus capitis posterior; *c*, rectus capitis lateralis; d, rectus capitis anterior minor; *e*, rectus capitis anterior major; *f*, longus colli; *g*, *g'*, scalenus; *h*, transversalis costarum; *i*, longissimus dorsi; *k*, spinalis et semispinalis; *l*, multifidus dorsi; *m*, multifidus cervicis; *n*, intertransversales; *o*, *o'*, rectus capitis posterior major; p, rectus capitis posterior minor; *q*, tendon of insertion of complexus; *1*, lamellar part, *1'*, funicular part of ligamentum nuchæ; *2*, occipital crest; *3*, paramastoid process; *4*, edge of wing of atlas; *5*, transverse, and *6*, articular, processes of cervical vertebræ; *7*, nerves of brachial plexus (cut); *8*, first rib. (Ellenberger-Baum, Anat. d. Haustiere.)

superficial and deep. The former blends somewhat with the terminal part of the complexus. The deep portion may be termed the rectus capitis posterior medius.

Relations.—Superficially, the anterior oblique, splenius, and complexus; internally, the ligamentum nuchæ; deeply, the atlas, the occipito-atlantal articulation, and the rectus capitis posterior minor. The dorsal branch of the first cervical nerve appears between this muscle and the small oblique.

Blood-supply.—Occipital artery.

Nerve-supply.—Dorsal branch of the first cervical nerve.

12. **Rectus capitis posterior minor** (s. dorsalis minor) (small posterior straight muscle of the head).—This small muscle lies under cover of the preceding.

Origin.—The dorsal surface of the atlas.

Insertion.—The occipital bone beneath the preceding muscle.

Action.—To assist the preceding muscle.

Structure.—It is fleshy and varies a good deal in volume, being sometimes small and difficult to recognize.[1] On the other hand, it is sometimes double.

Relations.—Superficially, the preceding muscle and the small oblique; deeply, the atlas and the occipito-atlantal articulation.

Blood-supply.—Occipital artery.

Nerve-supply.—Dorsal branch of the first cervical nerve.

The Fasciæ and Muscles of the Back and Loins

The **superficial fascia** presents no special features. The **lumbo-dorsal fascia** (Fascia lumbo-dorsalis) closely invests the muscles, but is easily stripped off the longissimus. It is attached medially to the supraspinous ligament and the spinous processes of the vertebræ; laterally, it divides into two layers. The superficial layer is practically the aponeurosis of the latissimus dorsi. The deep layer gives origin to the serratus anticus and posticus, the lumbar part of the obliquus externus abdominis, the transversus abdominis, and the retractor costæ. Its lateral edge curves under the longissimus and is attached to the ribs and lumbar transverse processes. Posteriorly, it is continuous with the gluteal fascia. At the withers it forms an important structure, the **dorso-scapular ligament.** This is a strong tendinous sheet, attached to the third, fourth, and fifth thoracic spines. Its upper part is very thick and gives origin by its superficial surface to the rhomboideus dorsi, by its anterior part to the splenius. The lower part is thin and elastic, and furnishes numerous lamellæ which intersect the scapular part of the serratus and are attached with it to the scapula. Three lamellæ are detached from the deep face of the ligament. The deepest of these passes between the longissimus and spinalis and is attached to the transverse processes of the first seven thoracic vertebræ; it gives attachment to the complexus. The middle one dips in between the longissimus and transversalis costarum. The superficial one gives origin to the serratus anticus. A strong fascial layer, the ilio-lumbar ligament, extends from the last rib to the external angle of the ilium.

There are nine pairs of muscles in this region, arranged in four layers.

First Layer

1. **Trapezius thoracalis.**
2. **Latissimus dorsi.**

Second Layer

3. **Rhomboideus thoracalis.**

The foregoing are described with the other muscles which attach the thoracic limb to the trunk (p. 251).

4. **Serratus anticus** (M. serratus dorsalis inspiratorius).—This is a thin quadrilateral muscle, named from its toothed ventral border. It lies beneath the rhomboideus, serratus magnus, and latissimus dorsi.

Origin.—The lumbo-dorsal fascia and dorso-scapular ligament.

Insertion.—The external surfaces of the fifth to the eleventh or twelfth ribs inclusive.

Action.—To draw the ribs on which it is inserted forward and outward, thus assisting in inspiration.

[1] This seems due to pressure produced by pathological changes in the supra-atloid bursa, which are frequently extensive in dissecting-room subjects.

Structure.—The muscle arises by means of a thin aponeurosis which blends with the lumbo-dorsal fascia and the aponeurosis of the latissimus dorsi. The muscle-fibers pass downward and backward to be attached to the ribs by seven or eight digitations below the outer edge of the transversalis costarum.

Relations.—Superficially, the rhomboideus, serratus magnus, latissimus dorsi, and serratus posticus; deeply, the longissimus dorsi, transversalis costarum, external intercostal muscles, and the ribs.

Blood-supply.—Intercostal arteries.

Nerve-supply.—Thoracic nerves.

5. **Serratus posticus** (M. serratus dorsalis exspiratorius).—This muscle resembles the preceding one, which it partly covers.

Origin.—The lumbo-dorsal fascia.

Insertion.—The outer surfaces of the last seven or eight ribs.

Action.—To draw the ribs backward, thus assisting in expiration.

Structure.—Similar to the preceding muscle. The fibers are directed downward and forward and terminate in seven or eight digitations, one or two of which cover the posterior teeth of the anticus. The aponeurosis blends with that of the latissimus dorsi.

Relations.—Superficially, the latissimus dorsi and external oblique; deeply, the longissimus dorsi, transversalis costarum, external intercostals, serratus anticus, and the ribs.

Blood-supply.—Intercostal and lumbar arteries.

Nerve-supply.—Thoracic nerves.

Third Layer

6. **Transversalis costarum** (M. ilio-costalis).—This long, segmental muscle extends, as its name indicates, across the series of ribs, in contact with the outer edge of the longissimus dorsi.

Origin.—(1) The transverse processes of the second and third lumbar vertebræ and the deep layer of the lumbo-dorsal fascia. (2) The anterior borders and external surface of the last fifteen ribs.[1]

Insertion.—The posterior borders of the ribs and the transverse processes of the last two or three cervical vertebræ.

Action.—Chiefly to depress and retract the ribs and so help in expiration. Acting together, they may assist in extending this spine, acting singly in inclining it laterally.

Structure.—This muscle presents a distinct segmental arrangement. It is composed of a series of bundles, the fibers of which are directed forward and a little downward and outward. From these are detached two sets of tendons. The superficial tendons spring from the outer edge of the muscle. They are flat and are about half an inch in width. Each crosses two or three intercostal spaces, to be inserted on the posterior border of a rib. The deep tendons are detached from the dorsal part of the deep face of the muscle. Each passes backward across one or two intercostal spaces to its origin on the anterior border or outer surface of a rib. Small bursæ may be found between the ribs and tendons.

Relations.—Superficially, the dorsal serrati and the complexus; deeply, the external intercostals and the ribs. The lumbar origin is covered by the longissimus. The superior (deep) cervical and dorsal vessels cross the surface of the muscle at the first and second intercostal spaces respectively, and branches of the intercostal vessels and nerves emerge between the transversalis and longissimus; here a fascial layer dips in between the two.

[1] The lumbar part of this muscle is subject to variation. It may, in quite exceptional cases, extend as far as the ilium.

Blood-supply.—Intercostal arteries.

Nerve-supply.—Dorsal branches of the thoracic nerves.

7. Longissimus.[1]—This is the largest and longest muscle in the body. It extends from the sacrum and ilium to the neck, filling up the space between the spinous processes medially and the lumbar transverse processes and the upper ends of the ribs below; consequently it has the form of a three-sided prism.

Origin.—(1) The internal angle, crest, and adjacent part of the ventral surface of the ilium; (2) the first three sacral spines; (3) the lumbar and thoracic spines and the supraspinous ligament.

Insertion.—(1) The lumbar transverse and articular processes; (2) the thoracic transverse processes; (3) the spinous and transverse processes of the last four cervical vertebræ; (4) the outer surfaces of the ribs, except the first.

Action.—Acting with its fellow, it is the most powerful extensor of the back and loins; by its cervical attachment it assists in extending the neck. By its costal attachment it may also assist in expiration. Acting singly, it flexes the spine laterally.

Structure.—This is quite complex. The posterior part of the muscle is greatly developed and constitutes the common mass of the loins. This is covered by a strong aponeurosis which blends with the supraspinous and sacro-iliac ligaments, and is attached to the crest and inner (sacral) angle of the ilium and the first and second sacral spines; it furnishes origin to the lumbar portion of the middle gluteus. In its course further forward the muscle receives fasciculi from the lumbar and thoracic spines, but diminishes somewhat in volume. At the withers it divides into two parts. The dorsal division (spinalis et semispinalis), reinforced by bundles from the first four thoracic spines, passes forward under the complexus to be inserted into the spines of the last four cervical vertebræ. The ventral division passes forward and downward underneath the serratus magnus to be inserted into the ribs and the transverse processes of the last four cervical vertebræ. Three sets of fasciculi may be distinguished, viz.: (1) spinal, which are superficial and internal; (2) transverse, attached to the transverse and articular processes, which are internal and deep; (3) costal, which are external.

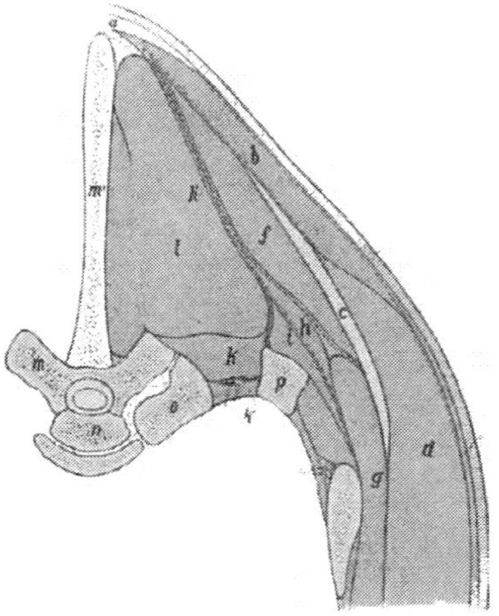

FIG. 181.—RIGHT PORTION OF CROSS-SECTION OF BACK OF HORSE. SECTION IS CUT THROUGH SEVENTH THORACIC VERTEBRA.

a, Ligamentum nuchæ; *b*, trapezius muscle; *c*, cartilage of scapula; *d*, latissimus dorsi; *e*, panniculus carnosus; *f*, rhomboideus dorsi; *g*, serratus magnus; *h*, serratus anticus; *h'*, lumbodorsal fascia, which divides below into three layers; *i*, transversalis costarum; *k*, levator costæ; *k'*, internal intercostal muscle; *l*, longissimus dorsi; *m*, *m'*, seventh thoracic vertebra; *n*, head of eighth thoracic vertebra; *o*, head of eighth rib; *p*, seventh rib; *r*, intercostal artery and nerve; *s*, skin. The fasciæ are indicated by dotted lines. (After Ellenberger, in Leisering's Atlas.)

Relations.—Superficially, the middle gluteus, the lumbo-dorsal fascia, the latissimus dorsi, dorsal serrati, serratus magnus, and complexus; deeply, the multifidus, intertransversales, external intercostals, levatores costarum, the ligamentum nuchæ, and its fellow of the opposite side (in the neck).

Blood-supply.—Dorsal, superior cervical, intercostal, and lumbar arteries.

Nerve-supply.—Dorsal branches of the thoracic and lumbar nerves.

[1] The muscle as here described includes the spinalis and semispinalis components, as the separation of these is largely artificial in the horse.

8. **Multifidus** dorsi (semispinalis of the back and loins).—This is a long segmental muscle which covers the sides of the spinous processes of the vertebræ from the sacrum to the neck.

Origin.—(1) The lateral portion of the sacrum; (2) the articular processes of the lumbar vertebræ; (3) the transverse processes of the thoracic vertebræ.

Insertion.—The spinous processes of the first two sacral, the lumbar, thoracic, and last cervical vertebræ.

Action.—Acting with its fellow, it is an extensor of the spine; acting singly, it flexes it laterally.

Structure.—It is composed of a series of bundles which are directed obliquely forward and upward. Each fasciculus passes over several vertebræ to its insertion. In the posterior part of the series the bundles cross two or three vertebræ and are inserted into the summits of the spines. Anteriorly, the bundles have a more horizontal direction, cross three to five vertebræ, and are inserted into the sides of the spines considerably below their summits. A further complication consists in the fusion of several bundles into a common insertion.

Relations.—Superficially, the longissimus; deeply, the vertebral spines.

Blood-supply.—Intercostal and lumbar arteries.

Nerve-supply.—Dorsal branches of the thoracic and lumbar nerves.

9. **Intertransversales lumborum.**—These are very thin muscular and tendinous strata, which occupy the spaces between the transverse processes of the lumbar vertebræ except the fifth and sixth.

Action.—To assist in flexing the loins laterally.

Relations.—Superficially, the longissimus; deeply, the quadratus lumborum.

Blood-supply.—Lumbar arteries.

Nerve-supply.—Lumbar nerves.

THE FASCIA AND MUSCLES OF THE TAIL

The muscles of the tail are inclosed in the strong coccygeal fascia, which is continuous in front with the gluteal fascia and blends with the lateral sacro-iliac ligament. At the root of the tail it is loosely attached to the subjacent muscles, but further back it is intimately adherent to them. From its deep face are detached septa which pass between the muscles to become attached to the vertebræ.

1. Coccygeus (Compressor coccygis; ischio-coccygeus).—This is a flat, triangular muscle which lies chiefly between the sacro-sciatic ligament and the rectum.

Origin.—The pelvic surface of the sacro-sciatic ligament near the ischiatic spine.

Insertion.—The first four coccygeal vertebræ and the coccygeal fascia.

Action.—Acting together, to depress (flex) the tail, compressing it over the perineum; acting singly, to depress and incline it to the same side.

Structure.—The origin of the muscle is aponeurotic. Becoming fleshy, its fibers pass upward and backward and divide into two layers. The outer layer is attached to the vertebræ, the inner to the fascia; included between the two lie the intertransversales. When the tail is raised, the ventral edges of the muscles produce a distinct ridge at either side of the anus.

Relations.—Outwardly, the sacro-sciatic ligament and the semimembranosus; inwardly, the rectum and the sacro-coccygeus ventralis muscle. The internal pudic artery crosses the outer face of the origin of the muscle.

2. Sacro-coccygeus superior (M. sacrococcygeus dorsalis medialis; erector s. extensor coccygis).—This muscle lies along the dorso-median aspect of the tail, in contact with its fellow.

Origin.—The last three sacral spines and some of the coccygeal spines.

Insertion.—The dorsal surface of the coccygeal vertebræ.

Action.—Acting together, to elevate (extend) the tail; acting singly, to elevate and incline it laterally.

Structure.—The muscle has a strong rounded belly. It is inserted by means of short tendons which fuse with those of the next muscle.

Relations.—Superficially, the coccygeal fascia; internally, its fellow; laterally, the sacro-coccygeus lateralis; deeply, the vertebræ.

3. **Sacro-coccygeus lateralis** (M. sacro-coccygeus dorsalis lateralis; curvator coccygis).—This muscle lies immediately lateral to the preceding.

Origin.—The sides of the sacral spines, with the multifidus, and the transverse processes of the sacral and coccygeal vertebræ.

Insertion.—The lateral surface of the coccygeal vertebræ, except the first four.

Action.—Acting with its fellow, to assist the preceding muscle in elevating the tail; acting singly, to incline it to the same side.

Structure.—This muscle appears to be a direct continuation of the multifidus dorsi. The belly is fusiform and receives reinforcing fasciculi from the transverse processes of the sacrum. This is succeeded by bundles of tendons, as many as four lying alongside of each other.

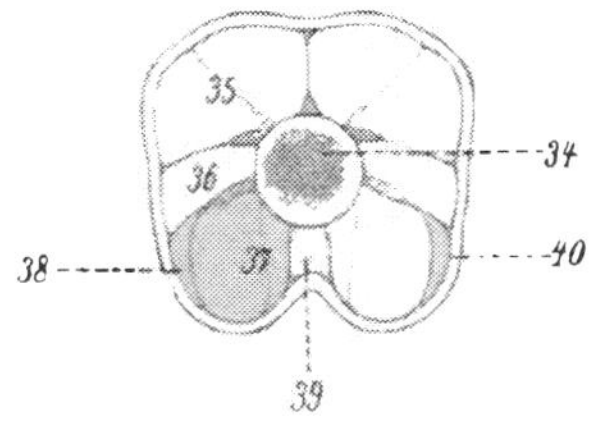

FIG. 182.—CROSS-SECTION OF TAIL OF HORSE CLOSE TO ANUS.

34, Coccygeal vertebra; *35*, sacro-coccygeus superior; *36*, intertransversalis; *37*, sacro-coccygeus inferior; *38*, coccygeus; *39*, recto-coccygeus; *40*, coccygeal fascia. (After Ellenberger-Baum, Anat. für Künstler.)

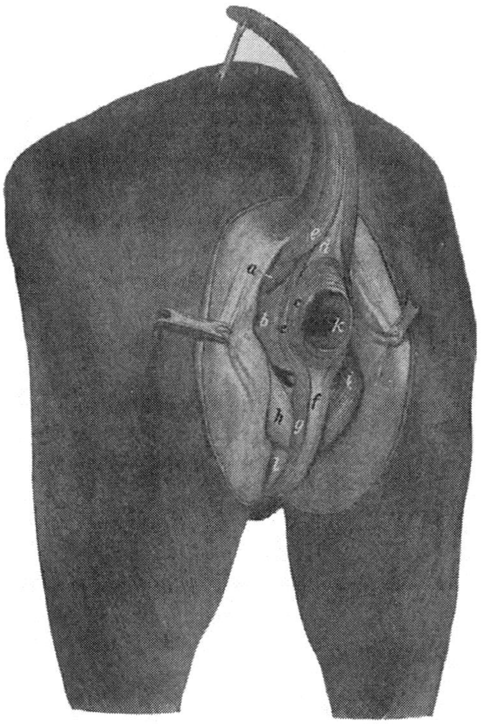

FIG. 183.—MUSCLES OF PERINEUM OF HORSE.

a, Coccygeus; *b*, retractor ani; *c*, *c'*, sphincter ani externus; *d*, recto-coccygeus; *e*, sacro-coccygeus inferior lateralis; *f*, retractor penis; *g*, bulbo-cavernosus; *h*, ischio-cavernosus; *i*, internal pudic artery; *k*, anus; *l*, penis. (After Ellenberger-Baum, Top. Anat. d. Pferdes.)

Relations.—Superficially, the lateral sacro-iliac ligament and the coccygeal fascia; dorsally, the sacro-coccygeus superior; ventrally, the intertransversales; deeply, the vertebræ and a branch of the lateral coccygeal artery and accompanying vein and nerve.

4. **Intertransversales** caudæ (Mm. intertransversarii caudæ).—These consist of muscular bundles which lie on the lateral aspect of the tail, between the preceding muscle and the sacro-coccygeus inferior. They begin on the lateral edge

of the sacrum and occupy the spaces between the transverse processes, to which they are attached. They are, however, not arranged in a strict segmental manner.

Action.—Acting together, to fix the coccygeal vertebræ; acting singly, to assist in lateral flexion.

5. **Sacro-coccygeus inferior** (Mm. sacro-coccygei ventrales; depressor coccygis).—This muscle lies on the ventral aspect of the sacrum and coccyx. It is composed of two portions, described by Bourgelat and the German anatomists as separate muscles.

(*a*) The **outer portion** (M. coccygeus ventralis lateralis) is much the larger of the two. It arises from the outer part of the ventral surface of the sacrum, about as far forward as the third foramen, and is inserted into the transverse processes and ventral surface of the coccygeal vertebræ.

(*b*) The **inner portion** (M. sacro-coccygeus ventralis medialis) arises from the ventral surface of the sacrum internal to the preceding muscle and the first eight coccygeal vertebræ, and is inserted into the ventral surfaces of the coccygeal vertebræ.

Action.—Acting together, to depress (flex) the tail; acting singly, to incline it laterally also.

Structure.—The outer portion has a somewhat compressed belly, and receives bundles from the transverse processes of the coccygeal vertebræ. The inner portion is much smaller and shorter, reaching only about to the middle of the tail.

Relations.—Ventrally, the pelvic and coccygeal fasciæ; dorsally, the sacrum, coccygeal vertebræ, and the intertransversales; laterally, the sacro-sciatic ligament, the coccygeus, and the coccygeal fascia; medially, its fellow, the recto-coccygeus, and the middle coccygeal vessels. Branches of the lateral coccygeal vessels and nerves lie between the outer division of the muscle and the intertransversales.

Blood-supply.—Middle and lateral coccygeal arteries.

Nerve-supply.—Coccygeal nerves.

The Muscles of the Thorax

These consist of seven muscles or sets of muscles, which are attached to the thoracic vertebræ, to the ribs and their cartilages, and to the sternum. Functionally, they are muscles of respiration.

1. **Levatores costarum.**—These constitute a series of small muscles which occupy and overlie the upper ends of the intercostal spaces.

Origin.—The transverse processes of the thoracic vertebræ.

Insertion.—The external surfaces of the upper ends of the ribs posterior to the vertebral origin.

Action.—To draw the ribs forward in inspiration.

Structure.—Arising by tendinous fibers, each muscle passes backward and outward and expands at its insertion. Some fibers pass over one rib and are inserted on a succeeding one. At the first and last spaces the muscle cannot be distinguished from the external intercostal, of which it is in reality only a specially developed part.

Relations.—Superficially, the longissimus dorsi; deeply, the ribs, internal intercostal muscles, and the intercostal vessels and nerves.

Blood-supply.—Intercostal arteries.

Nerve-supply.—Intercostal nerves.

2. **External intercostals** (Mm. intercostales externi).—Each of these occupies an intercostal space, from the levatores to the sternal extremity of the rib. They do not occupy the intercartilaginous spaces.

Origin.—The posterior borders of the ribs.

Insertion.—The anterior borders and external surfaces of the succeeding ribs.

Action.—To draw the ribs forward in inspiration.

Structure.—The fibers are directed downward and backward. There is a considerable admixture of tendinous tissue. The thickness of the muscles gradually diminishes toward the lower ends of the spaces.

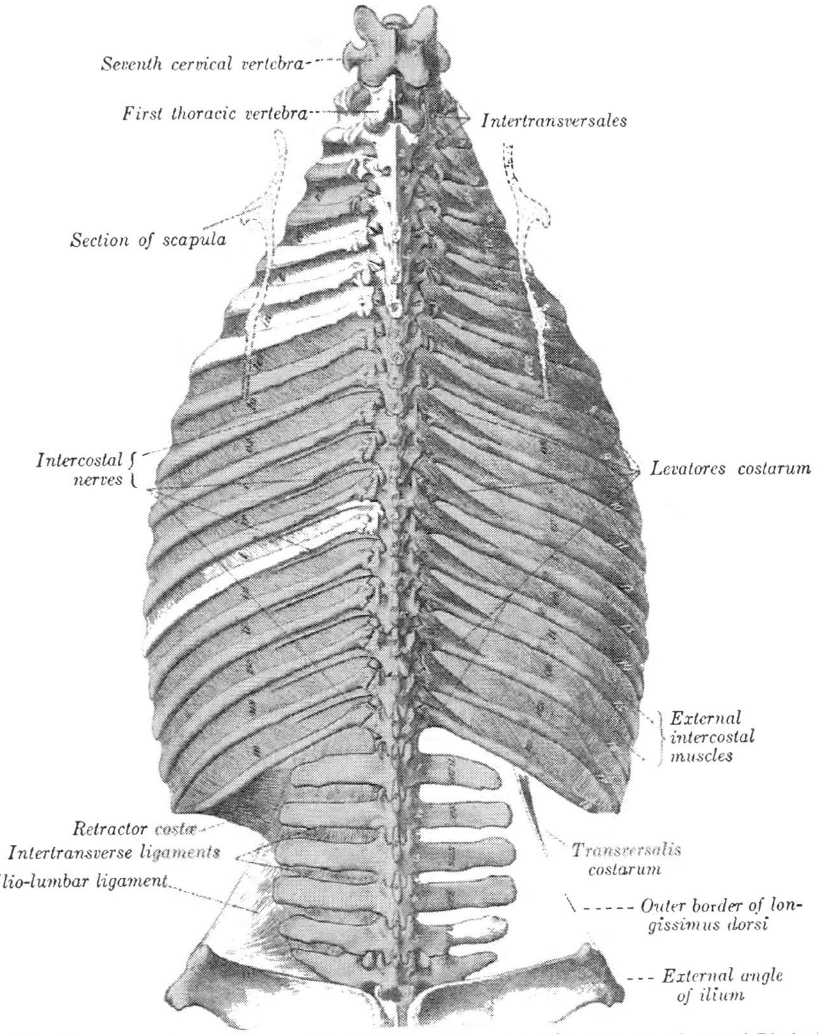

FIG. 184.—DORSAL AND LUMBAR REGIONS OF HORSE, DORSAL VIEW. (After Schmaltz, Atlas d. Anat. d. Pferdes.)

Relations.—Superficially, the serratus magnus, latissimus dorsi, serratus anticus and posticus, longissimus dorsi, transversalis costarum, rectus thoracis, deep pectorals, obliquus abdominis externus, and panniculus; deeply, the internal intercostals and (in the upper part of the spaces) the intercostal vessels and nerves.

Blood-supply.—Intercostal and internal thoracic arteries.

Nerve-supply.—Intercostal nerves.

3. Internal intercostals (Mm. intercostales interni).—These occupy the entire length of the intercostal spaces, including their interchondral portion.

Origin.—The anterior borders of the ribs and their cartilages.

Insertion.—The posterior borders of the preceding ribs and cartilages.

Action.—To draw the ribs backward in expiration. It seems probable, however, that the intercartilaginous portion is inspiratory.[1]

Structure.—The direction of the fibers is oblique downward and forward. There is a smaller amount of tendinous tissue than in the external set, and the thickness diminishes from below upward. In the upper part of the spaces fibers sometimes cross a rib in a fashion similar to the subcostals of man. A thin aponeurosis separates the internal from the external intercostal muscle in each space.

Relations.—Superficially, the levatores costarum and the external intercostals; deeply, the endothoracic fascia and pleura, the transversus thoracis, diaphragm, transversus abdominis, and the internal thoracic and asternal vessels. In the upper part of the intercostal spaces the intercostal vessels and nerves lie between the internal and external intercostal muscle, but below they lie chiefly on the deep face of the inner muscle.

Blood-supply.—Intercostal and internal thoracic arteries.

Nerve-supply.—Intercostal nerves.

4. **Retractor costæ.**—This is a small triangular muscle which lies behind the last rib, chiefly under cover of the serratus posticus.

Origin.—The transverse processes of the first three or four lumbar vertebræ by means of the lumbar fascia.

Insertion.—The posterior border of the last rib.

Action.—To retract the last rib.

Structure.—The muscle arises by a thin aponeurosis. Its fibers are parallel to those of the adjacent internal oblique.

Relations.—Superficially, the serratus posticus and external oblique; deeply, the transversus abdominis.

Blood-supply.—Lumbar arteries.

Nerve-supply.—Lumbar nerves.

5. Rectus thoracis (M. transversus costarum; lateralis sterni).—This is a thin muscle which lies under cover of the deep pectoral muscles. It is directed obliquely backward and downward, and crosses the lower part of the first three intercostal spaces.

Origin.—The outer surface of the first rib, below the scalenus.

Insertion.—The cartilage of the third or fourth rib. The aponeurosis usually joins the rectus abdominis. It may reach the sternum.

Action.—It may assist in inspiration or concur with the rectus abdominis.

Relations.—Superficially, the deep pectoral muscles; deeply, the intercostal muscles and the ribs.

6. Transversus thoracis (Triangularis sterni).—This is a flat muscle situated on the thoracic surface of the sternum and the cartilages of the sternal ribs.

Origin.—The sternal ligament.

Insertion.—The cartilages of the ribs, from the second to the eighth inclusive.

Action.—It draws the costal cartilages inward and backward, thus assisting in expiration.

Structure.—Each muscle has the form of a scalene triangle, of which the base is the strongly serrated external border. The muscle contains a good deal of tend inous tissue. The anterior bundles are directed forward and outward; the posterior backward and outward.

[1] The function of the intercostal muscles is still a subject of much discussion. The statements made above seem to represent the view most commonly held in regard to their action.

Relations.—Superiorly, the endothoracic fascia and pleura; inferiorly, the costal cartilages, the internal intercostal muscles, and the internal thoracic vessels.

Blood-supply.—Internal thoracic artery.

Nerve-supply.—The intercostal nerves.

7. **Diaphragm.**—This is a broad, unpaired muscle which forms a partition between the thoracic and abdominal cavities.[1] In outline it has some resemblance to a palm-leaf fan. In form it is dome-shaped, compressed laterally. On a median section it is seen to have a general direction downward and forward from the lumbar vertebræ to the xiphoid cartilage. The thoracic surface is strongly convex, and is covered by the pleura. The abdominal surface is deeply concave, and is covered for the most part by the peritoneum. The muscle consists of a peripheral fleshy portion, two muscular crura, and a tendinous center.

Attachments.—(1) **Costal part:** The cartilages of the ninth to the fifteenth ribs, and the last three ribs at an increasing distance from their sternal ends.

(2) **Sternal part:** The upper surface of the xiphoid cartilage.

(3) **Lumbar part:** (*a*) The **right crus** is attached to the inferior common ligament, and by this means to the first four or five lumbar vertebræ. (*b*) The **left crus** is attached in a similar fashion to the first and second lumbar vertebræ.

Action.—It is the principal muscle of inspiration and increases the longitudinal diameter of the chest. The contraction produces a general lessening of the curvature of the diaphragm. In the expiratory phase the costal part and crura lie directly on the body walls, so that the bases of the lungs are in contact with the tendinous center and sternal portion only. In ordinary inspiration the fleshy rim recedes from the chest-wall, so that the bases of the lungs move backward to a line about parallel with the curve formed by the cartilages of the asternal ribs, and about four or five inches (ca. 10 to 12 cm.) therefrom. It is stated that the inspiratory movement affects the tendinous center much less than the fleshy part, since the posterior vena cava is firmly attached to the former. It should be noted, however, that the direction of the thoracic part of the vena cava in the expiratory phase is oblique upward and backward. Thus it would seem that there is no anatomical reason why the diaphragm should not move as a whole in ordinary inspiration at least.

Structure.—The **costal part** (Pars costalis) consists of a series of digitations which meet, or are separated by a very narrow interval from, the transversus abdominis; between the two are the asternal vessels. From the tenth rib backward the attachments are to the ribs at an increasing distance above the costo-chondral junctions. Thus at the last rib the attachment is four to five inches (10 to 12 cm.) from the lower end. Anteriorly, the origin extends along the ninth costal cartilage to the xiphoid cartilage. From these points of origin the fibers curve inward and forward to join the tendinous center. The **right crus** (Crus dextrum) is about twice as thick as the left one and is also longer. It arises by a strong tendon from the lumbar vertebræ (by means of the inferior common ligament). The tendon is succeeded by a rounded belly which leaves the vertebral column, at the last thoracic vertebra. Passing downward and forward, its fibers spread out and join the tendinous center. The **left crus** (Crus sinistrum) arises by a thin tendon from the inferior common ligament at the first and second lumbar vertebræ. This is succeeded by a triangular belly which joins the central tendon. Between the crura and the attachment to the last rib the edge of the muscle crosses the ventral surface of the psoas muscles without attachment, forming the so-called lumbo-costal arch; here the thoracic and abdominal cavities are separated only by the serous membranes and some areolar tissue. The tendinous center (Centrum tendineum) resembles the periphery in outline, but is more elongated. It is par-

[1] It should be noted, however, that in the embryo the diaphragm appears as a paired structure, extending from the lateral walls of the cœlom to fuse with the septum transversum.

tially divided into right and left halves by the descent of the crura into it. It is composed largely of radiating fibers, but many interlace in various directions; this is specially evident around the foramen venæ cavæ, which is encircled by fibers. A strong tendinous layer extends across below the hiatus œsophageus.

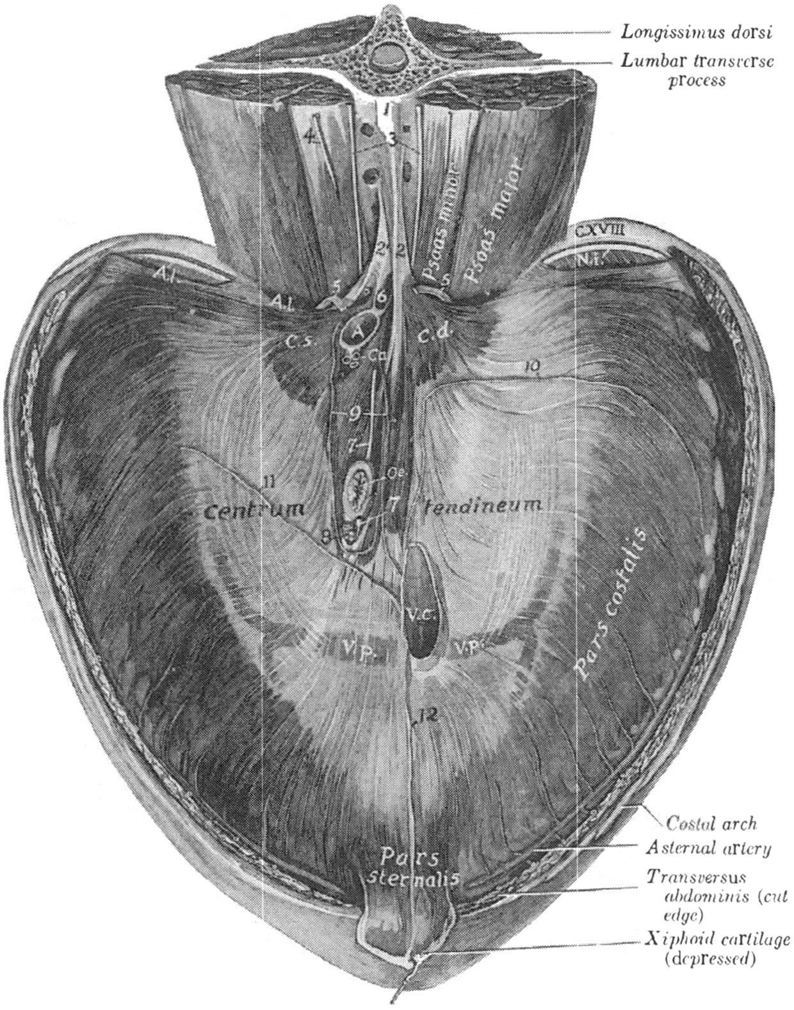

Fig. 185.—Diaphragm of Horse, Abdominal Surfac

1, inferior common ligament; *2*, *2'*, tendons of crura; *3*, lumbar sympathetic trunks; *4*, external spermatic nerve; *5*, *5*, great splanchnic nerves; *6*, cisterna chyli (opened); *7*, *7*, œsophageal continuations of vagus nerves; *8*, lymph-gland; *9*, coronary ligament of liver (cut); *10*, right lateral ligament of liver (cut); *11*, left lateral ligament of liver (cut); *12*, falciform ligament of liver (cut); *A.l.*, lumbo-costal arch; *N.i.*, intercostal nerve; *C.d.*, right crus; *C.s.*, left crus; *A*, aorta; *Ca*, cœliac artery; *Oe.*, œsophagus; *V.c.*, posterior vena cava; *V.p.*, phrenic veins. (After Schmaltz, Atlas d. Anat. d. Pferdes.)

The diaphragm is pierced by three foramina. (1) The **hiatus aorticus** is an interval between the two crura and below the last thoracic vertebra. It contains the posterior aorta, vena azygos, and cisterna chyli. (2) The **hiatus œsophageus** (or foramen sinistrum) perforates the right crus near its junction with the tendinous center. It is situated a little to the left of the median plane and two or three inches below the thirteenth thoracic vertebra (in expiration). It transmits the œsophagus, the vagus nerves, and the œsophageal branch of the gastric artery. (3) The **foramen venæ cavæ** (s. dextrum) pierces the tendinous center about an inch to the right of the median plane, and about six inches below the twelfth thoracic vertebra (in expiration). The vena cava is firmly attached to the margin of the opening.[1]

Relations.—The thoracic surface is related to the endothoracic fascia, pleuræ, pericardium, the bases of the lungs, and the ribs in part. The abdominal surface is in great part covered by the peritoneum, and is related chiefly to the liver, stomach, spleen, pancreas, kidneys and adrenals, and the anterior flexures of the colon. The sympathetic and splanchnic nerves pass between the crus and the psoas muscles on each side. The asternal vessels perforate the edge of the muscle at the ninth costo-chondral joint.

Blood-supply.—Phrenic and asternal arteries.

Nerve-supply.—Phrenic nerves (from the fifth, sixth, and seventh cervical nerves).

The Abdominal Muscles

The **superficial fascia** covering the lateral and ventral walls of the abdomen is continuous dorsally with the lumbo-dorsal fascia, in front with the thoracic fascia, and behind with the gluteal fascia. In the inguinal region it forms part of the fascia of the penis or of the mammary glands. At the lower part of the flank it forms a fold which is continuous with the fascia of the thigh near the stifle joint. In this fold are the precrural lymph-glands. Medially it blends with the linea alba. It contains the abdominal portion of the panniculus carnosus.

The **abdominal panniculus** (M. cutaneus maximus) covers a large part of the lateral surface of the abdomen and thorax. The general direction of its fibers is longitudinal. Its posterior extremity forms the basis of the fold of the flank. Its anterior extremity is inserted by a thin tendon into the internal tuberosity of the humerus, with the posterior deep pectoral muscle. Its dorsal edge may be indicated by a line drawn from the upper end of the thirteenth rib to the fold of the flank. Its ventral limit corresponds to a line drawn from the fold to a point about a hand-breadth external to the umbilicus, and from here to a point a little above the level of the elbow. Behind the shoulder the fibers become oblique and blend with the scapular portion. The aponeurosis extends ventrally to the linea alba, dorsally to the supraspinous ligament. The muscle is intimately adherent to the skin, so that special care is necessary in removing the latter. Its deep face, on the other hand, is loosely attached to the underlying structures by a quantity of areolar tissue which is more or less loaded with fat (panniculus adiposus) in animals in good condition. The large external thoracic ("spur") vein is partially embedded in the lower part of the muscle. Its action is to twitch the skin.

The **deep fascia** is represented chiefly by the **abdominal tunic** (Tunica flava abdominis). This is a sheet of elastic tissue which assists the muscles in supporting the great weight of the abdominal viscera. It is practically coextensive with the obliquus externus, which it covers. Ventrally it is thick, and is intimately adherent to the aponeurosis of the muscle. Laterally it becomes thinner and is more easily separated, although fibers from it dip in between the muscle-bundles. It is continued for some distance upon the intercostals and serratus magnus.

[1] In order to get a clear idea of the relative positions of these foramina and of the form of the diaphragm, the thoracic surface of the latter should be examined while the abdominal viscera remain *in situ*.

Traced forward, it passes as a thin layer beneath the posterior deep pectoral muscle. Posteriorly it is attached to the external angle of the ilium. In the inguinal region it forms the deep fascia of the prepuce or of the mammary glands.

The **linea alba** is a median fibrous raphé which extends from the xiphoid cartilage to the symphysis pubis. It is formed chiefly by the junction of the aponeuroses of the oblique and transverse muscles, but partly by longitudinal fibers. A little behind its middle is a cicatrix which indicates the position of the umbilical opening of the fœtus.

1. **Obliquus abdominis externus** (great oblique; external oblique of the abdomen).—This is the most extensive of the abdominal muscles. It is a broad sheet, irregularly triangular in shape, widest behind. Its fibers are directed chiefly downward and backward.

Origin.—(1) The outer surfaces of the last fourteen ribs, and the fascia over the external intercostal muscles; (2) the lumbo-dorsal fascia.

Insertion.—(1) The linea alba and the prepubic tendon; (2) the external angle and shaft of the ilium; (3) the internal femoral fascia.

Action.—(1) To compress the abdominal viscera, as in defecation, micturition, parturition, and expiration; (2) to flex the trunk (arch the back); (3) acting singly, to flex the trunk laterally.

Structure.—The muscle is composed of a fleshy portion and an aponeurosis. The **muscular portion** lies on the lateral wall of the thorax and abdomen. It arises by a series of digitations, the anterior four of which alternate with those of the serratus magnus. The origin may be indicated by a slightly curved line (concave above) drawn from the lower part of the fifth rib to the external angle of the ilium. The fibers are directed downward and backward and terminate on the aponeurosis, except in the flank, where they are almost horizontal in direction. The line of junction is a curve (concave above) extending from the upper edge of the posterior deep pectoral muscle toward the external angle of the ilium. The **aponeurosis** is intimately attached to the abdominal tunic, and its fibers are largely interwoven ventrally with those of the aponeurosis of the internal oblique. By this fusion is formed the outer sheath of the rectus abdominis, which blends at the linea alba with that of the opposite side. In the inguinal region the aponeurosis divides into two chief layers; one of these curves upward and backward and is inserted into the external angle of the ilium and the prepubic tendon. Between these points the aponeurosis is much strengthened and is called the **inguinal** (Poupart's) **ligament** (Ligamentum inguinale). This curves upward and somewhat forward, becomes thin, and blends with the iliac fascia. It forms the posterior wall of the inguinal canal. About an inch (ca. 2 to 3 cm.) in front of the pubis and about two inches (ca. 4 to 5 cm.) from the median plane the aponeurosis is pierced by a slit-like opening,[1] the **external inguinal ring** (Annulus inguinalis subcutaneus). This is the external orifice of the inguinal canal. Its long axis is directed outward and forward, and is about four inches (ca. 10 cm.) in length. The inner angle is rounded and is well defined by the junction of the inguinal ligament with the prepubic tendon, but the outer angle is not so sharply defined. The borders or pillars are constituted by arciform fibers of the aponeurosis of the external oblique (Crus mediale, laterale). The **femoral layer** of the aponeurosis (Lamina femoralis) passes on to the inner surface of the thigh, where it blends with the femoral fascia. A thin **iliac layer** (Lamina iliaca) passes over the outer margin of the iliacus to the external border of the ilium.

Relations.—Superficially, the skin, the panniculus carnosus, the abdominal tunic, and the posterior deep pectoral muscle; deeply, the ribs and their cartilages, the intercostal muscles, the internal oblique, the contents of the inguinal canal, and the sartorius and gracilis.

[1] It is narrow and slit-like in the natural condition, but may appear oval in the dissecting-room, especially if the hind limb is drawn back and abducted.

Blood-supply.—Intercostal and lumbar arteries.
Nerve-supply.—Intercostal and lumbar nerves.

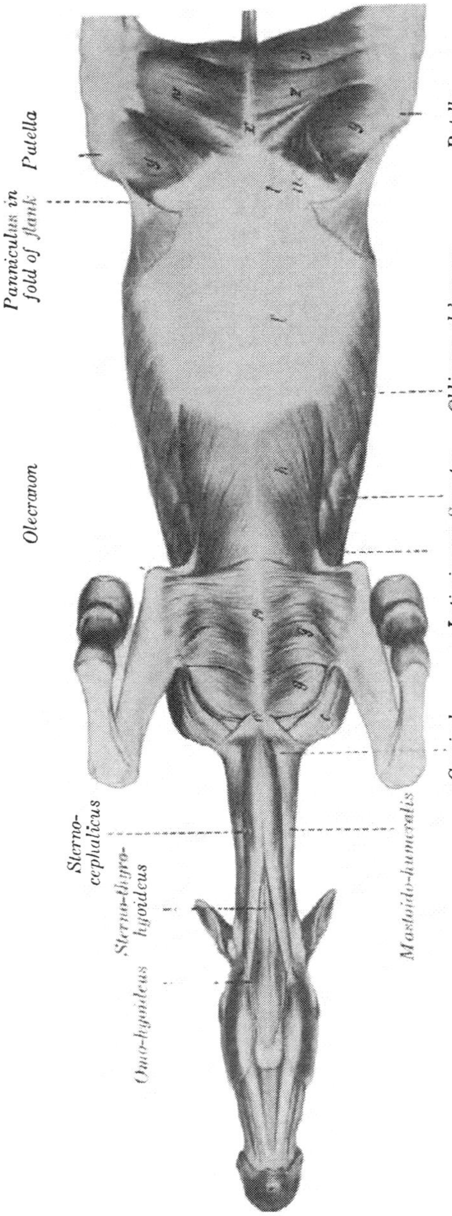

FIG. 186.—VENTRAL MUSCLES OF HORSE, AFTER REMOVAL OF GREATER PART OF PANNICULUS CARNOSUS AND ABDOMINAL TUNIC. SARTORIUS AND GRACILIS REMOVED FROM RIGHT THIGH.

c, Mastoido-humeralis; *g*, anterior superficial pectoral; *g'*, posterior superficial pectoral; *h*, posterior deep pectoral; *l'*, aponeurosis of obliquus abdominis externus; *t*, pectineus; *u*, ilio-psoas; *v*, semimembranosus; *w*, gracilis; *x*, sartorius; *y*, vastus internus; *z'*, adductor; *14*, sternum; *14'*, cariniform cartilage. (After Ellenberger-Baum, Anat. f. Künstler.)

2. **Obliquus abdominis internus** (small oblique; internal oblique of the abdomen).—This muscle is situated under the preceding one. Its fibers are directed downward, forward, and inward. It forms a triangular curved sheet with the base behind.

Origin.—The external angle of the ilium and the adjacent part of the inguinal (Poupart's) ligament.

Insertion.—(1) The cartilages of the last four or five ribs; (2) the linea alba and the prepubic tendon.

Action.—Similar to that of the preceding muscle.

Structure.—Like the external oblique, it is composed of a fleshy portion and an aponeurosis. The **fleshy portion** is fan-shaped, and is situated chiefly in the flank. At its iliac origin it is covered by a glistening aponeurosis. Traced inward and downward along the abdominal surface of the inguinal ligament, the muscular origin is found to become much thinner, and also becomes loosely attached to the ligament. About four or five inches (ca. 10 to 12 cm.) from the linea alba the muscle separates from the ligament and forms the anterior wall of the inguinal canal. The abdominal orifice of the canal, the **internal inguinal ring**[1] (Annulus inguinalis abdominalis), is found here. It is normally a narrow slit, bounded in front by the edge of the internal oblique, and behind by the inguinal ligament. The **aponeurosis** is to a great extent blended with that of the external oblique, being, indeed, considerably interwoven with it ventrally. Where it covers the rectus abdominis it is attached to the tendinous inscriptions of that muscle.

Relations.—Superficially, the external oblique; deeply, the rectus abdominis, transversus abdominis, and the peritoneum.

Blood-supply.—Circumflex iliac, lumbar, and intercostal arteries.

Nerve-supply.—Ventral branches of the lumbar nerves.

3. **Rectus Abdominis.**—This muscle is confined to the ventral part of the abdominal wall; it extends from the lower part of the chest-wall to the pubis.

Origin.—The cartilages of the fifth to the ninth ribs inclusive, and the adjacent surface of the sternum.

Insertion.—The pubis, by means of the prepubic tendon.

Action.—Similar to that of the oblique muscles. It is specially adapted to flex the lumbo-sacral joints and the lumbar and thoracic parts of the spine.

Structure.—The fibers of the muscle are directed longitudinally. Nine to eleven transverse bands of fibrous tissue extend in an irregular manner across the muscle. These are termed **inscriptiones tendineæ.** They strengthen the muscle and serve to prevent separation of its fibers. The width of the muscle is greatest about its middle.

Relations.—Superficially, the aponeuroses of the oblique muscles (which constitute the external rectus sheath), and the posterior deep pectoral; deeply, the transversus, intercostals, the cartilages of the ribs, and the sternum. The posterior abdominal artery runs along the outer edge of the muscle posteriorly, and the anterior abdominal artery on or in its anterior part.

Blood-supply.—Anterior and posterior abdominal arteries.

Nerve-supply.—Intercostal and lumbar nerves.

4. **Transversus abdominis.**—This muscle, named from the general direction of its fibers, is a triangular curved sheet. Its lateral part is muscular, its ventral aponeurotic.

Origin.—(1) The inner surfaces of the distal ends or the cartilages of the asternal ribs, meeting the costal attachment of the diaphragm; (2) the transverse processes of the lumbar vertebræ, by means of the deep layer of the lumbo-dorsal fascia.

Insertion.—The xiphoid cartilage and the linea alba.

[1] It must be admitted that the term "ring" is rather misleading as applied to the abdominal opening of the canal, since normally it is a mere dilatable slit. The ring-like constriction which exists here in the male is constituted by the peritoneum, which descends into the canal to form the tunica vaginalis. This peritoneal ring is termed the **vaginal ring** (Annulus vaginalis), and must not be confused with the subperitoneal ring, *i. e.*, the internal inguinal ring.

Action.—Similar to that of the oblique muscles.

Structure.—The **muscular part** is a sheet of parallel bundles of fibers, directed downward and inward. It is thickest over the cartilages of the ribs, and from here it thins out greatly toward the aponeurosis and the lumbar region. The fibers of the **aponeurosis** directly continue those of the fleshy part. Posteriorly it becomes extremely thin and blends with the aponeuroses of the oblique muscles. It covers the deep face of the rectus, so forming the internal rectus sheath.

Relations.—Superficially, the oblique and straight muscles, the retractor costæ, the cartilages of the asternal ribs, and the internal intercostal muscles; deeply, the transversalis fascia and the peritoneum. The **transversalis fascia** is little developed in the horse, and is very thin in emaciated subjects, but in animals in good condition it contains a good deal of fat. It blends with the iliac fascia and descends into the inguinal canal. The asternal artery runs along the interval between the origin of the transversus and the costal part of the diaphragm. The intercostal nerves pass down over the external surface of the muscle, to which they give branches. Branches of the first three lumbar nerves are similarly disposed further back.

Blood-supply.—Intercostal, lumbar, and asternal arteries.

Nerve-supply.—Intercostal and lumbar nerves.

5. **Cremaster externus.**—This small muscle may be regarded as a detached portion of the internal oblique, with which it blends at its origin (Figs. 272, 450).

Origin.—The iliac fascia, near the origin of the sartorius.

Insertion.—The tunica vaginalis communis.

Action.—To raise the tunica vaginalis, and with it the testicle.

Structure.—The muscle arises by a thin aponeurosis which is succeeded by a flat muscular belly about one and a half to two inches (ca. 4 to 5 cm.) in width.[1] It passes down the inguinal canal on the postero-external surface of the tunica vaginalis, to which it is rather loosely attached. On reaching the point where the tunic is reflected on to the tail of the epididymis, the muscle is firmly attached to the outer surface of the tunic by short tendinous fibers.

Relations.—The muscle lies between the peritoneum and the fascia transversalis in front and the iliac fascia and inguinal ligament behind. On reaching the internal ring it descends the inguinal canal on the postero-external surface of the tunica vaginalis communis.

Blood-supply.—External spermatic or cremasteric artery.

Nerve-supply.—External spermatic nerve.

The Inguinal Canal.—This term (Canalis inguinalis) is applied to an oblique passage through the posterior part of the abdominal wall.[2] It begins at the internal inguinal or abdominal ring, and extends obliquely downward, inward, and somewhat forward, to end at the external inguinal or subcutaneous ring. Its anterior wall is formed by the fleshy posterior part of the internal oblique muscle, and the posterior wall by the strong tendinous inguinal (Poupart's) ligament. The average length of the canal, measured along the spermatic cord, is about four inches (ca. 10 cm.). The **internal inguinal ring** (Annulus inguinalis abdominalis) is bounded in front by the thin margin of the internal oblique muscle, and behind by the inguinal ligament. It is directed approximately from the edge of the prepubic tendon toward the external angle of the ilium. Its length is about four or five inches (ca. 10 to 12 cm.). The edge of the muscle is attached to the

[1] As might be expected, the cremaster usually undergoes more or less atrophy, and is paler in the castrated subject. In the mare the muscle is small, and ends in the connective tissue in the lower part of the inguinal canal.

[2] The term canal is somewhat misleading; it is rather a slit-like passage or space between the two oblique muscles, since the inguinal ligament is that part of the aponeurosis of the external oblique muscle which stretches between the external angle of the ilium and the prepubic tendon.

surface of the ligament here by delicate connective tissue, except where structures intervene between the walls of the canal. Consequently the limits of the ring are not very clearly defined. The **external inguinal ring** (Annulus inguinalis subcutaneus) is a well defined slit in the aponeurosis of the external oblique muscle, situated lateral to the prepubic tendon. Its long axis is directed from the edge of the prepubic tendon outward and forward, and its average length is about four inches (ca. 10 cm.). The canal contains in the male the spermatic cord, the tunica vaginalis, the external cremaster muscle, the external pudic artery and a small satellite vein, and the inguinal lymph-vessels and nerves. In the female it contains the mammary vessels and nerves; in the bitch it also lodges the round ligament of the uterus, inclosed in a tubular process of peritoneum.

The two rings do not correspond in direction, so that the length of the canal varies greatly when measured at different points. The inner angle of the internal ring lies almost immediately above that of the external ring, but the outer angle is situated five to six inches (ca. 12 to 15 cm.) from that of the external ring. The inner angles of the external rings are well defined and distinctly palpable in the living subject; they are about three to four inches (ca. 8 to 10 cm.) apart.

The Prepubic Tendon.—The **prepubic tendon** is essentially the tendon of insertion of the two recti abdominis, but also furnishes attachment to the obliqui, the graciles, and the pectinei. It is attached to the anterior borders of the pubic bones, including the ilio-pectineal eminences. It has the form of a very strong thick band, with concave lateral borders which form the inner boundaries of the external inguinal rings. Its direction is oblique upward and backward.[1] Its structure is somewhat complex. Most of the fibers of the posterior part extend from one ilio-pectineal eminence to the other. The fibers which belong to the recti curve in to the median line. The aponeuroses of the internal oblique muscles are inserted into its abdominal surface, and the inguinal ligaments are attached to and continue across it in arciform fashion. The anterior part of the tendon of origin of the gracilis is fused with it ventrally, and many of the fibers of the pectineus arise from it. It gives off on either side a strong round band, the so-called **pubo-femoral** or **accessory ligament,** which is inserted into the fossa of the head of the femur with the round ligament (*vide* hip joint).

MUSCLES OF THE THORACIC LIMB

I. THE MUSCLES OF THE SHOULDER GIRDLE (Figs. 177, 178, 179, 186)

This group consists of those muscles which connect the thoracic limb with the head, neck, and trunk. The group naturally falls into two divisions—dorsal and ventral.[2]

A. DORSAL DIVISION

This division consists of two layers which overlie the proper muscles of the neck and back.

FIRST LAYER

1. **Trapezius.**—This is a flat, triangular muscle, the base of the triangle corresponding with the spine. It is divided by an aponeurotic portion into two divisions:

(a) **Trapezius cervicalis.**—*Origin.*—The funicular portion of the ligamentum nuchæ, from the second cervical to the third thoracic vertebra.

Insertion.—The spine of the scapula and the fascia of the shoulder and arm.

[1] The obliquity of the tendon and the angle which it forms with the pelvic floor are of clinical importance in regard to manipulation of the fœtus in obstetrical cases. The slope varies in different subjects. In some cases the tendon forms about a right angle with the pubic bones.

[2] The terms dorsal and ventral are here used in the topographic and not in the morphological sense. All the muscles of the group are ventral in the latter sense.

(b) **Trapezius thoracalis s. dorsalis.**—*Origin.*—The supraspinous ligament, from the third to the tenth thoracic vertebra.

Insertion.—The tubercle of the spine of the scapula.

Action.—Acting as a whole, to elevate the shoulder; the cervical portion draws the scapula forward and upward and the thoracic portion draws it backward and upward.

Structure.—The muscle arises by a short, thin aponeurosis, from which the fibers of the flat fleshy portion converge to the spine of the scapula and the aponeurosis which separates the two portions. The cervical fascia joins the ventral edge of the cervical portion to the mastoido-humeralis, or the two muscles may unite here.

Relations.—Superficially, the skin and fascia; deeply, the rhomboideus, latissimus dorsi, supraspinatus, infraspinatus, deltoid, splenius, serratus magnus, and anterior deep pectoral muscles, and the cartilage of the scapula.

Blood-supply.—Deep cervical and intercostal arteries.

Nerve-supply.—Spinal accessory nerve.

Second Layer

This consists of two muscles—the rhomboideus and the latissimus dorsi.

2. **Rhomboideus.**—This consists of two portions:

(a) **Rhomboideus cervicalis s. cervicis.**—*Origin.*—The funicular portion of the ligamentum nuchæ, from the second cervical to the second thoracic vertebra.

Insertion.—The internal surface of the cartilage of the scapula.

(b) **Rhomboideus thoracalis s. dorsalis.**—*Origin.*—The spinous processes of the second to the seventh thoracic vertebra by means of the dorso-scapular ligament.

Insertion.—The inner surface of the cartilage of the scapula.

Action.—To draw the scapula upward and forward. When the limb is fixed the cervical portion will elevate the neck.

Structure.—The cervical portion is narrow, pointed at its anterior extremity, and lies along the funicular part of the ligamentum nuchæ, to which it is attached by short tendon bundles. The fibers are directed for the most part longitudinally. The thoracic portion is quadrilateral in shape, and its fibers are nearly vertical. Its deep face is intimately attached to the dorso-scapular ligament.

Relations.—Superficially, the skin and fascia (over a small area), the trapezius, and the cartilage of the scapula; deeply, the dorso-scapular ligament, the splenius, complexus, longissimus dorsi, and serratus anticus.

Blood-supply.—Dorsal and superior cervical arteries.

Nerve-supply.—Sixth cervical nerve.

3. **Latissimus Dorsi.**—This is a wide muscle which has the form of a right-angled triangle. It lies for the most part under the skin and panniculus, on the lateral wall of the thorax, from the spine to the arm.

Origin.—The lumbo-dorsal fascia—and by this means from the lumbar and thoracic spines as far forward as the highest point of the withers.

Insertion.—The internal tubercle of the humerus, in common with the teres major.

Action.—To draw the humerus upward and backward and flex the shoulder-joint. If the limb is advanced and fixed, it draws the trunk forward.

Structure.—The muscle arises by a wide aponeurosis, which fuses with that of the serratus posticus and with the lumbo-dorsal fascia. The muscular portion is at first rather thin, but by the convergence of its fibers becomes thicker as it approaches the arm. The anterior fibers pass almost vertically downward over the dorsal angle of the scapula and its cartilage. The posterior fibers are directed downward and forward. The thick belly formed by the convergence of these passes under the triceps to end on the flat tendon of insertion, which is common to this muscle and the teres major.

Blood-supply.—Subscapular, intercostal, and lumbar arteries.

Nerve-supply.—Brachial plexus (eighth cervical and dorsal roots).

B. Ventral Division

1. Mastoido-humeralis (M. brachiocephalicus; levator humeri).—This muscle extends along the side of the neck from the head to the arm. It is incompletely divisible into two portions.

Origin.—(1) The mastoid process of the petrous temporal bone and the occipital crest; (2) the wing of the atlas and the transverse processes of the second, third, and fourth cervical vertebræ.

Insertion.—The deltoid tuberosity and the curved rough line which extends from this to the distal extremity of the humerus.

Action.—When the head and neck are fixed, to draw the limb forward, extending the shoulder joint. When the limb is fixed, to extend the head and neck, if the muscles act together; acting separately, to incline the head and neck to the same side.

Structure.—As already mentioned, the muscle is capable of incomplete division into two parts, the line of division being indicated by the emergence of superficial branches of the ventral divisions of the cervical nerves. The mastoid portion (M. cleido-mastoideus) partly overlaps the other portion (M. cleido-transversarius), which lies dorsal to it. The former is attached to the mastoid process and the occipital bone by a broad tendon which fuses with that of the splenius and trachelo-mastoideus; it is also attached to the tendon of insertion of the sterno-cephalicus by aponeurosis. The dorsal portion is attached to the transverse processes by four fleshy digitations. The belly of the muscle is adherent superficially to the cervical fascia and the panniculus, and deeply to the subscapulo-hyoideus. In front of the shoulder its deep face is marked by a tendinous intersection of variable development.[1] Here the muscle becomes wider, covers the shoulder joint, passes between the brachialis and biceps, and is inserted by means of a wide tendon which it shares with the superficial pectoral muscle.

Relations.—Superficially, the skin, cervical fascia, the parotid gland, the panniculus, brachialis, and branches of the cervical nerves; deeply, the splenius, trachelo-mastoideus, rectus capitis anterior major, omo-hyoideus, serratus magnus, anterior deep pectoral and biceps muscles, the inferior cervical artery, the prescapular lymph-glands, and branches of the cervical nerves. The ventral edge of the muscle forms the dorsal boundary of the jugular furrow. The dorsal border may be in contact with the cervical trapezius, or separated from it by a variable interval.

Blood-supply.—Inferior cervical, carotid, and vertebral arteries.

Nerve-supply.—Spinal accessory and cervical nerves.

The **pectoral fascia** is a thin membrane covering the surface of the pectoral muscles, to which it is, for the most part, pretty intimately attached. It detaches a layer which passes between the superficial and deep pectorals. At the posterior edge of the triceps another layer is given off, which passes on the outer surface of this muscle to blend with the scapular fascia; the deeper layer becomes continuous with the subscapular and cervical fasciæ.

The **pectoral muscles** form a large fleshy mass which occupies the space

[1] This is regarded as a vestige of the clavicle. On this basis the portion of the muscle from the vestige to the arm represents the clavicular part of the deltoid of man.

between the ventral part of the chest-wall and the shoulder and arm. They are clearly divisible into a superficial and a deep layer. The superficial layer may be subdivided into two portions by careful dissection; the deep layer is clearly made up of two muscles.

2. **Superficial pectoral** (M. pectoralis superficialis).

(a) **Anterior superficial pectoral** (portio clavicularis s. descendens; pectoralis anticus).—This is a short, thick, somewhat rounded muscle, which extends between the anterior part of the sternum and the front of the arm. It forms a distinct prominence on the front of the breast, which is easily recognized in the living animal.

Origin.—The cariniform cartilage of the sternum.

Insertion.—(1) The curved line of the humerus with the mastoido-humeralis; (2) the fascia of the arm.

Action.—To adduct and advance the limb.

Structure.—The belly of the muscle is convex on its superficial face, but deeply it is flattened where it overlaps the posterior superficial pectoral. Here the two muscles are usually pretty intimately attached to each other, and care must be exercised in making the separation. The tendon of insertion blends with that of the mastoido-humeralis and with the fascia of the arm. At the middle line of the breast a furrow occurs between the two muscles; laterally, another furrow, containing the cephalic vein, lies between the muscle and the mastoido-humeralis.

Relations.—Superficially, the skin, fascia, and panniculus; deeply, the posterior division, the deep pectoral, and the biceps. The cephalic vein lies in the groove between this muscle and the mastoido-humeralis.

(b) **Posterior superficial pectoral** (portio sternocostalis; pectoralis transversus).—This is a wide muscular sheet which extends from the ventral edge of the sternum to the fascia on the inner surface of the forearm.

Origin.—(1) The ventral edge of the sternum as far back as the sixth cartilage; (2) a fibrous raphé common to the two muscles.

Insertion.—(1) The fascia on the proximal third of the forearm; (2) the curved line of the humerus with the preceding muscle.

Action.—To adduct the limb and to tense the fascia of the forearm.

Structure.—It is thin and pale, and mixed with a good deal of fibrous tissue. The right and left muscles fuse at a median fibrous raphé. The tendon of insertion unites with the fascia on the inner side of the forearm for the most part; only a small part in front, about an inch in width, is attached to the humerus.

Relations.—Superficially, the skin, fascia, and the preceding muscle; deeply, the deep pectoral, the biceps, and the brachialis; at the elbow, the posterior radial vessels, the median nerve, and the inner and middle flexors of the carpus.

3. **Deep pectoral** (M. pectoralis profundus).—This muscle is much thicker and more extensive in the horse than the superficial pectoral. It consists of two distinct portions.

(a) **Anterior deep pectoral** (portio prescapularis; pectoralis parvus).—This division is prismatic and extends from the anterior part of the lateral surface of the sternum to the cervical angle of the scapula.

Origin.—The anterior half of the lateral surface of the sternum and the cartilages of the first four ribs.

Insertion.—The aponeurosis which covers the supraspinatus at its dorsal end, and the scapular fascia.

Action.—To adduct and retract the limb; when the limb is advanced and fixed, to draw the trunk forward.

Structure.—The muscle is almost entirely fleshy. It describes a curve (convex anteriorly), passing at first forward, then upward over the front of the shoulder, a little to its inner side, and finally upward and backward along the anterior border of the supraspinatus. It is loosely attached to the latter muscle, and terminates in a pointed end which becomes more firmly attached near the cervical angle of the scapula.

Relations.—Superficially, the skin and fascia, the panniculus, superficial pectoral, trapezius, and mastoido-humeralis muscles, the cephalic vein, and the inferior cervical artery; deeply, the posterior deep pectoral, biceps, supraspinatus, omo-hyoideus, and serratus magnus muscles, the brachial vessels, and the branches of the brachial plexus of nerves.

(b) **Posterior deep pectoral** (portio humeralis s. ascendens; pectoralis magnus).—This is much the largest of the pectoral group in the horse. It is somewhat triangular or fan-shaped.

Origin.—(1) The abdominal tunic; (2) the xiphoid cartilage and ventral aspect of the sternum; (3) the cartilages of the fourth to the ninth ribs.

Insertion.—(1) The internal tuberosity of the humerus; (2) the external lip of the bicipital groove; (3) the tendon of origin of the coraco-brachialis.

Action.—To adduct and retract the limb; if the limb is advanced and fixed, to draw the trunk forward.

Structure.—This muscle is also almost entirely fleshy. Its posterior part is wide and thin, but as the muscle is traced forward, it becomes narrower and much thicker. It passes forward and slightly upward in a gentle curve to its insertion. The humeral insertion is just below that of the inner division of the supraspinatus. Part of the fibers are inserted by means of a tendinous band which binds down the tendon of the biceps and is attached to the external lip of the bicipital groove, and a small part is attached to the tendon of origin of the coraco-brachialis.

Relations.—Superficially, the skin, panniculus, and superficial pectoral; deeply, the abdominal tunic, the external oblique, the rectus abdominis et thoracis, the brachial vessels, and branches of the brachial plexus of nerves. The external thoracic vein lies along the outer or upper border.

Blood-supply.—Internal and external thoracic, inferior cervical, anterior circumflex, and intercostal arteries.

Nerve-supply.—Pectoral (or thoracic) nerves, from the brachial plexus.

4. **Serratus magnus** (M. serratus ventralis).—This is a large, fan-shaped muscle, situated on the lateral surface of the neck and thorax. It derives its name from the serrated ventral edge of its thoracic portion. It consists of a cervical and a thoracic portion.

(a) **Cervical part** (M. serratus cervicis; levator scapulæ hominis).

Origin.—The transverse processes of the last four or five cervical vertebræ.

Insertion.—The anterior triangular area on the costal surface of the scapula and the adjacent part of the cartilage.

(b) **Thoracic part** (M. serratus thoracis; serratus anterior hominis).

Origin.—The external surfaces of the first eight or nine ribs.

Insertion.—The posterior triangular area on the costal surface of the scapula and the adjacent part of the cartilage.

Action.—The two muscles form a sort of sling in which the trunk is suspended. Contracting together, they raise the thorax; contracting singly, the weight is shifted to the limb on the side of the muscle acting. The two parts can contract separately and are antagonistic in their action on the scapula. The cervical part draws the base of the scapula toward the neck, while the thoracic part has the opposite action; these effects concur in the backward and forward swing of the limb respectively. With the limb fixed, the cervical part extends (raises) the neck or inclines it laterally. The thoracic part may act as a muscle of forced inspiration.

Structure.—In the domesticated animals there is no such clear division of the muscle as is found in man and the apes. On account of the difference in action, however, it seems desirable to distinguish the two portions. The cervical part is thick and almost entirely fleshy. The thoracic part has on its superficial face a thick, tendinous layer which may sustain the weight of the trunk when the muscle substance relaxes. The ventral edge presents distinct digitations, the last four of which alternate with those of the obliquus externus abdominis, and are covered by the abdominal tunic. The fourth, fifth, and sixth digitations extend nearly to the distal ends of the ribs. The last digitation is small and may be absent. Exceptionally additional digitations may be attached to the tenth or eleventh rib or to the fascia over the intercostal muscles. The fibers converge to the insertion, which is thick and is intersected by elastic lamellæ derived from the dorso-scapular ligament.

Relations.—Superficially, the mastoido-humeralis, trapezius, deep pectoral, subscapularis, teres major, latissimus dorsi, panniculus carnosus, the abdominal tunic, the brachial vessels, and the long thoracic nerve; deeply, the splenius, complexus, longissimus, transversalis costarum, the ribs and external intercostal muscles, and branches of the superior cervical and dorsal arteries.

Blood-supply.—Superior cervical, dorsal, vertebral, and intercostal arteries.

Nerve-supply.—Brachial plexus.

II. THE MUSCLES OF THE SHOULDER

Under this head will be described those muscles which arise on the scapula and end on the arm; they may be divided into two groups—one covering the dorsum, the other the venter of the scapula.

The **superficial fascia** of the shoulder and arm contains the panniculus carnosus of this region, and may be considered to be continued on the inner side of the limb by the subscapular fascia.

The **thoracic** or **scapulo-humeral portion** of the **panniculus** (M. cutaneus scapulæ et humeri) arises by a thin aponeurosis from the ligamentum nuchæ at the withers. The fleshy portion begins over the upper part of the scapula and extends to the elbow. Its fibers have in general a dorso-ventral direction. It is continuous behind with the abdominal portion.

The **deep fascia** of the shoulder and arm (Fascia omobrachialis) is much more developed and important. It is strong and tendinous, and is intimately adherent to the muscles on the outer surface of the scapula, between which it detaches **intermuscular septa,** which are attached to the spine and borders of the scapula. The brachial portion is, for the most part, only loosely attached to the underlying muscles, for which it forms sheaths; it is attached to the humerus, especially to the lips of the bicipital groove and the deltoid tuberosity. It blends distally with the tendon of insertion of the biceps, and is continued by the antibrachial fascia.

A. External Group (Figs. 178, 179)

1. **Deltoid** (M. deltoideus; long abductor of the arm; scapular portion of the deltoid of man).—This lies partly on the triceps in the angle between the scapula and humerus, partly on the infraspinatus and teres minor.

Origin.—(1) The upper part of the posterior border of the scapula; (2) the spine of the scapula, by means of the strong aponeurosis which covers the infraspinatus.

Insertion.—The deltoid tuberosity of the humerus.

Action.—To flex the shoulder joint and abduct the arm.

Structure.—The origin of the muscle is partly aponeurotic, partly fleshy. The aponeurosis fuses with that of the infraspinatus; the posterior part is attached to the scapula immediately in front of the origin of the long head of the triceps. The belly of the muscle lies for the most part in a cavity formed in the triceps. It is widest about its middle.

Relations.—Superficially, the skin, fascia, panniculus, and mastoido-humeralis; deeply, the infraspinatus, teres minor, triceps, and brachialis muscles, and branches of the posterior circumflex artery and axillary nerve.

Blood-supply.—Subscapular artery (chiefly through the posterior circumflex).

Nerve-supply.—Suprascapular and axillary nerves.

2. **Supraspinatus.**—This muscle occupies the supraspinous fossa, which it fills, and beyond which it extends, thus coming in contact with the subscapularis.

Origin.—The supraspinous fossa, the spine, and the lower part of the cartilage of the scapula.

Insertion.—The inner and outer lips of the bicipital groove.

Action.—To extend the shoulder joint. It also assists in preventing dislocation.

Structure.—The surface of the muscle is covered by a strong aponeurosis, from the deep face of which many fibers arise. The muscle is thin at its origin from the cartilage, but becomes considerably thicker below. At the neck of the scapula it divides into two branches, between which the tendon of origin of the biceps emerges. These branches, fleshy superficially, tendinous deeply, are inserted into the lips of the bicipital groove. They are united by a fibrous membrane already mentioned in connection with the deep pectoral muscle; some fibers are attached to this membrane and the capsule of the shoulder joint.

Relations.—Superficially, the skin, fascia, panniculus, trapezius, and mastoido-humeralis; deeply, the scapula and its cartilage, the subscapularis muscle, and the suprascapular vessels and nerve; in front, the anterior deep pectoral muscle; behind, the spine of the scapula and infraspinatus muscle.

Blood-supply.—Suprascapular and posterior circumflex arteries.

Nerve-supply.—Suprascapular nerve.

3. **Infraspinatus.**—This muscle occupies the greater part of the infraspinous fossa.

Origin.—The infraspinous fossa and the scapular cartilage.

Insertion.—(1) The outer tuberosity of the humerus, distal to the outer insertion of the supraspinatus; (2) the posterior eminence of the outer tuberosity.

Action.—To abduct the arm and rotate it outward.[1] It also plays the part of a lateral ligament.

Structure.—This muscle is also covered by a strong aponeurosis, from which many fibers arise, and by means of which the deltoid is attached to the spine of the scapula. A thick tendinous layer partially divides the muscle into two strata, and, coming to the surface at the shoulder joint, constitutes the chief means of insertion. This tendon, an inch or more (3 cm.) in width, passes over the posterior eminence of the external tuberosity of the humerus; it is bound down by a fibrous sheet, and a synovial bursa is interposed between the tendon and the bone. When the long insertion is cut and reflected, the short insertion, partly tendinous, partly fleshy, is exposed.

Relations.—Superficially, the skin, fascia, panniculus, trapezius, and deltoid; deeply, the scapula and its cartilage, the shoulder joint and capsule, the long head of the triceps, the teres minor, and the nutrient artery of the scapula.

Blood-supply.—Subscapular artery.

Nerve-supply.—Suprascapular and axillary nerves.

4. **Teres minor.**—This is a much smaller muscle than the foregoing. It lies chiefly on the triceps, under cover of the deltoid and infraspinatus.

Origin.—(1) The rough lines on the distal and posterior part of the infra-

[1] Günther states that this muscle assists in extension or flexion according to the position of the head of the humerus relative to the glenoid cavity.

spinous fossa; (2) a small part of the posterior border of the scapula, about its middle; (3) a tubercle near the rim of the glenoid artery.

Insertion.—The deltoid tuberosity and a small area just above it.

Action.—To flex the shoulder joint and to abduct the arm; also to assist in outward rotation.

Structure.—The muscle is not rounded in the horse and ox, but flat and triangular. Its origin from the posterior border of the scapula is by means of an aponeurosis which also gives origin to fibers of the infraspinatus and triceps. A **bursa** is commonly found between the terminal part of the muscle and the capsule of the shoulder joint, and is often continuous with that of the infraspinatus.

Relations. — Superficially, the deltoid and infraspinatus muscles; deeply, the scapula, the shoulder joint, and the triceps muscle.

Blood-supply. — Subscapular artery (circumflex branches).

Nerve-supply. — Axillary nerve.

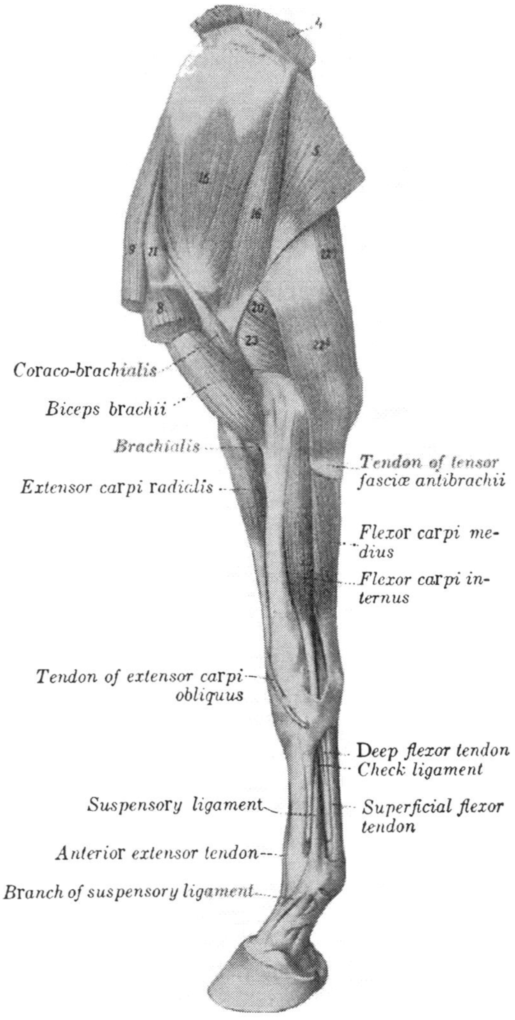

FIG. 187.—MUSCLES OF THORACIC LIMB OF HORSE, INTERNAL VIEW.
3, 4, Rhomboideus; 5, latissimus dorsi; 8, posterior deep pectoral; 9, anterior deep pectoral; 11, supraspinatus; 15, subscapularis; 16, teres major; 20, long head of triceps; 22a, 22b, tensor fasciæ antibrachii; 23, internal head of triceps. (After Ellenberger, in Leisering's Atlas.)

B. INTERNAL GROUP

1. Subscapularis.—This muscle occupies the subscapular fossa, beyond which, however, it extends both before and behind.

Origin.—The subscapular fossa.

Insertion.—The posterior eminence of the internal tuberosity of the humerus.

Action.—To adduct the humerus.

Structure.—The muscle is flat and triangular, with the base upward. The latter is thin and interdigitates with the scapular attachments of the serratus. Below this the belly thickens and becomes narrower. It is covered by an aponeurosis, and contains a considerable amount of tendinous tissue. The tendon of insertion is crossed by the tendon of origin of the coracobrachialis; it is intimately adherent to the capsule of the shoulder joint, and may be regarded as replacing the internal ligament of the latter. A small bursa may occur here.

Relations.—Superficially, the scapula and shoulder joint, the supraspinatus, triceps, and teres major muscles; deeply, the serratus magnus muscle, the brachial vessels, and the chief branches of the brachial plexus. The subscapular vessels run along or near the posterior edge of the muscle.

Blood-supply.—Subscapular artery.

Nerve-supply.—Subscapular nerves (from the brachial plexus).

2. **Teres major** (Teres internus; adductor of the arm).—This muscle is flat, widest about its middle, and lies chiefly on the deep face of the triceps.

Origin.—The dorsal angle and the adjacent part of the posterior border of the scapula.

Insertion.—The tubercle on the inner surface of the shaft of the humerus, in common with the latissimus dorsi.

Action.—To flex the shoulder joint and adduct the arm.

Structure.—It is for the most part fleshy, but the origin consists of an aponeurosis which blends with that of the tensor fasciæ antibrachii. The insertion is by a flat tendon which fuses with that of the latissimus dorsi.

Relations.—Superficially, the triceps, infraspinatus, and deltoid muscles; deeply, the serratus magnus muscle. The subscapular vessels lie in a groove between the anterior edge of this muscle and the posterior border of the subscapularis; near the shoulder joint the posterior circumflex artery and the axillary nerve emerge between the two muscles. The deep face of the muscle is crossed by the thoracic branches of the brachial plexus, and by the branch of the subscapular artery which supplies the latissimus dorsi.

Blood-supply.—Subscapular artery.

Nerve-supply.—Axillary nerve.

3. **Coraco-brachialis** (Coraco-humeralis).—This muscle lies on the inner surface of the shoulder joint and the arm.

Origin.—The coracoid process of the scapula.

Insertion.—(1) A small area above the internal tubercle of the humerus; (2) the middle third of the anterior surface of the humerus.

Action.—To adduct the arm and to flex the shoulder joint.

Structure.—The long tendon of origin emerges between the subscapularis and the inner branch of the supraspinatus. It passes over the terminal part of the subscapularis and is provided with a synovial sheath. The muscular part spreads out and divides into two portions. The smaller and shorter portion is inserted into the proximal third of the shaft of the humerus, close to the origin of the lateral head of the triceps; the larger and longer portion is inserted into the middle third of the humerus, in front of the internal tubercle and the inner head of the triceps.

Relations.—Externally, the subscapularis muscle and the humerus; internally, the deep pectoral and brachialis muscles. The anterior circumflex artery and the nerve to the biceps usually emerge between the two insertions, and the brachial vessels lie along the posterior border of the muscle.

Blood-supply.—Anterior circumflex artery.

Nerve-supply.—Musculo-cutaneous nerve.

4. **Capsularis** (Scapulo-humeralis posticus s. gracilis).—This is a very small muscle, which lies on the back of the capsule of the shoulder joint.

Origin.—The scapula, close to the rim of the glenoid cavity

Insertion.—The posterior surface of the shaft of the humerus, a short distance below the head.

Action.—It may perhaps tense the capsule of the shoulder joint and prevent its being pinched during flexion.

Structure.—It is fleshy and usually about the breadth of a finger. It may, however, consist of only a few bundles of fibers; sometimes it is double. Its attachment to the joint capsule is slight. It passes through the brachialis muscle to reach its insertion.

Relations.—Superficially, the teres minor and triceps muscles; deeply, the teres major and subscapularis muscles, and the capsule of the joint.

Blood-supply.—Posterior circumflex artery.

Nerve-supply.—Axillary nerve.

III. THE MUSCLES OF THE ARM

This group consists of five muscles which are grouped around the humerus. They arise from the scapula and the humerus, and are inserted into the forearm. They act on the elbow joint and the fascia of the forearm.

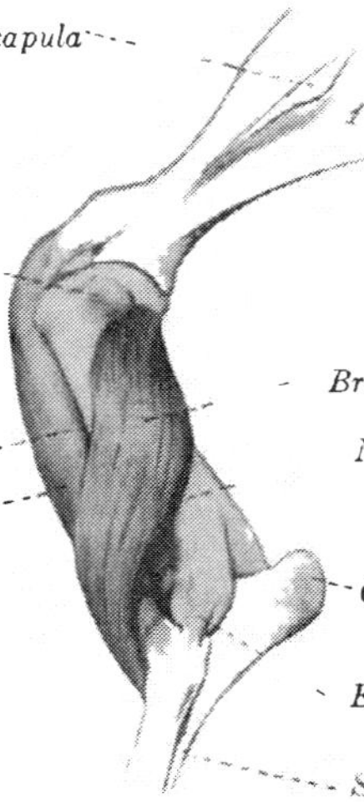

FIG. 188.—BICEPS AND BRACHIALIS MUSCLES OF HORSE. (After Ellenberger-Baum, Anat. für Künstler.)

1. **Biceps brachii** (Coraco-radialis; flexor brachii).—This is a strong, somewhat rounded muscle, which lies on the anterior surface of the humerus.

Origin.—The tuberosity of the scapula.

Insertion.—(1) The bicipital tuberosity of the radius; (2) the internal lateral ligament of the elbow joint; (3) the fascia of the forearm and the tendon of the extensor carpi radialis.

Action.—To flex the elbow joint, to fix the shoulder, elbow, and carpus in standing, and to tense the fascia of the forearm.

Structure.—The muscle is inclosed in a double sheath of fascia, which is attached to the lips of the bicipital groove and the deltoid ridge of the humerus. The tendon of origin is moulded on the bicipital groove; it is very strong and dense and is partly cartilaginous. Its play over the groove is facilitated by the large **bicipital bursa** (Bursa intertubercularis). The synovial membrane covers not only the deep face of the tendon, but extends somewhat over the edges to the superficial face. A well-marked tendinous intersection runs through the belly of the muscle and divides distally into two portions. Of these, the short, thick one is inserted into the bicipital tuberosity and detaches fibers to the internal lateral ligament. The long tendon (Lacertus fibrosus) is thinner, blends with the fascia of the forearm, and ends by fusing with the tendon of the extensor carpi radialis.

Relations.—Externally, the mastoido-humeralis and brachialis muscles; internally, the posterior deep pectoral and the superficial pectoral muscles; in front, the anterior deep pectoral muscle; behind, the humerus, the coraco-brachialis muscle, the anterior circumflex and anterior radial vessels, and the musculo-cutaneous nerve.

Blood-supply.—Branches of the brachial and anterior radial arteries.

Nerve-supply.—Musculo-cutaneous nerve.

2. **Brachialis** (Humeralis obliquus s. externus; brachialis anticus).—This muscle occupies the musculo-spiral groove of the humerus.

Origin.—The proximal third of the posterior surface of the humerus.

Insertion.—The inner surface of the neck of the radius (under cover of the lateral ligament) and the arciform ligament.

Action.—To flex the elbow joint.

Structure.—The peculiar spiral course of this muscle gave rise to the name often applied to it—humeralis obliquus. Beginning on the posterior surface of the shaft, close to the head of the humerus, it winds over the lateral surface, crosses the biceps very obliquely, and finally reaches the inner side of the forearm by passing between the biceps and the extensor carpi. It is entirely fleshy, with the exception of its relatively slender tendon of insertion.

Relations.—Externally the skin and fascia, the teres minor, deltoid, triceps (lateral head), biceps, and mastoido-humeralis muscles. The anterior radial artery crosses the deep face of the muscle in its distal third, and the radial nerve accompanies the muscle in the distal half of the musculo-spiral groove.

Blood-supply.—Brachial artery.

Nerve-supply.—Radial nerve.

3. **Tensor fasciæ antibrachii** (Fig. 187)[1] (Scapulo-ulnaris; long extensor of the forearm; accessory anconeus of the latissimus dorsi).—This is a thin muscle which lies on the inner surface of the triceps.

Origin.—The tendon of insertion of the latissimus dorsi and the posterior border of the scapula.

Insertion.—(1) The fascia of the forearm; (2) a small eminence on the posterior border of the olecranon.

Action.—(1) To tense the fascia of the forearm and to extend the elbow joint.

Structure.—The origin consists of a very thin aponeurosis which blends with those of the caput longum and the latissimus dorsi. The muscular portion is quite thin in its anterior part, somewhat thicker behind, and is narrower than the aponeurotic origin. It is succeeded by an aponeurotic insertion, which ends chiefly by blending with the fascia of the forearm a little below the elbow. There is, however, a small but constant tendinous attachment to the olecranon.

Relations.—Externally, the panniculus, triceps (long and internal heads), the inner and middle flexors of the carpus, and the ulnar vessels and nerve; internally, the latissimus dorsi, serratus magnus, and posterior pectoral muscles.

Blood-supply.—Subscapular, ulnar, and deep brachial arteries.

Nerve-supply.—Radial nerve.

4. **Triceps brachii** (Figs. 178, 179, 187) (Brachial triceps; triceps extensor cubiti).—This, together with the preceding muscle, constitutes the large muscular

[1] M'Fadyean and Vaughan term this muscle the scapulo-ulnaris, while Arloing and Lesbre term it "Ancone accessoire du grand dorsal." The above name seems to agree best with the chief insertion and action, although it certainly arises largely from the tendon of insertion of the latissimus dorsi.

mass which fills the angle between the posterior border of the scapula and the humerus. It is clearly divisible into three heads, as described below.

(a) **Long head** (Caput longum tricipitis; anconeus longus; caput magnum) —This, the largest and longest of the three heads, is a powerful, thick, triangular muscle, which extends from the posterior border of the scapula to the olecranon.

Origin.—The posterior border of the scapula.

Insertion.—The outer and posterior part of the summit of the olecranon.

Action.—(1) To extend the elbow joint; (2) to flex the shoulder joint.

Structure.—The muscle arises by a wide, strong aponeurosis from the posterior border of the scapula. From this the bundles of the fleshy portion converge to the short, strong tendon of insertion. A careful examination will show that the muscle is penetrated by a tendinous intersection from which many fibers take origin obliquely. The superficial face is covered by an aponeurosis which is specially developed at its distal part. A small bursa occurs under the tendon of insertion.

Relations.—Externally, the panniculus, deltoid, infraspinatus, teres minor, and the external head; internally, the tensor fasciæ antibrachii, teres major, latissimus dorsi, and posterior deep pectoral muscles, and the subscapular vessels; in front, the brachialis, and the inner head, the deep brachial and posterior circum flex vessels, and the axillary and radial nerves; behind, the skin and fascia.

Blood-supply.—Subscapular and deep brachial arteries.

Nerve-supply.—Radial nerve.

(b) **External head** (Caput laterale tricipitis s. anconeus lateralis s. externus; caput medium).—This is a strong, quadrilateral muscle, which lies on the outer surface of the arm. Its proximal third is covered by the deltoid and teres minor muscles; the remainder only by the thin panniculus and the skin.

Origin.—The deltoid tuberosity and the curved rough line which extends from it to the neck of the humerus.

Insertion.—(1) A small prominent area on the outer surface of the olecranon; (2) the tendon of the long head.

Action.—To extend the elbow joint.

Structure.—The origin consists of short tendinous fibers. The belly is thick, and is composed of parallel bundles which are directed obliquely downward and backward. They are inserted partly into the tendon of the long head and partly into the olecranon below and in front of that tendon.

Relations.—Externally, the deltoid, teres minor, and panniculus muscles; internally, the long and inner heads and the brachialis muscle. Branches of the circumflex vessels and axillary nerve emerge between the posterior edge of the muscle and the long head. The deep face of the muscle is related to the branches of the deep brachial artery and of the radial nerve.

Blood-supply.—Posterior circumflex and deep brachial arteries.

Nerve-supply.—Radial nerve.

(c) **Internal head** (Fig. 193) (Caput mediale tricipitis; anconeus medialis s. internus; caput parvum).—This is much the smallest of the three heads. It is situated on the inner surface of the arm, and extends from the middle third of the humerus to the olecranon.

Origin.—The middle third of the inner surface of the shaft of the humerus, behind and below the internal tubercle.

Insertion.—The inner and fore part of the summit of the olecranon, between the insertion of the long head and the origin of the ulnar head of the flexor perforans.

Action.—To extend the elbow joint.

Structure.—The muscle is fleshy except at its insertion, where it has a flat tendon, under which a small bursa may be found.

Relations.—Externally, the humerus, brachialis, anconeus, and the external head; internally, the posterior deep pectoral, coraco-brachialis, teres major, latissimus dorsi, and tensor fasciæ antibrachii muscles, the brachial and deep brachial vessels, and the median and ulnar nerves; behind, the long head, branches of the deep brachial vessels, and the radial nerve.

Blood-supply.—Deep brachial and ulnar arteries.

Nerve-supply.—Radial nerve.

5. **Anconeus** (M. anconeus parvus s. subanconeus).—This is a small fleshy muscle which covers the olecranon fossa and is covered by the triceps. It is somewhat difficult to separate from the outer head.

Origin.—The distal third of the posterior surface of the humerus.

Insertion.—The outer surface of the olecranon.

Action.—To extend the elbow joint, and to raise the capsule of the joint and prevent its being pinched during extension.

Structure.—It is almost entirely fleshy, and is adherent by its deep face to the joint capsule.

Relations. — Superficially, the triceps muscle; deeply, the humerus and the elbow joint.

Blood-supply. — Deep brachial artery.

Nerve-supply.—Radial nerve.

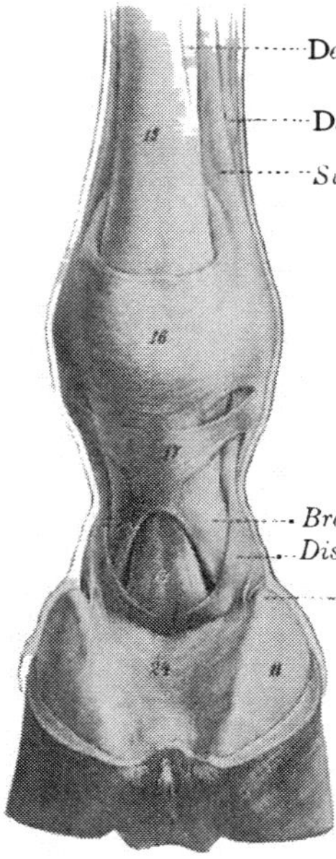

FIG. 189.—DIGIT OF HORSE, POSTERIOR VIEW.

14, Deep flexor tendon; *15*, superficial flexor tendon; *16*, posterior annular ligament of fetlock; *17*, proximal annular or vaginal ligament of digit; *11*, lateral cartilage; *24*, plantar cushion. (After Ellenberger-Baum, Anat. für Künstler.)

IV. FASCIÆ AND MUSCLES OF THE FOREARM AND MANUS

The forearm is covered on three sides by the muscles of this group, leaving the inner surface of the radius for the most part subcutaneous. The extensors of the carpus and digit lie on the anterior (dorsal) and external part of the region, while the flexors occupy the posterior (volar) surface.

The **fascia of the forearm** (Fascia antibrachii) forms a very strong and complete investment for all the muscles of the region. The **superficial fascia** is thin, and disappears at the carpus by fusing with the deep fascia. The **deep fascia** is very strong and tendinous in character. It furnishes insertion at its upper and inner part to the tensor fasciæ antibrachii and posterior superficial pectoral muscles; at its upper anterior and outer part, to aponeuroses from the mastoido-humeralis and biceps. It is attached at the elbow by its deep face to the outer tuberosities of the humerus and radius, to the ulna, and to the lateral ligaments. On the inner surface of the forearm it blends with the periosteum on the subcutaneous surface of the radius. It is closely adherent to the surface of the extensor muscles, but is rather loosely attached to the flexors. From its deep face are detached **intermuscular septa,** which form sheaths for the muscles and are attached to the underlying bones. The principal septa are: (*a*) One which passes between the common extensor (in front) and the lateral extensor and flexor carpi externus (behind); (*b*) one between the common extensor and the extensor carpi radialis; (*c*) one between the inner and middle flexors of the carpus.

The **carpal fascia** (Fascia carpi) is a direct continuation of that of the forearm. It is attached chiefly to the tuberosities at the distal end of the radius, to the accessory carpal (pisiform) bone, and to the lateral ligaments. In front it forms the so-called **anterior annular ligament** (Ligamentum carpi dorsale), bridging over the grooves and binding down the extensor tendons and their synovial sheaths. Behind it is greatly thickened and forms the **posterior annular** or **transverse ligament** of the carpus (Ligamentum carpi transversum). This stretches across from the accessory carpal bone to the internal lateral ligament and the proximal extremity of the inner metacarpal bone. It thus completes the carpal canal, in which lie the flexor tendons, their synovial sheath, and the principal vessels and nerves of the region.

The **fascia** of the **metacarpus** and **digit** (Fascia metacarpea et digitalis) is, in general, thinner than the preceding. It is attached to the tendons, ligaments, and the exposed bony prominences—especially to the small metacarpal bones. On the flexion surface of the fetlock joint it is much thickened by fibers passing transversely from one sesamoid bone to the other, forming an **annular ligament** which binds down the flexor tendons in the sesamoid groove or canal. Distal to this is a second thick quadrilateral sheet (Ligamentum vaginale) which covers and is adherent to the tendon of the flexor perforatus. It is attached on either side by two bands to the borders of the first phalanx, thus firmly binding down the flexor tendons. A little further down a crescentic **fibro-elastic sheet** covers the terminal expansion of the deep flexor tendon. It is attached on either side by a strong band to the side of the first phalanx about its middle.

A. Extensor Division

1. **Extensor carpi radialis** (M. extensor carpi radialis s. radialis dorsalis; extensor metacarpi magnus; anterior extensor of the metacarpus).—This is the largest muscle of the extensor division, and lies on the anterior (dorsal) surface of the radius.

Origin.—(1) The external condyloid crest of the humerus; (2) the coronoid fossa.

Insertion.—The tuberosity on the anterior (dorsal) surface of the proximal extremity of the large (third) metacarpal bone.

Action.—To extend and fix the carpal joint and to flex the elbow joint.

Structure.—The belly of the muscle is rounded, and runs out to a point at the distal third of the forearm. The tendon, which runs nearly the whole length of the fleshy portion, appears on the surface of the latter about its middle; here the muscle shows a distinctly pennate arrangement. The tendon passes through the middle groove at the distal extremity of the radius and over the capsule of the carpal joint, bound down by the anterior annular ligament and invested with a **synovial sheath.** The latter begins three to four inches (ca. 8 to 10 cm.) above the carpus and extends almost to the insertion of the tendon. In the lower half of the forearm the deep fascia blends with the tendon, and here the latter is joined by the long tendon of the biceps.

Relations.—Superficially, the skin, fascia, and the oblique extensor; deeply, the capsule of the elbow joint, the biceps tendon, the radius, the carpal joint capsule, the anterior radial artery, and the radial nerve; externally, the anterior or common extensor; internally, at the elbow, the brachialis and biceps.

Blood-supply.—Anterior radial artery.

Nerve-supply.—Radial nerve.

2. **Anterior** or **common digital extensor** (M. extensor digitalis communis;

anterior extensor of the phalanges; extensor pedis).—This muscle lies external to the foregoing, which it resembles in general form, although less bulky.

Origin.—(1) The front of the distal extremity of the humerus, just external to the coronoid fossa; (2) the external tuberosity on the proximal extremity of the radius, the external lateral ligament of the elbow, and the external border of the

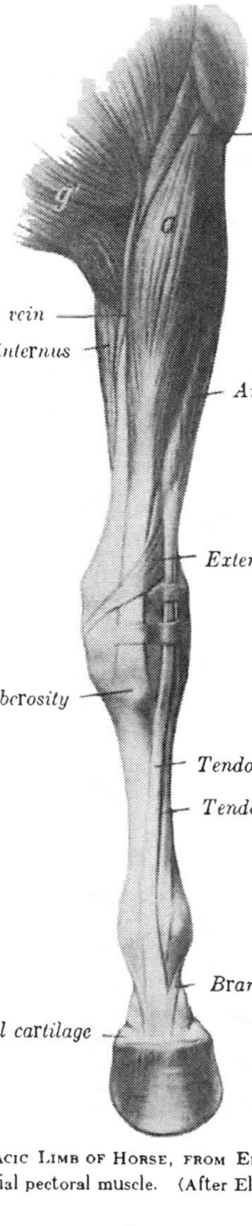

FIG. 190.—MUSCLES OF LEFT THORACIC LIMB OF HORSE, FROM ELBOW DOWNWARD, ANTERIOR VIEW. *a*, Extensor carpi radialis; *g'*, superficial pectoral muscle. (After Ellenberger-Baum, Anat. für Künstler.)

radius at the junction of its proximal and middle thirds; (3) the external surface of the shaft of the ulna; (4) the fascia of the forearm.

Insertion.—(1) The extensor (or pyramidal) process of the third phalanx; (2) the anterior surface of the proximal extremities of the first and second phalanges.

Action.—To extend the digital and carpal joints, and to flex the elbow joint.

Structure.—The muscle is a compound one, representing the common extensor, together with vestiges of the proper extensors of the digits. Usually at least **two heads** may be distinguished. The principal or humeral head (Caput humerale) arises from the front of the extensor epicondyle of the humerus in common with the extensor carpi. Its belly is fusiform, and terminates in a point near the distal third of the radius. The tendon appears on the surface of the muscle about the middle of the belly, the arrangement being pennate. The tendon passes downward through the outer of the two large grooves on the front of the distal end of the radius, and over the capsule of the carpal joint. Passing down over the front of the metacarpus, it inclines gradually inward, reaching the middle line of the limb near the fetlock. A little below the middle of the first phalanx it is joined by the branches of the suspensory ligament, and the tendon thus becomes much wider. Two **synovial membranes** facilitate the play of the tendon. The proximal one is a **sheath** which begins about three inches (ca. 7 to 8 cm.) above the carpus, and terminates at the proximal end of the metacarpus. At the fetlock a **bursa** occurs between the tendon and the joint capsule, but otherwise the two are adherent. The smaller head, arising chiefly from the radius and ulna, is often divisible into two parts (Fig. 443). The larger of these (Caput radiale, muscle of Phillips)[1] arises from the outer tuberosity and outer border of the radius, and from the lateral ligament of the elbow joint. The flat belly is succeeded by a delicate tendon, which accompanies the principal tendon over the carpus (included in the same sheath), and then passes outward to fuse with the tendon of the lateral extensor. Usually a slip is detached which is inserted on the proximal extremity of the first phalanx, or ends in the fascia here. The smaller and deeper division (Caput ulnare, muscle of Thiernesse)[2] is usually somewhat difficult to isolate. It arises from the ulna close to the interosseous space. It has a small rounded belly and is provided with a delicate tendon which may fuse with the principal tendon or may be inserted into the capsule and the fascia in front of the fetlock joint.

Relations.—The chief relations of the belly of the muscle are: superficially, the skin and fascia; deeply, the elbow joint, the radius and ulna, the extensor carpi obliquus, and the anterior radial vessels and radial nerve; in front and internally, the extensor carpi radialis; behind, the lateral extensor and the interosseous vessels

Blood-supply.—Radial and interosseous arteries.

Nerve-supply.—Radial nerve.

3. **Lateral digital extensor** (M. extensor digitalis lateralis s. digiti quinti proprius; lateral extensor of the phalanges; extensor suffraginis).—This muscle is much smaller than the preceding, behind which it is situated.

Origin.—The external tuberosity of the radius and the lateral ligament of the elbow joint, the shaft of the ulna, the outer border of the radius, and the intermuscular septum.

Insertion.—An eminence on the front of the proximal extremity of the first phalanx.

Action.—To extend the digit and carpus.

Structure.—The muscle is pennate, and is inclosed in a sheath formed by the deep fascia, from which many fibers arise. The belly is thin and fusiform and terminates at the lower third of the forearm. From here the tendon (at first small and round) passes downward through the groove on the outer tuberosity of the distal end of the radius, then over the carpus, and, gradually inclining toward the front, but not reaching the middle line of the limb, it passes over the metacarpus and fetlock to its insertion. Two **synovial membranes** occur in connection

[1] This is considered to represent the part of the common extensor for the fourth and fifth digits.

[2] Martin considers that this muscle represents the extensor indicis proprius and the part of the common extensor for the second digit.

with the tendon. A sheath envelops the tendon, beginning about three inches (ca. 6 to 8 cm.) above the carpus, and reaching to the proximal end of the metacarpus. At the fetlock a small bursa lies between the tendon and the joint capsule, but otherwise the tendon is adherent to the capsule. The tendon becomes flat and

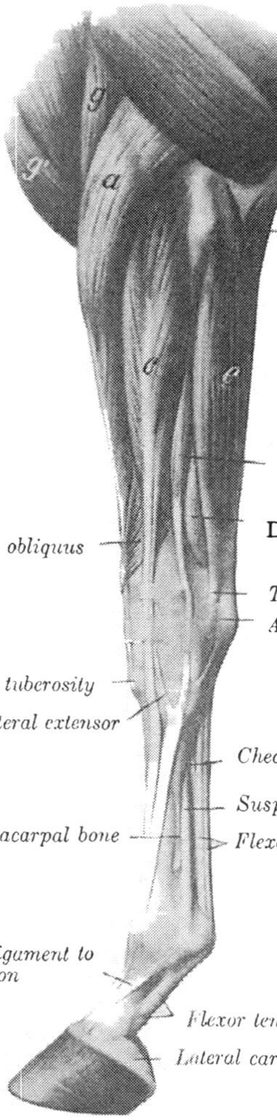

FIG. 191.—MUSCLES OF LEFT THORACIC LIMB OF HORSE FROM ELBOW DOWNWARD; EXTERNAL VIEW. *a*, Extensor carpi radialis; *g*, brachialis; *g'*, anterior superficial pectoral; *c*, anterior or common digital extensor; *e*, flexor carpi externus. (After Ellenberger-Baum, Anat. für Künstler.)

much larger below the carpus, having received the tendon of the radial head of the anterior extensor and a strong band from the accessory carpal bone.

Relations.—Superficially, the skin and fascia; deeply, the outer face of the radius and ulna; in front, the common extensor, the oblique extensor, and the interosseous artery; behind, the external flexor of the carpus and the deep flexor of the digit.

Blood-supply.—Interosseous artery.

Nerve-supply.—Radial nerve.

4. **Extensor carpi obliquus** (M. abductor pollicis longus et extensor pollicis brevis; oblique extensor of the metacarpus; extensor metacarpi obliquus).—This is a small muscle which curves obliquely over the distal half of the radius and the carpus.

Origin.—The external border and adjacent part of the anterior surface of the radius (the attachment area beginning at a point above the middle of the bone and extending down to its lower fourth).

Insertion.—The head of the inner (second) metacarpal bone.

Action.—To extend the carpal joint.

Structure.—The muscle is pennate and has a flat belly which curves downward, forward, and inward over the distal part of the radius. The tendon continues the direction of the muscle, crossing obliquely over the tendon of the extensor carpi radialis; it then occupies the oblique groove at the distal end of the radius, and crosses the inner face of the carpus. It is provided with a **synovial sheath.**

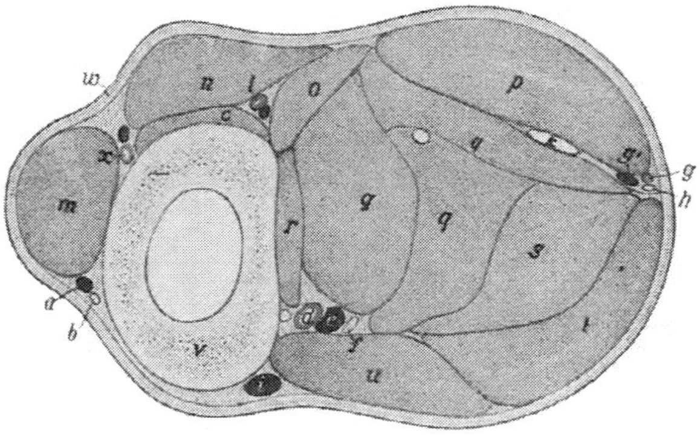

FIG. 192.—CROSS-SECTION OF MIDDLE OF RIGHT FOREARM OF HORSE

a, Accessory cephalic vein; *b*, cutaneous branch of median nerve; *c*, extensor carpi obliquus; *d*, posterior radial artery; *e*, satellite vein; *f*, median nerve; *g*, *g'*, ulnar vessels; *h*, ulnar nerve; *i*, cephalic vein; *k*, tendon of ulnar head of deep flexor; *l*, interosseous artery; *m*, extensor carpi radialis; *n*, anterior digital extensor; *o*, lateral digital extensor; *p*, flexor carpi externus; *q*, *q*, *q*, humeral heads of deep digital flexor; *r*, radial head of same; *s*, superficial digital flexor; *t*, flexor carpi medius; *u*, flexor carpi internus; *v*, radius; *w*, skin; *x*, anterior radial artery. (After Ellenberger, in Leisering's Atlas.)

Relations.—Superficially, the skin and fascia, the lateral extensor, and the common extensor; deeply, the radius, the extensor carpi radialis, the carpal capsule, and the internal lateral ligament.

Blood-supply.—Interosseous and anterior radial arteries.

Nerve-supply.—Radial nerve.

B. FLEXOR DIVISION

1. **Flexor carpi internus** (M. flexor carpi radialis s. radialis volaris; internal flexor of the metacarpus).—This muscle lies on the inner surface of the forearm, immediately behind the inner border of the radius.

Origin.—The flexor (internal) epicondyle of the humerus, below and behind the lateral ligament.

Insertion.—The proximal end of the internal (second) metacarpal bone.

Action.—To flex the carpal joint and to extend the elbow.

Structure.—The muscle has a short tendon of origin, which is succeeded by a somewhat flattened, fusiform belly. The tendon of insertion begins near the distal fourth of the radius. It is provided with a synovial sheath which begins two or three inches (ca. 5 to 8 cm.) above the carpus and extends almost to the insertion of the tendon.

Relations.—Superficially, the skin and fascia, the posterior superficial pectoral and the tensor fasciæ antibrachii; deeply, the elbow joint, the radius, the deep flexor, the flexor carpi medius, the posterior radial vessels, and the median nerve. At the elbow the artery and nerve lie in front of the muscle, but below they dip beneath it.

Blood-supply.—Posterior radial artery.

Nerve-supply.—Median nerve.

On removing the deep fascia on the inner surface of the elbow the student may notice a small muscle lying along the lateral ligament. This is the pronator teres, which is usually not present or a mere vestige in the horse. It arises by a small, flat tendon from the flexor epicondyle of the humerus, and is inserted into the internal lateral ligament of the elbow. On account of its small size and the fact that the forearm is fixed in the position of pronation, the muscle can have no appreciable function. It is usually represented by the long portion of the internal lateral ligament.

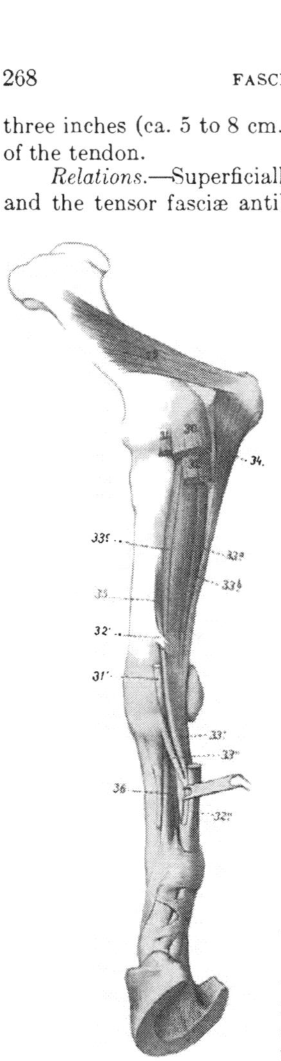

Fig. 193.—Deeper Muscles of Forearm of Horse, Internal View.

23, internal head of triceps; *30*, flexor carpi medius; *31*, flexor carpi internus; *31'*, tendon of *31*; *32*, superficial digital flexor; *32'*, radial check ligament; *32''*, tendon of superficial flexor; *33a*, *33b*, *33c*, humeral heads of deep flexor; *33'*, deep flexor tendon; *33''*, subcarpal check ligament; *34*, ulnar head of deep flexor; *35*, radial head of deep flexor; *36*, suspensory ligament. (After Ellenberger, in Leisering's Atlas.)

2. **Flexor carpi medius** (M. flexor carpi ulnaris s. ulnaris medialis; oblique or middle flexor of the metacarpus).—This muscle lies on the inner and posterior aspect of the forearm partly under, partly behind, the preceding muscle. It arises by two heads—humeral and ulnar.

Origin.—(1) The flexor (internal) epicondyle of the humerus just behind the preceding muscle; (2) the inner surface and posterior border of the olecranon.

Insertion.—The upper edge of the accessory carpal (pisiform) bone.

Action.—To flex the carpal joint, and to extend the elbow.

Structure.—The humeral head is much the larger, constituting, in fact, the bulk of the muscle. It is flattened, curved, and tapers at both ends. The ulnar head, much smaller and very thin, is covered by an aponeurosis from which many of its fibers arise. It joins the large head a little above the middle of the forearm. The tendon of insertion is short and strong; it blends with the posterior annular ligament of the carpus.

Relations.—Superficially, the tensor fasciæ antibrachii, superficial pectoral, and flexor carpi internus, the skin and fascia, and cutaneous branches of the ulnar nerve; deeply, the superficial and deep flexors of the digit. In the distal half of the forearm the ulnar vessels and nerve lie between the outer edge of this muscle and the external flexor of the carpus.

Blood-supply.—Ulnar and posterior radial arteries.

Nerve-supply.—Ulnar and median nerves.

3. **Flexor carpi externus** (M. extensor carpi ulnaris[1] s. ulnaris lateralis; external flexor of the metacarpus).—This muscle lies on the outer face of the forearm, behind the lateral extensor of the digit.

[1] In man the muscle is an extensor of the hand.

Origin.—The extensor (external) epicondyle of the humerus, behind and below the lateral ligament.

Insertion.—(1) The outer surface and upper edge of the accessory carpal bone; (2) the proximal extremity of the outer (fourth) metacarpal bone.

Action.—To flex the carpal joint and to extend the elbow.

Structure.—The belly of the muscle is flattened and is intersected by a good deal of tendinous tissue. There are two tendons of insertion. The short tendon is inserted into the accessory carpal bone. The long tendon is detached just above the carpus; it is smaller and rounded; it passes downward and a little forward through a groove on the outer surface of the accessory carpal bone, enveloped by a synovial sheath, to reach its insertion on the outer metacarpal bone. A synovial

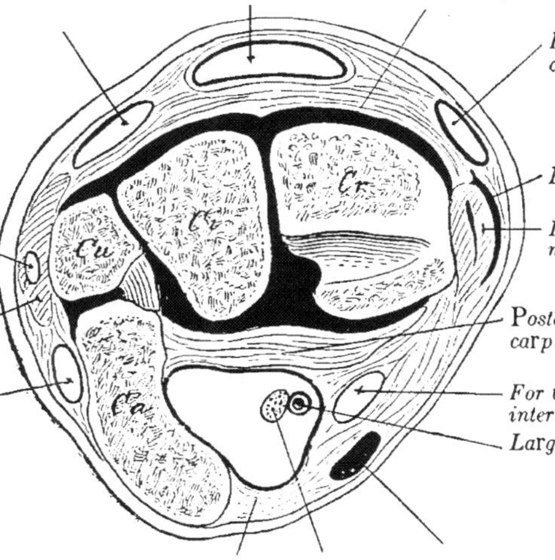

FIG. 194.—CROSS-SECTION OF PROXIMAL PART OF LEFT CARPUS OF HORSE.

The tendons have been removed to show the canals in which they lie. The joint cavity is black. By an oversight the carpal canal for the two flexor tendons behind the posterior ligament of the carpus is not marked. *Cr* Radial, *Ci*, intermediate, *Cu*, ulnar, *Ca*, accessory carpal bones.

pouch lies under the origin of the muscle at the elbow joint, with the cavity of which it communicates.

Relations.—Superficially, the skin, fascia, and cutaneous branches of the ulnar nerve; deeply, the elbow joint, the ulna, and the flexors of the digit; in front, the lateral extensor of the digit; behind, the middle flexor of the carpus, the ulnar head of the deep flexor, and the ulnar vessels and nerve.

Blood-supply.—Interosseous, ulnar, and median arteries.

Nerve-supply.—Radial nerve.

4. **Superficial digital flexor** or **flexor perforatus** (M. flexor digitalis sublimis; superficial flexor of the phalanges).—This muscle is situated in the middle of the flexor group, chiefly under cover of the middle flexor of the carpus.

Origin.—(1) The flexor epicondyle of the humerus, between the flexor carpi internus and the deep flexor of the digit; (2) a ridge on the posterior surface of the radius, below its middle and near the internal border.

Insertion.—(1) The eminences on the proximal extremity of the second phalanx behind the lateral ligaments; (2) the distal extremity of the first phalanx, also behind the lateral ligaments.

Action.—To flex the digit and carpus, and to extend the elbow.

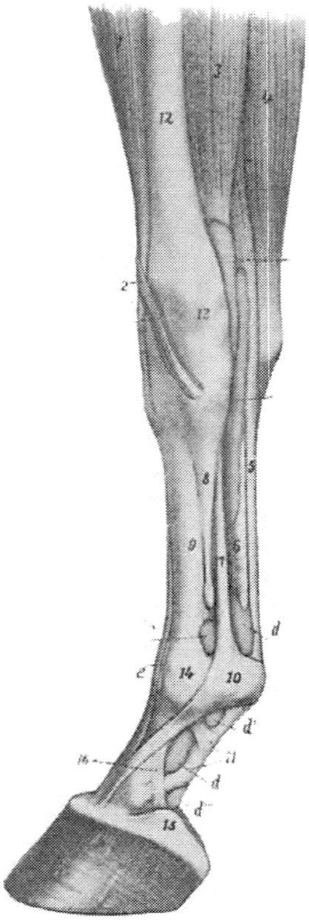

FIG. 195.—SYNOVIAL SHEATHS AND BURSÆ OF LOWER PART OF RIGHT FORE LIMB OF HORSE, INTERNAL VIEW.

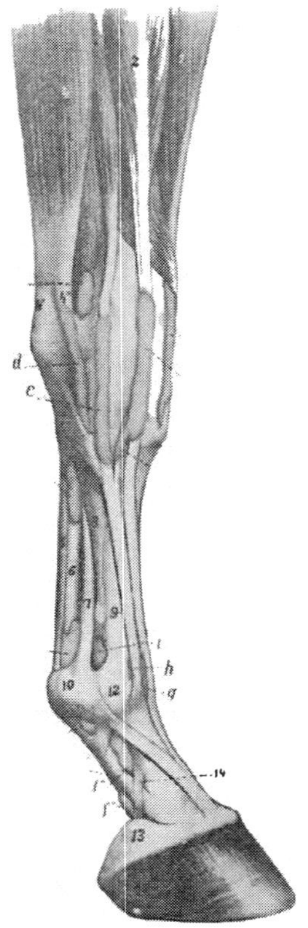

FIG. 196.—SYNOVIAL SHEATHS AND BURSÆ OF LOWER PART OF RIGHT FORE LIMB OF HORSE, EXTERNAL VIEW.

The synovial sheaths (colored yellow) and the joint capsules (colored pink) are injected.

a, Sheath of extensor carpi obliquus; *b*, sheath of flexor carpi internus; *c*, carpal sheath; *d*, *d'*, *d''*, *d'''*, digital sheath; *e*, bursa under anterior extensor tendon; *f*, capsule of fetlock joint; *1*, extensor carpi radialis; *2*, tendon of extensor carpi obliquus; *3*, flexor carpi internus; *4*, flexor carpi medius; *5*, superficial flexor tendon; *6*, deep flexor tendon; *7*, suspensory ligament; *8*, small metacarpal bone; *9*, large metacarpal bone; *10*, posterior annular ligament of fetlock; *11*, proximal digital annular ligament; *12*, radius; *13*, radiocarpal joint; *14*, fetlock joint; *15*, lateral cartilage; *16*, band from first phalanx to lateral cartilage. (After Ellenberger, in Leisering's Atlas.)

a, Sheath of extensor carpi radialis; *b*, sheath of anterior extensor; *c*, sheath of lateral extensor; *d*, sheath of outer tendon of flexor carpi externus; *e*, *e'*, carpal sheath; *f*, *f'*, *f''*, digital sheath; *g*, bursa under anterior extensor tendon; *h*, bursa under lateral extensor tendon; *i*, capsule of fetlock joint; *1*, extensor carpi radialis; *2*, anterior digital extensor; *3*, lateral digital extensor; *4*, flexor carpi externus; *4'*, *4''*, tendons of *4*; *5*, superficial flexor tendon; *6*, deep flexor tendon; *7*, suspensory ligament; *8*, external metacarpal bone; *9*, large metacarpal bone; *10*, posterior annular ligament of fetlock; *11*, digital annular ligament; *12*, fetlock joint; *13*, lateral cartilage; *14*, band from first phalanx to lateral cartilage. (After Ellenberger, in Leisering's Atlas.)

Structure.—The fleshy portion of the muscle or humeral head takes origin from the humerus. The radial head (Caput tendineum) consists of a strong fibrous band, usually termed the radial or superior check ligament, which fuses with the tendon near the carpus. The belly of the muscle is intersected by tendinous strands, and fuses more or less with that of the deep flexor. Near the carpus it is succeeded by a strong, thick tendon which passes down through the carpal canal, formed by the posterior ligament of the carpus, the accessory carpal bone, and the posterior annular ligament (Ligamentum carpi transversum). Here it is enveloped by a synovial sheath, in common with the deep flexor. This **carpal** sheath (Vagina carpea) begins three or four inches (8 to 10 cm.) above the carpus, and extends downward nearly to the middle of the metacarpus. Below the carpus the tendon becomes flattened and broader. Near the fetlock it forms a ring through which the tendon of the deep flexor passes (Fig. 150). Here the two tendons are bound down in the sesamoid groove by the posterior annular ligament, which fuses more or less with the superficial flexor tendon. At the distal end of the first phalanx the tendon divides into two branches which diverge to reach their points of insertion, and between these branches the tendon of the deep flexor emerges (Fig. 189). A second synovial **sheath,** the digital or **sesamoidean** (Vagina

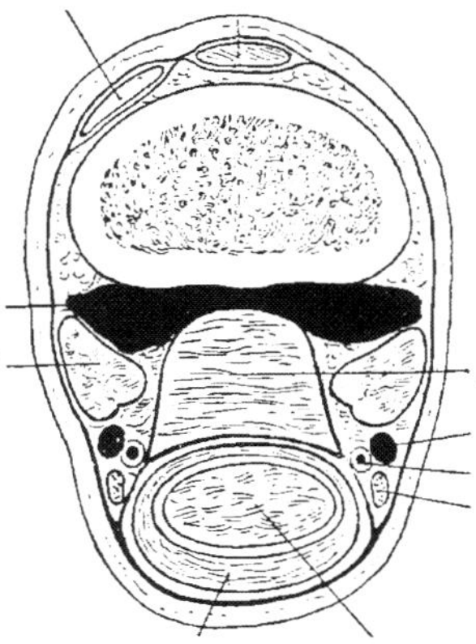

Fig. 197.—Cross-section of Distal Part of Left Metacarpus of Horse, Just Above Sesamoids.

digitalis), begins at the distal third of the metacarpus, three to four inches (8 to 10 cm.) above the fetlock, and extends to the middle of the second phalanx.

Relations.—The belly of the muscle is related superficially to the ulnar head of the deep flexor, the flexor carpi medius, and, at its origin, to the ulnar vessels and nerve; deeply to the humeral head of the deep flexor. The tendon is related superficially to the skin and fascia; deeply to the deep flexor tendon.

Blood-supply.—Posterior radial artery.

Nerve-supply.—Median nerve.

5. Deep **digital flexor** or **flexor** perforans (M. flexor digitalis profundus; deep flexor of the phalanges).—The fleshy part of this muscle lies on the posterior surface of the radius, under cover of the preceding muscles. It is the largest muscle of the flexor group.

Origin.—(1) The flexor (internal) epicondyle of the humerus; (2) the inner surface of the olecranon; (3) the middle of the posterior surface of the radius and a small adjacent area of the ulna.

Insertion.—The semilunar crest of the third phalanx, and the adjacent surface of the lateral cartilage.

Action.—To flex the digit and carpus, and to extend the elbow.

Structure.—This muscle consists of three principal heads. The **humeral head** (Caput humerale) constitutes the bulk of the muscle. It is marked by tendinous intersections, and is separable into three secondary heads. The **ulnar head** (Caput ulnare, ulnaris accessorius) is much smaller, and is at first superficially situated between the outer and middle flexors of the carpus. The **radial head** (Caput radiale, radialis accessorius) is the smallest, and is not always present; it is situated on the distal two-thirds of the posterior surface of the radius, under the humeral head. Each of these heads is provided with a tendon. The principal tendon—that of the humeral head—begins about three or four inches (8 to 10 cm.) above the carpus. It is soon joined by the small tendon of the ulnar head, which begins about the middle of the forearm. The tendon of the radial head fuses with the principal tendon close to the carpus. The conjoined tendon passes downward through the carpal canal, being included in the **carpal synovial sheath** with the superficial flexor tendon, as previously described. Continuing downward, it is joined about the middle of the metacarpus by a strong fibrous band, the so-called **inferior** or **subcarpal check ligament** (Caput tendineum). This is a direct continuation of the posterior ligament of the carpus. Below this the tendon passes through the ring formed by the perforatus, then in succession over the sesamoid groove, the inferior sesamoidean ligaments, and the tendon surface of the third sesamoid, to its insertion (Figs. 150 and 151). Its terminal part is much widened. From the distal third of the metacarpus to the distal end of the second phalanx it is inclosed in the **digital synovial sheath** described in connection with the perforatus. The **navicular bursa** or **bursa podotrochlearis** is found between the tendon and the third sesamoid or navicular bone. The terminal part of the tendon is bound down by the fibrous sheet described with the fascia.

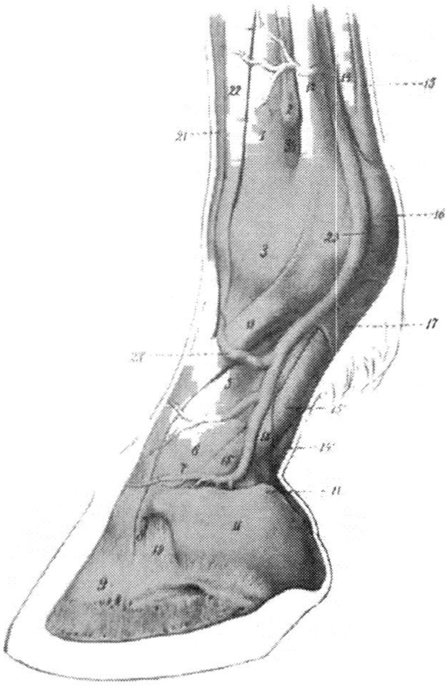

FIG. 198.—DIGIT OF HORSE, LATERAL VIEW.

1, Large metacarpal bone; *2*, distal end of small metacarpal bone; *3*, fetlock joint; *5*, first phalanx; *6*, pastern joint; *7*, second phalanx; *8*, coffin joint; *9*, third phalanx; *11*, lateral cartilage; *11′*, upper (subcutaneous) border of cartilage; *12*, suspensory ligament; *13*, branch of *12* to extensor tendon; *14*, deep flexor tendon; *15*, superficial flexor tendon; *15′*, branch of *15*; *16*, posterior annular ligament of fetlock; *17*, proximal annular or vaginal ligament of digit; *18*, distal annular ligament or reinforcing sheath of deep flexor tendon; *19*, lateral ligament of coffin joint; *21*, tendon of common or anterior extensor; *22*, tendon of lateral extensor; *23*, digital vein. (After Ellenberger-Baum, Anat. für Künstler.)

Relations.—The belly of the muscle is related posteriorly to the perforatus and the middle flexor of the carpus; internally, to the internal carpal flexor, the radial check ligament, and the posterior radial vessels and median nerve; externally, to the external flexor of the carpus; anteriorly, to the radius and ulna and branches of the posterior radial artery and median nerve. Below the carpus the tendon is accompanied by the vessels and nerves of the digit. It may also be noted that the muscle is not entirely covered by the other flexors; it comes in contact with the skin and fascia on the postero-external aspect of the proximal half of the forearm, and also on the outer aspect of the distal fourth.

Blood-supply.—Posterior radial and ulnar arteries.

Nerve-supply.—Median and ulnar nerves.

METACARPAL MUSCLES

The five muscles of this group are either reduced to vestiges or modified greatly in structure.

1, 2. **Lumbricales** (internus et externus).—These are two small muscles which lie on either side of the flexor tendons above the fetlock. They arise from the deep flexor tendon, and are lost in the fibrous tissue which lies under the nodule of horn or ergot at the fetlock (Fig. 447). Their action is inappreciable. The size of these muscles is subject to much variation. Often very little muscular tissue can be found, but the small tendon is constantly present.

Blood-supply.—Metacarpal arteries.

Nerve-supply.—Median and ulnar nerves.

3, 4, 5. **Interossei.**—These are three in number in the horse, and are situated chiefly in the metacarpal groove. Two, the **internus** and **externus,** are very small muscles, each of which arises from the corresponding small metacarpal bone near its proximal extremity, and is provided with a delicate tendon which is usually lost in the fascia at the fetlock (Fig. 150). They have no appreciable action. Their blood- and nerve-supply is the same as that of the preceding muscles.

The **interosseus medius** is so much modified that it is usually termed the **suspensory,** or **superior sesamoidean ligament.** It contains little muscular tissue, being transformed very largely into a strong tendinous band, bifurcate below, and having for its chief function the supporting of the fetlock. It has been described, in deference to common usage, with the ligaments.

FASCIÆ AND MUSCLES OF THE PELVIC LIMB

THE FASCIÆ

The **iliac fascia** (Fascia iliaca) covers the ventral surface of the iliacus and psoas muscles, over which it is tightly stretched (Fig. 450). It is attached internally to the tendon of the psoas minor, externally to the inguinal (Poupart's) ligament and the external angle of the ilium. Its anterior part is thin. Posteriorly, it is in part attached to the ilium, in part becomes continuous with the pelvic fascia. It furnishes surfaces of origin for the sartorius, cremaster externus, and transversus abdominis muscles.

The **pelvic fascia** (Fascia pelvis) lines the cavity (parietal layer) and is reflected on the viscera at the pelvic outlet (visceral layer). Laminæ are detached from it to strengthen the various peritoneal folds.

The **superficial fascia** of the gluteal region is continuous with the aponeurosis of the panniculus. It covers and partly blends with the deep fascia. The **gluteal fascia** (Fascia glutea) covers the superficial muscles of the region, and detaches intermuscular septa, which pass between the muscles. It is attached to the sacral spines, the dorsal sacro-iliac ligament, and the angles of the ilium, and is continuous in front with the lumbo-dorsal fascia, behind with the coccygeal fascia. Its deep face gives origin to fibers of the superficial and middle glutei, the biceps femoris, and the semitendinosus, so that care is necessary in dissecting it off these muscles. The chief **intermuscular septa** are: (1) One which passes between the superficial gluteus and the biceps femoris; (2) one between the biceps and semitendinosus, from which a lamella is detached which passes between the middle and posterior portions of the biceps and is attached to the tuber ischii; (3) one between the semitendinosus and semimembranosus, which is attached to the sacro-sciatic ligament and tuber ischii; it furnishes origin for fibers of the long head of the semimembranosus.

The **fascia lata** is continuous with the preceding, and covers the muscles on the outer surface and front of the thigh. It is tendinous and very strong, and for the most part easily separable from the underlying muscles. It furnishes insertion to the tensor fasciæ latæ and to the biceps femoris (in part), by both of which it is tensed. At the stifle it is attached to the patella and the inner and outer straight ligaments. Internally it is continuous with the internal femoral fascia. It furnishes the following **intermuscular septa**: (1) One which passes between the vastus externus and biceps femoris to be attached to the external trochanter of the femur; (2) two which pass between the three branches of the biceps femoris; (3) a fourth between the biceps femoris and semitendinosus.

The **internal femoral fascia** (Fascia femoralis medialis) covers the superficial muscles on the inner surface of the thigh. At its upper part it is joined by part of the aponeurosis of the external oblique muscle (Lamina femoralis) (Fig. 450). The posterior part is thin. It is continuous with the fascia lata in front and the crural fascia below. At the stifle it fuses with the tendons of the sartorius and gracilis.

The **crural fascia**, or fascia of the leg (Fascia cruris), consists of three layers. Two of these invest the entire region and may, therefore, be termed the **common fasciæ**. The superficial layer is a continuation of the fasciæ of the thigh, while the second layer may be regarded chiefly as a continuation of the tendons of the superficial muscles of the hip and thigh (biceps femoris, semitendinosus, tensor fasciæ latæ, sartorius, and gracilis). The two layers frequently fuse, and are attached chiefly to the patellar ligaments and the crest and internal surface of the tibia. About the middle of the leg the two layers unite behind the deep flexor of the digit and form a strong band which passes downward in front of the tendons of the gastrocnemius and superficial flexor, to be attached with the latter to the anterior and inner part of the tuber calcis. This may be regarded as an accessory or tarsal tendon of insertion of the biceps femoris and semitendinosus. The third layer forms sheaths for the muscles, furnishing origin in part to their fibers. Two important **intermuscular septa** are detached, viz.: (1) One which passes between the anterior and lateral digital extensors to be attached to the fibula and the external border of the tibia; (2) one between the lateral extensor and the deep flexor.

The **tarsal fascia** (Fascia tarsi) fuses with the ligaments and bony prominences of the region. It is strong and tendinous in front, and joins the tendon of the anterior extensor below the joint. Laterally, it is thin and fuses with the ligaments. Posteriorly, it is very thick and strong, forming an annular ligament which stretches from the internal lateral ligament to the fibular tarsal bone and the plantar ligament. This converts the groove at the back of the hock into a canal, in which are the deep flexor tendon with its synovial sheath and the plantar nerves. In front of the tarsus and above and below it there are three **annular ligaments** (Ligamenta transversa). The proximal one binds down the tendons of the anterior extensor, peroneus tertius, and tibialis anterior on the distal end of the tibia. The middle one stretches from the fibular tarsal bone to the outer tendon of the peroneus tertius, forming a loop around the tendon of the anterior extensor. The distal band stretches across the proximal extremity of the large metatarsal bone and incloses the tendons (and sheaths) of the two extensors of the digit.

The metatarsal and **digital fasciæ** do not differ materially from those of the corresponding regions of the thoracic limb.

The Muscles

I. The Sublumbar Muscles (Figs. 450, 456)

The muscles of this group are not confined to the sublumbar region, but extend beyond it both before and behind. Their chief function is to flex the hip joint. Two, however,—the psoas minor and the quadratus lumborum,—have not this action.

1. **Psoas minor** (s. parvus).—This is a fusiform, flattened, pennate muscle, which lies along the ventro-lateral aspect of the bodies of the last three thoracic and the lumbar vertebræ.

Origin.—The bodies of the last three thoracic and first four or five lumbar vertebræ, and the vertebral ends of the sixteenth and seventeenth ribs.

Insertion.—The psoas tubercle on the shaft of the ilium.

Action.—To flex the pelvis on the loins, or to incline it laterally.

Structure.—The muscle arises by a series of digitations which pass backward and outward to be inserted at an acute angle on the tendon. The latter lies along the outer border of the fleshy portion and is flattened. It appears on the surface of the muscle at the third lumbar process and increases gradually in width until it reaches the pelvic inlet, where it becomes narrower.

Relations.—The ventral surface of the thoracic portion of the muscle is related to the pleura, crura of the diaphragm, and sympathetic nerve. In the abdomen, the chief ventral relations are the peritoneum, the vena cava (right side), the aorta and left kidney (left side), the sympathetic nerves, and the ureters. Dorsally, the chief relations are the vertebræ, the psoas major, and lumbar nerves. Near its insertion the tendon is crossed internally by the external iliac artery, and externally by the femoral nerve.

Blood-supply.—Intercostal and lumbar arteries.

Nerve-supply.—Lumbar nerves.

2. **Psoas major** (s. magnus).—This is much larger than the preceding muscle, by which it is partly covered. It is triangular, with the base anterior.

Origin.—The ventral surfaces of the vertebral ends of the last two ribs and the transverse processes of the lumbar vertebræ.

Insertion.—The internal trochanter of the femur, by a common tendon with the iliacus.

Action.—To flex the hip joint and to rotate the thigh outward.

Structure.—The origin of the muscle is fleshy, the belly being in general flattened, thick in its middle, thin at its edges. The thoracic portion is small, the abdominal part much thicker and wider, extending laterally beyond the extremities of the lumbar transverse processes. From the lumbo-sacral articulation it lies in a deep groove formed in the iliacus (with which it is partly united), becomes smaller and rounded, and passes downward and backward to terminate by a strong tendon common to it and the iliacus.[1]

Relations.—Dorsally, the last two ribs and thoracic vertebræ, the lumbar vertebræ, the internal intercostals, quadratus lumborum, longissimus dorsi, and iliacus, and the lumbar vessels and nerves; ventrally, the pleura and peritoneum, the iliac fascia, inguinal ligament, the diaphragm, psoas minor, and sartorius, the kidneys, the spleen, the intestine (duodenum, cæcum, etc.) and the circumflex iliac vessels.

Blood-supply.—Lumbar and circumflex iliac arteries.

Nerve-supply.—Lumbar and femoral nerves.

3. **Iliacus.**—This muscle covers the ventral surface of the ilium external to the sacro-iliac articulation, and extends outward beyond the external border of the bone, underneath the middle gluteus.

Origin.—The ventral surface of the ilium external to the ilio-pectineal line, the ventral sacro-iliac ligament, the wing of the sacrum, and the tendon of the psoas minor.

Insertion.—The internal trochanter of the femur, by a common tendon with the psoas major.

[1] On account of the intimate union between the psoas major and iliacus they are frequently considered a single muscle, to which the name ilio-psoas is applied; some anatomists include the psoas minor also under this term.

Action.—To flex the hip joint and to rotate the thigh outward.

Structure.—The belly of the muscle is so deeply grooved for the psoas major as to give the appearance of being completely divided into outer and inner portions. When the psoas is removed, it is seen, however, that the two heads are not entirely separated. The outer, larger head arises from the wing of the ilium chiefly; the inner, smaller head arises chiefly from a small area on the shaft of the ilium, between the psoas tubercle and the depression for the inner tendon of the rectus femoris, and from the tendon of the psoas minor. The two portions inclose the psoas major in front of the hip joint.

Relations.—Dorsally, the ilium, sacrum, sacro-iliac articulation, the gluteus medius, the ilio-lumbar and external circumflex vessels; ventrally, the iliac fascia, inguinal ligament, the psoas major, sartorius, and abdominal muscles. At the hip joint the chief relations are: internally, the femoral vessels, the femoral nerve, and the sartorius muscle; externally, the rectus femoris and tensor fasciæ latæ; in front, the abdominal muscles; behind, the hip joint.

Blood-supply.—Lumbar, circumflex iliac, and deep femoral arteries.

Nerve-supply.—Lumbar and femoral nerves.

4. **Quadratus lumborum.**—This thin muscle lies on the outer part of the ventral surfaces of the lumbar transverse processes.

Origin.—The ventral surface of the upper part of the last two ribs and the lumbar transverse processes.

Insertion.—The ventral surface of the wing of the sacrum and the ventral sacro-iliac ligament.

Action.—Acting together, to fix the last two ribs and the lumbar vertebræ; acting singly, to produce lateral flexion of the loins.

Structure.—The muscle is pennate, and is curved with the convexity outward. It is thin, largely mixed with tendinous fibers, and is, in general, little developed in the horse in comparison with some of the other animals (*e. g.*, dog, sheep).

Relations.—Ventrally, the psoas major and the last intercostal and first three lumbar nerves; dorsally, the last two ribs, the lumbar transverse processes, and the lateral branches of the lumbar arteries.

Blood-supply.—Lumbar arteries.

Nerve-supply.—Lumbar nerves.

5. **Intertransversales lumborum** (M. intertransversarii lumborum).—These are described with the other spinal muscles. (See p. 238.)

II. THE EXTERNAL MUSCLES OF THE HIP AND THIGH

Under this head will be described the muscles of the outer surface of the pelvis and thigh, and those which form the posterior contour of the latter. They are given in the order in which they may be conveniently examined.

1. Tensor fasciæ latæ (Fig. 178).—This is the most anterior muscle of the superficial layer. It is triangular in form, with its apex at the external angle of the ilium.

Origin.—The external angle of the ilium.

Insertion.—The fascia lata, and thus indirectly to the patella, the external straight ligament, and the crest of the tibia.

Action.—To tense the fascia lata, flex the hip joint, and extend the stifle joint.

Structure.—The muscle arises by a rather small head, about two inches (ca. 5 cm.) wide, on the antero-inferior eminence of the external angle of the ilium. Below this the belly spreads out and terminates about midway between the point of the hip and the stifle in the aponeurosis. The belly fuses to a considerable extent with the superficial gluteus. The aponeurosis fuses with the fascia lata, and detaches a lamina which passes with the tendon of insertion of the superficial gluteus to the external border of the femur.

Relations —Externally, the skin and fascia; internally, the obliquus abdominis externus, the iliacus, superficial gluteus, rectus femoris, and vastus externus, branches of the circumflex iliac, ilio-lumbar, and iliaco-femoral arteries, and the anterior gluteal nerve; anteriorly, the precrural lymph-glands. A considerable quantity of connective tissue is found between the deep face of the muscle and the abdominal wall.

Blood-supply.—Circumflex iliac, ilio-lumbar, and iliaco-femoral arteries.

Nerve-supply.—Anterior gluteal nerve.

2. **Gluteus superficialis** (Figs. 178, 199) (Superficial gluteus; gluteus externus).—This muscle lies behind and partly underneath the tensor fasciæ latæ. It is triangular and consists of an anterior and a posterior head united by the gluteal fascia.

Origin.—(1) The external angle and the adjacent part of the external border of the ilium (anterior head); (2) the gluteal fascia (posterior head).

Insertion.—The third (external) trochanter of the femur.

Action.—To abduct the limb, flex the hip joint, and tense the gluteal fascia.

Structure.—The anterior head of the muscle is not completely separable (except artificially) from the tensor fasciæ latæ. The attachment to the border of the ilium is by means of an intermuscular septum, which passes beneath the thick outer border of the gluteus medius. The posterior head arises from the deep face of the gluteal fascia, and so indirectly from the dorsal sacro-iliac ligament. The two heads unite and terminate on a strong flat tendon, which is inserted into the edge of the third trochanter of the femur, beneath the biceps femoris.

Relations.—Superficially, the skin, fascia, and biceps femoris; deeply, the gluteus medius, iliacus, rectus femoris, and branches of the iliaco-femoral artery; in front, the tensor fasciæ latæ; behind, the biceps femoris.

Blood-supply.—Gluteal and iliaco-femoral arteries.

Nerve-supply.—Anterior gluteal nerve.

3. **Gluteus medius** (Figs. 178, 179) (Middle gluteus; gluteus maximus).—This is a very large muscle which covers the dorsal surface of the ilium and the greater part of the lateral wall of the pelvis, and extends forward also on the lumbar part of the longissimus.

Origin.—(1) The aponeurosis of the longissimus, as far forward as the first lumbar vertebra; (2) the gluteal or dorsal surface and internal and external angles of the ilium; (3) the dorsal and lateral sacro-iliac and sacro-sciatic ligaments, and the gluteal fascia.

Insertion.—(1) The summit of the trochanter major of the femur; (2) the crest below the trochanter; (3) the outer aspect of the trochanteric ridge.

Action.—To extend the hip joint and abduct the limb. By its connection with the longissimus a muscular mass is formed which is one of the chief factors in rearing, kicking, and propulsion.

Structure.—The anterior extremity of the muscle is relatively thin, and lies in a depression on the surface of the longissimus, from the strong aponeurosis of which the fibers take origin. The pelvic portion of the muscle is very voluminous, and forms the bulk of the muscular mass which gives the haunch its rounded contour. This part of the muscle is intersected by several tendinous sheets. One of these is particularly distinct, and is attached to the gluteal line on the ilium. This divides the muscle incompletely into superficial and deep strata. The superficial part is inserted by a strong tendon into the summit of the great trochanter, and by a pointed fleshy mass with a tendinous border into the trochanteric ridge. The deep part (Gluteus accessorius) is smaller, and arises entirely from the ilium between the gluteal line and the external angle (Fig. 455). It has a strong flat tendon which passes over the convexity of the trochanter to be inserted into the crest below it. The convexity is covered with cartilage, and the **trochanteric bursa** (Bursa trochanterica) is interposed between the tendon and the cartilage.[1]

Relations.—Superficially, the skin, lumbo-dorsal and gluteal fasciæ, the tensor fasciæ latæ, gluteus superficialis, and biceps femoris; deeply, the longissimus, the ilium, sacro-iliac and sacro-sciatic ligaments, the gluteus profundus, iliacus and rectus femoris, the iliaco-femoral artery, the gluteal and internal pudic vessels and nerves, and the great sciatic nerve.

Blood-supply.—Gluteal, ilio-lumbar, lumbar, and iliaco-femoral arteries.

Nerve-supply.—Gluteal nerves.

4. **Gluteus profundus** (Deep gluteus; gluteus internus; scansorius).—This much smaller, quadrilateral muscle lies under the posterior part of the preceding muscle, and extends over the hip joint, from the superior ischiatic spine to the anterior part of the great trochanter (Fig. 455).

Origin.—The superior ischiatic spine and the adjacent part of the shaft of the ilium.

Insertion.—The edge of the anterior part or convexity of the trochanter major of the femur.

Action.—To abduct the thigh and to rotate it inward.

Structure.—The muscle is short and thick and contains numerous tendinous intersections. The fibers are directed almost transversely outward over the capsule of the hip joint and converge at the convexity of the trochanter.

Relations.—Superficially, the gluteus medius and branches of the gluteal vessels and nerves; deeply, the shaft of the ilium, the hip joint, and the rectus femoris and capsularis.

Blood-supply.—Gluteal artery.

Nerve-supply.—Anterior gluteal nerve.

5. **Biceps femoris** (Gluteo-biceps s. paramero-biceps).—This large muscle lies behind and in part upon the superficial and middle glutei. It extends in a curved direction from the sacral and coccygeal spines to the outer surface of the stifle and leg (Figs. 178, 199, 200, 201, 202).

Origin.—(1) The dorsal sacro-iliac ligament, the gluteal and coccygeal fasciæ, and the intermuscular septum between this muscle and the semitendinosus; (2) the tuber ischii.

Insertion.—(1) A tubercle on the posterior surface of the femur near the external trochanter; (2) the anterior surface and external straight ligament of the patella; (3) the tibial crest; (4) the anterior and internal surface of the tuber calcis.

Action.—The action is somewhat complex, because the muscle is composed of three portions, has several points of insertion, and acts on all the joints of the limb except those of the digit. The general action is to extend the limb, as in propelling the body, rearing or kicking, and to abduct it. The anterior part, by its attachment to the posterior surface of the femur and to the patella, would extend the stifle and hip joints and abduct the limb. The middle part, being inserted chiefly on the tibial crest and the external straight ligament, would extend the hip, and, with the semitendinosus, flex the stifle. The posterior part, by virtue of its attachment to the tuber calcis, assists in extending the hock.

Structure.—The muscle has two heads of origin:[2] The long or vertebral head arises chiefly from the dorsal and lateral sacro-iliac ligaments, the coccygeal fascia,

[1] By some anatomists the portion inserted into the crest is termed the gluteus accessorius, but Lesbre considers this the deep gluteus, homologous with the gluteus minimus of man. The portion inserted into the trochanteric ridge apparently represents the piriformis of man.

[2] Apparently the muscle represents the biceps, together with part of the gluteus superficialis of man. Hence the names gluteo-biceps and paramero-biceps have been suggested.

and the intermuscular septum. There is often a large bursa between this head and the trochanter major. The short or ischiatic head arises by a strong tendon from the ventral spine on the tuber ischii. They unite, and a short tendon is detached from the deep face of the muscle, to be inserted into the posterior surface of the

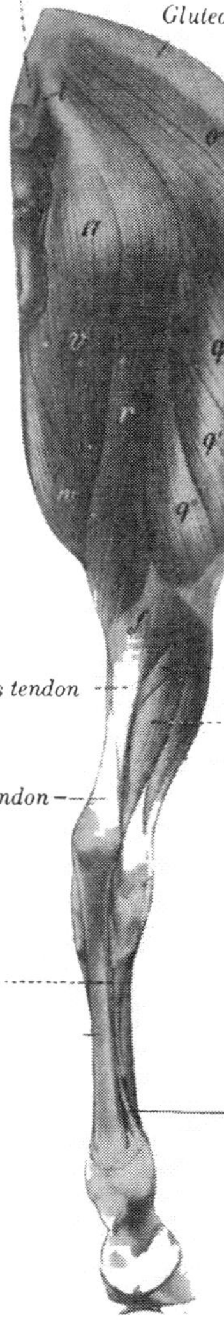

FIG. 199.—MUSCLES OF PELVIC LIMB OF HORSE, POSTERO-EXTERNAL VIEW.
17, Position of tuber ischii; *o''*, superficial gluteus; *q*, *q'*, *q''*, biceps femoris; *r*, semitendinosus; *t*, sacro-coccygeus lateralis; *v*, semimembranosus; *w*, gracilis; *f*, gastrocnemius. (After Ellenberger-Baum, Anat. f. Künstler.)

femur near the third trochanter (Fig. 455), a bursa being interposed between the tendon and the bone. The muscle then divides into three portions, which terminate on a strong aponeurosis over the junction of the thigh and leg. The anterior branch is directed toward the patella, the middle toward the tibial crest, while the posterior one assists in the formation of the posterior contour of the limb. The aponeurosis blends with the deep layer of the fascia cruris, as already described. A synovial **bursa** occurs under the patellar insertion.

Relations.—Superficially, the skin and fascia; deeply, the sacro-iliac and sacro-sciatic ligaments, the coccygeal fascia, the femur, the obturator, gemellus, quadratus femoris, adductor, semimembranosus, vastus externus, and gastrocnemius muscles, branches of the lateral sacral, gluteal, obturator, femoral and deep femoral vessels, the great sciatic, tibial, peroneal, and posterior gluteal nerves; in front, the superficial and middle glutei; behind and internally, the semitendinosus.

Blood-supply.—Gluteal, obturator, and femoro-popliteal arteries.

Nerve-supply.—Posterior gluteal and great sciatic nerves.

6. **Semitendinosus** (Biceps rotator tibialis).—This is a long muscle which extends from the first two coccygeal vertebræ to the proximal third of the inner surface of the tibia. It lies at first behind the biceps, then passes downward on the back of the thigh, between that muscle and the semimembranosus (Figs. 178, 179, 199). It has two heads of origin.

Origin.—(1) The transverse processes of the first and second coccygeal vertebræ, the coccygeal fascia, and the intermuscular septum between this muscle and the biceps femoris; (2) the ventral surface of the tuber ischii.

Insertion.—(1) The tibial crest; (2) the crural fascia and the tuber calcis.

Action.—To flex the stifle and rotate the leg inward; also to extend the hip and hock joints, acting with the biceps and semimembranosus in propulsion of the trunk, rearing, etc.

Structure.—The long or vertebral head is small at its origin, but becomes larger by the accession of fibers arising on the intermuscular septum. Below the tuber ischii it is joined by the short head, which arises partly by fleshy fibers, partly by a common tendon with the biceps. The muscle then passes downward on the back of the thigh, and terminates on a wide tendon on the inner surface of the proximal third of the leg. A distinct band passes forward to be inserted on the tibial crest (a **bursa** lying between the tendon and the tibia), part fuses with the fascia of the leg, while the remainder joins the biceps tendon and concurs in the formation of the tendinous band, which, as before described, terminates on the tuber calcis (Fig. 458). A **bursa** may occur under the long head where it passes over the tuber ischii.

Relations.—Externally, the skin and fascia, the biceps, and the internal head of the gastrocnemius; internally, the coccygeal fascia, the sacro-sciatic ligament, the semimembranosus; anteriorly, the biceps femoris, branches of the femoral artery, and the great sciatic nerve.

Blood-supply.—Posterior gluteal, obturator, and femoro-popliteal arteries

Nerve-supply.—Posterior gluteal and great sciatic nerves.

7. **Semimembranosus**[1] (Figs. 179, 186, 199, 451).—This muscle lies on the inner surface of the preceding muscle and the gastrocnemius, and has two heads of origin.

Origin.—(1) The posterior border of the sacro-sciatic ligament; (2) the ventral surface of the tuber ischii.

Insertion.—The internal epicondyle of the femur, behind the lateral ligament.

Action.—To extend the hip joint and to adduct the limb.

Structure.—The long head, small and pointed above, extends toward the root of the tail, fusing with the sacro-sciatic ligament. Passing downward, it becomes larger and covers in part the posterior aspect of the tuber ischii. A **bursa** may be found here. Below this it joins the short head, which is much larger. The large belly so formed passes downward and forward, covered in great part by the gracilis, and terminates on a short, flat tendon of insertion at the distal end of the femur.

Relations.—The upper part of the muscle assists in forming the lateral boun-

[1] This muscle was incorrectly designated the adductor magnus by Percivall and Strangeways. Its name, however, is not at all descriptive of its structure in the domesticated animals.

dary of the pelvic outlet. It is related posteriorly and externally to the skin and fascia and the semitendinosus; internally, to the anus and its muscles, the vulva in the female, and the internal pudic artery and nerve (Figs. 452, 453). Below the pelvis the chief relations are: externally, the semitendinosus, biceps, and gastrocnemius, branches of the obturator, femoral, and femoro-popliteal arteries, and the great sciatic nerve and its chief branches; internally, the crus penis and ischio-cavernosus muscle (in the male), and the gracilis; in front, the adductor and the femoral vessels; behind, the skin and fascia.

Blood-supply.—Obturator and femoral arteries.

Nerve-supply.—Great sciatic nerve.

IV. THE INTERNAL MUSCLES OF THE THIGH

The muscles of this group are arranged in three layers.

First Layer

1. **Sartorius** (Figs. 186, 202, 203).—This long and rather narrow muscle is the most anterior one of the first layer. It extends from the sublumbar region to the lower and inner part of the stifle.

Origin.—The iliac fascia and the tendon of the psoas minor.

Insertion.—The internal straight ligament of the patella and the adjacent part of the tuberosity of the tibia.

Action.—To flex the hip joint and adduct the limb.

Structure.—The muscle is very thin at its origin, but becomes thicker and narrower as it passes downward and a little backward. It terminates near the stifle joint on an aponeurosis which blends with that of the gracilis and with the fascia of the leg.

Relations.—Superficially, the inguinal (Poupart's) ligament, the abdominal muscles, the skin and fascia, and the saphenous vessels and nerve; deeply, the ilio-psoas, quadriceps femoris, and adductor. It forms the anterior boundary of the femoral canal, in which the femoral artery and vein and the deep inguinal lymph glands are situated (Fig. 451).

Blood-supply.—Femoral artery.

Nerve-supply.—Femoral and saphenous nerves.

2. **Gracilis** (Figs. 186, 199, 202, 203).—This is a wide, flat, quadrilateral muscle, situated behind the sartorius, which it exceeds greatly in extent.

Origin.—The middle third of the pelvic symphysis, the prepubic tendon and pubo-femoral ligament, and the ventral surface of the pubis behind the prepubic tendon.

Insertion.—The internal straight ligament of the patella, the internal surface of the tibia in front of the lateral ligament of the stifle joint, and the fascia of the leg.

Action.—To adduct the limb. It may also rotate it inward.

Structure.—The muscle arises by a strong tendon, chiefly in common with the opposite muscle. Its direct attachment to the ventral surface of the pelvis is not so extensive as a superficial inspection would suggest. The origin of the muscle presents anteriorly a round perforation for the passage of the external pudic vein. The belly is composed of parallel bundles, and is marked by a superficial furrow which, however, does not indicate a muscular division. It terminates on the inner surface of the stifle on a thin wide tendon which blends in front with that of the sartorius, below with the crural fascia.

Relations.—Superficially, the skin and fascia, the penis or mammary gland, and the saphenous vessels and nerve; deeply, the pectineus, adductor, semimembranosus and semitendinosus, and, at the middle of the femur, the femoral vessels; anteriorly, the sartorius. In the upper third of the thigh the sartorius and gracilis are separated by a triangular interval (femoral triangle), in which lie the deep inguinal lymph glands and the femoral vessels.

Blood-supply.—Femoral and deep femoral arteries.

Nerve-supply.—Obturator and saphenous nerves.

Second Layer

1. **Pectineus** (Figs. 186, 451, 456).—This muscle is fusiform and extends from the anterior border of the pubis to the middle of the inner border of the femur.

Origin.—The prepubic tendon, the pubo-femoral ligament, and the anterior border of the pubis.

Insertion.—The middle of the internal border of the femur, near the nutrient foramen.

Action.—To adduct the limb and flex the hip joint.

Structure.—The belly is cylindrical and contains little fibrous tissue. Its origin is perforated by the pubo-femoral ligament, and is thus divided into two unequal parts. The large upper part arises mainly from the prepubic tendon —only a very small part gaining direct attachment to the pubis. The small lower part does not reach the bone. The insertion is pointed and tendinous.

Relations.—Superficially, the gracilis; deeply, the femur, the vastus internus, the terminal tendon of the psoas major and iliacus, and the deep femoral artery; anteriorly, the sartorius, the femoral vessels, the saphenous nerve, and the deep inguinal lymph glands; posteriorly, the adductor, obturator externus, and quadratus femoris, and the obturator nerve (anterior division).

Blood-supply.—Femoral and deep femoral arteries.

Nerve-supply.—Femoral and obturator nerves.

The *femoral canal* is exposed in the dissection of the preceding muscles (Figs. 200, 451). It is bounded anteriorly by the sartorius, posteriorly by the pectineus, and externally by the iliacus and vastus internus. Its internal wall is formed by the femoral fascia and the gracilis. Its upper or abdominal opening (Lacuna vasorum) lies behind and a little internal to the internal inguinal ring and is bounded anteriorly by the inguinal ligament, posteriorly by the anterior border of the pubis, and externally by the tendon of the psoas minor. The canal terminates below at the insertion of the pectineus. It contains the deep inguinal lymph glands, the femoral artery and vein, and the saphenous nerve.

2. **Adductor**[1] (Figs. 179, 186, 451) (Great and small adductors of the thigh).—This fleshy, prismatic muscle lies behind the pectineus and vastus internus. It extends downward and forward from the ventral surface of the pelvis to the internal condyle of the femur.

Origin.—The ventral surface of the pubis and ischium and the tendon of the gracilis.

Insertion.—(1) The posterior surface of the femur from the level of the external trochanter to the groove for the femoral vessels; (2) the internal epicondyle of the femur and the internal lateral ligament of the stifle joint.

Action.—To adduct the limb and assist in extending the hip joint. It may also rotate the femur outward.

Structure.—It is almost entirely fleshy, and is composed of parallel bundles united rather loosely. It is usually possible to separate from the principal mass a small anterior short portion,[2] which is inserted into the femur behind the pectineus. The principal mass[3] is perforated below its middle by the femoral vessels, and is

[1] It has been customary to describe two adductors—a parvus or brevis, and a longus or magnus. This division is largely artificial, and has been abandoned in the new nomenclature—a return to the views of Bourgelat and Girard.

[2] This has been termed by various authors the adductor parvus or brevis.

[3] Termed by various authors the adductor magnus or longus.

thus divided into two branches. The outer branch is inserted into the back of the femur with the short portion, while the inner branch is attached to the internal epicondyle and lateral ligament. There is often a superficial slip which reaches the internal straight patellar ligament. Some fibers pass under the lateral ligament and end on the tendon of the semimembranosus.

Relations.—Internally, the gracilis, and branches of the femoral artery and of the obturator nerve; externally, the femur, the obturator externus, quadratus femoris, biceps femoris, and gastrocnemius, and the femoral, deep femoral, and obturator arteries; anteriorly, the pectineus, vastus internus, and a large branch of the obturator nerve; posteriorly, the semimembranosus and the great sciatic nerve.

Blood-supply.—Femoral, deep femoral, and obturator arteries.

Nerve-supply.—Obturator nerve.

3. **Semimembranosus.**—Described on p. 280.

Third Layer

1. **Quadratus femoris** (Ischio-femoralis).—This is a narrow, flat muscle, which lies under cover of the upper part of the adductor (Figs. 455, 456).

Origin.—The ventral surface of the ischium, just in front of the semimembranosus.

Insertion.—An oblique line on the posterior surface of the femur, near the lower part of the internal trochanter.

Action.—To extend the hip joint, and to adduct the thigh and rotate it outward.

Structure.—It is composed of parallel bundles of fibers directed downward, forward, and outward.

Relations.—Internally, the adductor, semimembranosus, and the obturator vessels; externally, the obturator externus and biceps femoris, the deep femoral artery, and the great sciatic nerve.

Blood-supply.—Deep femoral and obturator arteries.

Nerve-supply.—Great sciatic nerve.

2. **Obturator Externus** (Fig. 456).—This is a pyramidal muscle which extends across the back of the hip joint from the obturator foramen to the trochanteric fossa.

Origin.—The ventral surface of the pubis and ischium, and the margin of the obturator foramen.

Insertion.—The trochanteric fossa.

Action.—To adduct the thigh and to rotate it outward.

Structure.—It is almost entirely fleshy, the muscle-bundles being rather loosely connected. The insertion is pointed, flattened, and partly tendinous. The origin is perforated by the obturator vessels and nerve.

Relations.—Internally, the adductor and quadratus femoris and the deep femoral vessels; externally, the gemellus, the tendon of the obturator internus, the biceps femoris, and the great sciatic nerve; anteriorly, the hip joint, the pectineus, and the external pudic vein.

Blood-supply.—Deep femoral and obturator arteries.

Nerve-supply.—Obturator nerve.

3. **Obturator internus** (Fig. 451).—This arises by two heads within the pelvic cavity, the tendon emerging through the lesser sciatic foramen.

Origin.—(1) The pelvic surface of the pubis and ischium around the obturator foramen; (2) the pelvic surface of the shaft of the ilium and the wing of the sacrum.

Insertion.—The trochanteric fossa.

Action.—To rotate the femur outward.

Structure.—The ischio-pubic head lies on the pelvic floor and covers the obturator foramen. It is thin and fan-shaped. The iliac head extends along the lateral wall of the pelvis, and is pennate, with a central tendon throughout. Both terminate on a flat tendon which passes outward through the lesser sciatic foramen to be inserted into the trochanteric fossa. A synovial **bursa** facilitates the play of the tendon over the external border of the ischium.[1]

Relations.—The pelvic surface is covered by the pelvic fascia and the peritoneum. The obturator vessels and nerve lie between the two heads, and the internal pudic vessels and nerve lie along the dorsal edge of the iliac head.

Blood-supply.—Obturator and internal pudic arteries.

Nerve-supply.—Great sciatic nerve.

4. **Gemellus**[2] (Fig. 455).—This is a thin, triangular muscle, which extends from the external border of the ischium to the trochanteric fossa.

Origin.—The external border of the ischium near the ischiatic spine.

Insertion.—The trochanteric fossa.

Action.—To rotate the femur outward.

Structure.—Fleshy, some fibers being inserted into the tendon of the obturator internus.

Relations.—Dorsally, the tendon of the obturator internus and the gluteus profundus; ventrally, the obturator externus.

Blood-supply.—Obturator artery

Nerve-supply.—Sciatic nerve.

III. ANTERIOR MUSCLES OF THE THIGH

This group consists of the sartorius, quadriceps femoris, and capsularis.

1. **Sartorius.**—This is described on p. 281.

2. **Quadriceps femoris** (Figs. 179, 186, 200) (Crural triceps).—This constitutes the large muscular mass which covers the front and sides of the femur. It has four heads, one of which, the rectus, arises from the ilium; the other three arise from the femur. All are inserted into the patella.

(1) **Rectus femoris.**—This is fusiform and rounded. It arises by two tendons.

Origin.—Two depressions on the shaft of the ilium above and in front of the acetabulum.

Insertion.—The base and anterior surface of the patella.

Action.—To extend the stifle joint and to flex the hip joint.

Structure.—It has two short strong tendons of origin; beneath the outer one is a **bursa.** The belly is rounded and rests in a groove formed by the other portions of the quadriceps. Its sides are covered by a strong tendinous layer which furnishes insertion to fibers of the vasti. The tendon of insertion is formed by the fusion of these tendinous layers on the lower part of the muscle. The lower portion of the muscle is pennate, the fibers on either side converging on the tendon at an acute angle.

Relations.—Internally, the iliacus, sartorius, and vastus internus; externally, the tensor fasciæ latæ, glutei, and vastus externus; posteriorly, the hip joint and the vastus intermedius; anteriorly, the fascia lata and the skin. The anterior

[1] The iliac head is described by some authors as a separate muscle, and termed the pyriformis. This does not seem desirable, especially since it is at least probable that the homologue of the pyriformis of man is that portion of the middle gluteus which is inserted into the back of the trochanteric ridge.

[2] The name is based on the arrangement in man, in whom the muscle consists of two fasciculi forming a groove between them for the tendon of the obturator internus. In the horse it is undivided, and is grooved for the obturator tendon, so that at first sight it appears to be double. The gemellus may be regarded as the extrapelvic head of the obturator internus (Gegenbaur).

femoral artery and branches of the femoral nerve descend into the interspace be tween the upper part of the rectus and the vastus internus; similarly, the iliaco femoral artery dips in between the rectus femoris and vastus externus.

Blood-supply.—Femoral and iliaco-femoral arteries.

Nerve-supply.—Femoral nerve.

(2) **Vastus externus** (s. lateralis).—This lies on the outer surface of the thigh, extending from the great trochanter to the patella. It is thick and wide in its upper part, and becomes much thinner and narrow below.

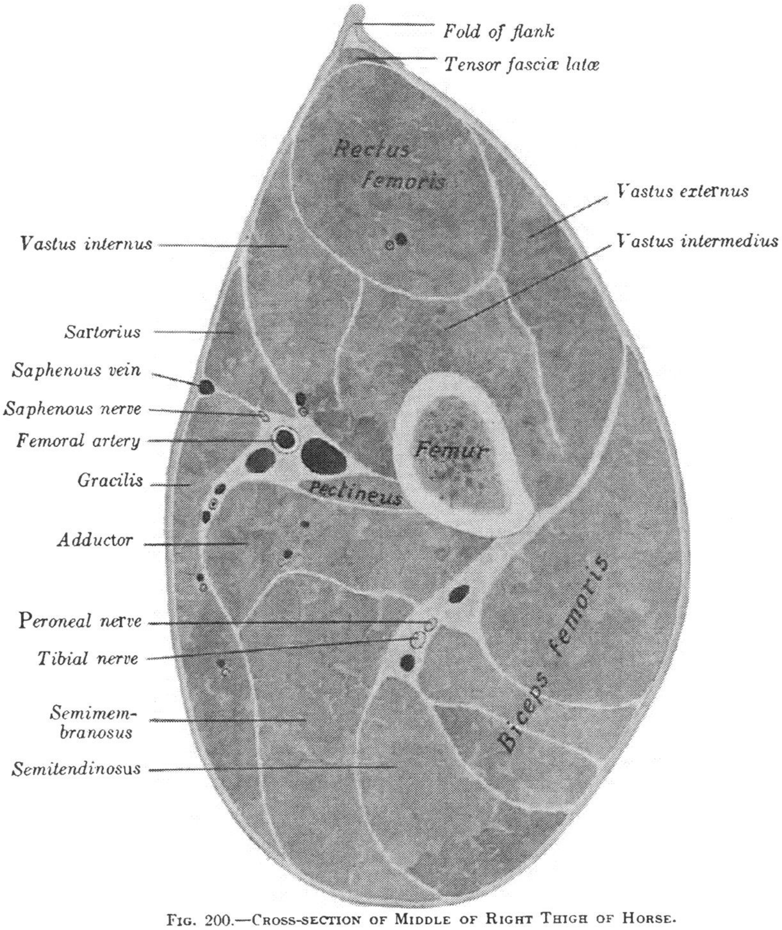

FIG. 200.—CROSS-SECTION OF MIDDLE OF RIGHT THIGH OF HORSE.

Origin.—The external border and surface of the femur, from the great trochanter to the supracondyloid fossa.

Insertion.—(1) The outer part of the anterior surface of the patella; (2) the tendon of the rectus femoris.

Action.—To extend the stifle joint.

Structure.—The fibers are directed downward and forward, many being inserted into the tendinous sheet which covers the side of the rectus. A bursa is often found between the distal end and the patella.

Relations.—Externally, the fascia lata and skin, tensor fasciæ latæ, superficial gluteus, and biceps femoris; internally, the femur and femoro-patellar joint capsule, the rectus femoris, vastus intermedius, and the iliaco-femoral artery.

Blood-supply.—Iliaco-femoral artery.

Nerve-supply.—Femoral nerve.

(3) **Vastus internus** (s. medialis).—This is smaller than the preceding muscle and lies in a similar position on the inner side of the thigh.

Origin.—The internal surface of the femur, from the neck to the distal third.

Insertion.—(1) The upper part of the inner border of the patella and its carti lage; (2) the tendon of the rectus femoris.

Action.—To extend the stifle joint.

Structure.—This is very similar to that of the vastus externus. It is, however, more difficult to separate from the intermedius, because many fibers of the latter arise on the tendinous sheet which covers the contact surface of the inner vastus. Its insertion into the patella is chiefly by means of a broad strong tendon. From the deep face fleshy fibers are inserted also into the femoro-patellar capsule.

Relations.—Internally, the skin and fascia lata, the iliacus, sartorius, pectineus, and adductor, the femoral vessels and saphenous nerve; externally, the femur, femoro-patellar joint capsule, rectus femoris, and vastus intermedius, the anterior femoral artery, and branches of the femoral nerve.

Blood-supply.—Femoral and anterior femoral arteries.

Nerve-supply.—Femoral nerve.

(4) **Vastus intermedius** (Crureus).—This muscle is deeply situated on the anterior face of the femur, and is entirely covered by the preceding heads.

Origin.—(1) The anterior and external surfaces of the femur, from the proximal to the distal fourth; (2) the aponeurosis of the vastus internus.

Insertion.—(1) The base of the patella; (2) the femoro-patellar joint capsule.

Action.—(1) To extend the stifle joint; (2) to tense (raise) the femoro-patellar capsule during extension of the joint.

Structure.—The muscle is usually quite difficult to isolate from the other vasti, so that many since Günther have declared it an artefact.[1] It is entirely fleshy, and is small at its proximal end, but when traced downward increases in bulk by the accession of fibers arising on the femur and the tendinous covering of the vastus internus. The terminal part is intimately adherent to the femoro-patellar joint capsule, where the latter bulges upward above the level of the patella.

Relations.—Internally, the vastus internus; externally, the vastus externus; anteriorly, the rectus; posteriorly, the femur and femoro-patellar capsule.

Blood-supply.—Iliaco-femoral and anterior femoral arteries.

Nerve-supply.—Femoral nerve.

The straight ligaments of the patella are to be regarded as tendons of the quadriceps which communicate the action of the latter to the tibia, the patella being intercalated as a sesamoid bone.

3. **Capsularis** (Fig. 154) (Rectus parvus).—This is a small muscle (scarcely as large as one's finger), which arises on the ilium immediately above the outer tendon of the rectus femoris, and passes down between the vastus internus and externus to be inserted into the anterior surface of the femur. It passes over the front of the hip joint, to the capsule of which some fibers are attached. Sometimes the muscle has two distinct heads, in which case the additional head arises between the two tendons of origin of the rectus femoris. Its action may be to raise the capsule during flexion of the joint.

[1] While it is true that the separation of the intermedius is probably never entirely a natural one in the horse, it varies in individual cases, and is usually clear on cross-sections. In some subjects it is possible to separate another slip which may represent the articularis genu of man.

IV. THE MUSCLES OF THE LEG AND FOOT

The muscles of this region cover almost all of the tibia except its internal face, which is largely subcutaneous. As in the forearm, the muscles fall into two groups,

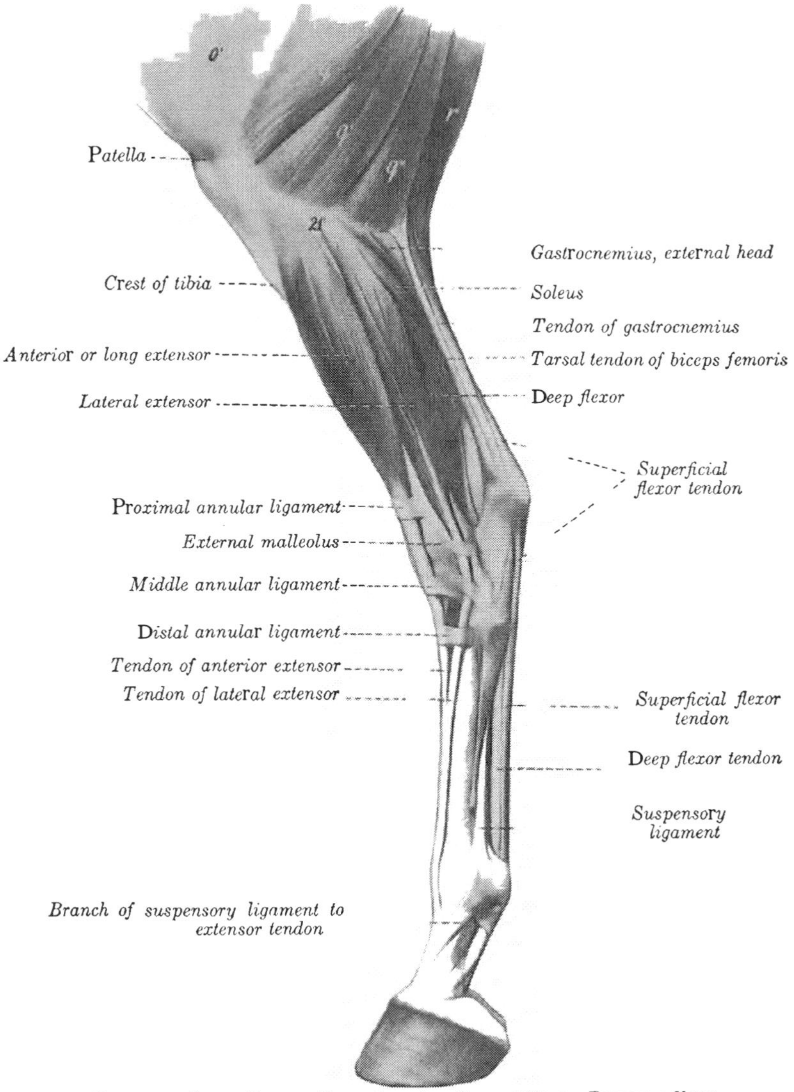

Fig. 201.—Muscles of Lower Part of Thigh, Leg, and Foot of Horse, External View.
o' Fascia lata; q, q', q'', biceps femoris; r, semitendinosus; 21', external condyle of tibia. (After Ellenberger-Baum, Anat. für Künstler.)

an anterior or dorso-lateral, and a posterior or plantar. The muscles of the first group are extensors of the digit and flexors of the hock, those of the second have the opposite action.

A. Anterior Group

1. **Anterior or long digital extensor** (M. extensor digitalis longus; extensor pedis; anterior extensor of the phalanges).—This muscle is situated superficially on the antero-external aspect of the leg, and is provided with a long tendon which passes down over the front of the tarsus, metatarsus, and digit.

Origin.—The small fossa (Fossa extensoria) between the external condyle and the trochlea of the femur.

Insertion.—(1) The extensor process of the third phalanx; (2) the anterior surface of the proximal extremities of the first and second phalanges.

Action.—To extend the digit and flex the hock. It also assists in fixing the stifle joint.

Structure.—The origin is by means of a strong tendon in common with the peroneus tertius, on which also many fibers arise. The common tendon passes downward in the groove between the outer condyle and the tuberosity of the tibia, where a pouch from the femoro-tibial capsule descends four or five inches (ca. 10 to 12 cm.) beneath the tendon. The belly is fusiform and somewhat flattened. The long tendon of insertion begins in the belly about its middle, and is clear of the fleshy part near the tarsus. It passes downward over the front of the hock, bound down by the three annular ligaments already described (see crural fascia), and enveloped by a **synovial sheath** which begins a little above the level of the external malleolus, and extends nearly to the junction with the lateral extensor tendon. This union occurs usually about a hand's breadth below the tarsus. In the angle of union the extensor brevis also joins the principal tendon. Beyond this point the arrangement is the same as in the fore limb.

Relations.—Superficially, the skin and fascia; deeply, the femoro-tibial capsule, peroneus tertius, and tibialis anterior; behind, the lateral extensor and the superficial and deep peroneal nerves. In front of the tarsus the anterior tibial artery crosses the deep face of the tendon (Fig. 460).

Blood-supply.—Anterior tibial artery.

Nerve-supply.—Peroneal nerve.

2. **Lateral digital extensor** (M. extensor digitalis lateralis; peroneus; lateral extensor of the phalanges).—This muscle lies on the outer surface of the leg, behind the preceding one.

Origin.—The external lateral ligament of the stifle joint, the fibula, the external border of the tibia, and the interosseus ligament.

Insertion.—The tendon of the anterior extensor, about a third of the way down the metatarsus.

Action.—To assist the anterior extensor.

Structure.—The belly is fusiform, flattened, and pennate. The tendon runs through the entire length of the belly and becomes free from it at the lower fourth of the tibia. It passes downward through the groove on the external malleolus, bound down by an annular ligament, and, inclining forward, blends (usually) with the tendon of the anterior extensor. It is provided with a **synovial sheath,** which begins about one inch (ca. 2 to 3 cm.) above the external malleolus and ends about one and one-half inches (ca. 3 to 4 cm.) above the junction. Sometimes the fusion does not occur, and the tendon then passes down the metatarsus, alongside of that of the long extensor, to be inserted into the first phalanx like the corresponding muscle of the thoracic limb.

Relations.—Externally, the skin and fascia and the superficial peroneal nerve; internally, the tibia and fibula; anteriorly, the intermuscular septum, the long extensor, and the tibialis anterior; posteriorly, the deep flexor and the soleus.

Blood-supply.—Anterior tibial artery.

Nerve-supply.—Peroneal nerve.

3. **Peroneus tertius** (Tendinous part of the flexor metatarsi; tendo femorotarseus [Schmaltz]).—This consists in the horse of a strong tendon which lies between the anterior extensor and the tibialis anterior.

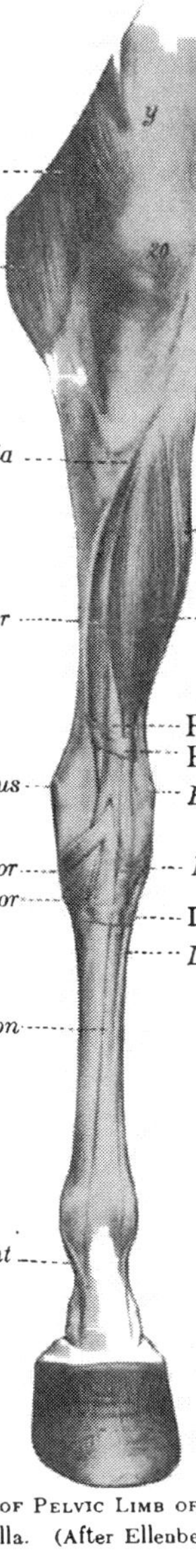

FIG. 202.—MUSCLES OF PELVIC LIMB OF HORSE, ANTERIOR VIEW.
y, Rectus femoris; *20*, patella. (After Ellenberger-Baum, Anat. für Künstler.)

Origin.—The fossa extensoria (between the external condyle and the trochlea of the femur), in common with the anterior extensor.

[1] It seems inadvisable to retain the old nomenclature, since it is inapplicable to other domesticated animals in which the muscle is well developed (*e. g.*, ox, pig).

Insertion.—(1) The proximal extremities of the large (third) and external small (fourth) metatarsal bones, and the third tarsal bone; (2) the fibular and fourth tarsal bones.

Action.—Mechanically to flex the hock when the stifle joint is flexed.

Structure.—This is entirely tendinous. The proximal end and the underlying prolongation of the synovial membrane of the femoro-tibial joint have been mentioned in the description of the anterior extensor. Fibers of the latter muscle and of the tibialis anterior arise on the tendon as it passes downward to the front of the hock. At the distal end of the tibia the tendon divides into two branches, between which the tendon of the tibialis anterior emerges. The anterior branch is attached to the third tarsal and third and fourth metatarsal bones, while the outer one curves outward, bifurcates, and is inserted into the fibular and fourth tarsal bones (Fig. 460).

Relations.—Superficially, the anterior extensor; deeply, the tibialis anterior. The anterior tibial vessels cross the deep face of the outer branch.

4. **Tibialis anterior** (Muscular portion of the flexor metatarsi).—This lies on the antero-external face of the tibia; it is wide and flattened above, pointed below.

Origin.—The external condyle and border of the tibia and a small area on the external surface of the tuberosity.

Insertion.—(1) The metatarsal tuberosity; (2) the first and second tarsal bones.

Action.—To flex the hock joint.

Structure.—The origin is fleshy, and is divided by the groove in which lie the common tendon of the long extensor and peroneus tertius and a synovial pouch. Passing downward on the tibia, the belly is united by tendinous and fleshy fibers with the peroneus tertius, and terminates close to the tarsus in a point on the tendon of insertion. The latter emerges between the branches of the peroneus tertius and bifurcates, the anterior branch being inserted into the metatarsal tuberosity, the inner one (cunean tendon) into the fused first and second tarsal bones (cuneiform parvum). The tendon is provided with a **synovial sheath** at its emergence, and a bursa (cunean bursa) is interposed between the inner branch and the internal lateral ligament.

Relations.—Superficially, the anterior and lateral extensors, the peroneus tertius, and the deep peroneal nerve; deeply, the tibia, the deep flexor, and the anterior tibial vessels.

Blood-supply.—Anterior tibial artery.

Nerve-supply.—Peroneal nerve.

B. Posterior Group

1. **Gastrocnemius** (Figs. 179, 201, 203).—This muscle extends from the lower third of the femur to the point of the hock. It arises by two heads.

Origin.—(1) Outer head, from the external rough margin of the supracondyloid fossa (Fossa plantaris); (2) inner head, from the supracondyloid crest.

Insertion.—The posterior part of the tuber calcis.

Action.—To extend the hock.

Structure.—The two bellies are thick, fusiform, and somewhat flattened. They are covered by a strong aponeurosis and contain tendinous intersections. They terminate toward the middle of the leg on a common tendon (Tendo calcaneus s. Achillis), which at first lies posterior to that of the superficial flexor, but, by a twist in both, comes to lie in front of the latter. The deep fascia blends with the tendon throughout its length, and the soleus muscle is inserted into its anterior edge. A small **bursa** (Bursa tendinis calcanei) lies in front of the insertion on the tuber calcis, and a large **bursa** is interposed between the two tendons from the twist downward. The superficial flexor lies between the two heads and is adherent to the outer one (Fig. 459).

Relations.—Anteriorly, the stifle joint, the superficial flexor, popliteus, deep flexor, popliteal vessels, and tibial nerve; internally (above), the semitendinosus,

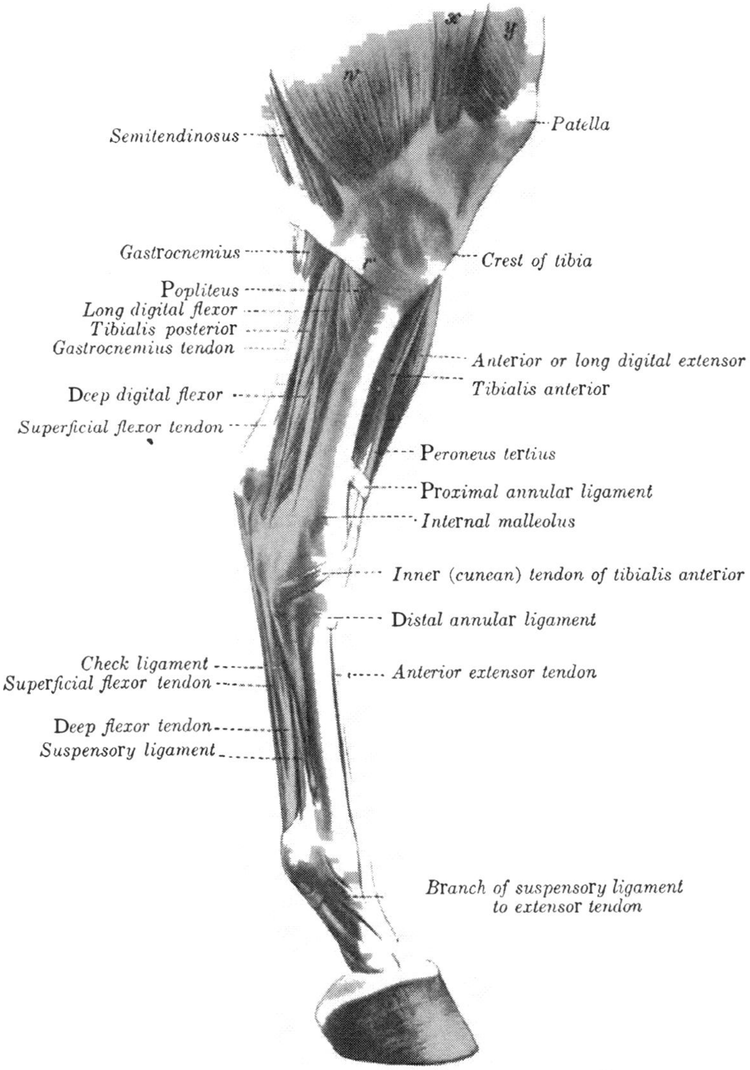

FIG. 203.—MUSCLES OF LEG AND FOOT OF HORSE, INTERNAL VIEW.
r' Tendon of semitendinosus; w, gracilis; x, sartorius; y, vastus internus. (After Ellenberger-Baum, Anat. für Künstler.)

semimembranosus, and adductor, (below) the fascia and skin; externally (above), the biceps femoris and peroneal (anterior tibial) nerve, (below) the fascia and skin.

Blood-supply.—Popliteal artery.

Nerve-supply.—Tibial nerve.

2. **Soleus** (Fig. 201).—This muscle is very small in the horse. It lies immediately under the deep fascia, on the proximal half of the outer surface of the leg, and is directed obliquely downward and backward.

Origin.—The head of the fibula.

Insertion.—The tendon of the gastrocnemius, about the middle of the leg.

Action.—To assist the gastrocnemius.

Structure.—It is a thin, fleshy band, about an inch (ca. 2 to 3 cm.) in width, terminating on a thin tendon which fuses with that of the gastrocnemius.[1]

Relations.—Superficially, the skin, fascia, and peroneal nerve; deeply, the lateral extensor and deep flexor.

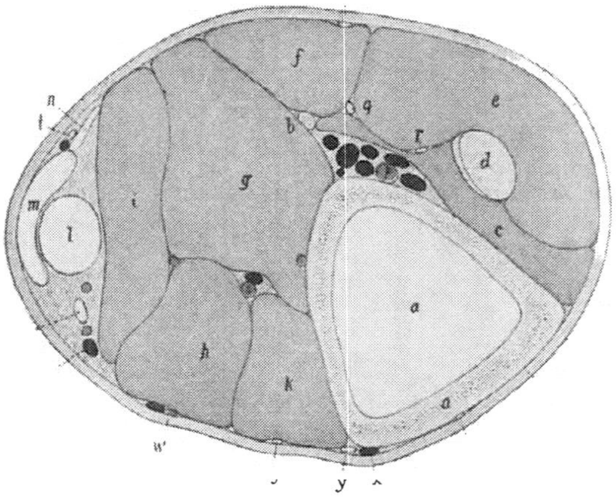

FIG. 204.—CROSS-SECTION OF LEFT LEG OF HORSE; SECTION IS CUT A LITTLE ABOVE MIDDLE OF REGION.

a, Tibia; *b*, fibula; *c*, tibialis anterior; *d*, peroneus tertius; *e*, anterior or long digital extensor; *f*, lateral extensor; *g*, deep head of deep flexor (flexor hallucis longus); *h*, inner head of deep flexor (flexor accessorius s. digitorum longus); *i*, superficial head of deep flexor (tibialis posterior); k, popliteus; *l*, superficial flexor tendon; *m*, gastrocnemius tendon; *n*, soleus; *o*, skin; *p*, anterior tibial artery; *q*, superficial peroneal nerve; *q'*, deep peroneal nerve; *r*, branch of q; *s*, posterior tibial artery; *t*, cutaneous nerve; *u*, tibial nerve; *v*, recurrent tibial vein; *w*, saphenous artery; *x*, saphenous vein; *y*, branches of saphenous nerve. (After Ellenberger, in Leisering's Atlas.)

Blood-supply. — Posterior tibial artery.

Nerve-supply.—Tibial nerve.

3. **Superficial digital flexor or flexor pedis perforatus** (Figs. 199, 201, 203) (M. flexor digitalis pedis sublimis; superficial flexor of the phalanges).—The proximal part of this muscle lies between and under cover of the two heads of the gastrocnemius (Fig. 459). It consists almost entirely of a strong tendon, the belly being very little developed.

Origin.—The supracondyloid fossa (Fossa plantaris) of the femur.

Insertion.—(1) The front and sides of the tuber calcis; (2) the eminences on the proximal extremity of the second phalanx, and the distal extremity of the first phalanx behind the lateral ligament.

Action.—To flex the digit and extend the hock joint. On account of the exceedingly small amount of muscular tissue the action is to be regarded chiefly as a mechanical effect, resulting from the action of other muscles on the stifle joint.

Structure.—The origin is by means of a strong round tendon which is incompletely covered with fleshy fibers as far as the upper third of the leg. It is pretty intimately attached to the gastrocnemius, especially to the outer head. At the distal third of the tibia it winds around the inner surface of the gastrocnemius tendon, and then occupies a position behind the latter. At the point of the hock it widens out, forming a sort of cap over the tuber calcis, detaching on either side a strong band which is inserted into the tuber calcis with the tarsal tendon of the biceps and semitendinosus. It then passes downward over the plantar (Calcaneometatarsal) ligament, becomes narrower, and is arranged below as in the thoracic limb. A large synovial bursa lies under the tendon from the distal fourth of the

[1] The soleus may, therefore, be included with the two heads of the gastrocnemius under the name triceps suræ.

tibia to the middle of the tarsus. A subcutaneous bursa is sometimes found on the wide part of the tendon at the point of the hock. (Either or both of these bursæ may be involved in so-called "capped hock.")

Relations.—Posteriorly, the gastrocnemius, fascia, and skin; anteriorly, the femoro-patellar capsule, the popliteus, the deep flexor, and the popliteal vessels; internally, the tibial nerve.

Blood-supply.— Femoro-popliteal artery.

Nerve-supply.—Tibial nerve.

4. **Deep digital flexor or flexor pedis perforans** (M. flexor digitalis pedis pro-

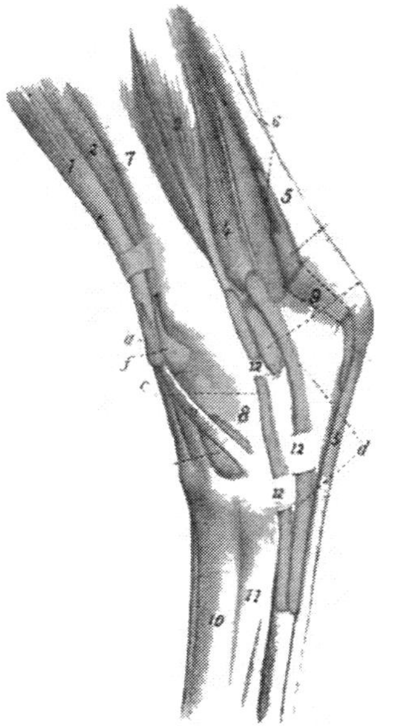

FIG. 205.—INJECTED SYNOVIAL SHEATHS AND BURSÆ OF TARSAL REGION OF HORSE, INNER VIEW.

a, Synovial sheath of peroneus tertius and tibialis anterior; *b*, bursa under inner (cunean) tendon of tibialis anterior; *c*, synovial sheath of flexor longus s. accessorius; *d*, tarsal sheath of deep flexor; *e*, *e'*, bursa under superficial flexor tendon; *f*, *f'*, tibio-tarsal joint capsule; *1*, anterior extensor; *2*, tibialis anterior; *2'*, inner (cunean) tendon of *2*; *3*, flexor longus; *4*, deep digital flexor; *5*, superficial flexor tendon; *6*, gastrocnemius tendon; *7*, tibia; *8*, tarsus; *9*, tuber calcis; *10*, large metatarsal bone; *11*, inner small metatarsal bone; *12*, *12'*, fascial bands. (After Ellenberger, in Leisering's Atlas.)

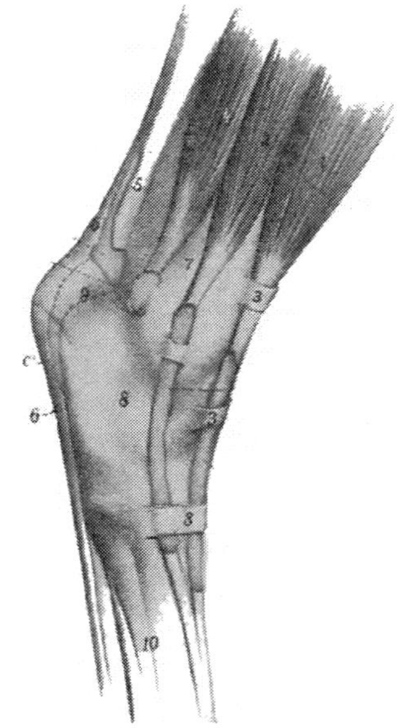

FIG. 206.—INJECTED SYNOVIAL SHEATHS AND BURSÆ OF TARSAL REGION OF HORSE, EXTERNAL VIEW.

a, Synovial sheath of anterior or long digital extensor; *b*, synovial sheath of lateral digital extensor; *c*, *c'*, bursa under superficial flexor tendon; *d*, capsule of hock joint; *1*, anterior or long extensor; *2*, lateral extensor; *3*, *3*, *3*, annular ligaments; *4*, deep digital flexor; *5*, tendon of gastrocnemius; *6*, superficial flexor tendon; *7*, tibia; *8*, tarsus; *9*, tuber calcis; *10*, metatarsus. (After Ellenberger, in Leisering's Atlas.)

fundus; deep and oblique flexors of the phalanges).—The belly of this muscle lies on the posterior surface of the tibia, and is divisible into three parts or heads, which, however, finally unite on a common tendon of insertion.

Origin.—(1) The posterior edge of the external condyle of the tibia; (2) the external border of the external condyle of the tibia, just behind the facet for the fibula; (3) the middle third of the posterior surface and the upper part of the external border of the tibia, the posterior border of the fibula, and the interosseous ligament.[1]

[1] The origins of these heads are given in the order in which they may be most conveniently dissected, not in order of size and importance.

Insertion.—The semilunar crest of the third phalanx and the adjacent surface of the lateral cartilage.

Action.—To flex the digit and to extend the hock joint.

Structure.—(1) The inner head (M. flexor digitalis longus s. flexor accessorius) is easily isolated (Figs. 203, 459). It has a fusiform belly, which crosses the leg obliquely and lies in a groove formed by the other heads and the popliteus. This terminates near the lower third of the tibia on a round tendon which passes downward, partly embedded in the internal lateral ligament of the hock, and joins the common tendon about a third of the way down the metatarsus. In its course over the inner surface of the hock the tendon lies in a canal formed by the strong tarsal fascia, the tibia, and the lateral ligament, and is provided with a synovial sheath which extends from the distal fourth of the tibia to the junction with the principal tendon. (2) The superficial head (M. tibialis posterior) is only partially separable. It has a flattened belly, terminating near the lower third of the tibia on a flat tendon which soon fuses with the principal tendon. (3) The deep head (M. flexor hallucis longus) is much the largest. It lies on the posterior surface of the tibia, from the popliteal line outward and downward. The belly contains much tendinous tissue, and terminates behind the distal end of the tibia on a strong round tendon. The latter receives the tendon of the tibialis posterior, passes downward in the tarsal groove, bound down by the strong tarsal fascia (Ligamentum laciniatum) and enveloped in a synovial sheath, receives the tendon of the inner head below the hock, and, a little further down, the so-called check ligament (Caput tendineum [Schmaltz]). The tarsal sheath (Vagina tarsea) begins about two to three inches (ca. 5 to 7.5 cm.) above the level of the internal malleolus, and extends about one-fourth of the way down the metatarsus. (Distention of the sheath, as in "thoroughpin," affects chiefly its proximal end.) The check ligament resembles that of the fore limb, except that it is longer and very much weaker; it may be absent. The remainder of the tendon is arranged like that of the thoracic limb.

Relations.—Anteriorly, the tibia and fibula, the popliteus, lateral extensor, tibialis anterior, and the tibial vessels; posteriorly, the gastrocnemius, superficial flexor, and the tibial nerve; externally, the fascia, skin, and the soleus; internally, the fascia and skin.

Blood-supply.—Posterior tibial artery.

Nerve-supply.—Tibial nerve.

5. **Popliteus** (Fig. 203).—This thick and triangular muscle lies on the posterior surface of the femoro-tibial articulation and the posterior surface of the tibia above the popliteal line.

Origin.—A small depression on the external epicondyle of the femur, close to the articular surface and under the lateral ligament.

Insertion.—A triangular area on the posterior surface of the tibia, above and internal to the popliteal line; also the proximal half of the inner border and a narrow adjacent part of the internal surface of the tibia.

Action.—To flex the femoro-tibial joint and to rotate the leg inward.

Structure.—The strong tendon of origin lies at first under the lateral ligament, and curves backward and inward over the external condyle of the tibia and its semilunar cartilage, being invested by a reflection of the synovial capsule of the joint (Fig. 459). The tendon is succeeded by a thick triangular belly, the fibers of which are directed obliquely downward and inward.

Relations.—Superficially, the fascia and skin, semitendinosus, gastrocnemius, superficial flexor; deeply, the femoro-tibial joint, the tibia, the popliteal vessels and their divisions. The saphenous vessels and nerve lie along the inner border of the muscle, separated from it, however, by the deep fascia.

Blood-supply.—Popliteal and posterior tibial arteries.

Nerve-supply.—Tibial nerve.

MUSCLES OF THE METATARSUS AND DIGIT

Extensor pedis brevis (M. extensor digitalis brevis).—This small muscle lies in the angle of union of the long and lateral extensors of the digit. (Shown in Fig. 201, but not marked.)

Origin.—The outer tendon of the peroneus tertius, the middle annular ligament, and the outer lateral ligament of the hock.

Insertion.—The tendon of the anterior or long extensor.

Action.—To assist the anterior or long extensor.

Structure.—It is principally fleshy, having a superficial origin from the annular ligament, and a deep one (by a thin tendon) from the outer tendon of the peroneus tertius. The insertion is by a thin tendon.

Relations.—Superficially, the skin and fascia and the tendons of the anterior and lateral extensors; deeply, the joint capsule, the great metatarsal artery, and the deep peroneal nerve.

Blood-supply.—Great metatarsal artery.

Nerve-supply.—Deep peroneal nerve.

The interossei and **lumbricales** are arranged like those of the thoracic limb, the only noticeable difference being the greater development of the lumbricales in the pelvic limb.

THE MUSCLES OF THE OX

MUSCLES OF THE FACE

The **panniculus** is much more developed than in the horse, presenting as a special feature the extensive **frontalis** muscle, which covers the frontal and nasal regions.

The **orbicularis oris** does not form a complete ring, the defect being in the middle of the upper lip.

The **levator nasolabialis** is extensive, thin, and not very distinct from the frontalis; it divides into two layers, between which the levator labii superioris proprius and the lateral dilator of the nostril pass. The superficial layer ends in the nostril and upper lip, the deep layer on the accessory (lateral) nasal cartilages and on the nasal process of the premaxilla.

The **levator labii superioris proprius** arises on and before the facial tuberosity and terminates by several tendons in the muzzle. It passes between the two layers of the preceding muscle, blending in part with the deep layer.

The **zygomaticus** is much stronger than in the horse. It arises on the masseteric fascia, and ends chiefly in the upper lip.

The **depressor labii superioris** does not resemble the muscle of the same name in the horse. It arises just in front of the facial tuberosity, and divides usually into two branches, which terminate in a number of tendons that form a network in the muzzle and upper lip.

The **incisivus inferior** is a small, rounded muscle, which arises on the body of the mandible below the second and third incisors, and ends in the lower lip, blending with the orbicularis.

The **depressor labii inferioris** is thin, and does not extend as far backward as in the horse; only the anterior end is distinct from the buccinator.

The **buccinator** shows no marked variation, but its superficial layer is well developed.

The **dilatator naris lateralis** arises in front of the facial tuberosity, passes forward between the branches of the levator nasolabialis, and terminates in the outer wing of the nostril.

The dilatator naris transversus is replaced by the **dilatator naris apicalis,** which is situated in the muzzle and joins its fellow at a median raphé. It arises on the border and upper surface of the body of the premaxilla, the fibers passing obliquely upward and outward to the inner wing of the nostril.

The dilatator naris superior arises from the alar cartilage of the nostril and ends in the inner wing of the nostril.

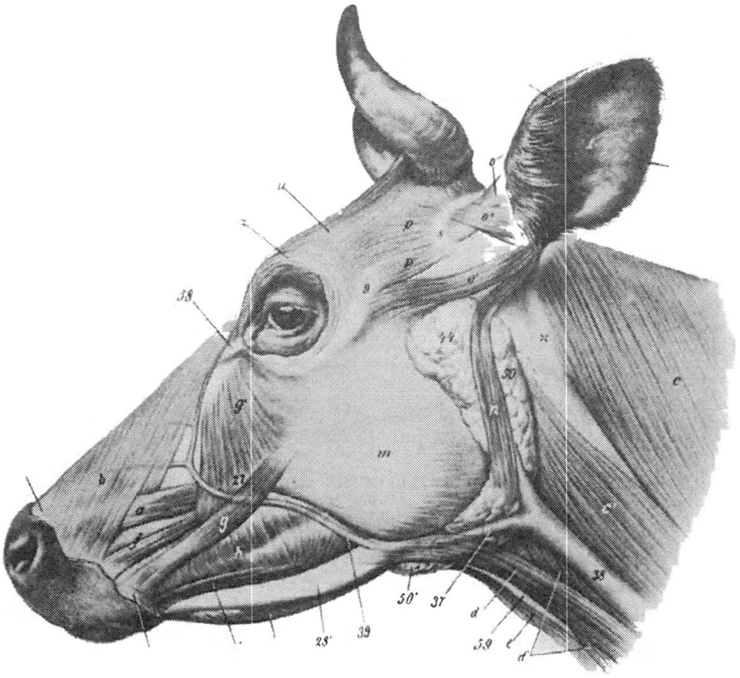

Fig. 207.—Muscles of Head of Ox, Lateral View.

a, Levator labii superioris proprius; *b*, levator nasolabialis; *c*, trapezius; *c'*, mastoido-humeralis; *d*, *d'*, sterno-cephalicus; *e*, omo-hyoideus; *f*, dilatator naris lateralis; *g*, zygomaticus; *g'*, malaris; *h*, buccinator; *i*, depressor labii inferioris; *k*, orbicularis oris; *m*, masseter; *n*, parotido-auricularis; *o'*, zygomatico-auricularis and scutulo-auricularis superficialis inferior; *o''*, scutulo-auricularis superficialis superior; *o'''*, scutulo-auricularis superficialis accessorius; p, p', scutularis; *u*, frontalis; *w*, mylo-hyoideus; *1*, concha; *2*, *3*, posterior and anterior borders of *1*; *8*, scutiform cartilage; *9*, zygomatic arch; *28'*, ramus of mandible; *37*, external maxillary vein; *38*, jugular vein; *39*, facial vein; *44*, parotid gland; *60*, *60'*, submaxillary gland; dotted line at *60* indicates position of large lymph gland, and another lies partly under parotid gland, just in front of *44*; *68*, internal palpebral ligament; *69*, laryngeal prominence. (After Ellenberger-Baum, Anat. für Künstler.)

The **dilatator naris inferior** consists of two layers which arise on the nasal process of the premaxilla and the lateral nasal cartilage and end in the outer wing of the nostril.

The **orbicularis oculi** is well developed.

The corrugator supercilii is not present as a separate muscle, its place and function being taken by the frontalis.

The **malaris** is broad, and spreads out below on the fascia over the buccinator and masseter; it is divided into two parts.

MUSCLES OF MASTICATION

The masseter is not so large as in the horse; a considerable part of it arises on the facial tuberosity and is directed obliquely backward and downward, so that it would draw the lower jaw forward as well as upward.

The temporalis conforms to the temporal fossa, and is therefore longer and entirely lateral in position.

The pterygoidei are not quite clearly separated; their direction is more oblique, and the origin of the pterygoideus internus is nearer the median plane than in the horse.

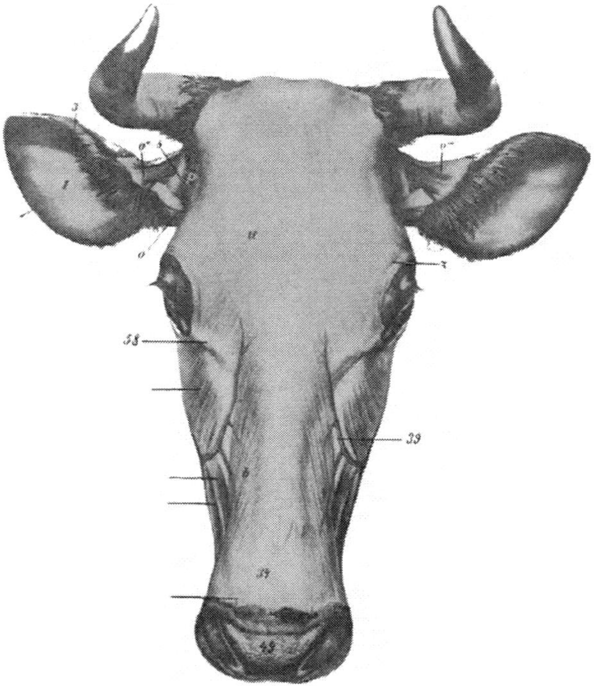

Fig. 208.—Muscles of Head of Ox, Dorsal View.

a, a', Levator labii superioris proprius; *b*, levator nasolabialis; *f*, dilatator naris lateralis; *g'*, malaris; *o*, zygomatico-auricularis and scutulo-auricularis superficialis inferior; *o''*, scutulo-auricularis superficialis superior; *o'''*, scutulo-auricularis superficialis accessorius; p, scutularis; *u*, frontalis; *z*, orbicularis oculi; *1*, concave surface of concha; *3*, *2*, anterior and posterior borders of concha; *8*, scutiform cartilage; *34*, parietal cartilage; *39*, facial vein; *49*, muzzle; *58*, internal palpebral ligament. (After Ellenberger-Baum, Anat. für Künstler.)

The **stylo-mandibularis** is absent.

The **digastricus** has a tendinous origin on the paramastoid or styloid process of the occipital bone; its bellies are short and thick. It does not perforate the stylo-hyoideus. The two digastrici are connected beneath the root of the tongue by a layer of transverse muscle-fibers (Transversus mandibulæ).

HYOID MUSCLES

The **mylo-hyoideus** is thicker and more extensive than in the horse.

The **stylo-hyoideus** has a long thin tendinous origin and is not perforated by the digastricus.

The genio-hyoideus is more developed.

The kerato-hyoideus has an additional attachment on the middle cornu of the hyoid bone.

The hyoideus transversus is bifid.

The sterno-thyro-hyoideus has no intermediate tendon and is thicker.

The omo-hyoideus arises as a thin band from the fascia over the third and fourth cervical vertebræ. It blends here with the rectus capitis anterior major. The occipito-hyoideus is thick.

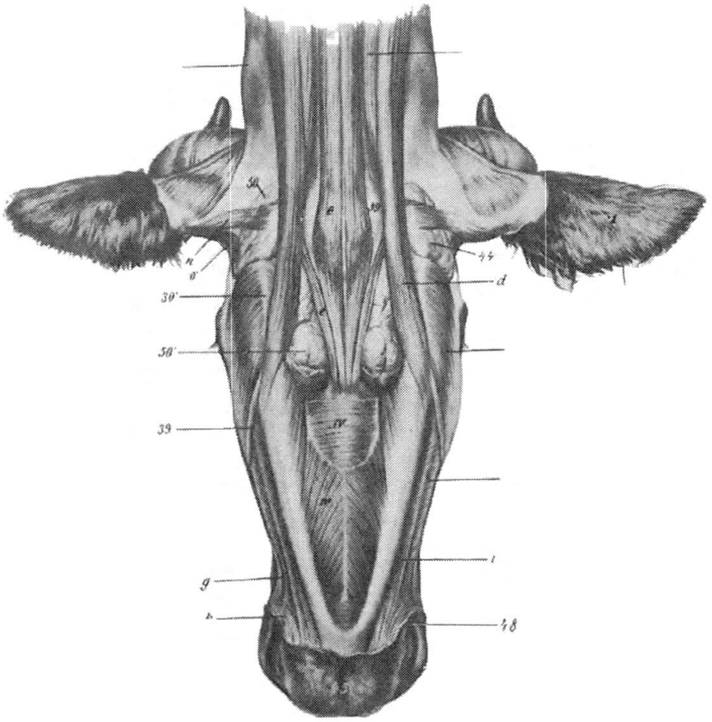

FIG. 209.—MUSCLES OF HEAD OF OX, VENTRAL VIEW.

d, d', Sterno-cephalicus; *e*, omo-hyoideus; *g*, zygomaticus; *h*, buccinator; *i*, depressor labii inferioris; *k* orbicularis oris; *m*, masseter; *n*, parotido-auricularis; *o'*, zygomatico-auricularis; *w*, mylo-hyoideus; *1*, concha, convex surface; *2*, anterior border of concha; *30'*, angle of jaw; *39*, facial vein; *44*, parotid gland; *45*, lower lip; *48*, angle of mouth; *60*, *60'*, submaxillary gland; *59*, larynx; *x*, wing of atlas. (After Ellenberger-Baum, Anat. für Künstler.)

MUSCLES OF THE NECK

A. VENTRAL GROUP

The sterno-cephalicus consists of two muscles. They arise from the manubrium sterni and first rib. The superficial muscle (Sterno-mandibularis) is inserted on the anterior border of the masseter, the ramus of the mandible, and the buccal fascia. The deep muscle (Sterno-mastoideus) crosses under the preceding and ends on the mastoid process, the mandible, and, in common with the rectus capitis anterior major, on the basilar process of the occipital bone.

There are two scaleni. The scalenus ventralis (s. primæ costæ) arises on the first rib and ends on the transverse processes of the third to the seventh cervical

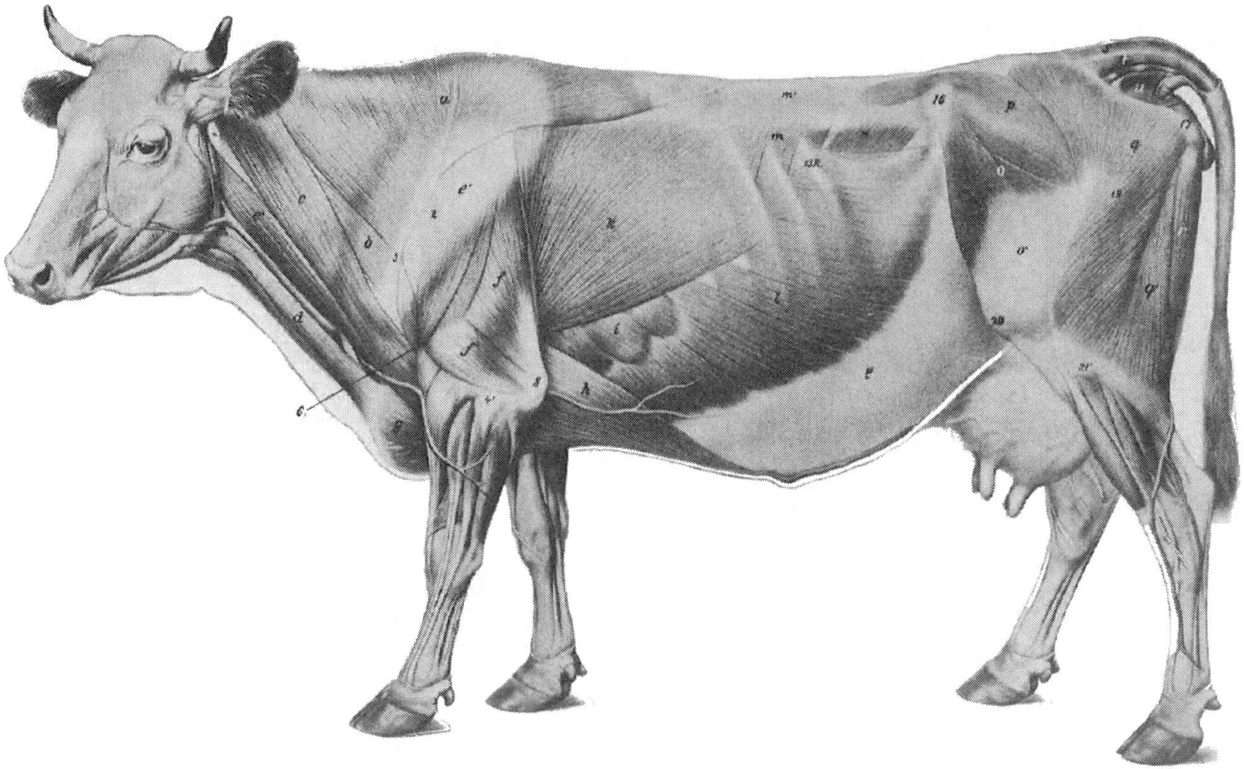

Fig. 210.—Superficial Muscles of Ox, After Removal of Panniculus.

a, trapezius; *b*, omo-transversarius; *c*, *c′*, mastoid-humeralis (*c*, cleido-mastoideus; *c′*, cleido-occipitalis); *d*, sterno-cephalicus; *e*, deltoid; *f*, long head, *f′* external head of triceps; *g*, superficial pectoral; *h*, posterior deep pectoral; *i*, serratus magnus; *k*, latissimus dorsi; *l*, obliquus abdominis externus; *l′*, aponeurosis of *l*; *m*, serratus posterior; *m′*, lumbo-dorsal fascia; *n*, obliquus abdominis internus; *o*, tensor fasciæ latæ; *o′*, fascia lata; *p*, gluteus medius; *q*, *q′*, biceps femoris; *r*, semitendinosus; *s*, sacro-coccygeus superior; *t*, sacro-coccygeus lateralis; *u*, coccygeus. (After Ellenberger-Baum, Anat. f. Künstler.)

vertebræ. It is traversed by the roots of the brachial plexus, which partially divide it into a small dorsal and a large ventral part. The brachial vessels lie below the latter. The scalenus dorsalis (s. supracostalis) arises usually on the second, third, and fourth ribs, and ends on the transverse processes of the third to the sixth cervical vertebræ.

The rectus capitis anterior major arises on the third to the sixth cervical transverse processes, and blends at its insertion with the sterno-mastoideus and the mastoid portion of the mastoido-humeralis.

The rectus capitis anterior minor is larger than in the horse.

The rectus capitis lateralis and longus colli resemble those of the horse.

The intertransversales are large. From the sixth cervical vertebra forward they form a muscular mass (M. intertransversarius longus) which is inserted into the wing of the atlas.

B. LATERAL GROUP

The splenius is thin. It arises directly from the first three or four thoracic spines, and ends by a thin tendon on the occipital bone, the wing of the atlas, and the transverse process of the axis, blending with the mastoido-humeralis, trachelo-mastoideus, and omo-transversarius. The remaining muscles present no very marked differential features.

MUSCLES OF THE THORAX

The levatores costarum number ten or eleven pairs.

The diaphragm presents several important differential features. Its slope is much steeper and its width is greater than in the horse. The costal attachment extends almost in a straight line from the upper fourth of the last rib to the junction of the eighth rib with its cartilage, and along the latter to the sternum. The mid-line slopes from the twelfth thoracic vertebra obliquely as far as the vena cava, beyond which it is almost vertical. The right crus divides into two branches, which circumscribe the œsophageal opening, unite below, and then spread out in the tendinous center. The left crus is small. The œsophageal opening is situated about four to five inches (10 to 12 cm.) below the eighth thoracic vertebra, a little to the left of the median plane. The foramen venæ cavæ is a little more ventral and almost in the median plane. The other muscles resemble those of the horse.

MUSCLES OF THE BACK AND LOINS

The serratus anticus is very thin. It is inserted on the fifth to the eighth ribs. It may be reduced to two or three digitations or may be absent. The serratus posticus is usually inserted on the last three or four ribs.

The transversalis costarum (Iliocostalis) has a distinct lumbar portion which is attached to the lumbar transverse processes and the external angle of the ilium.

The longissimus resembles that of the horse, but it is more fleshy anteriorly, and the spinalis dorsi is clearly distinguishable from the common mass. In the lumbar region the tendons meet across the summits of the spines.

Intertransversales are present in the back, and interspinales in the back and loins.

MUSCLES OF THE TAIL

These resemble those of the horse; the coccygeus is, however, much more developed.

Abdominal Muscles

The **obliquus abdominis externus** is somewhat thinner and has a less extensive origin, which begins at the lower part of the fifth intercostal space and ends on the last rib above its middle. The direction of the fibers in the flank is horizontal, and they do not reach to the external angle of the ilium, nor as high as the lumbar transverse processes. (In this region the abdominal tunic has a strong attachment to the point of the hip and the lumbo-dorsal fascia.) The aponeurosis is intimately united with the abdominal tunic, and does not detach a layer on the inner surface of the thigh.

The **obliquus abdominis internus** is more developed and has an additional

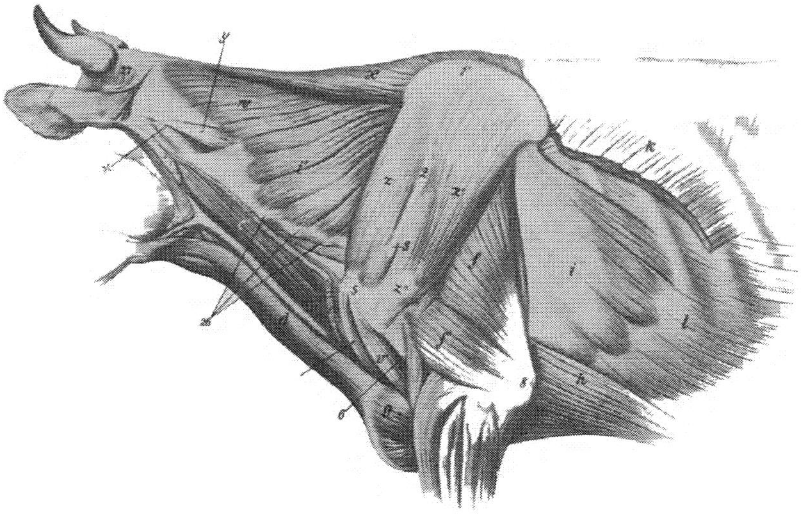

Fig. 211.—Deeper Muscles of Neck, Shoulder, and Thorax of Ox.

c', Cleido-occipitalis muscle; *d*, sterno-cephalicus; *f, f'*, long and external heads of triceps; *g*, superficial pectoral muscle; *h, h'*, posterior and anterior deep pectoral muscles; *i, i'*, serratus magnus; *k*, latissimus dorsi; *l*, obliquus abdominis externus; *v'*, biceps brachii; *w*, splenius; *x*, rhomboideus; *y*, trachelo-mastoideus; *z*, supraspinatus; *z'*, infraspinatus; *z''*, tendon of insertion of *z'*; *1'*, cartilage of scapula; *2*, tuberosity of spine of scapula; *3*, acromion; *5*, external tuberosity of humerus; *6*, deltoid tuberosity; *8*, olecranon; *26*, transverse processes of cervical vertebræ; *27*, posterior auricular muscles; ×, wing of atlas. (After Ellenberger-Baum, Anat. für Künstler.)

origin from the lumbo-dorsal fascia. The aponeurosis blends with that of the external oblique near the linea alba, and detaches a layer which assists in the formation of the internal sheath of the rectus.

The **rectus abdominis** arises on the lateral border of the sternum as far forward as the third costal cartilage. The two muscles are separated, except near the pelvis, by an interval varying from two to four inches (ca. 5 to 10 cm.), so that this part of the abdominal wall is entirely fibrous. (The umbilicus is in a transverse plane through the third lumbar vertebra.) There are five tendinous inscriptions, on the third of which is a foramen for the passage of the subcutaneous abdominal vein (milk vein). The prepubic tendon has, in addition to branches inserted into the ilio-pectineal eminences, a strong attachment to the median common tendon of the adductors of the thigh, so that the abdominal wall is strongly retracted and almost vertical at its junction with the pelvis.

The transversus abdominis presents no striking differential features. The transversalis fascia is strong and distinct except over the diaphragm.

Muscles of the Thoracic Limb

I. MUSCLES OF THE SHOULDER GIRDLE

The trapezius is much thicker and broader than in the horse, and is undivided. It arises on the ligamentum nuchæ and supraspinous ligament, from the atlas to the twelfth thoracic vertebra.

The omo-transversarius is a muscle (not present in the horse) which arises on the wing of the atlas, and, inconstantly, the transverse process of the second cervical vertebra, and is inserted into the scapular spine and fascia.

The rhomboideus is clearly divided into cervical and dorsal portions, the latter extending further than in the horse.

The latissimus dorsi has a broad tendon of origin, which blends with the lumbo-dorsal fascia; it is also attached to the eleventh and twelfth ribs, the fascia over the external intercostal and oblique abdominal muscles, and by a tendinous slip to the deep pectoral muscle.

The mastoido-humeralis has two distinct parts. The dorsal division (M. cleido-occipitalis) arises on the occipital bone and the ligamentum nuchæ. The ventral part (M. cleido-mastoideus) is smaller and arises by a round tendon on the mastoid process and the rectus capitis anterior major, and by a thin tendon on the mandible. At the shoulder a small muscle which arises on the first rib blends with the deep face of the mastoido-humeralis.[1]

The superficial pectoral muscle does not present any striking difference.

The deep pectoral arises as far forward as the second rib and is undivided. However, the scapular portion may be considered to be represented by a small branch extending over the lower part of the supraspinatus. A tendon is detached from the dorsal edge, which blends with the latissimus dorsi and coraco-brachialis.

The serratus magnus is clearly divided into cervical and thoracic portions. The former is large and extends from the third (or second) cervical vertebra to the fifth rib, being overlapped behind by the thoracic part. The thoracic part is relatively thin and is covered by a very strong aponeurosis; it is attached to the fourth to the ninth ribs by six digitations, and is inserted by a flat tendon into the inner face of the dorsal angle of the scapula.

II. MUSCLES OF THE SHOULDER

The deltoid is clearly divided into acromial and scapular portions. The former arises on the acromion, the latter on the posterior border of the scapula and the aponeurotic covering of the infraspinatus. The scapular part of the muscle is largely inserted into the fascia covering the triceps.

The supraspinatus, infraspinatus, and teres minor do not differ materially from those of the horse.

The subscapularis consists of three portions with a common tendon of insertion.

The teres major and coraco-brachialis resemble those of the horse.

III. MUSCLES OF THE ARM

The biceps is smaller and less tendinous, and is situated more internally than in the horse. The tendon of origin is flat, and is bound down in the bicipital groove

[1] This is probably the homologue of the subclavius of man.

by a fibrous band. (In the sheep the tendon is round and passes through the shoulder joint.)

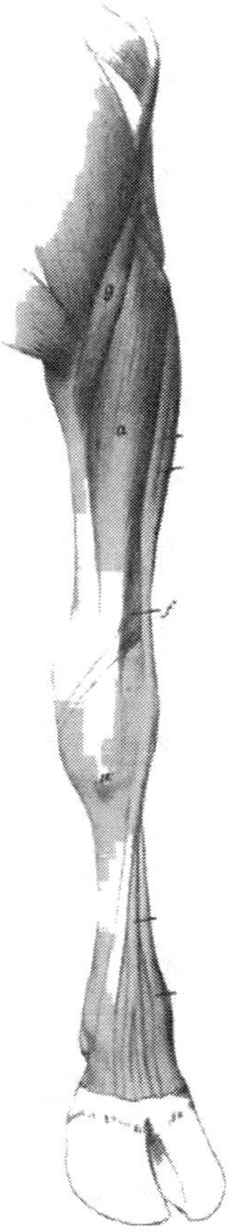

FIG. 212.—MUSCLES OF ANTIBRACHIUM AND MANUS OF OX, ANTERIOR VIEW.

a, Extensor carpi radialis; *b*, extensor digiti tertii; *c*, extensor digitalis communis; *d*, extensor digiti quarti (tendon); *f*, extensor carpi obliquus; *g*, brachialis; *12'*, metacarpal tuberosity. (After Ellenberger-Baum, Anat. für Künstler.)

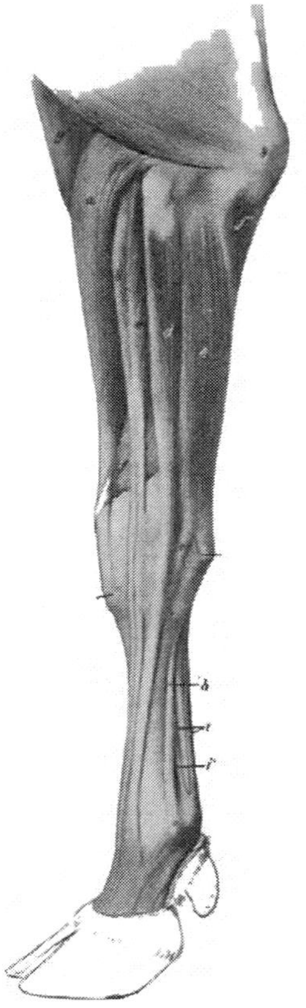

FIG. 213.—MUSCLES OF ANTIBRACHIUM AND MANUS OF OX, EXTERNAL VIEW.

a, Extensor carpi radialis; *b*, extensor digiti tertii; *c*, common or anterior digital extensor; *d*, extensor digiti quarti; *e*, flexor carpi externus; *f*, extensor carpi obliquus; *f'*, ulnar head of flexor carpi medius; *g*, brachialis; *h*, interosseus medius or suspensory ligament; *i*, flexor tendons; *i'*, branch of *h*, to superficial flexor tendon; *8*, olecranon; *11*, accessory carpal bone; *12'*, metacarpal tuberosity. (After Ellenberger-Baum, Anat. für Künstler.)

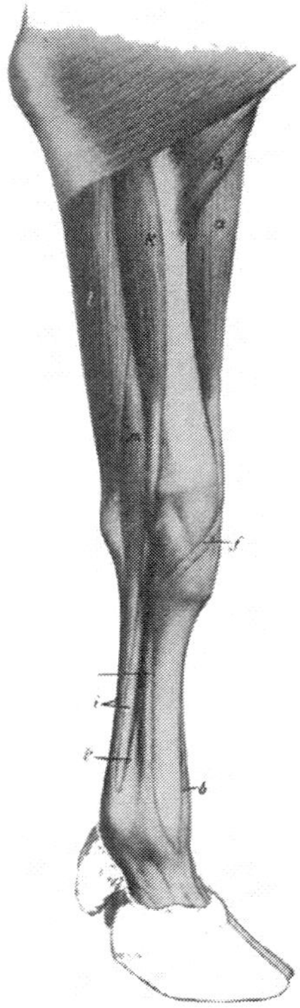

FIG. 214.—MUSCLES OF ANTIBRACHIUM AND MANUS OF OX, INTERNAL VIEW.

a, Extensor carpi radialis; *b*, tendon of extensor digiti tertii; *f*, tendon of extensor carpi obliquus; *g*, brachialis; *h*, interosseus medius or suspensory ligament; *i*, flexor tendons; *i'*, branch of *h*; *k*, flexor carpi internus; *l*, flexor carpi medius; *m*, superficial digital flexor. (After Ellenberger-Baum, Anat. für Künstler.)

The internal head of the triceps is more developed than in the horse. The tensor fasciæ antibrachii is a slender muscle.

IV. MUSCLES OF THE FOREARM

A. Extensor Division

The extensor carpi radialis is like that of the horse. There is sometimes a small muscle lying along its inner border, which may represent the extensores pollicis.

There are three digital extensors: 1. The common or anterior digital extensor (M. extensor digitalis communis) arises by two heads from the extensor epicondyle and the ulna. The heads fuse about the middle of the forearm, and terminate soon on a tendon which passes over the carpus and metacarpus, gradually inclining

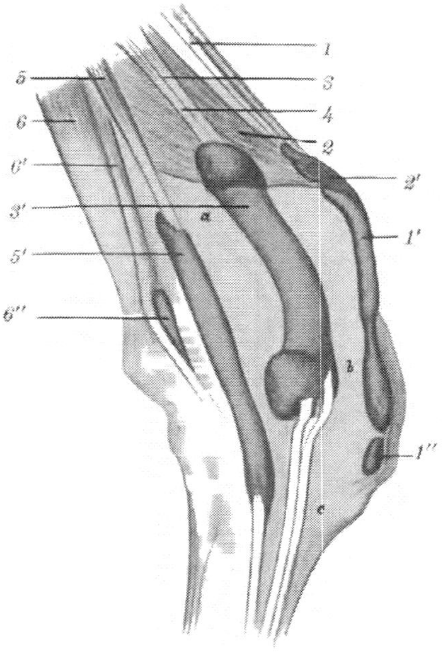

Fig. 215.—Right Carpus of Ox with Bursæ and Synovial Sheaths Injected, External View.

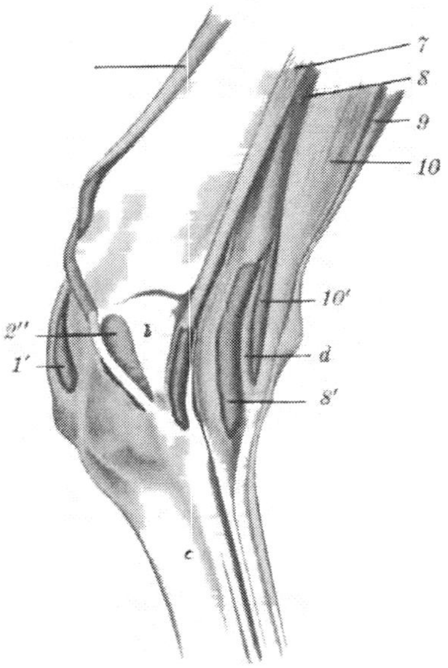

Fig. 216.—Right Carpus of Ox with Bursæ and Synovial Sheaths Injected, Internal View.

1, Extensor carpi radialis, with synovial sheath (*1'*) and bursa (*1''*); *2*, extensor carpi obliquus, with synovial sheath (*2'*) and bursa (*2''*); *3*, extensor digiti tertii proprius; *4*, extensor digitalis communis; *3'*, common synovial sheath of *3* and *4*; *5*, extensor digiti quarti proprius, with synovial sheath (*5'*); *6*, *6'*, flexor carpi externus, with bursa (*6''*); *7*, flexor carpi internus, with synovial sheath; *8*, deep digital flexor, with synovial sheath (*8'*); *9*, flexor carpi medius; *10*, superficial digital flexor, with synovial sheath *10'*; *a*, radius; *b*, carpus; *c*, metacarpus; *d*, cut edge of annular ligament. (After Schmidtchen.)

forward. At the fetlock joint it divides into two branches, which are inserted into the third phalanges. 2. The internal digital extensor (M. extensor digiti tertii proprius) arises on the extensor epicondyle, and is inserted by two branches into the second and third phalanges of the inner digit. The tendon receives two reinforcing slips from the suspensory ligament. 3. The lateral digital extensor (M. extensor digitalis lateralis s. digiti quarti proprius) arises from the external lateral ligament of the elbow joint, the external tuberosity of the radius, and the ulna. The tendon terminates like that of the preceding muscle.

The extensor carpi obliquus resembles that of the horse.

The extensor tendons are bound down at the carpus by an annular ligament, and are furnished with synovial sheaths (Figs. 215, 216).

B. Flexor Division

The three **flexors of the carpus** are like those of the horse.

The **superficial digital flexor** is somewhat blended at its origin with the middle flexor of the carpus. It divides into two bellies, superficial and deep, terminating on tendons at the distal part of the forearm. The superficial tendon passes over the posterior annular ligament (Ligamentum carpi transversum), perforates the metacarpal fascia, and joins the deep tendon about the middle of the metacarpus. The deep belly is connected with the deep flexor by a strong fibrous band. Its tendon passes under the annular ligament in a groove on the deep flexor, from which it receives fibers. The conjoined tendon soon bifurcates, each branch receiving a reinforcing band from the suspensory ligament, and forming near the fetlock a ring for the corresponding branch of the deep flexor tendon. Passing under two digital annular ligaments, they are inserted into the volar surfaces of the second phalanges by three slips.

The **deep digital flexor** has the same heads as in the horse, the humeral head, as before mentioned, being connected with the deep portion of the superficial flexor. The tendon divides near the distal end of the metacarpus into two branches which are inserted into the volar surfaces of the third phalanges.

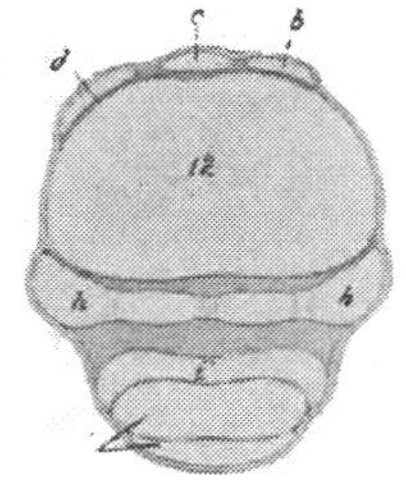

Fig. 217.—Cross-section of Distal Third of Metacarpus of Ox.

b, Tendon of extensor digiti tertii; *c*, tendon of common extensor; *d*, tendon of extensor digiti quarti; *h*, interosseus medius or suspensory ligament; *i*, tendons of digital flexors; *i'*, branch of *h*; *12*, metacarpal bone. (After Ellenberger-Baum, Anat. für Künstler.)

The synovial sheaths at the carpus present the following special features: One is found in connection with the tendon of the superficial part of the superficial flexor of the digits. There is a common sheath for the tendons of the common extensor and the inner extensor.

*B*ursæ may occur under the tendons of the proper extensors of the digits at the fetlock; they are constant only in old animals (Schmidtchen). The branches of the tendon of the common extensor are provided with synovial sheaths from their origin to the middle of the second phalanx. There are two digital synovial sheaths for the flexor tendons; they may communicate at their upper part, and extend from the distal third of the metacarpus nearly to the distal sesamoids. *B*ursæ occur between the latter and the branches of the deep flexor tendon.

METACARPAL MUSCLES

The **lumbricales** are absent, unless we regard as such the muscular bundles which arise on the deep flexor and are inserted into the superficial flexor tendon at the carpus.

The **interosseus medius** or suspensory ligament is somewhat more muscular than in the horse; indeed, in the young subject it may be almost entirely fleshy. Its arrangement is somewhat complex. Single at its origin, it detaches about the middle of the metacarpus a band which joins the tendon of the superficial flexor and concurs near the fetlock in the formation of the ring for the deep flexor tendon. A little lower down it divides into three and then into five branches. The lateral branches (two pairs) are attached to the corresponding sesamoids and tendons of the proper extensors, while the middle branch passes through the sulcus at the distal end of the metacarpus and bifurcates, each division fusing with the tendon of the corresponding proper extensor.

It is to be noted that the fascia on the posterior face of the metacarpus and digit is very thick. It is continuous above with the ligamentum carpi transversum, and is attached on either side to the metacarpal bone. At the fetlock it forms the fibrous basis for the small claws, and below this it detaches two strong bands which diverge to be inserted into the second and third phalanges, blending with the lateral ligaments.

The Muscles of the Pelvic Limb

I. The Sublumbar Muscles

The psoas minor begins at the disc between the twelfth and thirteenth thoracic vertebræ.

The psoas major has a fleshy origin on the posterior border of the last rib, and a thin tendon attached to the twelfth rib.

The iliacus begins under the body of the sixth lumbar vertebra, and is more closely united with the psoas major than in the horse.

The quadratus lumborum extends as far forward as the body of the tenth or eleventh thoracic vertebra.

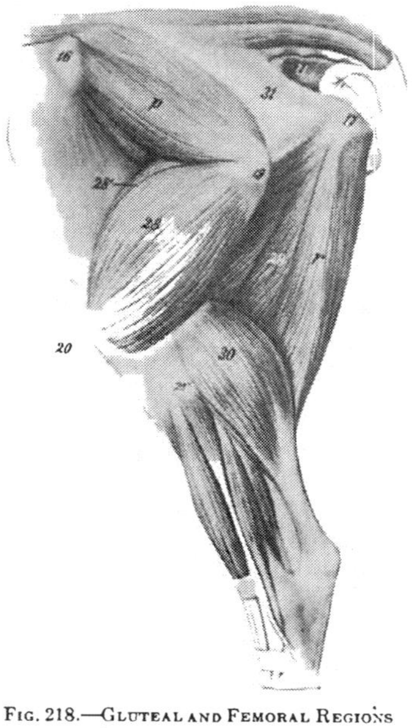

Fig. 218.—Gluteal and Femoral Regions of Ox, After Removal of Superficial Muscles.

p, Gluteus medius; *r*, semitendinosus; *u*, coccygeus; *28*, vastus externus; *28'*, rectus femoris; *29*, semimembranosus; *30*, gastrocnemius; *31*, sacro-sciatic ligament; *16*, tuber coxæ; *17*, tuber ischii; *19*, trochanter major; *20*, patella; *21'*, external condyle of tibia. (After Ellenberger-Baum, Anat. für Künstler.)

II. External Muscles of the Hip and Thigh

The tensor fasciæ latæ is large, and the fleshy part extends further down than in the horse.

The gluteus superficialis is not present as such; apparently its anterior part has fused with the tensor fasciæ latæ and its posterior with the biceps femoris.

The gluteus medius is small, the lumbar portion being insignificant and extending forward only to the fourth lumbar vertebra. Its deep portion (Gluteus accessorius) is easily separable, and its strong tendon is inserted into the femur below the trochanter major, under cover of the upper part of the vastus externus.

The gluteus profundus is thin, but extensive, arising as far forward as the external angle of the ilium, and from the lower part of the sacro-sciatic ligament. The fibers converge on a tendon which passes under the upper part of the vastus externus, and is inserted into a tubercle a short distance below the great trochanter.

The biceps femoris is very wide at its upper part, having apparently absorbed the posterior part of the superficial gluteus. It is divided in the thigh into two portions, which end on a wide aponeurosis. There is no femoral attachment. A large bursa occurs between the muscle and the great trochanter in the adult. The part of the tendon which fuses with the external patellar ligament presents a fibro-cartilaginous thickening, and an extensive bursa is interposed between it and the external condyle of the femur.

The semitendinosus and semimembranosus arise on the ischium only. The latter has a branch attached to the internal condyle of the tibia.

III. ANTERIOR MUSCLES OF THE THIGH

The **quadriceps** femoris resembles that of the horse; the vastus intermedius is more clearly separable, and consists of two parts. *Bursæ* occur under the insertions of the internal and external vasti, and often under the end of the biceps in the adult.

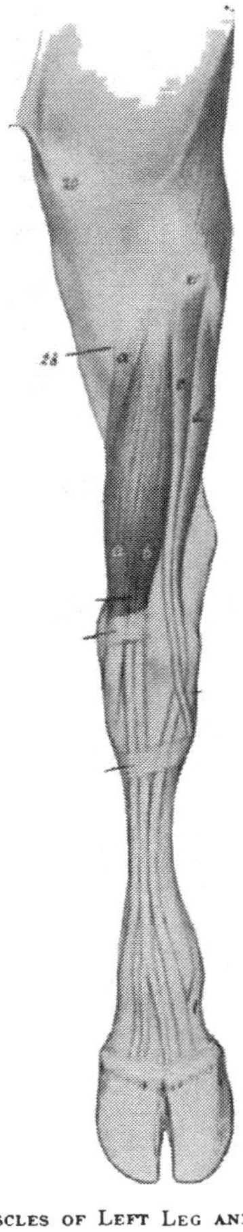

FIG. 219.—MUSCLES OF LEFT LEG AND FOOT OF OX, ANTERIOR VIEW.

a, Peroneus tertius; *a'*, tibialis anterior; *b*, anterior or long digital extensor; *b'*, extensor digiti tertii; *c*, peroneus longus; *d*, extensor digiti quarti; *i*, *i*, annular ligaments; *k*, external lateral ligament of hock joint; *l*, branch of suspensory ligament; *20*, patella; *21'*, external condyle of tibia; *28*, tuberosity of tibia. (After Ellenberger-Baum, Anat. für Künstler.)

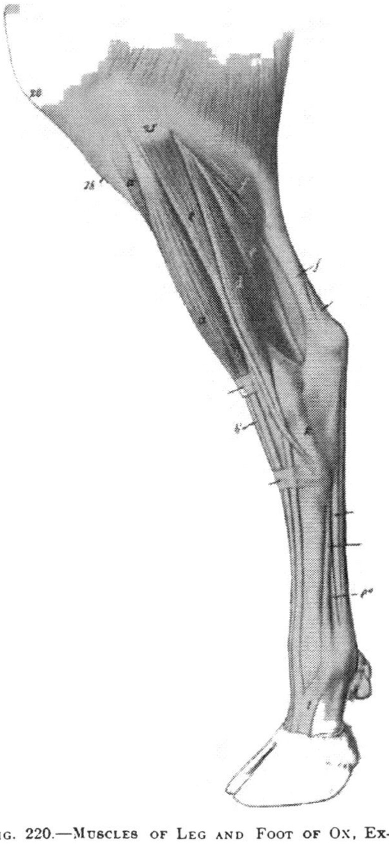

FIG. 220.—MUSCLES OF LEG AND FOOT OF OX, EXTERNAL VIEW.

a, Peroneus tertius; *a'*, tibialis anterior; *b*, anterior or long digital extensor; *b'*, tendon of *b*; *c*, peroneus longus; *d*, extensor digiti quarti; *e*, deep digital flexor; *e'*, tendon of *e*; *e''*, branch of interosseus medius or suspensory ligament; *f*, gastrocnemius (the soleus lies just in front of *f*); *f'*, tendon of *f*; *g*, tendon of superficial digital flexor; *h*, interosseus medius or suspensory ligament; *i*, *i*, annular ligaments; *20*, patella; *21'*, external condyle of tibia; *28*, crest of tibia. (After Ellenberger-Baum, Anat. für Künstler.)

The **articularis genu** or subcrureus is a small muscle which lies under the lower part of the vastus intermedius, and is inserted on the suprapatellar cul-de-sac of the synovial membrane.

The **capsularis** is absent.

IV. INTERNAL MUSCLES OF THE THIGH

The sartorius arises by two heads, one from the tendon of the psoas minor and the iliac fascia, the other from the shaft of the ilium. The femoral vessels pass between them.

The gracilis is more extensively united with its fellow than in the horse.

The pectineus is large, and arises by a single head from the pubic crest and

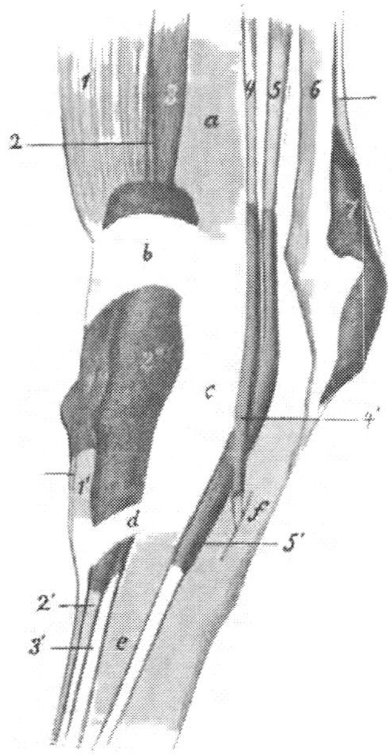

FIG. 221.—LEFT TARSUS OF OX WITH SYNOVIAL SHEATHS AND BURSÆ INJECTED, EXTERNAL VIEW.

1, Peroneus tertius; *1′*, tendon of *1* and its sheath, *1″*; *2*, extensor digiti tertii proprius; *2′*, tendon of *2*; *2″*, common sheath of tendons of extensor digiti tertii and extensor digitalis longus (*3*, *3′*); *4*, peroneus longus and its sheath, *4′*; *5*, extensor digiti quarti and its sheath, *5′*; *6*, tendon of gastrocnemius; *7*, superficial digital flexor and its sheath, *7′*; *8*, tendon of tibialis anterior; *a*, tibia; *b*, proximal annular ligament; *c*, tarsus; d, distal annular ligament; *e*, metatarsus; *f*, external lateral ligament. (After Schmidtchen.)

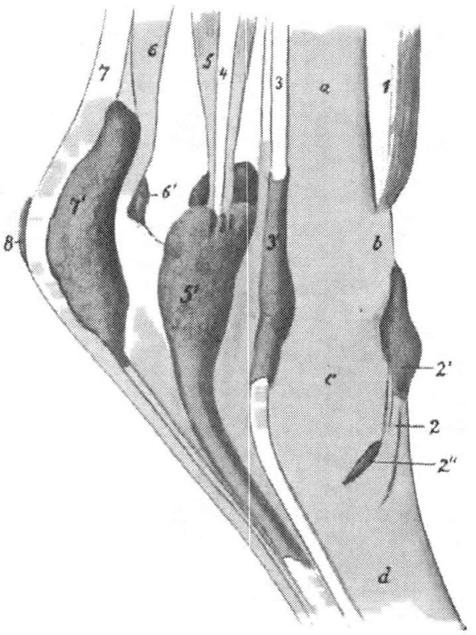

FIG. 222.—LEFT TARSUS OF OX WITH SYNOVIAL SHEATHS AND BURSÆ INJECTED, INTERNAL VIEW.

1, Peroneus tertius; *2*, tendon of tibialis anterior with sheath, *2′*, and bursa, *2″*; *3*, long digital flexor and *3′*, its sheath; *4*, tibialis posterior; *5*, deep digital flexor and its sheath, *5′*; *6*, tendon of gastrocnemius and bursa, *6′*; *7*, superficial digital flexor and its sheath, *7′*; *8*, subcutaneous bursa; *a*, tibia; *b*, proximal annular ligament; *c*, tarsus; d, metatarsus. (After Schmidtchen.)

prepubic tendon. It divides into two branches, one of which is inserted as in the horse, while the other extends to the internal epicondyle of the femur.

The adductor resembles that of the horse, but does not reach to the internal condyle.

The quadratus femoris and obturator externus resemble those of the horse.

The obturator internus arises from the ischium only, and its tendon passes through the obturator foramen.

The gemellus is large.

V. MUSCLES OF THE LEG AND FOOT

There are four **digital extensors,** two of which are fused with each other and the peroneus tertius in the upper third of the leg.

1. The **anterior** or **long digital extensor** (M. extensor digitalis longus) arises by the common tendon in the extensor fossa of the femur, and separates from the other muscles near the middle of the leg. At the distal end of the tibia it termi-

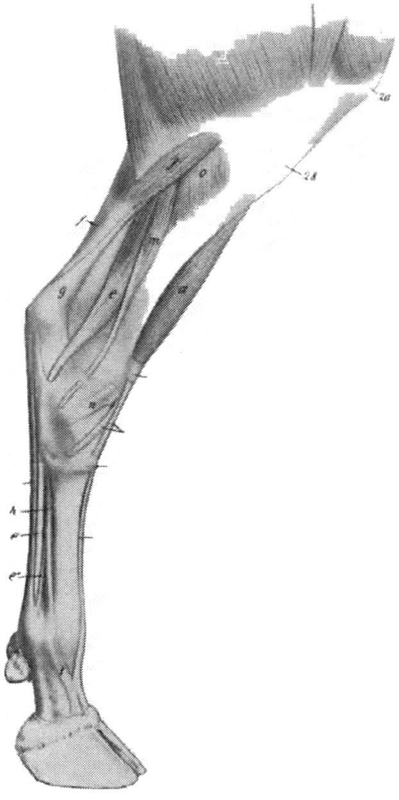

FIG. 223.—MUSCLES OF LEG AND FOOT OF OX, INNER VIEW.

a, Peroneus tertius; *b'*, tendon of anterior or long extensor; *e*, deep digital flexor; *e'*, tendon of *e*; *e''*, branch of *h* to superficial flexor tendon; *f*, gastrocnemius; *g*, tendon of superficial digital flexor; *h*, interosseus medius or suspensory ligament; *i*, annular ligaments; *l*, branch of *h*; *m*, long digital flexor; *o*, popliteus; *20*, patella; *28*, tuberosity of tibia. (After Ellenberger-Baum, Anat. für Künstler.)

nates on a tendon which passes down over the hock (bound down by two annular ligaments) and ends like that of the thoracic limb.

2. The **internal digital extensor** (M. extensor digiti tertii proprius) arises in common with the preceding muscle and the peroneus tertius, and is covered by them to the distal third of the tibia. Its tendon passes under the annular ligaments between those of its cogeners and ends on the second phalanx of the inner digit.

3. The **lateral digital extensor** (M. extensor digitalis lateralis s. digiti quarti proprius) arises on the external lateral ligament of the stifle joint and the external condyle of the tibia. Its tendon passes over the outer surface of the hock, and terminates on the anterior surface of the second phalanx of the external digit.

The reinforcing bands from the suspensory ligament are arranged as in the fore limb.

4. The **extensor brevis** resembles that of the horse, but is inserted on the tendon of the anterior extensor only.

The **peroneus longus** (not present in the horse) is situated in front of the lateral extensor. It arises on the external condyle of the tibia and the fibrous band which represents the shaft of the fibula. Its tendon passes downward and backward over the outer surface of the hock, crosses over that of the lateral extensor and under

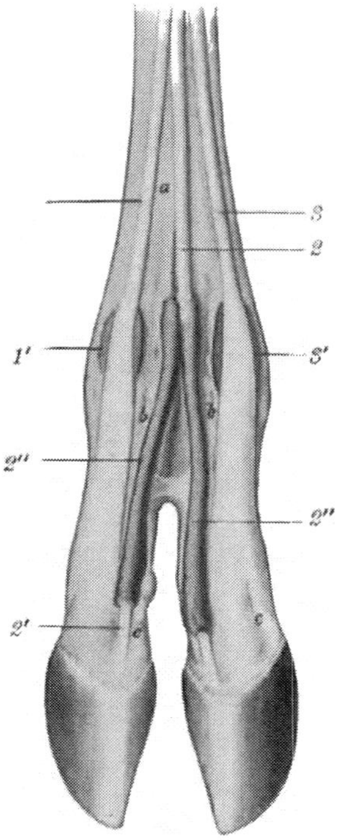

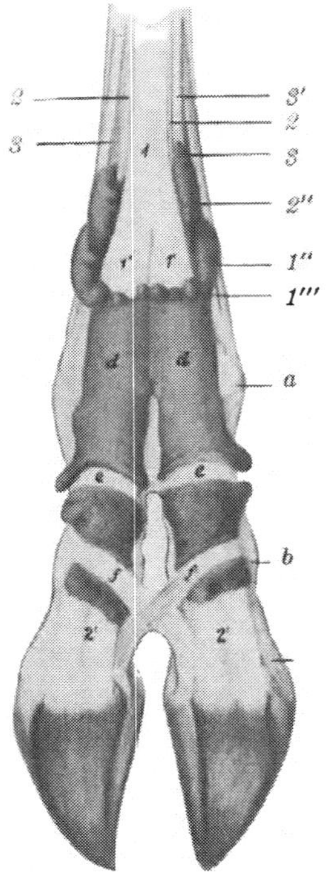

Fig. 224.—Distal Part of Limb of Ox with Synovial Sheaths and Bursæ Injected Anterior View.

1, Tendon of extensor digiti tertii, with bursa (*1'*); *2*, tendon of anterior extensor; *2'*, branch of *2*, with synovial sheath (*2''*); *3*, tendon of extensor digiti quarti, with bursa (*3'*); *a*, metatarsus; *b*, first phalanx; *c*, second phalanx. (After Schmidtchen.)

the lateral ligament, and ends on the first tarsal bone (Cuneiform parvum). It is enveloped by a synovial sheath. It would apparently act as an inward rotator at the hock joint.

The **peroneus tertius** is a well-developed muscle which arises on the common tendon with the long and internal extensors. It has a large, fusiform belly, which is superficially situated on the front of the leg. Close to the tarsus it ends on a flat tendon, which is perforated by that of the tibialis anterior, and ends on the large metatarsal and second and third (fused) tarsal bones (Cuneiform magnum).

The **tibialis anterior** is smaller, and arises by two heads. The larger head springs from the outer surface of the tuberosity of the tibia; the outer, smaller one (M. extensor hallucis longus), from the upper part of the external border of the tibia and the fibrous band which replaces the shaft of the fibula. The tendon perforates that of the preceding muscle and ends on the metatarsal and second and third tarsal bones.

B. Posterior Group

The gastrocnemius and soleus resemble those of the horse. The **superficial flexor** is more fleshy than in the horse. Its tendon terminates as in the fore limb.

The **deep flexor** has in its upper part a close resemblance to that of the horse, but the superficial head (tibialis posterior) is larger and distinct. The tendon ends like that on the fore limb.

MUSCLES OF THE PIG

Muscles of Head

The facial **panniculus** is pale, thin, and difficult to separate from the skin.

The orbicularis oris is little developed.

The **levator nasolabialis** is thin and pale, and is undivided.

The levator labii superioris proprius may well be termed the levator rostri. It has a large penniform belly, which arises in the fossa on the lacrimal bone and maxilla. The tendon ends on the anterior part of the os rostri. A muscular slip connects it with the premaxilla.

The zygomaticus arises on the fascia over the masseter and ends at the angle of the mouth.

The **depressor** labii **inferioris** separates from the buccinator only near the angle of the mouth; it ends by a number of tendinous branches in the lower lip.

The dilatator **naris lateralis** is well developed. It arises under the levator rostri and ends by a tendinous network around the nostril.

The dilatator **naris transversus** is represented only by a few fibers which cross over the os rostri.

The **depressor** rostri arises on the facial crest. It has a long strong tendon which passes below the nostril and turns up and inward to meet the tendon of the opposite side and end in the skin of the snout. It depresses the snout and contracts the nostril.

The malaris is absent, and the other palpebral muscles present no special features.

MUSCLES OF MASTICATION

The **digastricus** has only one belly. It ends on the inner and lower surface of the mandible, in front of the groove for the facial vessels.

The other muscles have no important differential features.

The same is true of the oral hyoid muscles.

Muscles of the Neck

The **panniculus carnosus** consists of two layers which cross each other obliquely. The fibers of the superficial layer are directed nearly vertically, those of the deep layer toward the face, on which they are continued to form the facial portion.

The **mastoido-humeralis** is described on p. 314.

The **sterno-cephalicus** (Sterno-mastoideus) arises on the sternum and is inserted by a long round tendon on the mastoid process.

The thyroid portion of the **sterno-thyro-hyoideus** has a peculiar arrangement. It arises (separately from the opposite muscle) on the manubrium sterni. About the middle of the neck it has an oblique tendinous intersection, beyond which it divides into two branches: one of these is inserted in the usual fashion, the other ends on the laryngeal prominence. The hyoid portion is well developed.

The **omo-hyoideus** is thin. It arises as in the horse, but has no connection with the mastoido-humeralis nor with the opposite muscle.

The **omo-transversarius** arises on the first or second cervical vertebra (under cover of the mastoido-humeralis), and is inserted into the lower part of the scapular spine.

There are two **scaleni.** The **scalenus ventralis** (s. primæ costæ) resembles

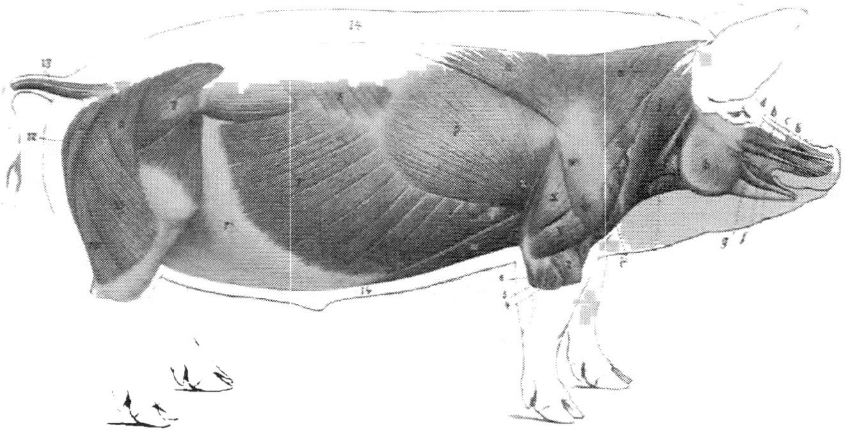

FIG. 226.—SUPERFICIAL MUSCLES OF PIG, AFTER REMOVAL OF PANNICULUS CARNOSUS.

a, Levator nasolabialis; *b*, levator labii superioris proprius; *b'*, fleshy slip of *b* which comes from premaxilla; *c*, dilatator naris lateralis; *d*, depressor rostri; *e*, orbicularis oris; *f*, depressor labii inferioris; *g*, zygomaticus; *h*, masseter; *i*, *i'*, *i''*, brachio-cephalicus (cleido-occipitalis, cleido-mastoideus, pars clavicularis); *k*, sterno-cephalicus; *l*, sterno-hyoideus; *m*, omo-transversarius; *n*, *n'*, trapezius; *o*, anterior deep pectoral; *p*, latissimus dorsi; *q*, lumbo-dorsal fascia; *r*, obliquus abdominis externus; *r'*, aponeurosis of *r*; *s*, serratus posticus; *t*, serratus magnus; *u*, posterior deep pectoral; *v*, supraspinatus; *w*, *w'*, deltoideus; *x*, long head of triceps; *y*, external head of triceps; *z*, tensor fasciæ antibrachii; *1*, brachialis; *2*, extensor carpi radialis; *3*, extensor digiti quarti; *4*, extensor digiti quinti; *5*, extensor carpi ulnaris; *6*, ulnar head of deep flexor; *7*, gluteus medius; *8*, tensor fasciæ latæ; *9*, *10*, *10'*, biceps femoris; *11*, semitendinosus; *12*, semimembranosus; *13*, caudal muscles; *14*, panniculus adiposus in section. (After Ellenberger, in Leisering's Atlas.)

that of the ox, is attached to the last four cervical vertebræ, and is perforated by the nerves of the brachial plexus. The **scalenus dorsalis** (s. supracostalis) arises on the transverse processes of the third to the sixth cervical vertebra, and ends on the third rib.

The **straight muscles** of the head present no special features.

The **longus colli** is separated from the opposite muscle, so that part of the bodies of the cervical vertebræ is exposed as in man.

The **intertransversales** resemble those of the ox.

The **splenius** is thick and extensive. It ends in three parts on the occipital, the temporal, and the wing of the atlas (inconstant).

The **trachelo-mastoideus** is small, and its atlantal portion is blended with the longissimus.

The **complexus** is large, and is clearly divided into two portions: the dorsal portion (Biventer cervicis) is marked by several tendinous intersections; the ventral part is the complexus proper.

The obliquus **capitis posterior** is relatively thin.

The **recti capitis** are thick and more or less fused.

MUSCLES OF THE THORAX

The levatores **costarum** and rectus thoracis present no special features.

The **external intercostal** muscles are absent under the serratus anticus and posticus and the digitations of the external oblique.

The **internal intercostals** are thick between the cartilages of the sternal ribs.

The **retractor costæ** and the **transversus** thoracis resemble those of the horse; the latter extends back to the eighth cartilage and fuses with the transversus abdominis.

The **diaphragm** has seven costal digitations on each side, the posterior ones being attached to the ribs at some distance (ca. one-third to one-fourth of rib-length) from the costo-chondral junction. The line of attachment reaches the latter at the tenth rib, and passes along the eighth cartilage to the xiphoid process. The tendinous center is more rounded than in the horse. The crura are well developed. The right crus is very large, and is perforated by the extensive slit-like opening for the œsophagus, which is median in position, and lies about two and one-half to three inches (ca. 6 to 8 cm.) below the twelfth thoracic vertebra. The hiatus aorticus is between the crura.

ABDOMINAL MUSCLES

The **abdominal tunic** is little developed.

The obliquus **abdominis externus** has an extensive fleshy portion and a correspondingly narrow aponeurosis; the latter does not detach a femoral lamina, but is reflected in toto to form the inguinal (Poupart's) ligament.

The obliquus **abdominis internus** resemblessthat of the ox; a small fusiform muscle, which crosses the inguinal canal obliquely and is attached on the abdominal surface of the inguinal ligament, is apparently a detached slip of the internal oblique.

The **rectus abdominis** is extensive and thick. It has seven to ten intersections. Its tendon of insertion fuses largely with the common tendon of the gracilis, and does not give off an accessory band to the head of the femur.

The fleshy part of the **transversus abdominis** is well developed. It blends in front with the transversus thoracis.

The **cremaster externus** is present in the female as well as in the male.

MUSCLES OF THE BACK AND LOINS

The **serratus anticus** is inserted into the fifth to the eighth ribs inclusive, the serratus posticus into the last four or five ribs. There are usually no digitations attached to the ninth and tenth ribs.

The **transversalis costarum** (Iliocostalis) extends to the wing of the atlas.

The **spinalis et semispinalis** can be separated without much difficulty from the longissimus dorsi, the division from the common mass of the loins beginning about the first lumbar vertebra.

The **multifidus** resembles that of the horse.

Interspinales are present, as well as distinct **intertransversales** of the back and loins.

MUSCLES OF THE TAIL

The superior and lateral **sacro-coccygei** arise as far forward as the last lumbar vertebra. Gurlt explains the twist of the tail as being due to the spiral arrangement of the insertions of the tendons.

MUSCLES OF THE THORACIC LIMB

MUSCLES OF THE SHOULDER GIRDLE

The **trapezius** is very wide, its line of origin extending from the occipital bone to the tenth thoracic vertebra. There is no clear division between its two parts, which are both inserted into the scapular spine.

The **omo-transversarius** resembles that of the ox.

The **rhomboideus** consists of three portions. The **cervical portion** (Rhomboideus cervicalis) is greatly developed, its origin extending from the second cervical to the sixth thoracic vertebra. The **cephalic portion** (Rhomboideus capitis) arises with the splenius on the occipital bone, and is inserted with the cervical part. The **dorsal portion** (Rhomboideus thoracalis) extends as far back as the ninth or tenth thoracic vertebra.

The **latissimus dorsi** is attached to the four ribs preceding the last. It is inserted into the internal lip of the bicipital groove.

The **mastoido-humeralis** divides into two parts, the **cleido-mastoideus** and **cleido-occipitalis**, which arise on the mastoid process and occipital crest respectively, and unite at the fibrous vestige of the clavicle.

The **anterior superficial pectoral** is thin. The **posterior superficial pectoral** is divided into parts, one of which ends on the humerus, the other on the fascia of the forearm.

The **deep pectoral** is clearly divided into two parts. The **scapular portion** resembles that of the horse, but its origin does not extend behind the first two chondro-sternal joints. The **posterior deep pectoral** is very long.

The cervical portion of the **serratus magnus** is greatly developed, its origin extending from the wing of the atlas to the upper part of the fifth rib, and passing under the thoracic portion; the latter resembles that of the ox.

MUSCLES OF THE SHOULDER

The **deltoid** is undivided; it arises from the aponeurosis covering the infraspinatus, and it ends largely on the deltoid ridge, but partly on the fascia of the arm.

The **supraspinatus** is large; it ends chiefly on the external tuberosity of the humerus.

The **infraspinatus** is inserted into a depression below the posterior division of the external tuberosity.

The **teres minor** is well developed; it ends on a tubercle between the external and deltoid tuberosities of the humerus.

The **subscapularis** and **teres major** have no remarkable features.

The **coraco-brachialis** is short and undivided.

The **capsularis** is very small and frequently absent.

MUSCLES OF THE ARM

The **biceps brachii** is fusiform and not greatly developed. Its tendon of origin is rounded and passes through the capsule of the shoulder joint. The tendon of insertion is bifid, ending on the radius and ulna.

The **brachialis** is well developed, and also ends on the radius and ulna.

The tensor fasciæ **antibrachii** resembles that of the horse.

The long **head** of **the triceps** is divided into two parts, except at its distal end, under which there is a synovial bursa. The **external head** is inserted into a crest on the outer surface of the olecranon by a thin tendon, under which there is a bursa. The **internal head** arises near the head of the humerus, beneath the coracobrachialis.

There are two **anconei.**

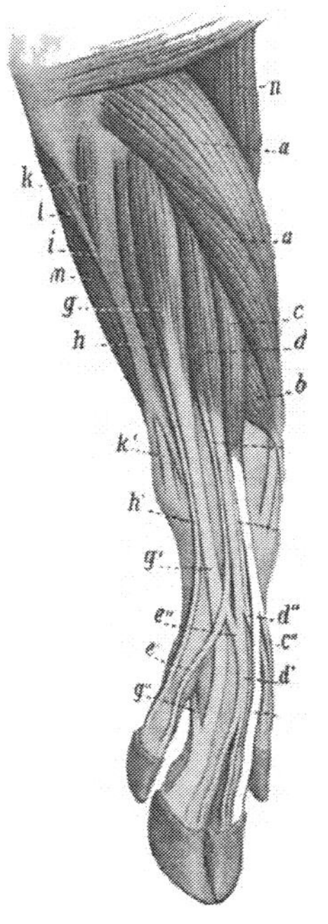

FIG. 227.—MUSCLES OF ANTIBRACHIUM AND MANUS OF PIG, ANTERO-EXTERNAL VIEW.

a, *a'*, Extensor carpi radialis; *b*, extensor carpi obliquus (s. abductor pollicis longus); *c*, *d*, *e*, common or anterior digital extensor; *c'*, *c''*, tendons of insertion of *c*; *d'*, *d''*, tendons of *d*; *e'*, *e''*, tendons of *e*; *f*, tendon of extensor indicis; *g*, extensor digiti quarti; *h*, extensor digiti quinti; *h'*, tendon of *h*; *i*, tendinous, and k, fleshy part of flexor carpi externus; k', tendon of k; *l*, ulnar head of deep digital flexor; *m*, superficial digital flexor; *n*, brachialis. (After Ellenberger, in Leisering's Atlas.)

MUSCLES OF THE FOREARM AND DIGITS

The **extensor carpi radialis** is a strong, fleshy muscle, the tendon of which is inserted into the proximal end of the third metacarpal bone. It may be divided into two parts (M. extensor carpi radialis longus, brevis).

The **extensor carpi obliquus** is well developed; it ends on the second metacarpal bone.

There are three (or four) **digital extensors.**

1. The **common** or **anterior digital extensor** (M. extensor digitalis communis) arises on the extensor epicondyle of the humerus and the lateral ligament of the elbow, and divides into three parts. The tendon of the **inner part** divides into two branches which end on the **second** and **third digits;** the tendon to the second digit is small and often absent. The tendon of the **middle part** divides lower down into two branches for the **third** and **fourth** (chief) **digits;** above this bifurcation it detaches a small branch to the **second digit,** which usually unites with the tendon of the extensor indicis. The tendon of the **deep head** divides into two branches, the inner one joining the tendon of the middle head, while the outer one ends on the **fifth digit.**

2. The **extensor** of **the second digit** (M. extensor indicis proprius) is covered by the preceding muscle, with which it is partially fused. It arises on the ulna. Its delicate tendon usually unites with the tendon of the middle head of the common extensor which goes to the **second digit.**

3. The **lateral digital extensor** (M. extensor digitalis lateralis) consists of two distinct parts: (1) The large **dorsal** (anterior) **muscle** (M. extensor digiti quarti proprius) has a long tendon which ends on the **fourth digit,** and often sends a slip to the fifth digit. (2) The small **volar** (posterior) **muscle** (M. extensor digiti quinti proprius) ends by a long tendon on the lateral aspect of the **fifth digit.**

The **supinator** has been found by Arloing and Lesbre, but is usually absent in the pig.

The **pronator teres** is a small muscle which lies on the internal lateral ligament of the elbow. It arises from the internal epicondyle of the humerus, and reaches about to the middle of the inner border of the radius.

The **flexor carpi internus** is well developed. It arises on the flexor epicondyle of the humerus, and is inserted into the third metacarpal bone.

The **flexor carpi medius** is narrow and has no ulnar head.

The **flexor carpi externus** (M. extensor carpi ulnaris) is covered by a thick, tendinous band, which extends from the extensor epicondyle to the accessory carpal bone and outer aspect of the carpus. The tendon of the muscle perforates this band in the distal part of the forearm and ends on the proximal end of the fifth metacarpal bone.

The **superficial digital flexor** has two bellies. The tendon of the **superficial head** passes down behind the posterior annular ligament of the carpus (bound down by a special annular ligament), forms a ring at the fetlock for a tendon of the deep flexor, and ends by two branches on the second phalanx of the fourth digit. The tendon of the **deep head,** after detaching a slip to the tendon of the deep flexor, passes down with the latter (for which it forms a ring), and ends on the third digit.

The **deep digital flexor** has three heads—humeral, ulnar, and radial. The common tendon divides into four branches, the larger central pair ending on the third phalanges of the principal digits, the smaller pair on the accessory digits. The latter are bound down by a peculiar spiral band. There is no check ligament.

The **lumbricales** are represented by bundles which extend from the deep flexor tendon to the tendon of the deep head of the superficial flexor.

The third and fourth **interossei** are present. Each sends two slips to the corresponding sesamoid bones and extensor tendon.

There are **flexors, adductors,** and **abductors** of the **second** and **fifth digits.**

Muscles of the Pelvic Limb

SUBLUMBAR MUSCLES

The **psoas minor** is intimately united with the psoas major in front and has a long small tendon which ends on the psoas tubercle. It has no thoracic part.

The **psoas major** is large and rounded. It begins at the last rib.

The **quadratus lumborum** is well developed, and extends forward as far as the twelfth rib.

MUSCLES OF THE HIP AND THIGH

The **tensor fasciæ latæ** is broad, and its fleshy part reaches almost to the patella.

The **gluteus superficialis** has a sacral head only; it blends with the biceps femoris.

The **gluteus medius** has a small lumbar part which does not extend so far forward as in the horse. The deep part (Gluteus accessorius) is pretty clearly marked.

The **gluteus profundus** is extensive, reaching nearly to the external angle of the ilium.

The **biceps femoris** has a narrow origin from the sacro-sciatic ligament and tuber ischii. It ends below like that of the ox.

The **semitendinosus** resembles that of the horse.

The **semimembranosus** has two insertions as in the ox.

The **sartorius** has two heads of origin, between which the external iliac vessels are situated. The inner arises from the tendon of the psoas minor, the outer one from the iliac fascia.

The **graciles** are united at their origin even more than in the ox.

The **pectineus** is well developed and is flattened from before backward.

The **adductor** shows no division and is partially fused with the gracilis. It ends on the femur just above the origin of the gastrocnemius.

The **quadratus femoris** is large.

The **obturator externus** resembles that of the horse.

The **obturator internus** is extensive and strong; its tendon emerges through the obturator foramen.

The **gemellus** is fused in part with the obturator internus.

The **quadriceps femoris** is more clearly divided than in the horse, and its action is transmitted by a single patellar ligament.

The **capsularis** is absent.

MUSCLES OF THE LEG AND FOOT

The **peroneus tertius** resembles that of the ox, but its tendon is not perforated by that of the tibialis anterior, and ends on the inner (second) large metatarsal bone, detaching a strong branch to the first and second tarsal bones.

The **tibialis anterior** arises on the tibial crest. Its tendon passes over the hock along the inner border of the tendon of the peroneus tertius (both being bound down by an annular ligament), and is inserted into the inner (second) metatarsal and first tarsal bones.

The **peroneus longus** lies partly on the outer surface of the peroneus tertius. Its tendon crosses those of the lateral extensor, passes along a groove on the plantar surface of the fourth tarsal bone, and ends on the first tarsal and second metatarsal bones.

The **anterior** or **long digital extensor** arises with the peroneus tertius and is largely covered by it and the peroneus longus. It divides into three parts. The tendon of the **inner division** (M. extensor digiti tertii) ends on the **inner chief** (third) digit; that of the **middle division** by two branches on the **principal digits**; and that of the **outer division** by three branches on the **second, fourth, and fifth digits.**

The **lateral digital extensor** divides into proper extensors of the fourth and **fifth digits** (Extensores digiti quarti et quinti).

The **extensor hallucis longus** arises on the fibula and ends on the **inner small** (second) digit.

The **extensor digitalis brevis** is well developed and consists of three parts. The inner and outer tendons end on the first phalanges of the chief digits, the middle one joins the common extensor tendon of the same.

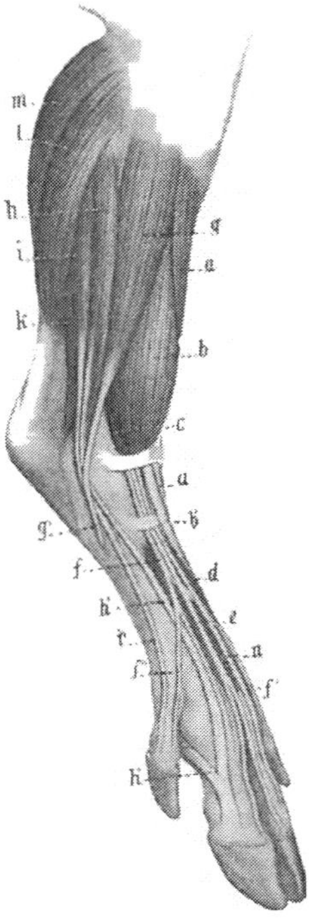

FIG. 228.—MUSCLES OF LEG AND FOOT OF PIG, ANTERO-EXTERNAL VIEW.

a, Tibialis anterior; *a'*, tendon of preceding; *b*, peroneus tertius; *b'*, tendon of *b*; *c*, anterior or long digital extensor; *d*, *e*, *f*, *f'*, *f''*, tendons of *c*; *g*, peroneus longus; *g'*, tendon of *g*; *h*, extensor digiti quarti; *h'*, tendon of *h*, which receives *h''*, from the interosseus medius; *i*, extensor digiti quinti; *k*, deep digital flexor; *l*, soleus; *m*, gastrocnemius; *n*, extensor brevis. (After Ellenberger, in Leisering's Atlas.)

The **gastrocnemius** presents nothing special.

The **soleus** is wide, and is partly blended with the external head of the gastrocnemius.

The **superficial digital flexor** has a large belly. Its tendon ends on the two chief digits, and is also connected with the ligaments of the accessory digits.

The **inner head** of the **deep digital flexor** (flexor digitalis longus) is relatively small. The common tendon ends as in the thoracic limb.

The **popliteus** presents no special features.

The **plantar muscles** resemble their homologues of the fore limb, except that the adductors of the accessory digits and the lumbricales are absent.

THE MUSCLES OF THE DOG

MUSCLES OF THE FACE

The **panniculus carnosus** is well developed and presents two distinct bands, one of which is inserted into the lower lip, the other into the scutiform cartilage of the ear.

The **orbicularis oris** is poorly developed. In the upper lip it is divided centrally, and in the lower it is distinct only near the angles of the mouth.

The **levator nasolabialis** is wide and undivided, and ends in the upper lip.

The **levator labii superioris proprius** arises behind the infraorbital foramen, runs forward under the preceding muscle, and ends in numerous small tendons around the nostril, some blending with those of the opposite side.

The **zygomaticus,** long and narrow, arises on the scutiform cartilage, and ends at the angle of the mouth.

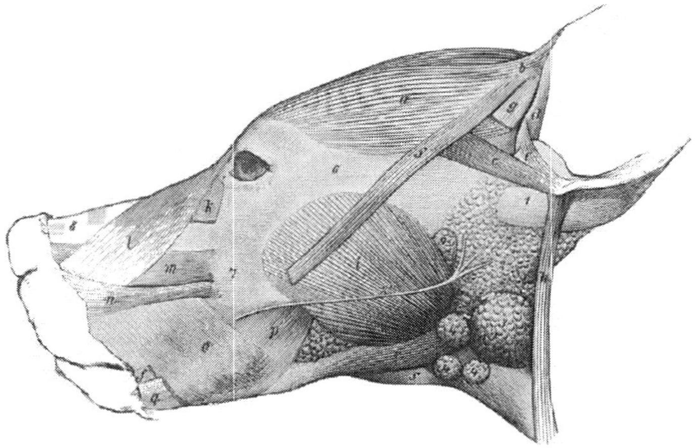

FIG. 229.—MUSCLES OF HEAD OF DOG

a, Scutularis; *b*, *c*, anterior auricular muscles; *d*,*helicis; *e*, antitragicus; *f*, *f*, zygomaticus, out of which a portion is cut; *g*, slip of panniculus; *h*, parotido-auricularis; *i*, masseter; k, malaris; *l*, levator nasolabialis; *m*, levator labii superioris proprius; *n*, dilatator naris lateralis; *o*, *p*, buccinator (buccalis, molaris); q, retractor anguli oris; *r*, digastricus; *s*, mylo-hyoideus; *1*, base of concha; *2*, parotid gland; *2'*, parotid duct; *3*, submaxillary gland; *4*, submaxillary lymph glands; *5*, buccal glands; *6*, zygomatic arch; *7*, maxilla; *8*, dorsum nasi; *9*, parotid lymph gland. (Ellenberger-Baum, Anat. d. Hundes.)

The **depressor labii inferioris** is absent, unless we recognize as such a thin stratum arising on the body of the mandible and spreading out in the orbicularis.

There are no special **nasal muscles,** the homologue of the lateral dilator ending almost entirely in the upper lip.

The **buccinator** is wide and very thin, and the two planes of fibers cross each other.

The **palpebral muscles** present no very noteworthy special characters.

MUSCLES OF MASTICATION

The **masseter** is large. It arises from the zygomatic arch, and extends beyond the branch of the jaw below and behind. Three strata may be recognized in its structure.

The **temporalis** is very large and strong, and contains much tendinous tissue. It arises from the temporal fossa and the orbital ligament.

The **digastricus** is usually not digastric, but is a strong, round, fleshy muscle, which arises on the paramastoid or styloid process and is inserted into the border and inner surface of the ramus at the level of the last molar teeth.

The stylo-mandibularis is absent.

HYOID MUSCLES

The **mylo-hyoideus** is well developed.

The **stylo-hyoideus** is very slender, and is inserted into the body of the hyoid bone: it is not perforated by the digastricus.

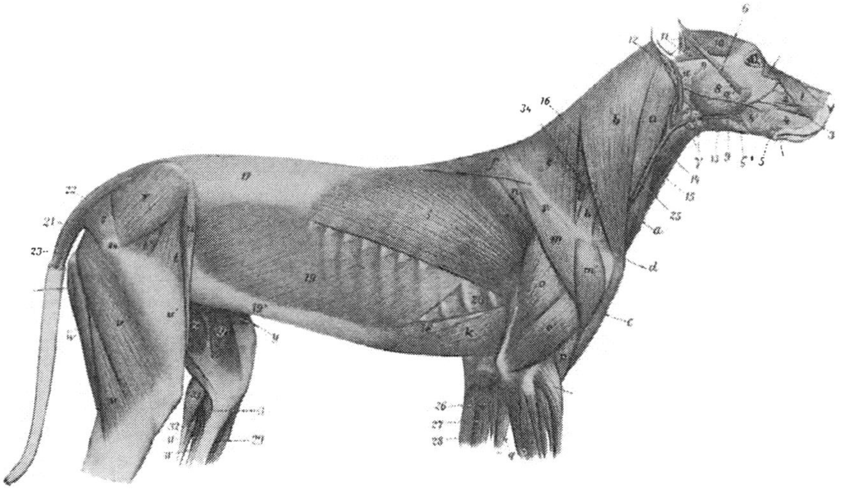

FIG. 230.—SUPERFICIAL MUSCLES OF DOG, AFTER REMOVAL OF PANNICULUS CARNOSUS.

1, Levator nasolabialis; *2*, levator labii superioris proprius; *3*, dilatator naris lateralis; *4*, *4'*, buccinator; *5*, retractor anguli oris s. risorius; *6*, zygomaticus; *7*, malaris; *8*, masseter; *9*, digastricus; *10*, scutularis; *11*, other auricular muscles; *12*, parotido-auricularis; *13*, mylo-hyoideus; *14*, sterno-hyoideus; *15*, sterno-thyroideus; *16*, splenius; *17*, lumbo-dorsal fascia; *18*, rectus abdominis; *19*, obliquus abdominis externus; *19'*, aponeurosis of preceding; *20*, intercostal muscle; *21*, sacro-coccygeus accessorius; *22*, sacro-coccygeus superior; *23*, sacro-coccygeus inferior; *24*, great trochanter; *25*, jugular vein; *a*, *b*, *c*, brachio-cephalicus; *d*, clavicle; *e*, *f*, trapezius; *g*, serratus cervicis; *h*, omo-transversarius; *i*, latissimus dorsi; k, posterior deep pectoral; *l*, supraspinatus; *m*, *m'*, deltoid; *n*, infraspinatus; *o*, triceps, long head; *o'*, triceps, external head; *p*, brachialis; *q*, extensor carpi radialis; *r*, gluteus medius; *s*, gluteus superficialis; *t*, *t'*, tensor fasciæ latæ; *u*, sartorius; *v*, biceps femoris; *v'*, fascia lata; *w*, semitendinosus; *x*, semimembranosus; *y*, sartorius; z, gracilis; *26*, pronator teres; *27*, flexor carpi radialis; *28*, flexor carpi ulnaris; *29*, tibialis anterior; *30*, popliteus; *31*, *31'*, deep digital flexor; *32*, superficial digital flexor; *33*, gastrocnemius; *34*, spine of scapula; α, parotid gland, with α', its duct; β, submaxillary gland; δ, submaxillary lymph glands; η, parotid lymph gland; ζ, inferior buccal glands. (After Ellenberger, in Leisering's Atlas.)

The hyoideus transversus and omo-hyoideus are absent.

The **sterno-thyro-hyoideus** is large and arises chiefly on the first costal carti lage.

MUSCLES OF THE THORACIC LIMB

The **trapezius** is thin, and is not clearly divided into cervical and thoracic portions. Its line of origin extends from about the middle of the neck to the ninth or tenth thoracic spine, the right and left muscles meeting on a median fibrous raphé.

The **omo-transversarius** arises by a tendon on the lower part of the spine of the scapula (often partially blended with the trapezius), and is inserted into the wing of the atlas.

The rhomboideus consists of three parts. The dorsal portion (Rhomboideus thoracalis) is small; it arises from the fourth to the sixth or seventh thoracic spine, and is inserted into the inner surface (chiefly) of the dorsal angle of the scapula. The cervical portion (Rhomboideus cervicalis) arises from the ligamentum nuchæ as far forward as the second or third cervical vertebra, and is inserted into the inner surface of the cervical angle of the scapula. The cephalic portion (Rhomboideus capitis) is a continuation of the preceding which is inserted into the occipital crest.

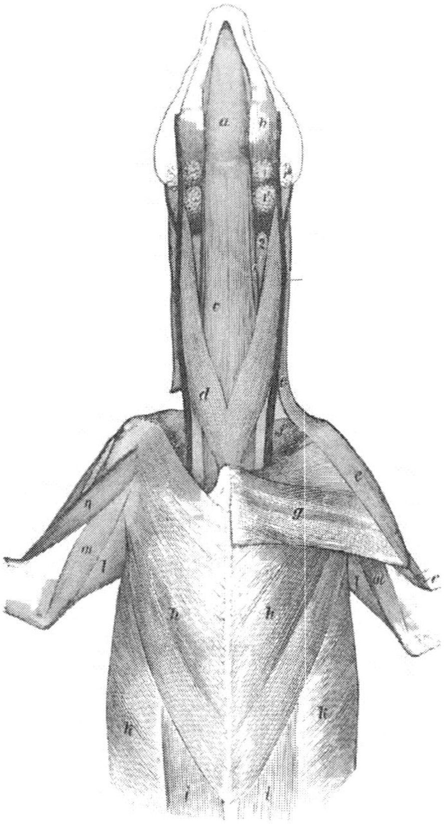

FIG. 231.—VENTRAL MUSCLES OF HEAD, NECK, AND THORAX OF DOG.

a, Mylo-hyoideus; *b*, digastricus; *c*, sterno-hyoideus; *c'*, sterno-thyroideus; *d*, sterno-cephalicus; *e*, brachio-cephalicus; *f*, subscapularis; *g*, superficial pectoral; *h*, deep pectoral; *i*, rectus abdominis; k, obliquus abdominis externus; *l*, long head of triceps; *m*, internal head of triceps; *n*, biceps brachii; *o*, brachialis; *1*, *1'*, *1''*, submaxillary lymph glands; *2*, thyroid gland; *3*, external jugular vein. (Ellenberger-Baum, Anat. d. Hundes.)

The latissimus dorsi is extensive, and has a fleshy attachment to the last two ribs. Its lower edge blends near the shoulder with the panniculus.

The mastoido-humeralis contains in front of the shoulder a fibrous mass in which the clavicle is embedded. Anterior to this it separates into two diverging portions. The dorsal portion (M. cleido-cervicalis) is attached to the median raphé of the neck and to the occipital bone. The ventral portion (M. cleido-mastoideus) is attached to the mastoid process. The common mass posterior to the clavicle and the fibrous intersection, which is attached to the humerus, is homologous with the clavicular portion of the deltoid of man.

The superficial pectoral muscle is small. It arises on the sternum from the first to the third costal cartilage, and is inserted into the anterior surface of the humerus. A superficial slip detached from it is inserted into the fascia of the forearm. The deep pectoral has no prescapular portion. It arises on the sternum and costal cartilages from the second costal to the xiphoid cartilage. It is inserted chiefly into the internal tuberosity of the humerus, but also by small slips into the external tuberosity and the fasela of the arm.

The serratus magnus shows no clear division into cervical and thoracic portions. It arises from the last five cervical vertebræ and the first seven or eight ribs, and is inserted into the upper part of the costal surface of the scapula.

The deltoid is clearly divided into scapular and acromial parts, the former arising on the spine, the latter on the acromion of the scapula. Both end on the deltoid tuberosity.

The **supraspinatus** ends chiefly on the external tuberosity of the humerus, but has a small attachment to the internal tuberosity also.

The **infraspinatus** is inserted into the outer surface of the external tuberosity of the humerus.

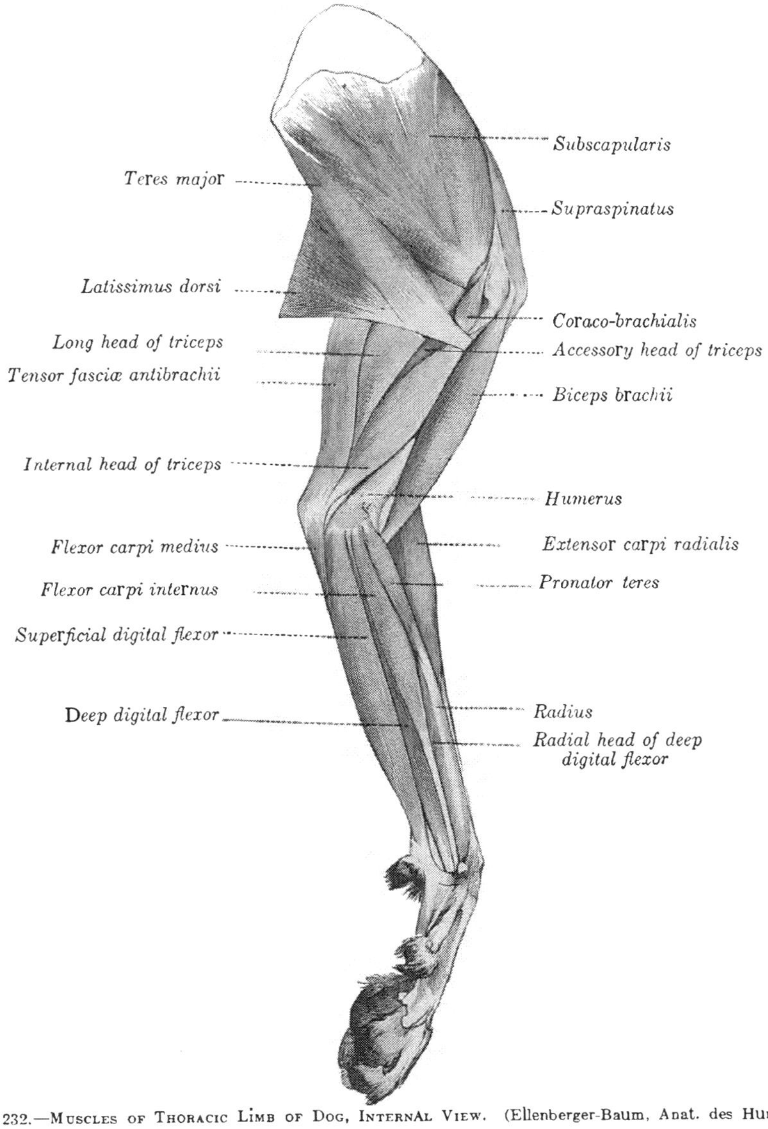

FIG. 232.—MUSCLES OF THORACIC LIMB OF DOG, INTERNAL VIEW. (Ellenberger-Baum, Anat. des Hundes.)

The **teres minor** arises on a tubercle on the posterior border of the scapula, just above the glenoid cavity, and is inserted into the deltoid ridge.

The **subscapularis** is wide and is somewhat multipennate in structure, being intersected by fibrous septa which are attached to the rough lines on the costal surface of the scapula.

The **teres major** is thick. It arises on the upper part of the posterior border of the scapula and on the subscapularis.

The **coraco-brachialis** is short and undivided, and is inserted into the upper part of the postero-internal surface of the humerus.

The capsularis is absent.

The **biceps brachii** lies almost entirely on the inner surface of the humerus. It is long and fusiform. The tendon of origin is round, and passes through the capsule of the shoulder joint. The tendon of insertion is bifid, one branch being attached to the ulnar, the other to the radial tuberosity.

The **brachialis** is very little curved, and is inserted chiefly into the tuberosity and inner border of the ulna.

The **tensor fasciæ antibrachii** is thin and narrow. It arises on the outer surface of the latissimus dorsi, and ends on the olecranon and the fascia of the forearm.

The **triceps** has an additional deep head (Caput accessorium), which arises just below the head of the humerus.

The **brachio-radialis** is a long, narrow, delicate muscle, situated superficially on the anterior surface of the forearm. It arises with the extensor carpi on the crest above the extensor epicondyle of the humerus, and is inserted into the distal part of the inner border of the radius. It is often much reduced, and is sometimes absent. It rotates the forearm and paw outward.

The **extensor carpi** divides into two parts. The larger outer part, the **extensor carpi radialis brevis,** ends on the proximal end of the third metacarpal bone. The inner and more superficial part, the **extensor carpi radialis longus,** ends on the second metacarpal bone. (A tendon to the fourth metacarpal may occur.)

The **extensor carpi obliquus** or **abductor pollicis longus** arises from the outer border and anterior surface of the ulna, the interosseous ligament, and the outer border of the radius. It is inserted into the first metacarpal bone by a tendon which contains a small (sesamoid?) bone. It abducts the first digit.

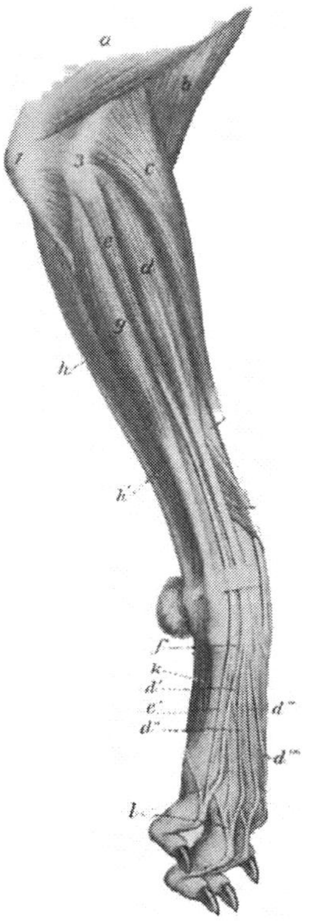

FIG. 233.—MUSCLES OF ANTIBRACHIUM AND MANUS OF DOG, EXTERNAL VIEW.

a, Triceps brachii; *b*, brachialis; *c*, extensor carpi radialis; *d*, common or anterior digital extensor; *d'*, *d''*, *d'''*, *d''''*, tendons of preceding; *e*, lateral digital extensor; *e'*, *f*, tendons of preceding; *g*, extensor carpi ulnaris; *h*, *h'*, flexor carpi ulnaris; *i*, extensor carpi obliquus (s. abductor pollicis longus); k, interossei; *l*, branches from preceding to extensor tendons; *1*, olecranon; *2*, radius; *3*, extensor epicondyle of humerus. (After Ellenberger, in Leisering's Atlas.)

There are three (or four) **extensors of the digits.**

1. The **common digital extensor** (M. extensor digitalis communis) arises on the extensor epicondyle of the humerus and the lateral ligament of the elbow joint. It has four bellies, each terminating in a tendon. These are inserted into the third phalanges of the second, third, fourth, and fifth digits.

2. The **extensor of the first and second digits** M. extensor pollicis longus et extensor indicis proprius) is small, and is covered by the common and lateral extensors. It arises on the proximal part of the ulna. Its tendon passes down with that of the common extensor and divides into two branches. The delicate inner branch ends on the first digit, while the other blends with the tendon of the common extensor for the second digit.

3. The **lateral digital extensor** (M. extensor digitalis lateralis) consists of two

muscles which are not rarely fused. They arise on the extensor epicondyle of the humerus and the lateral ligament of the elbow joint.. The larger, **superficial** belly (M. extensor digiti tertii et quarti) terminates on a tendon which divides at or near the carpus into two branches, which are inserted into the third phalanges of the third and fourth digits, blending with the corresponding tendons of the common extensor. The **posterior belly** (M. extensor digiti quinti) terminates by a tendon which fuses with that of the common extensor for the fifth digit.

The **ulnaris lateralis** or **extensor carpi ulnaris** corresponds to the flexor carpi externus of the horse, but is an extensor of the carpus. It is a large flat muscle which lies on the outer surface of the ulna. It arises on the extensor epicondyle of the humerus, and is inserted into the proximal end of the fifth metacarpal and the accessory carpal bone.

The **ulnaris medialis** or **flexor carpi medius** (s. ulnaris) consists of two quite distinct heads. The larger, **humeral head** arises on the flexor epicondyle, while the smaller, superficial **ulnar** head arises on the posterior border of the ulna. The tendons of the two end together on the accessory carpal bone.

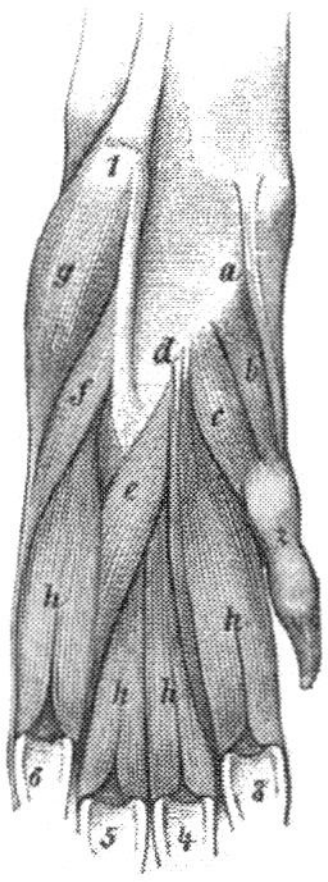

FIG. 234.—VOLAR MUSCLES OF FORE PAW OF DOG.

a, Abductor pollicis brevis et opponens pollicis; *b*, flexor pollicis brevis; *c*, adductor pollicis; *d*, adductor digiti secundi; *e*, adductor digiti quinti; *f*, flexor digiti quinti brevis; *g*, abductor digiti quinti; *h*, interossei; *1*, accessory carpal bone; *2*, first digit; *3–6*, sesamoids of metacarpo-phalangeal joints. (Ellenberger-Baum, Anat. d. Hundes.)

The **radialis volaris** or **flexor carpi internus** (s. radialis) arises on the flexor epicondyle of the humerus and is inserted by a bifid tendon into the second and third metacarpal bones.

The tendons of the foregoing muscles are provided with synovial sheaths at the carpus.

The **pronator teres** is a round muscle, which is situated superficially on the inner border of the proximal part of the radius. It arises on the flexor epicondyle of the humerus, and is inserted into the internal border of the radius. Its action is to flex the elbow and rotate the forearm inward.

The **superficial digital flexor** is situated superficially on the posterior and inner surfaces of the forearm. It arises on the flexor epicondyle of the humerus and terminates near the carpus on a tendon which passes downward outside of the carpal canal and receives below the carpus two reinforcing bands, one from the accessory carpal, the other from the sesamoid bone at the inner side of the carpus. Below this it divides into four branches, which are inserted into the second phalanges of the second, third, fourth, and fifth digits.

The **deep digital flexor** has **humeral, ulnar,** and **radial heads,** the latter arising from the inner border of the radius. They unite on a common tendon which passes down through the carpal canal, gives off a branch to the first digit, and divides into four branches. These perforate the tendons of the superficial flexor and are inserted into the third phalanges of the second to the fifth digits. The tendons are provided with synovial sheaths from the middle of the metacarpus downward, and are held in place by three digital annular ligaments.

The **palmaris longus accessorius** (?) is a small muscle which arises from the deep flexor below the middle of the forearm and ends by two tendons which unite with those of the superficial flexor for the third and fourth digits.

The **supinator** is a short, wide muscle which arises on the humerus beneath the external lateral ligament, crosses the anterior surface of the radius, and is inserted into the inner border of the radius. (A pouch of the capsule of the elbow joint lies under the tendon of origin.) Its action is to rotate the forearm outward (supination).

The **pronator quadratus** consists of fibers which cross the inner surface of the interosseous ligament of the forearm, except at the two extremities of the latter. It is attached to the inner border of the ulna and the anterior surface of the radius. It rotates the forearm inward (pronation).

The **palmaris brevis** (?) is a very small muscle, which arises on the tendon of the superficial digital flexor for the fifth digit, and is inserted at the fifth metacarpo-phalangeal joint into the sheath and annular ligament of the deep flexor.

The **lumbricales** are three very delicate muscles, which arise on the tendons of the deep flexor, and are inserted into the first phalanges of the third, fourth, and fifth digits.

The **abductor pollicis brevis et opponens pollicis,** a very small pale muscle, arises on the fibrous band which connects the superficial flexor tendon with the inner carpal sesamoid, and ends on the distal end of the first metacarpal bone and the first phalanx of the first digit. It abducts the first digit.[1]

The **flexor pollicis brevis** arises on the posterior carpal ligament over the second metacarpal bone, and ends on the volar sesamoid of the first digit.

The **adductor pollicis,** situated externally to the preceding, is the largest of the thumb muscles. It arises between the preceding and the second interosseous muscle, and is inserted into the first phalanx of the first digit.

The **adductor digiti secundi** is situated between the second interosseous muscle and the adductor digiti quinti. It arises on the carpal ligament, and ends on the first phalanx of the second digit.

The **adductor digiti quinti** arises close to the preceding muscle, and passes outward to end on the first phalanx of the fifth digit.

The **flexor digiti quinti** arises on the ligament connecting the accessory carpal to the third and fourth metacarpal bones, crosses the corresponding interosseous muscle, and ends on the fifth digit with the next muscle.

The **abductor digiti quinti** is larger than the two preceding muscles; it arises on the accessory carpal bone, and ends on the outer sesamoid of the fifth digit and on the lateral ligament.

There are four **interossei** which lie on the volar (posterior) surface of the metacarpus. They are well developed and fleshy. They arise on the distal row of the carpus and on the proximal ends of the metacarpals. Each divides distally into two branches, which are inserted by small tendons on the corresponding sesamoid bones, and detach slips to the extensor tendons.

Muscles of the Neck

The **sterno-cephalicus** is well developed. It arises on the manubrium sterni and ends on the mastoid process, blending with the cleido-cervicalis.

The **scalenus ventralis** (s. primæ costæ) arises on the last four cervical transverse processes, and is inserted into the first rib.

The **scalenus dorsalis** (s. supracostalis) is large. Anteriorly it blends with the preceding muscle, while posteriorly it divides into two parts. The upper part is inserted on the third and fourth ribs, the lower part by a long, thin tendon on the eighth rib.

The **longus colli** resembles that of the horse.

The **rectus capitis anterior major** arises on the transverse processes of the second to the sixth cervical vertebræ and ends as in the horse. The **rectus minor** and **lateralis** resemble those of the horse.

The **intertransversales** resemble those of the ox.

The **splenius** is strong and extensive. It arises on the first four or five thoracic

[1] Movements of individual digits are specified with regard to the axis of the manus (hand, paw), and not to the median plane of the body.

spines and the median raphé of the neck, and is inserted into the occipital crest and mastoid process.

The **complexus** is composed of two parts—the biventer cervicis and the complexus major proper. The **biventer cervicis** arises from the transverse processes of the fifth and sixth, and the spines of the second to the fifth (or sixth) thoracic vertebræ, from the ligamentum nuchæ, and the median raphé. It has four tendinous intersections. The **complexus major** arises on the transverse processes of the first three or four thoracic vertebræ and the articular processes of the last five cervical. Both end on a strong common tendon which is inserted into the occipital crest and the depression below it.

The **trachelo-mastoideus** consists of two unequal portions. The large **dorsal part** (M. longissimus capitis) arises on the transverse processes of the first four thoracic and the articular process of the last three or four cervical vertebræ, and ends with the splenius on the mastoid process of the temporal bone. The small **ventral part** (M. longissimus atlantis) arises on the articular processes of the third, fourth, and fifth cervical vertebræ, and ends on the wing of the atlas.

The other muscles present no striking differential features,but it may be noted that distinct **interspinales** are present.

Muscles of the Thorax

There are twelve pairs of **levatores costarum.**

The **external intercostals** do not occupy the spaces between the costal cartilages.

The **diaphragm** has a small tendinous center. The œsophageal opening is between the pillars. The fleshy rim is attached at the costo-chondral junctions from the eighth backward, and along the thirteenth rib nearly its entire length.

Muscles of the Back and Loins

The **serratus anticus** arises from the median raphé of the neck and the first six or seven thoracic spines, and is inserted into the second to the ninth ribs. It is well developed. The **serratus posticus**—much weaker—arises on the lumbodorsal fascia, and is inserted into the last three or four ribs. Thus one or two ribs intervene between the two.

The **transversalis costarum** (Ilio-costalis) is well developed, and extends from the ilium to the sixth, fifth, or fourth cervical vertebra.

The **longissimus** resembles that of the other animals, but the spinalis et semispinalis separates clearly at the sixth or seventh thoracic vertebra. It is inserted into the articular and spinous processes of the last six cervical vertebræ. It has no depression in the lumbar region for the gluteus medius.

The **intertransversales** are fleshy, as in the ox.

The **interspinales** are distinct, especially in the lumbar region.

Muscles of the Tail

These present the same general arrangement as in the horse. The **sacrococcygei,** however, arise on the lumbar vertebræ also, and the **coccygeus** on the ischiatic spine. There is found a **sacro-coccygeus accessorius,** which arises on the internal border of the ilium, the edge of the sacrum, and the transverse processes of the first coccygeal vertebræ, and is inserted between the superior and lateral sacro-coccygei. It is homologous with the intertransversales.

MUSCLES OF THE ABDOMEN

The abdominal tunic is practically absent.

The **obliquus abdominis externus** has an extensive fleshy portion. It arises from the last eight or nine ribs and the lumbo-dorsal fascia.

The **obliquus abdominis internus** arises from the external angle of the ilium and the lumbo-dorsal fascia. The fibers have an almost vertical direction, and there is a fleshy attachment to the last rib.

The **rectus abdominis** is attached by a long tendon on the first five or six costal cartilages, and by fleshy fibers on the xiphoid cartilage. It has three to six indistinct tendinous inscriptions.

The **transversus abdominis** presents no special features except that the posterior part of its aponeurosis splits into two layers which include the rectus between them.

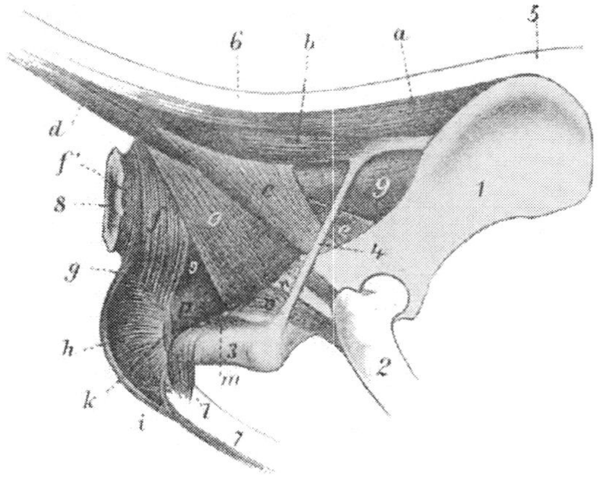

FIG. 235.—MUSCLES OF TAIL, ANUS, AND GENITAL ORGANS OF DOG. *1*, ilium; *2*, femur; *3*, tuber ischii; *4*, sacro-sciatic lig.; *5*, sacral region; *6*, tail; *7*, penis; *8*, anus; *9*, rectum; *a*, sacro-coccygeus superior; *b*, sacro-coccygeus accessorius; *c*, coccygeus; *d*, sacro-coccygeus inferior; *e*, retractor ani; *f*, *f'*, sphincter ani externus; *g*, retractor penis; *h*, bulbo-cavernosus; *i*, transversus perinei (?); k, *m*, ischio-urethrales; *l*, ischio-cavernosus; *n*, tendon of obturator internus; *o*, gemellus; *p*, urethral muscle. (After Ellenberger, in Leisering's Atlas.)

MUSCLES OF THE PELVIC LIMB

The **psoas minor** arises on the last thoracic and first four or five lumbar vertebræ, and is inserted into the ilio-pectineal line.

The **psoas major** is short, arising from the last four lumbar vertebræ.

The outer head of the **iliacus** is small, while the inner head is large and fuses with the psoas major.

The **quadratus lumborum** is well developed, and extends laterally beyond the outer edge of the ilio-psoas. It arises from the last four ribs and the lumbar transverse processes, and ends on the pelvic surface of the wing of the ilium.

The **tensor fasciæ latæ** consists of two parts. The anterior part is long and rounded; the posterior is shorter and fan-like.

The **gluteus superficialis** is small. It arises on the sacrum, first coccygeal vertebræ, and sacro-sciatic ligament. It is inserted below and behind the trochanter major of the femur, on the outer branch of the linea aspera.

The **gluteus medius** has no lumbar portion. It is inserted into the trochanter major by a strong tendon.

The **gluteus profundus** is broad and fan-shaped. It arises on the superior ischiatic spine and on the ilium as far forward as the gluteal line, and is inserted into the trochanter major below the medius.

The **pyriformis** is not blended with the gluteus medius. It arises from the border of the sacrum and from the sacro-sciatic ligament, and ends on the trochanter major.

The **biceps femoris** has two heads of origin which soon fuse. The larger head arises from the sacro-sciatic ligament and tuber ischii, the smaller one from the tuber ischii. The aponeurosis of insertion ends on the patella, the patellar ligament, and the tibial crest. There is also a tendinous band, which comes from the deep face of the muscle and terminates at the tarsus, as in the horse.

The **abductor cruris posterior** may be regarded as an accessory head of the biceps femoris. It is a thin, muscular band which arises on the sacro-sciatic ligament, passes downward between the biceps and semimembranosus, and ends by blending with the former.

The **semitendinosus** arises from the tuber ischii only. It ends as in the horse.

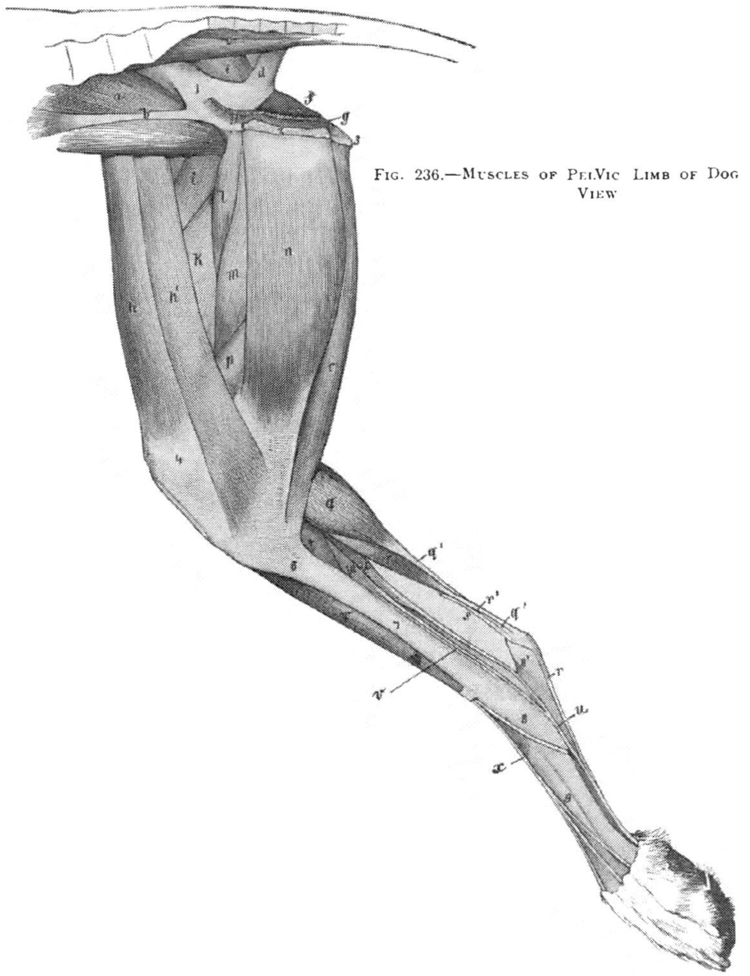

FIG. 236.—MUSCLES OF PELVIC LIMB OF DOG INTERNAL VIEW

The **semimembranosus** is large and arises from the ischium only. It divides into two portions: the anterior portion ends on the tendon of the pectineus, on the femur above the internal condyle, and on the inner (Vesalian) sesamoid bone; the posterior portion ends on the internal condyle of the tibia, the tendon passing under the internal lateral ligament of the stifle joint.

The **rectus femoris** has only one tendon of origin. The single patellar ligament acts as the tendon of insertion of the quadriceps.

The **capsularis** is usually present, but is small and pale.

The **sartorius** consists of two portions. It arises from the external angle and border of the ilium. The anterior portion ends on the patella, the posterior on the internal surface of the tibia, its tendon blending with that of the gracilis.

The **graciles** are not so much fused at their origin as in the other animals.

The **pectineus** is long and slender. It arises from the ilio-pectineal eminence and ends on the internal branch of the linea aspera above the distal end of the femur.

There are two distinct **adductors.** The small anterior one ends on the proximal third of the femur, the posterior one on the distal part of the femur and on the inner face of the stifle joint.

The **quadratus femoris** is short and strong. The other external rotators of the thigh present no special features.

The **peroneus tertius** is represented by a tendinous band which arises on the internal surface of the tibia below the crest. It passes downward on the inner surface of the tibialis anterior, blends with the annular ligament above the tarsus, and is attached to the joint capsule and the proximal end of the third metatarsal bone.

Arloing and Lesbre say: "The third peroneus is a proper extensor of the fifth digit; it is a very feeble, fleshy band, situated behind the peroneus brevis, which it partially covers. It is attached to the upper part of the fibula, and is continued by a long, delicate tendon which passes in the same malleolar groove with the muscle mentioned; it then crosses behind the tendon of the peroneus longus and extends to the phalanges of the outer digit, where it joins one of the branches of the common extensor."

The **tibialis anterior** is large and superficial. It arises on the external condyle and crest of the tibia, and is inserted into the first metatarsal bone, or into the first tarsal and second metatarsal.

There are four **extensors of the digits.**

1. The **anterior or long digital extensor** (M. extensor digitalis longus) is fusiform, and lies largely under the preceding muscle. It arises from the extensor fossa of the femur. The tendon is bound down by two annular ligaments, and divides below the tarsus into four branches, which end on the distal phalanges of the digits (second to fifth).

2. The **lateral digital extensor** (M. extensor digitalis lateralis) is feeble and semipennate. It arises on the fibula below the head. The tendon passes under the lateral ligament of the tarsus and joins the branch of the tendon of the long extensor for the fifth digit.

3. The **extensor hallucis longus** is a very thin muscle which arises from the fibula under the long extensor. Its delicate tendon accompanies that of the tibialis anterior to the first metatarsal bone, or becomes lost in the fascia.

4. The **extensor digitalis brevis** has three divisions. It arises on the fibular tarsal bone and the adjacent ligaments. The three tendons are inserted into the second, third, and fourth digits, blending with the interossei. (Sometimes there is found a tendon to the rudimentary first digit, which may represent the extensor hallucis brevis. There may be a fourth belly for the tendon to the second digit.)

The **peroneus longus** arises on the external condyle of the tibia, the head of the fibula, and the lateral ligament. The long tendon passes down the leg parallel to the fibula, crosses the plantar (posterior) surface of the tarsus transversely, and ends on the first metatarsal bone. A short branch is detached to the external metatarsal bone.

The **peroneus brevis** is semipennate and arises from the distal half or more of the outer face of the tibia and the fibula. Its tendon accompanies that of the lateral extensor over the external malleolus of the tibia, and ends on the proximal end of the fifth metatarsal bone.

The soleus is absent. (It is present and large in the cat.)

The **gastrocnemius** arises on the rough lines above the condyles of the femur. The heads of origin each contain a bone about the size of a pea—the sesamoid of Vesal—which articulates with the corresponding condyle of the femur. The tendon comports itself as in the horse.

The **superficial digital flexor** has a large round belly. It arises in common with the outer head of the gastrocnemius from the external rough line and Vesalian sesamoid bone, and from the aponeurosis of the vastus externus. The tendon winds around that of the gastrocnemius, passes over the tuber calcis (where it is arranged as in the horse), and divides below the tarsus into two branches. Each of these divides into two branches which end as in the fore limb. The outer and inner branches detach slips to the suspensory ligaments of the large digital pad. Muscle-fibers often occur in the tendon in the metatarsal region.

The **deep digital flexor** has two heads. The large outer head, the **flexor hallucis longus,** arises from the tibia and fibula, filling the interosseous space. The small inner head, **flexor digitalis pedis longus,** also arises from the tibia and fibula, its tendon joining that of the large head below the tarsus. The common tendon detaches a branch to the large digital pad and terminates as in the fore limb.

The **tibialis posterior** is a small but distinct muscle, which arises on the proximal part of the fibula. The thin tendon accompanies that of the flexor longus and ends on the internal lateral ligament of the tarsus.

The tendon of the **popliteus** contains a small sesamoid bone.

The **adductors of the second and fifth digits,** the **lumbricales,** and the **interossei** are arranged as in the thoracic limb.

The **quadratus plantæ** arises on the outer surface of the distal end of the fibular tarsal bone and on the lateral tarsal ligament, passes downward and inward, and terminates on a thin tendon which fuses with that of the deep flexor.

The **abductor digiti quinti** is a very small muscle which consists of two parts. One of these is a tendinous slip which extends from the posterior surface of the proximal part of the fibular tarsal bone to the head of the fifth metatarsal bone; the other part arises from the inner surface of the fibular tarsal bone (or from the tendinous part) and ends on the first phalanx of the fifth digit.

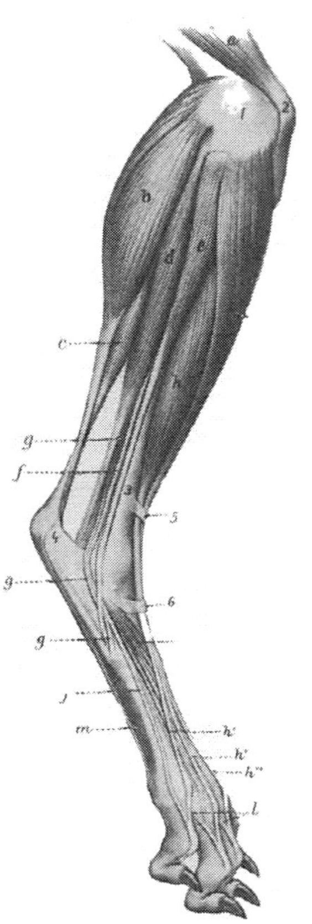

FIG. 237.—MUSCLES OF LEG AND FOOT OF DOG, EXTERNAL VIEW.

a, Quadriceps femoris; *b*, gastrocnemius, external head; *c*, superficial digital flexor; *d*, deep digital flexor; *e*, peroneus longus; *f*, tendon of lateral extensor; *g*, peroneus brevis; *h*, long or anterior digital extensor; *h'*, *h''*, *h'''*, tendons of preceding; *i*, tibialis anterior; k, extensor brevis; *l*, slips from interossei (*m*); *1*, external condyle of femur; *2*, patella; *3*, tibia; *4*, tuber calcis; *5*, *6*, annular ligaments. (After Ellenberger, in Leisering's Atlas.)

In case the skeleton of the first digit is well developed, there are found three muscles homologous with those of the same digit in the fore limb. These are the **abductor hallucis, adductor hallucis,** and **flexor hallucis brevis.**

THE DIGESTIVE SYSTEM

This system consists of the organs directly concerned in the reception and digestion of the food, its passage through the body, and the expulsion of the unabsorbed portion. These organs are conveniently grouped under two heads, viz.: (1) the **alimentary canal**; (2) the **accessory organs.**

The **alimentary canal** (Tractus alimentarius) is a tube, about 100 feet (ca. 30 m.) in length in the horse, and extends from the lips to the anus. It has a complete lining of mucous membrane, external to which is an almost continuous muscular coat. The abdominal portion of the tube is largely covered with a serous membrane—the visceral peritoneum. The canal consists of the following consecutive segments:

1. Mouth.
2. Pharynx.
3. Œsophagus.
4. Stomach.
5. Small intestine.
6. Large intestine.

The **accessory organs** are the teeth, tongue, salivary glands, liver, and pancreas.

DIGESTIVE SYSTEM OF THE HORSE

THE MOUTH

The **mouth**[1] (Cavum oris) is the first part of the alimentary canal. In the horse it is a long cylindrical cavity, and when closed, it is almost entirely filled up by the contained structures. The entrance to it (Rima oris) is closed by the lips. Laterally it is bounded by the cheeks; above, by the hard palate; below, by the body of the mandible and the mylo-hyoid muscles; behind, by the soft palate.

The **cavity** of the mouth is subdivided into two parts by the teeth and alveolar processes. The space external to these and inclosed externally by the lips and cheeks is termed the vestibule of the mouth (Vestibulum oris). In the resting state of the parts the walls of this cavity are in contact, and the space is practically obliterated. Its existence becomes very evident in facial paralysis, when the food tends to collect in it laterally, pouching out the cheeks. The space within the teeth and alveolar processes is termed the mouth cavity proper (Cavum oris proprium). When the teeth are in contact, it communicates with the vestibule only by the interdental spaces and the intervals behind the last molar teeth. Posteriorly it communicates with the pharynx through the isthmus of the fauces.

The **mucous membrane** lining the mouth (Tunica mucosa oris) is continuous at the margin of the lips with the common integument, and behind with the mucous lining of the pharynx. During life it is chiefly of a pink color.

The **lips** (Labia oris) are two musculo-membranous folds which surround the orifice of the mouth. Their angles of union (Anguli oris s. commissuræ labiorum) are situated near the first cheek tooth and are rounded. Each lip presents two surfaces and two borders. The outer surface is covered by the skin, which presents long tactile hairs in addition to the ordinary fine hair. The upper lip shows

[1] The term "mouth" is commonly used to signify either the oral cavity (Cavum oris) or the entrance to it (Rima oris).

a shallow median furrow (Philtrum), the lower a rounded prominence, the chin (Mentum). The inner or oral surface is covered with mucous membrane which is

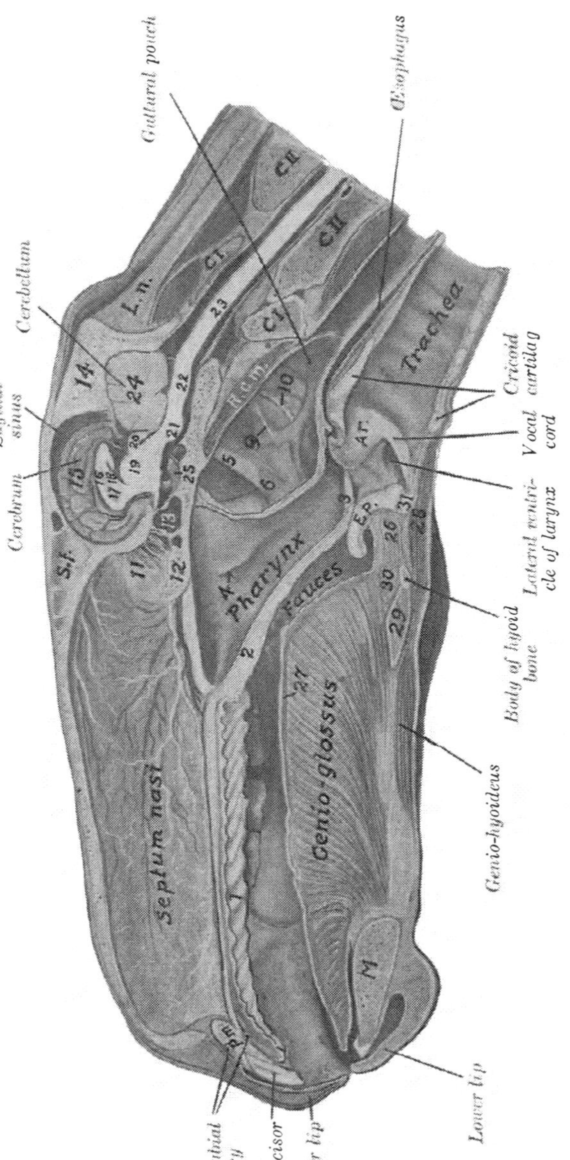

FIG. 238. SAGITTAL SECTION OF HEAD OF HORSE. THE SECTION IS ABOUT 1 [illegible] TO THE LEFT OF THE MEDIAN PLANE.
[illegible]; 2, [illegible]; 3 posterior pillar of soft palate; 4, Eustachian opening; [illegible] oid bone; 6, stylo-pharyngeus muscle; 9, glosso-haryn[illegible]; [illegible] ; 11, perpendicular plate of ethmoid; 12, presphe[illegible]id; [illegible] sin[illegible]; 14, occipital bone; 15, median surface o[illegible] cerebral [illegible] is [illegible] m; 17, septum lucidum; 18, fornix; 19, thalamus; [illegible] corpo[illegible] gemina; 21, pons; 22, medulla oblongata; 23, spinal cord; [illegible] pituitary body; 26, hyo-epiglottic muscle; 27, superior l[illegible] gi[illegible] muscle o[illegible] gue; 28, omo-hyoideus; 29, hyo-glossus; 30, hyoideu[illegible] cartilage (body); S. f., frontal sinus; L. n., lig. nuchæ; [illegible] I, atlas; C II, axis; [illegible] c. m., rectus cap. ant. major and minor; E[illegible]., ep[illegible]tis; [illegible] tilage; P m., premaxilla; M., mandible. The leader line [illegible]r the guttural pouch points to the external carotid artery.

commonly more or less pigmented. The small papillæ on this surface show on their summits the openings of the ducts of the labial glands. Small folds of mucous membrane which pass from the lip to the gum represent the frænula labii (superioris, inferioris). The free border of the lip is dense and presents short, very stiff hairs. The attached border is continuous with the surrounding structures, and is adherent to the alveolar borders of the bones of the jaws.

Structure.—The lips are covered externally by the skin, and are lined by mucous membrane; between these are muscular tissue and glands. The skin lies directly on the muscles, many fibers of which are inserted into the former. The muscles have been described (page 214). The **labial glands** (Glandulæ labiales) form a compact mass near the angles; they are numerous in the upper lip, fewer in the lower. The mucous membrane is often pigmented, and is reflected upon the bones of the jaws to form the gums.

Blood-vessels and Nerves.—The arteries are derived from the superior and inferior labial and palato-labial arteries. The sensory nerves come from the trigeminus, and the motor from the facial nerve.

The **cheeks** (Buccæ) form the sides of the mouth, and are continuous in front with the lips. They are attached above and below to the alveolar borders of the bones of the jaws.

Structure.—This comprises: (1) The skin; (2) the muscular and glandular layer; (3) the mucous membrane. The skin offers nothing in particular to notice. The muscular tissue is formed mainly by the buccinator, but also by parts of the panniculus, zygomaticus, dilatator naris lateralis, levator nasolabialis, and depressor labii inferioris. The **buccal glands** (Glandulæ buccales) are arranged in two rows. The upper row (superior buccal or molar glands) is found on the outer surface of the buccinator muscle, near its upper border. The anterior part of the row consists of scattered lobules; the posterior part, which lies under cover of the masseter muscle, is more developed and compact. The lower row (inferior buccal or molar glands), less voluminous than the upper, is situated in the submucous tissue at the lower border of the buccinator muscle. The mucous membrane is reflected above and below upon the gums, and is continuous behind with that of the soft palate. It is reddish in color and frequently shows pigmented areas. Opposite the third upper cheek tooth is the opening of the parotid (Stenson's) duct, surrounded by a circular fold of the mucous membrane. A linear series of small papillæ above and below indicates the orifices of the small ducts from the buccal glands.

Blood-vessels and Nerves.—The blood-supply is derived from the facial and buccinator arteries. The sensory nerves come from the trigeminus and the motor from the facial nerve.

The **gums** (Gingivæ) are composed of a dense fibrous tissue intimately united with the periosteum of the alveolar processes, and blending at the edges of the alveoli with the alveolar periosteum, which fixes the teeth in their cavities. They are covered by a smooth mucous membrane, destitute of glands, and of a low degree of sensibility.

The **hard palate** (Palatum durum) is bounded in front and on the sides by the alveolar arches; behind it is continuous with the soft palate. Its osseous basis is formed by the premaxilla, maxilla, and palate bones. The mucous membrane is smooth, and is attached to the bones by a submucosa which contains in its anterior part an exceedingly rich venous plexus, constituting an erectile tissue. A central raphé (Raphé palati) divides the surface into two equal portions. Each of these presents about eighteen transverse curved ridges (Rugæ palatini) which have their concavity and their free edges directed backward. They are further apart and more prominent anteriorly. There are no glands in the submucosa.

Vessels and Nerves.—The blood-supply is derived chiefly from the palatine arteries and the nerves from the trigeminus.

The **soft palate** (Palatum molle) is a musculo-membranous curtain which separates the cavity of the mouth from that of the pharynx. It slopes downward and backward from its junction with the hard palate. The oral **surface** faces downward and forward, and is covered with a mucous membrane continuous with that of the hard palate. It is corrugated and presents numerous small orifices (of gland-ducts) and two sagittal ridges. On each side a short, thick fold passes to join the base of the tongue; this is the **anterior pillar** of the soft palate (Arcus glossopalatinus). The **pharyngeal surface** looks upward and backward and is covered by a mucous membrane continuous with that of the nasal cavity. The **free border** (Arcus palatinus) is concave and thin; it is in contact (except during deglutition) with the epiglottis. It is continuous with a fold of the mucous membrane, which passes on each side along the lateral wall of the pharynx and unites with its fellow over the beginning of the œsophagus; this fold is termed the **posterior pillar** of the soft palate (Arcus pharyngopalatinus). The space between the diverging anterior and posterior pillars (Sinus tonsillaris) is occupied by the faucial tonsil. In the horse, however, there is not a compact tonsil, as in man, dog, etc., but a somewhat extended group of mucous glands and masses of lymphoid tissue. These cause elevations of the surface, on which are seen numerous depressions (crypts) in which the gland-ducts open. The soft palate is greatly developed in equidæ, its length being five to six inches (12 to 15 cm.). Its length and contact with the epiglottis account for the fact that in these animals mouth-breathing does not occur under normal conditions, and that in vomiting the ejected matter escapes usually through the nasal cavity.[1]

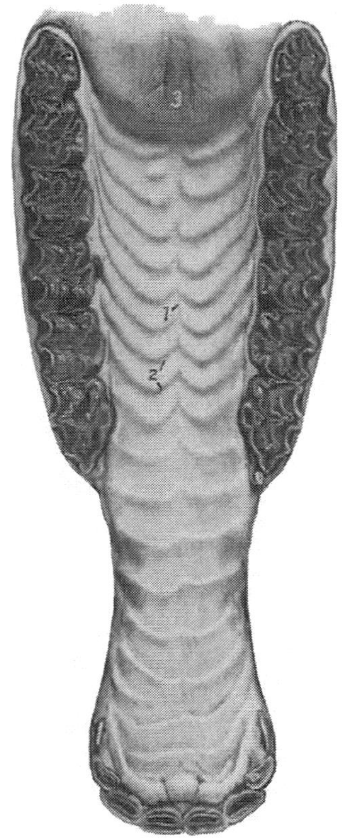

FIG. 239.—HARD PALATE AND PART OF SOFT PALATE OF HORSE.

1, Raphé palati; *2*, ridges of palate; *3*, anterior end of soft palate, showing orifices of ducts of palatine glands.

Structure.—The soft palate consists of: (1) The oral mucous membrane, continuous with that of the hard palate; (2) the **palatine glands** (Glandulæ palatinæ), which form a layer about half an inch in thickness; (3) the aponeurotic and muscular layer; (4) the pharyngeal mucous membrane, continuous with that of the nasal cavity.

The **muscles** proper to the soft palate are the azygos uvulæ, the levator palati, and the tensor palati.

The **azygos uvulæ** (M. palatinus) consists of two small muscular bundles which lie together at the median line. It is attached through the medium of the palatine aponeurosis to the palatine arch, and terminates near the free edge of the soft palate. Its action is to shorten and raise the soft palate.

The **levator palati** (M. levator veli palatini) arises from the muscular process of the petrous temporal bone and from the Eustachian tube, and passes forward and downward externally to the latter, to spread out on the pharyngeal surface of the soft palate. It raises the soft palate, thus closing the posterior nares during deglutition.

The **tensor palati** (M. tensor veli palatini) is larger than the levator, and is fusiform and flattened. It arises from the muscular process of the petrous temporal bone and the Eustachian tube, and passes forward external to the levator.

[1] The epiglottis may be either in front of or behind the soft palate; most often it is prevelar.

Its tendon is then reflected around the hamulus of the pterygoid bone, being held in position by a fibrous band and lubricated by a bursa. It turns inward and expands in the aponeurosis of the soft palate. It tenses the soft palate.

Vessels and Nerves.—The blood-supply of the soft palate is derived from the internal and external maxillary arteries. The nerves come from the trigeminus, vagus, and glosso-pharyngeal nerves.

The floor of the mouth in its anterior part is free and is formed by the body of the mandible, covered by mucous membrane. The remainder is concealed by the attached portion of the tongue, with the exception of a narrow space on each side

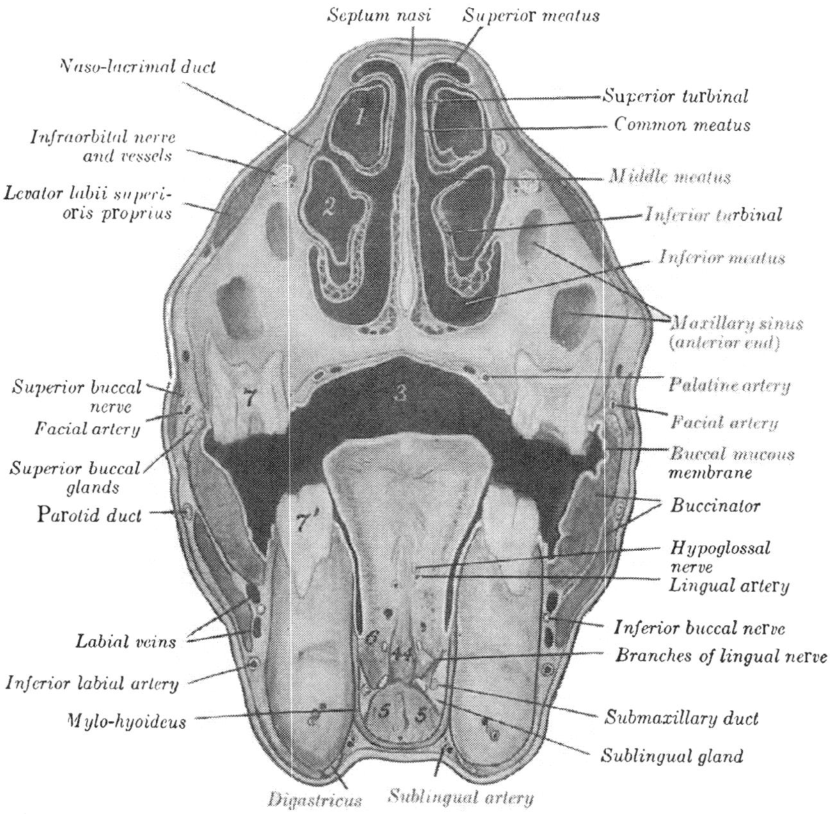

FIG. 240.—CROSS-SECTION OF HEAD OF HORSE JUST IN FRONT OF FACIAL CREST.
1, Cavity of superior turbinal; *2*, cavity of inferior turbinal; *3*, cavum oris; *4*, *4*, genio-glossi; *5*, *5*, genio-hyoidei; *6*, hyo-glossus; *7*, upper, *7'*, lower fourth cheek tooth. Line to facial artery crosses zygomaticus.

of the latter. About opposite the canine tooth on each side is a papilla, the **caruncula sublingualis,** through which the duct of the submaxillary gland opens. Just behind these papillæ is a median fold of mucous membrane which passes to the under surface of the tongue, constituting the **frenum linguæ.** On either side are the sublingual crests, which extend from the frenum to the level of the fourth cheek tooth. The crest presents numerous small papillæ, through which open the ducts from the subjacent sublingual gland.[1] Behind the last tooth a vertical fold

[1] In the undisturbed state of the parts there is no space between the tongue and the rami of the lower jaw; consequently the tongue must be drawn aside to see the sublingual crest.

of the mucous membrane passes from upper to lower jaw. This is termed the plica pterygomandibularis: it contains a ligament of like name.

The **isthmus faucium** is the orifice of communication between the mouth and the pharynx. It is bounded above by the soft palate, below by the root of the tongue, and laterally by the anterior pillars of the soft palate. It is long, relatively small, and not very dilatable in the horse, and is closed by the soft palate under normal conditions, except during deglutition.

THE TONGUE

The tongue (Lingua) is situated on the floor of the mouth, between the rami of the mandible, and is supported mainly in a sort of sling formed by the mylohyoid muscles. Its posterior portion, the root (Radix linguæ), is attached to the hyoid bone, soft palate, and pharynx. Only the upper surface of this part is free, and slopes downward and backward. The middle portion, the body (Corpus linguæ), has three free surfaces. The upper surface or **dorsum** (Dorsum linguæ) is rounded. The lateral surfaces are nearly flat for the most part, but anteriorly become rounded and narrower. The lower surface is attached to the mandible. The **apex** or tip (Apex linguæ) is free, spatula-shaped, and presents superior and inferior surfaces and a rounded border.

Structure.—The tongue consists of: (1) The mucous membrane; (2) the glands; (3) the muscles.

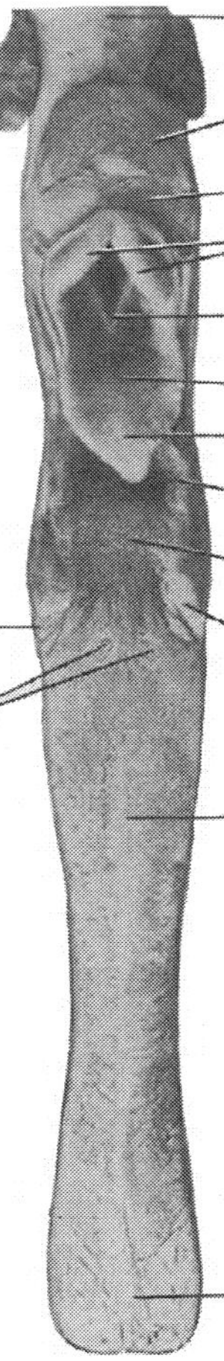

Fig. 241.—Tongue of Horse, Dorsal Aspect.

The **mucous membrane** (Tunica mucosa linguæ) adheres intimately to the subjacent tissue, except on the lower part of the lateral surfaces of the body and the under surface of the tip. It varies considerably in thickness. On the dorsum it is very thick and dense. Underneath this portion there is a dense fibrous cord, which extends medially a distance of five or six inches forward from the vallate papillæ. On the sides and under surface of the tongue the membrane is much thinner and smooth, and can more readily be dissected off the muscular tissue. From the under surface of the free part of the tongue a fold of the mucous membrane passes to the floor of the mouth, forming the **frenum linguæ.** This contains the anterior edges of the genio-glossi muscles. Posteriorly a fold passes on each side from the edge of the dorsum to join the soft palate, forming the anterior pillars of the latter. A central glosso-epiglottic fold (Plica glossoepiglottica) passes from the root to the base of the epiglottis. The mucous membrane presents numerous **papillæ,** which are of four kinds—filiform, fungiform, vallate, and foliate. The **filiform papillæ** (Papillæ filiformes) are fine, pointed projections. They cover the upper surface of the body and tip, to which they give a distinct pile. The **fungiform papillæ** (Papillæ fungiformes) are rounded at the free end, which is supported by a neck. They occur principally on the lateral part of the tongue, but are also found scattered over the dorsum and upper surface of the free portion. The **vallate papillæ** (Papillæ vallatæ) are usually two or three in number. The two constant ones have a diameter of about 7 mm., and are found on the posterior part of the dorsum, one on each side of the median plane, about an inch (ca. 3 cm.) apart.

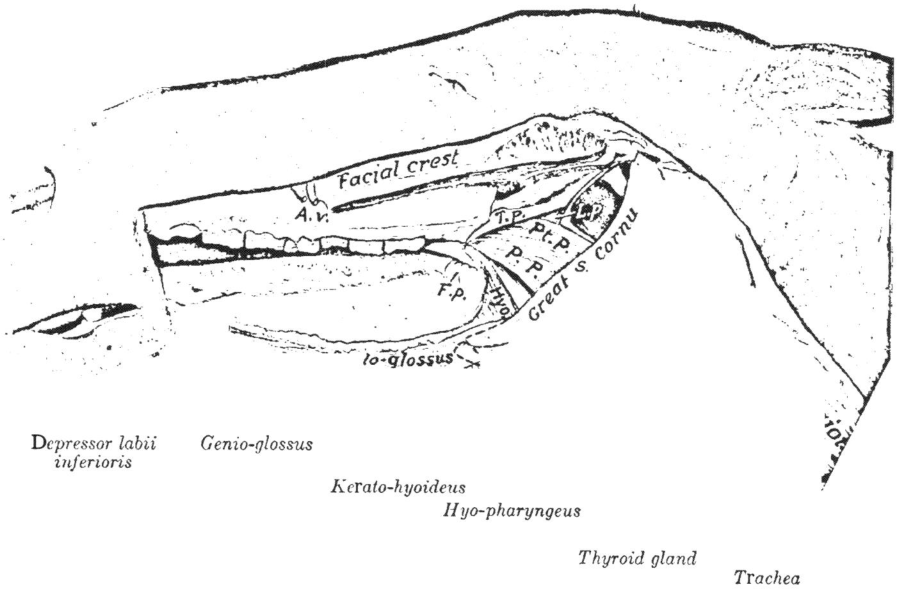

FIG. 242.—MUSCLES OF TONGUE, HYOID BONE, PHARYNX, ETC., OF HORSE.

T. p., Tensor palati; *L. p.*, levator palati; *Pt. p.*, pterygo-pharyngeus; *P. p.*, palato-pharyngeus; *S. p.*, stylo-pharyngeus; *Th. p.*, thyro-pharyngeus; *C. p.*, crico-pharyngeus; *Th. h.*, thyro-hyoideus; *Hyo. gl.*, hyo-glossus; *G. p.*, guttural pouch; *F. p.*, foliate papilla; *A. v.*, facial artery and vein. The concealed parts of the hyoid bone are indicated by dotted line.

The third, when present, is behind these, is centrally situated, and is always smaller. Rarely a fourth may be seen. They are rounded, broader at their exposed than at their attached surfaces, and are situated in a cup-shaped cavity. The **foliate papillæ** (Papillæ foliatæ) are situated just in front of the anterior pillars of the soft palate, where they form a rounded eminence about an inch (ca. 2 to 3 cm.) in length, marked by transverse fissures. The last three varieties are covered with microscopic secondary papillæ and are furnished with taste-buds. The mucous membrane of the root of the tongue presents numerous folds and depressions. Into the latter open the ducts from the **lingual glands** (Glandulæ linguales), which constitute a thick layer in the loose submucous tissue. Mucous glands are found also on the dorsum and sides of the tongue. In the submucosa of the root is found also a large quantity of lymph follicles (Folliculi tonsillares) and diffuse lymphoid tissue.

The **muscular tissue** may be divided into intrinsic and extrinsic. The intrinsic musculature consists, not of distinct muscles, but rather of systems of fibers which run longitudinally, vertically, and transversely, blending with the extrinsic muscles, which are now to be described.

1. **Stylo-glossus.**—This is a long, thin muscle, which lies on the lateral part

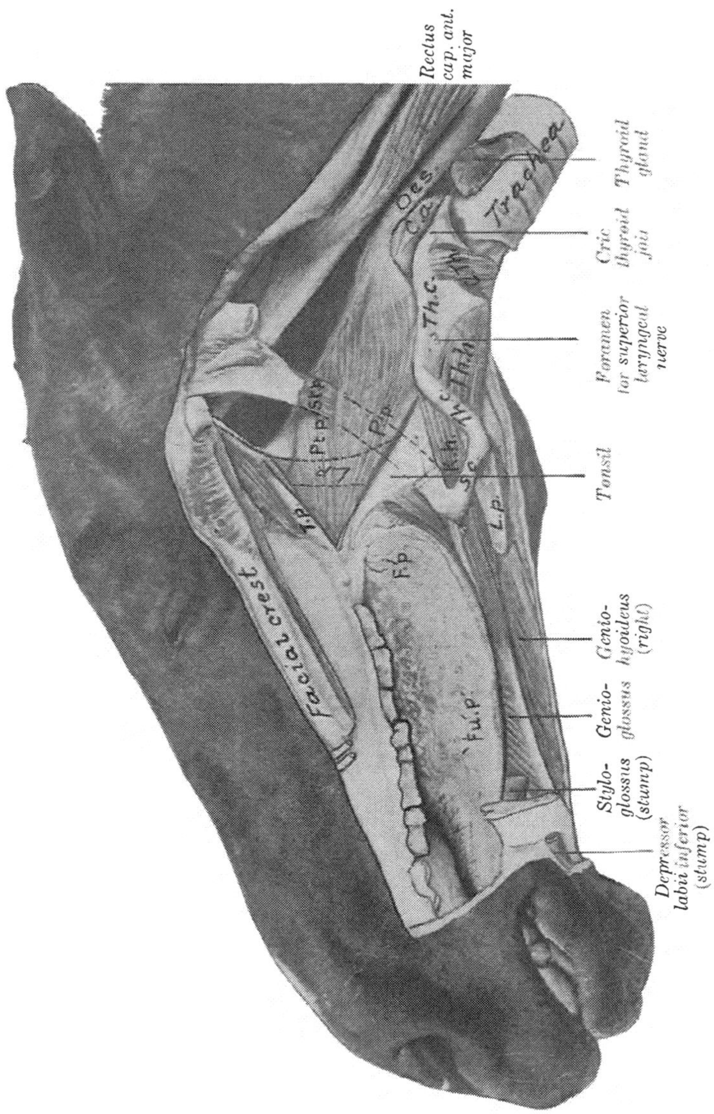

FIG. 243. MUSCLES OF [illegible] ETC., DEEP DISSECTION.

[illegible] ati; [illegible] concealed part indicated by dotted lin[illegible]; *Pt. p.*, pterygo-pharyngeus; *P. p.*, palato-pharyngeus; *St. p.*, [illegible] post.; *C. th.*, crico-thyroideus; *Th. c.*, thyroid cartilage (wing); *Th. h.*, thyro-hyoideus; *K. h.*, kera[illegible]; [illegible] c., t[illegible] id[illegible] u; [illegible] c., small cornu; *L. p.*, lingual [illegible]rocess; *F. p.*, foliate papilla; *Fu. p.*, fungiform papillæ. Part of great corn[illegible] is r[illegible] ndi[illegible] line.

of the tongue. It arises by a thin tendon from the outer surface of the great cornu of the hyoid bone, near the articulation with the small cornu. It terminates near the tip of the tongue by blending with its fellow of the opposite side and with the intrinsic musculature. The action is to retract the tongue. Unilateral contraction would also draw the tongue toward the side of the muscle acting.

2. **Hyo-glossus.**—This is a wide, flat muscle, somewhat thicker than the preceding. It lies on the lateral part of the root and body of the tongue, partly under cover of the preceding muscle. Its deep face is related to the genio-glossus. It arises from the lateral aspect of the hyoid bone, from the lingual process to the oral extremity of the great cornu, and from the thyroid cornu. The fibers pass obliquely forward and upward, and for the most part turn toward the median plane of the dorsum of the tongue. Its action is to retract and depress the tongue.

(It is usually possible to recognize in this muscle three portions, which would correspond to the baseo-, kerato-, and chondro-glossus of human anatomy.)

3. **Genio-glossus.**—This is a fan-shaped muscle, which lies parallel to the median plane of the tongue. It is separated from the muscle of the opposite side by a quantity of fat and connective tissue. It arises from the inner surface of the ramus of the mandible near the symphysis. From the tendon the fibers pass in a radiating manner, some toward the tip, others toward the dorsum, and others toward the root of the tongue; some fibers pass from the posterior end of the tendon to the body and small cornu of the hyoid bone. The muscle as a whole is a depressor of the tongue, and especially of its middle portion; when both muscles act, a median groove is formed on the dorsum. The posterior fibers protrude the tongue, the middle fibers depress the tongue, and the anterior fibers retract the tip of the tongue.

Vessels and Nerves.—The arteries of the tongue are the lingual and sublingual branches of the external maxillary artery. The sensory nerves are the lingual and glosso-pharyngeal, and the muscles are innervated by the hypoglossal nerve.

THE TEETH

The teeth are hard white or yellowish-white structures, implanted in the alveoli of the bones of the jaws—premaxilla, maxilla, and mandible. Morphologically they are large calcified papillæ. Functionally they are organs of prehension and mastication, and may serve as weapons of offense and defense. They are classified according to form and position as follows:

1. **The incisor teeth** (Dentes incisivi) are situated in front and are implanted in the premaxilla and mandible.

2. **The canine teeth** (Dentes canini) are situated a little further back, at or near the premaxillary suture in the upper jaw; in the lower jaw they are nearer the incisors.

3. **The cheek teeth** (Dentes premolares et molares), the remaining teeth, occupy the sides of the dental arch. The space between the incisors and cheek teeth is termed the interdental or interalveolar space. It is customary to divide the cheek teeth into an anterior series, termed **premolars,** which appear as temporary, deciduous, or milk teeth, and are replaced by permanent successors, and a posterior series, the **molars,** which appear only as permanent teeth without deciduous predecessors.

As the teeth of the two sides of the jaws are alike in number and character (in normal cases), the complete dentition may be briefly indicated by a **dental formula** such as the following:

$$2\left(I\frac{2}{2}\ C\frac{1}{1}\ P\frac{2}{2}\ M\frac{3}{3}\right) = 32.$$

In this formula the letters indicate the kinds of teeth, and the figures above and below the lines give the number of teeth of one side in the upper and lower jaw respectively in man.

The individual teeth of each group are designated numerically, the starting-point being the middle line; thus the incisor on either side of the middle line is the first incisor, and may be conveniently indicated by the notation I^1. The temporary or deciduous teeth may be designated in a similar manner, prefixing D (for deciduous) to the letter indicating the kind of tooth. In addition to the above systematic method of notation other terms have received the sanction of popular usage. Thus the first incisors are commonly called "pinchers," or "nippers"; the second, intermediate; and the third, corner teeth. The canines, when highly developed, may be termed tusks or fangs. The vestigial and inconstant first premolar of the horse is popularly termed the "wolf tooth."

Each tooth presents for description a portion coated with enamel, termed the **crown** (Corona dentis), and a portion covered with cement, termed the root (Radix dentis). The line of union of these parts is the **neck** (Collum dentis).[1] In many teeth the neck is distinct and is embraced by the gum, *e. g.*, the teeth of the dog and the temporary incisors of the horse. In other teeth no constriction is seen, as in the permanent incisors of the horse. Between these extremes may be noted the molars of the horse, in which the neck is seen only in advanced age.

The **surface** of a tooth directed toward the lips is termed **labial**; toward the cheek, **buccal**; and toward the tongue, **lingual** (Facies labialis, buccalis, lingualis). The surface opposed to a neighboring tooth of the same dental arch is termed the **contact surface** (Facies contactus). The grinding or **masticatory** or "table" surface (Facies masticatoria) is that which comes in contact with a tooth or teeth of the opposite jaw.

Structure.—Teeth are composed of four tissues, which are considered here from within outward. The **pulp** (Pulpa dentis) is a soft gelatinous tissue, which occupies a space in the central part of the tooth termed the **pulp cavity** (Cavum dentis). The pulp is well supplied with blood-vessels and nerves. It occupies a relatively large space in young growing teeth, but later the dentine deposited on its surface gradually encroaches on it until, in advanced age, the cavity is obliterated or much reduced. The **dentine** (Substantia eburnea) forms the bulk of most teeth, covering the surface of the pulp. It is very hard, and is yellowish-white in color. The **enamel** (Substantia adamantina) constitutes a layer of varying thickness covering the dentine of the crown of the tooth. It is easily distinguished by its clear bluish-white appearance and its extreme density. The **cement** (Substantia ossea) is always the outermost tooth substance. In simple teeth it forms usually a thin layer on the surface of the dentine of the root only, but in complex teeth it exists in considerable quantity, tending to fill in the spaces between the enamel folds of the crown also. Its structure is practically the same as that of bone without Haversian canals, and even these occur where the cement forms a very thick layer. The embedded part of the tooth is attached to the alveolus by a vascular layer of connective tissue, the **alveolar periosteum** (Periosteum alveolare), which constitutes the periosteum at once of tooth and alveolus.

The **blood-supply** to the pulp is derived from the alveolar or dental branches of the internal artery; the **nerve-supply** comes from branches of the trigeminus.

[1] It will be noted that this definition of crown and root does not agree exactly with the popular view that the crown is the free portion and the root the embedded portion. The objection to the latter statement lies in the fact that it is not capable of general application. Thus the morphological crown of the permanent molars in the horse is extremely long, and is, for the most part, embedded in the bone in the young animal. The root proper begins to form at four or five years of age, and continues its growth for about eight years. As the exposed part of the crown wears down, the embedded part pushes out of the alveolus, thus preventing deficiency of length. On the old basis we should have to say that successive portions of the root become crown, while in point of fact it is only in very extreme age that the true root comes into wear.

THE TEETH OF THE HORSE

THE PERMANENT TEETH

The formula of the permanent teeth of the horse is:

$$2\left(I\frac{3}{3}\ C\frac{1}{1}\ P\frac{3\text{ or }4}{3}\ M\frac{3}{3}\right) = 40 \text{ or } 42$$

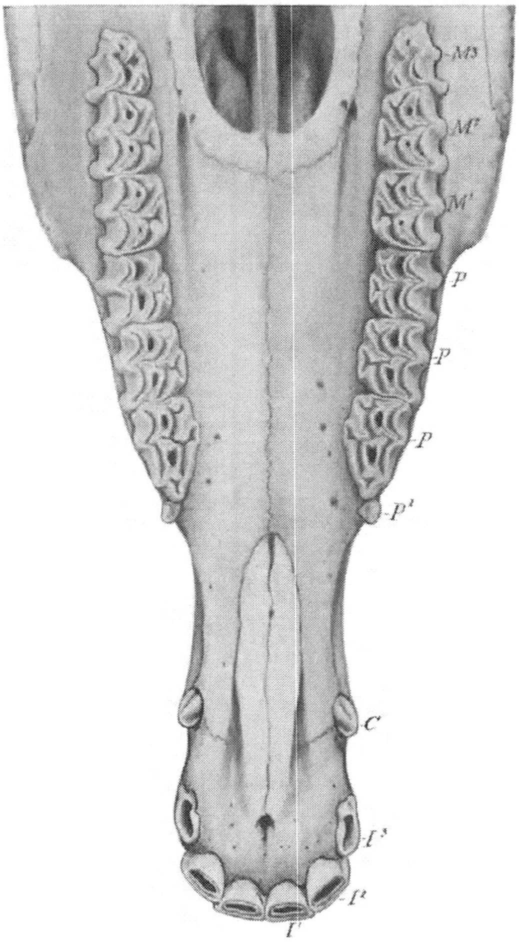

FIG. 244.—UPPER TEETH OF HORSE, ABOUT FOUR AND ONE-HALF YEARS OLD.

I^1, I^2, I^3, incisors; C, canine; P^1, P^2, P^3, P^4, premolars; M^1, M^2, M^3, molars.

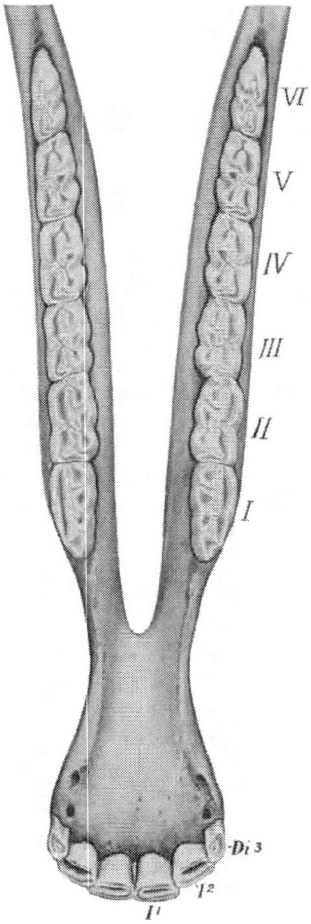

FIG. 245.—LOWER TEETH OF HORSE, FOUR YEARS OF AGE.

I^1, I^2. First and second permanent incisors; Di^3, third deciduous incisor. The cheek teeth are numbered according to popular usage.

In the mare the canines usually are very small and do not erupt, reducing the number to 36 or 38.[1]

[1] Ellenberger found, as the result of extensive observations (8000 subjects), that about 2 to 3 per cent. of mares have erupted canines in both jaws; that 6 to 7 per cent. have them in the upper jaw; while 20 to 30 per cent. have them in the lower jaw.

Incisor Teeth.—These are twelve in number. The six in each jaw are placed close together, so that their labial edges form almost a semicircle. They have the peculiarity (not found in existing mammals other than the equidæ) of presenting, instead of the simple cap of enamel on the crown, a deep invagination, the **infundibulum,** which becomes partly filled up with cement. Hence as the tooth wears the table surface has a central ring of enamel surrounding this cavity in addition to the peripheral enamel. The cavity becomes darkened by deposits from the food, and is commonly termed the "cup" or "mark." Each tooth is curved so that the labial surface is convex and the roots converge. The average length of the incisors at five or six years of age is about two and a half to three inches (ca. 7 cm.). They taper regularly from crown to root, without any constriction, and in such a manner that in young horses the exposed crown is broad transversely; toward the middle, the two diameters of a cross-section are about equal; near the root the antero-posterior diameter is considerably greater than the transverse.

This fact is of value in the determination of age by the teeth, since the table surface at different ages represents a series of such cross-sections. As the exposed crown wears down the embedded part (reserve crown) pushes up out of the alveolus, so that the tables of the first and second lower incisors are at first oval, with the long diameter transverse; later—at about fourteen years usually for the first lower incisors—the tables are triangular, with the base at the labial edge. At the same time the infundibulum or cup becomes smaller, approaches the lingual border, and finally disappears; it remains longer on the upper incisors, as it is deeper in them. Another marked feature in old age is the progressive approach to a horizontal direction as seen in profile; at the same time the teeth become parallel and finally convergent.

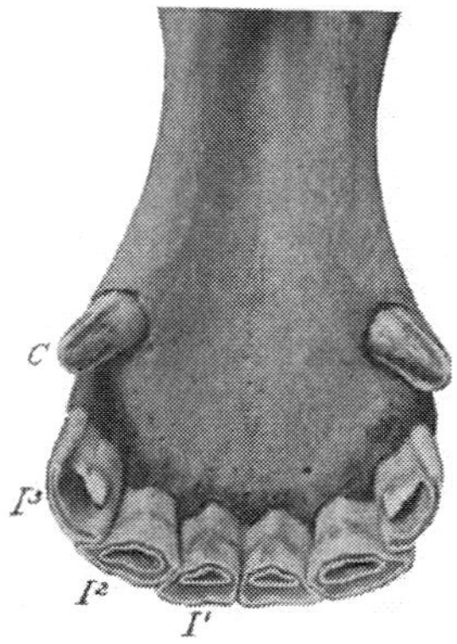

FIG. 246.—LOWER INCISOR AND CANINE TEETH OF HORSE, FIVE YEARS OLD.

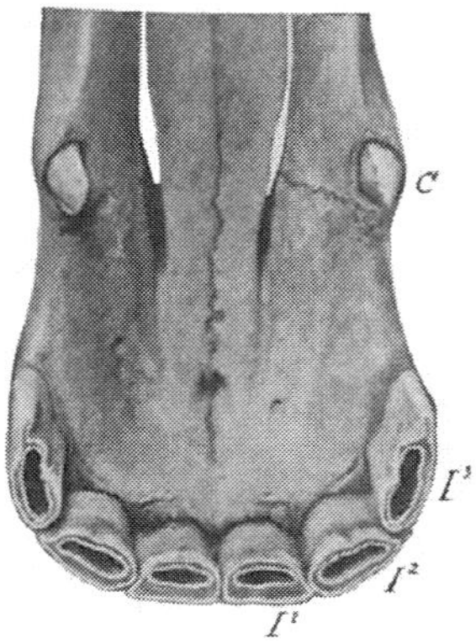

FIG. 247.—UPPER INCISOR AND CANINE TEETH OF HORSE, FIVE YEARS OLD.

I^1, I^2, I^3, incisors; C, canine.

Canine Teeth.—These are four in number in the male; in the mare they are usually absent or rudimentary.[1] They interrupt the interdental space, dividing it into two unequal parts. The upper canine is situated at the junction of the premaxilla and the maxilla; the lower canine is placed nearer the corner incisor. The canines are simple teeth, smaller than the incisors, and are curved with the concavity directed backward. The crown is compressed, convex, and smooth

[1] It is interesting to notice that vestigial canines are not at all uncommon in mares, especially in the lower jaw. They are very small, and do not usually erupt; their presence is indicated in the latter case by a prominence of the gum. This is in conformity with the fact that they were present in both sexes in Eocene and Miocene ancestors of existing equidæ.

externally; concave with a median ridge internally; its edges are sharp, and the apex is pointed in the unworn tooth. The root is round and the pulp cavity is large, persisting to advanced age.

Cheek Teeth (Premolars and Molars).[1]—The constant number of these is twenty-four – twelve in each jaw. Quite commonly, however, the number is increased by the presence in the upper jaw of the so-called wolf-tooth. This tooth is usually situated just in front of the first well-developed tooth; it is a much-reduced vestige, not often more than one-half or three-fourths of an inch (ca. 1 to 2 cm.) in length. (It is interesting as being the remnant of a tooth which was well developed in the Eocene ancestors of the horse.) It may erupt during the first six months, and is often shed about the same time as the milk-tooth behind it, but may remain indefinitely. The occurrence of a similar tooth in the lower jaw—which rarely erupts—increases the dental formula to 44, which is considered the typical number for mammals. They may be regarded as belonging to the permanent set, having no predecessors. The cheek teeth are very large, prismatic in form, and quadrilateral in cross-section, except the first and last of the series, which are triangular. The crown is remarkably long, most of it being embedded in the bone or situated in the maxillary sinus in the young horse. As the exposed part wears down the embedded part pushes up to replace it, so that a functional crown of about four-fifths of an inch (ca. 2 cm.)

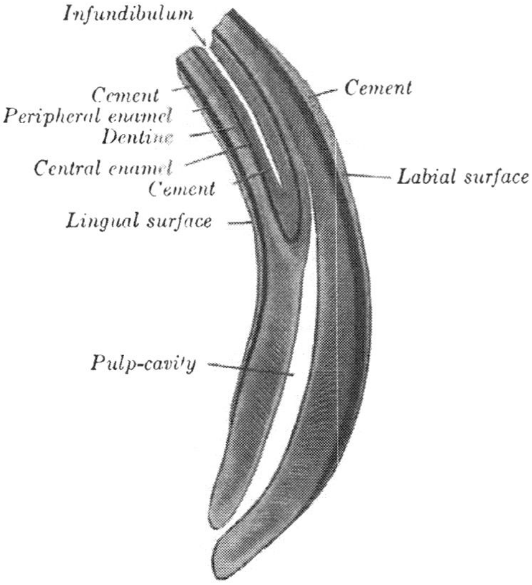

Fig. 248.—Longitudinal Section of Permanent Incisor Tooth of Horse, About Natural Size.

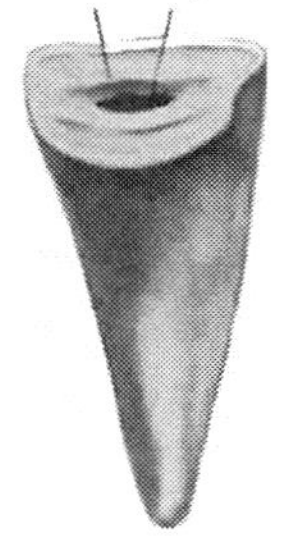

Fig. 249.—Incisor Tooth of Horse, Lingual Aspect. (After Ellenberger-Baum, Anat. für Künstler.)

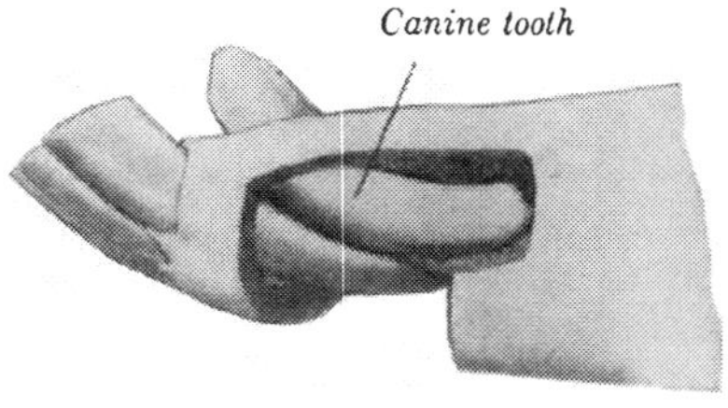

Fig. 250.—Canine and Incisor Teeth of Horse. The bone has been removed to show the embedded parts of the teeth. (After Ellenberger-Baum, Anat. für Künstler.)

[1] It is common in veterinary works to call all the cheek teeth molars, since, in the horse particularly, the premolars are molariform, *i. e.*, do not differ materially from the true molars in size or form. The term cheek teeth conveniently includes the premolars and molars.

is maintained. The root begins to grow at four or five years of age, and is complete at twelve to fourteen, although the deposition of cement may continue indefinitely.

The upper or **maxillary teeth** are embedded in the alveolar processes of the

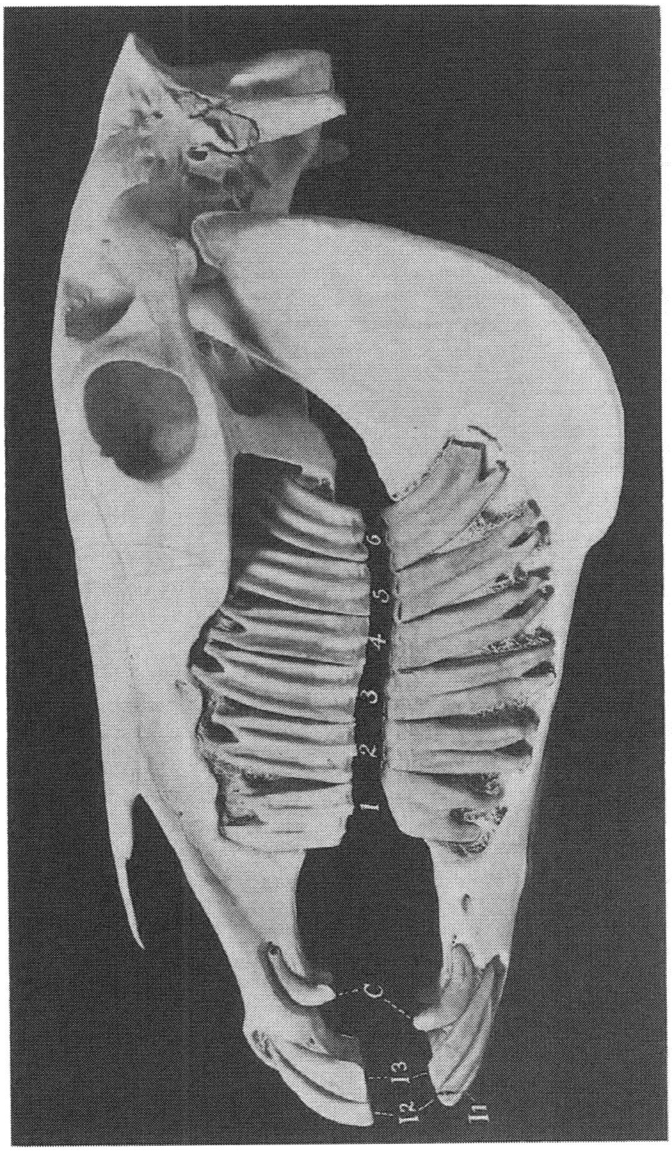

FIG. 251.—SKULL OF ADULT HORSE SCULPTURED TO EMBEDDED PARTS OF TEETH.
to show the embedded parts of the teeth I^1 I^2, I^3, Incisors; *C*, canines. The cheek teeth are numbered.

maxilla. The exposed parts of the crowns are normally in close contact, forming a continuous row which is slightly curved, with the convexity toward the cheek. The embedded parts diverge in the manner shown in the annexed figures (Figs. 251, 253). Thus the long axis of the first is directed upward and a little forward, that of the second is almost vertical, while in the remainder it is curved backward in an increasing degree. The average **length** at six years of age is about three to three and a half inches (ca. 7 to 9 cm.). The **buccal** (or outer) **surface** presents a central ridge running lengthwise, and separating two grooves; the first tooth has, in addition, a less prominent ridge in front of the primary one. The **lingual** (or inner) **surface** is marked by a wide, rounded ridge, the accessory pillar or column, which separates two very shallow grooves. The **masticatory** or **table surface** presents two infundibula, an anterior and a posterior. It slopes obliquely downward and outward, so that the outer edge is prominent and sharp. The first and last teeth have three roots, the remainder four or three.

The position of the embedded crowns and roots of the last four varies at different ages and in different subjects. Two factors in this variation may be noted. All these teeth are developed in the maxillary sinus close to the orbital fossa. As growth proceeds the teeth move forward, so that commonly only the last three, but sometimes also the third, remain (except as to their free crowns) in the sinus. The second cause of variation is the fact that the anterior limit of the maxillary sinus may be at the extremity of the facial ridge, or more than an inch beyond it. In the latter case the third tooth projects into the sinus.[1]

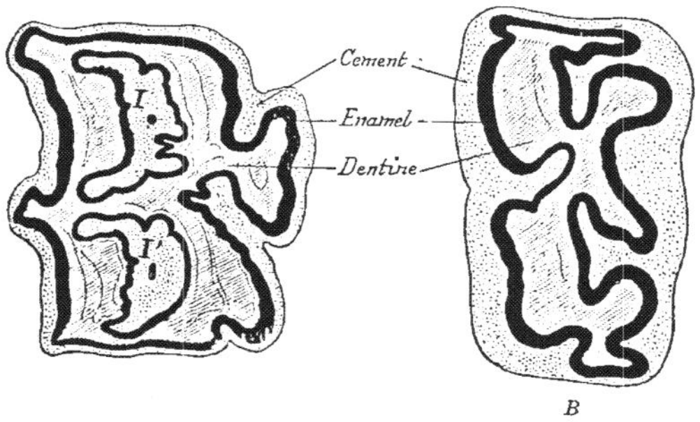

FIG. 252.—CROSS-SECTIONS OF CHEEK TEETH OF HORSE.
Buccal (outer) surfaces face to left. *A*, Upper tooth, *B*, lower tooth; *I*, anterior, *I'*, posterior infundibulum, both almost filled up with cement.

The **structure** is quite complex. Two infundibula run vertically through the entire length of the crown; these become filled with cement. There are five main divisions of the pulp-cavity and five enamel folds, four of which are arranged symmetrically, while the fifth is an outgrowth from the inner side of the antero-internal fold. On the exposed crown of the unworn tooth the enamel folds form rounded ridges covered with a thin layer of cement. After the tooth comes into wear the enamel on the masticatory surface stands out in the form of sharp prominent ridges. Progressive cementation of the periphery of the tooth takes place, thus leveling up the irregularities of surface to a considerable extent.

The lower or **mandibular cheek teeth** are implanted in the rami of the mandible, forming two straight rows which diverge behind. The space between the rows is considerably less than that separating the upper teeth, especially in the middle of the series. The length of the lower teeth is about the same as that of the upper set. Their direction is also similar, but the embedded portions diverge even more, with the exception of the first and second. The long axis of the first is vertical; the remainder project downward and backward in a gradually increasing obliquity. The **buccal** (outer) **surface** has a longitudinal furrow; the last molar has a secon-

[1] The student is advised to amplify these very general statements by the examination of heads of subjects of varying ages. It may also be noted that the position of the septum between the two divisions of the sinus varies much.

dary, shallower furrow in addition. The **lingual** (inner) **surface** is uneven, but the grooves are not regular; there are usually three on the first and last tooth. The **masticatory** or **table surface** is oblique, sloping upward and inward in corre-

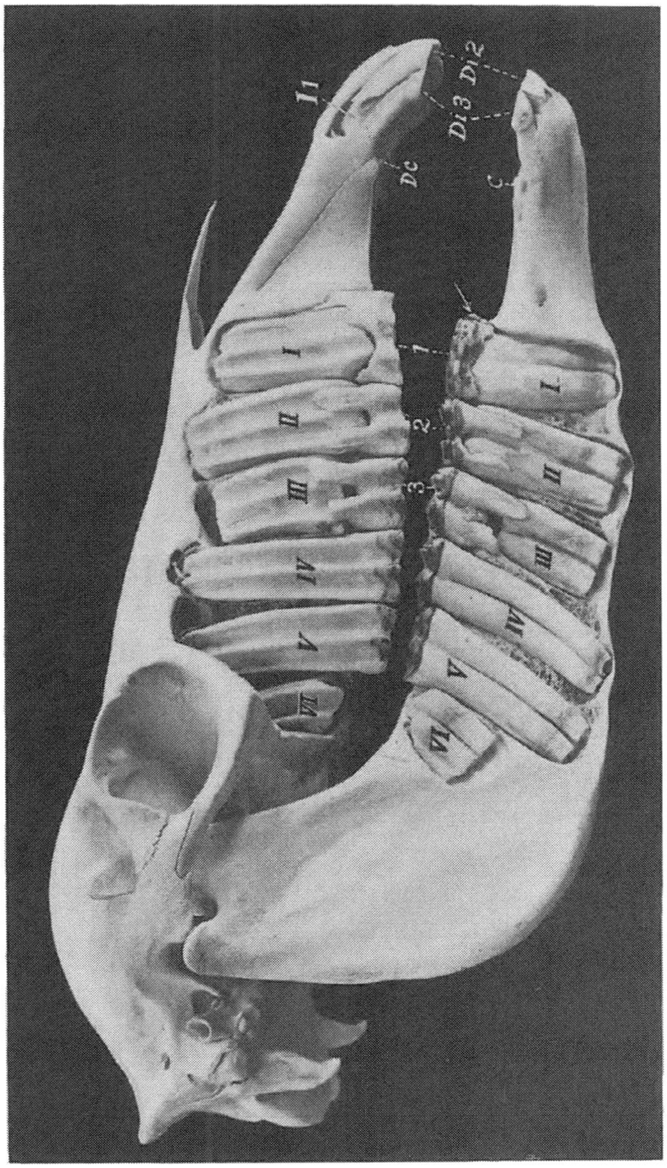

Fig. 3.—S ... Sculptu

spondence with the opposing tooth; thus the inner edge is prominent. The first five have two roots, while the sixth commonly has three. The width of the lower molars is a little more than half that of the upper. There are two infundibula, which are open along the inner face of the tooth until closed by cement. The pulp-cavity has two principal divisions, and four or three secondary diverticula. The enamel folds correspond, forming a pattern even more complicated than on the upper teeth.

The Temporary Teeth

The deciduous, temporary, or "milk" teeth (Dentes decidui) are smaller and fewer than those of the permanent set. The formula is:

$$2\left(\text{Di}\ \frac{3}{3}\ \text{Dc}\ \frac{0}{0}\ \text{Dp}\ \frac{3}{3}\right) = 24.$$

The deciduous incisors are much smaller than the permanent ones. They have a distinct neck at the junction of the crown and root. The crown is short, white in color, and its labial surface is smooth. The infundibulum is shallow. The root is flattened; it undergoes absorption as the permanent tooth develops behind it.

The deciduous canines are quite vestigial. They occur in both sexes as slender spiculæ about a quarter of an inch in length, but do not erupt. The lower one develops close to the corner incisor. They are not usually included in the formula, as they are never functional.

The deciduous cheek teeth differ from the permanent set chiefly in that they have much shorter crowns than the latter. The roots form early, so that a distinct neck occurs.

The subjoined table indicates the average periods of the eruption of the teeth:

Teeth		Eruption
A. *Deciduous:*		
1st incisor	(Di 1)	Birth or first week.
2nd "	(Di 2)	4–6 weeks.
3rd "	(Di 3)	6–9 months.
Canine	(Dc)	
1st premolar	(Dp 2)	Birth or first two weeks.
2nd "	(Dp 3)	
3rd "	(Dp 4)	
B. *Permanent:*		
1st incisor	(I 1)	2½ years.
2nd "	(I 2)	3½ years.
3rd "	(I 3)	4½ years.
Canine	(C)	4–5 years.
1st premolar (or wolf-tooth)	(P 1)	5–6 months.
2nd "	(P 2)	2½ years.
3rd "	(P 3)	3 years.
4th "	(P 4)	4 years.
1st molar	(M 1)	10–12 months.
2nd "	(M 2)	2 years.
3rd "	(M 3)	3½–4 years.

(The periods given for P 3 and 4 refer to the upper teeth; the lower ones may erupt about six months earlier.)

THE SALIVARY GLANDS

This term is usually restricted to the three pairs of large glands situated on the sides of the face and the adjacent part of the neck—the parotid, submaxillary, and sublingual. Their ducts open into the mouth.

The parotid gland (Glandula parotis) (Fig. 172)—so named from its proximity to the ear—is the largest of the salivary glands in the horse. It is situated chiefly in the space between the ramus of the mandible and the wing of the atlas. It is somewhat triangular in shape, the apex partially embracing the base of the external ear. Its length is about eight to ten inches (ca. 20 to 25 cm.), and its average thickness nearly an inch (ca. 2 cm.). Its average weight is about seven ounces (ca. 200 to 225 g.).

It presents for description two surfaces, two borders, a base, and an apex. The **external** (or superficial) **surface** is covered by the parotid fascia, the panniculus, and the parotido-auricularis muscle. It is crossed obliquely by the jugular vein, which is embedded in the gland tissue to a varying extent. It is also related to the great auricular vein, the cervical branch of the facial nerve, and branches of the second cervical nerve. The **internal** (or deep) **surface** is very uneven, and has numerous important relations. Some of these are: the guttural pouch, and the great cornu of the hyoid bone; the masseter, stylo-maxillaris, digastricus, and occipito-hyoideus muscles; the tendons of the mastoido-humeralis and sterno-cephalicus (which separate the parotid from the underlying submaxillary gland); the external carotid artery and some of its branches; the facial nerve; the pharyngeal lymph glands. The **anterior** (or facial) **border** is closely attached to the ramus of the mandible and the masseter muscle; it overlaps the latter to a varying extent. (In some cases there is a well-marked triangular facial process, which covers the temporo-mandibular joint, the facial nerve, and the transverse facial vessels.) The **posterior** (or cervical) **border** is somewhat concave, and is loosely attached to the underlying muscles. The **base** or **ventral border** is related to the external maxillary vein. The **apex** is attached to the base of the external ear, which it partially embraces.

The gland has a yellowish-gray color and is distinctly lobulated. It is inclosed in a capsule formed by the parotid fascia. The **parotid duct** (Ductus parotideus Stenonis) is formed at the lower part of the gland, near the facial edge, by the union of three or four radicles. It leaves the gland about an inch (ca. 2 to 3 cm.) above the external maxillary vein, crosses the tendon of the sterno-cephalicus, and gains the inner face of the pterygoideus internus. It then runs forward in the submaxillary space below the external maxillary vein and winds around the lower border of the mandible behind the vein, passes upward between the vein and the masseter muscle for about two inches (ca. 5 cm.), turns forward underneath the facial vessels, and perforates the cheek obliquely opposite the third upper cheek tooth. Before piercing the cheek it is somewhat dilated, but its termination is small, and is surrounded by a circular mucous fold (Papilla salivalis).

Blood-supply.—Branches of the carotid and maxillary arteries.

Nerve-supply.—Trigeminal, facial, and sympathetic nerves.

The **submaxillary gland** (Glandula submaxillaris) is much smaller than the parotid. It is long, narrow, and curved, the dorsal edge being concave. It extends from the fossa below the wing of the atlas to the body of the hyoid bone, so that it is covered partly by the parotid gland, partly by the lower jaw. Its length is about eight to ten inches (ca. 20 to 25 cm.), its width an inch to an inch and a half (ca. 2.5 to 3 cm.), and its thickness about half an inch (ca. 1 cm.). It weighs about one and a half to two ounces (ca. 45 to 60 g.). It is often divisible into two parts.

It presents for description two surfaces, two borders, and two extremities. The **external surface** is covered by the parotid gland, the stylo-maxillaris, digastricus, and pterygoideus internus muscles. The tendon of the sterno-cephalicus crosses this surface, and is a useful guide in separating the parotid gland from it. The **internal surface** is related chiefly to the flexor muscles of the head; the guttural pouch; the larynx; the division of the carotid artery; and the tenth, eleventh, and sympathetic nerves. The **superior border** is concave and thin. It is related to the guttural pouch and the duct of the gland. The **inferior border** is convex and thicker. It is related to the thyroid gland and the external maxillary vein. The **posterior extremity** is loosely attached in the fossa atlantis. The **anterior extremity** lies at the side of the root of the tongue, and is crossed externally by the external maxillary artery.

The **submaxillary duct** (Ductus submaxillaris Whartoni) is formed by the union of small radicles which emerge along the concave edge. It runs forward along this border, and, after leaving the anterior extremity, crosses the intermediate tendon of the digastricus, passes between the hyo-glossus and mylo-hyoideus, and gains the inner surface of the sublingual gland. Its terminal part lies on the body of the mandible, under the mucous membrane, which it pierces opposite the canine tooth. The orifice is at the end of a flattened papilla (Caruncula sublingualis).

Blood-supply.—Occipital, external carotid, and external maxillary arteries.

Nerve-supply.—Chorda tympani and sympathetic nerves.

The **sublingual gland** (Glandula sublingualis) is situated beneath the mucous membrane of the mouth, between the body of the tongue and the ramus of the mandible. It extends from the symphysis to the third or fourth lower cheek tooth. Its length is about five or six inches (ca. 12 to 15 cm.) and its weight about half an ounce (ca. 15 to 16 g.).

It is flattened laterally, and has a thin **upper border** which causes an elevation of the mucous membrane of the floor of the mouth, termed the **sublingual crest** (Plica sublingualis). The **external surface** is related to the mylo-hyoideus muscle, and the **internal surface** to the genio-glossus and stylo-glossus, the submaxillary duct, and branches of the lingual nerve. The **inferior border** is related to the genio-hyoid muscle.

The **sublingual ducts** (Ductus sublinguales minores), about thirty in number, are small, short, and twisted; they open on small papillæ on the sublingual crest.

Blood-supply.—Sublingual artery.

Nerve-supply.—Trigeminal and sympathetic nerves.

THE PHARYNX

The pharynx is a musculo-membranous sac which belongs to the digestive and respiratory tracts in common. It is funnel-shaped, the base joining the mouth and nasal cavity, while the apex is continued by the œsophagus. Its long axis is directed obliquely downward and backward, and has a length of about six inches (ca. 15 cm.).

The pharynx is attached by its muscles to the palate, pterygoid, and hyoid bones, and to the cricoid and thyroid cartilages of the larynx.

Its principal **relations** are: dorsally, the base of the cranium and the guttural pouches; ventrally, the larynx; laterally, the internal pterygoid muscle, the great cornu of the hyoid bone, the internal and external maxillary arteries, the glosso-pharyngeal, superior laryngeal, and hypoglossal nerves, the submaxillary salivary gland, and the pharyngeal lymph glands.

It presents **seven openings.** The **posterior nares** (Choanæ) communicate dorsally with the nasal chambers. The pharyngeal orifices (Ostia pharyngea) of the two **Eustachian** tubes are situated on the lateral wall behind the nares and a little below the level of the inferior nasal meatus. They are slit-like openings, slightly oblique downward and backward, and are a little more than an inch (ca. 3 cm.) in length. They are bounded internally by a valvular flap formed by the expanded extremity of the cartilaginous Eustachian tube. The **isthmus faucium** is situated below and in front. It is closed by the soft palate except during swallowing. The **laryngeal orifice** (Aditus laryngis) occupies the greater part of the ventral wall or floor of the pharynx. Behind this is the **œsophageal opening.**

The wall of the pharynx comprises from without inward: the muscles, the pharyngeal aponeurosis, and the mucous membrane.

The **muscles** (Figs. 243, 244) are covered by the pharyngeal fascia, which is attached to the base of the skull, the great cornu of the hyoid bone, and the thyroid cartilage of the larynx. They are as follows:

1. The **stylo-pharyngeus** arises from the inner surface of the dorsal third of the great cornu of the hyoid bone, passes downward and inward, and enters the wall of the pharynx by passing between the pterygo-pharyngeus and palato-pharyngeus. Its fibers radiate, many passing forward, others inward beneath the hyo-pharyngeus. It raises and dilates the pharynx to receive the bolus in swallowing.

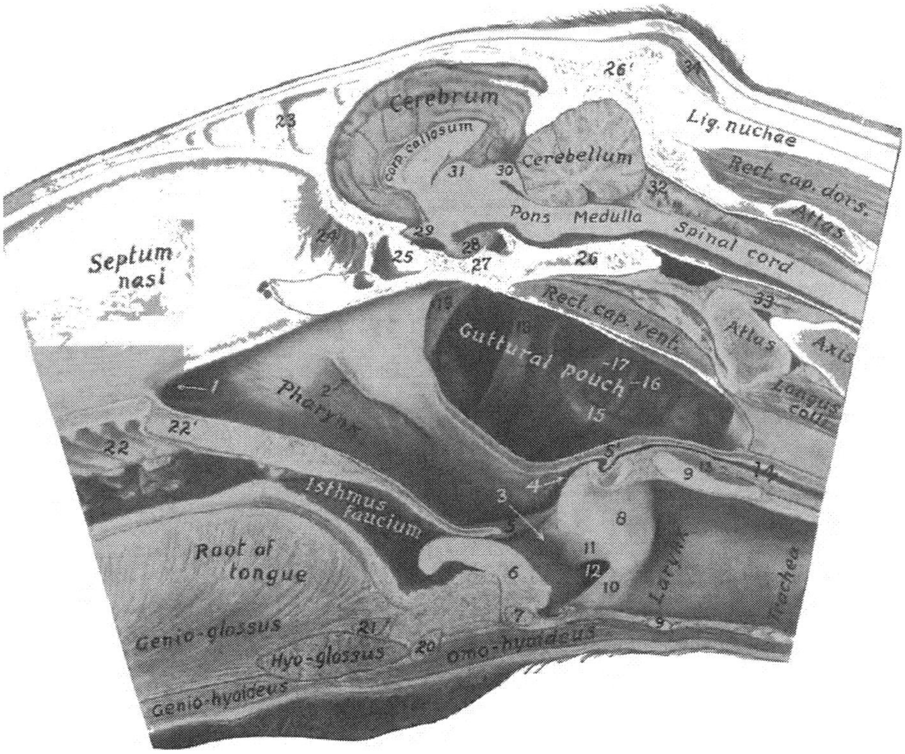

FIG. 254.—POSTERIOR PART OF A SAGITTAL SECTION OF HEAD OF HORSE, CUT ABOUT CM. TO THE LEFT OF THE MEDIAN PLANE.

1, Posterior nares; *2*, pharyngeal orifice of Eustachian tube; *3*, aditus laryngis; *4*, entrance to œsophagus; *5*, posterior pillar of soft palate; *5'*, junction of *5* with its fellow over entrance to œsophagus; *6*, epiglottis; *7*, body of thyroid cartilage; *8*, arytenoid cartilage; *9, 9*, cricoid cartilage; *10*, true vocal cord; *11*, false vocal cord; *12*, lateral ventricle of larynx; *13*, crico-arytenoideus post. s. dorsalis; *14*, œsophagus; *15*, external carotid artery; *16*, hypoglossal nerve; *17*, glosso-pharyngeal nerve; *18*, great cornu of hyoid bone; *19*, Eustachian tube; *20*, body of hyoid bone; *21*, hyoideus transversus; *22*, ridges of hard palate; *22'*, soft palate; *23*, septum between frontal sinuses; *24*, olfactory mucous membrane; *25*, sphenoidal sinus; *26*, basilar part of occipital bone; *26'*, supraoccipital; *27*, body of sphenoid bone; *28*, pituitary body; *29*, chiasma opticum; *30*, corpora quadrigemina; *31*, thalamus; *32*, arachnoid; *33*, odontoid ligament; *34*, posterior auricular muscles.

2. The **palato-pharyngeus** arises by means of the aponeurosis of the soft palate from the palate and pterygoid bones. Its fibers pass backward on the lateral wall of the pharynx, and are inserted in part into the upper edge of the thyroid cartilage, in part turn inward to end at the median fibrous raphé. Its action is to shorten the pharynx, and to draw the larynx and œsophagus toward the root of the tongue in swallowing.

3. The **pterygo-pharyngeus** is flat and triangular. It lies on the anterior part of the lateral wall of the pharynx. It arises from the pterygoid bone above the

preceding muscle—from which it is not distinctly separated—crosses the levator palati, and is inserted into the median raphé. Its action is similar to the preceding.

4. The **hyo-pharyngeus** may consist of two portions:

(*a*) The **kerato-pharyngeus** is a small and inconstant muscle which arises from the inner surface of the great cornu of the hyoid bone near its lower end. It passes upward and backward, turns inward toward the raphé, and spreads out under the next muscle.

(*b*) The **chondro-pharyngeus,** broad and fleshy, arises from the thyroid cornu of the hyoid bone and by a thin fasciculus from the wing of the thyroid cartilage and ends at the median raphé.

5. The **thyro-pharyngeus** arises from the lateral surface of the wing of the thyroid cartilage. Its fibers pass forward and inward to the median raphé.

6. The **crico-pharyngeus** arises from the cricoid cartilage and ends at the raphé. The fibers are directed upward, forward, and inward; they blend behind with the longitudinal fibers of the œsophagus.

The last three muscles are constrictors of the pharynx.

The **pharyngeal aponeurosis** is attached to the base of the cranium. It is well developed on the inner face of the palato-pharyngeus muscle and forms a median raphé (Raphé pharyngis) dorsally, which is wide in its posterior part.

The **mucous membrane** of the pharynx is continuous with that of the several cavities which open into it. It is thin and closely adherent to the base of the skull in the vicinity of the posterior nares, where the muscular wall is absent. Behind the Eustachian openings is a median cul-de-sac, the **pharyngeal recess.** The recess is somewhat variable, but is usually about an inch in depth and will admit the end of the finger. In the ass and mule it is much deeper. Here also the muscular wall is absent and the mucous membrane lies against the guttural pouches. From the Eustachian opening a fold of the mucous membrane (Plica salpingo-pharyngea) passes toward but does not reach the laryngeal opening. Below, a horizontal fold, the **posterior pillar of the soft palate** (Arcus pharyngo-palatinus), passes along the lateral wall and unites with its fellow over the entrance to the œsophagus. The upper part of the cavity (the naso-pharynx) is lined with a ciliated epithelium, while the lower part (oro-pharynx) has a stratified squamous epithelium. The communication between the two is oval and is bounded by the free edge of the soft palate and its posterior pillars; it is termed the **pharyngeal isthmus.** On either side of the laryngeal opening is a narrow deep depression, the **pyriform sinus** (Recessus piriformis).

The submucous tissue contains numerous mucous glands (Glandulæ pharyngeæ). In the young subject the lymph follicles are numerous and form a collection dorsally and between the Eustachian openings, known as the pharyngeal tonsil.

Blood-supply.—External carotid, external maxillary, and thyro-laryngeal arteries.

Nerve-supply.—Glosso-pharyngeal, vagus, and sympathetic nerves.

THE ŒSOPHAGUS

The œsophagus is a musculo-membranous tube, about 50 to 60 inches (ca. 125 to 150 cm.) in length, which extends from the pharynx to the stomach. It begins in the median plane above the cricoid cartilage of the larynx. In its course it shows several changes of direction. At the level of the fourth cervical vertebra it inclines to the left side of the trachea, and continues this relation to the level of the third thoracic vertebra. Here it again gains the dorsal surface of the trachea, and passing backward, crosses the left bronchus, being here almost in the median plane. It continues in the mediastinum between the lungs backward, upward, and a little to the left, to reach the hiatus œsophageus of the diaphragm. Passing through this it terminates at once at the cardiac orifice of the stomach, at the level of the fourteenth thoracic vertebra, a little to the left of the median plane, and about four or five inches (ca. 10 to 12 cm.) ventral to the vertebral column.

Viewed with reference to the frontal plane, its course is downward and back ward till it enters the thorax and passes upward to gain the dorsal face of the trachea. For a short distance (*i. e.*, to the root of the lung) its direction is almost horizontal;

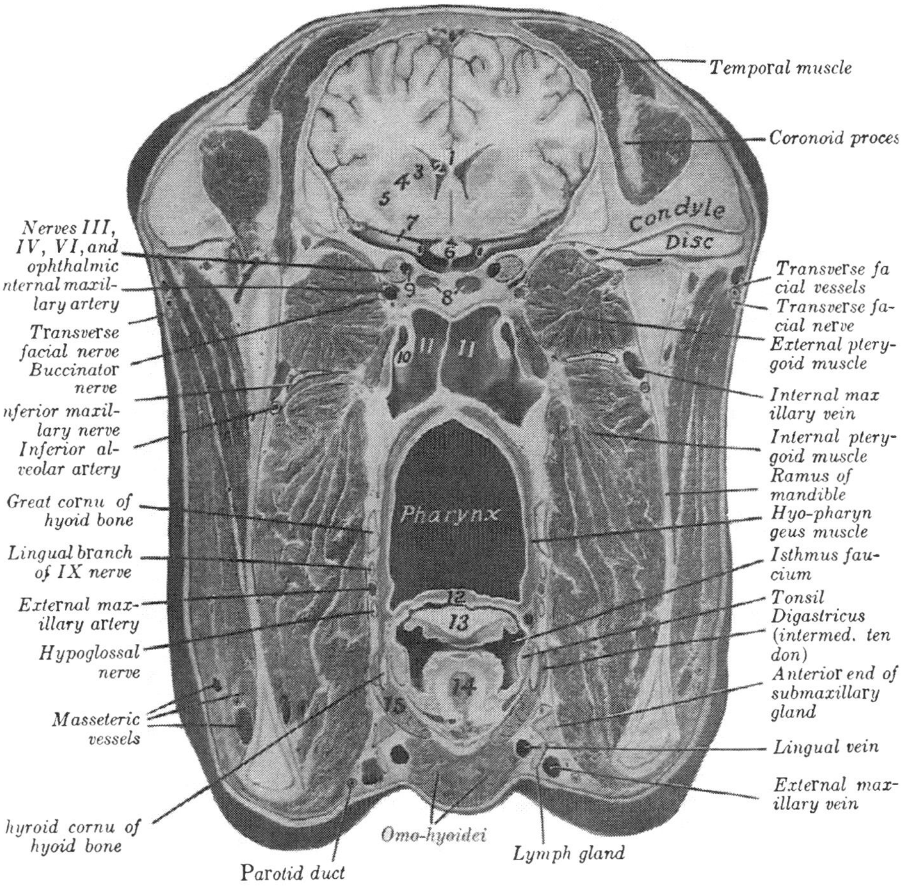

FIG. 255.—CROSS-SECTION OF HEAD OF HORSE.

The section passes through the temporo-mandibular articulation, but is slightly oblique. *1*, Corpus callosum; *2*, lateral ventricle of brain; *3*, caudate nucleus; *4*, internal capsule; *5*, lenticular nucleus; *6*, optic chiasma; *7*, middle cerebral artery; *8*, sphenoidal sinuses; *9*, cavernous sinus; *10*, Eustachian tube, inner lamina; *11, 11*, guttural pouches; *12*, soft palate; *13*, epiglottis; *14*, hyo-epiglottic muscle; *15*, thyro-hyoid muscle.

behind this it passes somewhat upward to its termination. The **cervical part** of the tube is about four to six inches (10 to 15 cm.) longer than the **thoracic part,** while the so-called abdominal part is about an inch (2 to 3 cm.) long.[1]

[1] Careful observations (especially on frozen subjects and those in which the organs have been hardened *in situ*) show that there is no abdominal part of the œsophagus in the strict sense of the term. The stomach here lies directly on the diaphragm, so that the last inch or so of the œsophagus is placed obliquely in the hiatus œsophageus, and is partly covered by the pleura, but not by peritoneum. In soft subjects the weight of the stomach, or traction on it, draws part of the œsophagus into the abdomen, inclosed in a collar of peritoneum.

The principal **relations** of the œsophagus at its origin are: to the cricoid cartilage below; to the guttural pouches and the ventral straight muscles above; and to the carotid arteries laterally. In the middle of the neck the relations are: to the left longus colli muscle above; to the trachea internally; to the left carotid artery, vagus, sympathetic, and recurrent nerves externally. At its entrance into the thorax it has the trachea on its inner side; the first rib, the roots of the brachial plexus of nerves and the inferior cervical ganglion externally. After gaining the upper surface of the trachea, it has the aorta on its left and the vena azygos and right vagus nerve on its right side. In its course through the posterior mediastinum the œsophageal trunks of the vagus nerves lie above and below it, and the œsophageal artery is dorsal to it.

Structure.—The wall is composed of four coats: (1) A fibrous sheath; (2) the muscular coat; (3) a submucous layer; (4) the mucous membrane. The **muscular coat** is of the striped variety as far as the base of the heart, where it rapidly changes to the unstriped type. In addition to this change, the muscular coat becomes much thicker and firmer, while the lumen is diminished.[1] The outer fibers are arranged longitudinally, beginning in two bundles attached in the interval between the arytenoid and cricoid cartilages. The inner fibers run in two spiral strata to the terminal part of the tube, where the arrangement is an outer longitudinal and an inner circular layer.[2] The **mucous membrane** is pale, and is covered with squamous stratified epithelium. It is loosely attached to the muscular coat by an abundant submucosa, and lies in longitudinal folds which obliterate the lumen except during deglutition.

Blood-supply.—Carotid, broncho-œsophageal, and gastric arteries.

Nerve-supply.—Vagus, glosso-pharyngeal, and sympathetic nerves.

THE ABDOMINAL CAVITY

The abdominal cavity (Cavum abdominis) is the largest of the body cavities. It is separated from the thoracic cavity by the diaphragm and is continuous behind with the pelvic cavity.

It is ovoid in form but somewhat compressed laterally. Its long axis extends obliquely from the center of the pelvic inlet to the sternal part of the diaphragm. Its dorso-ventral diameter is greatest at the first lumbar vertebra, while its greatest transverse diameter is a little nearer the pelvis.

The **dorsal wall** or roof is formed by the lumbar vertebræ, the lumbar muscles, and the lumbar part of the diaphragm.

The **lateral walls** are formed by the oblique and transverse abdominal muscles, the abdominal tunic, the anterior parts of the ilia, the cartilages of the asternal ribs, and the parts of the posterior ribs which are below the attachment of the diaphragm.

The **ventral wall** or floor consists of the two recti, the aponeuroses of the oblique and transverse muscles, the abdominal tunic, and the xiphoid cartilage.

The **anterior wall** is formed by the diaphragm, which is very deeply concave, thus greatly increasing the size of the abdomen at the expense of the thorax.

It should be noted that the diaphragm also concurs practically in the formation of a considerable part of the lateral walls, since its costal portion even during ordinary inspiration lies directly on the ribs over a width of four or five inches (ca. 10 to 12 cm.); in expiration this area

[1] The potential lumen is difficult to determine at all accurately. When distended, its diameter (according to Ruheli) varies from 5.7 cm. at its origin to 4 cm. at its cardiac end. The thickness of the wall varies (inversely as the lumen) from 4 mm. to 1.2 cm. or more.

[2] At the origin of the tube muscular bundles arise on the raphé pharyngis and blend with the crico-pharyngeus. Ventrally fibers come from the depression between the cricoid and arytenoid cartilages. Bundles of striped fibers may be continued in the superficial part of the muscular coat as far as the cardia.

of contact would be about twice as wide, including about all of the fleshy rim. This fact is of clinical importance, with reference to auscultation and percussion, and penetrating wounds. The cupola of the diaphragm extends as far forward as a plane through the sixth intercostal space to the right of the heart.

There is no wall between the abdominal and pelvic cavities. The line of demarcation here is the **terminal line** (Linea terminalis) or brim of the pelvis; it is formed by the base of the sacrum, the ilio-pectineal lines, and the anterior borders of the pubic bones.

The muscular walls are lined by a layer of fascia, distinguished in different parts as: (1) the diaphragmatic fascia; (2) the transversalis fascia; (3) the iliac fascia; (4) the deep layer of the lumbo-dorsal fascia.

The subperitoneal or extraperitoneal connective tissue (Tela subserosa) unites the fascia and peritoneum. It is composed of areolar tissue, more or less loaded with fat according to the condition of the subject, except over the diaphragm. It sends laminæ into the various peritoneal folds.

The peritoneum, the serous membrane which lines the cavity, will be described later.

The abdominal walls are pierced in the adult by **five apertures.** These are: the three openings in the diaphragm which transmit the aorta, posterior vena cava, and the œsophagus; the inguinal canals, which contain the spermatic cord or the round ligament (in female carnivora). In the fœtus there is the umbilical opening also.

The cavity contains the greater part of the digestive and urinary organs, part of the internal generative organs, numerous nerves, blood-vessels, lymph vessels and glands, ductless glands (spleen and adrenal bodies), and certain fœtal remains.

For topographic purposes the abdomen is divided into nine regions by imaginary planes.[1] Two of these planes are sagittal, and two are transverse. The sagittal planes cut the middles of the inguinal (Poupart's) ligaments; the transverse planes pass through the last thoracic and fifth lumbar vertebræ, or the lower end of the fifteenth rib and the external angle of the ilium respectively. The transverse planes divide the abdomen into three zones, one behind the other, viz., **epigastric, mesogastric,** and **hypogastric:** these are subdivided by the sagittal planes as indicated in the subjoined table.

Left parachondriac	Xiphoid..................	Right parachondriac
Left lumbar.......	Umbilical.................	Right lumbar
Left iliac.........	Prepubic..................	Right iliac.

Other useful regional terms are: sublumbar, diaphragmatic, inguinal. The first two require no explanation. The inguinal regions (right and left) lie in front of the inguinal (Poupart's) ligament. The flank is that part of the lateral wall which is formed only of soft structures. The depression on its upper part is termed the paralumbar fossa.

THE PERITONEUM[2]

The peritoneum is the thin serous membrane which lines the abdominal and (in part) the pelvic cavity, and covers to a greater or less extent the viscera contained therein. In the male it is a completely closed sac, but in the female there are two small openings in it; these are the abdominal orifices of the Fallopian tubes, which at their other ends communicate with the uterus, and so indirectly with the exterior. The peritoneal cavity is only a potential one, since its opposing walls

[1] This method of division, although long in use, is of very little value for accurate description. It is mentioned here chiefly because agreement on a more useful topographic method has not been arrived at.

[2] Only a general account of the arrangement of the peritoneum is given in this section, since a detailed description cannot be understood without a knowledge of the viscera concerned.

are normally separated only by the thin film of serous fluid (secreted by the membrane) which acts as a lubricant.

The free surface of the membrane has a glistening appearance and is very smooth. This is due to the fact that this surface is formed by a layer of flat endothelial cells, and is moistened by the peritoneal fluid. Friction is thus reduced to a minimum during the movements of the viscera. The outer surface of the peritoneum is related to the subperitoneal tissue, which attaches it to the abdominal wall or the viscera.

In order to understand the general disposition of the peritoneum, we may imagine the abdominal cavity to be empty and lined by a simple layer of peritoneum, termed the **parietal** layer (Lamina parietalis). We may regard the organs as beginning to develop in the subperitoneal tissue, enlarging, and migrating into the cavity to a varying extent. In doing so they carry the peritoneum before them, producing introversion of the simple sac, and forming folds which connect them with the wall or with each other. The viscera thus receive a more or less complete covering of peritoneum, termed the **visceral** layer (Lamina visceralis). The connecting folds are termed **omenta, mesenteries, ligaments,** etc. They contain a varying quantity of connective tissue, fat and lymph glands, and furnish a path for the vessels and nerves of the viscera. Some contain unstriped muscular tissue. An **omentum** is a fold which passes from the stomach to other viscera. There are three of these, namely: (1) the **small** or **gastro-hepatic omentum** (Omentum minus), which passes from the lesser curvature of the stomach to the liver; (2) the **gastro-splenic omentum** (Ligamentum gastrolienale), which extends from the greater curvature of the stomach to the spleen; (3) the **great omentum** (Omentum majus), which passes from the greater curvature of the stomach and from the spleen to the terminal part of the great colon and the origin of the small colon. It does not pass directly from one organ to the other, but forms an extensive loose sac (Figs. 278, 279). A **mesentery** (Mesenterium) is a fold which attaches the intestine to the dorsal wall of the abdomen. There are two mesenteries, namely: (1) the **great mesentery** which connects the greater part of the small intestine with the dorsal abdominal wall; (2) the **colic mesentery,** which attaches the small colon to the dorsal abdominal wall. **Ligaments** are folds which pass between viscera other than parts of the digestive tube, or connect them with the abdominal wall. The term is also applied to folds which attach parts of the digestive tract to the abdominal wall, but do not contain their blood-vessels and nerves. In some cases (*e. g.*, the lateral and coronary ligaments of the liver) they are strengthened by fibrous tissue; in other cases (*e. g.*, the broad ligaments of the uterus) they contain also unstriped muscular tissue.

THE PELVIC CAVITY

The pelvis is the posterior part of the trunk. It incloses the pelvic cavity (Cavum pelvis), which communicates in front with the abdominal cavity, the line of demarcation being the pelvic brim or terminal line.

The dorsal wall or roof is formed by the sacrum and first three coccygeal vertebræ. The **lateral walls** are formed by the parts of the ilia behind the ilio-pectineal lines and the sacro-sciatic ligaments. The **ventral wall** or floor is formed by the pubic and ischial bones. The boundary of the outlet is formed by the third coccygeal vertebra dorsally, the ischial arch ventrally, and the posterior edges of the sacro-sciatic ligaments and the semimembranosus muscles laterally. The outlet is closed by the perineal fascia; this consists of superficial and deep layers, which are attached around the margin of the outlet and centrally to the organs at the outlet—the anus and its muscles, the vulva (in the female), and the root of the penis (in the male).

The cavity contains the rectum, parts of the internal generative and urinary organs, some fœtal remnants, muscles, vessels, and nerves. It is lined by the fascia pelvis, and in part by the peritoneum.

The **pelvic peritoneum** is continuous in front with that of the abdomen. It lines the cavity as far back as the third or fourth sacral vertebra in the horse, where it is reflected on to the viscera, and from one organ to another. We may therefore distinguish an anterior, peritoneal, and a posterior, retroperitoneal part of the cavity. Along the mid-dorsal line it forms a continuation of the colic mesentery, the **mesorectum,** which attaches the first or peritoneal part of the rectum to the roof. In animals in fair condition a considerable quantity of subperitoneal and retroperitoneal fat is found on the walls and in the various interstices.

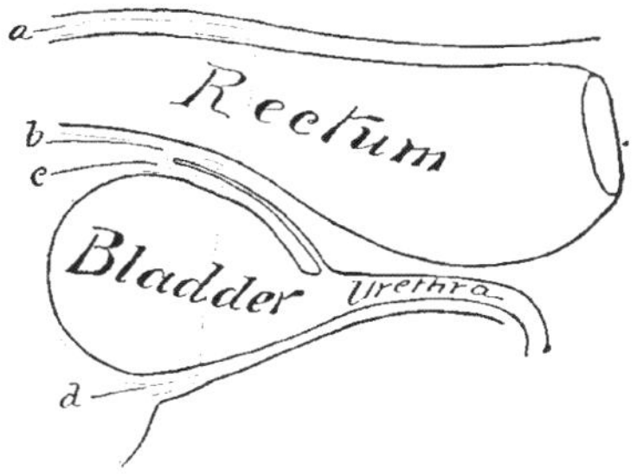

Fig. 256.—Diagram of Sagittal Section of Male Pelvis to show Disposition of Peritoneum.

a, Pouch between rectum and roof of cavity, continuous laterally with *b*, recto-genital pouch; *c*, vesico-genital pouch; *d*, pouch below bladder and its lateral ligaments. The lateral line of reflection of the peritoneum is dotted. The area of rectum covered by peritoneum varies widely. When the rectum is empty, the reflection dorsally may be at the posterior end of the sacrum; when the rectum is very full, the reflection may occur a short distance behind the promontory.

In the male the general disposition of the peritoneum here is as follows. If traced along the dorsal wall, it is reflected at the third or fourth sacral vertebra on to the rectum, forming the visceral peritoneum for the first part of that tube. Laterally it is reflected in a similar fashion. If the rectum be raised, it will be seen

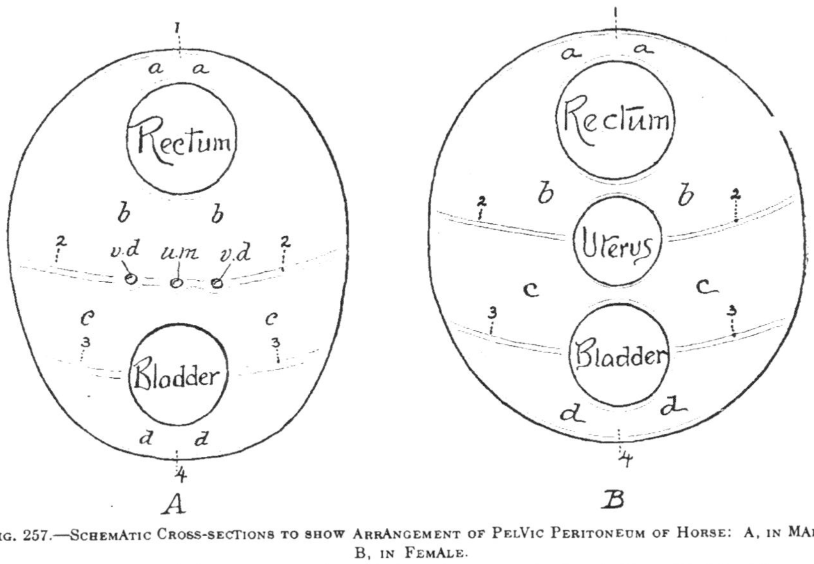

Fig. 257.—Schematic Cross-sections to show Arrangement of Pelvic Peritoneum of Horse: A, in Male; B, in Female.

A: a, b, Recto-genital pouch; *c, c*, vesico-genital pouch; *d, d*, pouch below bladder and its lateral ligaments; *1*, mesorectum; *2, 2*, urogenital fold; *3, 3*, lateral, *4*, median ligaments of bladder; *v. d.*, vas deferens; *u m.*, uterus masculinus. *B: a, b*, recto-genital pouch; *c, c*, vesico-genital pouch; *d, d*, pouch below bladder and its lateral ligaments; *1*, mesorectum; *2, 2*, broad ligaments of uterus; *3, 3*, lateral, *4*, median ligaments of bladder.

that the peritoneum passes from its ventral surface and forms a transverse fold which lies on the dorsal surface of the bladder (Fig. 272). This is the **urogenital** fold (Plica urogenitalis). Its concave free edge passes on either side into the inguinal canal. The ventral layer of this fold is reflected on to the dorsal surface of the bladder near its neck. Thus there is formed a pouch between the rectum and bladder—the **recto-vesical pouch** (Excavatio recto-vesicalis), which is partially subdivided by the urogenital fold into recto-genital and vesico-genital cavities. The fold contains the vasa deferentia, part of the vesiculæ seminales, and the uterus masculinus (a fœtal remnant). The space on either side of the rectum is occupied by coils of the small colon and the pelvic flexure of the great colon usually. If the bladder is now raised, it is seen that the peritoneum passes from its ventral surface on to the pelvic floor, forming a median fold, the so-called **middle ligament** (Plica umbilicalis media). It also forms on each side a lateral fold, the **lateral**

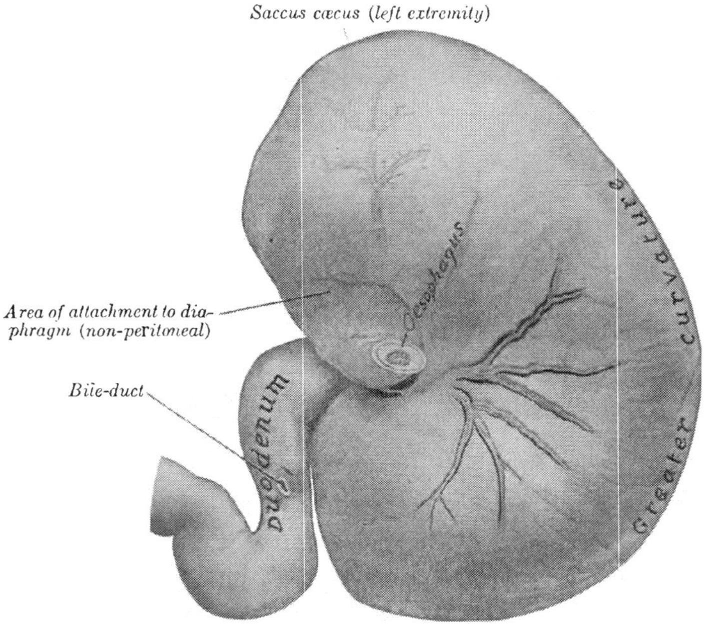

FIG. 258.—STOMACH OF HORSE, PARIETAL SURFACE, WITH FIRST PART OF DUODENUM.
Fixed *in situ* when full but not distended. The larger branches of the anterior gastric artery with two satellite veins are shown.

ligament (Plica umbilicalis lateralis), which contains in its edge the so-called **round ligament** (Ligamentum teres)—the partially occluded umbilical artery, which is a large vessel in the fœtus.

In the female the arrangement is modified by the presence of the uterus; the urogenital fold is very large, so as to inclose the uterus and a small part of the vagina. It forms two extensive folds, the **broad ligaments of the uterus** (Ligamenta lata uteri), which attach that organ to the sides of the pelvic cavity and the lumbar part of the abdominal wall (Fig. 271). It thus divides the recto-vesical pouch completely into dorsal and ventral compartments—the **recto-genital pouch** (Excavatio recto-uterina), and the **vesico-genital** pouch (Excavatio vesico-uterina).

Further details will be given in the description of the pelvic viscera.

THE STOMACH

The stomach (Ventriculus) is the large dilatation of the alimentary canal between the œsophagus and the small intestine. It is a sharply curved, U-shaped sac, the right branch being, however, much shorter than the left one. The convexity is directed ventrally. When moderately distended, there is often a slight constriction which indicates the division into right and left sacs. It is relatively small, and is situated in the dorsal part of the abdominal cavity behind the diaphragm and liver, mainly to the left of the median plane.

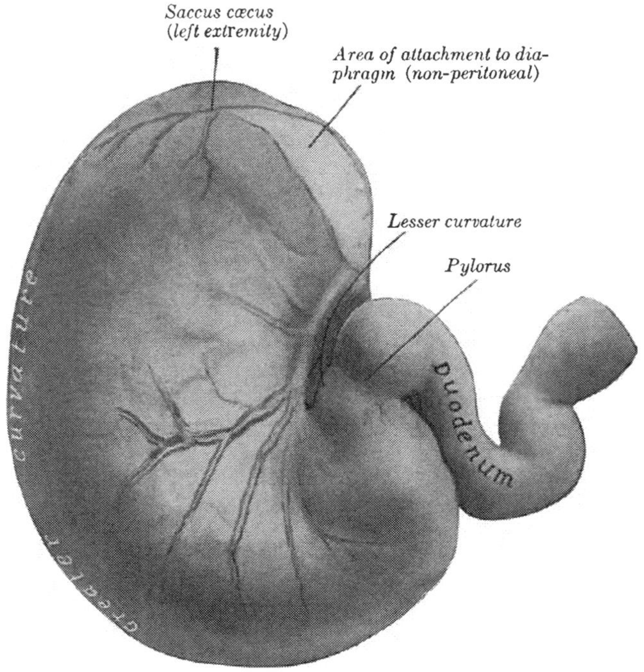

FIG. 259.—STOMACH OF HORSE, VISCERAL SURFACE, WITH FIRST PART OF DUODENUM. Fixed *in situ* when full but not distended. The posterior gastric artery and its larger branches with two satellite veins are shown.

It presents for description two surfaces, two curvatures, and two extremities. The **parietal surface** (Facies parietalis) is convex and is directed forward, upward, and toward the left; it lies against the diaphragm and liver. The **visceral surface** (Facies visceralis), also convex, faces in the opposite direction; it is related to the terminal part of the large colon, the pancreas, the small colon, and the small intestine. The **lesser curvature** (Curvatura minor) is very short, extending from the termination of the œsophagus to the junction with the small intestine. When the stomach is *in situ*, its walls are here in contact, and the cardia and pylorus close together. The **greater curvature** (Curvatura major) is very extensive. From the cardia it is first directed upward and curves over the left extremity; it then descends, passes to the right, crosses the median plane, and curves upward to end at the pylorus. Its left portion is related to the spleen, while its ventral portion rests on the left divisions of the great colon. The left **extremity** or **saccus cæcus** is a rounded cul-de-sac which lies under the upper ends of the fourteenth, fifteenth, and sixteenth ribs and the diaphragm.[1] It is related to the pancreas behind and the base of the spleen externally. The right or **pyloric extremity** is much smaller and is continuous with the duodenum, the junction being indicated by a marked constriction. It lies on the liver, a little to the right of the median plane, and a little lower than the cardiac opening. About two or three inches (ca. 5 to 8 cm.) from the pylorus there is a constriction which marks off the **antrum pylori** from the rest of the right sac. The **œsophageal orifice** or **cardia** is situated at the left extremity of the lesser curvature, but about eight to ten inches (ca. 20 to 25 cm.) from the left extremity. The œsophagus joins the stomach very obliquely. The opening is closed by the sphincter cardiæ and numerous folds of mucous membrane. The **pyloric orifice** communicates with the duodenum. Its position is indicated externally by a distinct constriction. Internally it presents a circular ridge produced by a ring of muscular tissue—the **sphincter pylori.**

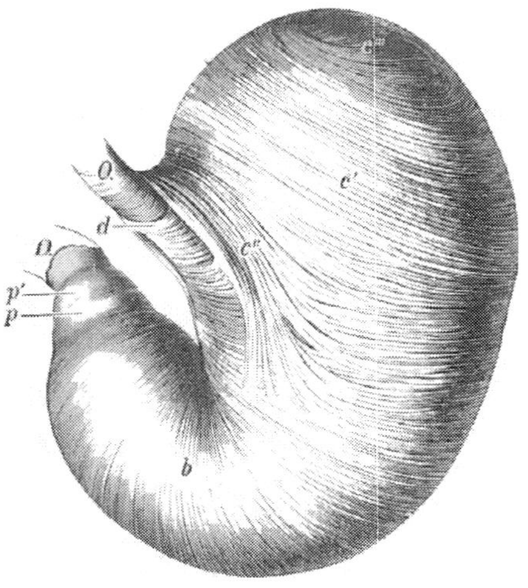

FIG. 260.—EVERTED STOMACH OF HORSE FROM WHICH THE MUCOUS MEMBRANE HAS BEEN REMOVED.

O, Œsophagus; *D*, duodenum; *b*, circular layer; *c'*, internal oblique fibers; *c''*, loop around cardia; *c'''*, transition of internal to external oblique fibers; *d*, fibers connecting the two branches of the cardiac loop; *p*, antral sphincter; *p'*, pyloric sphincter. (Ellenberger-Baum, Anat. d. Haustiere.)

The stomach is held in position mainly by the pressure of the surrounding viscera and by the œsophagus. The following peritoneal folds connect it with the adjacent parts:

1. The **gastro-phrenic ligament** (Lig. gastrophrenicum) connects the great curvature, from the cardia to the left extremity, with the crura of the diaphragm. This leaves a narrow area uncovered with peritoneum, and here the stomach is attached to the diaphragm by loose connective tissue.

2. The **small or gastro-hepatic omentum** (Omentum minus) connects the lesser curvature and the first part of the duodenum with the liver below the œsophageal notch and the portal fissure.

3. The **gastro-splenic omentum** (Lig. gastro-lienale) passes from the left part of the great curvature to the hilus of the spleen.

4. The **great or gastro-colic omentum** (Omentum majus) connects the ventral part of the great curvature and the first curve of the duodenum with the terminal part of the great colon and the initial part of the small colon.

5. The **gastro-pancreatic fold** (Plica gastro-pancreatica) extends from the left sac above the cardia to the duodenum. It is attached dorsally to the liver and vena cava, ventrally to the pancreas.

The stomach of the equidæ is relatively small, its capacity varying from two to four gallons (ca. 8 to 15 liters).

The size, form, and position of the stomach are subject to considerable variation. When the stomach is nearly empty the saccus cæcus contains only gas and is strongly contracted; the middle portion (physiological fundus) contains the ingesta and preserves its rounded character, while the pyloric portion is contracted. When distended the middle portion settles down some four or five inches, pushing back coils of the small colon and small intestine which may lie between the great curvature and the large colon, and also pushing to the left or right the left dorsal part of

[1] This is the position in the expiratory phase as usually seen in the dead subject. In inspiration the saccus cæcus lies under the upper parts of the sixteenth and seventeenth ribs.

the great colon; the spleen, small colon, and small intestines are pushed back by the distention of the left sac.

Structure.—The wall is composed of four coats—serous, muscular, submucous, and mucous.

The **serous coat** (Tunica serosa) covers the greater part of the organ and is closely adherent to the muscular coat except at the curvatures. It partially bridges over the lesser curvature, and covers here elastic tissue which assists in retaining the bent form of the stomach. The peritoneal folds have been described.

The **muscular coat** consists of three incomplete layers, an external of longitudinal, a middle of circular, and an internal of oblique fibers. The layer of **longitudinal fibers** (Stratum longitudinale) is very thin and exists only along the curvatures and at the antrum. At the lesser curvature it is continuous with the longi-

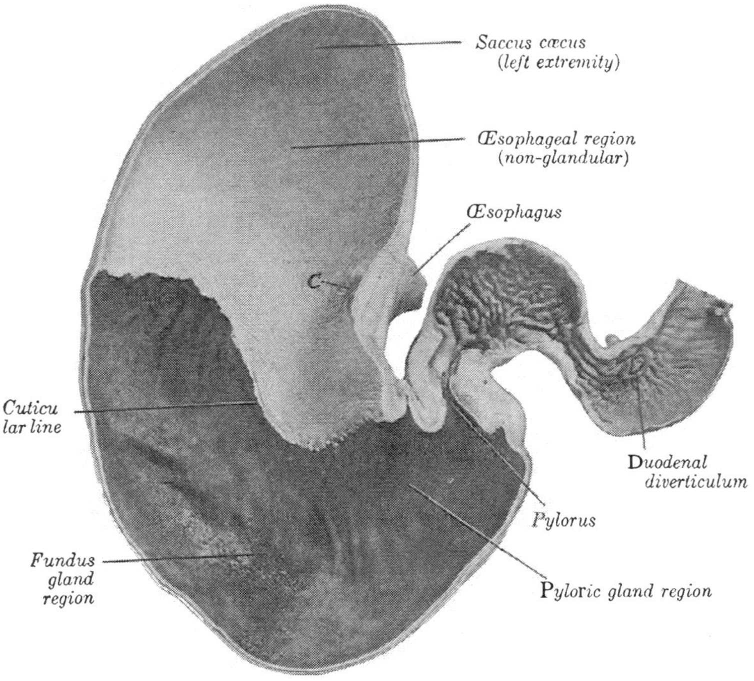

Fig. 261.—Frontal Section of Stomach and First Part of Duodenum of Horse. *C*, Cardiac orifice. Photograph of specimen fixed *in situ*.

tudinal fibers of the œsophagus. On the antrum pylori it forms a well developed complete layer. The layer of **circular fibers** (Stratum circulare) exists only on the right sac. At the pyloric orifice it forms a thick ring—the **pyloric sphincter.** Another ring, the antral sphincter, is found at the left end of the antrum pylori. The **oblique fibers** (Fibræ obliquæ) are arranged in two layers; the external stratum covers the left sac and is a continuation (in part) of the longitudinal fibers of the œsophagus; the internal stratum is found also on the left sac, and exchanges fibers with the circular and external oblique layers. It forms a remarkable loop around the cardiac orifice, constituting a powerful **cardiac sphincter** (Sphincter cardiæ).

The **submucous coat** is a layer of loose connective tissue which connects the muscular and mucous coats; in it the vessels and nerves ramify before entering the mucosa.

The **mucous coat** is clearly divided into two parts. That which lines the left sac resembles the œsophageal mucous membrane, and is termed **œsophageal** or **cuticular.** It is white in color, destitute of glands, and covered with a thick, squamous, stratified epithelium. At the cardiac orifice it presents numerous folds which occlude the opening.[1] It terminates abruptly at an elevated, denticulated, sinuous line, termed the **cuticular ridge** (Margo plicatus). Below and to the right of this line the mucous membrane has a totally different character, being soft and velvety to the touch, and covered by a mucoid secretion. It is glandular, and three zones may be recognized, although no sharp line of demarcation exists. A narrow zone next to the cuticular ridge has a yellowish-gray color, and contains short tubular **cardiac glands** (Cardiac gland region). Next to this is a large area which has a mottled reddish-brown color, and contains **fundus glands** (fundus gland region). This part of the mucous membrane is thick and very vascular, and corresponds to the fundus of the stomach in man and the dog. The remainder of the mucous membrane has a reddish-gray color and contains branched, tubular, **pyloric glands** (pyloric gland region); it corresponds to the pyloric portion of man and the dog.

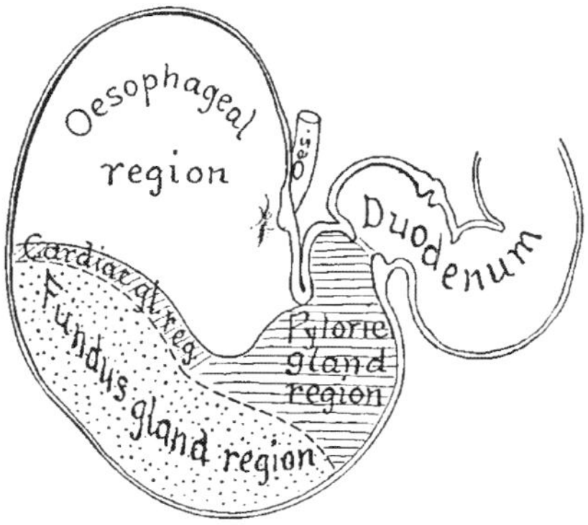

FIG. 262.—DIAGRAM OF ZONES OF MUCOUS MEMBRANE OF STOMACH OF HORSE.

The folding of the stomach wall at the lesser curvature produces a prominent ridge which projects into the cavity of the stomach. Circular ridges occur at the antral and pyloric sphincters.

Blood-vessels and Nerves.—The stomach receives blood from all the branches of the cœliac artery. The gastric veins drain into the portal vein. The nerves are derived from the vagus and sympathetic nerves.

THE SMALL INTESTINE

The **small intestine** (Intestinum tenue) is the tube which connects the stomach with the large intestine. It begins at the pylorus and terminates at the lesser curvature of the cæcum. Its average length is about seventy feet (ca. 22 meters). When distended, its diameter varies from two to four inches (5 to 10 cm.). Its capacity is about twelve gallons (40 to 50 liters).

It is clearly divisible into a **fixed** and a **mesenteric** or floating portion. The fixed portion is termed the duodenum, while the mesenteric portion (Intestinum tenue mesenteriale) is arbitrarily divided into parts termed the jejunum and ileum.[2]

The **duodenum** is about three to four feet (ca. 1 to 1.25 m.) long. Its shape is somewhat like a horseshoe, the convexity being directed toward the right. The **first part** is directed to the right and forms an ∽-shaped curve. The convexity of the first part of the curve is dorsal, of the second ventral. It lies on the middle and right lobes of the liver, and presents two dilatations (Ampullæ) with a constriction between them. The duodenal angle or head of the pancreas lies in the con-

[1] This occlusion is usually so complete that distention of the stomach by air or fluid forced in through the pylorus may be carried far enough to rupture the stomach without ligating the œsophagus.

[2] No natural line of demarcation exists, but there is a marked increase of the thickness of the wall toward the terminal part. Other differences will be noted in the further description.

cavity of the second curve, and here, five to six inches (ca. 12 to 15 cm.) from the pylorus, the pancreatic duct and the bile duct pierce the bowel wall. The **second part** passes upward and backward on the right lobe of the liver and, on reaching the right kidney and the base of the cæcum, it curves toward the median plane, opposite the last rib. The **third part** passes almost transversely from right to left behind the base of the cæcum, crosses the median plane under the third and fourth lumbar vertebræ, and turns forward to become continuous with the jejunum under the left kidney. The sacculations of the first part have a diameter of three to four inches (ca. 7.5 to 10 cm.).

It is attached by a short peritoneal fold termed the **mesoduodenum.** This fixes the first part of the duodenum closely to the liver and the right dorsal part of the colon; the remainder is somewhat less closely attached by it to the cæcum

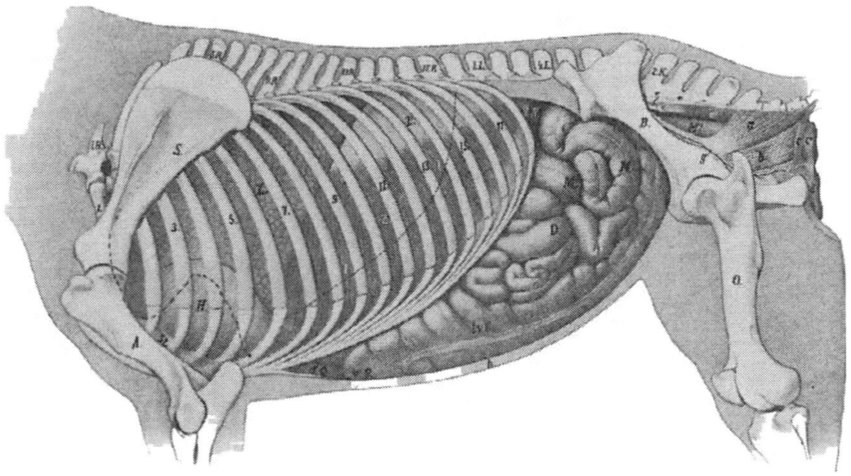

FIG. 263.—TOPOGRAPHY OF VISCERA OF HORSE, LEFT VIEW.

1.R., First thoracic vertebra; *1.L.*, first lumbar vertebra; *2.K.*, second sacral spine; *S.*, scapula; *A.*, humerus; *St.*, sternum; *B.*, ilium; *O.*, femur; *L.*, lung in complete expiration; *l.*, dotted line indicating contour of lung in inspiration; *H*, pericardium; *Z*, costal part of diaphragm; *Z'*, tendinous center of diaphragm; *l.N.*, left kidney; *l.v.C.*, left ventral colon; *v.Q.*, sternal flexure of colon; *d.Q.*, diaphragmatic flexure of colon; *D.*, small intestine; *M.*, small colon; *M'*, rectum; *a*, coccygeus muscle; *b*, retractor ani; *c, c*, sphincter ani externus; *d*, constrictor vulvæ; *e*, sacro-coccygeus inferior; *f*, anterior gluteal artery; *g*, internal pudic artery; *h*, abdominal wall in section. (After Ellenberger, in Leisering's Atlas, reduced.)

and right kidney, the sublumbar muscles, and (more closely) to the terminal part of the great colon and the first part of the small colon.[1]

The **jejunum** and **ileum** together (Jejuno-ileum) constitute the mesenteric or floating portion of the small intestine. No distinct point exists at which to make the demarcation. With the exception of the last two or three feet, the mesenteric part of the intestine varies so much in position that only a general statement can be made. It lies in numerous coils (Ansæ) mingled with those of the small colon, chiefly in the dorsal part of the left half of the abdomen, from the visceral surface of the stomach to the pelvis. It may insinuate itself between the left portions of the colon and the abdominal wall; also between the ventral portions of the colon, reaching the floor of the abdomen. The terminal part of the intestine (ileum) ascends almost vertically, a little to the right of the median plane, to open into the

[1] It will be noticed that the mesoduodenum is not continuous with the great mesentery, but ends by a free edge. The mesentery begins on the opposite surface of the end of the duodenum, so that the bowel is attached by two peritoneal folds at this point.

cæcum at the lesser curvature of its base. The average diameter of the jejuno-ileum is about two and a half to three inches (ca. 6 to 7 cm.). In the cadaver one finds most of the tube presenting irregular constricted and dilated parts. The last three or four feet (ca. 1 meter) are usually tightly contracted, resembling somewhat the terminal part of the œsophagus. This part may be termed the ileum.

The mesenteric part is connected with the dorsal abdominal wall by the **great mesentery.** This is a wide fan-shaped fold, consisting of two layers of peritoneum, between which the vessels and nerves reach the bowel; it also contains the mesenteric lymph glands and some fat. The visceral border of the mesentery contains the intestine, while the parietal border or root (Radix mesenterii) is attached to a small area around the great mesenteric trunk under the first and second lumbar vertebræ. The root is thick, as it contains a large number of vessels and nerves placed close together. The mesentery is short at first, but soon reaches a length of one and a half to two feet (ca. 50 cm.)—sufficient to allow coils of the intestine to reach the abdominal floor, the pelvic cavity, or even to descend into the scrotum through the inguinal canal. Near its termination the intestine (ileum) leaves the border of the mesentery, so that the latter has a free edge which passes to the cæcum.

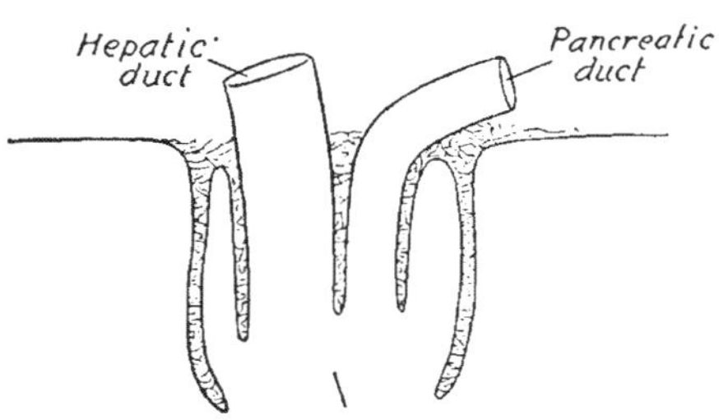

FIG. 264.—DIAGRAM OF SECTION OF DIVERTICULUM DUODENI OF HORSE.
Solid line indicates mucous membrane.

Structure.—The wall consists of four coats—serous, muscular, submucous, and mucous, enumerated from without inward.

The **serous coat** is complete except at the mesenteric edge, where the vessels and nerves reach the bowel.

The **muscular coat** consists of an outer longitudinal and an inner circular layer, the latter being the thicker. In the last few feet of the intestine the muscular coat is very thick, and being usually firmly contracted in the dead subject, gives the impression that this part of the bowel is of smaller caliber; such, however, is not the case during life.

The **submucous coat** is a layer of areolar tissue in which the vessels and nerves ramify. It contains also the duodenal glands and the bases of the solitary glands and Peyer's patches.

The **mucous membrane** is soft and velvety. It has a grayish or yellowish-red color and is very vascular. About five or six inches from the pylorus it forms a pouch, the **diverticulum duodeni,** in which the pancreatic and hepatic ducts open. On a small papilla opposite this is the termination of the accessory pancreatic duct. At the ileo-cæcal opening the mucous membrane projects slightly into the cavity of the cæcum, forming the **ileo-cæcal valve.** The free surface is thickly beset with **villi,** small projections of the mucous membrane which can be seen well by placing a piece of the membrane in water. They are relatively short and thick and have a distinct neck in the horse. Each contains a central lymph-vessel (lacteal), and around this a plexus of capillaries, lymphoid tissue, and unstriped muscle-fibers. They are important agents in absorption from the contents of the intestine. The epithelium is columnar, with many goblet cells. Underneath the basement membrane is a layer of unstriped muscle-fibers, the **muscularis mucosæ.**

The glands of the small intestine are of three kinds:

1. The **intestinal glands** (Glandulæ intestinales Lieberkuehni) are found throughout. They are simple tubular glands which open between the villi.

2. The **duodenal glands** (Glandulæ duodenales Brunneri) are found in the first twenty feet (ca. 6 meters) of the bowel. They are racemose glands, and are situated in the submucosa, so that their ducts perforate the muscularis mucosæ and the mucous membrane.

3. The **lymph follicles** (Noduli lymphatici) are found either scattered or in groups. In the former case they are termed **solitary glands** (Noduli lymphatici solitarii), in the latter **Peyer's patches** (Noduli lymphatici aggregati). The solitary glands are about the size of a millet-seed or a small sago grain. Peyer's patches are situated chiefly along the surface opposite to the mesenteric attachment and begin about three or four feet from the pylorus. They number one to two hundred, and are usually one to two inches (2 to 5 cm.) long and a quarter of an inch to one-half inch (ca. 2 to 14 mm.) wide. Larger ones occur in the terminal part, where one patch may have a length of seven to fifteen inches (ca. 17 to 38 cm.) and a width of half an inch to one inch (ca. 5 to 25 mm.) in young horses (Ellenberger). They undergo atrophy in old subjects.

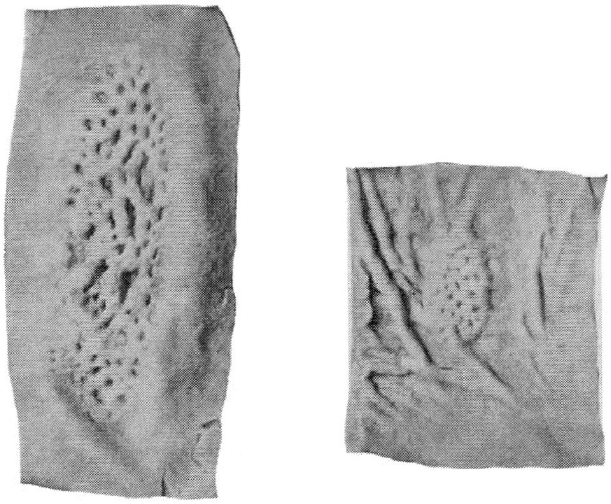

Fig. 265.—Peyer's Patches of Small intestine of Horse.

Vessels and Nerves.—The **arteries** of the small intestine come from the cœliac and anterior mesenteric arteries. The **veins** go to the portal vein. The **lymph-vessels** are numerous and go to the mesenteric lymph glands. The **nerves** are derived from the vagus and sympathetic through the solar plexus.

THE LARGE INTESTINE

The large intestine (Intestinum crassum) extends from the termination of the ileum to the anus. It is about twenty-five feet (ca. 7.5 to 8 m.) in length. It differs from the small intestine in its greater size, in being sacculated, for the most part, possessing longitudinal bands, and having a more fixed position. It is divided into cæcum, great colon, small colon, and rectum.

The Caecum

The **cæcum** (Intestinum cæcum) is a great cul-de-sac intercalated between the small intestine and the colon. It has a remarkable size, shape, and position in the horse. Its length is three to four feet (ca. 1 to 1.25 m.), and its capacity about seven to eight gallons (ca. 25 to 30 liters). It is conical in form, and is curved somewhat like a reversed comma. It is situated almost entirely to the right of the median plane, extending from the right iliac and sublumbar regions to the abdominal floor behind the xiphoid cartilage. Both extremities are blind, and the two orifices are placed close together on the concave curvature. It presents for description a base, a body, and an apex.

The **base** (Saccus cæcus) extends from about the thirteenth intercostal space backward almost to the pelvic inlet. Its greater curvature is dorsal, its lesser ventral; connected with the latter are the termination of the ileum and the origin of the colon. The body (Corpus cæci) extends downward and forward from the base and rests largely on the ventral wall of the abdomen. Its lesser curvature is about parallel with the costal arch and about five to six inches (10 to 15 cm.) below it. The **apex** (Apex cæci) lies usually on the abdominal floor about a hand's length behind the xiphoid cartilage.

The base is attached dorsally by connective tissue and peritoneum on the ventral surface of the pancreas and right kidney, the psoas muscles, and the iliac fascia; internally, it is attached to the terminal part of the great colon, and ventrally to the origin of the great colon. The body is attached dorsally to the first part of the colon by the cæco-colic fold. The apex is free, and consequently may vary in position.

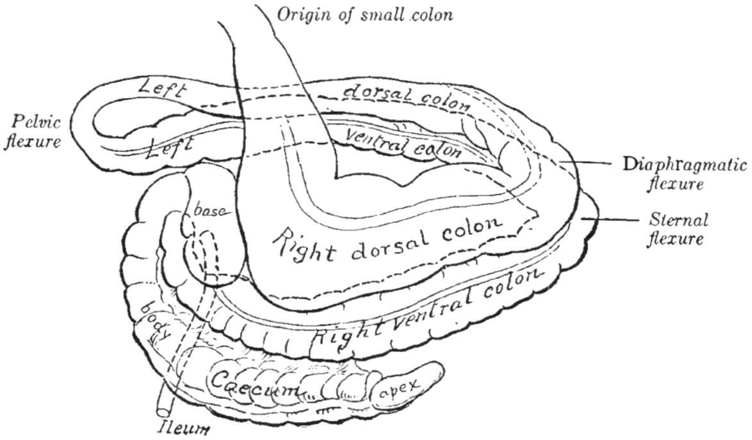

FIG. 266.—DIAGRAM OF CÆCUM AND LARGE COLON OF HORSE.

The cæcum has four **longitudinal bands** (Tæniæ), situated on the dorsal, ventral, right, and left surfaces; these cause four rows of **sacculations** (Haustra). The ventral band is entirely exposed or free (Tænia libera); the dorsal band is free on the apex. The cæcal arteries are placed on the other two. The right or parietal surface of the cæcum is related chiefly to the right abdominal wall, the diaphragm, duodenum, and liver. The left or visceral surface lies against the left divisions of the colon, the root of the great mesentery, and the small intestine.

The **ileo-cæcal orifice** (Ostium ileocæcale) is situated in the lesser curvature of the base, about four or five inches (ca. 10 to 12 cm.) to the right of the median plane and about opposite the lower end of the last rib. The end of the ileum is partially telescoped into the cæcum, so that the orifice is surrounded by a fold of mucous membrane, forming the **ileo-cæcal valve** (Valvula ileocæcalis). The peritoneum and longitudinal muscle-fibers do not take part in its formation.

The **cæco-colic orifice** (Ostium cæcocolicum) is placed above and external to the preceding one; the interval between them is only about two inches (ca. 5 cm.), and they are separated by a distinct ridge which projects into the interior of the cæcum. The orifice is slit-like and is small in relation to the size of the cæcum and colon. It has a **valvular fold** (Valvula cæcocolica) at its lower margin and a

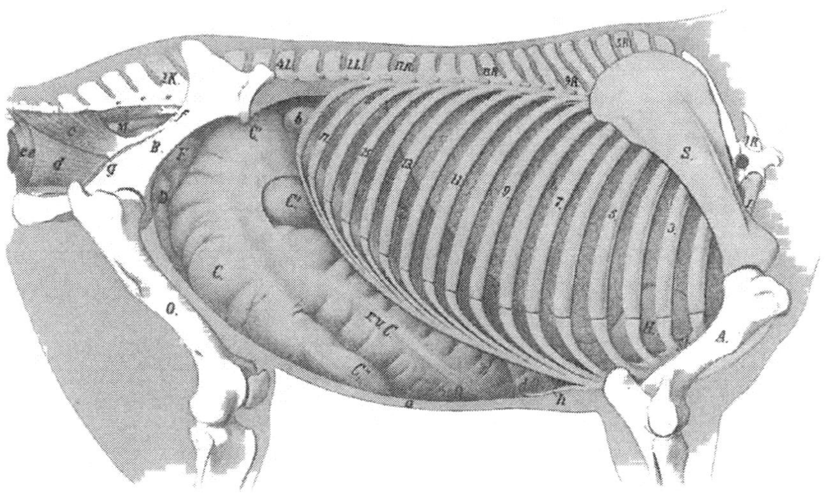

FIG. 267.—TOPOGRAPHY OF VISCERA OF HORSE, RIGHT VIEW.

1R., First thoracic vertebra; *1L.*, first lumbar vertebra; *2K.*, second sacral spine; *S.*, scapula; *A.*, humerus; *St.*, sternum; *B.*, ilium; *O.*, femur; *L.*, right lung; *H.*, pericardium; *Z.*, diaphragm (pars costalis); *r.v.C.*, right ventral colon; *v.Q.*, sternal flexure of colon; *d.Q.*, diaphragmatic flexure of colon; *C.*, body of cæcum; *C'.*, base of cæcum; *C''.*, apex of cæcum; *D.*, small intestine; *F.*, pelvic flexure of colon; *M.*, rectum; *a.*, abdominal wall in section; *b*, duodenum; *c*, coccygeus muscle; *d*, retractor ani; *e, e'*, sphincter ani externus; *f*, anterior gluteal artery; *g*, internal pudic artery; *h*, xiphoid cartilage. (After Ellenberger, in Leisering's Atlas.)

muscular ring (Sphincter cæci). Large crescentic or semilunar folds (Plicæ cæci) project into the cavity of the bowel, and between these are large pouches (Cellulæ cæci).

Vessels and Nerves.—The cæcal arteries come from the great mesenteric artery. The veins go to the portal vein. The nerves are derived from the great mesenteric plexus of the sympathetic.

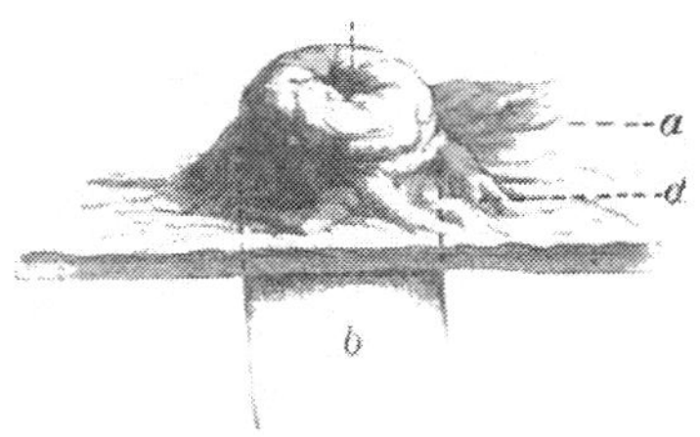

FIG. 268.—ILEO-CÆCAL ORIFICE OF HORSE.

a, Mucous membrane of cæcum; *b*, ileum; *c*, ileo-cæcal orifice; *d*, fold of mucous membrane. (After P. Schumann.)

THE GREAT COLON

The **great colon** (Colon crassum) begins at the cæco-colic orifice, and terminates by joining the small colon behind the saccus cæcus of the stomach. It is ten to twelve feet (ca. 3 to 3.7 m.) long, and its average diameter (exclusive of its narrowest part) is about eight to ten inches (ca. 20 to 25 cm.). Its capacity is more than double that of the cæcum. When removed from the abdomen, it consists of two parallel portions, which are connected by peritoneum and partially by areolar tissue also. *In situ*, it is folded so that it consists of four parts, which are designated according to their position or numerically. The three bent connecting parts are termed the flexures. The first, **right ventral part** (Colon ventrale dextrum), begins at the cæco-colic orifice about opposite the middle of the last rib, passes downward and forward along the right costal arch, and reaches the floor of the abdomen. Over the xiphoid cartilage it bends sharply to the left and backward, forming the **sternal flexure** (Flexura diaphragmatica ventralis). The second, **left ventral part** (Colon ventrale sinistrum), passes backward on the left part of the abdomi-

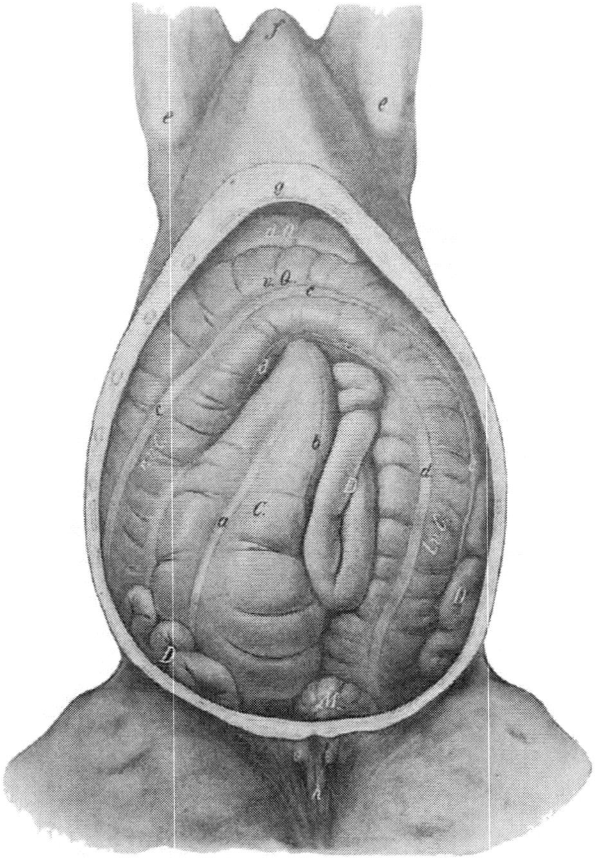

Fig. 269.—Abdominal Viscera of Horse, Ventral View.

The ventral wall and part of the lateral walls of the abdomen are removed. *C*, Cæcum; *r.v.C.*, right ventral part of colon; *v.Q.*, sternal flexure of colon; *l.v C.*, left ventral part of colon; *d.Q.*, diaphragmatic flexure of colon; *D*, small intestine; *M*, small colon; *a*, ventral free band of cæcum; *b*, inner band of cæcum; *c*, lateral band of ventral part of colon; *d*, ventral band of ventral part of colon; *e*, point of elbow; *f*, anterior end of sternal region; *g*, xiphoid cartilage; *h*, teats. (After Ellenberger-Baum, Top. Anat. d. Pferdes.)

nal floor, and, on reaching the pelvic inlet, bends sharply dorsally and forward, forming the **pelvic flexure** (Flexura pelvina). This is continued by the third, **left dorsal part** (Colon dorsale sinistrum), which passes forward above the left ventral portion. On reaching the stomach, diaphragm, and left lobe of the liver, it turns to the right, forming the **diaphragmatic** or **gastro-hepatic flexure** (Flexura diaphragmatica dorsalis). The fourth or right dorsal **part** (Colon dorsale dextrum) passes backward above the first portion, and on reaching the inner or left surface of the base of the cæcum it turns upward and to the left behind the left sac of the stomach; here it becomes constricted, and joins the small colon below the left kidney.

The **caliber** of the great colon varies greatly at different points. At its origin it is only about two to three inches (ca. 5 to 7.5 cm.) in diameter. This soon increases to about eight to ten inches (ca. 20 to 25 cm.) for the ventral portions. Beyond the pelvic flexure the diameter is reduced to about three or four inches (ca. 8 to 9 cm.). Near the diaphragmatic flexure the caliber rapidly increases, and reaches its maximum in the last division, where it may be about twenty inches (50 cm.) in its widest part. This is succeeded by a somewhat funnel-shaped terminal contraction.

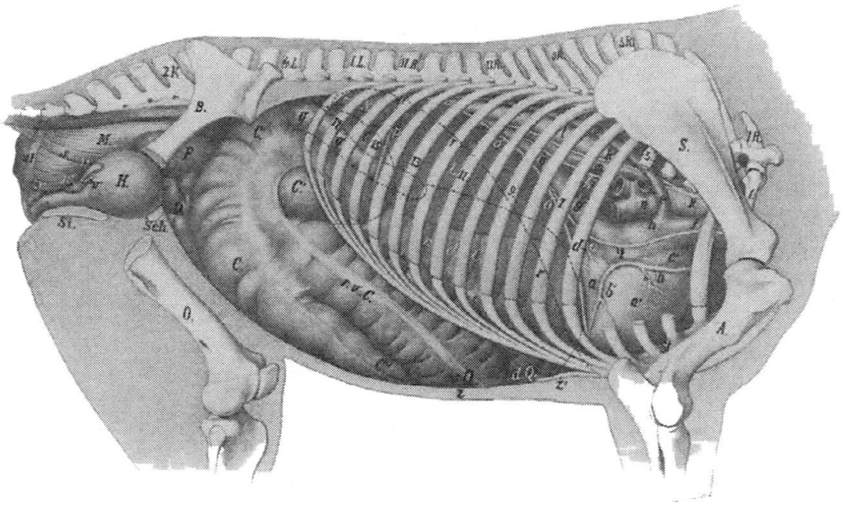

FIG. 270.—TOPOGRAPHY OF VISCERA OF HORSE, RIGHT SIDE, DEEPER VIEW.

1.R., First thoracic vertebra; *1.L.*, first lumbar vertebra; *2.K.*, second sacral spine; *S*, scapula; *A*, humerus; *B*, ilium; *O.*, femur; *Sch.*, pubis; *Si.*, ischium; *St.*, sternum; *L.*, right lobe of liver; *r.N.*, right kidney; *C.*, body, *C'.*, base, *C''.*, apex of cæcum; *r.v.C.*, right ventral colon; *v.Q.*, sternal flexure of colon; *d.Q.*, diaphragmatic flexure of colon; *r.d.C.*, right dorsal colon; *F.*, pelvic flexure of colon; *D.*, small intestine; *H.*, urinary bladder; *M.*, rectum; *a*, left ventricle; *a'*, right ventricle; *b*, *b'*, right coronary artery; *c*, left atrium; *c'*, right atrium; *d*, small (left) coronary vein; *e*, vena azygos; *f*, anterior vena cava; *g*, posterior vena cava; *h*, sinus venosus; *i*, right phrenic nerve; k, right vagus, with its dorsal (*k'*) and ventral (*k''*) divisions; *l*, aorta; *m*, œsophagus; *n*, trachea; *o*, diaphragm (median section); *p*, right lateral ligament of liver; q, duodenum; *r*, dotted line indicating position in median section of diaphragm in inspiratory phase; *s*, recto-coccygeus; *t*, suspensory ligament of rectum; *u*, sphincter ani; *v*, vesicula seminalis; *w*, prostate; *x*, bulbo-urethral (Cowper's) gland; *y*, urethra; z, abdominal wall; *z'*, xiphoid cartilage. (After Ellenberger, in Leisering's Atlas, reduced.)

The first part of the great colon is attached to the lesser curvature of the cæcum by two layers of peritoneum which form the **cæco-colic fold.** The ventral parts of the colon are similarly connected to the dorsal parts of the same side by the mesocolon. The right portions are united also by areolar tissue and muscular fibers, the surface of contact being about four or five inches (ca. 10 to 12 cm.) wide; the left portions are attached to each other by a peritoneal fold wide enough to allow them to be drawn apart five or six inches (ca. 12 to 15 cm.) near the pelvic flexure. The terminal part of the colon is attached by peritoneum and areolar tissue to the ventral surface of the pancreas dorsally and to the base of the cæcum externally. It is connected indirectly with the diaphragm and liver by means of a fold derived from the right lateral ligament of the liver.

The **relations** are complex, but the more important facts are as follows: The ventral portions (first and second) have extensive contact with the abdominal wall ventrally and laterally. On the right side the colon is almost entirely excluded from contact with the flank by the cæcum; on the left side it has no contact with the upper part of the flank, being excluded here by coils of the small colon and small intestine. Dorsally the chief relations are to the stomach, duodenum, liver, pancreas, small colon, small intestine, aorta, vena cava, and portal vein. Since there are no transverse attachments of the right and left portions, and the latter have no attachment to the wall, they are subject to considerable displacement.[1]

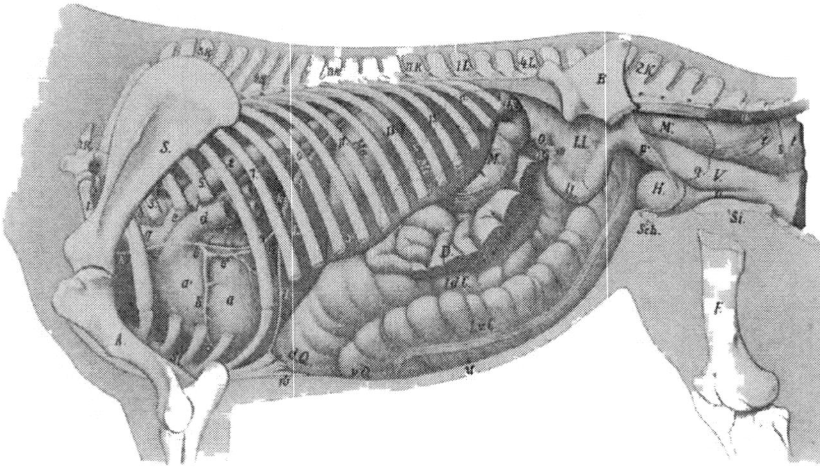

FIG. 271.—TOPOGRAPHY OF VISCERA OF HORSE, LEFT DEEP VIEW.

1R., First thoracic vertebra; *1L.*, first lumbar vertebra; *2K.*, second sacral spine; *S.*, scapula; *A.*, humerus; *B.*, ilium; *F.*, femur; *Sch.*, pubis; *Si.*, ischium; *L.*, liver (left lobe); *Ma.*, stomach, the posterior contour of which is indicated by dotted line *x*; *Mi*, spleen; *l. N.*, left kidney, concealed part indicated by dotted line; *M.*, small colon; *D.*, small intestine, parts of which have been removed; *l. d. C.*, left dorsal colon; *l.v.C.*, left ventral colon; *v.Q.*, sternal flexure; *d.Q.*, diaphragmatic flexure; *O.*, left ovary; *U.*, cornu uteri; *L.l.*, broad ligament *M'.*, rectum; *V.*, vagina; *H.*, bladder; *a*, left ventricle; *a'*, right ventricle; *b*, left coronary artery with descending (*b'*) and circumflex (*b''*) branches; *c*, left auricle; *d*, pulmonary artery (cut); *e*, aorta; *f*, ligamentum arteriosum; *g*, brachiocephalic trunk (anterior aorta); *h*, trachea; *i*, œsophagus; k, left phrenic nerve; *l*, diaphragm in median section; *m*, Fallopian tube; *n*, bursa ovarica; *o*, urethra; *p*, cut edge of broad ligament; q, line of reflection of pelvic peritoneum; *r*, recto-coccygeus; *s*, so-called suspensory ligament of rectum; *t*, sphincter ani internus; *u*, sacro-coccygeus inferior; *v*, abdominal wall in section; *w*, xiphoid cartilage. (After Ellenberger, in Leisering's Atlas.)

The pelvic flexure is variable in position, but usually it is directed to the right across the pelvic inlet.

The ventral portions of the colon have four longitudinal **muscular bands** (Tæniæ) which produce four rows of sacculations (Haustra). On the first part the external and internal bands are free; the dorsal band is covered by the adhesion to the overlying dorsal division, while the ventral band is largely covered by the adhesion to the cæcum. On the left ventral part the external and ventral bands are free; of the two dorsal bands, the inner one is concealed by the mesocolon, the outer one is chiefly free. The pelvic flexure has a band on its lesser curvature, which is continued on to the third part, concealed by the peritoneal attachment; these parts are practically non-sacculated. Near the diaphragmatic flexure two

[1] Abnormal displacement, *e. g.*, torsion of the left parts, is not rare, and is liable to produce death if not promptly reduced.

other bands appear, so that the flexure has three bands; two of these are dorsal and free, the third is ventral and concealed. The last part has three bands, of which the inner and outer ones are free, the ventral one covered.

THE SMALL COLON

The **small** colon (Colon tenue) begins at the termination of the great colon, behind the saccus cæcus of the stomach and below the left kidney, and is continued by the rectum at the pelvic inlet. Its length is about ten to twelve feet (ca. 3.5 m.), and its diameter about three to four inches (ca. 7.5 to 10 cm.).

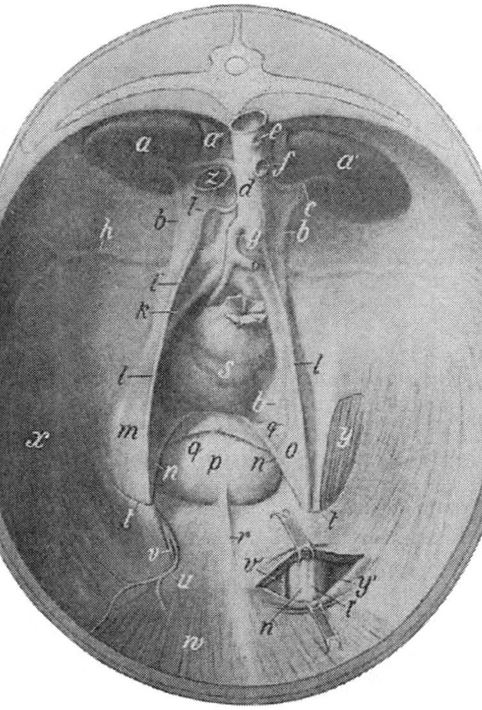

Fig. 272.—Pelvic Inlet and Posterior Part of Abdominal Wall of Horse, Viewed from the Front.

The left inguinal canal is partially opened. The peritoneum is retained except over a part of the left cremaster muscle. The sublumbar region is greatly foreshortened in this view. *a*, *a'*, Kidneys; *a''*, adrenal; *b*., ureter; *c*, renal artery; *d*, aorta; *e*, cœliac artery (cut); *f*, anterior mesenteric artery (cut); *g*, posterior mesenteric artery; *h*, circumflex iliac artery; *i*, external iliac artery; *k*, internal iliac artery; *l*, spermatic artery in peritoneal fold (plica vasculosa), *m*; *n*, vas deferens, inclosed in urogenital fold, *o*; p, urinary bladder; *q*, round ligament of bladder; *r*, middle ligament of bladder; *s*, rectum; t, margin of vaginal ring; u, posterior abdominal artery; *v*, external pudic artery; *w*, rectus abdominis muscle; *x*, transversus and obliquus internus abdominis; *y*, *y'*, cremaster externus; *z*, posterior vena cava (cut). (After Ellenberger-Baum, Top. Anat. d. Pferdes.)

Its coils lie in the space between the stomach and the pelvic inlet, dorsal to the left portions of the great colon. They are mingled with those of the small intestine, from which they are easily distinguished by the tæniæ and sacculation.

It is attached to the sublumbar region by the colic **mesentery,** and to the termination of the duodenum by a short peritoneal fold (Lig. duodeno-colicum). The great omentum is also attached to the origin of the bowel. The colic mesentery is narrow at its origin, but soon reaches a width of about three feet (ca.

80 to 90 cm.). Its parietal border is attached along a line extending from the ventral surface of the left kidney to the sacral promontory; it is continuous in front with the root of the great mesentery, and behind with the mesorectum.

There are two tæniæ and two rows of sacculations. Of the tæniæ, one is free, the other concealed by the mesentery. When the bowel is hardened *in situ* its lumen between the pouches is reduced to a narrow slit.

The Rectum

The rectum (Intestinum rectum) is the terminal part of the bowel; it extends from the pelvic inlet to the anus.[1] Its length is about one foot (ca. 30 cm.). Its direction may be straight or oblique. The first or peritoneal part of the rectum is like the small colon, and is attached by a continuation of the colic mesentery termed the mesorectum. The second or retroperitoneal part forms a flask-shaped dilatation termed the ampulla recti; it is attached to the surrounding structures by connective tissue and muscular bands.

The first part of the rectum is related to the small colon and the pelvic flexure of the great colon. It is frequently deflected to the left by the latter. The second part of the rectum is related dorsally and laterally to the pelvic wall. Ventrally the relations differ in the two sexes. In the male they are the bladder, the terminal parts of the vasa deferentia, the vesiculæ seminales, the prostate, the bulbo-urethral (Cowper's) glands, and the urethra. In the female they are the uterus, vagina, and vulva.[2]

Structure of the Large Intestine.—The serous coat covers the different parts in varying degrees. It does not cover (*a*) the opposed surfaces of the cæcum and colon which are between the layers of the cæco-colic fold and mesocolon; (*b*) the areas of attachment of the cæcum and colon to the pancreas, right kidney, and sublumbar region; (*c*) the second part of the rectum.

The muscular coat consists of longitudinal and circular fibers. The bulk of the former is in the bands already described. Some of the circular fibers pass from one part of the colon to another, where they are attached to each other, forming the fibræ transversæ coli. The muscular coat of the second part of the rectum presents special features. The longitudinal layer of fibers is very thick and consists of large bundles, loosely united. A large band, the recto-coccygeus, is detached from it on either side, and passes upward and backward to be inserted into the fourth and fifth coccygeal vertebræ.

The submucous tissue is abundant in the wall of the rectum, so that the mucous membrane is loosely attached to the muscular coat, and forms numerous folds when the bowel is empty.

The mucous membrane of the large intestine is thicker and darker in color than that of the small intestine. It forms large crescentic or semilunar folds corresponding to the external constrictions. It has no villi, Brunner's glands, or Peyer's patches. The intestinal glands (of Lieberkühn) are large and numerous. Solitary glands are also numerous, especially at the apex of the cæcum and in the left dorsal part of the colon.

Blood-supply.—Greater and lesser mesenteric and internal pudic arteries. The veins go to the portal vein.

Nerve-supply.—Mesenteric plexus of the sympathetic nerves.

[1] There is no natural line of demarcation between the small colon and rectum: the plane of the pelvic inlet is selected for convenience of description.

[2] The anterior part of the rectum is very variable in position and relations. It is not often median, but may be deflected either to right or left. Most often it is pushed to the left by the pelvic flexure of the colon. In other cases—especially when empty—it may lie against the right wall, and the space to the left is occupied by the small colon. The amount covered by peritoneum dorsally and laterally is very variable, and appears to be in inverse proportion to the fullness of the bowel.

The **anus** is the terminal orifice of the alimentary canal. It is situated below the root of the tail, where it forms a round projection, with a central depression when contracted. It is covered externally by an integument which is thin, hairless, and provided with numerous sebaceous and sweat glands. The mucous lining is pale, glandless, and covered with a thick, squamous, stratified epithelium.

There are three muscles of the anus.

1. The **sphincter ani internus** is merely a terminal thickening of the circular coat of the bowel.

2. The **sphincter ani externus** is a broad band of striped muscle-fibers outside the internal sphincter. Some fibers are attached to the coccygeal fascia above, others to the perineal fascia below. Its action is to close the anus.

3. The **retractor ani** (M. levator ani) is a flat muscle which lies between the rectum and the sacro-sciatic ligament. It arises from the superior ischiatic spine and the sacro-sciatic ligament, and ends under the external sphincter. Its action is to reduce the partial prolapse which the anus undergoes during defecation.

The suspensory ligament of the anus is a band of unstriped muscle which arises from the first coccygeal vertebra, passes downward over the retractor, and unites with its fellow below the anus. In the male it is largely continued by the retractor penis muscle; in the female it blends with the constrictor vulvæ. It may act as an accessory sphincter of the anus.

Blood-supply.—Internal pudic artery.

Nerve-supply.—Hæmorrhoidal and perineal nerves (for the sphincter ani externus and retractor ani).

THE PANCREAS

The **pancreas** is situated transversely on the dorsal wall of the abdomen, the greater part being to the right of the median plane. Its central part lies under the sixteenth and seventeenth thoracic vertebræ.

When fresh it has a reddish cream color, but if left in the unpreserved cadaver it rapidly decomposes and becomes dark. It resembles the salivary glands in appearance, but is softer, and its lobules are more loosely united. Its average weight is about twelve ounces (ca. 350 g.).

When hardened *in situ* its shape is very irregular. It is triangular in outline, and presents for description two surfaces, three borders, and three angles.[1]

The **dorsal surface** faces upward and forward. It is partially covered by peritoneum. It is related chiefly to the ventral surface of the right kidney and adrenal, the posterior vena cava, the portal vein, the cœliac artery and its divisions, the gastro-phrenic ligament and the saccus cæcus of the stomach, the right and caudate lobes of the liver, and the gastro-pancreatic fold. There are grooves for the divisions of the cœliac artery, and a large one for the splenic vein.

The **ventral surface** looks downward and backward; it is in general concave. It presents two impressions, separated by an oblique ridge. The smaller of these (Impressio cæcalis) lies to the right, and is caused by the pressure of the base of the cæcum; the larger one (Impressio colica) indicates the area of contact with the terminal part of the great colon and its junction with the small colon. It has usually no peritoneal covering except over a small area at the anterior angle.

The **right border** is nearly straight; it is related to the second part of the duodenum and the caudate lobe of the liver.

The left **border** is slightly concave, and is related to the first part of the duodenum, the left sac of the stomach, and the splenic vessels.

[1] A descriptive method based on that in use in human anatomy cannot be applied with clearness to the organ in the horse.

The posterior border presents a deep notch to the right of the median plane for the portal vein, which passes through the gland very obliquely. There is a thin bridge of gland tissue dorsal to the vein, thus forming the portal ring (Annulus portarum). The root of the great mesentery is in contact with the border just to the left of the median plane.

The anterior or duodenal angle (Caput pancreatis) is attached to the concavity of the second curve of the duodenum, and the adjacent part of the right lobe of the liver. The ducts leave at this extremity.

The left or splenic angle (Cauda pancreatis) corresponds to the tail of the pancreas in man. It is in contact with the base of the spleen, the left kidney and adrenal body, and the saccus cæcus of the stomach.

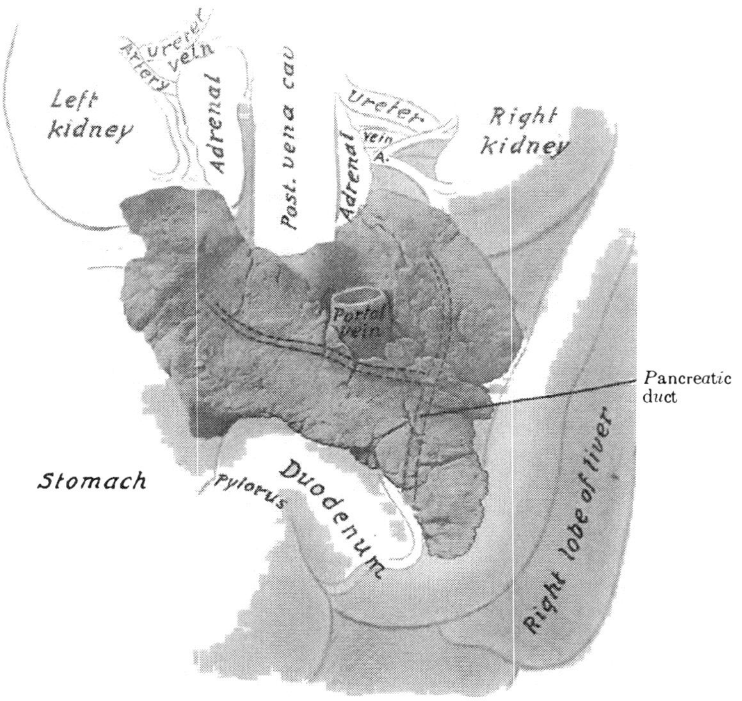

FIG. 273.—PANCREAS OF HORSE WITH CHIEF RELATIONS, VENTRAL VIEW.
The pancreatic duct and its two chief radicles are indicated by dotted lines, since they are in the substance of the gland.

The right angle is rounded, and lies on the ventral surface of the right kidney and adrenal body.

The pancreas is attached dorsally by connective tissue to the kidneys and adrenal bodies, the gastro-phrenic ligament and the suspensory ligament of the spleen, the posterior vena cava, the portal fissure, and the gastro-pancreatic fold. The ventral surface is mainly attached by areolar tissue to the base of the cæcum and the terminal part of the great colon.

There are almost invariably two ducts. The large one is termed the **pancreatic duct** (Ductus pancreaticus [Wirsungi]). It is formed by the union of two radicles which come from the right and left extremities, and passes through the duodenal angle to end at the duodenal diverticulum alongside of the bile-duct. The duct is nearly half an inch (ca. 1 cm.) wide, and is very thin-walled. It is situated in the substance of the gland near its dorsal surface; none of it is free. The accessory **pancreatic duct** (Ductus pancreaticus accessorius [Santorini]) arises either from the chief duct or its left radicle, and ends on a papilla in the duodenum opposite the chief duct.

Structure.—The pancreas belongs to the class of tubulo-alveolar glands, the alveoli being long, like those of the duodenal glands; in other respects it resembles the serous salivary glands very closely. It has no proper capsule and the lobules are rather loosely united.

Vessels and Nerves.—The arteries of the pancreas come from the branches of the cœliac and anterior mesenteric arteries. The nerves are derived from the cœliac and mesenteric plexuses of the sympathetic.

THE LIVER

The liver (Hepar) is the largest gland in the body. It is situated obliquely on the abdominal surface of the diaphragm. Its highest point is at the level of the right kidney, its lowest on the left side, usually about three or four inches (ca. 8 to 10 cm.) from the abdominal floor, opposite the lower end of the seventh or eighth rib. The greater part of it lies to the right of the median plane.

It is red-brown in color and is rather friable. Its average weight is about ten to twelve pounds (ca. 5 kg.). When in the body, or if hardened *in situ,* it is strongly curved and accurately adapted to the abdominal surface of the diaphragm. When removed in the soft state, it flattens out into a cake-like form quite different from its natural configuration. It presents for description two surfaces and a circumference, which may be divided into four borders.

The **parietal surface** (Facies diaphragmatica) is strongly convex, and lies against the diaphragm. It faces chiefly upward and forward. It presents, just to the right of the median plane, a sagittal groove for the posterior vena cava (Fossa venæ cavæ). The vein is partially embedded in the substance of the gland, and receives the hepatic veins.

The **visceral surface** (Facies visceralis) faces in general downward and backward; it is concave and irregular, being moulded on the organs which lie against it. It presents, a little to the right of the median plane, the **portal fissure** (Porta hepatis). Through this the portal vein, hepatic artery, and hepatic plexus of nerves enter, and the hepatic duct and lymph vessels leave the liver. The portal or hepatic lymph glands are also found here. The pancreas is attached at and to the right of the fissure, and the gastro-hepatic omentum to the left of it. Above the fissure is a ridge which represents the caudate lobe (Lobus caudatus Spigelii), and is continued to the right by the pointed caudate process (Processus caudatus). Further to the left there is a large depression (Impressio gastrica) for the stomach. To the right of this may be seen a groove passing to the right and dorsally; this is the duodenal impression (Impressio duodenalis). Ventral to these is a large depression for the great colon (Impressio colica). Dorsal to this is a smaller depression for the blind end of the base of the cæcum.[1] Coils of the small intestine may also lie on this surface, and the apex of the spleen may reach to it when the stomach is empty.

The **dorsal border** (Margo obtusus) is thick for the most part. It presents from right to left: (1) a depression for the right kidney (Impressio renalis); (2) a notch, which is the dorsal end of the fossa venæ cavæ; (3) a deep notch (Impressio

[1] These impressions are not evident on the soft organ. In hardened material they are clearly mapped out, although of course variable in size, in conformity with the degree of fullness of the various hollow viscera. The cæcal impression may not be evident if, as often happens in old horses, the right lobe of the liver is much atrophied.

œsophagea) which is mainly occupied by the thick margin of the œsophageal opening of the diaphragm.

The ventral border is thin, and is marked by two deep **interlobar fissures** or **incisures** (Incisuræ interlobares), which partially divide the organ into three principal lobes—**right, middle,** and **left.** The right lobe is the largest, except in old subjects, in which it is frequently much atrophied. The middle lobe is the smallest. It is marked by several small fissures, and by the **umbilical fissure** (Incisura umbilicalis); the latter contains the umbilical vein in the fœtus, which is transformed into the round ligament after birth.

The right border is thin and long. It is nearly vertical, and extends backward to about the middle of the sixteenth rib.

The left border is thin and short. It extends backward to a point opposite the lower part of the ninth or tenth rib. The ventral and lateral borders together constitute the margo acutus.

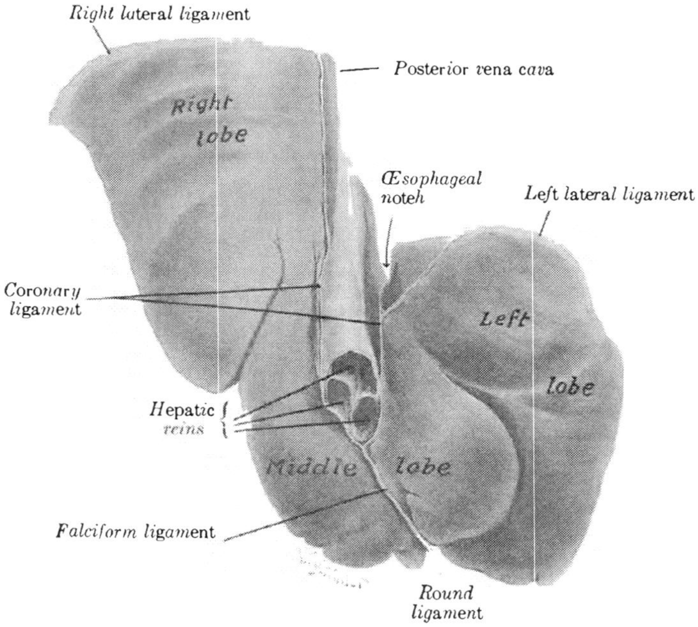

Fig. 274.—Liver of Young Horse, Hardened *in situ*, Parietal Surface.

The liver is held in position largely by the pressure of the other viscera and by its close application to the diaphragm. It has six ligaments.

1. The **coronary ligament** (Lig. coronarium hepatis) attaches it closely to the diaphragm. It consists of two laminæ. The right one is attached to the right of the fossa venæ cavæ; the left one begins to the left of the vena cava and passes upward and outward, becoming continuous with the left lateral ligament at the left margin of the œsophageal notch; it detaches a middle fold which extends to the notch and is continuous with the small omentum. The two laminæ unite below the vena cava to form the next ligament.

2. The **falciform ligament** (Lig. falciforme hepatis) is a crescentic fold which attaches the middle lobe to the sternal part of the diaphragm and to the abdominal floor for a variable distance. In its concave free edge is found

3. The **round ligament** (Lig. teres hepatis), a fibrous cord which extends from the umbilical fissure tó the umbilicus; it is the vestige of the umbilical vein, which in the fœtus carries the blood from the placenta to the liver.

4. The **right lateral ligament** (Lig. triangulare dextrum) is a wide fold which attaches the dorsal border of the right lobe to the costal part of the diaphragm.

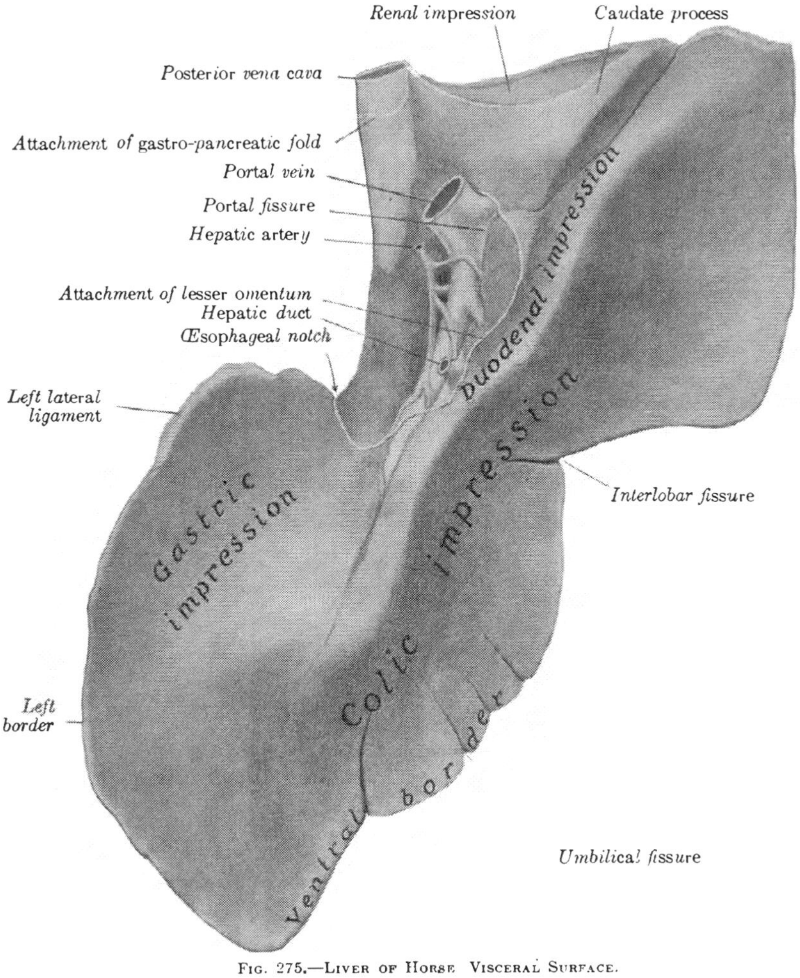

FIG. 275.—LIVER OF HORSE. VISCERAL SURFACE.
Specimen from middle-aged subject, hardened *in situ*.

5. The **left lateral ligament** (Lig. triangulare sinistrum) attaches the dorsal edge of the left lobe to the tendinous center of the diaphragm.

6. The **hepato-renal** or caudate ligament (Lig. hepatorenale) attaches the caudate process to the right kidney and the base of the cæcum. The gastro-hepatic omentum and the mesoduodenum have been described.

As stated above, the liver is divided by fissures into three principal lobes—right, middle, and left. The right lobe is the largest in the young subject and is irregularly quadrilateral in form. On its dorsal part is the caudate lobe, which ends in a pointed process directed outward, and assists in forming the cavity for the right kidney. The middle lobe is normally much the smallest. The left lobe is oval in outline and thickest centrally. In old or middle-aged subjects it often exceeds the right one in size. In some cases the atrophy of the right lobe is so extreme that the middle lobe may exceed it in size.[1]

The hepatic duct (Ductus hepaticus) is formed at the ventral part of the portal fissure by the union of right and left chief lobar ducts. It is two or three inches (ca. 5 to 8 cm.) long and about half an inch (ca. 1 to 1.5 cm.) wide. It passes between the two layers of the lesser omentum, and pierces the wall of the duodenum about five or six inches (ca. 12 to 15 cm.) from the pylorus, alongside of the pan-

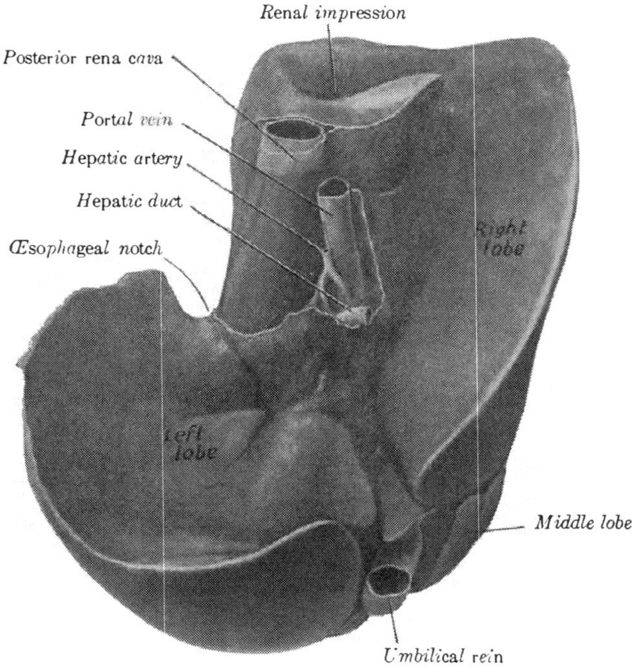

Fig. 276.—Liver of New-born Foal, Hardened *in situ*. Visceral Surface.
The differences, when compared with the organ in the adult, are very striking.

creatic duct. The ducts pass obliquely through the wall of the duodenum for about half an inch (ca. 1 cm.) before opening into the diverticulum duodeni. The arrangement forms an effective valve, which prevents regurgitation from the intestine. There is no gall-bladder.

Structure.—The liver is covered by an outer serous, and an inner fibrous coat. The serous coat covers the gland except at the attachment of the pancreas and at the portal fossa; it is reflected from it to form the ligaments and the lesser omentum. The fibrous capsule is in general thin; it sends laminæ into the ligaments, and also

[1] Flower and Ruge describe the mammalian liver as being primarily divided by the umbilical fissure into two parts, the right and left lobes. Secondary fissures on either side may subdivide each of these primary lobes. On this basis we may recognize in the liver of the horse right lateral, right central, left central, and left lateral lobes. In the young foal these four lobes are distinctly recognizable. The two central lobes would correspond to the middle lobe of the foregoing description, and the right central lobe would be the equivalent of the quadrate lobe of man.

delicate strands into the gland substance. At the portal fissure it is abundant and surrounds the vessels and ducts, which it accompanies in the portal canals of the gland substance.

The gland substance is composed of the parenchyma and the interstitial tissue. The **parenchyma** is made up of lobules, 1 to 2 mm. in diameter, which are held together by a small amount of interlobular connective tissue. On account of the very small amount of the latter, the lobulation of the horse's liver is not usually at all distinct to the naked eye; for the same reason the organ is also quite friable.[1]

Vessels and Nerves.—The **portal vein** enters at the portal fissure. It conveys blood from the digestive tract and the spleen, which contains various products of digestion and numerous white blood-cells. The **hepatic artery** also enters at the portal fissure; it may be termed the nutrient vessel. All the blood is returned from the liver to the posterior vena cava by the hepatic veins. The portal vein and the hepatic artery both divide into interlobular branches, which run together in the portal canals of the interlobular tissue. The branches of the portal vein (Venæ interlobulares) give off intralobular branches which form plexuses of capillaries in the lobules and give rise to a central vein (Vena centralis). The branches of the hepatic artery (Rami arteriosi interlobulares) are of relatively small size. They supply mainly (if not exclusively) the interlobular tissue, the capsule, and the walls of the vessels and ducts. The **hepatic veins**[2] (Venæ hepaticæ) empty into the vena cava as it lies in the fossa of the gland. Their ultimate radicles are the central lobular veins, which emerge from the bases of the lobules and join the sublobular veins (Venæ sublobulares); the latter unite to form the hepatic veins. The largest hepatic veins, three or four in number, join the posterior vena cava just before it leaves the liver to pass through the diaphragm.

The nerve-supply comes from the **hepatic plexus,** composed of branches from the vagus and sympathetic nerves.

THE SPLEEN

The **spleen** (Lien) is the largest of the ductless glands.[3] It is situated chiefly in the left parachondrium, in close relation to the left part of the great curvature of the stomach, to which its long axis corresponds. Its size and weight vary greatly in different subjects, and also in the same subject under different conditions, depending chiefly on the great variability of the amount of blood contained in it. The average weight is about 35 ounces (ca. 1 kg.), its length about 20 inches (ca. 50 cm.), and its greatest width about 8 to 10 inches (ca. 20 to 25 cm.). It is usually bluish-red or somewhat purple in color. In the natural state it is soft and yielding, but not friable.

The weight appears to vary ordinarily from about one to eight pounds, although in large horses the latter figure even may be exceeded without any apparent evidence of disease. There does not seem to be any constant relation to the body-weight. For example, the spleen of a colt about ten months old weighed three and a half pounds, while it often weighs less than two

[1] In the young foal the interlobular tissue is more abundant and the lobulation correspondingly distinct.

[2] The hepatic veins may be recognized on section from the fact that they remain open, being connected closely with the parenchyma.

[3] The ductless glands are organs which elaborate substances which pass directly into the veins or lymphatics, instead of being conveyed away by ducts. This process is termed internal secretion. The ductless glands include the lymph glands, which are described with the organs of circulation; the thyroid and thymus bodies, described usually with the respiratory organs; the adrenal or suprarenal bodies, described with the urinary organs; the pineal and pituitary bodies, described with the brain; and the spleen, described with the digestive system as a matter of convenience. The spleen is not, strictly speaking, a gland at all: it is not epithelial in origin or structure, but is mesenchymatous.

pounds in horses weighing 1000 to 1200 pounds. The chief variation in outline consists of increase of width, especially of the dorsal part.

It extends obliquely in a curved direction from the left crus of the diaphragm and the saccus cæcus of the stomach to the ventral third of the ninth or tenth rib. It presents for description two surfaces, two borders, and two extremities.

The **parietal** or **external** surface (Facies parietalis) is convex, and lies chiefly against the diaphragm, but is in direct contact with the upper parts of the last two ribs and to a small extent with the flank at the lumbo-costal angle.

The **visceral** or **internal** surface (Facies visceralis) is in general concave. It is divided into two unequal portions by a longitudinal ridge; on this is a groove, the **hilus**, in which the vessels and nerves are situated. The area in front of the ridge (Facies gastrica) is moulded on the great curvature of the stomach; it is about two inches (ca. 5 cm.) wide. The area behind the ridge (Facies intestinalis) is

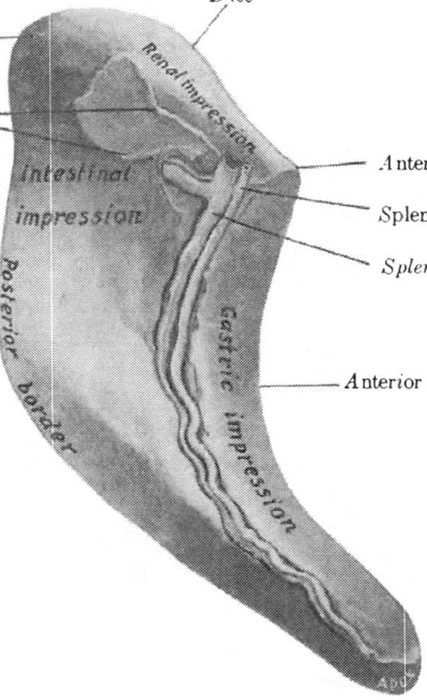

Fig. 277—Spleen of Horse, Hardened *in situ*. Visceral Surface.
The area marked intestinal impression is related to the first coil of the small colon.

much more extensive; it is related chiefly to the small colon, the small intestine, and the great omentum. It may be marked by one or two fissures.

The **anterior border** (Margo anterior) is concave and thin.

The **posterior border** (Margo posterior) is convex and thin.

The **base** or **dorsal extremity** is beveled, and fits into the interval between the left kidney and the left crus of the diaphragm and the psoas major. When hardened *in situ*, it shows an impression (Facies renalis) where it lies against the kidney. The left extremity of the pancreas touches it also. The anterior basal angle fits in between the saccus cæcus of the stomach and the left kidney; the posterior basal angle usually lies against the flank just behind the last rib.

The **apex** or **ventral extremity** is small; it lies—when the stomach is not full—between the left lobe of the liver and the left dorsal portion of the colon; when the stomach is full, the spleen is pushed further back and loses contact with the liver.

The spleen is attached by two peritoneal folds, the suspensory ligament and the gastro-splenic omentum. The **suspensory ligament** (Lig. suspensorium lienis) attaches the base to the left crus of the diaphragm and the left kidney; it contains a quantity of elastic tissue. The part which passes to the diaphragm is the ligamentum phrenico-lienale, and blends with the gastro-phrenic ligament; the part which goes to the kidney is termed the ligamentum renolienale. The **gastro-splenic omentum** (Lig. gastrolienale) passes from the hilus to the left part of the great curvature of the stomach. It is narrow above, where it joins the suspensory ligament; below it becomes much wider and is continuous with the great omentum.

Small globular or lenticular masses of splenic tissue may be found in the gastro-splenic omentum. They are termed **accessory spleens** (Lienes accessoriæ).

Structure.—The spleen has an almost complete serous **coat**. Subjacent to this and intimately united with it is a **capsule** of fibrous tissue (Tunica albuginea), which contains many elastic fibers and some unstriped muscular tissue. Numerous **trabeculæ** (Trabeculæ lienis) are given off from the deep face of the capsule and ramify in the substance of the organ to form a supporting network. In the interstices of this framework is the **spleen pulp** (Pulpa lienis), a dark red, soft, grumous material. This is supported by a delicate adenoid **reticulum,** and contains numerous leukocytes, the large splenic cells, red blood-corpuscles, and pigment. The pulp is richly supplied with blood. The branches of the splenic artery enter at the hilus and pass along the trabeculæ. The arteries which enter the pulp have a sheath of lymphoid tissue, which collects on the vessel wall at certain points, forming small **lymph nodules,** the so-called Malpighian corpuscles (Noduli lymphatici lienales). These are visible to the naked eye as white spots, about as large as the head of a pin. The blood passes into cavernous spaces lined by endothelium which is continuous with the cells of the reticulum of the pulp. From these the veins arise. The splenic vein runs in the hilus in company with the artery and nerves, and joins the posterior gastric vein to form a large radicle of the portal vein.

Blood-supply.—Splenic artery.

Nerve-supply.—Splenic plexus.

THE PERITONEUM

The general disposition of the peritoneum has been described, and other facts in regard to it were mentioned in the description of the viscera. It is now desirable to study it as a continuous whole.[1] (Figs. 256, 257, 278, 279.)

We may consider the peritoneum as consisting of two sacs—a greater and a lesser. The **greater sac** lines the greater part of the abdominal cavity, and covers most of the viscera which have a peritoneal investment. The **lesser sac** is an introversion or recess of the greater sac, formed during the development of the viscera. The two sacs communicate by a relatively narrow passage, termed the **epiploic foramen** of Winslow (Foramen epiploicum). This opening is situated on the visceral surface of the liver above the portal fissure. It can be entered by passing the finger along the caudate lobe of the liver toward its root. Its dorsal (or anterior) wall is formed by the caudate lobe and the posterior vena cava. Its ventral (or posterior) wall consists of the pancreas, the gastro-pancreatic fold, and the portal vein. The walls are normally in contact, and the passage merely a potential one. It is usually about four inches (ca. 10 cm.) in length. It is narrowest at the right

[1] The student is strongly recommended to study the peritoneum of a foal or other small subject when the opportunity occurs, as in these the viscera are easily handled, and the course of the peritoneum can be followed without difficulty.

extremity, where it is about an inch (ca. 2.5 to 3 cm.) wide.[1] If the finger is passed into the foramen from right to left, it enters the cavity of the lesser sac. If now an opening is made in the great omentum and the other hand introduced through it, the fingers of the two hands touch each other over the lesser curvature of the stomach. The formation and boundaries of the lesser sac should now be examined by spreading out the great omentum. It will be found that the latter now incloses a considerable cavity behind the stomach; this is termed the omental **cavity** (Bursa omentalis). Passing forward over the lesser curvature of the stomach, we enter another space, the **vestibule** of the omental cavity (Vestibulum bursæ omentalis). This space is closed on the left by the gastro-phrenic ligament, below and on the right by the lesser omentum, and dorsally by the gastro-pancreatic fold, which is attached to the dorsal border of the liver and to the posterior vena cava. Above the œsophageal notch the fingers can be passed around the border of the liver and the vena cava till the coronary ligament is encountered. Thus the vestibule is closed except (1) on the right, where it communicates with the cavity

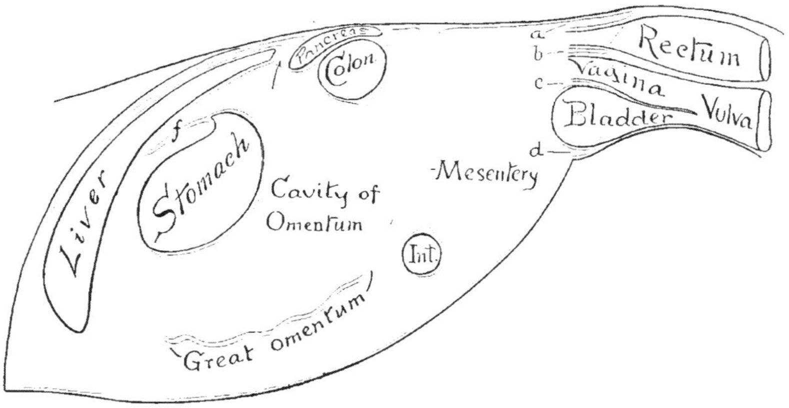

FIG. 278.—DIAGRAM OF GENERAL ARRANGEMENT OF PERITONEUM (OF MARE) IN SAGITTAL TRACING.

a, Pouch between rectum and roof of pelvis, continuous with *b*, recto-genital pouch; *c*, vesico-genital pouch; *d*, pouch below bladder and its lateral ligaments; *f*, lesser omentum; *Int.*, small intestine. The arrow points to the epiploic foramen (of Winslow).

of the greater sac by the epiploic foramen; and (2) behind, where it communicates with the cavity of the omentum.

The general arrangement of the great omentum has already been indicated. We may now trace its line of attachment, which would correspond to the mouth of the sac. Beginning at the ventral part of the great curvature of the stomach, the line passes to the ventral face of the pylorus, then crosses obliquely the first part of the duodenum to the point where the pancreas is adherent to it. Here it passes to the anterior face of the terminal transverse part of the great colon, runs along this transversely (from right to left), and continues for some ten or twelve inches (ca. 25 to 30 cm.) on the small colon. It then forms an acute angle, passes inward and forward along the small colon to the dorsal part of the hilus of the spleen, where it blends with the suspensory ligament of the latter, and forms a recess (Recessus lienalis) behind the saccus cæcus of the stomach. It now passes along the hilus of the spleen, and is continued to the great curvature of the stomach by the gastro-splenic omentum. It is convenient to regard the spleen as being intercal-

[1] The passage is subject to a good deal of variation in caliber and is sometimes completely occluded.

ated in the left part of the great omentum; on this basis the gastro-splenic omentum would be that part of the great omentum which connects the hilus of the spleen with the great curvature of the stomach. The great omentum is relatively small in the horse, and is usually not visible when the abdomen is opened. It is generally folded up in the space between the visceral surface of the stomach and the intestine.[1]

The lesser sac furnishes the peritoneal covering for: (1) the visceral surface of the stomach and a small area of the first curve of the duodenum; (2) a large part of the dorsal surface of the pancreas and portal vein; (3) a small part of the visceral surface of the liver above the attachment of the lesser omentum and the portal fossa; (4) the posterior vena cava, from the level of the epiploic foramen [of Winslow] to its passage through the diaphragm (in so far as it is not embedded); (5) the part of the parietal surface of the liver between the right and middle divisions of the coronary ligament; (6) the corresponding part of the diaphragm, and the right part of the right crus of the same; (7) part of the anterior surface of the terminal part of the great colon, and the origin of the small colon; (8) the left extremity of the pancreas (inconstant); (9) the spleen.

We may now trace the peritoneum in a longitudinal direction, beginning in front. It is reflected from the ventral abdominal wall and the diaphragm upon the liver, forming the ligaments and serous coat of the gland. It leaves the visceral surface of the liver as lesser omentum, and the crura of the diaphragm as the gastrophrenic ligament, reaches the saccus cæcus and lesser curvature of the stomach and the first curve of the duodenum, covers these organs, and is continued by the great omentum.

On the left it passes from the left crus of the diaphragm and the left kidney to form the suspensory ligament of the spleen, clothes that organ, and leaves it to be continued by the great omentum.

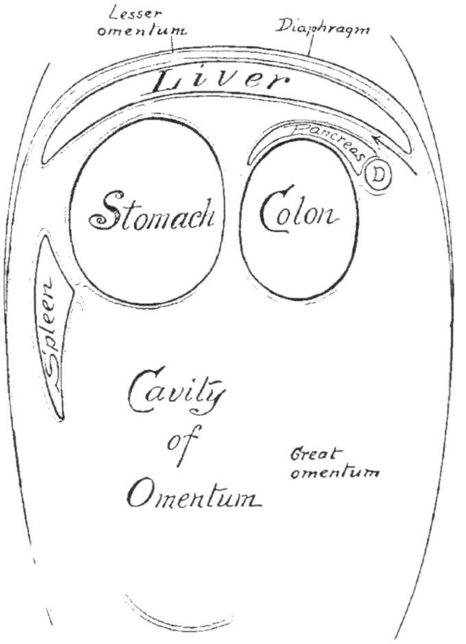

FIG. 279.—DIAGRAM OF ABDOMINAL PERITONEUM IN FRONTAL (HORIZONTAL) TRACING.

D, Duodenum. The arrow indicates the epiploic foramen (of Winslow). By an oversight the leader line to the great omentum is omitted, and the coronary ligament of the liver is erroneously marked lesser omentum; the latter extends from liver to stomach, but is not marked.

On the right it passes from the right crus of the diaphragm and the dorsal border of the liver to the concave border of the duodenum, forming the gastro-pancreatic fold (second part of the mesoduodenum), and covering part of the dorsal surface of the pancreas. From the margin of the pancreas, the right kidney, and a small area of the sublumbar region behind the latter, it passes on to the base of the cæcum and the terminal part of the great colon. From these it passes on the right to the duodenum, forming the third part of the mesoduodenum. On the left it clothes part of the ventral surface and the outer border of the left kidney, from which it passes to the base of the spleen, forming the ventral layer of the suspensory ligament of the latter. Behind the terminal part of the great colon it is reflected around the great mesenteric artery to form the great mesentery. Behind this it is reflected almost transversely from the roof of the cavity and from the origin of the small colon on to the duodenum, forming the terminal part of the mesoduo-

[1] In dissecting-room subjects (which are usually aged) the omentum often exhibits pathological changes, such as adhesions, rents, tumors, formation of twisted strands, etc.

denum. The line of origin of the colic mesentery begins on the inner part of the ventral surface of the left kidney, and extends to the sacral promontory, where the mesorectum begins. At the termination of the latter the peritoneum is reflected from the rectum on the dorsal and lateral walls of the pelvic cavity. Below the rectum it forms the urogenital fold, and passes on to the dorsal surface of the bladder, covers its anterior part, and is reflected on to the body-wall laterally and ventrally, forming the lateral and middle ligaments of the bladder. In the female the broad ligaments of the uterus replace the urogenital fold, with which they are homologous.

In the new-born foal certain folds are specially large. The falciform ligament of the liver extends to the umbilical opening, and contains in its free edge the large umbilical vein. The bladder—at this time an abdominal organ—has a ventral median fold, which connects it and the urachus with the abdominal floor. This is flanked on either side by a fold which also extends to the umbilicus, and contains the large umbilical artery.

DIGESTIVE SYSTEM OF THE OX

THE MOUTH

The cavity of the mouth is shorter and wider than that of the horse, and the vestibule is more capacious.

The **lips** are thick, wide, and comparatively immobile. The middle part of the upper lip and the surface between the nostrils is bare, and is termed the muzzle (Planum nasolabiale). It is smooth, and (in health) is kept cool and moist by a

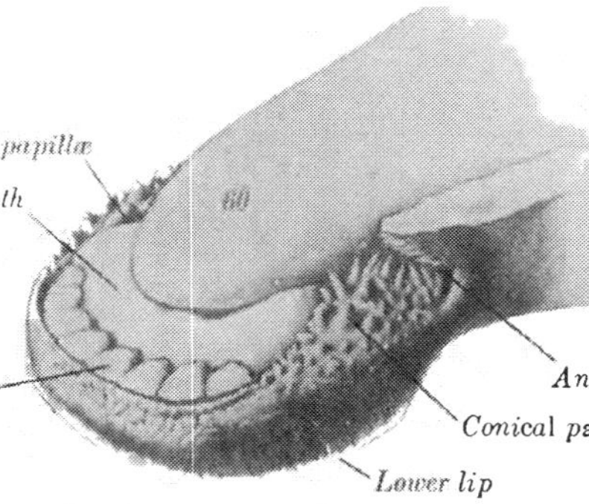

Fig. 280.—Anterior Part of Lower Jaw of Ox.
60, Tip of tongue. (After Ellenberger-Baum, Anat. für Künstler.)

clear fluid secreted by a layer of subcutaneous glands (Glandulæ nasolabiales) about half an inch (ca. 1.5 cm.) thick. It shows irregular lines, mapping out small polygonal areas on which the orifices of the gland ducts are visible. A narrow bare strip also exists along the edge of the lower lip. The remainder of the integument is provided with ordinary and tactile hairs. The free edge and the lining membrane present verrucose, horny papillæ. The labial glands form compact masses near the angles of the mouth.

The cheeks are more capacious than in the horse. The mucous membrane presents large conical pointed **papillæ,** which are directed toward the fauces and are covered with a horny epithelium. The largest of these have a length of about half an inch (ca. 1 to 1.5 cm.) and are situated around the angle of the mouth and parallel with the cheek teeth. The orifice of the parotid duct is opposite the fifth upper cheek tooth. (In the sheep and goat it is opposite the fourth tooth.) The **buccal** or **molar glands** are very well developed, and are arranged in three parts. The dorsal row extends from the maxillary tuberosity to the angle of the mouth. Its lobules are of a light yellow color. The ventral part consists of a compact

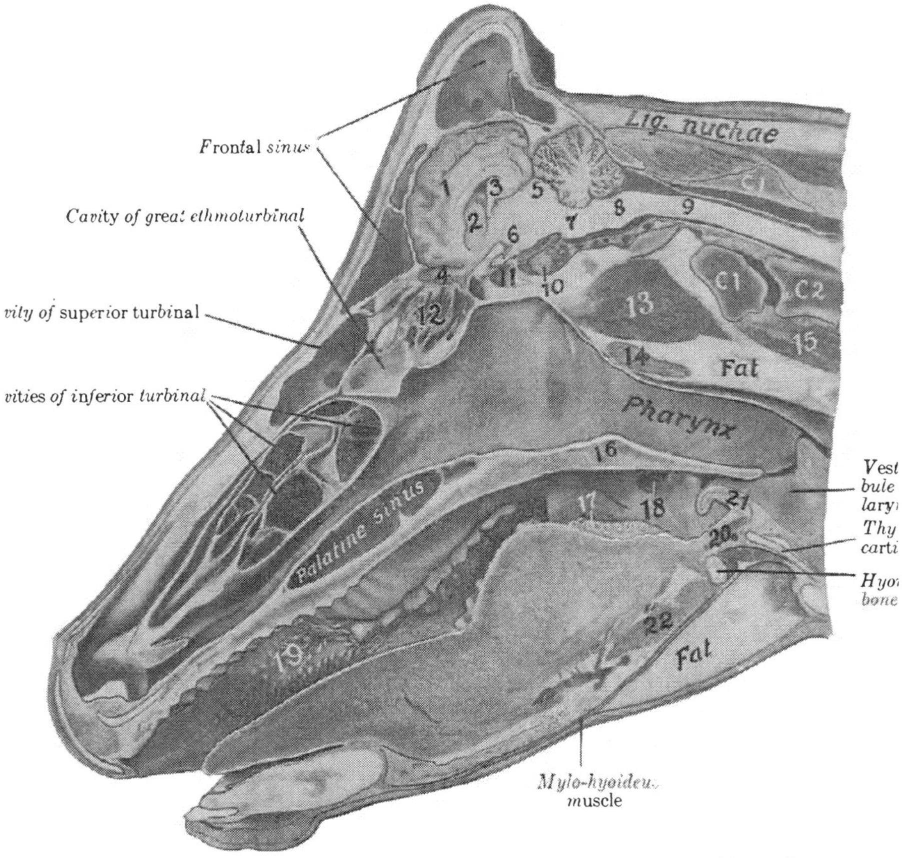

FIG. 281.—SAGITTAL SECTION OF HEAD OF COW, CUT A LITTLE TO THE RIGHT OF THE MEDIAN PLANE.

1, Cerebral hemisphere; *2*, corpus striatum; *3*, hippocampus; *4*, olfactory bulb; *5*, corpora quadrigemina; *6* optic nerve; *7*, pons; *8*, medulla oblongata; *9*, spinal cord; *10*, pituitary body; *11*, sphenoid sinus; *12*, lateral mass of ethmoid; *13*, ventral straight muscles; *14*, pharyngeal (retropharyngeal) lymph gland; *15*, longus colli; *16*, soft palate; *17*, vallate papillæ; *18*, tonsillar sinus; *19*, conical papillæ of cheek; *20*, hyo-epiglotticus muscle; *21*, epiglottis; *22*, hyo-glossus muscle; *C1*, *C2*, atlas, axis. Subject was hardened with mouth open.

brownish mass which reaches from the angle of the mouth a short distance under the masseter muscle. The middle part consists of loosely arranged yellow lobules.

A linear series of large papillæ exists on the floor of the mouth on each side of the frenum linguæ. Near these are found the openings of the small ducts of the sublingual gland. The papilla on which the submaxillary duct opens is wide, hard, and has a serrated edge.

The **hard palate** is wide, and is usually more or less pigmented. The body of the premaxilla is covered with a thick layer of dense connective tissue, which has a thick, horny epithelial covering—forming the so-called dental plate or pad. The palatine ridges extend from this backward about two-thirds of the length of the hard palate. They are nearly straight, and, for the most part, are serrated on the free edge. A median furrow extends between the ridges. The posterior third of the palate is smooth. Between the dental plate and the first ridge is the triangular papilla incisiva; on either side of this is a deep furrow, in which is the oral opening

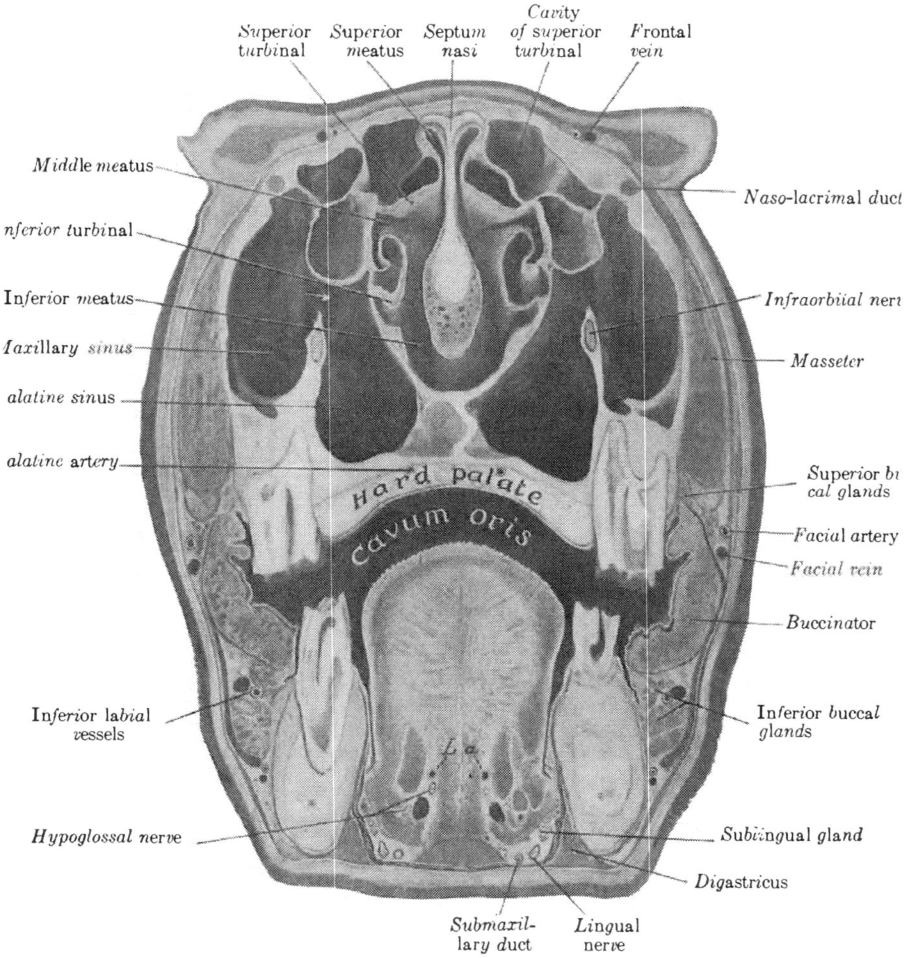

FIG. 282.—CROSS-SECTION OF HEAD OF OX.
The section passes through the internal canthi. *L.a.*, Lingual arteries. The arrow indicates the communication between the maxillary and palatine sinuses.

of the **naso-palatine canal.** This canal is two inches or more (ca. 5 to 6 cm.) in length and opens on the floor of the nasal cavity; it also communicates by a slit-like opening with the organ of Jacobson.

The **soft palate** is somewhat shorter than that of the horse, but is long enough to close the isthmus of the fauces. The posterior pillars do not extend to the entrance of the œsophagus. The azygos muscle is much better developed than in the horse. The fibrous aponeurosis is for the most part replaced by muscular tissue.

The **isthmus faucium** is wide and dilatable. On either side, behind the anterior pillar of the soft palate, is a deep depression, the **sinus tonsillaris**; external to this is the compact bean-shaped tonsil, which is about one to one and a half inches (ca. 3 to 4 cm.) in length. The tonsil does not project into the fauces, but outward instead: hence it does not occupy the tonsillar sinus, and is not visible internally, as is the case in most animals.

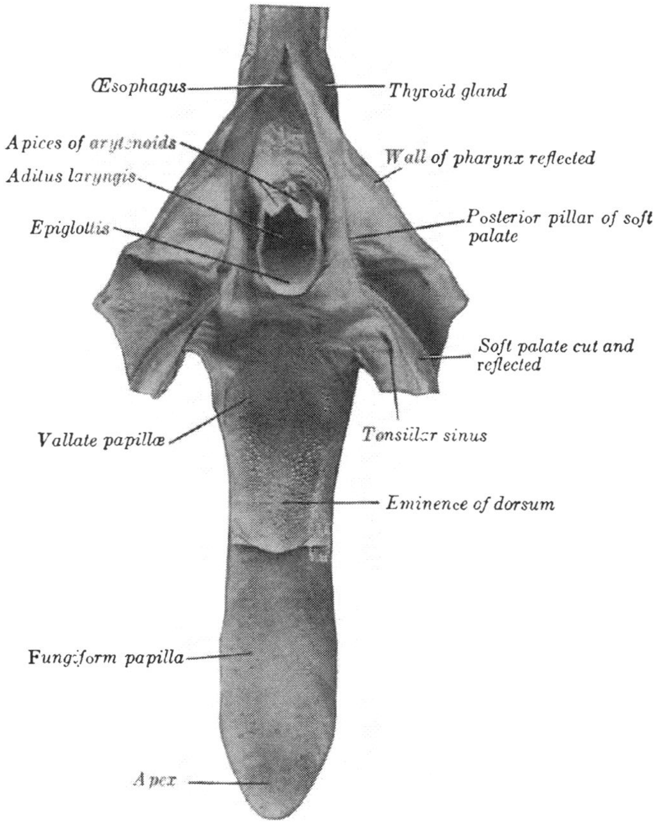

FIG. 283.—TONGUE OF OX, DORSAL ASPECT.
Pharynx, soft palate, and origin of œsophagus are cut dorsally and reflected.

THE TONGUE

The tongue of the ox is often variably pigmented. The root and body are wider than that of the horse, but the free part is more pointed. The posterior part of the dorsum forms a remarkable elliptical prominence, which is sharply defined in front. The filiform papillæ in front of this prominence are large and horny, with sharp points directed backward. They impart to the tongue its rasp-like roughness. The papillæ on the prominence are large, broad and horny; some have a blunt conical form, others are rounded or flattened. Behind the prominence, the papillæ are long and soft, *i. e.*, not horny. The fungiform papillæ are numerous and distinct; they are scattered more generally over the dorsum and edges of the free part. The vallate papillæ are about twenty or thirty in number; they are smaller than those of the horse, and are irregularly distributed on either side of the posterior part of the prominence of the dorsum. The foliate papillæ and the lingual fibrous cord are absent. The muscles are well developed; the hyo-glossus arises bv additional portions from the great and middle cornua of the hyoid bone. The tongue is highly protractile and is the chief organ of prehension.

THE TEETH

The dental formula of the ox is:

$$2\left(I\frac{0}{4}-C\frac{0}{0}-P\frac{3}{3}-M\frac{3}{3}\right)=32$$

The incisors are absent from the upper jaw. There are eight incisors in the lower jaw, arranged in a somewhat fan-like manner. They are simple teeth, without infundibulum. The crown is white, short, and shovel-shaped. The root is

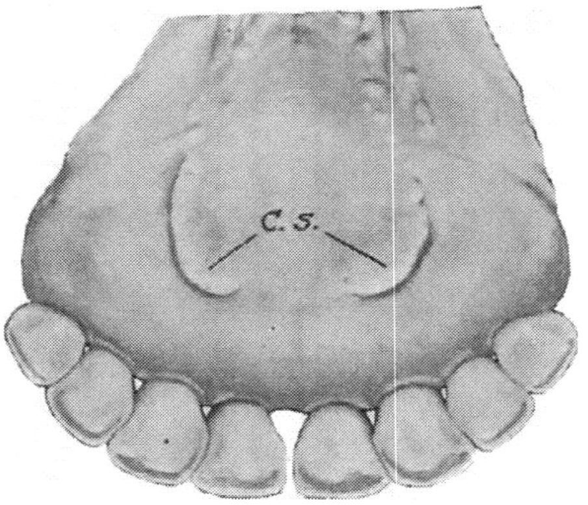

FIG. 284.—INCISOR TEETH OF OX, LINGUAL ASPECT. *C.s.*, Caruncula sublingualis.

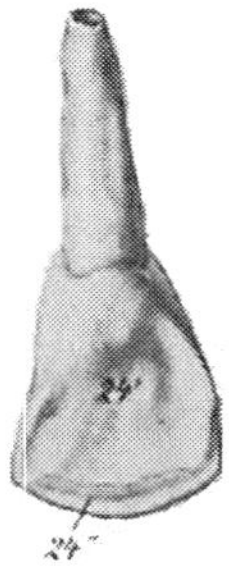

FIG. 285.—INCISOR TOOTH OF OX. *24'*, Lingual surface of crown; *24"*, masticatory surface. The crown is clearly marked off from the rounded root by a neck. (After Ellenberger-Baum, Anat. für Künstler.)

rounded, and is embedded in the jaw in such a manner as to allow a considerable degree of movement. There is a distinct neck. In addition to the simple numerical designation, the following terms are commonly applied to the individual teeth: pinchers or central, first intermediate, second intermediate, and corner incisors. It is probable that the latter are much modified canines. The incisors of the ox do not advance out of the alveoli, as is the case in the horse; in old age, however, the gum retracts so that the roots are partly exposed and may come into wear.[1]

The deciduous incisors differ from the permanent set chiefly in being much smaller. The crowns are narrower and diverge more.

The canines are absent (unless the fourth incisors be considered to represent them).

The cheek teeth (Fig. 286) resemble those of the horse in number and general arrangement. They are, however, smaller, and also differ in the fact that they

[1] The student will note here the difference between the structure and behavior of the brachydont (short-crowned) incisors of the ox and the hypsodont (long-crowned) type of the horse.

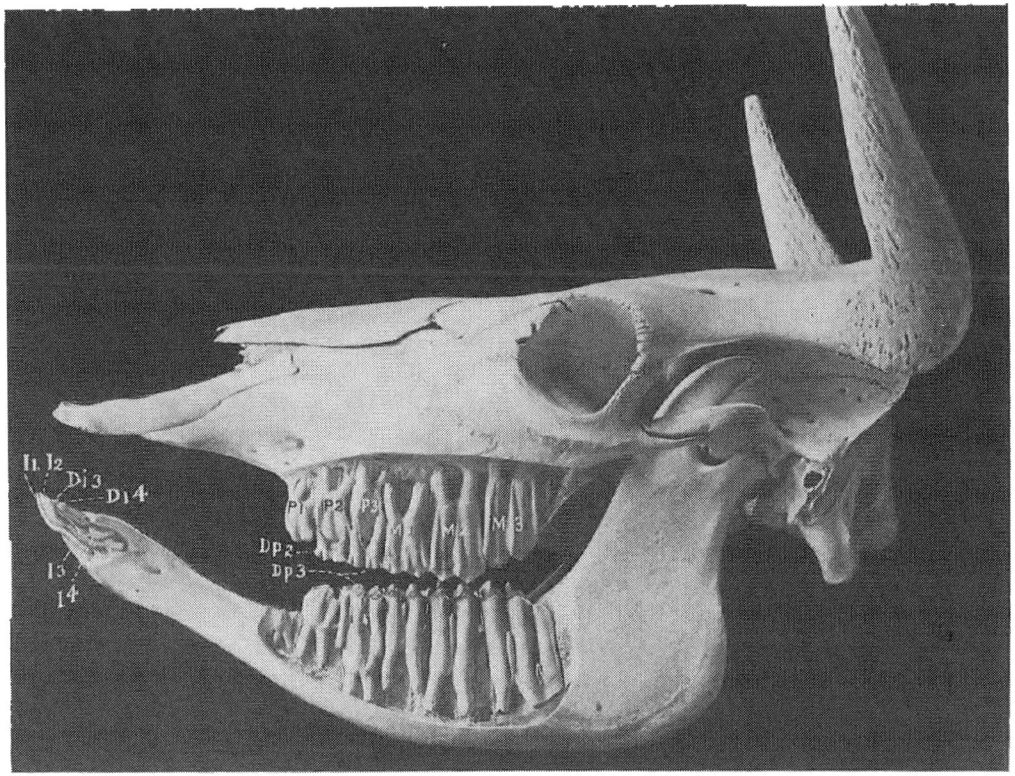

Fig. 286.—S ull of Ox Teeth.

I1-4, Permanen ncisor t *1-3*, upper permanen

progressively increase in size from before backward. This feature is so marked that the first tooth is quite small, and the space occupied by the first three (*i. e.*, the premolars) is only about one-half of that required for the posterior three (*i. e.*, the true molars). The enamel folds stand out even more prominently in relief on the masticatory surface than in the horse. The occurrence of wolf-teeth is rare.

The formula of the deciduous teeth is:

$$2\left(\text{Di}\frac{0}{4}\ \text{Dc}\frac{0}{0}\ \text{Dp}\frac{3}{3}\right) = 20$$

TABLE OF AVERAGE PERIODS OF ERUPTION OF THE TEETH IN THE OX

TEETH	ERUPTION
A. Temporary:	
First incisor (Di 1)	Birth to 3 weeks.
Second incisor (Di 2)	Birth to 3 weeks.
Third incisor (Di 3)	Birth to 3 weeks.
Fourth incisor (Di 4)	Birth to 3 weeks.
First cheek tooth (Dp 1)	Birth to 3 weeks.
Second cheek tooth (Dp 2)	Birth to few days.
Third cheek tooth (Dp 3)	Birth to few days.
B. Permanent:	
First incisor (I 1)	
Second incisor (I 2)	
Third incisor (I 3)	
Fourth incisor (I 4)	
First cheek tooth (P 1)	
Second cheek tooth (P 2)	
Third cheek tooth (P 3)	
Fourth cheek tooth (M 1)	
Fifth cheek tooth (M 2)	
Sixth cheek tooth (M 3)	

The eruption of the permanent teeth is subject to great variation. The above figures are the average of observations of improved breeds under favorable conditions.

THE SALIVARY GLANDS

The **parotid gland** is smaller than that of the horse, and is light red-brown in color. It has somewhat the form of a very narrow long triangle, and lies chiefly on the posterior part of the masseter muscle. The thick wide upper end partly covers a large subparotid lymph gland. The small lower end is bent forward and fits into the angle of union of the jugular and external maxillary veins; it lies on the submaxillary gland. The parotid duct leaves the lower part of the deep face; in its course it resembles that of the horse, but it pierces the cheek opposite the fifth upper cheek tooth.

The **submaxillary gland** is very large, and is pale yellow in color. It is covered to a small extent by the parotid. Its general form resembles that of the horse, but its lower (or anterior) end is large and rounded, and is separated by a small interval only from the gland of the other side. This part can be distinctly felt in the living animal, and is related externally to a large submaxillary lymph gland. The duct leaves the middle of the superficial face of the gland, crosses the stylohyoideus and the intermediate tendon of the digastricus, and is then disposed as in the horse.

The **sublingual gland** consists of two parts. The dorsal part (Glandula sublingualis parvicanalaris) is long, thin, and pale yellow in color. It extends from the anterior pillar of the soft palate about to the symphysis of the jaw. It has numerous small tortuous ducts (Ductus sublinguales minores), which open between the papillæ under the side of the tongue. The ventral part is shorter and thicker, and is salmon pink in color. It has a single duct (Ductus sublingualis major), which either opens alongside of or joins the submaxillary duct.

THE PHARYNX

The pharynx is short and wide. The vault (Fornix pharyngis) is divided into two cul-de-sacs by a median fold of mucous membrane (Septum nasi membranaceum), which is a continuation of that of the septum nasi; on the outer wall of each is the relatively small opening of the Eustachian tube, which is covered by a

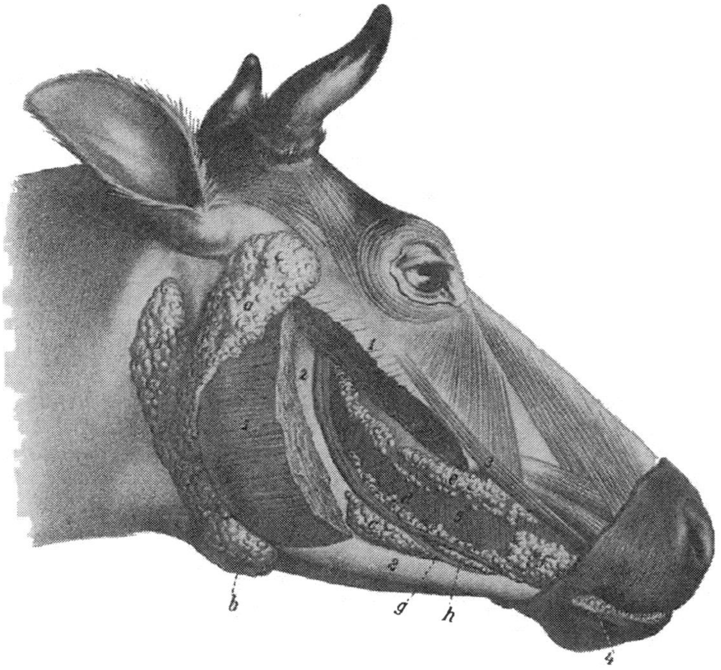

Fig. 287.—Salivary Glands of Ox.

a, Parotid gland; *b*, submaxillary gland; c, inferior, d, middle, and *e*, superior buccal glands; *f*, labial glands; *g*, buccinator nerve; *h*, buccinator vein; *1*, masseter (cut); *2*, ramus of mandible; *3*, zygomaticus muscle; *4*, conical papillæ of lip; *5*, buccinator muscle. (After Ellenberger, in Leisering's Atlas.)

simple fold of mucous membrane. The posterior nares are small. The entrance to the œsophagus is large.

On the dorsal wall of the pharynx are two large pharyngeal lymph glands, which, when enlarged, cause difficulty in swallowing and breathing (Fig. 281).

THE ŒSOPHAGUS

This is much shorter, wider, and more dilatable than that of the horse. Its average diameter (when moderately inflated) is about two inches (ca. 5 cm.), and its length in a large animal is about three to three and a half feet (ca. 90 to 100 cm.). The wall is relatively thin, and the muscular tissue is striped throughout. The latter consists of two strata of spiral fibers, except near the stomach, where they are longitudinal and circular. Fibers are continued into the wall of the stomach for some distance. There are submucous glands in the first part of the tube. There is no terminal dilatation, and no part in the abdominal cavity

A very large mediastinal lymph gland lies above the posterior part of the œsophagus and may, if enlarged, obstruct it (Fig. 289).

THE ABDOMINAL CAVITY

The abdominal cavity of the ox is very capacious, both absolutely and relatively, as compared with that of the horse. This is due to several factors. The lumbar portion of the spine is about one-fourth longer than that of the horse. The transverse diameter between the last ribs is greater. The costal attachment of the diaphragm is almost vertical in direction from the lower part of the ninth rib to the extreme upper part of the thirteenth; in fact, the attachment to the last rib is not constant. Thus the abdomen is increased at the expense of the thorax, and the last three or four ribs enter more largely into the formation of the abdominal wall than in the horse. The flank is also much more extensive. The ilia, on the other hand, do not extend forward beyond a transverse plane through the middle of the last lumbar vertebra. The epigastric and mesogastric regions would be separated by a plane through the lower end of the tenth pair of ribs, or through the last thoracic vertebra. The chief differential features in the arrangement of the peritoneum will be described with the viscera.

THE PELVIC CAVITY

The pelvic cavity is relatively long and narrow. The inlet is more oblique than that of the horse; it is elliptical in outline, and the transverse diameter is smaller than that of the horse. The anterior (pubic) part of the floor is about horizontal, but the posterior (ischial) part slopes upward and backward to a marked degree; this part is also deeply concave transversely. The roof is concave in both directions. The peritoneum extends backward as far as the first coccygeal vertebra, so that the retroperitoneal part of the cavity is short.

THE STOMACH

General Arrangement.—The stomach of the ox is very large, and occupies nearly three-fourths of the abdominal cavity. It fills all of the left half of the cavity (with the exception of the small space occupied by the spleen) and extends considerably over the median plane into the right half.

It is compound, being composed of four divisions, viz., **rumen, reticulum,** omasum, and **abomasum.**[1] The division is clearly indicated externally by furrows or constrictions. The first three divisions may be regarded as proventriculi or œsophageal sacculations, the fourth being the stomach proper (in the narrower sense of the term). The œsophagus opens into the stomach on a sort of dome formed by the rumen and reticulum, and is continued through the latter by the œsophageal groove. From the ventral end of the latter a groove traverses the ventral wall of the omasum, thus giving a direct path to the abomasum for finely divided or fluid food. The abomasum joins the small intestine.

Capacity.—The capacity of the stomach varies greatly, depending on the age and size of the animal. In cattle of medium size it holds 30 to 40 gallons, in large animals 40 to 60, in small 25 to 35. The relative sizes of the four parts vary with age. In the new-born calf the rumen and reticulum together are about half as

[1] In popular language these are conveniently regarded as so many stomachs, and termed accordingly "first," "second," etc. Other names are in common use, *e. g.*, paunch, honeycomb, manifold or manyplies, and rennet or true stomach.

large as the abomasum; in ten or twelve weeks this ratio is reversed. During this period the omasum appears to be contracted and functionless. At four months the rumen and reticulum together are about four times as large as the omasum and abomasum together. At about one and one-half years the omasum equals (or nearly so) the abomasum in capacity. The four divisions have now reached their definitive relative capacities, the rumen constituting about 80 per cent., the reticulum 5 per cent., the omasum 7 or 8 per cent., and the abomasum 8 or 7 per cent. of the total amount.

Exterior and Relations

The **rumen** occupies almost all of the left half of the abdominal cavity, and extends considerably over the median plane ventrally and in its middle. It is somewhat compressed laterally, and may be described as having two surfaces, two curvatures or borders, and two extremities. The **parietal** (or left) **surface** (Facies parietalis) is convex and is related to the diaphragm, spleen, and the left wall of the abdomen. It extends from the lower part of the seventh intercostal space

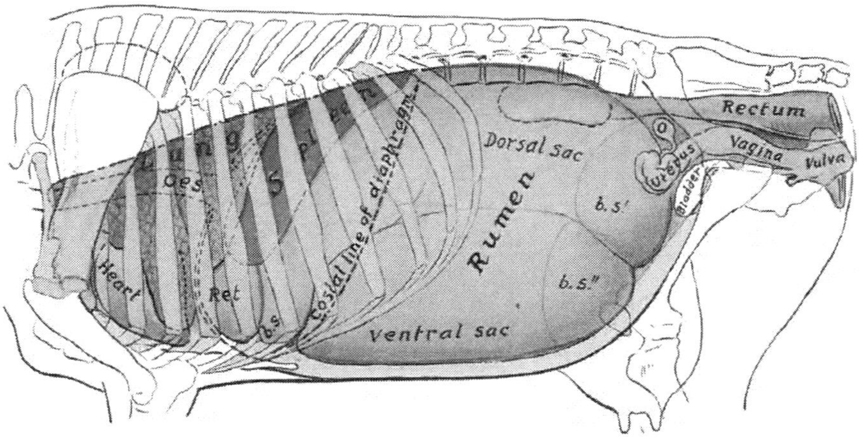

Fig. 288.—Projection of Viscera of Cow on Body-wall, Left Side.

Oes., Œsophagus; *Ret.*, reticulum; *b.s.*, anterior blind sac; *b.s.'*, *b.s''.*, posterior blind sacs of rumen; *O*, ovary. The left kidney, concealed by the dorsal sac of the rumen, is indicated by dotted line. The median line of the diaphragm is dotted.

almost to the pelvis. The **visceral** (or right) **surface** (Facies visceralis) is somewhat irregular, and is related chiefly to the omasum and abomasum, the intestine, the liver, pancreas, kidneys, the uterus in the female, and the posterior aorta and vena cava. The **dorsal curvature** (Curvatura dorsalis) is convex, following the curve formed by the diaphragm and sublumbar muscles. It is firmly attached to the left portion of the crura of the diaphragm and the sublumbar muscles by peritoneum and connective tissue. The **ventral curvature** is also convex and lies on the floor of the abdomen. The surfaces are marked by the right and left **longitudinal furrows** (Sulci longitudinales), which indicate externally the division of the rumen into dorsal and ventral sacs.[1] The **reticular** (or anterior) **extremity** (Extremitas reticularis) is divided ventrally by a transverse groove (Sulcus ruminis cranialis) into two sacs. The dorsal sac is the longer of the two, and curves ventrally over the round, blind end of the ventral sac. The former only is continuous

[1] It has been customary to term the sacs left and right respectively, but these do not represent the relations as they exist *in situ* and as they are presented on frozen sections.

with the reticulum, a ventral groove (Sulcus rumino-reticularis) being the only external line of demarcation. Dorsally no natural separation exists, the rumen and reticulum together forming a dome-like vestibule (Atrium ventriculi) on which the œsophagus terminates. The pelvic (or posterior) **extremity** (Extremitas pelvina) extends nearly to the pubis, and is related to the intestine and bladder, and the uterus in the cow. It is divided into dorsal and **ventral blind** sacs (Saccus cæcus caudalis dorsalis, ventralis) by a deep transverse groove (Sulcus ruminis caudalis) in which the longitudinal furrows terminate. The blind sacs are marked off from the remainder of the rumen by the **dorsal** and **ventral** coronary **grooves** (Sulcus coronarius dorsalis, ventralis).

The left longitudinal groove (Sulcus longitudinalis sinister) begins at the anterior transverse groove, passes somewhat dorsally and backward and divides into two grooves. The ventral one is the chief groove and passes backward to terminate in the angle of union of the posterior blind sacs. The dorsal (accessory) groove curves dorsally and then backward to terminate in the dorsal coronary sulcus. On the right surface there are two longitudinal grooves. The dorsal one is the chief sulcus (Sulcus longitudinalis dexter). It extends in a curved direction (the convexity being dorsal) and is continuous with the left longitudinal groove by means of the grooves between the dorsal and ventral blind sacs at each end. The ventral groove (Sulcus accessorius) curves somewhat ventrally and backward to rejoin the chief sulcus between the posterior blind sacs.

The **reticulum** is the smallest of the four divisions in the ox. It is also the most anterior, and lies on the concave surface of the diaphragm, so that the median plane divides it into two nearly equal portions. It is somewhat pyriform, but much compressed from before backward. The **parietal** or **phrenic** surface (Facies diaphragmatica) is convex and lies against the diaphragm and liver.[1] The **ruminal** (or posterior) **surface** (Facies ruminalis) is flattened by the pressure of the other three compartments; it ends dorsally by joining the wall of the rumen, the concave line of junction forming, in the interior of the stomach, the lower margin of the large rumino-reticular orifice. The omasal (or right) **surface** is narrow and concave, and is connected with the omasum. The dorsal **curvature** by its left portion joins the rumen to form the atrium, and by its right portion touches the liver. The ventral **curvature** lies on the sternal portion of the diaphragm, opposite the sixth and seventh ribs. The **right extremity** forms a rounded cul-de-sac, which is in contact with the liver, omasum, and abomasum.

The omasum (Fig. 294) is ellipsoidal in form and somewhat compressed laterally. It is very clearly marked off from the other divisions. It is situated almost entirely to the right of the median plane, opposite the seventh to the eleventh ribs. The parietal (right) surface (Facies dextra) lies against the diaphragm, liver, and lateral wall of the abdomen. The contact with the latter extends over a small area only (ventral part of seventh to ninth intercostal spaces). The visceral (left) **surface** (Facies sinistra) is in contact with the rumen and reticulum. The dorsal (greater) **curvature** is convex, and is related to the diaphragm, liver, and vena cava. The **ventral** (lesser) **curvature** is concave, and rests on the abomasum chiefly, the junction with the latter appearing as a constriction near the middle of the curvature; at its anterior part there is a **neck** (Collum omasi) which is the connection with the reticulum.

The abomasum (Fig. 294) is an elongated pyriform or flask-shaped sac, which lies for the most part on the abdominal floor, to the right of the ventral sac of the rumen. Its narrow posterior part is strongly curved, the concavity being dorsal. The parietal (right) **surface** lies against the abdominal wall from the seventh to the twelfth intercostal space. The visceral (left) **surface** is related chiefly to the ventral sac of the rumen. The dorsal (lesser) **curvature** is concave, and is in contact with the omasum; the junction of the two sacs is indicated by a constriction about four or

[1] It is important to notice that the reticulum is separated from the pericardium by an interval of about 1 to 1½ inches (ca. 2 to 4 cm.) only, since foreign bodies which are often swallowed by cattle lodge in the reticulum, and not rarely (if sharp) perforate the reticulum and diaphragm.

five inches (ca. 10 to 12 cm.) from the anterior extremity of the abomasum. The **ventral** (greater) **curvature** is convex, and rests on the abdominal wall from the xiphoid cartilage to the ventral part of the last (right) intercostal space. The **anterior extremity** forms a rounded blind sac which lies against the reticulum. The posterior (or pyloric) **extremity** is much smaller and bends upward and forward to join the duodenum. About six to eight inches (ca. 15 to 20 cm.) from the pylorus is a constriction which marks off the pyloric portion from the fundus.

The rumen is attached by peritoneum and connective tissue to the crura of the diaphragm and left psoas muscles, from the hiatus œsophageus backward to about the third or fourth lumbar vertebra.

The lesser omentum attaches the right face of the omasum and the pyloric portion of the abomasum to the visceral surface of the liver.

A small area of the anterior part of the right face of the rumen is adherent to the adjacent surface of the abomasum. The greater part of the ventral curvature of the omasum is attached by connective tissue to the dorsal face of the abomasum.

(Adhesion of the reticulum to the diaphragm is frequently present, but is pathological; the same is true in regard to adhesion to the liver.)

Interior

The cavity of the rumen is partially divided into dorsal and ventral sacs by the **pillars**; these are folds of the wall, strengthened by additional muscular fibers, and correspond with the grooves on the outside. The two most extensive ones project like shelves into the anterior and posterior ends of the cavity forming the blind sacs at either extremity; they are termed the **chief pillars**. The **anterior chief pillar** (Pila cranialis) projects obliquely backward and upward from the ventral wall, and has a thick concave free edge which is opposite to the tenth and eleventh ribs. Its width from the middle of the free edge to its anterior border is about eight to ten inches (ca. 20 to 25 cm.). It is continued on either side by the relatively narrow **longitudinal pillars**, which connect it with the posterior pillar. The **posterior pillar** (Pila caudalis) is more nearly horizontal than the anterior one, and separates the large dorsal and ventral posterior blind sacs. Its concave free border is about a hand's breadth in front of a transverse plane through the external angles of the ilia. From it are detached three **accessory pillars** on either side; of these, two pass around the blind sacs to meet the corresponding pillars of the opposite side. They thus mark off the posterior blind sacs from the general cavity, and are termed the **coronary pillars**. It will be noticed that the ventral coronary pillar is complete, while the dorsal one is not. The other accessory pillars join the right and left longitudinal pillars. The **right longitudinal pillar** is in part double; its ventral division fades out about the middle of the surface, while the dorsal one joins the posterior chief pillar. The distance between the middles of the anterior and posterior pillars is only about sixteen to eighteen inches (ca. 40 to 45 cm.) in a cow of medium size. In this space the dorsal and ventral sacs communicate freely.

The anterior dorsal blind sac of the rumen is separated from the reticulum by an almost vertical fold formed by the apposition of the walls of the two compartments. This **rumino-reticular fold** (Pila rumino-reticularis) is opposite to the seventh rib and intercostal space. Its free upper edge is concave and forms the lower and outer margin of the large, oval **rumino-reticular orifice** (Ostium rumino-reticulare). The inner margin of the fold if continued would end about at the cardia, but there is in this region no demarcation between rumen and reticulum; hence it is termed the **atrium ventriculi** or **vestibule**.

If the rumino-reticular fold and an imaginary completion of it be taken as the boundary between the rumen and reticulum, it will be seen that the cardia belongs to the latter. The outer border of the rumino-reticular fold ends above and behind the cardia, the inner one just behind the œsophageal groove and about four to five inches lower down. Undoubtedly food or water swallowed with a moderate degree of force passes first into the rumen. Foreign bodies (which are commonly swallowed by cattle) are, however, found in the reticulum.

The **cardiac orifice** is opposite the seventh rib, a little to the left of the median plane and about four inches (ca. 10 cm.) below the spine; it is not funnel-shaped.

The mucous membrane of the rumen is brown in color, except on the margins of the pillars, where it is pale. It is for the most part thickly studded with large papillæ, many of which are nearly half an inch (ca. 1 cm.) long. The edges of the chief pillars and a large part of the wall of the middle of the dorsal sac are, however, not papillated. The papillary arrangement is most marked in the blind sacs. The papillæ vary much in size and form; the largest are foliate, many are narrow or filiform, and others are conical or club-shaped. The mucous membrane on the inner wall of the atrium is finely wrinkled and non-papillated, while above and

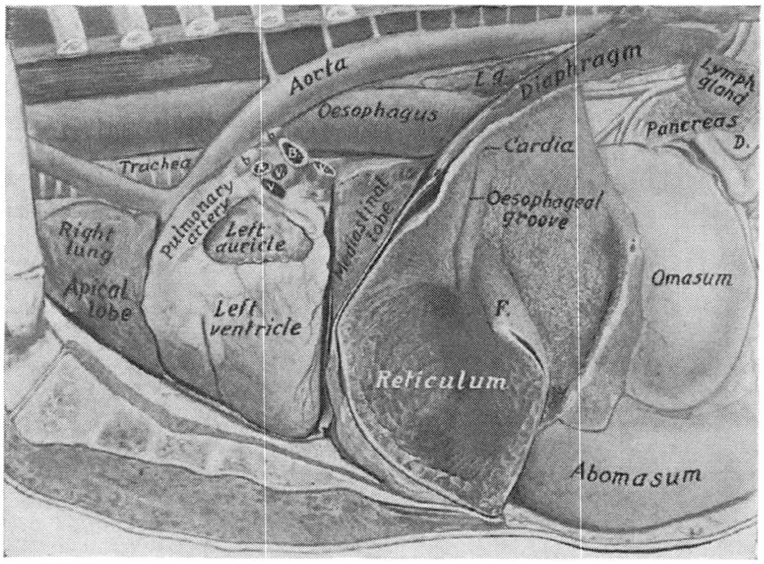

FIG. 289.—THORACIC AND ANTERIOR ABDOMINAL VISCERA OF OX, DEEP DISSECTION.

Most of the rumen has been removed and the left wall of the reticulum cut away. *A.*, Left pulmonary artery; *B.*, left bronchus; *V. V. V.*, pulmonary veins; *b. b.*, bronchial lymph glands; *L.g.*, posterior mediastinal lymph-gland; *D.*, termination of duodenum; *F*, rumino-reticular fold.

externally it is papillated. The papillary arrangement also extends over the edge of the rumino-reticular fold an inch or two (ca. 2 to 5 cm.).

The **œsophageal groove** (Sulcus œsophageus) is a semicanal which begins at the cardia and passes downward (ventrally) on the right wall of the reticulum to end at the reticulo-omasal orifice. It is about six or seven inches (ca. 15 to 18 cm.) in length. Its axial direction is practically vertical, but it is twisted in a spiral fashion; thus its thickened edges or lips project first backward, then to the left, and finally forward. The twist involves chiefly the left lip, and the relative positions of the lips is reversed at the ventral end.

The mucous membrane on the lips of the œsophageal groove is brown and wrinkled, like that of the atrium; in the bottom of the groove it is pale, like that of the œsophagus, marked by longitudinal folds, and presents pointed horny papillæ on the lower part.

The reticulo-omasal orifice (Ostium reticulo-omasicum) is situated in the right wall of the reticulum about five or six inches above the bottom of the latter. It is rounded, and is limited below and laterally by the junction of the lips of the œsophageal groove.

In the reticulum the mucous membrane is raised into folds about half an inch high, which inclose four-, five-, or six-sided spaces (Cellulæ reticuli); this peculiar arrangement suggested the scientific name, and also the popular term "honeycomb." These cells are subdivided by smaller folds, and the bottoms are studded with pointed horny papillæ. The cells grow smaller and gradually disappear near the œsophageal groove and the edge of the rumino-reticular fold; an inch or two from the latter the mucous membrane has the papillary arrangement of the rumen.

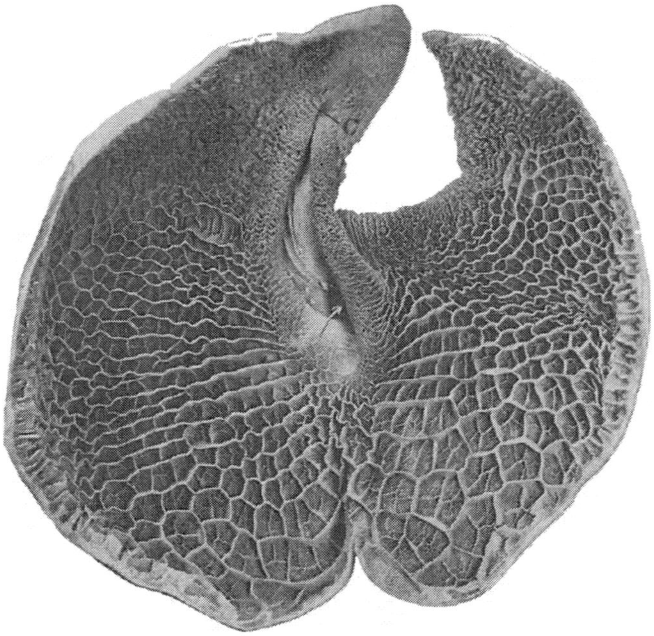

FIG. 290.—RETICULUM OF OX, FROM PHOTOGRAPH.

The specimen was cut along the greater curvature and laid open by reflecting the anterior wall. *C* is the cardia. The arrow points to the reticulo-omasal orifice. The spiral twist of the œsophageal groove was of necessity partly undone by reflecting the wall; its lips are drawn apart, showing some of the peculiar birdclaw-like papillæ in the lower part.

At the reticulo-omasal orifice there are peculiar horny papillæ, which are curved and resemble the claws of a small bird.

The cavity of the omasum is occupied to a considerable extent by about a hundred longitudinal folds, the **laminæ** (Laminæ omasi), which spring from the dorsal and lateral walls. The largest of these—a dozen or more in number—have a convex attached edge, and a ventral, free, slightly concave edge which reaches to within a short distance of the ventral wall of the sac. If these are drawn apart or a cross-section is made, it will be seen that there is a second order of shorter laminæ, and a third order still shorter; finally, there is a series of very low folds or lines. The food is pressed into thin layers in the narrow spaces between the laminæ (Recessus interlaminares), and reduced to a fine state of division by being ground down by the numerous rounded horny papillæ which stud the surfaces of the folds. The ventral wall of the omasum forms a groove (Sulcus omasi), which connects the reticulo-omasal opening with the omaso-abomasal opening; it is about three or four inches (ca. 8 to 10 cm.) long, and is directed backward and a little downward and to the right. It is free from leaves, but marked usually by slight folds and small papillæ; it forms a direct path from the reticulum to the abomasum for fluid and finely divided food. In the neck of the omasum there are thick folds, and a number of the peculiar papillæ already mentioned as occurring in the lower part of the œsophageal groove. The **omaso-abomasal orifice** (Ostium omaso-abomasicum) is oval, and is about four inches (ca. 10 cm.) long. It is bounded in front by a thick muscular pillar which fades out above on the lateral walls of the omasum. Laterally there are two folds (Valvulæ terminales), which probably prevent regurgitation of the contents of the abomasum.

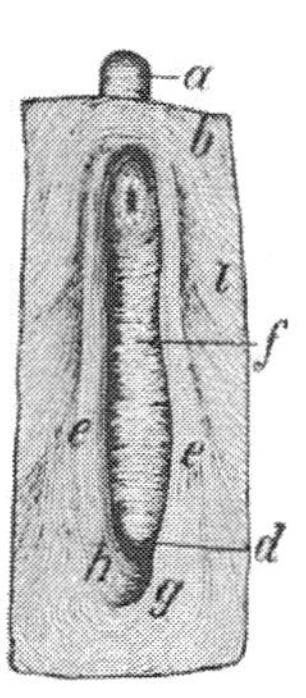

Fig. 291.—Musculature of Œsophageal Groove and Adjacent Part of Stomach of Ox, seen from within after Removal of Mucous Membrane.

a, Œsophagus; *b*, inner muscular layer of atrium; *d*, reticulo-omasal orifice; *e*, *e'*, muscle of lips of groove; *g*, lower end of muscle of larger lip, which curves around the reticulo-omasal orifice in part and spreads out in the inner muscular layer of the reticulum in part; *h*, lower end of muscle of smaller lip which in part curves around the reticulo-omasal orifice and is in part continuous with the inner muscular layer of the omasal groove and the omasum; *i*, inner muscular layer of reticulum. (Ellenberger-Baum, Anat. d. Haustiere.)

The cavity of the abomasum is divided by a constriction into two areas. The first of these (fundus gland region) is lined with a soft glandular mucous membrane, which forms about a dozen large, slightly spiral folds (Plicæ spirales). The second part (pyloric region) is much narrower and resembles in appearance the corresponding region of the horse's stomach. A small cardiac gland zone surrounds the omaso-abomasal orifice. The pyloric orifice is small and round.

Structure.—The **serous coat** invests all of the free surface of the stomach. The surface of the rumen which is attached to the dorsal abdominal wall is of course uncovered, as well as the adjacent area to which the spleen is attached. The furrows are bridged over by the peritoneum and superficial muscle-fibers, and contain fat and (in most cases) branches of the gastric arteries. The **lesser omentum** passes from the visceral surface of the liver to the right (parietal) face of the omasum and the pyloric portion of the abomasum. There is a fold between the ventral curvature of the omasum and the dorsal curvature of the abomasum. The **great omentum** is formed by the peritoneum leaving the stomach along the left longitudinal and posterior transverse furrows and the right surface of the rumen below the longitudinal furrow, also the ventral curvature of the abomasum. Its superficial (ventral) part is attached on the right to the duodenum, while the deep (dorsal) part blends with the mesentery. It conceals the greater part of the intestine on the right side, with the exception of the duodenum, and covers the ventral sac of the rumen almost entirely. It is not lace-like, as in the horse, and contains a large amount of fat in animals in good condition. The **epiploic foramen** (of Winslow) is almost sagittal in direction.

The **muscular coat of the rumen** consists of an external longitudinal, and a thicker internal circular layer. The latter forms the bulk of the chief pillars, where it is about one-half to one inch (ca. 1 to 2 cm.) thick. Scattered bundles of striped muscle-fibers radiate from the cardia in the wall of the atrium.

The **muscular coat of the reticulum** consists of two chief layers which begin and end at the œsophageal groove; they pass in a circular or oblique fashion around the sac, the fibers of the two layers crossing each other at an acute angle. The walls of the cells contain a central muscular layer. The lips of the œsophageal groove contain a thick layer of longitudinal fibers, which are largely continuous at or cross each other below the reticulo-omasal orifice. The bottom of the groove has two layers of oblique, unstriped muscle-fibers, with a variable outer layer of striped muscle continuous with that of the œsophagus.

The **muscular coat of the omasum** consists of a thin external longitudinal layer and a thick internal circular layer. At the omasal groove there is an additional inner layer of longitudinal fibers. The laminæ contain three muscular strata—a central layer of vertical fibers, flanked on either side by a layer of longitudinal fibers, which are continuous at the attached border with the muscularis mucosæ.

The **muscular coat of the abomasum** consists of longitudinal and circular layers; the latter forms a well-developed pyloric sphincter.

The **mucous membrane** of the first three divisions is destitute of glands, and is covered with a thick, stratified, squamous epithelium; the superficial part of the latter is horny, and is shed in large patches in the rumen and omasum. The corium (Tunica propria) is papillated. The mucous membrane of the abomasum is glandular, and corresponds to that of the right sac of the stomach of the horse. The short fundus glands occur in that part which presents the large folds, while the long pyloric glands are found in the remainder, except about the omaso-abomasal orifice, where cardiac glands occur. The mucosa of the fundus gland region is very thin as compared with that of the horse. There is a round prominence on the pyloric valve.

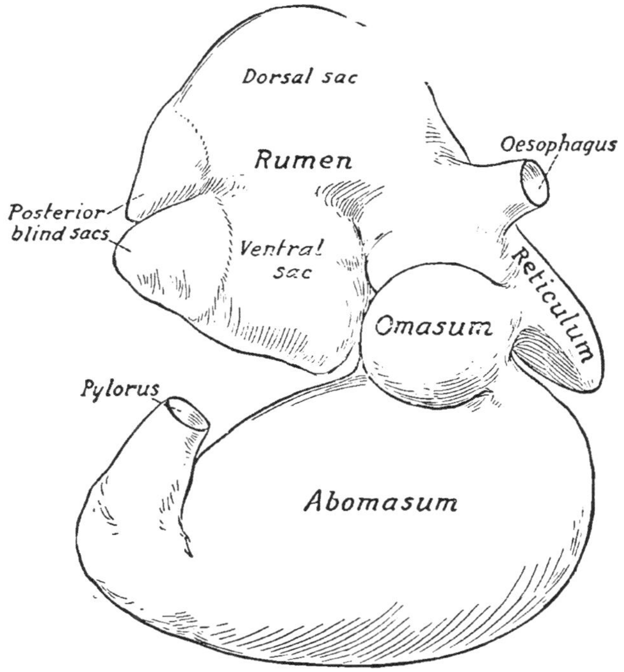

FIG. 292.—STOMACH OF NEW-BORN CALF, RIGHT VIEW.
The rumen is raised.

THE INTESTINE

The intestine of the ox lies almost entirely to the right of the median plane, chiefly in contact with the right face of the rumen. It is attached to the sublumbar region by a common mesentery.

The **small intestine** has an average length of about 130 feet (ca. 40 m.) and a diameter of about two inches (ca. 5 to 6 cm.).

The **duodenum** is about three or four feet (ca. 1 m.) in length. It passes forward to the visceral surface of the liver; here it forms, ventral to the right kidney, an S-shaped curve. Thence it runs backward almost to the external angle of the ilium, where it turns on itself, passes forward alongside of the terminal part of the colon, and joins the mesenteric part (jejunum) under the right kidney. It is attached to the liver by the lesser omentum, to the abomasum by the great omentum, and to the terminal part of the colon. The **bile duct** opens in the ventral part of the S-shaped curve, about two feet (ca. 60 cm.) from the pylorus. The **pancreatic duct** opens about a foot (ca. 30 cm.) further back.

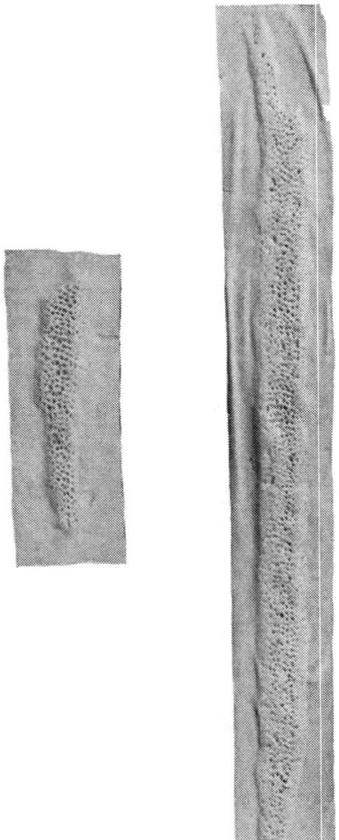

FIG. 293.—PEYER'S PATCHES OF SMALL INTESTINE OF OX (about ⅓ natural size).

The remainder of the small intestine is arranged in numerous very close coils, in contact chiefly with the right face of the ventral sac of the rumen, forming a sort of festoon at the edge of the mesentery. It is not subject to much variation in position, but a few coils may find their way behind the blind sacs of the rumen to the left side.

The orifices of the pancreatic duct and the bile duct are on papillæ, no diverticulum being present. There are permanent transverse folds of the mucous membrane (Plicæ circulares). Duodenal glands (of Brunner) occur in the first fifteen feet or more (4 to 5 m.), intestinal glands throughout. Peyer's patches are larger and more distinct than in the horse, and vary greatly in size and number; in adult cattle there are eighteen to forty; in calves, twenty to fifty-eight. They usually have the form of narrow bands. Close to the ileo-cæcal valve there is always a patch, and in most cases there is also a patch on the cæcal side of the valve.

The **large intestine** is much smaller in caliber than that of the horse, has no bands, and is not sacculated. Most of it is situated between the layers of the common mesentery.

The **cæcum** is about 20 to 30 inches (ca. 50 to 60 cm.) long, 4 to 5 inches (ca. 10 to 12 cm.) wide, and has a capacity of about 2½ gallons (ca. 9 to 10 liters). It begins opposite the lower part of the eleventh rib, and extends upward and backward against the right flank; its rounded blind end is free, and lies near or in the pelvic inlet.

The **colon** is about 35 feet (ca. 10 m.) long; its diameter is at first about the same as that of the cæcum, but diminishes to about two inches (ca. 5 cm.). Its capacity is about 6 to 8 gallons (ca. 25 to 30 liters). With the exception of its first and terminal parts, it is arranged in double elliptical coils between the layers of the mesentery; the adjacent parts are therefore alternately centripetal and centrifugal (Gyri centripetales et centrifugales). The first part (Ansa proximalis) is marked off from the cæcum only by the ileo-cæcal opening; it forms an S-shaped

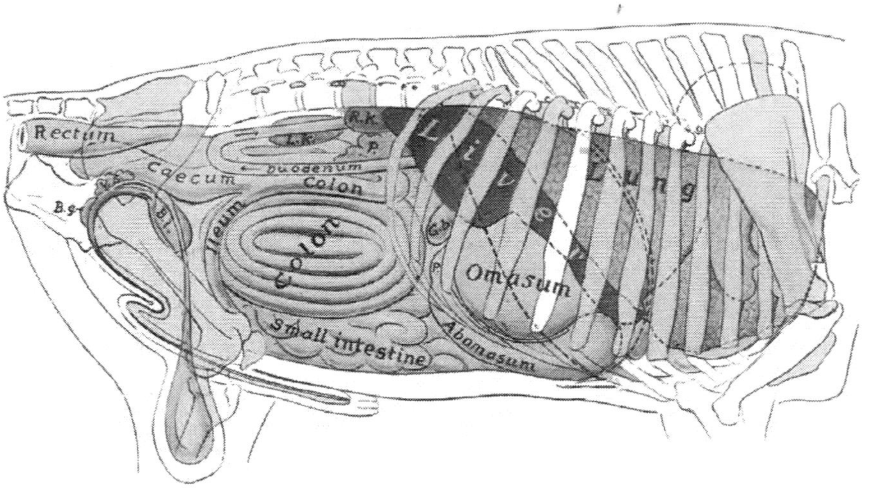

FIG. 294.—PROJECTION OF VISCERA OF BULL ON BODY-WALL, RIGHT SIDE.

P. Pylorus; *G.b.*, gall-bladder; *R.K.*, right kidney; *L.K.*, left kidney; *P.*, (above duodenum) pancreas; *Bl.*, urinary bladder; *V. s.*, vesicula seminalis; *B. g.*, bulbo-urethral (Cowper's) gland. Costal attachment and median line of diaphragm are indicated by dotted lines.

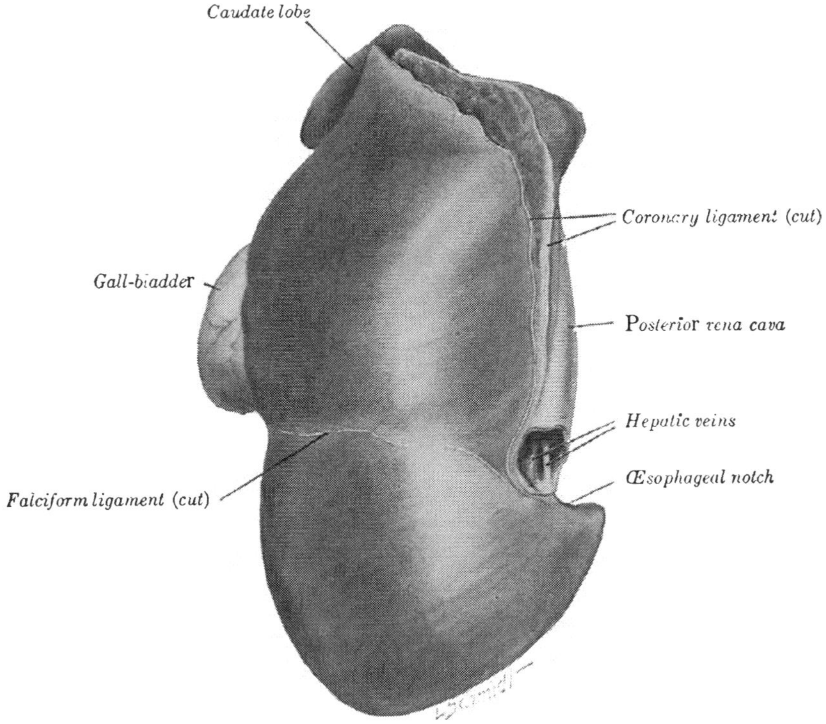

FIG. 295.—LIVER OF OX, PARIETAL SURFACE; HARDENED *in situ*.

curve and is continued by the spiral part (Ansa spiralis). The coils of this are attached to each other by connective tissue, and are best seen from the inner side. The bowel gradually diminishes in caliber, and the terminal part (Ansa distalis) leaves the spiral mass, passes forward to the great mesenteric artery and turns backward between the duodenum and the initial sigmoid part. From the ventral surface of the right kidney it passes backward, forms an **S**-shaped curve near the pelvic inlet, and joins the rectum; this part is attached to the sublumbar muscles by a short mesentery, and is also attached to the dorsal part of the duodenum.

The **rectum** is somewhat shorter than that of the horse, and is usually covered with peritoneum as far back as the first coccygeal vertebra. The retroperitoneal part is surrounded by a quantity of fat. The anus is not prominent.

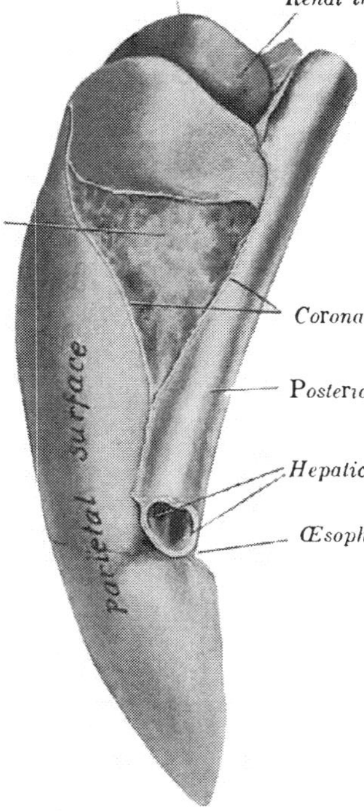

FIG. 296.—LIVER OF OX, LEFT MARGINAL VIEW; HARDENED *in situ*.

The **serous coat** is of course absent on the adherent surfaces of the spiral part of the colon. There is a large amount of fat in the mesentery. The **longitudinal muscular coat** is evenly distributed, consequently there is no sacculation of the bowel. There is a valvular mucous fold at the ileo-cæcal orifice. A Peyer's patch occurs in the beginning of the cæcum and one in the first part of the colon.

THE LIVER

The liver lies almost entirely to the right of the median plane. Its long axis is directed obliquely downward and forward, about parallel with the median plane, and corresponds to the curvature of the right portion of the diaphragm. It is less extensive, but thicker than that of the horse. Its average weight is about 10 to 12 pounds (ca. 4.5 to 5.5 kg.).

In small subjects the weight (according to Schmaltz) varies from 6½ to 10 pounds (ca. 3 to 4.5 kg.), in large subjects from 11 to 13 pounds (ca. 5 to 6 kg.). According to Schneider, the average weight is about 13 pounds (ca. 6 kg.)—a little over 1 per cent. of the live weight and about 2 per cent. of the dressed carcass.

When hardened *in situ*, its configuration adapts it accurately to the structures with which it is in contact.

The **parietal surface** is convex and is for the most part applied to the right part of the diaphragm, but a small part of it is in direct contact with the last two ribs and with the flank at the lumbo-costal angle. It faces upward, forward, and to the right.

The curvature of the parietal surface is not regular. It is marked, except in its ventral part, by a blunt oblique ridge which corresponds to the basal border of the right lung. This prominence divides the surface into two areas. Of these, the external one is directed outward,

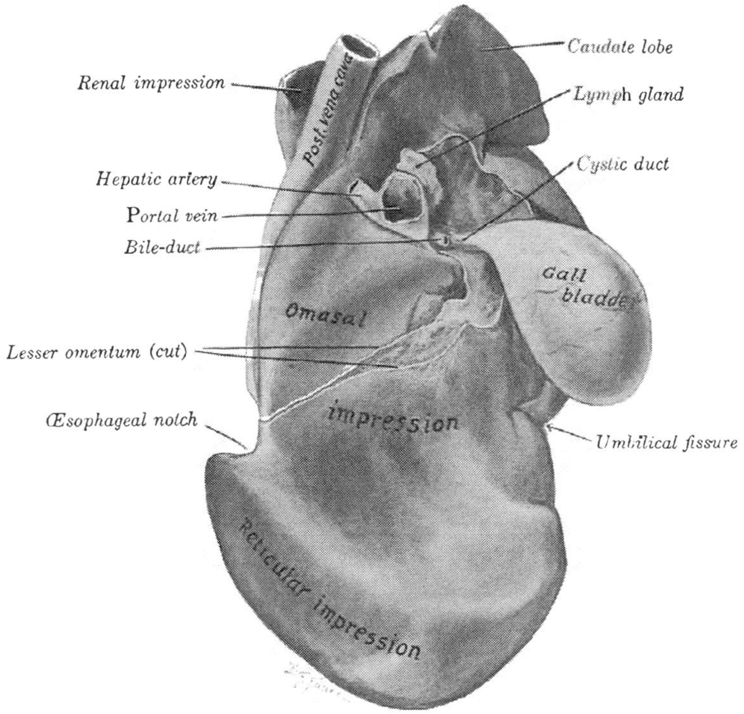

FIG. 297.—LIVER OF YOUNG OX, VISCERAL SURFACE; HARDENED *in situ*.

is only slightly convex, and often shows impressions of the last three ribs. The inner area presents a depression produced by the right crus of the diaphragm, and otherwise is regularly convex and adapted to the tendinous center and sternal portion of the diaphragm. The falciform ligament is attached to the surface from the œsophageal notch to the umbilical fissure.

The **visceral surface** is concave and very irregular; it presents impressions of the chief organs which are in contact with it—the omasum and reticulum. It is also related to the pancreas and duodenum.

The following markings are quite distinct on the visceral surface of well-hardened specimens: (1) The omasal impression (Impressio omasica) is a deep central cavity below the portal fissure. (2) The reticular impression (Impressio reticularis) is a smaller marginal depression below the œsophageal notch and the inner part of the preceding, from which it is separated by a rounded ridge. (3) The abomasal impression (Impressio abomasica), present only in the calf, is produced by the anterior part of the abomasum. It lies along the ventral part of the surface, and is separated by ridges from the preceding impressions. It disappears as the omasum and reticulum increase in size and displace the abomasum from contact with the liver. (4) Shallow grooves for the S-shaped portion of the duodenum (Impressio duodenalis) may be found above and external to the portal fissure. (5) The fossa of the gall-bladder (Fossa vesicæ felleæ) is distinct when that organ is full. In the calf the omasal impression is small, and the abomasal one large in correspondence with the relative sizes of these two sacs.

The **portal fissure** is a well-defined rounded depression, situated dorsal to the omasal impression. It contains, besides the vessels and duct, several large hepatic lymph glands. Above and external to it a part of the pancreas is attached.

The **dorsal** border is short and thick; it extends backward a short distance

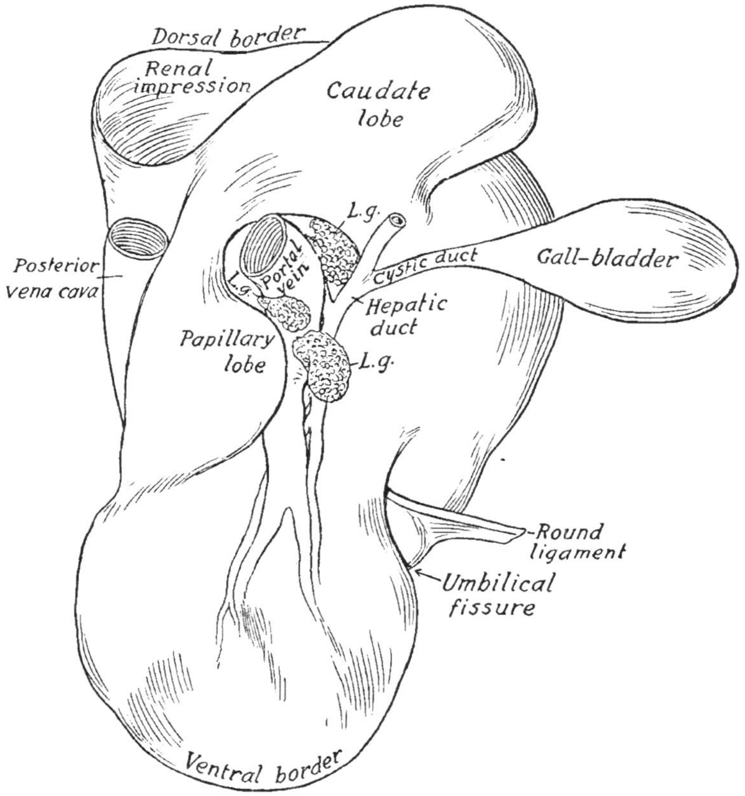

Fig. 298.—Line Drawing of Liver of Ox, Visceral Surface of Soft Specimen. *L.g.*, Hepatic lymph-glands at portal fissure.

beyond the upper part of the last rib. It presents the large, thick, quadrilateral **caudate lobe,** and a deep depression for the right kidney and adrenal.

The **ventral** border is short and thin and has no interlobar incisures.

The right (or external) border is marked by a small umbilical fissure, in which the ligamentum teres is attached in the young subject.

The **left** border presents the œsophageal notch below its middle. Above this it is practically median in position, and lodges the posterior vena cava, which is partially embedded in the gland. Below the notch the border extends an inch or two (ca. 2.5 to 5 cm.) to the left of the median plane opposite the ventral third of the sixth rib.

There is no left lateral ligament. The falciform ligament is usually present, but the ligamentum teres is found only in young subjects. The lesser omentum leaves the liver along a line extending from the œsophageal notch to the portal fissure. The only distinct lobe in the adult is the caudate (Processus caudatus).

A **gall-bladder** (Vesica feliea) is present. This is a pear-shaped sac, four to six inches (ca. 10 to 15 cm.) long, which lies partly on the visceral surface of the liver (to which it is attached), but largely on the abdominal wall at the lower part of the eleventh or twelfth intercostal space. It may be regarded as a diverticulum of the bile-duct, enlarged to form a reservoir for the bile. Its neck is continued by the **cystic duct** (Ductus cysticus), which joins the hepatic duct at an acute angle

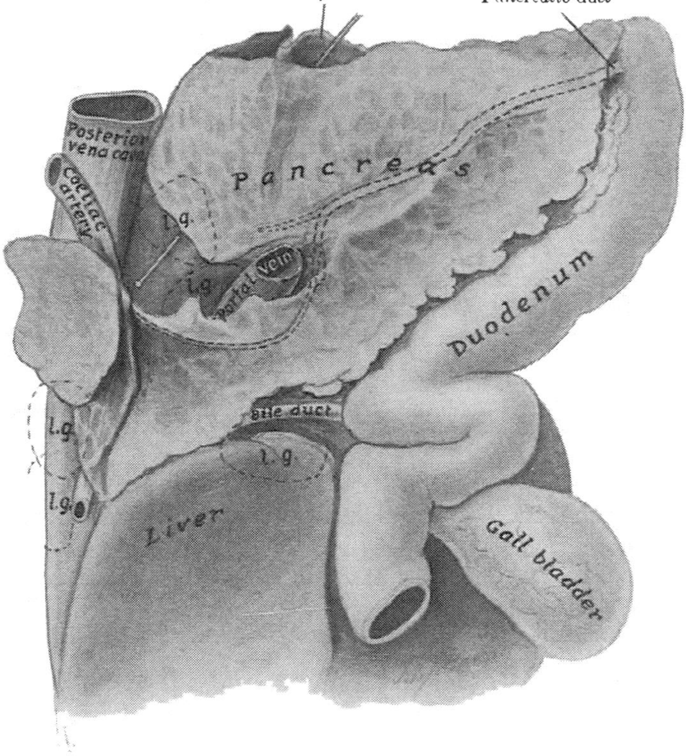

FIG. 299.—PANCREAS OF OX GASTRO-INTESTINAL SURFACE, WITH RELATED ORGANS.
The position of some of the larger lymph glands (*l.g.*) is indicated by dotted line; also the intraglandular course of the pancreatic duct. Probe is passed through epiploic foramen (of Winslow).

just outside of the portal fissure, to form with it the bile-duct (Ductus choledochus). The latter is short and enters the second bend of the **S**-shaped curve of the duodenum, *i. e.*, about two feet (ca. 60 cm.) from the pylorus. Several small ducts (Ductus hepato-cystici) open directly into the gall-bladder.

In the new-born calf the liver is relatively much larger than in the adult. The visceral surface presents, below the portal fissure, a large rounded eminence, which is caused by the presence in the underlying gland substance of a large venous sinus into which the umbilical and portal veins empty. A large vessel, the ductus venosus, leads from this sinus directly to the posterior vena cava. Just external to this elevation is a small but distinct lobe about two inches long (Processus papillaris?). The umbilical fissure is deep and partially divides the gland into two chief lobes.

THE PANCREAS

The pancreas of the ox is irregularly quadrilateral in form, and lies almost entirely to the right of the median plane. Its weight is about the same as that of the horse. Its dorsal surface is related to the crura of the diaphragm, the cœliac and anterior mesenteric arteries, and the liver. It is attached to the liver at and external to the portal fissure, and to the crura of the diaphragm. Between these adhesions it is free and forms the ventral wall of the epiploic foramen (of Winslow). On the right side it extends backward beyond the caudate lobe of the liver between the layers of the mesoduodenum; here it is in contact with the upper part of the flank at the lumbo-costal angle, and is related above to the right kidney and by its ventro-lateral border to the ventral part of the duodenum. The gastro-

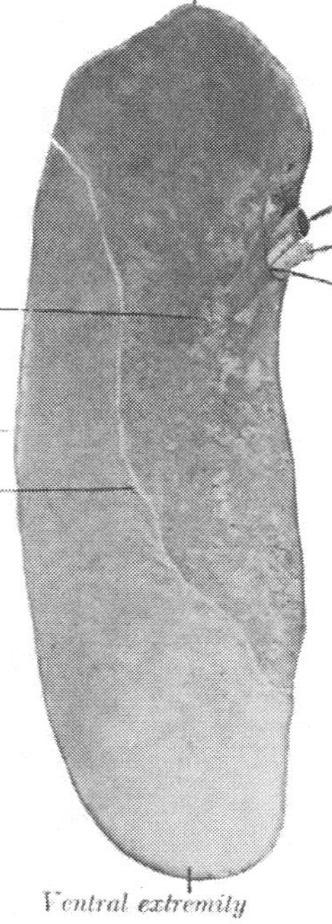

FIG. 300—SPLEEN OF OX; VISCERAL SURFACE.

intestinal or ventral surface is in contact with the dorsal curvature of the rumen and the intestine. The portal vein passes through the gland. The left extremity is small; the right or posterior is wide and thin and is often divided into two branches. The duct leaves the posterior part of the ventro-lateral (or right) border and enters the duodenum about twelve inches (ca. 30 cm.) further back than the bile-duct.

THE SPLEEN

The spleen has an elongated, elliptical outline, both extremities being thin, rounded, and similar in size.

Its average weight is about 30 ounces (ca. 800 to 900 gm.), or about $\frac{1}{6}$ per cent. of the body-weight. Its length is about 16 to 20 inches (ca. 40 to 50 cm.), its width about 5 to 6 inches (ca. 12 to 15 cm.), and in the middle its thickness is about an inch (ca. 2 to 3 cm.).

The **dorsal extremity** lies under the upper ends of the last two ribs; the ventral **extremity** is usually opposite the seventh or eighth rib, about a handbreadth above its junction with the cartilage. The **parietal surface** is convex, and is related to the diaphragm. The **visceral surface** is concave, and is related chiefly to the left face of the rumen, but also usually to a narrow adjacent area of the reticulum. The dorsal part is attached to the left crus of the diaphragm and the left surface of the rumen by peritoneum and connective tissue; the ventral part is free. The **hilus** is situated on the dorsal third of the visceral surface, near the anterior border.

About one-half of the visceral surface of the spleen is attached directly to the rumen and is not covered by peritoneum; the line of reflection of the latter crosses the surface obliquely, from the upper part of the posterior border to the anterior border a little below the middle. Similarly there is a narrow uncovered area on the upper part of the parietal surface along the anterior border. The hilus is not a groove, but a simple depression. When hardened *in situ*, the organ is seen to be somewhat twisted, so that the upper part of the parietal surface faces upward and forward, while below it is directed outward.

DIGESTIVE SYSTEM OF THE SHEEP

The **lips** are thin and mobile; the upper one is marked by a very distinct philtrum, and otherwise is not bare.

The anterior part of the **hard palate** is prominent and smooth; on the posterior part of this area there are two narrow depressions in the form of a V, at the deep anterior ends of which the naso-palatine ducts open. The ridges of the palate are irregular and their edges are smooth. The posterior third or rather more of the palate is not ridged and presents numerous orifices of ducts of the palatine glands. The mucous membrane is often more or less pigmented.

The mucous membrane of the **cheeks** is covered with large papillæ, many of which are long and sharp-pointed, while others are short and blunt. There is also a series of conical papillæ on the floor of the mouth under the lateral part of the tongue.

The **tongue** resembles that of the ox in form, but the tip is comparatively smooth; the papillæ here are very numerous, but short and blunt. This difference is in conformity with the dissimilarity in the mode of prehension. The prominence of the dorsum is commonly not so pronounced nor so sharply marked off in front as in the ox. The root is smooth. The mucous membrane of the dorsum is often pigmented in spots.

The dental formula is the same as that of the ox. The **incisor teeth** form a narrow and strongly curved arch. The crowns are long and narrow; their labial surfaces are strongly convex and end at a sharp edge which is used in cropping the grass. The roots are more firmly embedded than in the ox.

The **cheek teeth** resemble those of the ox. There is a thinner layer of cement, which is usually black.

The average periods of eruption of the teeth are indicated in the subjoined table.

Teeth	Temporary	
I_1	At birth or first week	
I_2	First or second week	
I_3	Second or third week	
I_4	Third or fourth week	
P_1, P_2, P_3	2 to 6 weeks	
M_1		months (upper)
M_2		
M_3		

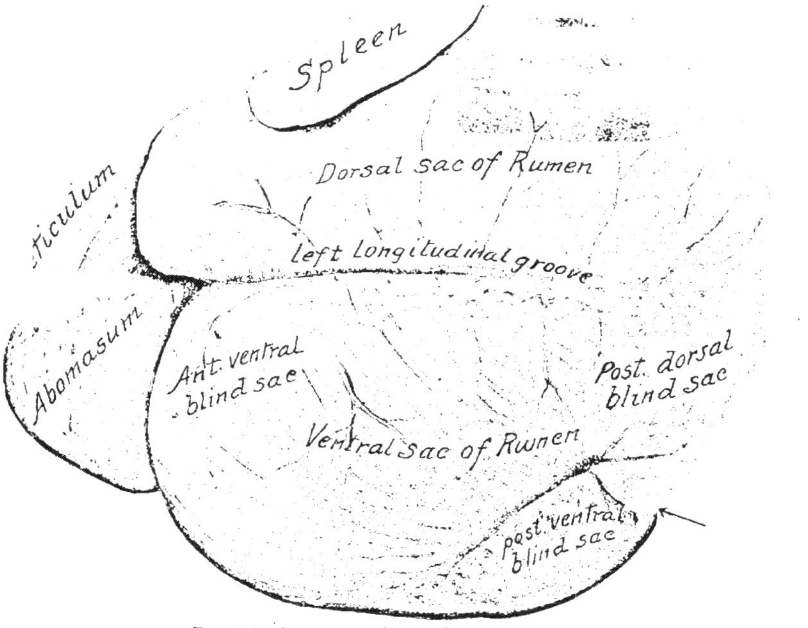

FIG. 301.—STOMACH OF SHEEP, LEFT VIEW.
From photograph of specimen hardened *in situ*. The reticulum is somewhat contracted. Arrow points to posterior furrow between blind sacs.

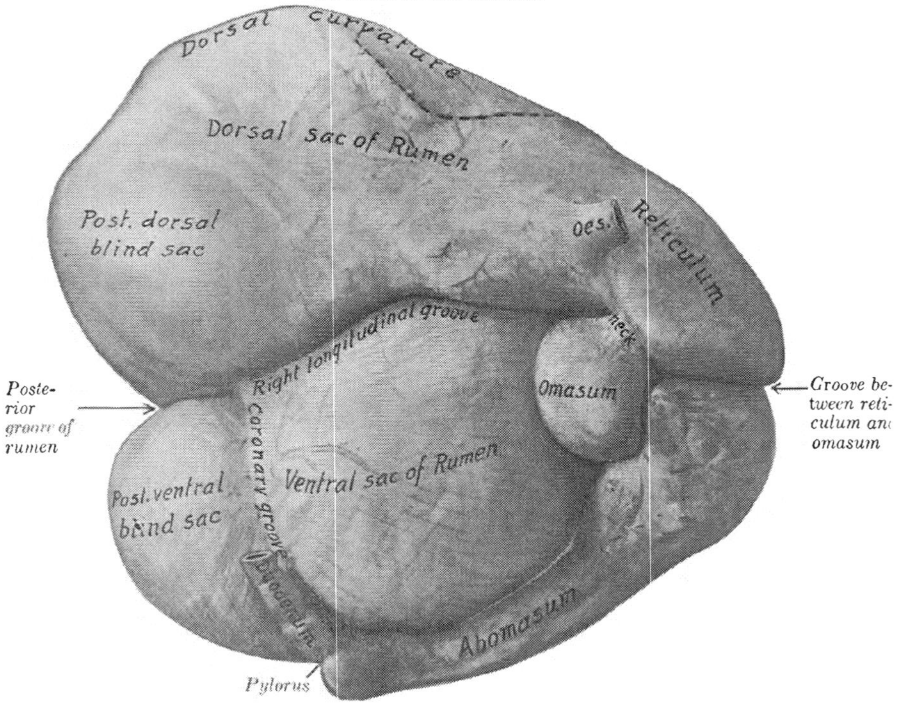

FIG. 302—STOMACH OF SHEEP, RIGHT VIEW
From photograph of specimen hardened *in situ*. Dotted line indicates position of spleen.

The **salivary glands** resemble those of the ox in general, but the parotid duct crosses the surface of the masseter muscle, and opens opposite the third or fourth cheek tooth.

The **tonsil** is bean-shaped and about half an inch (ca. 12 mm.) in length. It does not project into the fauces. The mucous membrane of the latter presents two deep and very narrow tonsillar sinuses on either side.

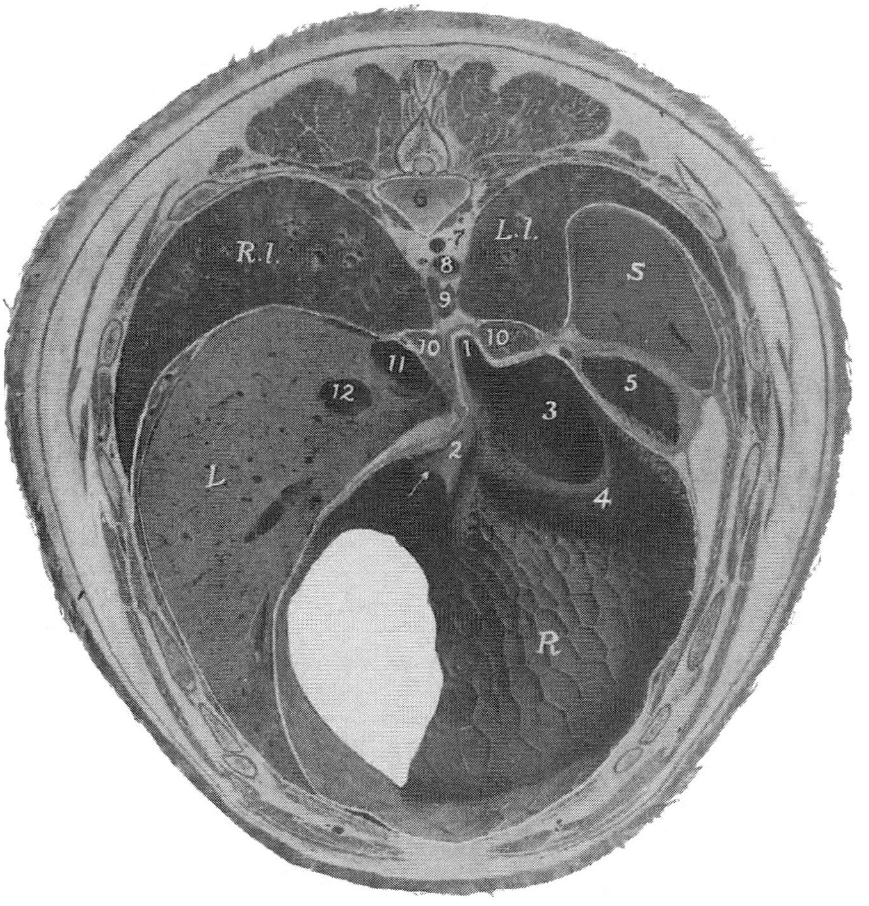

FIG. 303.—CROSS-SECTION OF SHEEP, THROUGH NINTH THORACIC VERTEBRA, ANTERIOR VIEW.

1, Cardiac orifice; *2*, œsophageal groove; *3*, rumino-reticular orifice; *4*, rumino-reticular fold; *5*, dorsal sac of rumen; *6*, body of ninth thoracic vertebra; *7*, vena hemiazygos; *8*, aorta; *9*, posterior mediastinal lymph gland; *10*, *10*, crura of diaphragm; *11*, posterior vena cava; *12*, portal vein; *R.l.*, right lung; *L.l.*, left lung; *S*, spleen (cut very obliquely); *L*, liver; *R*, reticulum (posterior wall). Arrow points to reticulo-omasal orifice.

The fornix of the **pharynx** presents a median plicated fold which is a continuation of the septum nasi. The pharyngeal orifice of the Eustachian tube has the form of a crescentic slit, placed about on a level with the inferior nasal meatus. There are two large lymph glands and a number of hæmolymph glands above the pharynx.

The **œsophagus** has a lumen of about an inch when moderately distended: otherwise it resembles that of the ox.

The stomach is like that of the ox in its general arrangement. Its average capacity is about four gallons (ca. 15 liters). The cardiac opening is opposite the middle of the eighth intercostal space; it is just to the left of the median plane and about two to three inches (ca. 5 to 7 cm.) below the vertebral column. The ventral sac of the rumen is relatively larger and extends further to the right of the median plane than in the ox. There are no coronary pillars in the dorsal sac, but its upper part is papillated. The papillæ of the rumen are relatively large and somewhat tongue-like; the largest are about a fourth of an inch (ca. 6 mm.) in length. The reticulum is relatively larger than in the ox. Its ventral part curves more backward and less to the right than in the ox. The parietal surface extends forward as

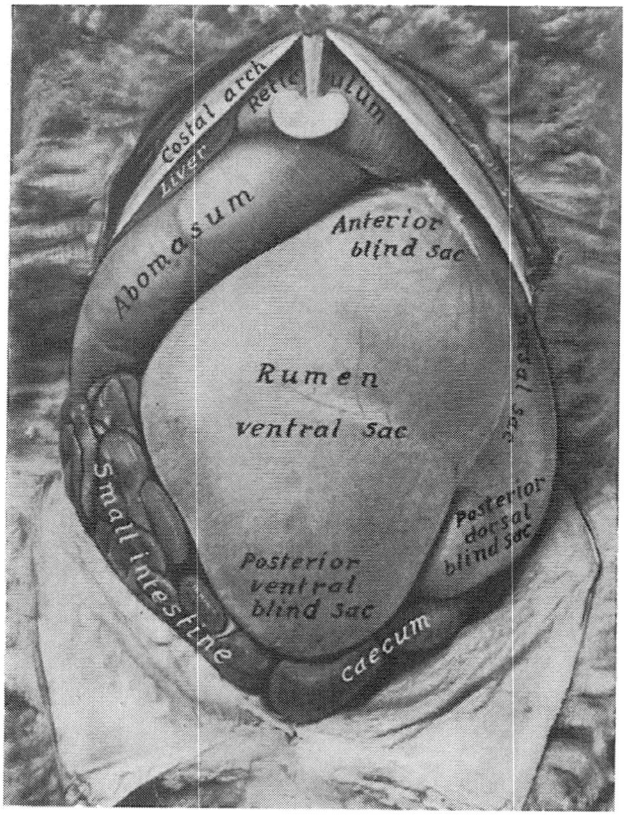

FIG. 304.—ABDOMINAL VISCERA OF SHEEP, SUPERFICIAL VENTRAL VIEW.

far as the sixth rib or intercostal space, and is related to the diaphragm and liver. The fundus lies on the sternal part of the diaphragm and in contact with the abomasum. The œsophageal groove is disposed much like that of the ox, and is about four to five inches (ca. 8 to 10 cm.) long. The omasum is much smaller than the reticulum, its capacity being only about one pint. It is oval and compressed laterally. It is situated almost entirely to the right of the median plane, opposite to the ninth and tenth ribs, higher than in the ox, and has no contact with the abdominal wall. It is related on the right to the liver and gall-bladder, on the left to the rumen, and below to the abomasum. The laminæ are less numerous than in the ox; in the neck which connects the omasum with the reticulum they have the form of low thick ridges, and bear long, pointed, horny papillæ. The abomasum is relatively larger and longer than in the ox. Its capacity is about twice that of the reticulum and averages about two quarts (ca. 1.75 to 2 liters). The blind anterior end lies almost centrally in the xiphoid region, in relation to the liver and reticulum. Its body extends backward a little below and almost parallel with the right costal arch. The pylorus is opposite the ventral end of the eleventh or twelfth intercostal space. The cells of the reticulum are much shallower than in the ox. At the reticulo-omasal opening and on the adjacent part of the laminæ of the omasum are large, pointed, horny papillæ. The number of laminæ is less than in the ox.

The general arrangement of the **intestine** is like that of the ox. The **small**

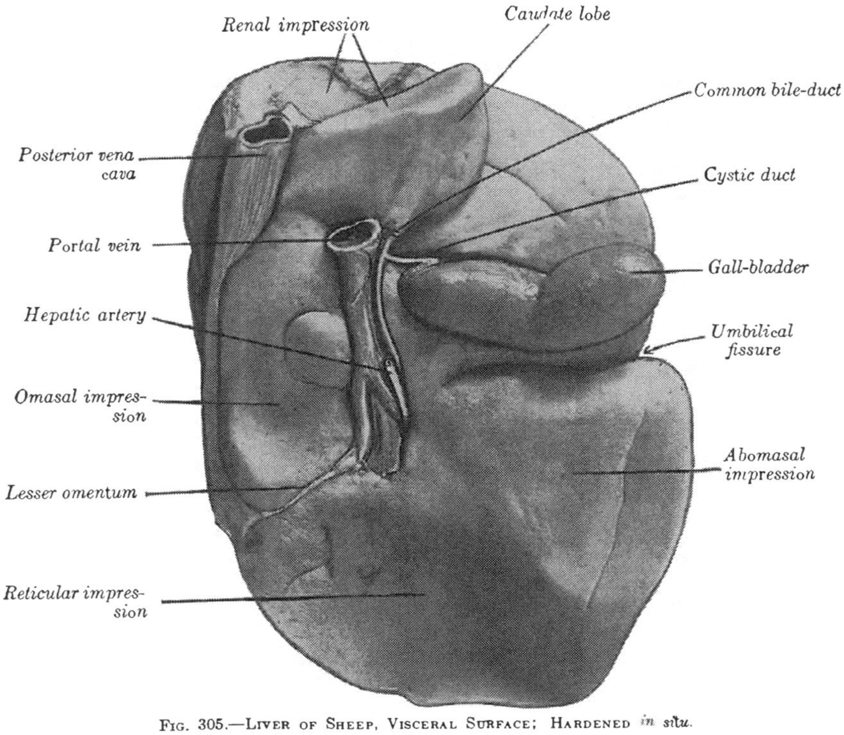

FIG. 305.—LIVER OF SHEEP, VISCERAL SURFACE; HARDENED *in situ*.

intestine is about 80 feet (ca. 24 to 25 m.) long; its average diameter is about an inch (ca. 2 to 3 cm.), the caliber increasing in its terminal part, where a very extensive Peyer's patch is found. The **cæcum** is about 10 to 12 inches (ca. 25 to 30 cm.) long, 2 inches (ca. 5 cm.) wide, and has a capacity of about a quart (ca. 1 liter). The **colon** is about 15 feet (ca. 4 to 5 m.) long. Its caliber is at first about the same as that of the cæcum, but diminishes to about the width of the small intestine.

The **liver** weighs about 20 to 25 ounces (ca. 550 to 700 gm.). It lies entirely to the right of the median plane. The parietal surface is related almost exclusively to the right part of the diaphragm. The visceral surface presents extensive reticular and abomasal impressions, and a small omasal impression internal to the portal fissure. The umbilical fissure is deep and partially divides the gland into two chief lobes. The caudate lobe is prismatic and blunt-pointed. The neck of the gall-bladder is long. The bile-duct joins the pancreatic duct to form a common duct (Ductus choledochus communis) which opens into the duodenum about one foot (ca. 30 cm.) from the pylorus.

The **pancreas** is arranged as in the ox. Its duct unites with the bile-duct.

The **spleen** (Fig. 301) is somewhat triangular, with the angles rounded off. It weighs about three or four ounces (ca. 100 grams). Its length is about five inches (ca. 12 to 13 cm.) and its greatest width about four inches (ca. 10 cm.). The parietal surface is convex and is related to the diaphragm, to which rather more than the anterior third is adherent. The visceral surface is concave and its anterior half is attached to the dorsal curvature of the rumen. The dorsal end or base is attached

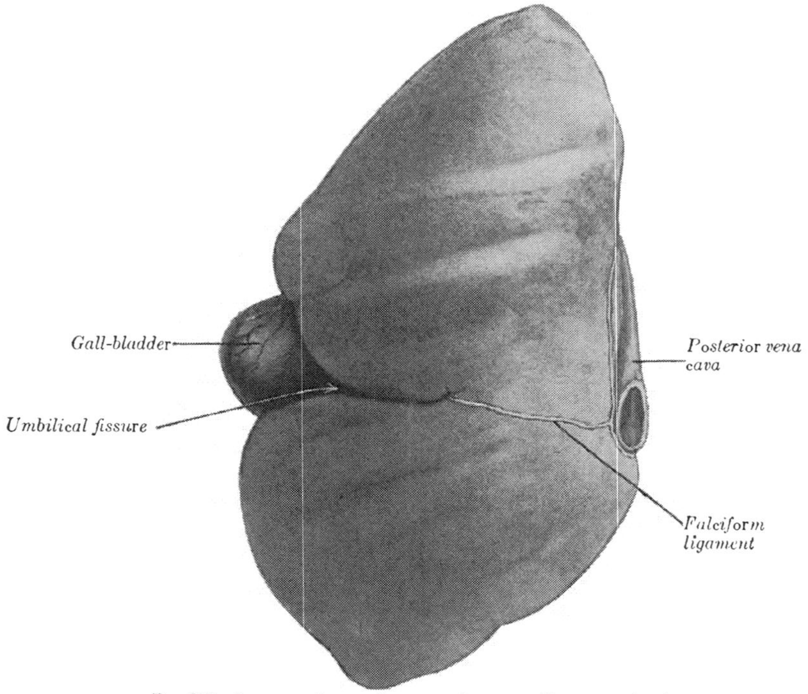

Fig. 306.—Liver of Sheep, Parietal Surface; Hardened *in situ*.

to the left crus of the diaphragm under the last two or three ribs. The hilus is at the posterior basal angle. The ventral end is narrower and thinner than the base; it is situated opposite the ninth and tenth ribs above their middles.

DIGESTIVE SYSTEM OF THE PIG

THE MOUTH

The **rima oris** is extensive, the angles of the mouth being situated far back. The upper lip is thick and short, and is blended with the snout; the lower **lip** is small and pointed. The labial glands are few and small.

The mucous membrane of the **cheeks** is smooth. The buccal glands are compactly arranged in two rows opposite the cheek teeth. The parotid duct opens opposite the fourth or fifth cheek tooth.

The **hard palate** is long and narrow; it is marked by a median furrow, on each side of which are twenty or more ridges. On its anterior part there is a triangular incisive papilla, at which the naso-palatine ducts open.

The **soft palate** is very thick. Its direction almost continues that of the hard palate, *i. e.*, it is nearly horizontal. It extends to the middle of the oral surface of the epiglottis.[1] It has a median prolongation termed the **uvula.** The oral surface presents a median furrow, on either side of which is an oval raised area,

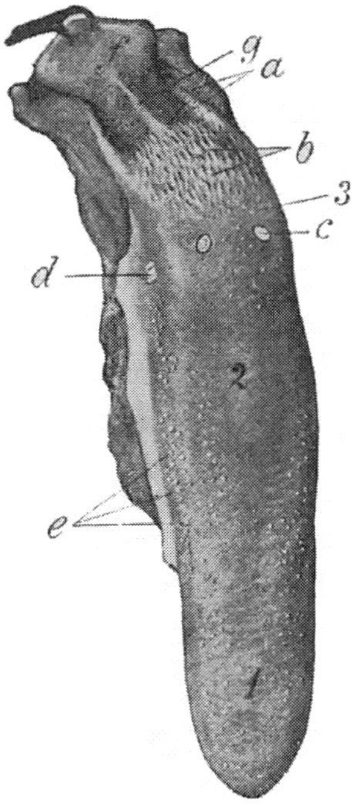

FIG. 307.—TONGUE OF PIG.

1, Apex; *2*, dorsum; *3*, root; *a*, orifices of ducts of lingual glands; *b*, papillæ of root; c, vallate papilla (not really so distinct as in figure); *d*, foliate papilla; *e*, fungiform papillæ; *f*, epiglottis (pulled back); *g*, median glosso-epiglottic fold. (Ellenberger-Baum, Anat. d. Haustiere.)

marked by numerous crypts; these elevations are the tonsils. Tonsillar tissue also occurs in the lateral walls of the fauces.

The **tongue** is long and narrow and the apex is thin. Two or three vallate papillæ are present. The fungiform papillæ are small and are most numerous laterally. The filiform papillæ are soft and very small. On the root there are soft, long, pointed papillæ, directed backward. Foliate papillæ are also present.

There is a well-marked median glosso-epiglottic fold, on either side of which is a depression (Vallecula epiglottica). The frenum linguæ is double.

The **dental formula** of the pig is:

$$2\left(I\frac{3}{3}-C\frac{1}{1}-P\frac{4}{4}-M\frac{3}{3}\right)=44$$

[1] The epiglottis in the pig seems to be constantly retrovelar. The pig frequently breathes through the mouth, and this is no doubt possible only when the soft palate is raised; it seems probable that it is also shortened.

The formula for the temporary teeth is:

$$2\left(Di\frac{3}{3}-Dc\frac{1}{1}-Dp\frac{4}{4}\right)=32$$

The **upper incisors** are small; they are separated from each other by spaces, and from the canines by a larger interval. The first incisors are the largest, are convergent, and have no distinct neck. The second are narrower and somewhat smaller. The third (corner) incisors are much smaller, are flattened laterally, and have three small eminences on the crown.

The **lower incisors** are almost horizontal and are convergent and close together. The first and second are about equal in size, prismatic, and deeply im-

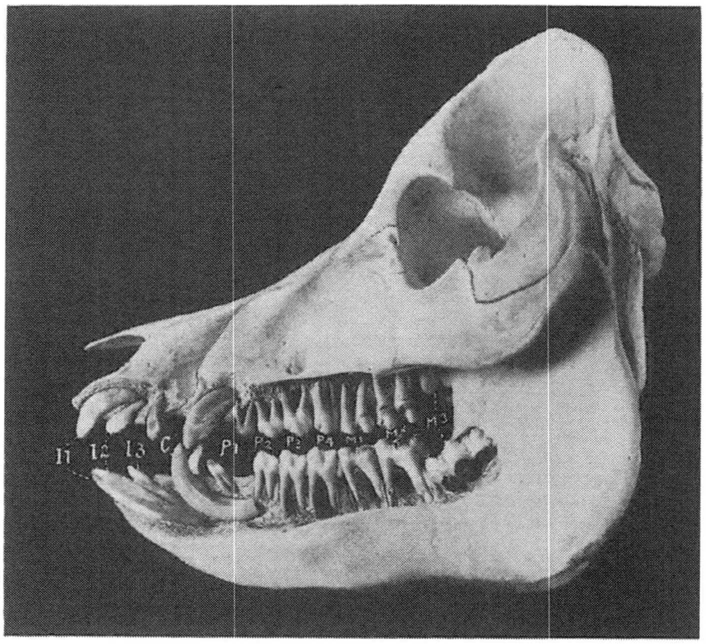

FIG. 308.—SKULL OF PIG ABOUT A YEAR AND A HALF OLD, SCULPTURED TO SHOW THE EMBEDDED PARTS OF THE TEETH.
I1–3, Incisors; C, canines; *P1–4*, premolars; *M1–3*, molars.

planted in the jaw. The labial surface is slightly convex, the lingual concave and marked near its extremity by a ridge. The third incisor is much smaller and has a short narrow crown and a distinct neck.

The **canine teeth** or tusks of the male are greatly developed and project out of the mouth. The upper canine of the boar may be about three or four inches (ca. 8 to 10 cm.) long. The crown is conical and is curved somewhat backward and outward; the embedded part is curved and has a large pulp cavity.[1] The lower canine may reach a length of eight inches or more (ca. 20 cm.); the crown is prismatic and is curved backward and outward in front of the upper one, so that the friction between the two keeps a sharp edge on the lower tooth. In the sow they are much smaller.

The **cheek teeth** increase in size from before backward. They have (with

[1] The canines of the pig are "permanent pulp" teeth and therefore capable of continued growth, and are without roots in the strict sense.

certain exceptions noted below) complex tuberculate crowns; the term bunodont is applied to this condition, as distinguished from the selenodont structure in horses and cattle, in which there are prominent ridges of enamel. They are short-crowned teeth with a distinct neck and root. The first tooth in each jaw is small, simple, and appears only once; in the lower jaw it is near the canine, in the upper near the second cheek tooth. The next two teeth are larger, laterally compressed, and sectorial. The fourth tooth below is larger, but otherwise like the preceding ones, while the upper one is much wider and is tuberculate.

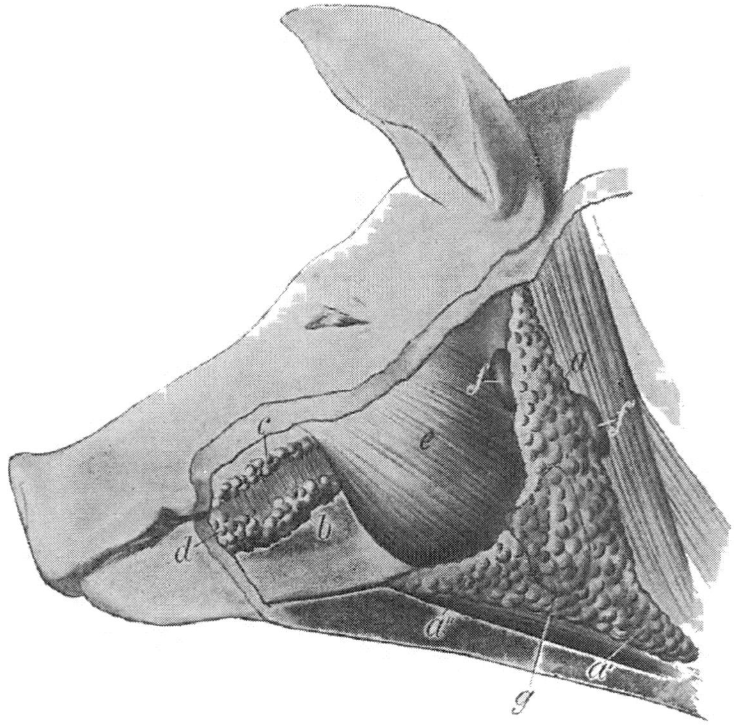

Fig. 309.—Superficial Glands of Head of Pig.

a, Parotid gland; *a'*, *a''*, cervical and submaxillary angles of *a*; *b*, *c*, ventral and dorsal buccal glands; *d* labial glands; *e*, masseter muscle; *f*, *f'*, lymph glands; *g*, dotted line indicating outline of submaxillary gland, which is concealed. (Ellenberger-Baum, Anat. d. Haustiere.)

The average periods of **eruption** of the teeth are given in the subjoined table.

Tooth	Eruption	Change
I_1	2 to 4 weeks	12 months
I_2	upper 2 to 3 months	
	lower 1½ to 2 months	16 to 20 months
I_3	Before birth	8 to 10 months
C	Before birth	9 to 10 months
P_1	5 months	
P_2	5 to 7 weeks	
P_3	upper 4 to 8 days	
	lower 2 to 4 weeks	12 to 15 months
P_4	upper 4 to 8 days	
	lower 2 to 4 weeks	
M_1	4 to 6 months	
M_2	8 to 12 months	
M_3	18 to 20 months	

The parotid gland is large and triradiate. It extends very little on to the masseter muscle and its upper angle does not quite reach the base of the ear. It is pale in color, and is embedded in fat in animals in good condition. On its deep face are several large subparotid lymph glands, some of which are only partially

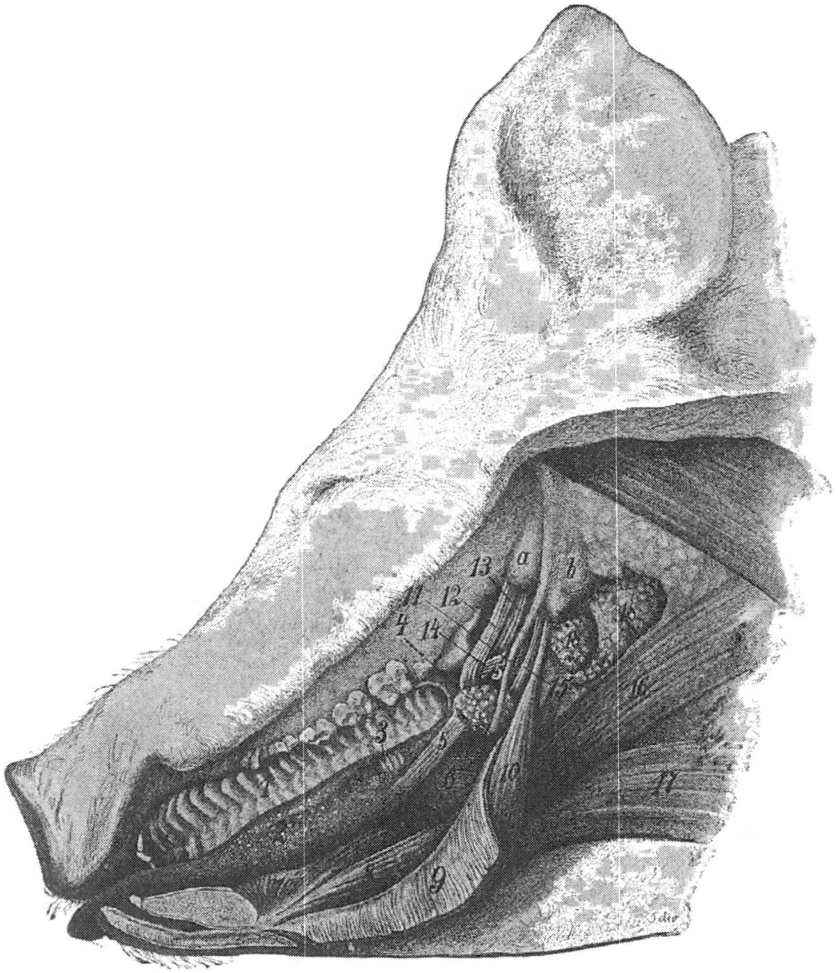

FIG. 310.—DISSECTION OF MOUTH AND PHARYNGEAL REGION OF PIG.

1, Hard palate; *2*, tongue showing distinctly fungiform papillæ; *3*, foliate papilla; *4*, lymph nodules of soft palate; *5*, stylo-glossus muscle, out of which a portion has been cut; *6*, hyo-glossus; *7*, genio-glossus; *8*, genio-hyoideus; *9*, mylo-hyoideus (reflected); *10*, stylo-hyoideus; *11*, great cornu of hyoid bone; *12*, tensor palati; *13*, levator palati; *14*, pterygo- et palato-pharyngeus; *15*, stylo-pharyngeus; *16*, chondro-pharyngeus; *17*, sterno- et omo-hyoideus; *18*, retropharyngeal lymph glands; *a*, bulla ossea; *b*, paramastoid process. (Ellenberger-Baum, Anat. d. Haustiere.)

covered by the parotid. The duct arises on the deep face, has a course similar to that of the ox, and perforates the cheek opposite the fourth or fifth upper cheek tooth. Small accessory glands (Glandulæ parotideæ accessoriæ) may be found along the course of the duct.

The **submaxillary gland** is small, reddish in color, and oval in outline; it is covered by the parotid. Its superficial face is convex, and is marked by rounded prominences. From its deep face a narrow process extends forward about two or

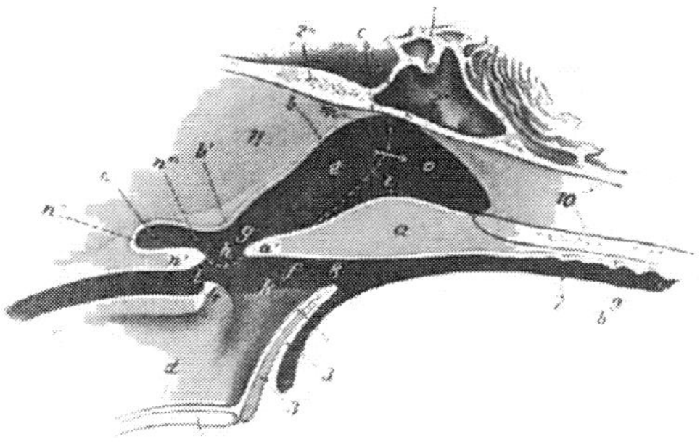

FIG. 311.—SAGITTAL SECTION OF PHARYNGEAL REGION OF PIG PARTLY SCHEMATIC.

1, Palate bone; *2*, sphenoid bone; *2'*, sphenoidal sinus; *2"*, occipital bone; *3*, epiglottis; *4*, arytenoid cartilage; *5*, thyroid cartilage; *6*, root of tongue; *7*, mouth cavity; *8*, isthmus faucium; *9*, hard palate; *10*, septum nasi; *11*, ventral muscles of head; *a*, soft palate; *a'*, free edge of *a*; *b*, dorsal wall of pharynx; c, fornix of pharynx; d, cavity of larynx; *e*, *g*, naso-pharynx; *f*, oro-pharynx; *h*, posterior pillar of soft palate; *i*, dotted line indicating lateral boundary between nasal cavity and pharynx; *k*, aditus laryngis; *l*, entrance to œsophagus; *m*, Eustachian orifice; *n*, pharyngeal recess; *o*, posterior naris. (After Ellenberger, in Leisering's Atlas.)

three inches (ca. 5 to 7.5 cm.) beneath the mylo-hyoideus muscle along with the duct. The latter opens near the frenum linguæ, but there is no papilla.

The **sublingual gland** has an arrangement similar to that of the ox. The pos-

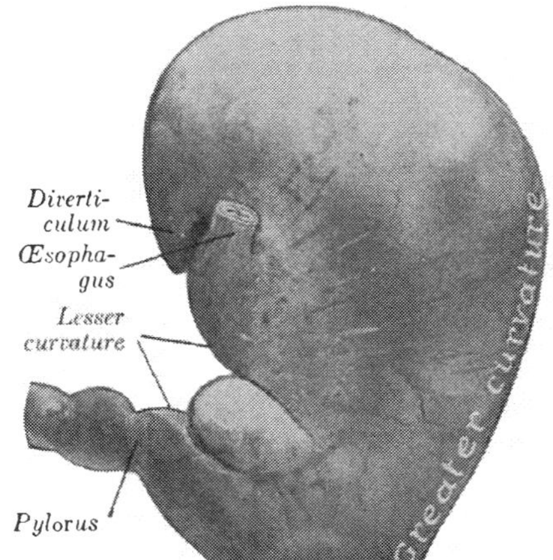

FIG. 312.—STOMACH OF PIG, PARIETAL SURFACE.
The organ contained a rather small amount of ingesta and hence is somewhat contracted.

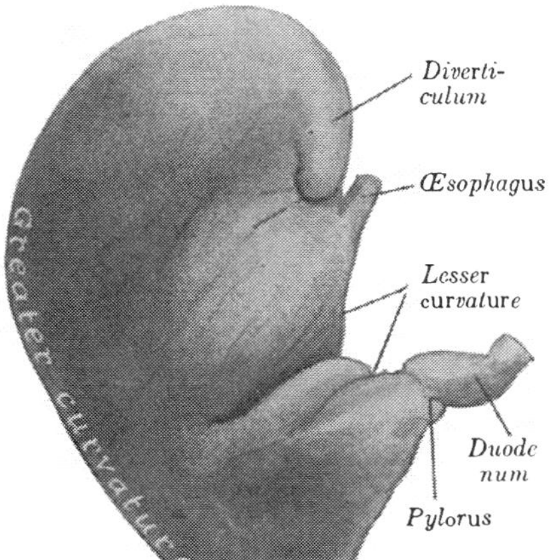

FIG. 313.—STOMACH OF PIG, VISCERAL SURFACE.
Organ was fixed *in situ* and is somewhat contracted.

terior part (Glandula sublingualis grandicanalaris) is reddish-yellow in color, and is about two inches (ca. 5 cm.) long, and half an inch wide; its posterior end is in relation to the submaxillary gland and its duct. The anterior part is much larger, being two or three inches (ca. 5 to 7 cm.) long and about twice the width and thickness of the posterior part. All or most of the ducts from the posterior

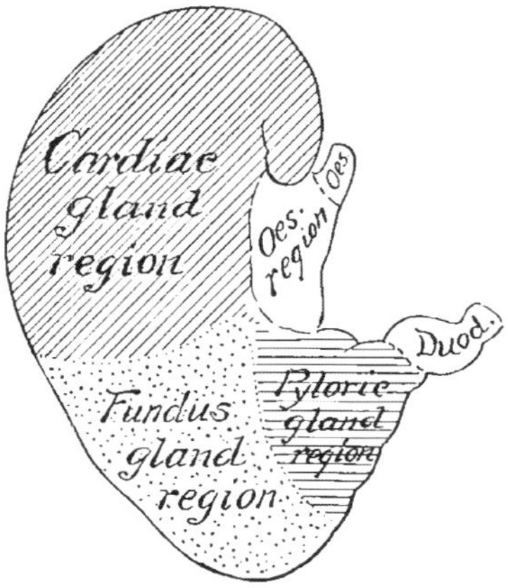

FIG. 314.—DIAGRAM OF ZONES OF MUCOUS MEMBRANE OF STOMACH OF PIG.

part unite to form the **ductus sublingualis major,** which opens near the ductus submaxillaris. Eight or ten **ductus sublinguales minores** convey the secretion from the anterior part through the floor of the mouth.

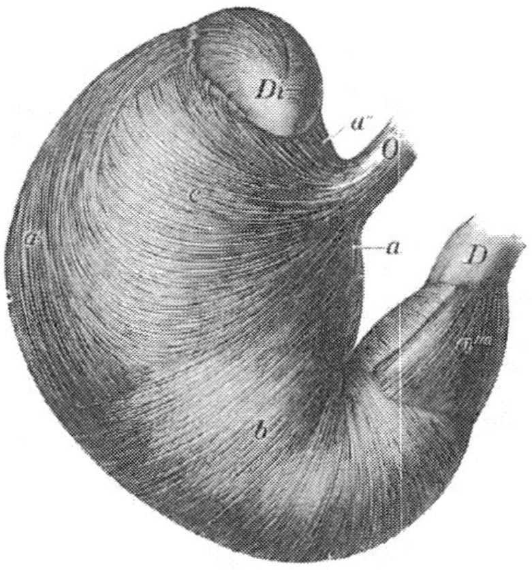

FIG. 315.—VISCERAL SURFACE OF STOMACH OF PIG FROM WHICH THE SEROUS COAT HAS BEEN REMOVED.

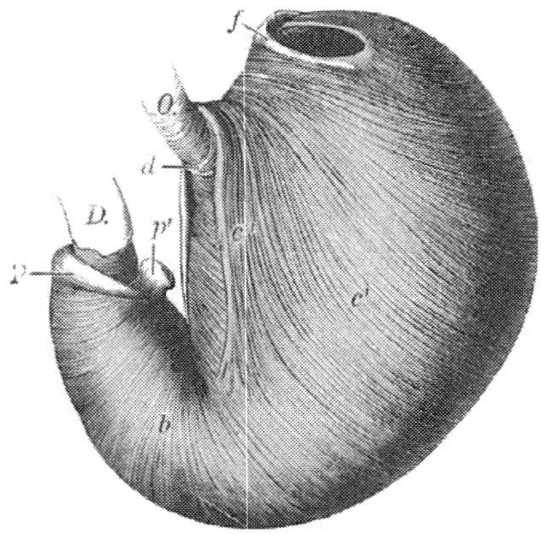

FIG. 316.—EVERTED STOMACH OF PIG, FROM WHICH THE MUCOUS MEMBRANE HAS BEEN REMOVED.

O, Œsophagus; *D*, duodenum; *Di*, diverticulum; *a*, *a'*, *a''*, *a'''*, longitudinal fibers; *b*, circular fibers; *c*, external oblique fibers; *c'*, internal oblique fibers; *c''*, cardiac loop; *d*, fibers which connect branches of cardiac loop; *f*, fold at entrance to diverticulum; *p*, pyloric sphincter; *p'*, pyloric prominence. (Ellenberger-Baum, Anat. d. Haustiere.)

THE PHARYNX

The **pharynx** presents in its posterior part a median cul-de-sac about an inch and a half (ca. 3 to 4 cm.) long, which is situated between the ventral straight muscles of the head and the origin of the œsophagus. Its lower margin is formed by the junction of the posterior pillars of the soft palate, which contain muscular tissue derived from the palatinus and palato-pharyngeus. The vault of the pharynx (Fornix pharyngis) is divided by a median fold of mucous membrane which is a direct continuation of the septum nasi. On either side of this is an infundibulum in which the Eustachian tube opens.

THE ŒSOPHAGUS

The **œsophagus** is short and nearly straight. It has (according to Ruheli) a potential caliber of nearly 3 inches (ca. 7 cm.) at either end, and about $1\frac{7}{10}$ inches (ca. 4.2 cm.) in its middle part.[1] The muscular coat, except near the cardia, is striated. There are mucous glands in the submucosa to about the middle of the tube.

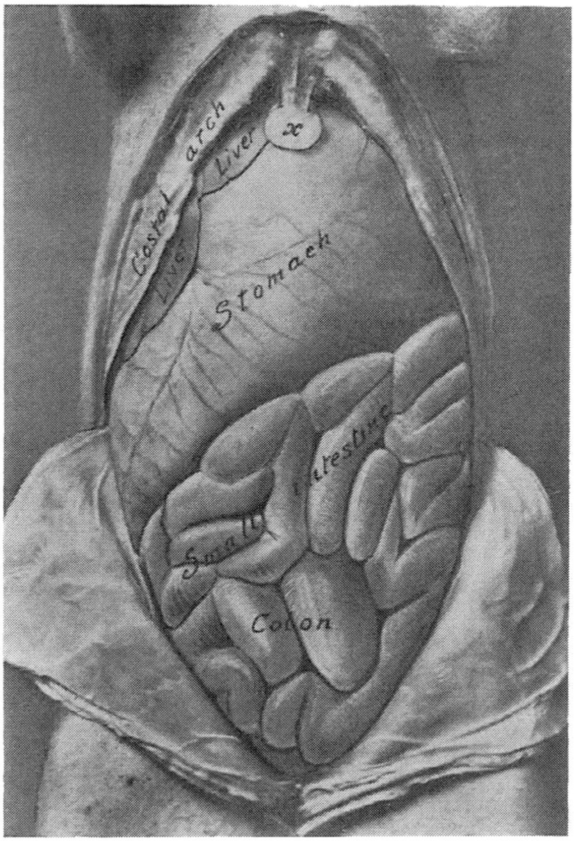

FIG. 317.—ABDOMINAL VISCERA OF YOUNG PIG, VENTRAL ASPECT.
The stomach was very large in this subject.

THE STOMACH

The **stomach** is large and pyriform. Its average capacity is about $1\frac{1}{2}$ to 2 gallons (ca. 5.7 to 8 liters). When full it extends backward to the last left inter-

[1] It is usually stated that the cardiac end is funnel-shaped, but it is not so in formalin hardened cadavers nor in frozen sections. The hiatus œsophagus is a long slit in the right crus of the diaphragm, and the terminal part of the œsophagus, which lies in it, is flattened transversely.

costal space laterally and the umbilicus ventrally. The left portion is large and rounded, while the right portion (Pars pylorica) is small, and bends sharply upward to join the small intestine. The parietal surface is related to the liver, gall-bladder,

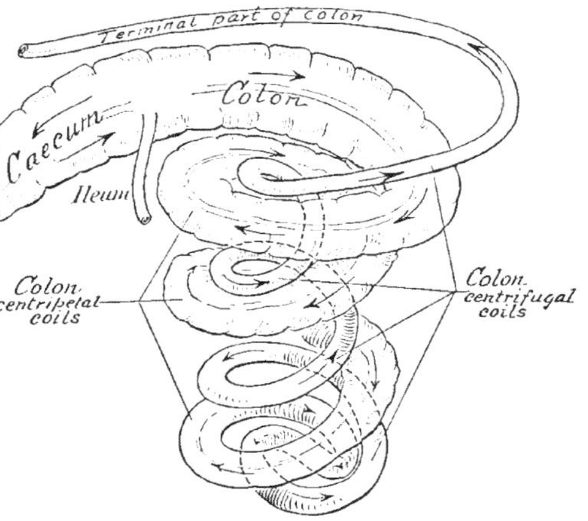

FIG. 318.—DIAGRAM OF CÆCUM AND COLON OF PIG.
Coils of colon have been pulled apart somewhat.

and diaphragm. The visceral surface is related to the intestine the mesentery, and the pancreas. The great curvature is related to the diaphragm, spleen, and abdominal floor. The pyloric end lies on the right lateral lobe of the liver. The

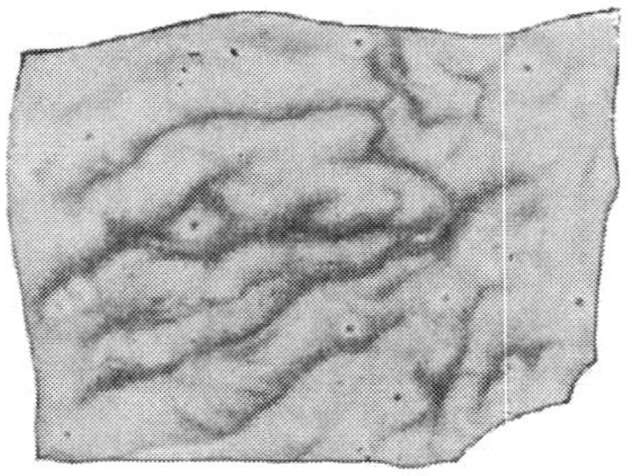

FIG. 319.—SOLITARY NODULES FROM LARGE INTESTINE OF PIG. (Ellenberger-Baum, Anat. d. Haustiere.)

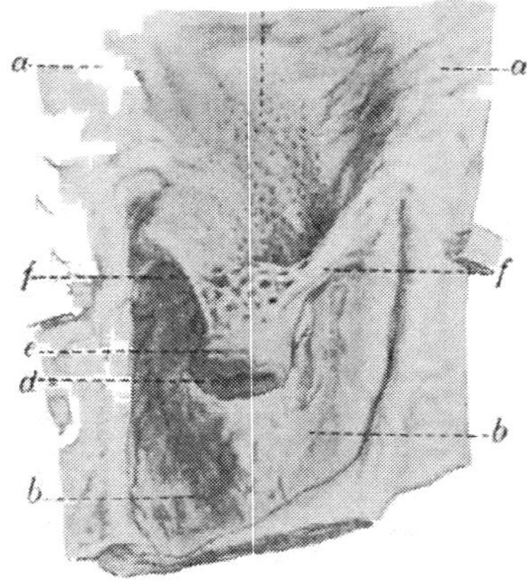

FIG. 320.—ILEO-CÆCAL OPENING AND ADJACENT PART OF CÆCUM AND COLON OF PIG.

a, Mucous membrane of colon; b, mucous membrane of cæcum; c, Peyer's patch; d, ileo-cæcal opening; e, end of ileum; f, folds (frenula) of ileum. (After P. Schumann.)

left extremity presents a flattened conical blind pouch, the **diverticulum ventriculi**, the apex of which projects backward. The œsophagus joins the stomach very obliquely, almost in the median plane, and about three or four inches (ca. 8 to 10 cm.) below the twelfth thoracic vertebra. The cardiac opening is slit-like and is bounded above and to the left by a fold which contains a thickening of the internal oblique layer of the muscular coat. The opening into the diverticulum is situated above and a little to the left of the cardia; it is transversely oval, and is bounded (except externally) by a thick fold which contains spirally arranged muscular fibers. The mucous membrane may be divided into four regions. Over a quadrilateral area around the cardia (about one inch on the right and two or three inches on the left side of the orifice) it is œsophageal in character, and presents a number of folds. A sharp line of demarcation separates this from the rest of the mucous membrane, which is soft and glandular. The second or cardiac gland region is pale gray in color and thin (ca. 0.5 to 1 mm.); it extends about to the middle of the stomach. The third or fundus gland region is readily distinguished by its thickness (ca. 3 mm.) and its brownish-red mottled appearance.[1] The fourth or pyloric region is pale, thinner than the preceding, and presents a number of irregular folds. At the pylorus there is a remarkable ridge which projects from the wall of the lesser curvature and diminishes considerably the size of the orifice. It is about an inch and a half (ca. 3 to 4 cm.) long and nearly half an inch (ca. 1 cm.) high. Sometimes it is grooved; in other cases it has the form of a rounded eminence attached by a pedicle to the wall. Fibers from the circular muscular coat extend into it.

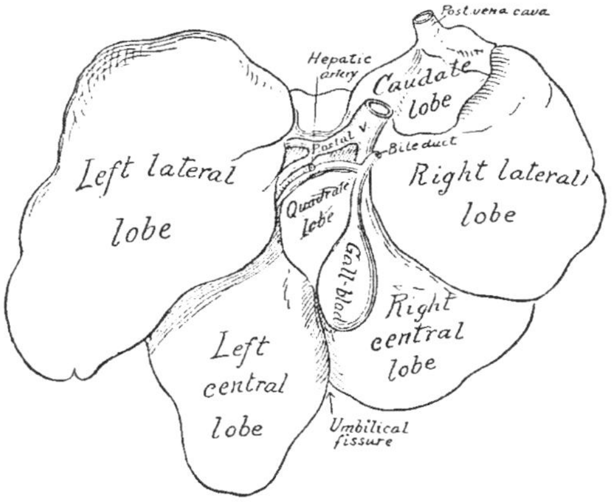

FIG. 321.—LIVER OF PIG, SOFT SPECIMEN SKETCHED WITH LOBES DRAWN APART.

THE INTESTINE

The **small intestine** is 50 to 65 feet (ca. 15 to 20 m.) long. The mesentery of about the first two feet (ca. 60 cm.) is two to two and a half inches (ca. 5 to 6 cm.) long; this part may be termed duodenum. The remainder (Jejuno-ileum) has a mesentery about six to eight inches (ca. 15 to 20 cm.) long, which is thick and contains a quantity of fat, and numerous large lymph glands at its root; the root is attached in the sublumbar region behind the stomach and blends here with the mesentery of the large intestine. The small intestine is arranged in close coils and lies mainly on the left side and floor of the abdomen, from the stomach to the pelvis; some coils, however, lie against the right flank. The opening of the **bile duct** is about one or two inches (ca. 2.5 to 5 cm.) from the pylorus, and that of the **pancreatic** duct about four or five inches (ca. 10 to 15 cm.) beyond it. **Peyer's**

[1] It will be noted that the fundus gland region does not extend up to the lesser curvature; here the cardiac mucosa joins the pyloric.

patches and **solitary glands** are numerous and very distinct; the patches are usually band-like and prominent; the solitary glands form projecting nodules marked by crypts.

The **large intestine** is about 15 feet (ca. 4 to 5 meters) in length, and is for the most part much wider than the small intestine; it is connected by a mesentery with the dorsal abdominal wall between the kidneys. The **cæcum** is cylindrical, about 8 to 12 inches (ca. 20 to 30 cm.) long, and 3 to 4 inches (ca. 8 to 10 cm.) wide. It lies against the upper part of the right flank, its blind end reaching to within about two inches (ca. 5 cm.) of the pelvic inlet. The ileum joins the cæcum obliquely and projects somewhat into its lumen. The **colon** has at first about the

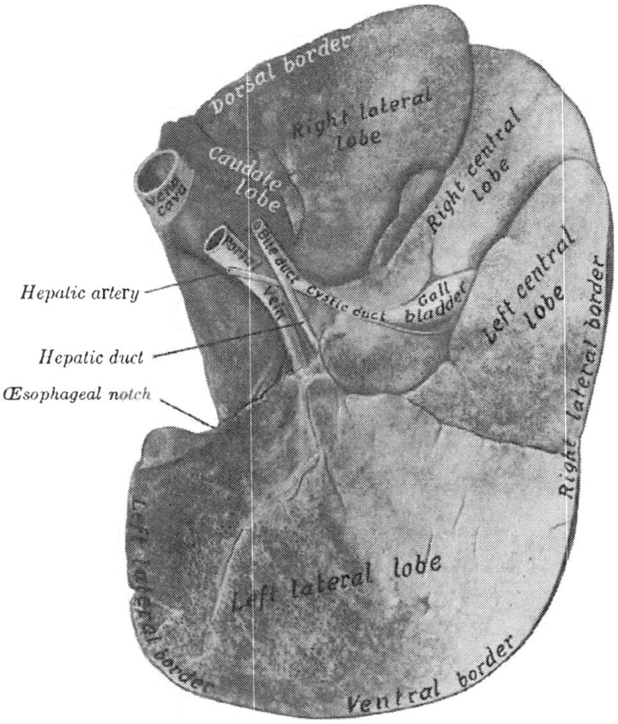

FIG. 322.—LIVER OF PIG, VISCERAL SURFACE.
Photograph of specimen hardened *in situ*.

same caliber as the cæcum, but becomes gradually smaller. Most of it is arranged in three close, double spiral coils in the mesentery, in relation chiefly to the right flank externally, and to the small intestine behind and to the left. On emerging from this spiral labyrinth, it passes forward to the stomach and pancreas and then turns backward; this terminal part is narrow, median in position, and closely attached by a short mesentery to the sublumbar region. The **rectum** is usually surrounded by a quantity of fat. The cæcum has three longitudinal muscular bands and three rows of sacculations, which are continued a short distance on the colon. The spiral colon has two bands and two series of sacculations, which, however, gradually disappear in the centrifugal part.

THE LIVER

The liver is relatively large, its average weight being about 4 to 4½ pounds (ca. 2 kg.). It is thick and very strongly curved.[1] It is divided by three deep interlobar incisures into four principal lobes — right lateral, right central, left central, left lateral; the last of these is usually considerably the largest. On the upper part of the right lateral lobe is the caudate lobe and its process. That part of the right central lobe which lies below the portal fissure and to the left of the gall-bladder and cystic duct is homologous with the quadrate lobe of man. The parietal surface is extremely convex, its most anterior part reaching to a plane through the lower part of the sixth or seventh intercostal space. The

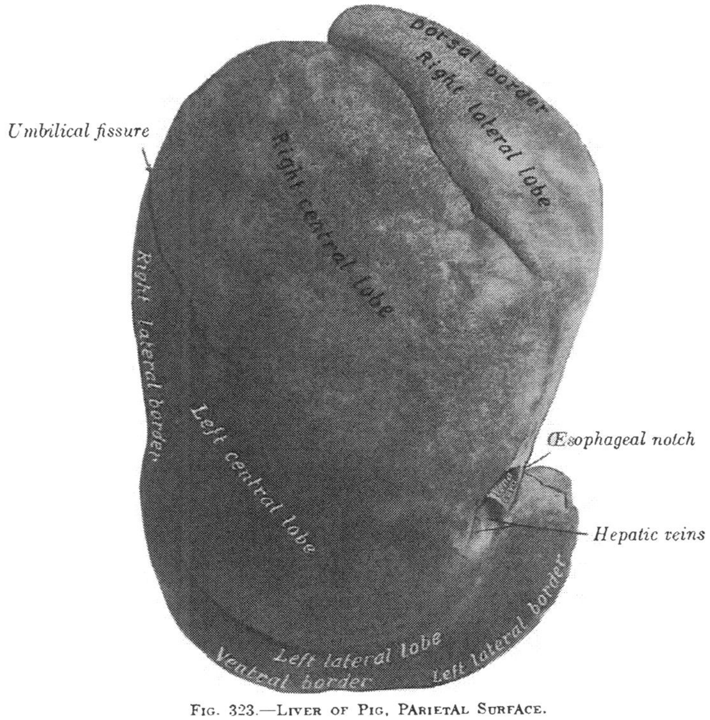

Fig. 323.—Liver of Pig, Parietal Surface.
Photograph of specimen hardened *in situ*.

visceral surface is deeply concave; most of it is related to the stomach, for which there is a correspondingly large and deep gastric impression. There is a duodenal impression on the upper part of the right lateral lobe, but no renal impression, as the right kidney does not touch the liver. The fossa for the gall-bladder is mainly on the right central lobe, but also in part on the adjacent surface of the left central lobe. The posterior vena cava enters the dorsal border of the caudate lobe and soon becomes entirely embedded in the gland-substance, emerging only at its passage through the diaphragm. The œsophageal notch is large and is occupied mainly by the large right crus of the diaphragm. The right

[1] The description here given is based mainly on the appearance of the organ as hardened *in situ*, which differs radically from that of the soft organ, as is seen on comparison of the annexed figure (Fig. 321).

lateral border extends backward to the upper part of the twelfth intercostal space or thirteenth rib. The left lateral border is opposite the eighth rib and intercostal space. The ventral border extends backward about as far as the umbilicus.

There are no lateral ligaments and the falciform ligament disappears early.

The gall-bladder is attached in the fossa vesicæ felleæ on the right central lobe, at a considerable distance from the ventral border. The cystic duct joins the hepatic duct at an acute angle immediately after the emergence of the latter from the portal fissure. The bile duct (Ductus choledochus) opens at the papilla duodeni about one or two inches (ca. 2.5 to 5 cm.) from the pylorus.

Owing to the large amount of interlobular tissue, the lobules are mapped out sharply; they are polyhedral in form and are 1 to 2.5 mm. in diameter. For the same reason the gland tissue is much less friable than that of the other animals, from which it is easily distinguished.

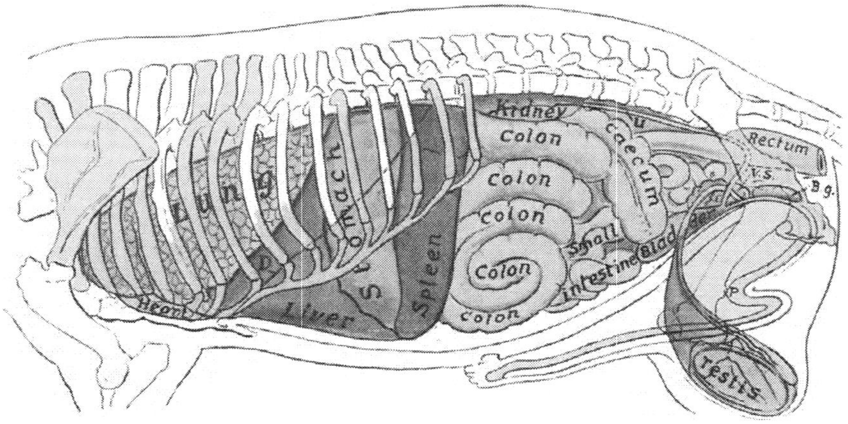

FIG. 324.—PROJECTION OF VISCERA OF PIG ON BODY-WALL, LEFT SIDE.
D, Costal line of diaphragm; *U*, ureter; *V. S.*, vesicula seminalis; *B. g.*, bulbo-urethral gland; *P*, penis.

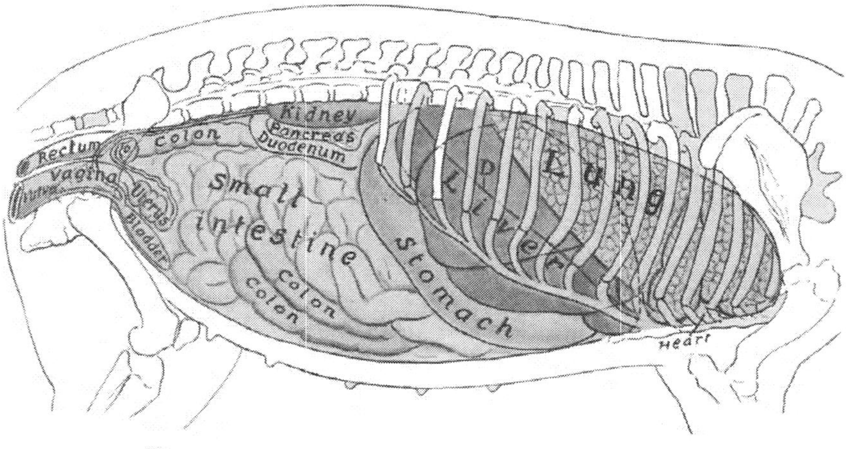

FIG. 325.—PROJECTION OF VISCERA OF PIG ON BODY-WALL, RIGHT SIDE.
D, Costal attachment of diaphragm; *O*, ovary.

THE PANCREAS

The **pancreas** is elongated, and is situated transversely on the dorsal abdominal wall, with its right extremity on the ventral surface of the right kidney, and the left end touching the dorsal end of the spleen and the left kidney. The right portion has two lobes; the posterior lobe bends around the great mesenteric artery and the portal vein; the anterior one is pointed, extends downward and forward about in the median plane, and is attached to the portal fissure and the duodenum. The left portion is prismatic and rests mainly on the left sac of the stomach, its left extremity being included between the left kidney and the dorsal end of the spleen. The pancreatic duct passes from the anterior lobe directly through the duodenal wall, opening about five or six inches (ca. 12.5 to 15 cm.) from the pylorus. The interlobular tissue usually contains a good deal of fat.

THE SPLEEN

The **spleen** is long and narrow. Its long axis is nearly dorso-ventral in direction, and is slightly curved to conform to the left part of the greater curvature of the stomach. The dorsal end lies under the vertebral ends of the last three ribs. The ventral end is smaller, reaches to the ventral abdominal wall, and lies against the left lobe of the liver. The visceral surface has a longitudinal ridge on which the hilus is situated; this divides the surface into nearly equal gastric and intestinal areas. The spleen is attached so loosely to the stomach that it may be regarded as being intercalated in the great omentum. In large subjects it may reach a length of 15 to 18 inches (ca. 38 to 45 cm.) and a width of 3 to 4 inches (ca. 8 to 10 cm.).

DIGESTIVE SYSTEM OF THE DOG

THE MOUTH

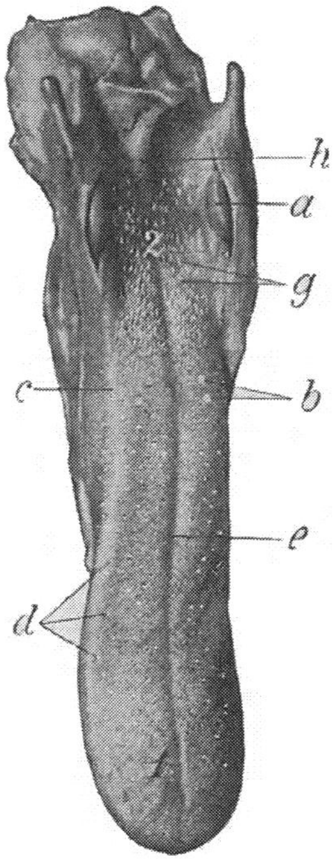

FIG. 326.—TONGUE OF DOG.

a, Tonsil; *b*, vallate papillæ; *c*, foliate papilla; *d*, fungiform papillæ; *e*, median groove of dorsum; *f*, epiglottis; *g*, soft papillæ of root; *h*, middle glosso-epiglottic fold; *1*, tip; *2*, root. (Ellenberger-Baum, Anat. d. Haustiere.)

The size and form of the mouth vary greatly in different breeds, the cavity being in some long and narrow, in others short and wide. The **rima oris** is very extensive, so that the labial commissure is opposite the third or fourth cheek tooth. The **lips** are thin and mobile, and present numerous tactile hairs. The upper lip has a small, central, bare area which forms part of the muzzle, and is marked by a central groove, the philtrum, or (as in the bull-dog) a fissure, giving the appearance of harelip. The lateral borders of the lower lip are flaccid and denticulated. The mucous membrane is usually pigmented and forms distinct frena labiorum. The labial glands are small and scanty.

The **cheeks** are loose and capacious, and their mucous lining is smooth and more or less pigmented. The **parotid duct** opens usually opposite the third upper cheek tooth. Near the last tooth are the openings of the four or five ducts from the orbital gland.

The **hard palate** is widest between the fourth pair of cheek teeth. It has eight to ten curved ridges on either side of the raphe. Behind the first pair of incisor teeth is the triangular incisive papilla, at which the naso-palatine ducts open. The mucous membrane is usually pigmented.

The **soft palate** is thick except at its margins. In the resting state of the parts it comes in contact with the oral surface of the epiglottis. Between its anterior and posterior pillars on either side is a marked tonsillar sinus, in which an elongated **tonsil** is situated; this is reddish in color, about an inch long, and projects somewhat into the fauces between two folds of mucous membrane.

The **tongue** is wide, thin, and very mobile. It is not pigmented, but has a bright red color. The upper surface is marked by a median groove (Sulcus medianus linguæ), and is thickly beset with short, pointed, filiform papillæ, the free ends of which are directed backward. On the root the papillæ are long and soft; similar papillæ occur on the lateral walls of the isthmus faucium. The fungiform papillæ are small, and are scattered over the dorsum and sides of the tongue, but are absent on the root. There are usually two or three vallate papillæ on either side. Small foliate papillæ are also present. In the inferior part of the tip of the tongue is the **lyssa,** a fusiform cord, composed of fibrous tissue, muscular tissue, and fat. In large dogs it is about two inches (ca. 4 to 5 cm.) long.

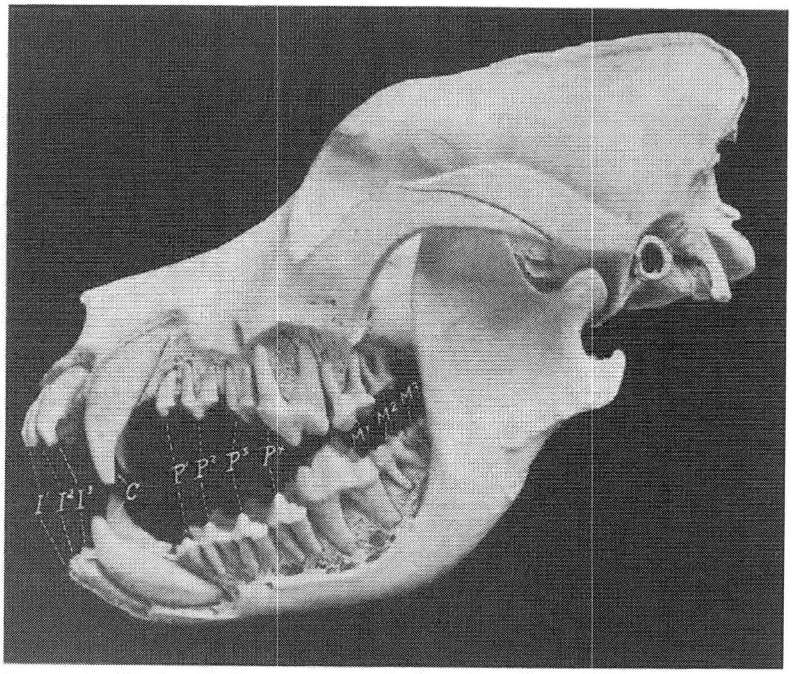

Fig. 327.—Skull of Adult St. Bernard Dog, Sculptured to Show the Embedded Parts of the Teeth. *I1–3*, incisors; *C*, canines; *P1–4*, premolars; *M1–3*, molars.

THE TEETH

The formula for the permanent teeth is:

$$2\left(I\frac{3}{3}\ C\frac{1}{1}\ P\frac{4}{4}\ M\frac{2}{3}\right) = 42$$

All of the teeth have short crowns and distinct necks; they erupt rapidly. The crowns are white, being destitute of cement.

The **incisors** are placed almost vertically and close together in the jaw-bones. They do not correspond to an opposing tooth, but rather to parts of two teeth of the other jaw. The crowns are trituberculate, the central projection being the largest. They increase in size from the first to the third. The labial surface is convex, the lingual slightly concave, and marked off from the neck by a V-shaped ridge, the cingulum. The roots are flattened transversely. The lower incisors are smaller than the upper ones. One or two supernumerary teeth may be present.

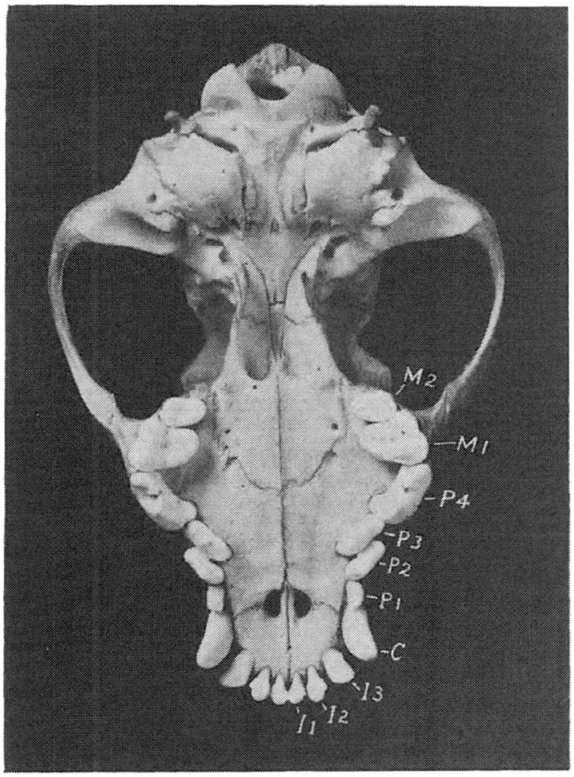

FIG. 328.—BASE OF SKULL OF COCKER SPANIEL.
I1–3 incisors; *C*, canine; *P1–4*, premolars; *M1–2*, molars. Note the crowding of the canines and premolars on account of the shortness of the jaw.

The **canine teeth** are large, conical, and curved. The upper canine is separated from the corner incisor by an interval into which the lower canine is received when the jaws are closed.[1] The lower canine is close to the corner incisor. The root is about an inch (ca. 2 to 3 cm.) long and is flattened laterally.

The **cheek teeth** are typically $\frac{6}{7}$, but in brachycephalic breeds they are commonly reduced to $\frac{5}{7}$, and in extreme cases even to $\frac{4}{5}$. The reduction occurs at either

[1] In the bull-dog, which is very prognathic ("undershot"), the lower canines are opposite to or slightly in front of the plane of the upper incisors, and the upper canines are about opposite to the first lower cheek teeth. In the epignathic ("overshot") dachshund the lower canines are under or slightly behind the upper ones.

end or at both ends of the series.[1] The first tooth appears only once. The fourth tooth of the upper row and the fifth of the lower row are much larger than the rest, and termed **sectorial** or **carnassial** teeth. From these the teeth diminish in size both forward and backward. The upper and lower teeth do not correspond, but rather dovetail. The teeth behind the sectorial ones are tuberculate, *i. e.*, have rounded eminences on the masticatory surface. The others are all sectorial in character, *i. e.*, have sharp-edged, pointed projections, the middle one being the most prominent. The premolars are laterally compressed, and are separated by intervals from the canines and from each other, except in the brachycephalic breeds. The upper molars have wide, somewhat quadrangular crowns, and three roots. The crown of the upper fourth premolar (Dens sectorius) is divided into two pointed lobes and has an antero-internal tubercle; it has three roots. The

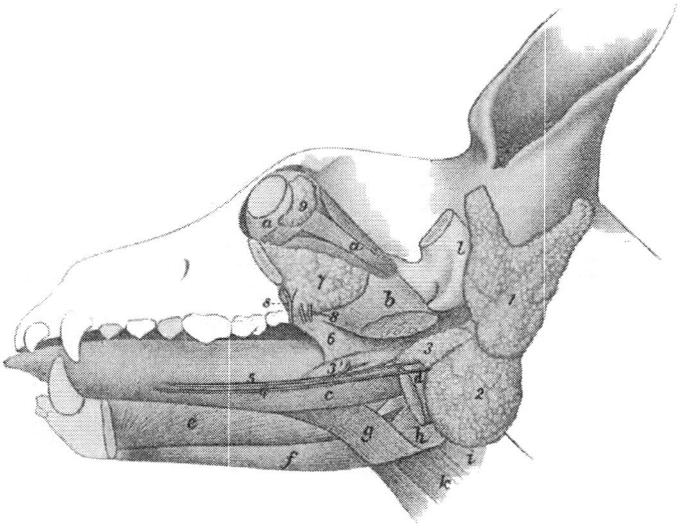

FIG. 329.—DISSECTION OF HEAD OF DOG, SHOWING SALIVARY GLANDS ETC.

a, Ocular muscles; *b*, pterygoideus internus (cut); *c*, stylo-glossus; *d*, digastricus (cut); *e*, genio-glossus; *f*, genio-hyoideus; *g*, hyo-glossus; *h*, thyro-pharyngeus; *i*, crico-pharyngeus; k, thyro-hyoideus; *l*, zygomatic process of temporal (sawn off); *1*, parotid gland; *2*, submaxillary gland; *3*, posterior part of sublingual gland; *3'*, anterior part of same; *4*, submaxillary duct; *5*, ductus sublingualis major; *6*, palatine glands; *7*, orbital or zygomatic gland; *8*, ducts of *7*; *9*, lacrimal gland. (Ducts colored red.) (After Ellenberger, in Leisering's Atlas.)

crown of the first lower molar (Dens sectorius) is compressed laterally and has two pointed, sharp-edged lobes, behind which are one or two tubercles; it has two roots.

The average periods of eruption are given below.

TOOTH	ERUPTION	CHANGE
I_1	4 to 5 weeks	
I_2	4 to 5 weeks	4 to 5 months
I_3	4 weeks	
C	3 to 4 weeks	4 to 5 months
P_1	4 to 5 months	
P_2	4 to 5 weeks	5 to 6 months
P_3	3 to 4 weeks	
P_4	3 to 4 weeks	
M_1	4 months	
M_2	upper 5 to 6 months; lower 4½ to 5 months	
M_3	6 to 7 months	

[1] Increase in number also occurs, the supernumerary teeth being at either end of the series.

THE SALIVARY GLANDS

The **parotid gland** is small. Its upper part is wide and is divided into two lobes by a deep notch into which the base of the ear is received. The lower end is small and overlaps the submaxillary gland. The duct leaves the gland at its anterior border, crosses the masseter muscle, and opens into the mouth opposite the third upper cheek tooth. Small accessory glands (Glandulæ parotidæ accessoriæ) are sometimes found along the course of the duct.

The **submaxillary gland** is usually larger than the parotid. In large dogs it is about two inches (ca. 5 cm.) long and an inch or more (ca. 3 cm.) wide. It is rounded in outline and of a pale yellow color. Its upper part is covered by the parotid, but it is otherwise superficial, and is palpable in the angle of junction of the jugular and external maxillary veins. The **duct** leaves the deep face of the gland, passes along the surface of the digastricus and stylo-glossus, and opens into the mouth near the frenum linguæ on a very indistinct papilla.

The **sublingual gland** is divided into two parts. The posterior part (Glandula sublingualis grandicanalaris) lies on the digastricus muscle in intimate relation with

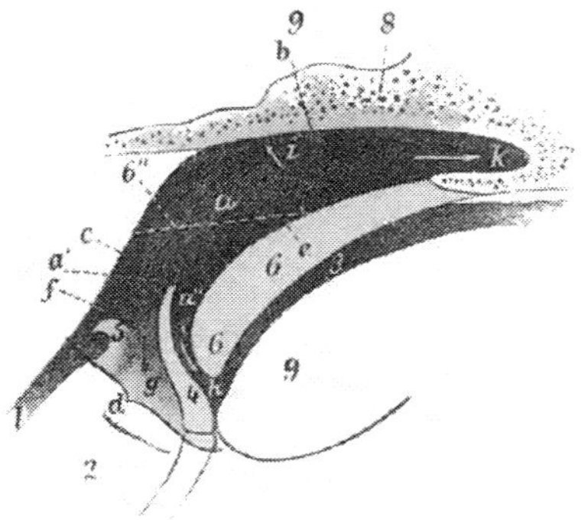

FIG. 330.—SAGITTAL SECTION OF PHARYNGEAL AND LARYNGEAL REGIONS OF DOG.

1, Œsophagus; *2*, larynx; *3*, mouth cavity; *4*, epiglottis; *5*, arytenoid cartilage; *6*, soft palate; *6″*, position of soft palate when raised; *7*, vomer; *8*, base of cranium; *9*, root of tongue; *a*, *a′*, *a″*, pharynx; *b*, fornix of pharynx; *c*, posterior wall of pharynx; *d*, floor of pharynx; *e*, pharyngeal surface of soft palate; *f*, origin of œsophagus; *g*, vestibule of larynx; *h*, isthmus faucium; *i*, Eustachian opening; k, posterior naris. (After Ellenberger, in Leisering's Atlas.)

the submaxillary gland, but clearly separable from it after removal of the common fibrous capsule. It has a pointed anterior process. The **duct** (Ductus sublingualis major) accompanies the submaxillary duct, and usually opens beside it, but in some cases joins it. The anterior part (Glandula sublingualis parvicanalaris) is long and narrow; it lies on the stylo-glossus muscle. It has a number (8 to 12) of small **ducts** (Ductus sublinguales minores), some of which open directly into the mouth, while others join the large duct.

The **orbital** or **zygomatic gland** (Glandula zygomatica) represents the superior molar glands of herbivora. It is prismatic and is situated in the orbital region, between the zygomatic arch and the internal pterygoid muscle, in contact with the periorbita. It has four or five **ducts** (Ductus zygomatici) which open near the last upper cheek tooth; one of them (canal of Nuck) is almost as large as the parotid duct; the others are small.

THE PHARYNX

The fornix is narrow. The orifices of the Eustachian tubes are small and slit-like; the end of the tube causes a rounded projection of the mucous membrane

(Torus tubarius). The œsophageal opening is relatively small and is encircled by a fold of the mucous membrane. The hyo-pharyngeus muscle is clearly divided into a kerato-pharyngeus and a chondro-pharyngeus.

THE ŒSOPHAGUS

The **œsophagus** is relatively wide and dilatable except at its origin. The constriction at its origin is termed the **isthmus œsophagi.** The cardiac end is slightly dilated; it joins the stomach under the tenth or eleventh thoracic vertebra, slightly to the left of the median plane. The muscular tissue is striated and consists mainly of two layers of spiral fibers which cross each other; near the cardia, however, the fibers are longitudinal and circular. There are mucous glands and lymph glands in the submucosa throughout.

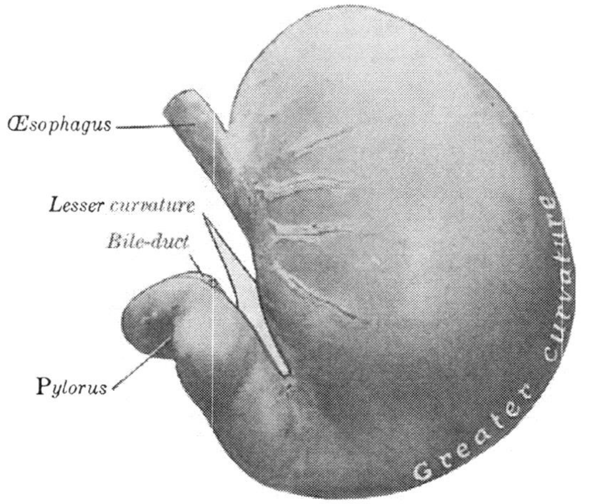

FIG. 331.—STOMACH OF DOG, PARIETAL SURFACE.
Organ fixed *in situ* when well filled.

THE STOMACH

The **stomach** is relatively large. Its capacity in a dog weighing about 40 pounds is about six to seven pints.

Colin estimates the average capacity at about 3 liters (ca. 6½ pints), with a range between 0.6 and 8 liters (ca. 1⅓ to 17½ pints). Neumayer gives the capacity as 100 to 250 c.c.per kilogram of body-weight (ca. 2.7 ounces per pound). The average capacity of the human stomach is estimated at 35 to 40 ounces—only about one-half of that of a dog of medium size.

When full it is irregularly pyriform. The left or cardiac part (Corpus ventriculi) is large and rounded, while the right or pyloric part (Pars pylorica) is small and cylindrical. When empty, or nearly so, the left sac is strongly contracted; the pyloric part is not materially affected by variations in the amount of ingesta.

The parietal surface of the full stomach is very extensive, strongly convex, and faces partly forward, but largely to the left. It is related to the liver, the left part of the diaphragm, and the left and ventral abdominal wall as far back as a transverse section through the second or third lumbar vertebra.

The visceral surface is much less extensive and is considerably flattened; it faces chiefly to the right, and is related to the intestine, pancreas, and left kidney.

The upper part of the lesser curvature is nearly straight and vertical, but the lower part forms a deep, narrow angle, due to the fact that the pyloric part is directed sharply forward and upward.

The greater curvature is nearly four times as long as the lesser curvature. In the full stomach it extends considerably behind the left costal arch (having carried the spleen backward); ventrally, it lies on the abdominal wall, almost midway from the xiphoid cartilage to the pubis.

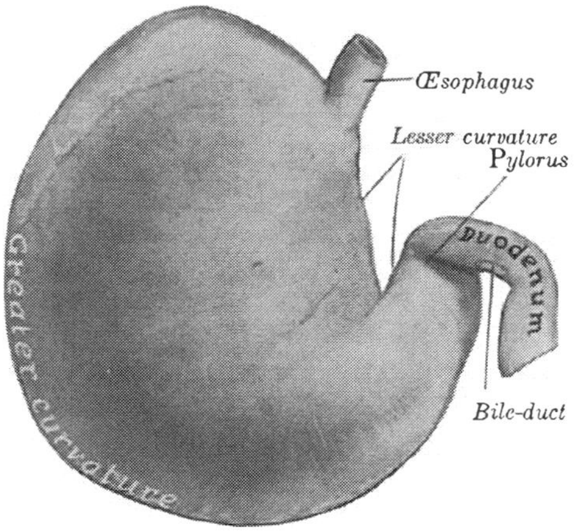

FIG. 332.—STOMACH OF DOG, VISCERAL SURFACE. Organ fixed *in situ* when well filled.

The left extremity or fundus is large and rounded; it is the most dorsal part of the organ, and lies under the dorsal ends of the eleventh and twelfth ribs.

The pyloric extremity is small and is directed forward and somewhat upward; it lies usually about an inch or two (ca. 3.5 to 5 cm.) below the cardia, a little to the right of the median plane. It is related to the portal fissure of the liver and to the pancreas.

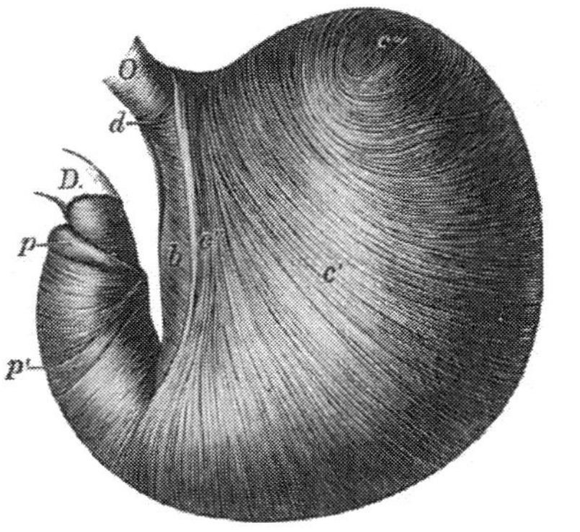

FIG. 333.—EVERTED STOMACH OF DOG FROM WHICH THE MUCOUS MEMBRANE IS REMOVED.

O, Œsophagus; *D*, duodenum; *b*, circular fibers; *c'*, internal oblique fibers; *c''*, cardiac loop; *c'''*, transition of internal to external oblique fibers; *d*, fibers uniting branches of cardiac loop; *p*, pyloric sphincter; *p'*, antral sphincter. (Ellenberger-Baum, Anat. d. Haustiere.)

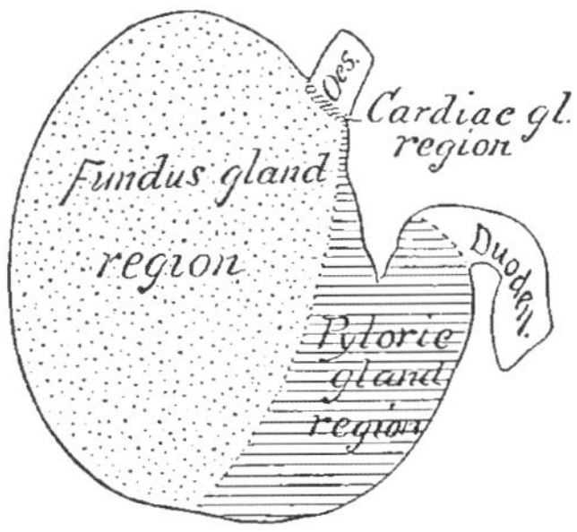

FIG. 334.—DIAGRAM OF ZONES OF MUCOUS MEMBRANE OF STOMACH OF DOG.

The cardia is situated about two to three inches (ca. 5 to 7 cm.) from the left extremity, and is oval; it lies a little to the left of the median plane, below the tenth or eleventh thoracic vertebra.

When empty, or nearly so, the stomach is separated from the ventral abdominal wall by the liver and small intestine, and the greater curvature extends back to the eleventh or twelfth rib. In this state there is not rarely a marked constriction between the right and left portions.

The longitudinal muscular fibers are found on the curvatures and on the pyloric part. The oblique fibers are arranged in two layers: the external layer is a continuation of the longitudinal fibers of the œsophagus onto the body and fundus. The circular layer covers the whole stomach except the fundus, and forms a pyloric sphincter and an antral sphincter. The internal oblique layer is arranged as in the horse, and forms a similar loop-like, cardiac sphincter.

Three regions of the mucous membrane exist. Cardiac glands are found in a very narrow pale zone around the cardiac opening, and also scattered along the lesser curvature. The fundus gland region has a thick, reddish-brown mucous mem-

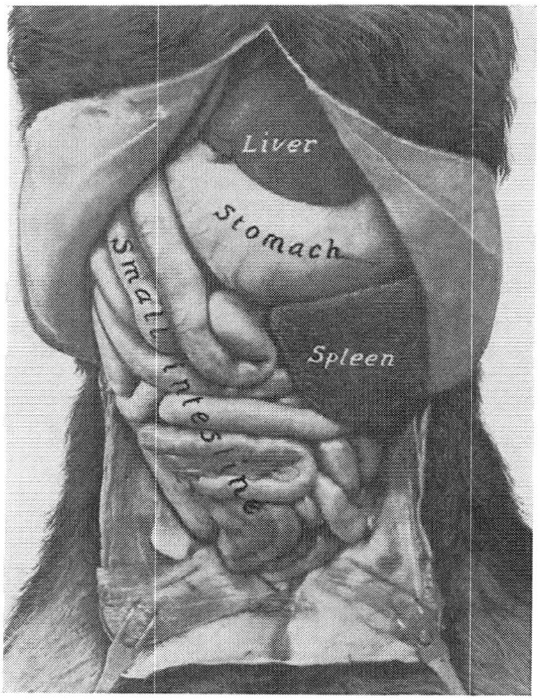

FIG. 335.—ABDOMINAL VISCERA OF DOG.
Superficial ventral View after removal of the great omentum. From photograph of formalin-hardened subject.

brane, which lines about two-thirds of the organ. The pyloric mucous membrane is thinner and pale; in the dead subject it is often stained by regurgitated bile.

THE INTESTINE

The intestine is short—about five or six times the length of the body.

The **small intestine** has an average length of about thirteen feet (ca. 4 meters). It occupies most of the abdominal cavity behind the liver and stomach. The duod enum begins at the portal fissure and passes backward and upward, at first on the visceral surface of the liver, then in contact with the right flank. Near the pelvis it turns inward and sharply forward, passes along the inner border of the left kidney, and joins the jejunum to the left of the root of the mesentery. The mesoduodenum is given off from the common mesentery; it is a relatively wide fold, except at the terminal part. Here there are two short folds, one of which joins the mesocolon; the other passes on to the terminal part of the colon. The first part of the mesoduodenum contains the right branch of the pancreas. Its root is blended with the mesocolon to form a common mesentery. The remainder of the small intestine forms numerous coils, and is attached by a wide mesentery to the sublumbar region. The **pancreatic** and **bile ducts** open into the duodenum about two or three inches (ca. 5 to 8 cm.) from the pylorus; the **accessory pancreatic duct** opens an inch or two (ca. 2.5 to 5 cm.) further back. The mucous membrane has very long villi. The duodenal (Brunner's) glands occur only near the pylorus. Peyer's patches are numerous (about twenty in young subjects), and begin in the duodenum. They are usually elliptical in outline, but the last one is band-like, reaches to the end

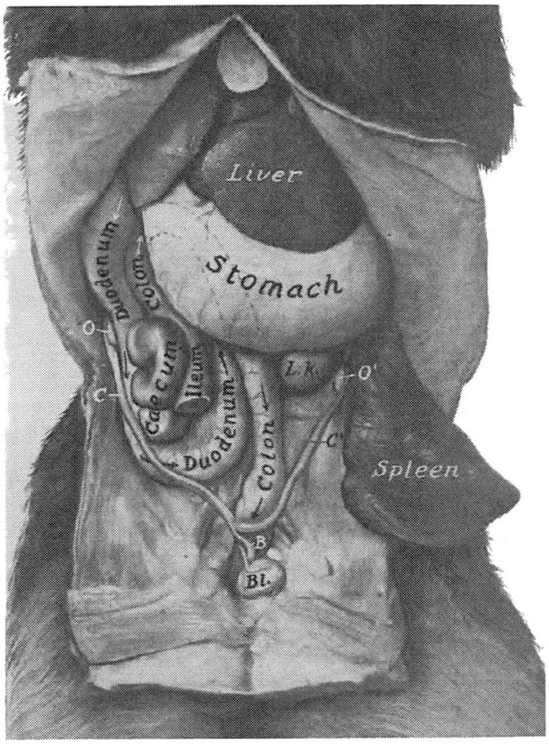

FIG. 336.—DEEP DISSECTION OF ABDOMINAL VISCERA OF DOG (FEMALE).
Bl., Bladder; *B*, body; *C, C'*, cornua of uterus; *O, O'*, ovaries; *L. K.*, left kidney. The concealed part of the colon is indicated by dotted lines. (From photograph of formalin-hardened subject.)

of the ileum and is four to sixteen inches (ca. 10 to 40 cm.) long in young dogs (Ellenberger). There is an ileo-cæcal valve.[1] The muscular coat is relatively thick.

The **large intestine** is two to two and a half feet (ca. 60 to 75 cm.) long. Its caliber is about the same as that of the small intestine, and it has neither longitudinal bands nor sacculations.

The **cæcum** is about three or four inches (ca. 8 to 10 cm.) long, and is twisted in a spiral fashion. The twist is maintained by the peritoneum, which attaches it

[1] The valve does not seem to be efficient, since experience shows that rectal injections can be made to pass beyond it. This may be partly due also to the fact that the terminal part of the ileum runs horizontally forward, and the ileo-cæcal orifice faces into the beginning of the colon.

to the ileum. It is situated usually against the middle of the upper part of the right flank, below the duodenum and the right branch of the pancreas.[1]

The **colon** is attached to the sublumbar region by a mesentery, the mesocolon. It presents three parts, which correspond to the ascending, transverse, and descending colon of man. The first or right part (Colon ascendens) is very short. It begins at the junction of the ileum and cæcum, and passes forward along the inner surface of the duodenum and the right branch of the pancreas till it reaches the pyloric part of the stomach; here it turns inward and crosses the median plane, forming the transverse part (Colon transversum). The third or left part (Colon descendens) passes backward in the sublumbar region along the inner border or ventral surface of the left kidney; then inclines toward the median plane and joins the rectum.[2] The caliber of the colon is about the same throughout. It has no bands nor sacculations.

The mucous membrane of the cæcum contains numerous solitary glands; they are found also in the first part of the colon.

The **rectum** is almost completely covered with peritoneum, the line of peritoneal reflection being under the second or third coccygeal vertebra. At the junction of the rectum and anus the mucous membrane has a stratified, squamous epithelium, and contains the **anal glands.** A small opening on either side leads into two lateral **anal sacs** (Sinus paranales); these are usually about the size of a hazelnut, and contain a dirty gray, fatty substance, which has a peculiar and very unpleasant odor. The skin which lines these pouches contains coil-glands. Further back the skin contains large sebaceous glands and peculiar **circumanal glands.**

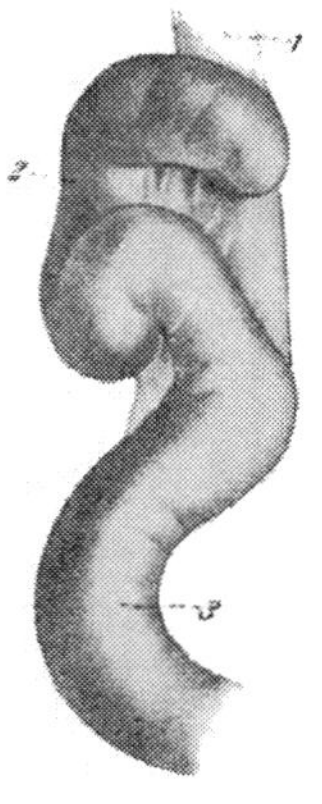

FIG. 337.—CÆCUM OF DOG.
1, ileum; *2*, cæcum; *3*, colon. (From Leisering's Atlas.)

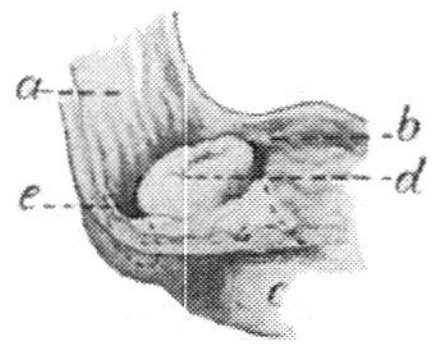

FIG. 338.—TERMINATION OF ILEUM OF DOG.
a, Colon; *b*, cæcum; *c*, ileum; *d*, ileo-cæcal opening; *e*, circular depression around end of ileum. (After P. Schumann.)

The retractor ani muscle is extensive. It arises from the shaft of the ilium, the pubis, and the symphysis pelvis, and passes upward and backward to end on the first coccygeal vertebræ and the sphincter ani externus. The retractors, together with the coccygei, form a sort of pelvic diaphragm, analogous to that of man.

THE LIVER

The liver is relatively large, weighing usually about 5 per cent. of the body-weight. It is divided into six or seven **lobes** by fissures which converge at the portal fissure. When the gland is examined in the soft condition, all the lobes are visible on the visceral surface, but usually only four on the parietal surface.

The left **lateral** lobe is the largest, and is oval in outline. The left **central lobe**

[1] Ellenberger and Baum state that the cæcum may reach a length of 20 cm. in very large dogs.

[2] When the stomach is very full, it pushes the left portion of the colon over to the right, producing an acute angle in place of a transverse branch. The terminal part of the colon is thus oblique in direction.

is much smaller and is prismatic. The **right central lobe** is second in size, and presents a somewhat tongue-shaped quadrate lobe, marked off by the deep fissure in which the gall-bladder lies. The **right lateral lobe** is third in size, and is oval in outline. On its visceral surface is the large **caudate lobe**; this consists of two parts

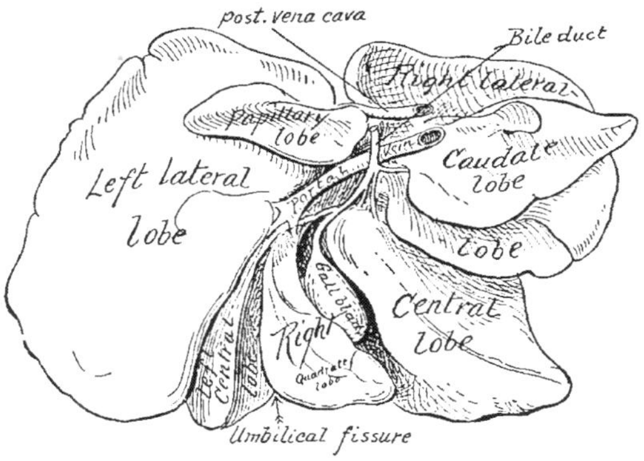

FIG. 339.—LIVER OF DOG.
Soft specimen sketched with lobes drawn apart.

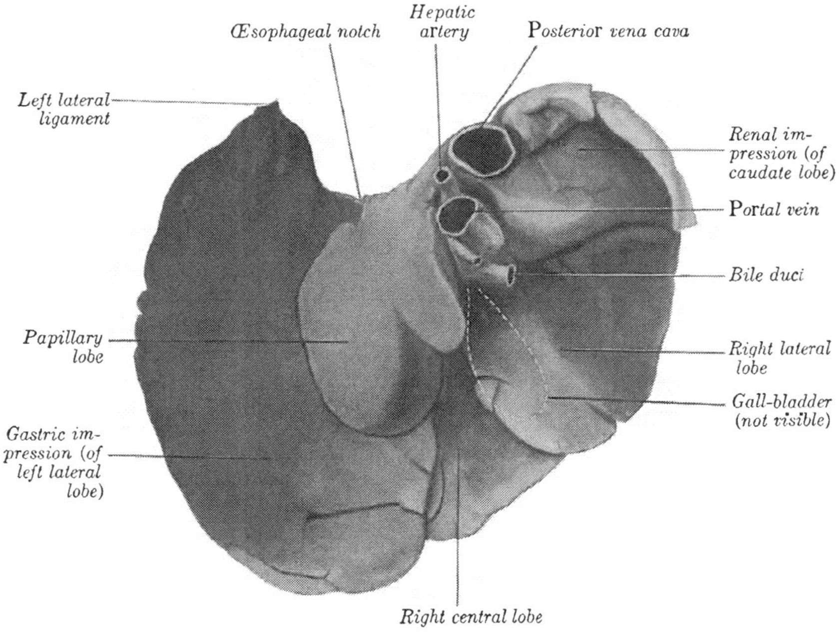

FIG. 340.—LIVER OF DOG, VISCERAL SURFACE; HARDENED *in situ*.
Left central lobe, gall-bladder, and great part of right central lobe not visible.

—on the right, the caudate process; on the left, the papillary process or lobe, both often being subdivided by fissures.

When hardened *in situ* (with the stomach full), the gland presents the following characters:

The visceral surface is marked by a somewhat oblique ridge (corresponding to the lesser curvature of the stomach), which separates two deep cavities. The depression to the left of the ridge is occupied by the body and fundus of the stomach. The depression on the right is smaller, and is occupied by the pyloric part of the stomach, the origin of the duodenum, and the right branch of the pancreas. The gall-bladder is not visible.

When the stomach is empty and contracted, the visceral surface of the liver is strikingly different. There is then a shallow impression for the left part of the stomach on the left lobe, and a large convex area, related to the small intestine and a mass of omentum. The pyloric and duodenal impressions are not much changed. The gall-bladder is visible.

The portal fissure is very deep and might well be termed a fossa. It is bounded on the right (externally) by the caudate process, on the left (internally) by the papillary process or lobe, which is directed ventrally. The hepatic artery enters at the dorsal end and the portal vein centrally, while the bile duct leaves at the ventral part. The left central lobe is not visible, and the right central one is largely concealed.

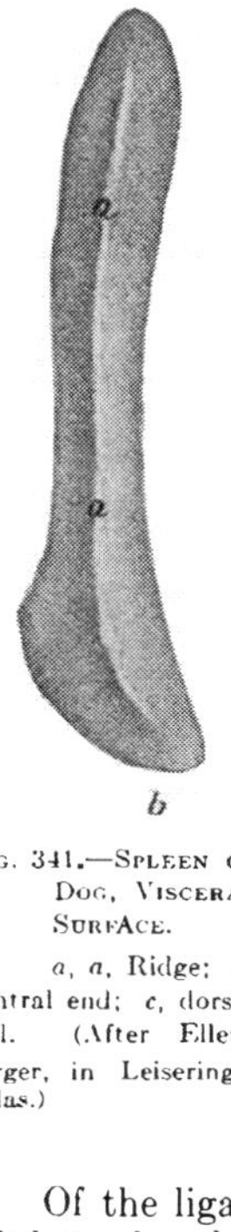

FIG. 341.—SPLEEN OF DOG, VISCERAL SURFACE.
a, a, Ridge; *b*, ventral end; *c*, dorsal end. (After Ellenberger, in Leisering's Atlas.)

The parietal surface is extremely convex, being adapted to the diaphragm and the adjacent part of the ventral wall of the abdomen. On it all the lobes except the papillary are completely or partially visible. The gall-bladder is visible in the fissure between the quadrate and chief portions of the right central lobe.

The dorsal border presents a renal impression on its right portion. The posterior vena cava passes downward and forward at first in a deep groove on the caudate lobe, then largely embedded in the parietal surface of the right lateral lobe; it receives two large hepatic veins just before piercing the diaphragm.

The œsophageal notch is large, and is occupied on the right by the thick margin of the hiatus œsophageus. The left border is opposite to the ninth and tenth ribs; it is thin and is marked by numerous indentations. The caudate process extends usually a little beyond the last right rib, between the right kidney and the right branch of the pancreas. The ventral border lies on the ventral abdominal wall a variable distance behind the xiphoid cartilage.

The **gall-bladder** lies in the fossa vesicæ felleæ, between the two parts of the right central lobe; it does not reach to the ventral border of the liver. The cystic duct joins the hepatic duct at the lower part of the portal fissure, forming with it the bile duct (Ductus choledochus); the latter passes to the right and opens into the duodenum, about two or three inches (ca. 5 to 8 cm.) from the pylorus.

Of the ligaments, the coronary and right lateral are well developed, but the left lateral and falciform are small.

THE PANCREAS

The **pancreas** is **V**-shaped, consisting of two long narrow branches, which meet at an acute angle above the pylorus. The right **branch** extends backward above the first part of the duodenum, below the caudate lobe of the liver and the right kidney, and ends usually a short distance behind the latter. The left **branch** passes inward and backward on the visceral surface of the stomach, and ends under the left kidney. There are two **ducts**: the larger one unites with the bile duct, while the smaller one enters the duodenum an inch or two (ca. 3 to 5 cm.) further back.

THE SPLEEN

The **spleen** is bright red in color in the fresh state. It is somewhat falciform, long, and narrow; the ventral part is the widest. Its position varies in accordance with the fullness of the stomach. When that organ is moderately full the long axis of the spleen corresponds to the direction of the last rib. Its parietal surface

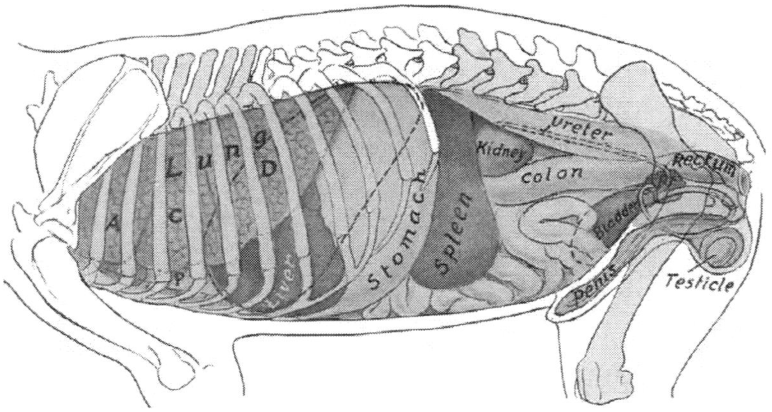

FIG. 342.—PROJECTION OF VISCERA OF DOG (MALE) ON BODY WALL, LEFT SIDE.
A, C, D, Apical, cardiac, and diaphragmatic lobes of lung; *P,* pericardium; *Pr,* prostate. Costal attachment and median line of diaphragm are dotted.

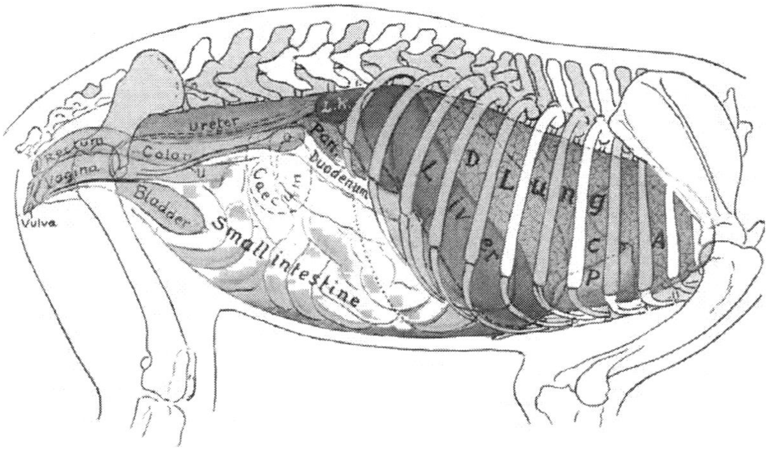

FIG. 343.—PROJECTION OF VISCERA OF DOG (FEMALE) ON BODY WALL, RIGHT SIDE.
A, C, D, Apical, cardiac, and diaphragmatic lobes of right lung; *P.,* pericardium; *L. K.,* right kidney; *Pan.,* right branch of pancreas; *O,* ovary; *U,* cornu of uterus. Costal attachment and median line of diaphragm are dotted; also posterior contour of stomach.

is convex and lies largely against the left flank. The visceral surface is concave in its length, and is marked by a longitudinal ridge, on which the vessels and nerves are situated. The dorsal end lies against the left kidney and left crus of the diaphragm. The ventral end is a little further back, and reaches to the ventral wall of the abdomen. It is so loosely attached by the great omentum as to be regarded as an appendage of the latter.

THE RESPIRATORY SYSTEM

The organs of respiration (Apparatus respiratorius) comprise the **nasal cavity**,[1] the **pharynx**, the **larynx**, the **trachea**, the **bronchi**, and the **lungs**. The lungs are the central organs in which the exchange of gases between the blood and the air takes place; the other parts of the system are passages by which the air passes to and from the lungs. The nasal cavity opens externally at the nostrils, and communicates behind with the pharynx through the posterior nares (Choanæ); it contains the peripheral part of the olfactory apparatus, which mediates the sense of smell. The pharynx is a common passage for the air and food—a remnant of the primitive embryonic arrangement; it has been described as a part of the digestive tube. The larynx is a complex valvular apparatus which regulates the volume of air passing through the tract; it is also the chief organ of voice. The trachea, and the bronchi formed by its bifurcation, are permanently open conducting tubes. The thorax, the pleural sacs which it contains, and the muscles which increase or diminish the size of the cavity are also parts of the system. The bones, joints, and muscles of the thorax have already been described.

For topographic reasons two ductless glands, the **thyroid** and the **thymus**, are usually described in this section, although they are in no sense a part of the respiratory system.

RESPIRATORY SYSTEM OF THE HORSE

THE NASAL CAVITY

The **nasal cavity** (Cavum nasi), the first segment of the respiratory tract, is a long, somewhat cylindrical passage, inclosed by all the facial bones except the mandible and hyoid. It is separated from the mouth ventrally by the palate. It opens externally at the nostrils, and communicates posteriorly with the pharynx through the posterior nares.

The **nostrils** or **anterior nares** (Nares) are somewhat oval in outline, and are placed obliquely, so that they are closer together below than above. They are bounded by two **alæ** or wings (Alæ nasi), which meet above and below, forming the **commissures**. The outer ala is concave; the inner one is convex above, concave below. The upper commissure is narrow, the lower one wide and rounded. If the finger is passed into the nostril at the upper commissure, it enters the so-called **false nostril**, which leads backward to a blind cutaneous pouch. This cul-de-sac, the **diverticulum nasi**, extends backward to the angle of junction of the nasal bone and the nasal process of the premaxilla. The posterior part of the diverticulum is blind, but the false nostril communicates below and internally with the vestibule of the nasal cavity. The external opening of the **naso-lacrimal duct** is seen when the nostril is dilated; it is situated on the floor of the vestibule, perforating the skin close to its junction with the mucous membrane, about two inches (ca. 5 cm.) from the lower commissure. (It is not rare to find one or two accessory orifices further back.)

Structure.—The **skin** around the nostrils presents long tactile hairs as well as the ordinary ones. It is continued around the alæ and lines the vestibule. In the

[1] An external nose (Nasus externus), such as exists in man, forming a projection distinctly marked off from the rest of the face, does not exist in the domesticated animals.

posterior part of the diverticulum the skin is thin and usually black, and is covered with exceedingly fine hairs; it is provided with numerous sebaceous glands. The inner wing is supported by the **alar cartilage** (Cartilago alaris), which is shaped somewhat like a comma, the convex margin being direct medially. The cartilages are attached by fibrous tissue to the extremity of the septal cartilage. Each consists of an upper, quadrilateral curved plate, the **lamina,** and a narrow **cornu** which curves downward and outward, supporting the inner wing and the lower commissure, but not entering into the formation of the outer wing. The lamina causes the projection of the upper part of the internal wing, from which the thick **alar fold** (Plica alaris) passes backward along the external wall of the nasal cavity to cover the cartilaginous prolongation of the inferior turbinal bone. This fold separates the true from the false nostril. The extremity of the cornu usually causes a slight projection of the skin a short distance behind and below the lower commissure.

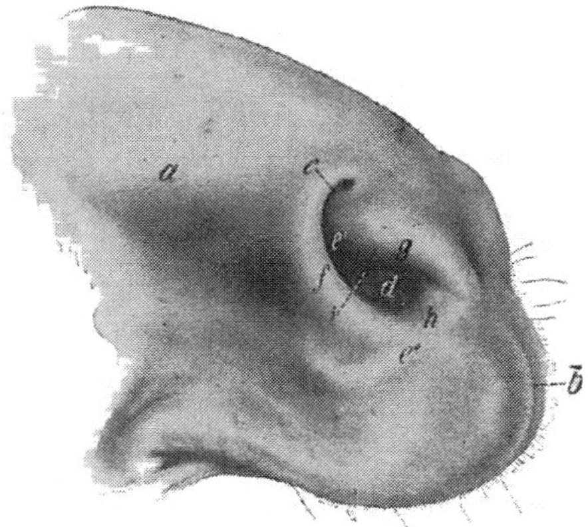

FIG. 344.—NOSTRILS OF HORSE.

a, Diverticulum nasi (shown as if distended); *b*, philtrum; *c*, false nostril; *d*, true nostril; *e'*, prominence caused by lamina of alar cartilage; *e''*, prominence over cornu of same; *f*, external wing of nostril; *g*, internal wing; *h*, lower commissure; *i*, orifice of naso-lacrimal duct. (Ellenberger-Baum, Anat. d. Haustiere.)

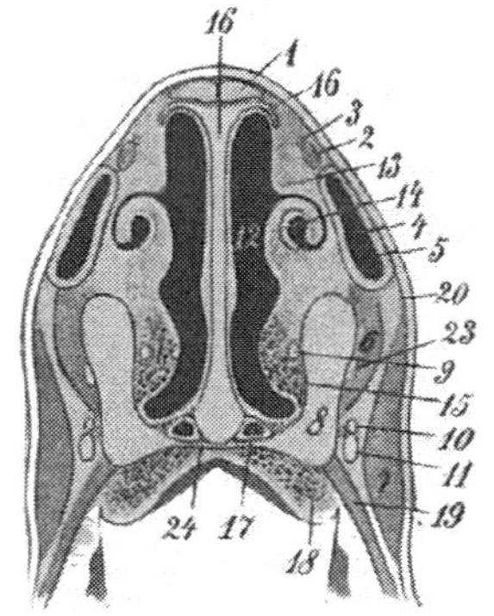

FIG. 345.—CROSS-SECTION OF NARIAL REGION OF HORSE.

1, Nasal bone; *2*, tendon of levator labii superioris proprius; *3*, external nasal nerve; *4*, nasal diverticulum; *5*, outer wall of *4*; *6*, dilatator naris inferior; *7*, levator nasolabialis + dilatator naris lateralis; *8*, maxilla and premaxilla; *9*, naso-lacrimal duct; *10*, *11*, chief branches of superior labial nerve, with superior labial artery at their inner side; *12*, nasal cavity; *13*, superior turbinal fold; *14*, inferior turbinal fold, inclosing cartilaginous prolongation of inferior turbinal bone; *15*, venous plexus; *16*, septum nasi; *16'*, parietal cartilage; *17*, vomero-nasal organ (of Jacobson); *18*, venous plexus of palate; *19*, buccinator; *20*, skin; *23*, anterior nasal nerve; *24*, palatine process of premaxilla. (After Ellenberger-Baum, Top. Anat. d. Pferdes.)

The muscles of the nostrils have been described.

Blood-supply.—Palato-labial, superior labial, and lateral nasal arteries.

Nerve-supply.—Trigeminal and facial nerves.

The nasal cavity is divided into two symmetrical halves by the median **septum nasi.** The osseous part of the septum (Septum osseum) is formed behind by the perpendicular plate of the ethmoid and below by the vomer. A few ridges on the former correspond to the ethmoidal meatuses. The major part of it, however, is formed by the **septal cartilage** (Cartilago septi nasi). The surfaces of the cartilage are marked by faint grooves for the vessels and nerves which course over it. The **dorsal border** is attached along the frontal and nasal sutures, and extends beyond the apices of the nasal bones about two inches (ca. 5 cm.). From this border a thin, narrow plate, the **parietal cartilage** (Cartilago parietalis) curves outward for a short distance on either side. Near the nostrils these plates are somewhat wider, partially making good the defect in the bony roof of the cavity in this situation. The **ventral** border is thick and rounded; it lies chiefly in the groove of the vomer, but anteriorly it occupies the space between the premaxillary bones. The **posterior border** is continuous with the perpendicular plate of the ethmoid bone.[1] The alar cartilages are attached to the anterior extremity by fibrous tissue in such a manner as to allow very free movement—in fact, an actual joint may be found. The ventral part of the cartilage is about half an inch (ca. 1 cm.), the middle part about one-tenth of an inch (ca. 2.5 mm.), and the dorsal part about a quarter to a third of an inch (ca. 6 to 8 mm.) in thickness.

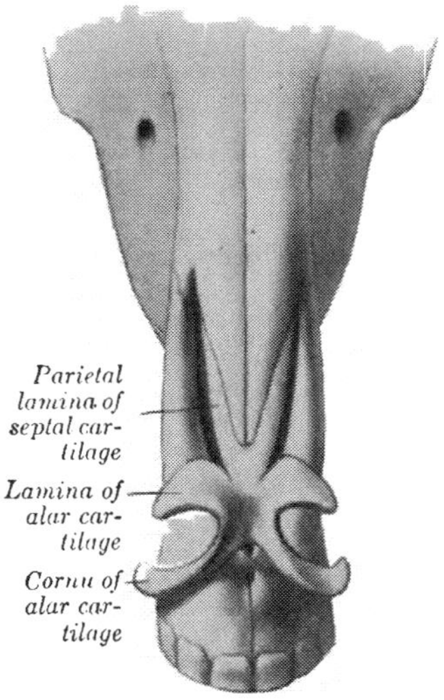

FIG. 346.—NASAL CARTILAGES OF HORSE, DORSAL VIEW. (After Ellenberger-Baum, Anat. für Künstler.)

The two **turbinal bones** (Conchæ nasales) project from the lateral wall, and divide the outer part of the cavity into three **meatuses**—superior, middle, and inferior.

The **superior meatus** (Meatus nasi dorsalis) is a narrow passage, bounded dorsally by the roof of the cavity, and ventrally by the superior turbinal bone; its posterior end is closed by the junction of the inner plate of the frontal bone with the cribriform plate and lateral mass of the ethmoid. It transmits air to the upper part of the olfactory region.

The **middle meatus** (Meatus nasi medius) is between the two turbinal bones. It is somewhat larger than the superior meatus, and does not extend back so far; it ends near the great ethmoturbinal and the ethmoidal meatuses.

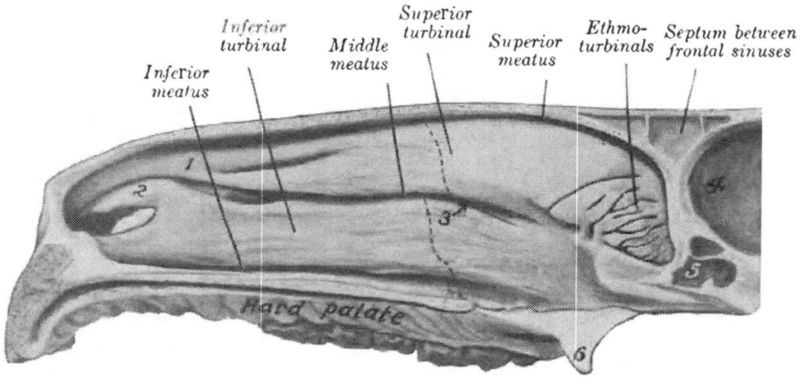

FIG. 347.—NASAL CAVITY OF HORSE, SAGITTAL SECTION WITH SEPTUM REMOVED.

1, Superior turbinal fold; *2*, alar fold, containing cartilaginous prolongation of inferior turbinal; *3*, arrow pointing to naso-maxillary fissure; *4*, cranial cavity; *5*, sphenoidal sinus; *6*, hamulus of pterygoid bone. The olfactory mucous membrane is shaded. Dotted lines indicate anterior limit of uncoiled parts of turbinal bones, which inclose parts of frontal and maxillary sinuses.

In its posterior part is found the extremely narrow, slit-like interval by which the

[1] The septal cartilage is to be regarded as an unossified part of the mesethmoid. It will be noted that the line of demarcation between the bone and the cartilage is irregular and varies with age; extensive ossification (or calcification) of the cartilage is commonly found in old animals. The process often results in the formation of calcareous islands in the cartilage.

maxillary sinus communicates with the nasal cavity—the **naso-maxillary fissure** (Aditus naso-maxillaris). The fissure is not visible from the nasal side, being concealed by the overhanging superior turbinal. A fine flexible probe, passed outward and somewhat backward between the turbinal bones, enters the maxillary sinus; if introduced a little further in the same direction, it usually passes through the orifice of communication between the maxillary and the frontal sinus and enters the latter.

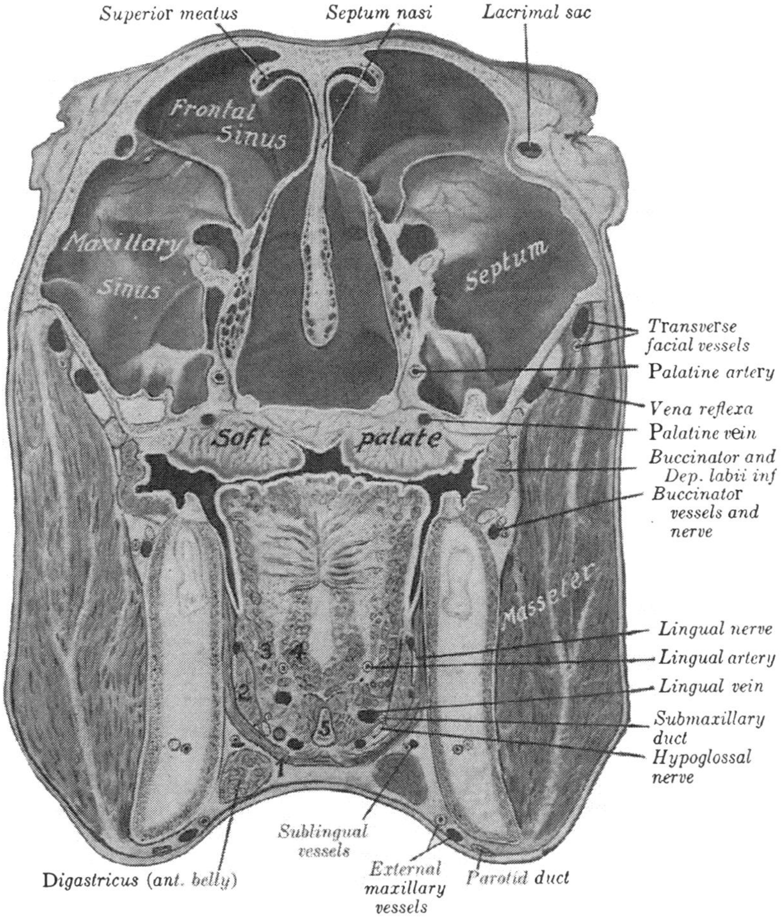

FIG. 348.—CROSS-SECTION OF HEAD OF HORSE. THE SECTION PASSES THROUGH THE INTERNAL CANTHI. *1*, Mylo-hyoideus; *2*, stylo-glossus; *3*, hyo-glossus; *4*, genio-glossus; *5*, lingual process of hyoid bone. An arrow points to the naso-maxillary fissure.

A small part of the fissure usually brings the anterior division of the maxillary sinus into communication with the nasal cavity. The spaces inclosed by the coiled portions of the turbinals also open into the middle meatus. This passage may be characterized as the sinus-meatus, but it also conducts air to the olfactory region.

The **inferior meatus** (Meatus nasi ventralis) is situated between the inferior turbinal and the floor of the cavity. It is much larger than the other two, and is the direct passage between the nostrils and the pharynx.

The **common meatus** (Meatus nasi communis) is situated between the septum and the turbinals, and is continuous externally with the other meatuses. It is very narrow dorsally, but widens ventrally.

The lateral masses of the ethmoid bone project forward into the posterior part (fundus) of the nasal cavity (Fig. 347). Between the ethmoturbinals of which each mass is composed there are three principal and numerous small passages, the **ethmoidal meatuses** (Meatus ethmoidales).

The **posterior nares** (Choanæ) are two elliptical orifices by which the nasal cavity and pharynx communicate. They are in the same plane as the floor of the nasal cavity, and are separated from each other by the vomer. They are, taken together, about two inches (ca. 5 cm.) wide and three to four inches (ca. 8 to 10 cm.) long.

The **nasal mucous membrane** (Membrana mucosa nasi) is thick, highly vascular, and is, in general, firmly attached to the underlying periosteum and perichondrium. It is continuous in front with the skin which lines the nostrils, and behind with the mucous membrane of the pharynx. It is also continuous at the naso-maxillary fissure with the very thin and only slightly vascular mucous membrane which lines the sinuses. In the anterior part of the cavity it forms prominent thick folds on the lateral wall, which extend from the turbinal bones to the nostril. There are usually two **superior turbinal folds** which unite anteriorly. The upper one incloses a thin plate of cartilage which is continuous with the superior turbinal bone. The **inferior turbinal fold** is curved, and incloses an ∽ shaped cartilaginous plate which prolongs the inferior turbinal bone; this fold is continuous with the alar fold of the nostril, and forms with it the upper margin of the entrance from the true nostril to the nasal cavity. Below this there is a rounded ridge produced by the nasal process of the premaxilla. The mucous membrane of the greater part of the cavity (Regio respiratoria) is red in color, and is covered with a stratified ciliated epithelium. It contains numerous acinous **nasal glands** (Glandulæ nasales). The submucosa contains rich venous plexuses which form in certain situations a sort of cavernous tissue (Plexus cavernosus), composed of several strata of freely anastomosing veins, between which there are unstriped muscle-fibers. This arrangement is most marked in the turbinal folds, on the lower part of the inferior turbinal bone, and the lower part of the septum. On the posterior part of the lateral masses of the ethmoid and the adjacent part of the superior turbinal and the septum (Regio olfactoria) the mucous membrane is brownish-yellow in color and thicker; it contains the olfactory nerve-endings in a special non-ciliated epithelium. In it are numerous **olfactory glands** (Glandulæ olfactoriæ); these are long, tubular, and often branched.

The **vomero-nasal organ** of Jacobson (Organon vomeronasale) is situated on the floor of the nasal cavity, on either side of the ventral border of the septum (Fig. 345.) It consists of a tubular cartilage lined with mucous membrane, to which fibers of the olfactory nerve may be traced. Its anterior part communicates with the nasal cavity by a slit-like orifice.

The **paranasal sinuses** are described in the Osteology.

THE LARYNX

The **larynx** is a short tube which connects the pharynx and trachea. It is a complex valvular apparatus, which regulates the volume of air in respiration, prevents aspiration of foreign bodies, and is the chief organ of voice.

It is situated partly between the internal pterygoid muscles, partly in the neck between the parotid glands.[1] Its long axis is practically horizontal when the head and neck are extended (Fig. 254).

It is related dorsally to the pharynx and the origin of the œsophagus. Ventrally it is covered by the skin, fascia, and sterno-hyoid and omo-hyoid muscles. Laterally it is related to the parotid and submaxillary glands and to the internal pterygoid, stylo-maxillaris, digastricus, stylo-hyoid, and pharyngeal constrictor muscles.

It is attached to the body and thyroid cornua of the hyoid bone, and thus indirectly to the base of the cranium.

Its cavity communicates anteriorly with the pharynx and (potentially) with the mouth; posteriorly, with the trachea.

The wall of the larynx consists of a framework of cartilages, connected by joints and ligaments or membranes, and moved by extrinsic and intrinsic muscles. The cavity is lined with mucous membrane.

Cartilages of the Larynx

There are three single cartilages and one pair; the single cartilages are the cricoid, thyroid, and epiglottis; the arytenoid cartilages are paired.

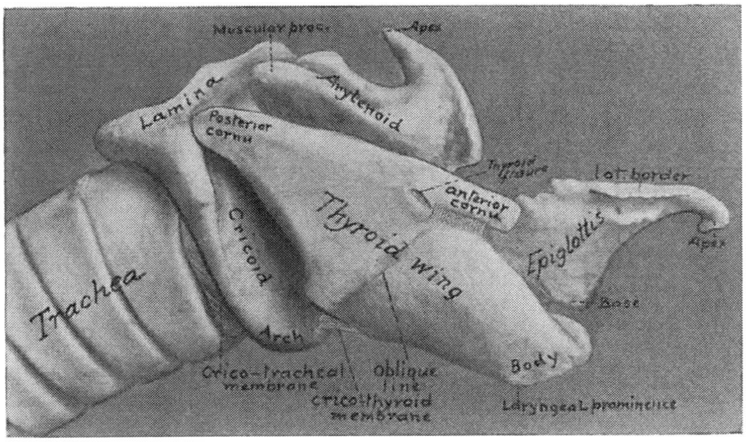

Fig. 349.—Laryngeal Cartilages of Horse, Right View.

The **cricoid cartilage** (Cartilago cricoidea) is shaped like a signet ring. The dorsal part is a broad, thick, quadrilateral plate termed the **lamina**; the outer (dorsal) surface of this is marked by a median ridge separating two shallow cavities, which give attachment to the posterior crico-arytenoid muscles. On either side of these depressions are two articular facets. The **anterior facets** (Facies articulares arytænoideæ) are placed at the anterior border, are oval and convex, and articulate with the arytenoid cartilages. The **posterior facets** (Facies articulares thyreoideæ) are situated on the front of a ridge, a short distance from the posterior border; they are concave, and articulate with the posterior cornua of the thyroid cartilage. The ventral and lateral parts of the ring are formed by a curved band, called the **arch** (Arcus), which is narrowest below. The lateral surfaces of the arch are grooved for the crico-thyroid muscle. The anterior border of the

[1] In the ordinary position of the head and neck, and while the parts are at rest, about half of the larynx lies between the branches of the mandible; when the head and neck are extended, proportionately more of the larynx lies behind a plane through the posterior borders of the rami. It is here described in the position it occupies when the head and neck are extended.

lamina is thick and slightly concave; the posterior border is thin and irregularly notched. The anterior border of the arch is concave ventrally and gives attachment to the crico-thyroid membrane; laterally it is thicker and gives attachment to the crico-arytenoideus lateralis muscle. The posterior border is attached to the first ring of the trachea by an elastic membrane. The inner surface is smooth and is covered with mucous membrane.

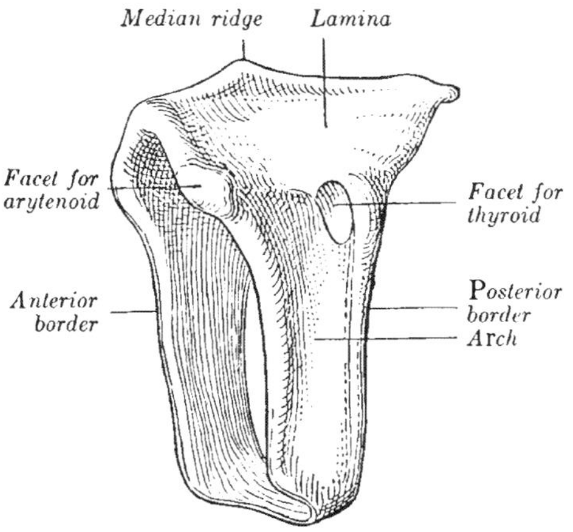

FIG. 350.—CRICOID CARTILAGE OF HORSE, LEFT LATERAL VIEW.

The **thyroid cartilage** (Cartilago thyreoidea) consists of a median thickened portion, termed the body, and two lateral laminæ or wings. The **body** forms ventrally a slight prominence (Prominentia laryngea), which can be felt, but is not visible in the living subject; it supports the base of the epiglottis, which is attached to it by an elastic ligament. The **wings** or **laminæ** spring from the body on either side and form a large part of the lateral wall of the larynx. Each is a rhomboid plate, presenting a slightly convex outer surface, which is divided into two areas by an oblique line (Linea obliqua), on which the thyro-hyoid and thyro-pharyngeus muscles meet. The superior (dorsal) border is nearly straight; it gives attachment to the pharyngeal fascia and the palato-pharyngeus muscle, and bears a cornu at each end. The **anterior cornu** (Cornu orale) is attached to the thyroid cornu of the hyoid bone; below it is a notch, which is converted into a foramen (Foramen thyreoideum) by a fibrous band, and transmits the superior laryngeal nerve to the interior of the larynx. The **posterior cornu** (Cornu caudale) articulates with the cricoid cartilage. The inferior (ventral) border is fused with the body in front; behind, it diverges from its fellow to inclose a triangular space (Incisura thyreoidea caudalis), which is occupied by the crico-thyroid membrane. The anterior border is slightly convex, and is attached to the hyoid bone by the thyro-hyoid membrane. The posterior border overlaps the arch of the cricoid cartilage, and gives attachment to the crico-thyroid muscle. The inner surface is concave, and is covered by mucous membrane to a small extent.

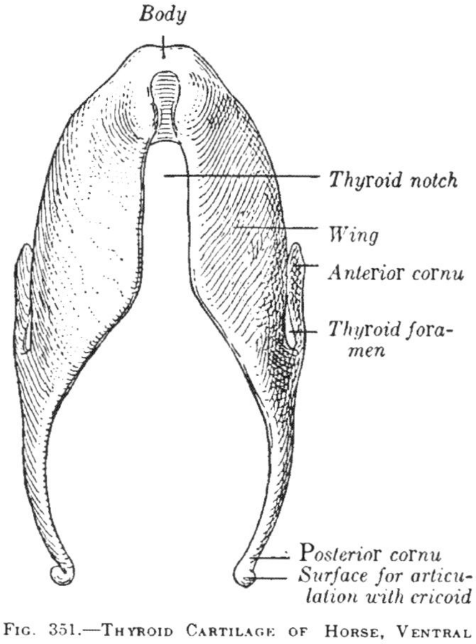

FIG. 351.—THYROID CARTILAGE OF HORSE, VENTRAL VIEW.

The **epiglottis** (Cartilago epiglottica) is situated above the body of the thyroid cartilage and curves toward the root of the tongue. It is shaped somewhat like a pointed ovate leaf, and presents two surfaces, two borders, a base, and an apex. The **oral** (or anterior) **surface** is concave in its length, convex transversely; the **pharyngeal** (or posterior) **surface** has the reverse configuration. The borders are thin, denticulated, and somewhat everted. The **base** is thick, and is attached to the dorsal surface of the body of the thyroid cartilage by elastic tissue. From each side of it a cartilaginous bar projects backward; these processes correspond to the cuneiform cartilages of man. The **apex** is pointed and curved ventrally. Nearly all of the epiglottis is covered with mucous membrane. It lies sometimes in front of, sometimes behind, the soft palate.

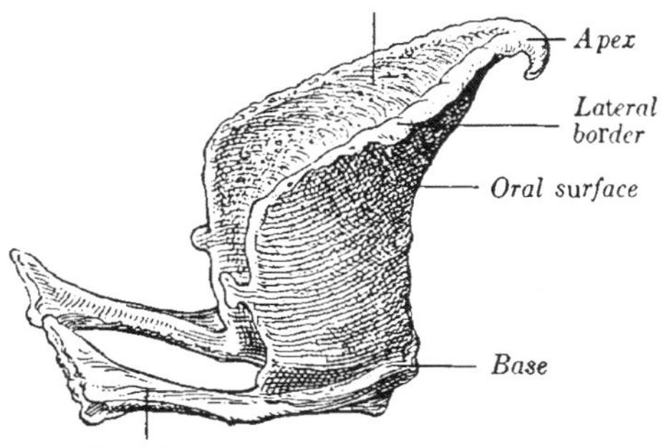

Fig. 352.—Epiglottis of Horse, Right Lateral View.

The **arytenoid cartilages** (Cartilagines arytenoideæ) are situated on either side, in front of the cricoid, and partly between the alæ of the thyroid cartilage. They are somewhat pyramidal in form, and may be described as having two surfaces, two borders, a base, and an apex. The **internal surface** is concavo-convex, smooth, and covered by mucous membrane. The **external surface** is divided by a ridge into two areas: the lower flat area faces outward, and is covered by the thyro-arytenoid and lateral crico-arytenoid muscles; the upper concave area faces chiefly forward, and is covered by the transverse arytenoid muscle. The **anterior border** is convex, and at the base of the cartilage forms a projection termed the **vocal process** (Processus vocalis); it is so named because it gives attachment to the vocal or thyro-arytenoid ligament, which forms the basis of the true vocal cord. The **posterior border** is straight, and extends from the vocal process to the facet on the base. The **dorsal border** forms a deep notch with the apex. The **base** is concave and faces chiefly backward; it presents an oval, concave facet for articulation with the anterior border of the lamina of the cricoid cartilage. The external angle of the base forms a strong eminence termed the **muscular process** (Processus muscularis), which gives attachment to the crico-arytenoid muscles. The internal angle is attached to its fellow by the transverse arytenoid ligament. The **apex** (Cartilago corniculata) curves upward and backward, forming with its fellow the pitcher-shaped lip, from which the cartilages derive their name.

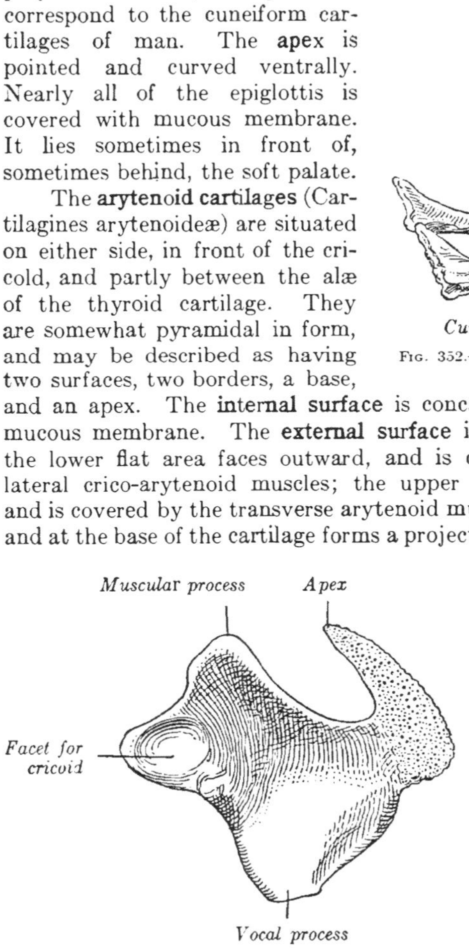

Fig. 353.—Left Arytenoid Cartilage of Horse, Inner View.

The cricoid and thyroid cartilages, and the greater part of the arytenoid cartilages, consist of hyaline cartilage. The apices and vocal processes of the arytenoid cartilages and the epiglottis (including the cuneiform processes) consist of elastic cartilage; they show no tendency toward ossification at any age. The thyroid and cricoid cartilages regularly undergo considerable ossification; the process begins in the body of the thyroid, and often involves the greater part of the cartilage.

Joints, Ligaments, and Membranes of the Larnyx

The **crico-thyroid joints** (Articulationes crico-thyreoideæ) are diarthroses formed by the apposition of the convex facets on the ends of the posterior cornua of the thyroid cartilage with corresponding facets on the sides of the cricoid cartilage. The **capsule** is thin, but is strengthened by accessory bands dorsally, externally, and internally. The movements are chiefly rotation around a transverse axis passing through the centers of the two joints.

The **crico-arytenoid joints** (Articulationes crico-arytænoidea) are also diarthrodial. They are formed by the apposition of the convex facets on the anterior border of the cricoid cartilages with the concave facets on the bases of the arytenoid cartilages. Each has a very thin, loose **capsule,** strengthened by accessory bundles dorsally and internally. The movements are gliding and rotation. In the former the arytenoid cartilage glides inward or outward; in the latter it rotates around a longitudinal axis, so that the vocal process swings outward or inward.

The **thyro-hyoid joints** (Articulationes hyo-thyreoideæ) are formed by the anterior cornua of the thyroid cartilage and the extremities of the thyroid cornua of the hyoid bone. They permit rotation around a transverse axis passing through the two joints.

The **crico-thyroid membrane** (Ligamentum crico-thyreoideum) occupies the thyroid notch and extends backward to the arch of the cricoid cartilage. It is triangular in form, and is attached by its base to the anterior border of the arch of the cricoid cartilage, while its borders are attached to the margins of the thyroid notch. It is strong, tightly stretched, and composed largely of elastic tissue. It is reinforced ventrally by longitudinal fibers, dorsally by fibers which stretch across the thyroid notch.

The **thyro-hyoid membrane** (Membrana hyo-thyreoidea) connects the anterior border of the thyroid cartilage with the body and thyroid cornua of the hyoid bone.

The **hyo-epiglottic ligament** (Ligamentum hyo-epiglotticum) attaches the lower part of the oral surface of the epiglottis to the body of the hyoid bone. It forms an elastic sheath for the hyo-epiglottic muscle. Ventrally it blends with the thyro-hyoid membrane, and dorsally it is not well defined.

The **thyro-epiglottic ligament** (Ligamentum thyreo-epiglotticum) is strong and thick; it is composed chiefly of elastic tissue. It connects the base of the epiglottis with the body and the adjacent inner surface of the laminæ of the thyroid cartilage. Other fibers attach the cuneiform processes somewhat loosely to the thyroid laminæ.

The **transverse arytenoid ligament** (Ligamentum arytænoideum transversum) is a slender band which connects the inner angles of the bases of the arytenoid cartilages.

The **vocal** (or inferior thyro-arytenoid) **ligament** (Ligamentum vocale) forms the basis of the true vocal cord (Fig. 254). It is elastic and is attached ventrally to the body of the thyroid cartilage and the crico-thyroid membrane close to its fellow of the opposite side, and ends dorsally on the processus vocalis of the arytenoid cartilage.

The **ventricular** (or superior thyro-arytenoid) **ligament** (Ligamentum ventriculare) is included in the false vocal cord. It consists of loosely arranged bundles which arise chiefly from the cuneiform process and end on the outer surface of the processus vocalis and adjacent part of the arytenoid cartilage.

The **crico-tracheal membrane** (Ligamentum crico-tracheale) connects the cricoid cartilage with the first ring of the trachea.

Muscles of the Larynx

A. Extrinsic Muscles

The **sterno-thyro-hyoideus** is described on p. 226.

The **thyro-hyoideus** (M. hyo-thyreoideus) is a flat, quadrilateral muscle, which lies on the outer surface of the thyroid lamina and the lateral part of the thyro-hyoid membrane. It arises from the thyroid cornu of the hyoid bone, and ends on the oblique line on the lamina of the thyroid cartilage. Its action is to draw the larynx toward the root of the tongue.

The **hyo-epiglotticus** (M. hyo-epiglotticus) is a feeble muscle which occupies a median position above the central part of the thyro-hyoid membrane, inclosed by an elastic sheath, the hyo-epiglottic ligament. It arises from the body of the hyoid

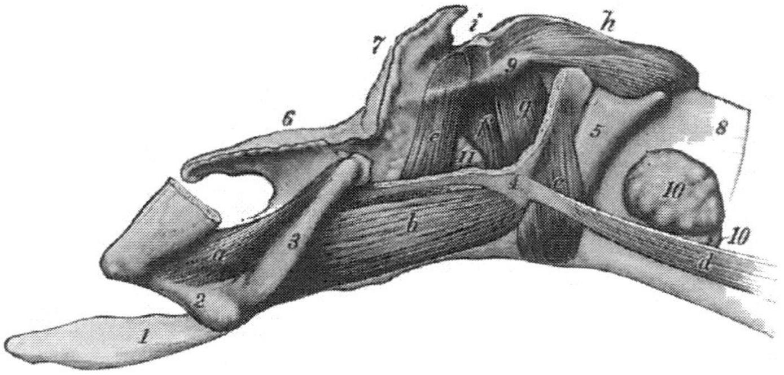

Fig. 354.—Laryngeal Muscles of Horse, Seen from Left Side After Removal of Major Part of Lamina of Thyroid Cartilage.

a, Kerato-hyoideus; *b*, thyro-hyoideus; *c*, crico-thyroideus; *d*, sterno-thyroideus; *e*, ventricularis; *f*, vocalis; *g*, crico-arytenoideus lateralis; *h*, crico-arytenoideus post. s. dorsalis; *i*, arytenoideus transversus; *1*, lingual process; *2*, small cornu; *3*, thyroid cornu, of hyoid bone; *4*, thyroid cartilage; *5*, cricoid cartilage; *6*, epiglottis; *7*, apex of arytenoid cartilage; *8*, trachea; *9*, muscular process of arytenoid; *10*, lateral lobe of thyroid gland; *10'*, isthmus of thyroid gland; *11*, laryngeal saccule. (Ellenberger-Baum, Anat. d. Haustiere.)

bone by two branches which unite and are inserted into the front of the base of the epiglottis. Its action is to draw the epiglottis toward the root of the tongue.

B. Intrinsic Muscles

The **crico-thyroideus** (M. crico-thyreoideus) is a short muscle which fills the groove on the lateral surface of the cricoid cartilage; its fibers are directed dorsally and somewhat forward. It arises on the lower half of the lateral surface and posterior edge of the cricoid cartilage, and is inserted into the posterior border and adjacent part of the surfaces of the lamina of the thyroid cartilage. Its action is to draw the thyroid cartilage and the ventral part of the cricoid cartilage together. In this action the cricoid cartilage is probably rotated, carrying the bases of the arytenoid cartilages with it and thus tensing the vocal cords.

The **crico-arytenoideus dorsalis s. posterior** (M. crico-arytænoideus dorsalis) is a strong, somewhat fan-shaped muscle, which, with its fellow, covers the dorsal surface of the lamina of the cricoid cartilage. It is partially divisible into two layers. It has a broad origin on half of the lamina of the cricoid cartilage, and its fibers converge to be inserted into the processus muscularis of the arytenoid cartilage.

Its action is to dilate the rima glottidis by rotating the arytenoid cartilage so as to carry the vocal process and cord outward.

The **crico-arytenoideus lateralis** (M. crico-arytænoideus lateralis) lies on the inner face of the thyroid lamina. It arises from the anterior border of the lateral part of the arch of the cricoid cartilage. The fibers pass in a dorsal direction and converge on the processus muscularis of the arytenoid cartilage. It closes the rima glottidis by rotating the arytenoid cartilage inward.

The **arytenoideus transversus** (M. arytænoideus transversus) is an unpaired muscle which stretches across the concave dorsal surface of the arytenoid cartilages. Its fibers are attached on either side to the processus muscularis and the ridge which extends forward from it. The right and left parts of the muscle meet at a fibrous

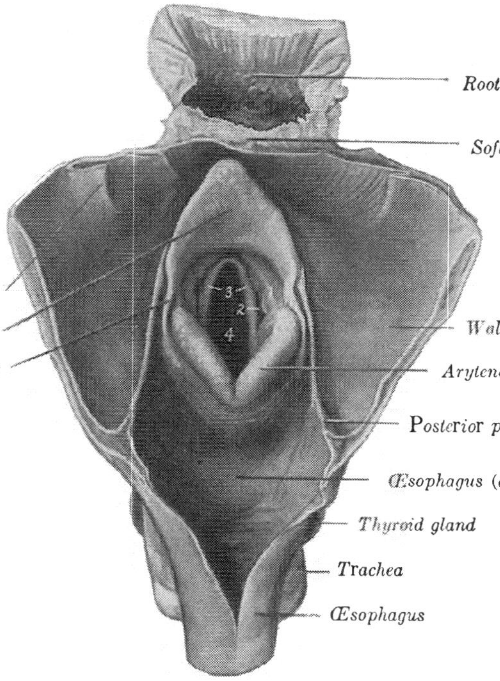

Fig. 355.—Aditus Laryngis of Horse Exposed by Opening Pharynx And Beginning of Œsophagus Along Median Dorsal Line.
1, False vocal cord; *2*, lateral ventricle; *3*, true vocal cords; *4*, rima glottidis.

raphé which is connected with the transverse arytenoid ligament. Fibers of the thyro-arytenoideus muscle overlap its anterior part. It narrows the rima by drawing the arytenoid cartilages together.

The **thyro-arytenoideus** (Mm. ventricularis et vocalis) is situated in the lateral wall of the larynx, covered by the lamina of the thyroid cartilage. It consists of two parts, between which the mucous membrane of the lateral ventricle pouches to form the saccule. The **anterior part** (M. ventricularis) arises from the anterior part of the cricothyroid membrane and the ventral border of the thyroid lamina. Its fibers pass upward and backward to end partly on the processus muscularis, partly on the arytenoideus transversus, meeting its fellow. The **posterior part** (M. vocalis) has a more extensive origin on the crico-thyroid membrane. Its direction corresponds with that of the true vocal cord. It is inserted into the outer surface of the arytenoid cartilage below the processus muscularis. The muscle closes the rima and slackens the vocal cords. With the arytenoideus transversus and crico-arytenoideus lateralis it forms a sphincter which closes the entrance to the larynx.

CAVITY OF THE LARYNX

The **cavity** of the larynx (Cavum laryngis) is smaller than one would expect from its external appearance. On looking into it through the pharyngeal end two folds are seen projecting from its láteral walls. These are termed the **vocal cords,** and they divide the cavity into two portions.

The **aditus laryngis,** or pharyngeal aperture, is a large, oblique, oval opening, which faces forward and upward into the ventral part of the pharynx. It is bounded in front by the epiglottis, behind by the arytenoid cartilages, and

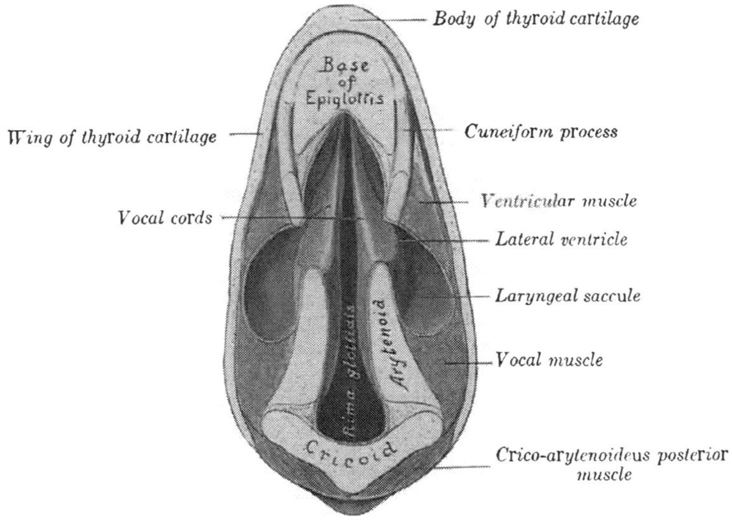

FIG. 356.—SECTION OF LARYNX OF HORSE.
The plane of the section is parallel with the vocal cords.

laterally by the **aryteno-epiglottic** folds of mucous membrane (Plicæ aryepiglotticæ), which stretch between the edges of the epiglottis and the arytenoid cartilages.

The **vestibule** of the larynx (Vestibulum laryngis) is that part of the cavity which extends from the aditus to the vocal cords. On its lateral walls are the **false vocal cords** (Plicæ ventriculares), each of which consists of a fold of mucous membrane covering the anterior part of the thyro-arytenoid ligament and the cuneiform process. Between the false and true vocal cord there is a pocket-like depression termed the **lateral ventricle** of the larynx (Ventriculus lateralis laryngis). This is the entrance to the **laryngeal saccule** (Appendix ventriculi laryngis), a cul-de-sac of the mucous membrane which is about one inch (ca. 2 to 3 cm.) long and extends upward and backward on the inner surface of the thyroid lamina. There is a small **middle ventricle** (Ventriculus laryngis medianus) at the base of the epiglottis.

The middle, narrow part of the cavity is termed the **glottis** or **rima glottidis.**[1]

[1] The term glottis is commonly used to designate the interval between the vocal bands and arytenoid cartilages or the structures that inclose that space.

It is bounded on either side by the true vocal cord and the inner surface of the arytenoid cartilage. The true vocal cords (Labia vocales) are situated behind the false cords and the lateral ventricles. They extend from the angle between the body and laminæ of the thyroid cartilage to the vocal processes of the arytenoid cartilages. They are prismatic in cross-section, and their free edges look forward and somewhat upward. The mucous membrane of the cord (Plica vocalis) is very thin and smooth, and is intimately attached to the underlying ligament. In ordinary breathing the rima is somewhat lanceolate in form; when dilated, it is diamond-shaped, the widest part being between the vocal processes. The narrow part of the glottis between the vocal cords is termed the glottis vocalis (Pars intermembranacea), while the wider part between the arytenoid cartilages is the glottis respiratoria (Pars intercartilaginea).

The posterior compartment of the laryngeal cavity is directly continuous with the trachea. It is inclosed by the cricoid cartilage and the crico-thyroid membrane. It is oval in form, the transverse diameter being an inch and a half to two inches (ca. 4 to 5 cm.), and the dorso-ventral diameter two to two and a half inches (ca. 5 to 6 cm.).

The mucous membrane which lines the larynx (Tunica mucosa laryngis) is reflected around the margin of the aditus to become continuous with that of the pharynx, and behind it is continuous with that which lines the trachea. It is closely attached to the pharyngeal surface of the epiglottis, but elsewhere in the aditus and vestibule it is loosely attached by submucous tissue which contains many elastic fibers.[1] It is thin and very closely adherent over the vocal cords and the inner surfaces of the arytenoid cartilages. The epithelium is of the stratified squamous type from the aditus to the glottis, beyond which it is columnar ciliated in character. There are numerous mucous glands (Glandulæ laryngeæ), except over the glottis and the pharyngeal surface of the epiglottis, in which situations they are scanty.

Blood-supply.—Thyro-laryngeal artery.

Nerve-supply.—Superior laryngeal and recurrent laryngeal nerves (from the vagus).

THE TRACHEA

The trachea extends from the larynx to the roots of the lungs, where it divides into the right and left bronchi. It is kept permanently open by a series of about fifty to fifty-five incomplete cartilaginous rings embedded in its wall. It occupies a median position, except near its termination, where it is pushed a little to the right by the arch of the aorta. It is approximately cylindrical, but its cervical portion is for the most part depressed dorso-ventrally by contact with the longus colli muscle, so that the dorsal surface is flattened. The average caliber is about two to two and one-half inches (ca. 5 to 6 cm.), but in the greater part of the neck the transverse diameter is greater and the dorso-ventral smaller. It is inclosed by a fascia propria.

In its cervical part the trachea is related dorsally to the œsophagus for a short distance, but chiefly to the longus colli muscle. Laterally it is related to the thyroid gland, the carotid artery, the jugular vein, the vagus, sympathetic, and recurrent laryngeal nerves, and the tracheal lymph ducts and cervical lymph glands. The œsophagus lies on its left face from the third cervical vertebra backward. The sterno-cephalicus muscles cross it very obliquely, passing from the ventral surface forward over its sides, and diverging to reach the angles of the jaw. The omo-hyoidei also cross it very obliquely, passing over the lateral surfaces of the tube, and converging ventrally to the body of the hyoid bone. The sterno-thyro-

[1] In so-called œdema glottidis this loose submucous tissue becomes infiltrated with fluid, in some cases causing occlusion of the vestibule.

hyoideus lies on the ventral surface.[1] The scaleni lie on either side near the entrance to the thorax.

The thoracic part of the trachea passes backward between the pleural sacs and divides into the two bronchi over the left atrium of the heart. It is related dorsally to the longus colli for a short distance, and beyond this to the œsophagus. Its left face is crossed by the aortic arch, the left brachial artery, and the thoracic duct. Its right face is crossed by the vena azygos, the dorso-cervical and vertebral vessels, and the right vagus nerve. Ventrally it is related to the anterior vena

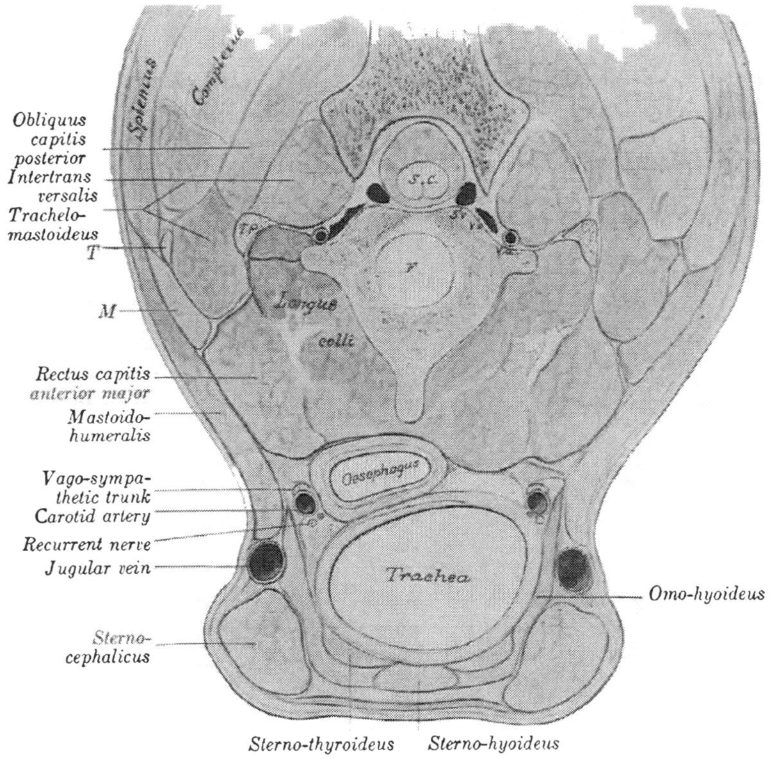

FIG. 357.—CROSS-SECTION OF VENTRAL PART OF NECK OF HORSE.

The section is cut at right angles to the long axis of the neck, passing through the junction of the second and third cervical vertebræ. *S.c.*, Spinal cord; *S.v.*, spinal vein; *V.v.*, *V.a.*, vertebral vein and artery; *T.p.*, transverse process (tip); *F*, intervertebral fibro-cartilage; *T*, atlantal tendon common to mastoido-humeralis, splenius, and lower part of trachelo-mastoideus; *M*, digitation of mastoido-humeralis inserted by *T*.

cava, the brachiocephalic and common carotid trunks, and the left recurrent nerve.

The **bifurcation** of the trachea (*Bifurcatio tracheæ*) is situated opposite to the fifth intercostal space, and about five or six inches (ca. 12 to 15 cm.) below the seventh and eighth thoracic vertebræ.

The trachea is composed of—(1) A fibro-elastic membrane in which are embedded (2) the cartilaginous rings; (3) a muscular layer; (4) the mucous membrane. The **elastic membrane** is intimately attached to the perichondrium

[1] The arrangement of the muscles should be noted, since the space inclosed by the divergence of the sterno-cephalici and the convergence of the omo-hyoidei is the area of election for the operation of tracheotomy.

of the rings. In the intervals between the latter it constitutes the annular ligaments (Ligamenta annularia). The rings of the trachea (Cartilagines tracheales) are composed of hyaline cartilage. They are incomplete dorsally, and when their free ends are drawn apart, resemble somewhat the letter C. In the cervical part the thin wide free ends overlap, while in the thoracic part they do not meet; here the deficiency is made up by thin plates of variable size and form, embedded in a membrana transversa. Ventrally the rings are about one-half inch (ca. 1 to 1.2 cm.) wide and much thicker than dorsally. The first ring is attached to the cricoid cartilage by the crico-tracheal membrane, and is usually fused dorsally with the second ring. Various irregularities, such as partial bifurcation or partial or complete fusion with an adjacent ring, are common. The arrangement in the terminal part is very irregular. The muscular layer (Musculus trachealis) consists of unstriped fibers which stretch across the dorsal part of the tube. It is separated from the ends of the rings and the membrana transversa by a quantity of areolar tissue. When it contracts the caliber of the tube is diminished. The mucous membrane is pale, normally, and presents numerous fine longitudinal folds, in which are bundles of elastic fibers. The epithelium is stratified columnar ciliated. Numerous tubular mucous glands (Glandulæ tracheales) are present.

Blood-supply.—Common carotid arteries.

Nerve-supply.—Vagus and sympathetic nerves.

THE BRONCHI

The two bronchi, right and left (Bronchus dexter, sinister), are formed by the bifurcation of the trachea. Each passes backward and outward to the hilus of the corresponding lung. The right bronchus is a little wider and less oblique in direction than the left. They are related ventrally to the divisions of the pulmonary artery, and dorsally to the branches of the bronchial artery and the bronchial lymph glands. Their structure is similar to that of the trachea.

THE THORACIC CAVITY

The thoracic cavity (Cavum thoracis) is the second in point of size of the body cavities. In form it is somewhat like a truncated cone, much compressed laterally in its anterior part, and with the base cut off very obliquely.

The dorsal wall or roof is formed by the thoracic vertebræ and the ligaments and muscles connected with them.

The lateral walls are formed by the ribs and the intercostal muscles.

The ventral wall or floor is formed by the sternum, the cartilages of the sternal ribs, and the muscles in connection therewith. It is about one-half as long as the dorsal wall.

The posterior wall, formed by the diaphragm, is very oblique and is strongly convex.

The anterior aperture or inlet (Apertura thoracis cranialis) is relatively small, and of narrow, oval form. It is bounded dorsally by the first thoracic vertebra and laterally by the first pair of ribs. It is occupied by the longus colli muscles, the trachea, œsophagus, vessels, nerves, and the prepectoral lymph glands.

The cavity is lined by the endothoracic fascia and by the pleuræ.

A longitudinal septum, termed the mediastinum (Septum mediastinale), extends from the dorsal wall to the ventral and posterior walls, and subdivides the cavity into two lateral chambers which contain the lungs. Each of these chambers is lined by a serous membrane called the pleura, and is called a pleural cavity (Cavum pleuræ). The mediastinum is, for the most part, not median in position; this is largely due to the fact that the largest organ contained in it, the heart, is placed more on the left side; consequently the right pleural cavity and lung are larger than the left. Practically all the organs in the thorax are in the mediastinal space with the exception of the lungs, the posterior vena cava, and the right phrenic nerve. The part in which the heart and the pericardium are situated, together with that above it, is usually called the middle mediastinal space; the parts before and behind this are termed the anterior and posterior mediastinal spaces respectively.

THE PLEURÆ

The **pleuræ** are two serous sacs which line the pleural cavities and are reflected at the roots of the lungs to invest those organs. We, therefore, distinguish **parietal** and **visceral** parts of the pleuræ.

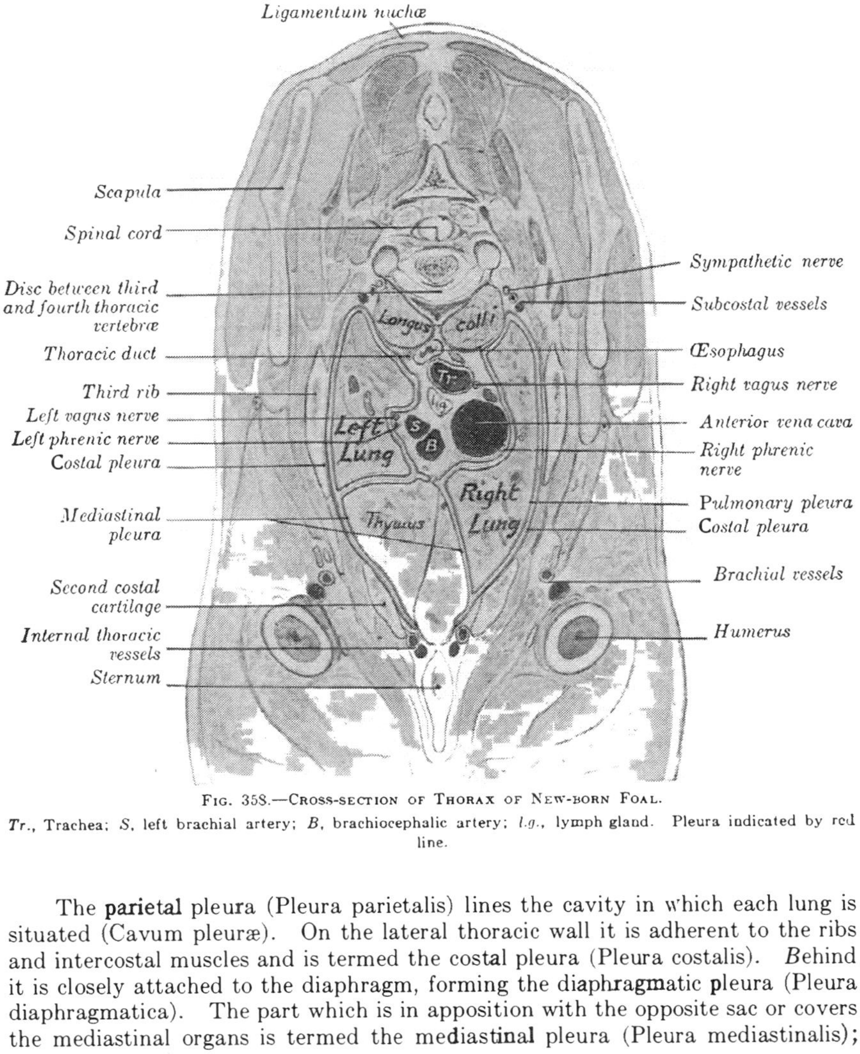

FIG. 358.—CROSS-SECTION OF THORAX OF NEW-BORN FOAL.
Tr., Trachea; *S*, left brachial artery; *B*, brachiocephalic artery; *l.g.*, lymph gland. Pleura indicated by red line.

The **parietal** pleura (Pleura parietalis) lines the cavity in which each lung is situated (Cavum pleuræ). On the lateral thoracic wall it is adherent to the ribs and intercostal muscles and is termed the costal pleura (Pleura costalis). Behind it is closely attached to the diaphragm, forming the **diaphragmatic** pleura (Pleura diaphragmatica). The part which is in apposition with the opposite sac or covers the mediastinal organs is termed the **mediastinal** pleura (Pleura mediastinalis);

where this layer is adherent to the pericardium, it is distinguished as **pericardiac pleura** (Pleura pericardiaca).[1]

The pleura is reflected at the root of the lung, which it covers, constituting the visceral or **pulmonary pleura** (Pleura pulmonalis). Behind the root of the lung a considerable triangular area is not covered by the pleura, the two lungs being attached to each other by connective tissue in this situation.

The **ligament of the lung** (Lig. pulmonale) is a fold formed by the reflection of the pleura from the mediastinum and the diaphragm to the lung, behind the

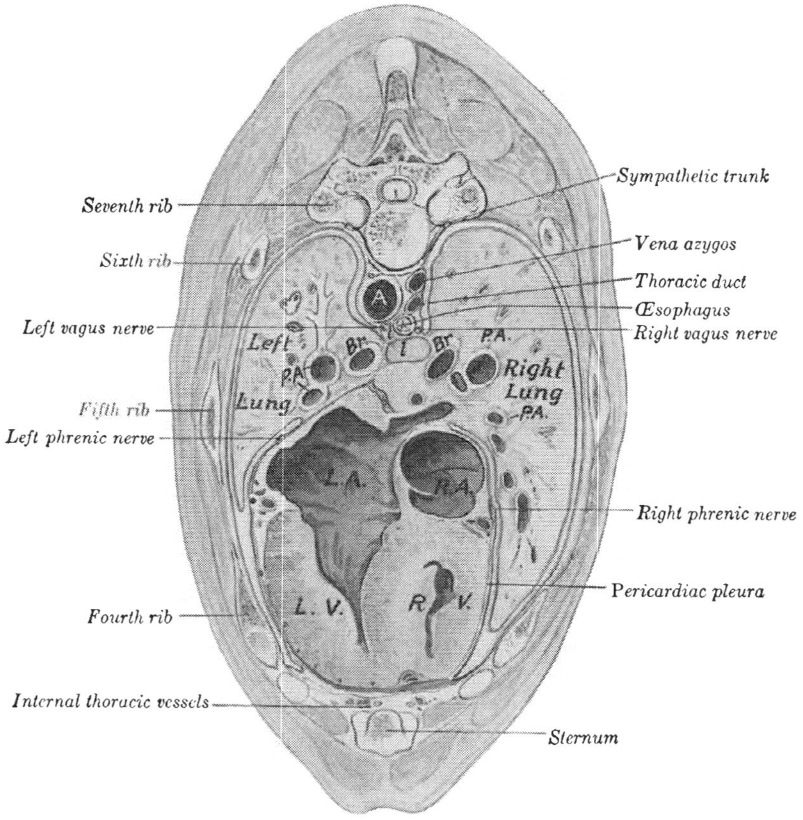

FIG. 359.—CROSS-SECTION OF THORAX OF NEW-BORN FOAL.
A Aorta; *Br.*, bronchi; *P.A.*, pulmonary arteries; *l*, lymph gland; *R.A.*, right atrium; *L.A.*, left atrium; *R.V.*, right ventricle; *L.V.*, left ventricle of heart.

triangular area of adhesion just mentioned. It is seen when the base of the lung is drawn outward. It contains elastic tissue, especially in its posterior part.

The right pleura forms a special sagittal fold (Plica venæ cavæ) about a handbreadth to the right of the median plane, which incloses the posterior vena cava in its upper edge and gives off a small accessory fold for the right phrenic nerve. The fold arises from the thoracic floor and from the diaphragm below the foramen venæ cavæ, and intervenes between the mediastinal lobe and the body of the right lung. It is delicate and lace-like.

[1] The student should bear in mind that these terms are employed simply as a matter of convenience in description; all the parts, though differently named, form a continuous whole.

The posterior mediastinum is very delicate below the œsophagus, and usually appears fenestrated; when these apertures are present, the two pleural cavities communicate with each other.[1]

The pleural sacs contain a serous fluid, the **liquor pleuræ**; in health there is only a sufficient amount to moisten the surface, but it accumulates rapidly after death.

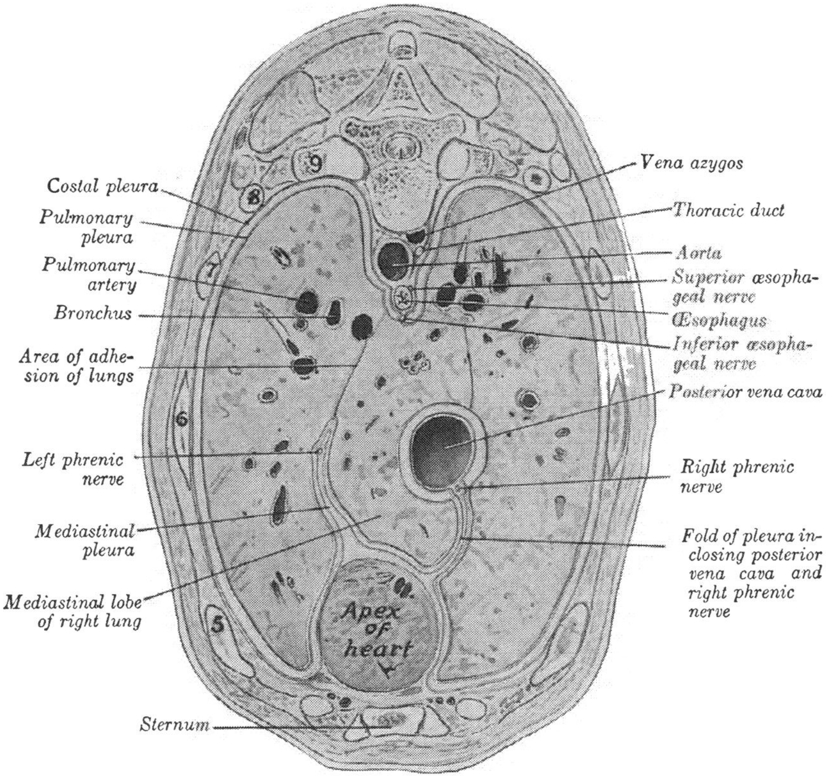

FIG. 360—CROSS-SECTION OF THORAX OF NEW-BORN FOAL.
Ribs are numbered.

THE LUNGS

The **lungs** (Pulmones) occupy much the greater part of the thoracic cavity. They are accurately adapted to the walls of the cavity and the other organs contained therein. The two lungs are not alike in form or size, the right one being considerably larger than the left; the difference is chiefly in width, in conformity with the projection of the heart to the left.

The lung is soft, spongy, and highly elastic. It crepitates when pressed between the finger and thumb, and floats in water. When the thoracic cavity of the unpreserved subject is opened, the lung collapses immediately to about one-third of its original size, and loses its proper form; this is due to its highly elastic character and the fact that the tension of the lung

[1] The apertures do not exist in the fœtus, and are sometimes absent in the adult subject. Some of them may be produced in dissection by the necessary disturbance of the parts. Clinicians state that a serous exudate formed in one pleural sac usually passes through to the other side in the horse.

tissue caused by the air pressure in its cavities has been relieved by the external air pressure.[1]

The color varies according to the amount of blood contained in the lung. During life the lung has a pink color, but in subjects which have been bled for dissection it is light gray or faintly tinged with red. In unbled subjects it is dark red; the depth of color varies, and is often locally accentuated by gravitation of blood to the most dependent parts (hypostasis).

The fœtal lung, since it contains no air and has a relatively small blood-supply, differs from that of an animal which has breathed in the following respects: (1) It is much smaller; (2) it is firmer and does not crepitate; (3) it sinks in water; (4) it is pale gray in color.

In form the lungs are like casts of the pleural cavities in which they are situated. When well hardened *in situ*, their surfaces present impressions and elevations

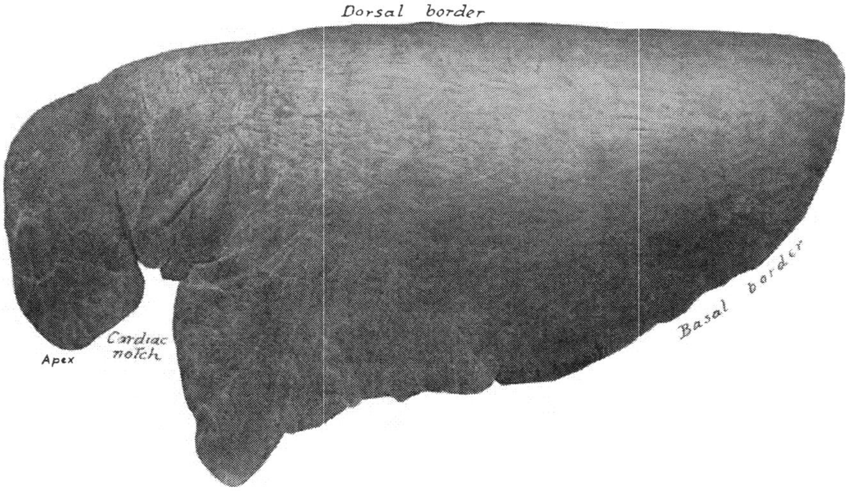

FIG. 361.—LEFT LUNG OF HORSE, COSTAL SURFACE.
Specimen hardened *in situ*.

corresponding exactly to the structures with which they are in contact. Each lung presents two surfaces, two borders, a base, and an apex.

The costal (or external) surface (Facies costalis) is convex, and lies against the lateral thoracic wall, to which it is accurately adapted.

The mediastinal (or internal) surface (Facies mediastinalis) is less extensive than the costal surface. It is molded on the mediastinum and its contents. It presents a large cavity adapted to the pericardium and heart; this is termed the cardiac impression (Impressio cardiaca), and is larger and deeper on the left lung than on the right. Above and behind this is the **hilus**, at which the bronchus, vessels, and nerves enter the lungs. The bronchial lymph glands are also found here. Behind this the two lungs are adherent to each other over a triangular area. Above this is a groove for the œsophagus (Sulcus œsophageus), which is deepest on the left lung. A groove for the aorta (Sulcus aortæ) curves upward and backward over the hilus, and passes backward near the dorsal border of the lung; the curved part of the groove for the aortic arch is absent on the right lung, on which there is a groove for the vena azygos. Anteriorly there

[1] A correct idea of the natural form and size of the lung cannot be obtained from a specimen in this state. The lungs should be hardened *in situ* for this purpose.

are grooves for the trachea, the anterior aorta, the anterior vena cava, and other vessels.

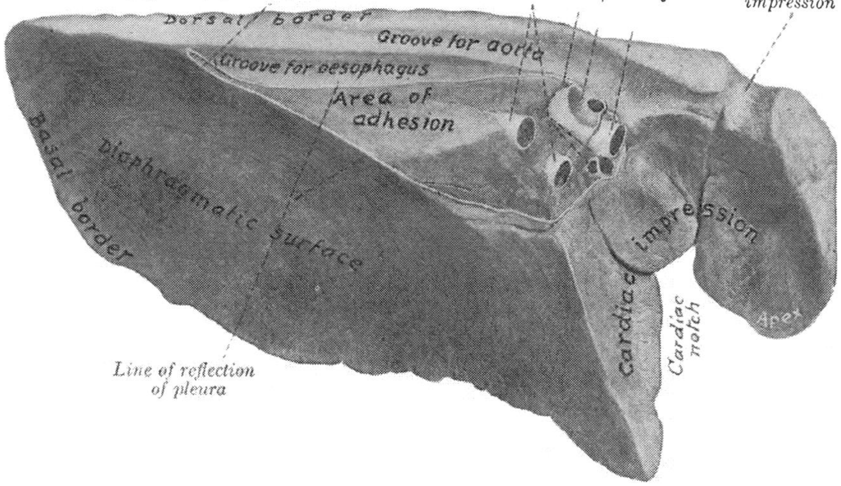

FIG. 362.—LEFT LUNG OF HORSE, MEDIASTINAL AND DIAPHRAGMATIC SURFACES. Organ hardened *in situ*. (Venous impression for common dorso-cervico-vertebral stem.)

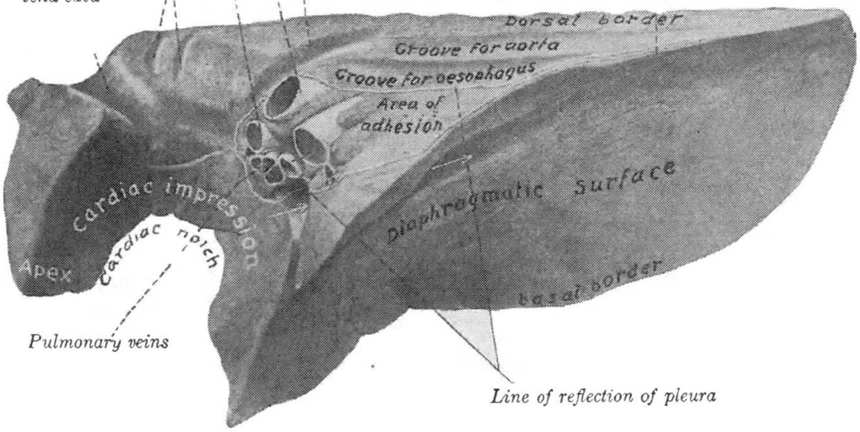

FIG. 363.—RIGHT LUNG OF HORSE, MEDIASTINAL AND DIAPHRAGMATIC SURFACES. Organ hardened *in situ*. *c, d*, Grooves for superior cervical and dorsal veins. Arrows indicate canal for posterior vena cava between mediastinal lobe and main part of lung.

The **dorsal** (or superior) **border** (Margo obtusus) is long, thick, and rounded; it lies in the groove alongside of the bodies of the thoracic vertebræ.

The **ventral** (or inferior) border (Margo acutus) is thin and short. It presents, opposite to the heart, the cardiac notch (Incisura cardiaca). On the left lung this notch is opposite to the third, fourth, and fifth ribs, so that a considerable area of the pericardium here lies in direct contact with the chest-wall. On the right lung the notch is less extensive, and is an intercostal space further forward.

The base of the lung (*B*asis pulmonis) is oval in outline; its surface (Facies diaphragmatica) is deeply concave in adaptation to the thoracic surface of the diaphragm. Laterally and posteriorly it is limited by a thin basal border which fits into the narrow recess (Sinus phrenico-costalis) between the diaphragm and the chest-wall. The position of this border, of course, varies during respiration. In the deepest inspiration it may reach the bottom of this recess; in ordinary inspiration it lies about four or five inches (ca. 10 to 12 cm.) from the costal arch, to which it is nearly parallel; in ordinary expiration it lies about twice as far from the costal arch.

The apex of the lung (Apex pulmonis) is prismatic, narrow, and flattened transversely. It is partially marked off from the rest of the lung by the cardiac notch. It curves downward, and is related internally to the anterior mediastinum and behind to the anterior part of the pericardium.

In the horse the lungs are not divided into distinct lobes by deep fissures, as in most mammals. In the case of the left lung there is no lobation, but the right lung presents a mediastinal lobe, separated from the body of the lung by a fissure which forms in its dorsal part a canal for the posterior vena cava and the right phrenic nerve, inclosed in a special fold of the right pleura.[1]

The root of the lung (Radix pulmonis) is composed of the structures which enter or leave the lung at the hilus on the mediastinal surface. These are: (1) The bronchus; (2) the pulmonary artery; (3) the pulmonary veins; (4) the bronchial artery; (5) the pulmonary nerves; (6) the lymph vessels, which open into the bronchial lymph glands. The bronchus is situated dorsally, with the bronchial artery on its upper surface and the pulmonary artery immediately below it. The pulmonary veins lie chiefly below and behind the artery.

The lobulation of the lungs is not very evident on account of the small amount of interlobular tissue. The lobules appear on the surface or on sections as irregular polygonal areas of different sizes.[2]

Bronchial Branches.—Each bronchus at its entrance into the lung gives off a branch to the apex of the lung. It is then continued backward as the main stem bronchus, parallel with the dorsal border of the lung, giving off branches (Rami bronchiales) in monopodic fashion; these branch similarly and reach all parts of the lung. The right bronchus gives off a special branch to the mediastinal lobe.

The arrangement of the larger bronchi is not the same in the two lungs. The right bronchus, after detaching the apical branch, gives off a large ventral branch which shortly bifurcates. One of the divisions passes ventrally into the part of the lung behind the cardiac notch (homologue of cardiac lobe), while the other passes downward and backward into the lower part of the base. The stem bronchus then gives off the branch to the mediastinal lobe, and divides, about six inches from the hilus of the lung, into two nearly equal branches; the dorsal branch is a direct continuation of the stem, the ventral one passes into the middle part of the base. The left bronchus, after a short course, divides into two nearly equal branches. The dorsal branch may be regarded as the continuation of the stem; it passes backward parallel with the dorsal border of the lung, giving off a ventral branch much further back than in the right lung. The ventral division of the stem bronchus divides, after a very short course, into two branches; the anterior one passes ventrally into the homologue of the cardiac lobe, while the posterior one passes downward and backward into the base of the lung.

The structure of the larger bronchial tubes is, in general, similar to that of the trachea. Their walls contain irregular plates of cartilage instead of rings. There is

[1] Some authors consider each lung to be divided into anterior and posterior lobes by the cardiac notch, so that the right lung would have three lobes and the left lung two lobes.

[2] In fœtal lung the lobulation is much more distinct. Pigmentation of the lung is sometimes seen in horses, and in such cases the pigment is deposited mainly in the interlobular tissue, thus mapping out the lobules.

a continuous layer of unstriped muscle, composed of circularly arranged bundles. The mucous membrane presents numerous longitudinal folds; it contains many elastic fibers, mucous glands, and lymph nodules, and is lined by ciliated columnar epithelium. As the tubes diminish in size the coats become thinner and the cartilages smaller; in tubes about 1 mm. in diameter the cartilages and mucous glands are absent.

By repeated branching the **interlobular bronchi** are formed, and from these arise the lobular **bronchioles.** The latter enter a lobule and branch within it, forming the respiratory **bronchioles;** these give off the **alveolar ducts,** the walls of which are pouched out to form hemispherical diverticula, the alveoli or **air-cells.**

A **lobule** of the lung, the unit of lung structure, is made up of a lobular bronchiole with its branches, and their air-cells, blood- and lymph-vessels, and nerves. Between the lobules is the **interlobular tissue,** which forms the supporting framework of the lung.

Vessels of the Lungs.—The branches of the **pulmonary artery** carry venous blood to the lungs. They accompany the bronchi, and form rich capillary plexuses on the walls of the alveoli. Here the blood is arterialized, and is returned to the heart by the **pulmonary veins.** The **bronchial arteries** are relatively small vessels which carry arterial blood for the nutrition of the lungs. The branches of these arteries accompany the bronchial ramifications as far as the alveolar ducts, but do not extend to the alveoli. The œsophageal artery also supplies pulmonary branches (in the horse) which reach the lung by way of the ligament of the latter. These branches vary much in size, and ramify chiefly in the subpleural tissue of the basal part of the lung.[1] The **lymph vessels** are numerous, and are arranged in two sets. The superficial set forms close networks in and under the pleura, while the deep set accompanies the bronchi and pulmonary vessels. All converge to the root of the lung and enter the **bronchial lymph glands.**

Nerve-supply.—The pulmonary nerves come from the vagus and sympathetic nerves. They enter at the hilus and supply branches to the bronchial arteries and the air-tubes.

THE THYROID GLAND

The **thyroid gland** (Glandula thyreoidea) is a very vascular ductless gland, situated on the trachea close to the larynx. It is red brown in color, and consists of two **lateral lobes** and a connecting **isthmus** (Fig. 354).

The **lateral lobes** are situated on either side of the first and second or second and third rings of the trachea, to which they are loosely attached. Each is about the size of a walnut, and has a convex superficial face which is related to the parotid gland and the omo-hyoid muscle, and a slightly concave, deep face, applied to the trachea.

The **isthmus** in the adult horse is usually very rudimentary. It may occur as a very narrow glandular band which connects the posterior extremities of the lateral lobes, extending across the ventral surface of the trachea, but it is frequently only a small strand of connective tissue, and sometimes is entirely absent. It may be represented by a small tail-like process of one lobe.

The lateral lobes vary in size and position, and are often dissimilar on the two sides. The anterior extremity is the larger; it is rounded and usually lies about a finger's breadth behind the larynx, but may be in contact with it. The posterior extremity is often produced to form a narrow tail-like process, which is continuous with the isthmus when one is present. In the ass and mule the isthmus is usually well developed. There is sometimes a narrow band of thyroid

[1] It must not be inferred from the necessarily brief account here given that the two sets of vessels are quite distinct. On the contrary, competent observers state that numerous small branches of the bronchial arteries anastomose with pulmonary vessels. Part of the blood conveyed to the lungs by the bronchial arteries is returned by the pulmonary veins. In the horse bronchial veins are absent or inconstant.

tissue which extends forward from the isthmus for a variable distance; this is termed the pyramidal lobe. The position of the lateral lobe is indicated approximately by the junction of the external maxillary and jugular veins.

Structure.—The gland is enveloped by a thin, fibrous **capsule,** from which **trabeculæ** pass into the gland, dividing it into lobules. The lobules consist of non-communicating alveoli or follicles of varying form and size. The alveoli are lined by cubical epithelium, and contain a viscid colloid substance.

Blood-supply.—The arteries are relatively very large; there are usually two thyroid arteries, which arise from the carotid and enter each extremity of the gland.

Nerve-supply.—The nerves are derived from the sympathetic system.

Nodules of thyroid tissue of variable size, sometimes as large as a pea, may be found near the anterior extremity of the lateral lobes, on the course of the anterior thyroid artery or on the trachea, even at a considerable distance from the thyroid region. They are termed accessory thyroids (Glandulæ thyreoidæ accessoriæ).

The parathyroids are small glandular bodies found in the thyroid region. They are paler and not so dense as the thyroid tissue, but often cannot be differentiated by their naked-eye appearance. In the horse there is usually only one on each side in the connective tissue over the anterior extremity of the lateral lobe of the thyroid. They resemble in structure embryonic thyroid tissue.

THE THYMUS GLAND

The **thymus** is a ductless gland which has a close resemblance to the lymphoid tissues. It is well developed only in late fœtal life and for a few months after birth. After this it undergoes rapid atrophy, fatty infiltration, and amyloid degeneration, so that in the adult it is represented by a thin remnant in the lower part of the anterior mediastinum or has entirely disappeared. In the new-born foal it is of a grayish-pink color, and consists of two **lateral lobes** (Fig. 358). The greater part of the gland is situated in the anterior mediastinum, but the two lobes are continued into the neck by a chain of lobules which lie along the course of the carotid artery, extending sometimes as far as the thyroid gland.[1]

Structure.—The thymus is inclosed in a thin, connective-tissue **capsule,** and consists of secondary lobules (Lobuli thymi), of varying shape and size, held together by areolar tissue and fat, and all attached to a cord of adenoid tissue termed the **tractus centralis.** These lobules are subdivided into polyhedral primary lobules, which are composed of lymphoid tissue, and present a dark vascular cortex, and a lighter medulla that contains Hassal's corpuscles.

Blood-supply.—Internal thoracic and carotid arteries.

Nerve-supply.—Sympathetic and vagus nerve.

RESPIRATORY SYSTEM OF THE OX

THE NASAL CAVITY

The nostrils, situated on either side of the muzzle, are relatively small, and are much less dilatable than those of the horse. The alæ are thick and firm. The superior commissure is narrow. There is no false nostril or diverticulum nasi. The skin is smooth, bare, and moist, and there is no clear line of demarcation be-

[1] The cervical part of the gland is very variable. The thoracic lobe of one side may have no cervical continuation; the other lobe may then give off a single prolongation which bifurcates. The thoracic part in the new-born foal occupies most of the space which is later taken up by the apices of the lungs. Its two lobes are in contact, and its deep surface is molded on the anterior part of the pericardium and the large vessels.

tween it and the nasal mucosa. The opening of the naso-lacrimal duct is not visible, as it is on the outer wall of the nostril, and is concealed by the cartilaginous prolongation of the inferior turbinal. There are two **parietal** or **lateral cartilages** on either side, united by fibrous tissue. The dorsal cartilages are thin laminæ which curve outward and downward from the dorsal margin of the septal cartilage; they are prolongations of the nasal bones, and carry the alar cartilages on their anterior extremities. The ventral pair are lateral continuations of the basal lamellæ of the inferior turbinals. They lie along the nasal processes of the premaxillæ; anteriorly, they become thicker, turn a little upward, and each blends with the cartilaginous prolongation of the upper coil of the inferior turbinal. The **alar cartilages** are of peculiar form. The lamina is oblong, and curves outward and downward from the anterior extremity of the dorsal parietal cartilage, with which it is connected. The cornu springs from the outer part of the lamina and curves outward and upward into the outer wing of the nostril; it carries on its extremity a small transverse bar, thus having some resemblance to the fluke of an anchor.

The **nasal cavity** is short, wide anteriorly, narrow behind. It is not completely divided by the septum, which in its posterior third is separated from the floor of the cavity by an interval that increases from before backward. The middle meatus is very narrow, and divides posteriorly into two branches; the upper division leads to the ethmoidal meatuses, and communicates with the frontal sinus and the cavity of the superior turbinal. Anterior to the division are communications with the upper cavity of the ventral turbinal and the maxillary sinus. The main facts in regard to the sinuses were stated in the osteology.

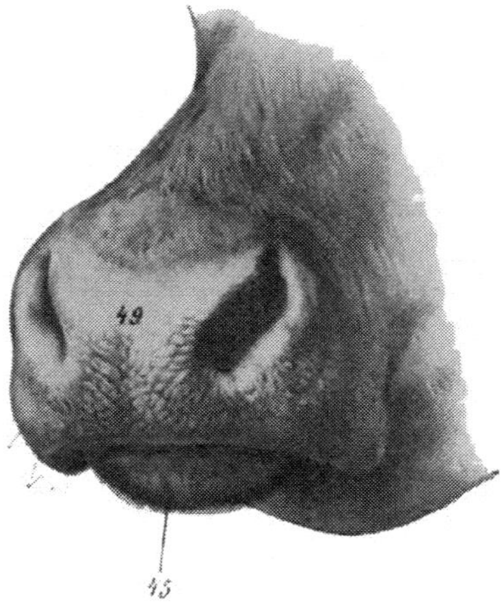

FIG. 364.—MUZZLE OF OX.
49, Naso-labial region; *45*, lower lip. (After Ellenberger-Baum, Anat. für Künstler.)

THE LARYNX

The **larynx** is more compact than in the horse, and presents numerous differential features. The **cricoid cartilage** is compressed laterally. The lamina is not distinctly marked off from the arch; it slopes downward and backward and has a large median ridge. The **thyroid cartilage** is complete ventrally, *i. e.*, the laminæ are united throughout to form a long plate which is notched in front and behind; the laryngeal prominence is small and is situated posteriorly. The height and thickness of the cartilage increase from before backward. The posterior cornua are about an inch long, and form syndesmoses with the cricoid cartilage; the short anterior cornua unite similarly with the hyoid bone. The **epiglottis** is oval in outline and its apex is rounded; its base rests on the thyro-hyoid membrane, to which it is rather loosely attached. The cuneiform cartilages are absent. The **arytenoid cartilages** present only slight differences. The muscular process is well developed, and the vocal process is narrow and long. The **vocal** cords project very little from the wall, so that the rima glottidis is wide; the vocal ligament is attached ventrally to the crico-thyroid membrane; it has the form of a half tube, open behind. The **lateral ventricles** are extremely shallow, and the saccules are absent. The thyro-arytenoideus muscle is not divided; it is fan-shaped, thick, and narrow dorsally; ventrally, it is attached to the base of the epiglottis, the angle of the union of the thyroid laminæ, and the crico-thyroid membrane. The hyo-epiglotticus muscle is large and bifid.

THE TRACHEA

The caliber of the trachea is relatively small, its width being about an inch and a half (ca. 4 cm.) and its height one and a half to two inches (ca. 4 to 5 cm.) The rings are smaller, and number about fifty. In the neck their free ends are sep-

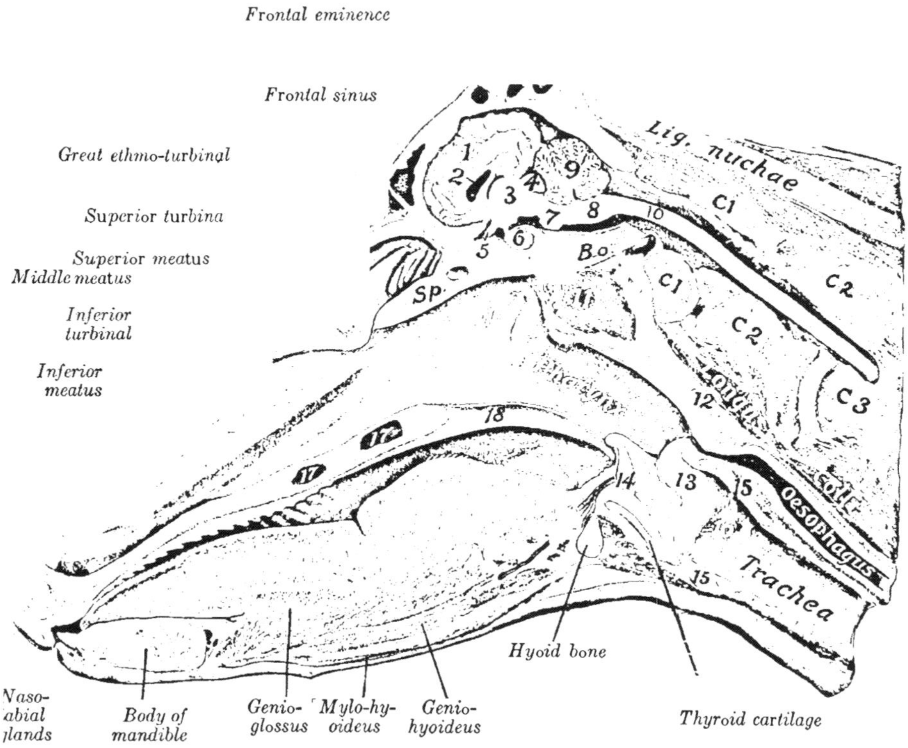

FIG. 365.—SAGITTAL SECTION OF HEAD OF COW.

1, Cerebral hemisphere; *2*, lateral ventricle; *3*, thalamus; *4*, corpora quadrigemina; *5*, optic chiasma; *6*, pituitary body; *7*, pons; *8*, medulla oblongata; *9*, cerebellum; *10*, spinal cord; *11*, ventral straight muscles; *12*, pharyngeal lymph gland; *13*, arytenoid cartilage; *14*, epiglottis; *15*, cricoid cartilage; *16*, vocal cord; *17*, palatine sinus; *18*, soft palate; *19*, Eustachian opening; C_1, C_2, C_3, first, second, and third cervical vertebræ; *B.o.*, basioccipital; *Sp.*, presphenoid.

arated by a varying interval, so that the tube is flattened and membranous dorsally. In the thorax the ends are in apposition, so that they form a ridge dorsally The trachea is adherent to the right lung from the second rib backward. The bifurcation is opposite the fourth intercostal space.

THE BRONCHI

There are three chief bronchi. The bronchus for the apical and the anterior cardiac lobe of the right lung is detached from the trachea at a considerable distance anterior to the bifurcation.

THE THORACIC CAVITY AND PLEURA

The thoracic cavity is relatively small; it is especially short dorsally, and is diminished laterally by the mode of attachment of the diaphragm to the ribs (*vide* Myology). The endothoracic fascia is better developed than in the horse, and is

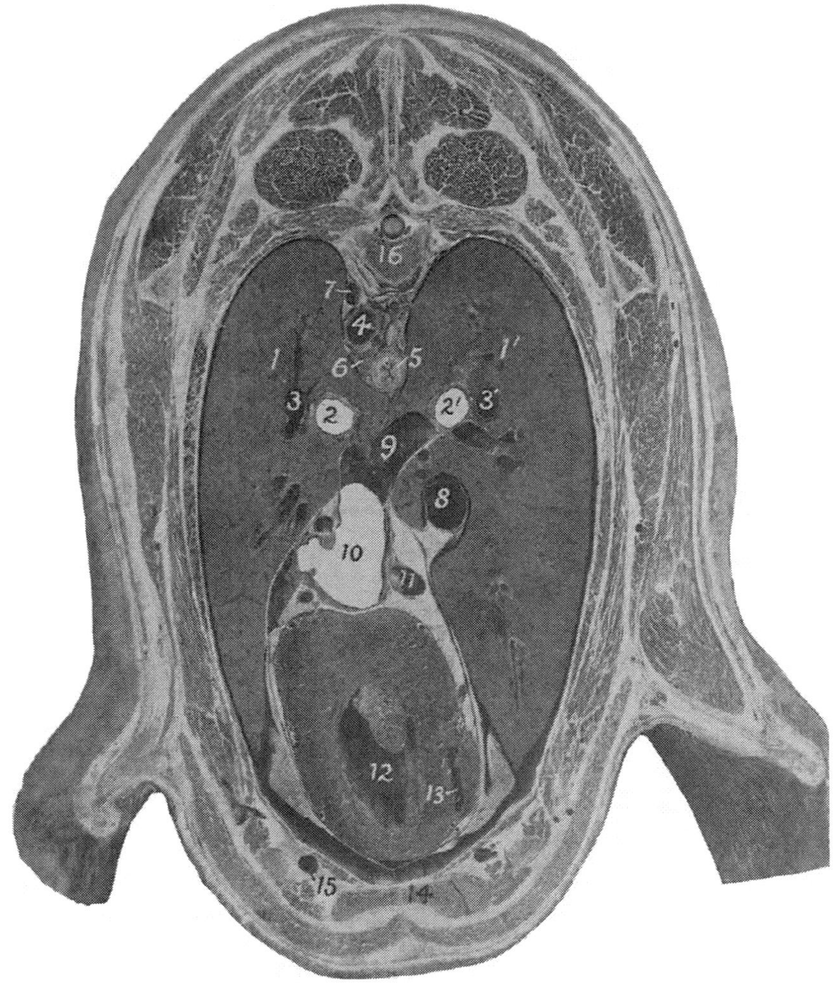

FIG. 366.—CROSS-SECTION OF THORAX OF SHEEP, PASSING THROUGH MIDDLE OF FIFTH PAIR OF RIBS, POSTERIOR VIEW.

1, 1', Lungs; *2, 2'*, bronchi; *3, 3'*, pulmonary arteries; *4*, thoracic aorta; *5*, œsophagus; *6*, lymph gland; *7*, vena hemiazygos; *8*, posterior vena cava; *9*, large pulmonary vein; *10*, left atrium, *11*, vena hemiazygos; *12*, left ventricle; *13*, right ventricle; *14*, sternum; *15*, internal thoracic vessels; *16*, sixth thoracic vertebra.

distinctly elastic. The pleura is also thick, and there are no perforations of the mediastinum. The pleural sacs are more unequal in extent than in the horse, and the ventral part of the mediastinum is further to the left; in front of the pericardium it lies for the most part on the left wall of the chest.

THE LUNGS

The difference in size between the two lungs is greater than in the horse, the right lung weighing about half as much again as the left one. The average weight

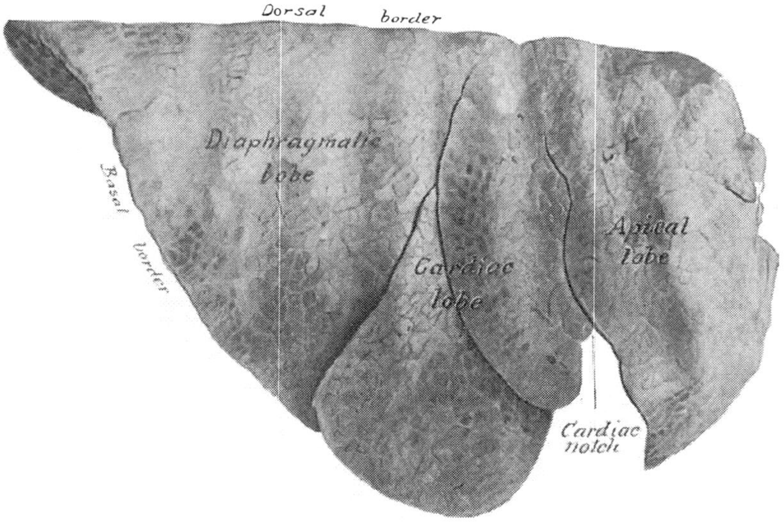

FIG. 367.—RIGHT LUNG OF OX, COSTAL SURFACE.
Organ hardened *in situ*.

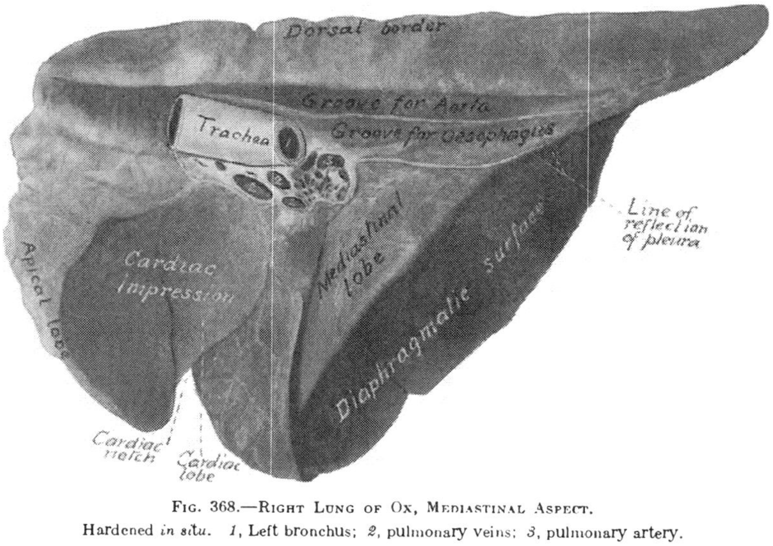

FIG. 368.—RIGHT LUNG OF OX, MEDIASTINAL ASPECT.
Hardened *in situ*. *1*, Left bronchus; *2*, pulmonary veins; *3*, pulmonary artery.

of the lungs is about 7½ pounds (ca. 3 to 4 kg.); they form about $\frac{1}{170}$ of the body weight.

They are divided into lobes by deep fissures (Incisuræ interlobares). The left lung is divided into three lobes, named from before backward apical, cardiac, and diaphragmatic. The right lung has four or five lobes; the apical lobe is much larger than that of the left lung, and occupies the space in front of the pericardium, pushing the mediastinum against the left wall;[1] the mediastinal lobe resembles that of the horse, while the cardiac lobe is often divided by a fissure into two parts. The apical lobe of the right lung receives a special bronchus from the trachea opposite the third rib. The right lung is adherent to the trachea from the second rib backward.

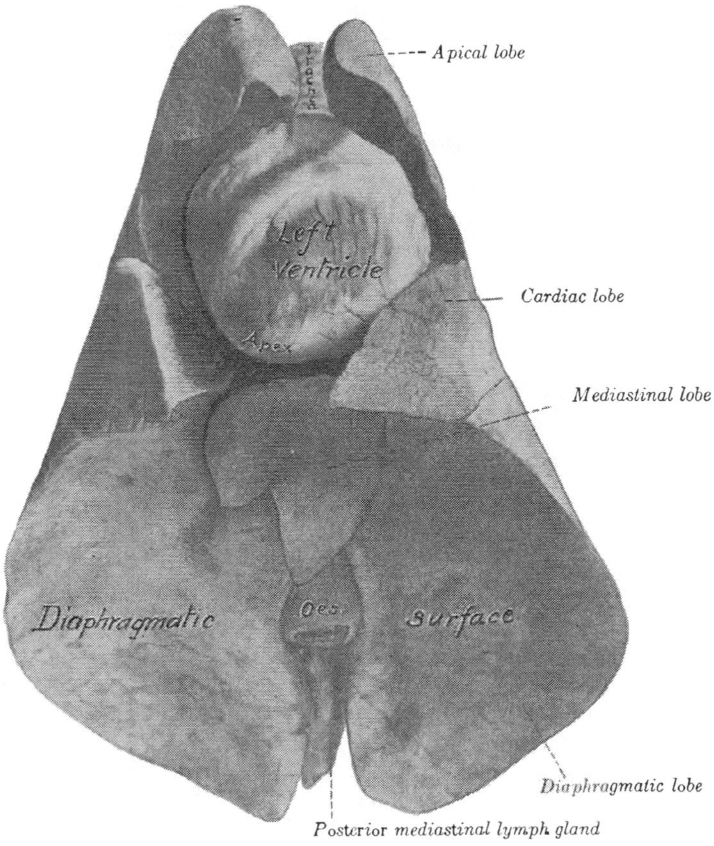

FIG. 369.—LUNGS AND HEART OF SHEEP, VENTRAL VIEW.
Specimen hardened *in situ*. Space between heart and lungs was occupied by pericardium and fat.

The interlobar fissures begin at the ventral margin of the lung and pass toward the root. Those of the left lung lie opposite to the fourth and sixth ribs. The diaphragmatic lobe is the largest, and has the form of a three-sided pyramid with its base resting on the diaphragm. The cardiac lobe is prismatic and forms the posterior margin of the cardiac notch; its long axis corresponds to the fifth rib. The apical lobe of the left lung is small and pointed; its ventral margin lies on the pulmonary artery and the anterior aorta; below this the space in front of the heart is occupied by the apical lobe of the right lung. The cardiac lobe of the right lung is much larger than that of the left lung, and covers the right face of the pericardium, so that the latter has no contact with the lateral wall of the thorax.

The lobulation is very distinct on account of the extremely large amount of interlobular tissue.

[1] It is therefore often termed the precardiac lobe.

In the **sheep** the costal attachment of the diaphragm resembles that of the horse, and the basal part of the lung corresponds thereto. The lobation of the lungs resembles that of the ox, but the lobulation is very indistinct. The pleural sacs extend under the first lumbar vertebra.

THE THYROID GLAND

The lobes of the thyroid gland are more extensive and paler in color than in the horse; they extend further forward, overlapping the crico-pharyngeus muscle to a small extent, and come in contact dorsally with the œsophagus. They are flattened, and have an irregular, lobulated surface. In the young subject the isth mus is well developed, being about half an inch (ca. 1 to 1.5 cm.) in width.

Accessory thyroids may be found, and parathyroids also occur near the posterior extremity or inner surface of the lateral lobes of the thyroid.

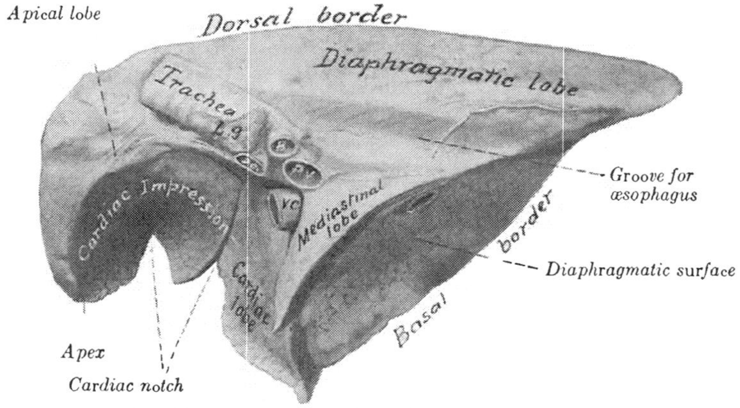

FIG. 370.—RIGHT LUNG OF SHEEP, MEDIASTINAL ASPECT.
Hardened *in situ*. *B*, Bronchus; *P.a.*, pulmonary artery; *P.v.*, pulmonary vein; *V.c.*, posterior vena cava; *L.g.*, bronchial lymph-gland.

THE THYMUS GLAND

The thymus is pale and distinctly lobulated. It is much larger in the calf than in the foal, weighing at five or six weeks about 15 to 25 ounces (ca. 425 to 600 grams). The cervical part is specially large, thick, and compact; it extends to the thyroid gland. It undergoes atrophy slowly and remnants of the thoracic part often remain even in advanced age.

RESPIRATORY SYSTEM OF THE PIG

THE NASAL CAVITY

The nostrils are small, and are situated on the flat anterior surface of the rostrum or snout (Rostrum suis). The latter is a short cylindrical projection, with which the upper lip is fused, and is circumscribed by a prominent circular margin. The skin on the snout is thin and highly sensitive; it presents small pores, and scattered over it are fine short hairs. In the snout between the nostrils is the **os rostri**, which is to be regarded as a special development of the extremity of the septum nasi in adaptation to the habit of rooting. A plate of cartilage, representing the lamina of the alar cartilage of the horse, curves outward and downward from the upper part of the os rostri and a pointed bar of cartilage curves upward from the lower part of the bone in the outer wing of the nostril. The notch between the nasal bone and the premaxilla is closed in by parietal cartilages which resemble those of the ox.

The **nasal** cavity is long and narrow. It is divided behind by a horizontal plate into an upper olfactory part, which leads to the ethmoidal meatuses, and a lower respiratory part, which is a direct continuation of the inferior meatus. The posterior part of the septum is membranous.

The **turbinal bones** resemble in general those of the ox. The superior **meatus** is exceedingly small. The **middle meatus** is a deep fissure between the two turbinals: it divides posteriorly into two branches; one of these extends upward and backward between the lateral mass of the ethmoid bone and the superior turbinal; the other widens and joins the inferior meatus. The opening between the maxillary sinus and the middle meatus lies in a plane through the last cheek teeth. The middle meatus is continuous with the space inclosed by the dorsal part of the inferior turbinal and with the cavity of the superior turbinal. The dorsal division of the middle meatus presents several openings into the frontal sinus. The **inferior** meatus is relatively roomy; it communicates with the space inclosed by the ventral coil of the inferior turbinal. The opening of the naso-lacrimal duct is found in the posterior part of the inferior meatus. The naso-palatine duct and the vomero-nasal organ (of Jacobson) resemble those of the ox.

THE LARYNX

The larynx is remarkable for its great length and mobility. The cartilages are more loosely attached to each other than in the other animals. The **cricoid cartilage** is thick and compressed laterally; its lamina is long and narrow; its arch is directed obliquely downward and backward. The **thyroid cartilage** is very long; its laminæ are united ventrally and form a median ridge. The anterior cornua being absent, there are no joints formed with the hyoid bone. The posterior cornua are broad, bent inward, and articulate with the cricoid cartilage. The **epiglottis** is relatively very large, and is more closely attached to the hyoid bone than to the rest of the larynx. The middle part of its base is turned forward, and rests on the thyro-hyoid membrane; it is closely connected with the body of the hyoid bone by the hyo-epiglottic ligament and the strong hyo-epiglottic muscle.[1] The apex of the **arytenoid cartilage** is very large, and is divided into two parts at its extremity; the inner part is fused with that of the opposite cartilage. There is a small **interarytenoid cartilage** in the transverse ligament. The **rima glottidis** is very narrow. The **vocal cords** are directed obliquely downward and backward; and each is pierced by a long, slit-like opening, which leads into the large laryngeal saccule. The thyro-arytenoid or vocal ligament is similarly divided into a larger anterior and a smaller posterior part. There is a middle ventricle near the base of the epiglottis. The thyro-arytenoid muscle is very strong and is undivided. The arytenoideus is very small. The crico-thyroid consists of two strata; the superficial layer corresponds to the muscle of the other animals; the deep part consists of transverse fibers.

[1] The arrangement here is one of the most striking features of the pig's larynx. The short, thick middle hyo-epiglottic ligament and the anterior part of the thyro-hyoid membrane are inelastic, while the posterior part of the membrane is thin and elastic and allows the epiglottis to be separated by a considerable interval from the thyroid cartilage. Morever, the borders of the epiglottis are connected with the thyroid cornua of the hyoid bone by lateral hyo-epiglottic ligaments.

TRACHEA AND BRONCHI

The trachea is circular in cross-section, and contains thirty or more rings which almost meet dorsally. A special bronchus is detached for the apical lobe of the right lung, as in the ox.

THE LUNGS (Figs. 324, 325)

The right lung has four or five lobes, according to whether the apical is subdivided or not. The left lung resembles that of the ox in form and lobation. The lobulation is distinct, but the interlobular septa are thinner than in the ox.

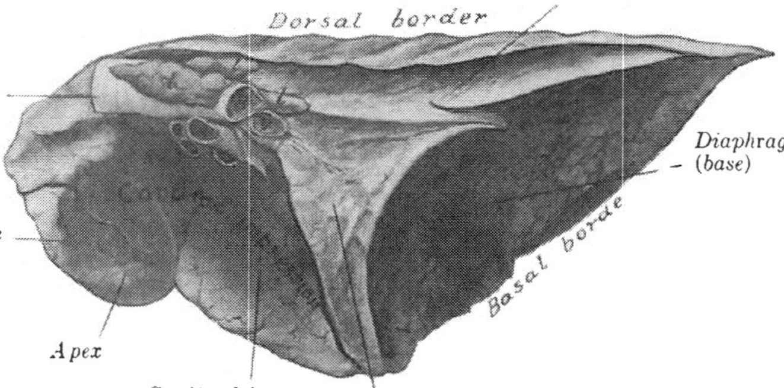

FIG. 371.—RIGHT LUNG OF PIG, MEDIASTINAL ASPECT.
Hardened *in situ*. *B* Left bronchus; *V*., pulmonary veins; *A*., pulmonary artery; *l*, lymph glands.

THE THYROID GLAND

The two lobes of the thyroid are long and flattened; they are situated close together, on the ventral surface of the trachea, extending as far forward as the cricoid cartilage. The gland is dark red in color.

THE THYMUS

The thymus is very large, extending to the larynx or even to the submaxillary space in young subjects.

RESPIRATORY SYSTEM OF THE DOG

THE NASAL CAVITY

The nostrils are situated on the muzzle, with which the upper lip blends. They are shaped somewhat like a comma, with the broad part next to the septum and the narrow part directed backward and outward. The skin around the nostrils is bare, usually black, and in health moist and cool. The muzzle is marked by a median furrow (philtrum) or a deep fissure in some breeds. The cartilaginous framework is formed essentially by the septal cartilage and the parietal cartilages which proceed from it. The septal cartilage projects beyond the premaxilla, and is much thickened at its extremity; it gives off from its upper and lower margins the two parietal cartilages, which curve laterally and toward each other. A grooved plate extends outward from the septal cartilage in the floor of the nostril, and another lamina supports the alar fold of the inferior turbinal bone.

The length of the nasal cavity varies greatly in different breeds, corresponding, of course, to the length of the face. The cavity is roomy, but is very largely occupied by the turbinals and the lateral masses of the ethmoid bone. The middle meatus is short and narrow, and divides posteriorly into two branches; the upper branch leads to the ethmoidal meatuses; the lower branch joins the inferior meatus. The inferior meatus is very small in its middle part, owing to the great development here of the inferior turbinal. The posterior part of the nasal cavity is divided by a horizontal plate, the lamina transversalis, into an upper olfactory part and a lower respiratory part. The sinuses have been described (*vide* Osteology).

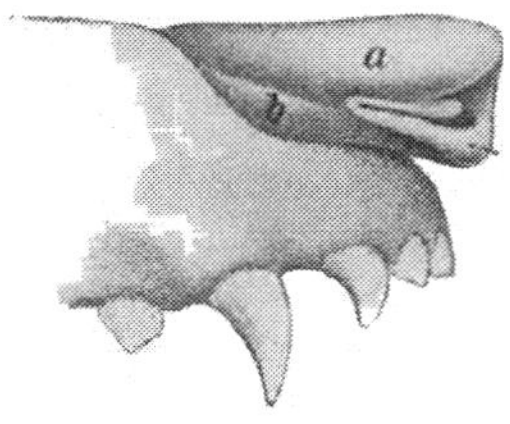

Fig. 372.—Nasal Cartilages of Dog.

a, Upper parietal cartilage; *b*, lower parietal cartilage; c, alar cartilage. (After Ellenberger, in Leisering's Atlas.)

THE LARYNX

The larynx is relatively short. The lamina of the cricoid cartilage is wide; the arch is grooved laterally. The laminæ of the thyroid cartilage are high, but short; they unite ventrally to form the body, on which there is anteriorly a marked prominence, and posteriorly a deep notch. The oblique line on the outer surface of the lamina is prominent. There is a rounded notch (Fissura thyreoidea) below the short anterior cornua for the passage of the superior laryngeal nerve. The posterior cornu is strong, and has a rounded surface for articulation with

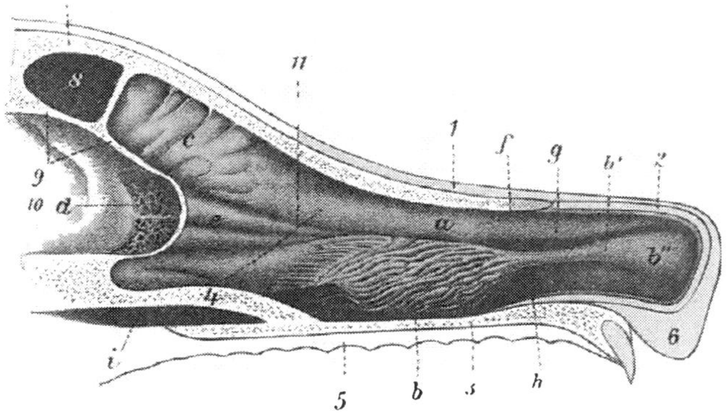

Fig. 373.—Sagittal Section of Nasal Region of Dog.

1, Skin; *2*, parietal cartilage; *3*, floor of nasal cavity; *4*, lamina transversalis; *5*, mucous membrane of hard palate; *6*, upper lip; *7*, frontal bone; *8*, frontal sinus; *9*, cranial plate of frontal bone; *10*, cranial cavity; *11*, dotted line indicating anterior limit of olfactory region; *a*, superior turbinal; *b*, inferior turbinal; *b'*, *b''*, inferior turbinal fold; c, *e*, ethmoturbinals; *d*, cribriform plate of ethmoid; *f*, superior meatus; *g*, middle meatus; *h*, inferior meatus; *i*, naso-pharyngeal meatus. (After Ellenberger, in Leisering's Atlas.)

the cricoid cartilage. The arytenoid cartilages are relatively small, and have between them a small interarytenoid cartilage. The epiglottis is quadrilateral; its lower part or stalk is narrow, fitting into the angle of the thyroid cartilage. The cuneiform cartilages are large and somewhat crescent-shaped; they are not blended with the epiglottis.

The false vocal cords extend from the cuneiform cartilages to the thyroid.

The **true vocal cords** are large and prominent. The entrance to the large lateral ventricle and saccule is a long slit parallel with the anterior margin of the true vocal cord.

The crico-thyroid muscle is thick. The hyo-epiglotticus is well developed, and is double at its hyoid attachment. The anterior part of the thyro-arytenoideus arises on the cuneiform cartilage. Hence Lesbre has suggested the name cuneo-arytenoideus for it.

THE TRACHEA AND BRONCHI

The trachea is very slightly flattened dorsally. It contains forty to forty-five U-shaped rings; the ends of the rings do not meet dorsally, so that here the wall of the trachea is membranous and is composed of a layer of transverse smooth muscle-fibers outside of the rings, the fibrous membrane, and the mucous membrane.

The stem bronchi diverge at an obtuse angle, and each divides into two branches before entering the lung. The anterior branch goes to the apical and cardiac lobes, the posterior one to the diaphragmatic lobe, supplying also the mediastinal lobe of the right lung. The anterior branch of the left bronchus crosses under the pulmonary artery.

THE LUNGS

The lungs (Figs. 342, 343) differ in shape from those of the horse and ox in conformity with the shape of the thorax, which is relatively very wide in the dog; the lateral thoracic walls are strongly curved, and the costal surface of the lungs is correspondingly convex. There is no cardiac notch on the left lung, although a small part of the pericardium is not covered by the lung at the lowest part of the fifth and sixth intercostal spaces. On the right side the cardiac notch is opposite the fourth and fifth intercostal spaces. Each lung is divided by deep fissures into **three** lobes—**apical, cardiac,** and **diaphragmatic**; the right lung has in addition a **mediastinal lobe.** The apical lobe of the right lung is considerably larger than that of the left. The latter is often more or less fused with the cardiac lobe. Variable accessory lobes may be found. On account of the small amount of interlobular tissue the lobulation is not distinct.

THE THYROID GLAND

The **lateral lobes** of the thyroid gland are long and narrow, and have a flattened, ellipsoidal form; they are placed on the lateral surfaces of the trachea near the larynx. The extremities are small, the posterior one often being pointed. The isthmus is inconstant and variable; in large dogs it usually has the form of a glandular band which may be nearly half an inch (ca. 1 cm.) wide; in small dogs it is usually absent.

Accessory thyroids are frequently present; three or four may be found on either side, as well as a median one near the hyoid bone.

The **parathyroids,** about the size of millet or hemp seed, are four in number usually. Two are placed on the deep face of the thyroid lobes; the others are placed laterally near the anterior extremity of the thyroid.

THE THYMUS

The thymus is relatively small, and is situated almost entirely in the thorax. The left lobe is much larger than the right, and extends back as far as the sixth rib at the time of its greatest size. According to Baum the gland increases in size during the first two weeks after birth, and atrophies rapidly in the next two or three months. Traces of it are present at two or three years of age, and may be found even in old subjects.

THE UROGENITAL SYSTEM

This system (Apparatus urogenitalis) includes two groups of organs, the urinary and the genital. The **urinary organs** elaborate and remove the chief excretory fluid, the urine. The **genital organs** serve for the formation, development, and expulsion of the products of the reproductive glands. In the higher vertebrates the two apparatus are independent except at the terminal part, which constitutes a urogenital tract, and includes the vulva in the female and the greater part of the urethra in the male.

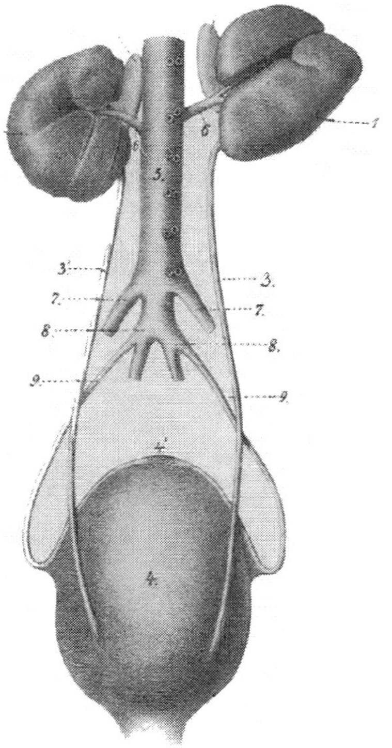

FIG. 374.—GENERAL DORSAL VIEW OF URINARY ORGANS OF HORSE.

1, Right kidney; *1'*, left kidney; *2*, *2'*, adrenal bodies; *3*, *3'*, ureters; *4*, urinary bladder; *4'*, anterior end of bladder with cicatricial remnant of urachus; *4''*, urethra; *5*, aorta; *6*, *6*, renal arteries; *7*, *7*, external iliac arteries; *8*, *8*, internal iliac arteries; *9*, *9*, umbilical arteries. (After Leisering's Atlas.)

THE URINARY ORGANS

The urinary organs (Organa uropoiëtica) are the kidneys, ureters, bladder, and urethra. The **kidneys** are the glands which secrete the urine; they are red-brown in color, and are situated against the dorsal wall of the abdomen, being in most animals almost symmetrically placed on either side of the spine. The **ureters** are tubes which convey the urine to the **bladder**. The latter is an ovoid or pyriform sac, situated on the pelvic floor when empty or nearly so; it is a reservoir for the urine. The urine accumulates in the bladder until that organ is full, and is then expelled through the **urethra**.

THE URINARY ORGANS OF THE HORSE

THE KIDNEYS

Each kidney (Ren) presents two surfaces, two borders, and two extremities or poles, but they differ so much in form and position as to require a separate description of each in these respects.[1]

The **right kidney** (Ren dexter) in outline resembles the heart on a playing card, or an equilateral triangle with the angles rounded off. It lies ventral to the

[1] The kidneys are soft, plastic organs, and hence an accurate knowledge of their form can be gained only from a study of specimens which have been hardened *in situ*. The description here given is based on this method. For this purpose subjects should be hardened in the standing position to avoid artefacts.

upper parts of the last two or three ribs and the tip of the first lumbar transverse process. The **dorsal (or superior) surface** (Facies dorsalis) is strongly convex; it is related chiefly to the diaphragm, but also to a small extent posteriorly to the psoas muscles. In well hardened specimens, especially those from thin subjects, impressions of the last two ribs and the tip of the first lumbar transverse process are usually visible. The **ventral (or inferior) surface** (Facies ventralis) is in general slightly concave, and is related to the liver, pancreas, cæcum, and right adrenal; it either has no peritoneal covering, or only a narrow area externally is so covered. The **internal border** (Margo medialis) is convex and rounded; it is related to the right adrenal and the posterior vena cava. It presents about its middle a deep notch, the hilus (Hilus renalis); this is bounded by rounded margins, and leads into a space termed the **renal sinus** (Sinus renalis). The vessels and nerves reach the kidney at the hilus, and the sinus contains the pelvis or dilated origin of the ureter. The **external border** (Margo lateralis) is rounded, and is thinner than the internal one. It consists of two parts, anterior and posterior, which meet at an external angle; the anterior part fits into the renal impression of the liver. The duodenum curves around the external border. The **anterior extremity** (Extremitas cranialis), thick and rounded, lies in the renal impression of the liver. The **posterior extremity** (Extremitas caudalis) is thinner and narrower

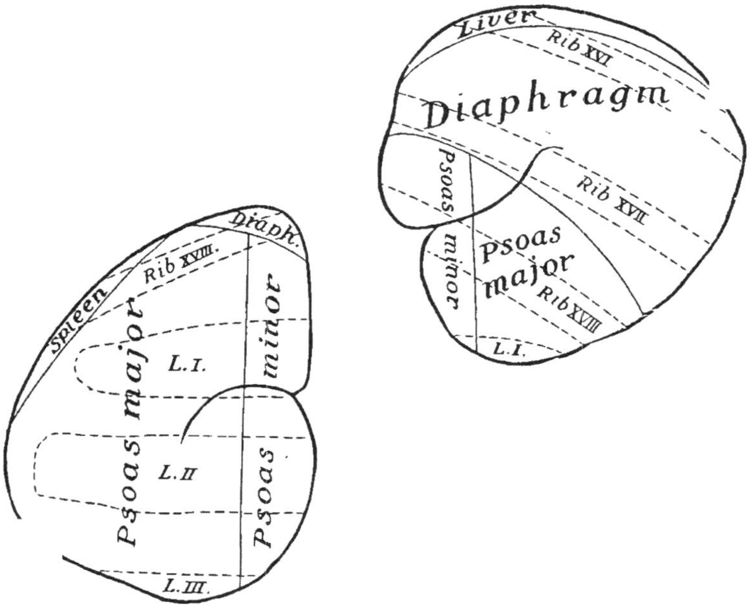

Fig. 375.—Diagram of Position and Dorsal Relations of Kidneys of Horse.
Areas of direct relations are inclosed by continuous lines; parts of skeleton which overlie the kidneys but are not in contact with them are indicated by dotted lines. *L.I–III*, lumbar transverse processes.

The **left kidney** (Ren sinister) is bean-shaped. It is considerably longer and narrower than the right one, and is situated nearer the median plane and further back, so that the hilus of the left kidney is about opposite to the posterior extremity of the right one. It lies usually under the upper part of the last rib and the first two or three lumbar transverse processes. The **dorsal surface** is convex, and is related to the left crus of the diaphragm, the psoas muscles, and the base of the spleen. The **ventral surface** is convex and irregular; the greater part of it is covered by the peritoneum. It is in relation with the origin of the small colon, the

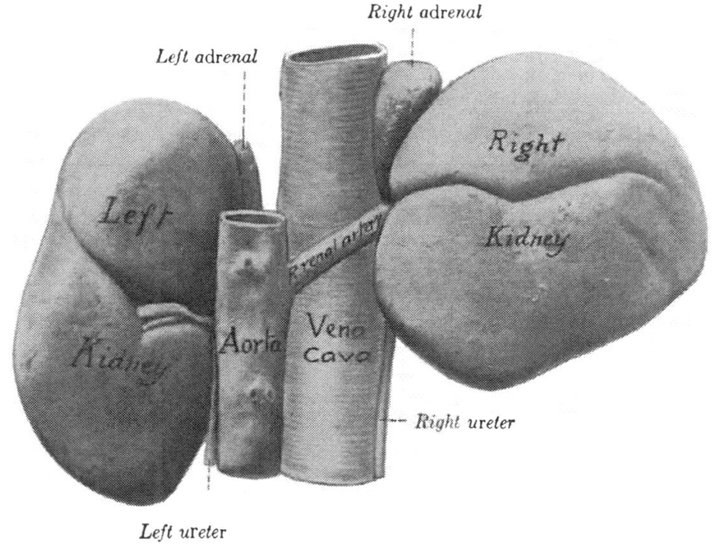

FIG. 376—KIDNEYS AND ADRENALS OF HORSE, DORSAL VIEW.
Hardened *in situ*. Impression of seventeenth rib on right kidney is indicated by small cross.

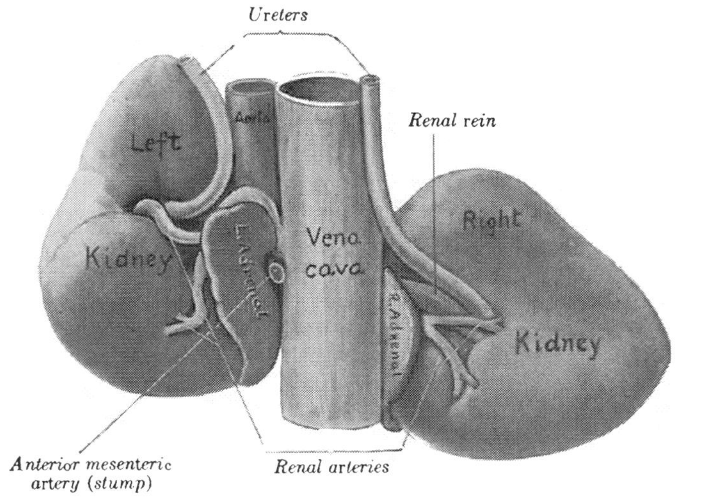

FIG. 377.—KIDNEYS AND ADRENALS OF HORSE, VENTRAL VIEW.
Hardened *in situ*. Left renal vein (not marked) is seen curving round posterior end of left adrenal.

terminal part of the duodenum, the left adrenal, and the left extremity of the pancreas. The **internal border** is longer, straighter, and thicker than that of the right kidney. It is related to the posterior aorta, the adrenal, and the ureter. The **external border** is related chiefly to the base of the spleen. The **anterior extremity** extends almost to the saccus cæcus of the stomach; it is related to the left end of the pancreas, and the splenic vessels. The **posterior extremity** is usually larger than the anterior one.

The form of the left kidney is variable. In some cases its outline is similar to that of the right kidney, but its ventral surface is convex and is often marked by several furrows which diverge from the hilus. In well-hardened specimens the three areas of the dorsal surface are often distinct. The psoas area is flat, parallel with the inner border, and widens behind. The diaphragmatic area is small and convex; it is crescentic and is confined to the anterior pole. The splenic area, convex and external, is often so extensive and distinct as really to constitute a third surface.

Fixation.—The kidneys are held in position chiefly by the pressure of adjacent organs and by the renal fascia. The latter is a special development of the subperitoneal tissue, which splits into two layers to inclose the kidney, together with the perirenal fat or capsula adiposa. On account of its relations with the liver,

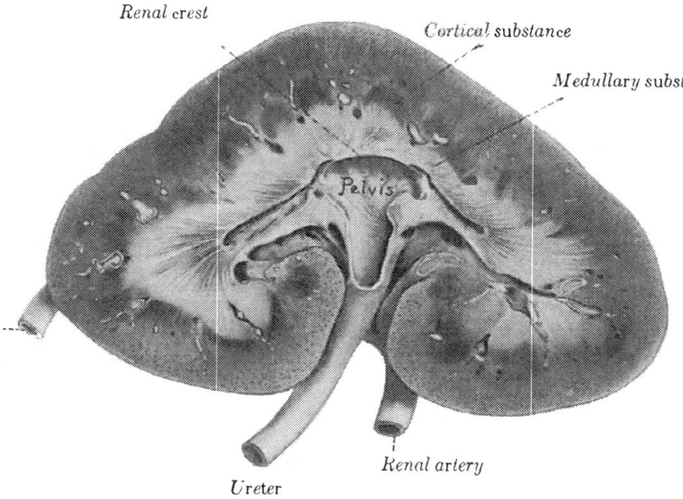

FIG. 378.—FRONTAL (HORIZONTAL) SECTION OF KIDNEY OF HORSE.
The renal vein is removed. A large accessory renal artery entered the posterior pole. Sections of arteries in limiting layer between cortical and medullary substance are white in figure.

pancreas, and the base of the cæcum, the right kidney is much more strongly attached than the left one. It is, therefore, not surprising that the latter varies somewhat in position; its posterior pole may be found ventral to the third or fourth lumbar transverse process. The position of the right kidney seems to be very constant, excluding its movements during respiration.

Weight and Size.—The right kidney is usually one or two ounces heavier than the left. The average weight of the right kidney is about 23 to 24 ounces (ca. 700 gm.); that of the left, about 22 to 23 ounces (ca. 670 gm.). The relation of the weight of both kidneys to the body-weight is about 1 : 300–350.

Chauveau gives as an average 750 grams for the right kidney, and 710 grams for the left. Ellenberger and Baum (24 cases) give the right kidney as varying between 430 and 840 grams; and the left between 425 and 780; this is an average of 635 grams (about 22½ ounces) for the right kidney, and 602.5 grams (about 21½ ounces) for the left. They give the relation of the weight of both kidneys to the body-weight as 1: 255–344. In a Percheron mare weighing about 2000 pounds the right kidney weighed 4 pounds 3 ounces, and the left one 4 pounds. In a horse of medium size the right kidney is about six inches (ca. 15 cm.) in length, about the same in width, and about two inches (ca. 5 cm.) thick. The left kidney is about seven inches (ca. 18 cm.) long, four to five inches (ca. 10 to 12 cm.) wide, and two to two and a half inches (ca. 5 to 6 cm.) thick.

Structure.—The surface of the kidney is covered by a thin but strong fibrous **capsule** (Tunica fibrosa), which is in general easily stripped off the healthy kidney. It is continued along the hilus and lines the renal sinus. Sections through the kidney show it to consist of an external cortical substance and an internal medullary substance.[1] The **cortical substance** (Substantia corticalis) is red brown in color and has a granular appearance. It is dotted over with minute dark points; these are the **renal** (or Malpighian) **corpuscles** (Corpuscula renis), each consisting of the dilated origin of a uriniferous tubule (Capsula glomeruli), with an invaginated tuft of capillaries (Glomerulus) inclosed by it. The **medullary substance** (Substantia medullaris) is more resistant and presents a distinct radial striation. Its central part is pale, but its periphery, the **intermediate zone,** is of a deep red color; in the latter are seen, at fairly regular intervals, sections of the relatively large arciform vessels, which are taken to represent the demarcation between the primitive lobes.[2] Between the vessels the medulla is prolonged somewhat toward the periphery, forming the bases of the renal (or Malpighian) **pyramids.** These are not very pronounced in the kidney of the horse, especially as the gland is not papillated.

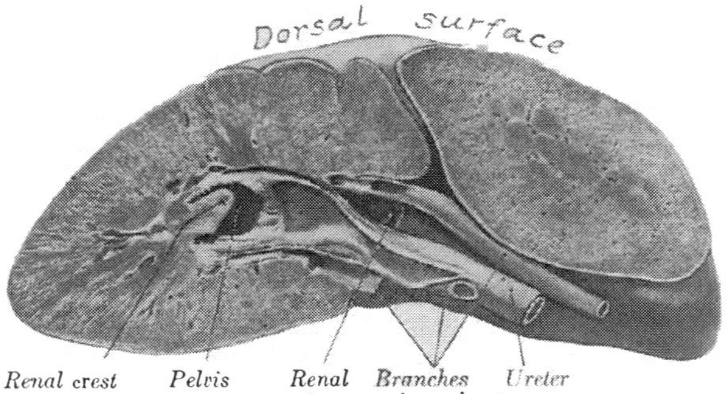

FIG. 379.—TRANSVERSE SECTION OF RIGHT KIDNEY OF HORSE THROUGH THE HILUS. Posterior portion of organ hardened *in situ*. Note curvature of dorsal surface.

Between the bases of the pyramids processes of the cortex dip in toward the sinus, forming the **renal columns.**[3] The inner central part of the medulla forms a concave ridge or crest which projects into the pelvis of the kidney; the crest is marked by numerous small openings at which the renal tubules terminate.

Examination with a pocket lens shows that the cortex is imperfectly divided into **lobules** (Lobuli corticales). Each lobule consists of an axial **radiate part** (Pars radiata), surrounded by a **convoluted part** (Pars convoluta). The former (formerly termed pyramids of Ferrein) appear as ray-like prolongations from the bases of the pyramids (hence also termed medullary rays), and consist largely of narrow, straight or slightly flexuous, tubules (limbs of the loops of Henle). The convoluted part (formerly termed the labyrinth) is granular in appearance, and consists largely of the renal corpuscles and convoluted tubules.

The **pelvis** of the kidney (Pelvis renalis) is the dilated origin of the excretory

[1] The most instructive sections are those made in the horizontal and transverse planes, through the pelvis in each case.

[2] The fœtal kidney is divided by furrows into a number of polygonal areas, each of which is the base of a pyramidal lobe or renculus. These furrows usually disappear before or soon after birth in the foal, although traces of them are sometimes seen in the adult.

[3] In the kidney of the horse the renal columns dip in between the pyramids very superficially as compared with the arrangement in the human kidney. Breuer states that the pyramids are 40 to 64 in number, and are arranged in four rows. Only the middle ones are distinct.

duct. It lies in the sinus of the kidney, and it is funnel-shaped, but flattened dorso-ventrally. The renal crest[1] (Papilla communis) projects into the outer part of the pelvis in the form of a horizontal ridge with a concave free edge. The tubules of the middle part of the medullary substance open on this crest into the pelvis. The tubules from each end of the kidney do not open into the pelvis proper (Recessus medius), but into two long, narrow diverticula (Recessus terminales), which proceed from it toward the poles of the kidney. The wall of the pelvis consists of three layers. The external fibrous coat or adventitia is continuous with the supporting tissue of the kidney. The muscular coat consists of longitudinal and circular fibers. The mucous coat does not cover the renal crest, nor is it continued

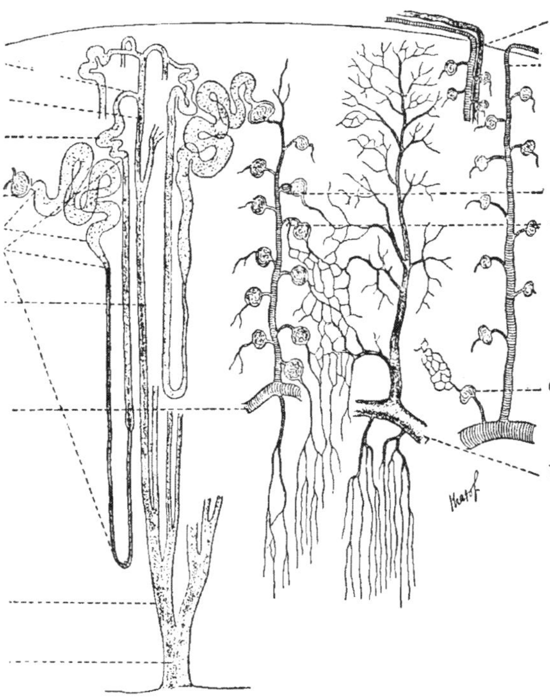

FIG. 380.—DIAGRAMMATIC SCHEME OF URINIFEROUS TUBULES AND BLOOD-VESSELS OF KIDNEY. Drawn in part from the descriptions of Golubew (Böhm, Davidoff, and Huber).

into the diverticula of the pelvis. It has a yellowish tinge, and presents numerous folds. It contains glands (Glandulæ pelvis renalis) which secrete the thick mucus always found in the pelvis.

Renal Tubules—The parenchyma or proper substance of the kidney is composed of the small renal or uriniferous tubules (Tubuli renales), which are very close together and have a complicated course. Each tubule begins in a thin-walled, spherical dilatation or capsule, which is invaginated to receive a tuft of looped capillaries termed a glomerulus; these two structures constitute a renal (or Malpighian) corpuscle; the corpuscles are visible as minute red or dark spots in the convoluted part of the cortex. Succeeding this is a short narrow neck, beyond which the tubule becomes wide and convoluted, forming the proximal convoluted tubule, and enters the radiate portion of the cortex. It then gradually narrows and enters the intermediate zone; becoming very narrow and nearly straight, it descends for a variable distance into the medullary substance, turns sharply upon itself, and returns to the cortex, forming thus the loop of Henle, with its descending and ascending limbs. In the convoluted part of the cortex, it widens

[1] The crest is the result of fusion of the papillæ or apices of the pyramids in the embryo.

and becomes tortuous, constituting the distal convoluted tubule. The tubule then narrows, enters a medullary ray, and opens with other tubules into a straight collecting tubule; this passes axially through a pyramid, and unites with other collecting tubules to form the relatively large papillary ducts, which open into the renal pelvis.

Stroma.—The interstitial tissue forms a reticulum throughout which supports the tubules and blood-vessels. It is very scanty in the cortex, much more abundant in the medulla, in which it increases in amount toward the pelvis.

Blood-supply.—The kidneys receive a large amount of blood through the **renal arteries.** Branches of these enter at the hilus and on the ventral surface of the gland, and reach the intermediate zone, where they form anastomotic arches (Arteriæ arciformes). From these arciform arteries branches pass into the cortex and medulla. The cortical branches (Arteriæ interlobulares) have in general a radial course between the cortical lobules, and give off short lateral branches, each of which ends as the **afferent vessel** (Vas afferens) of a renal corpuscle. The blood is carried from the glomerulus by a smaller **efferent vessel,** which breaks up immediately into capillaries which form networks around the tubules. The medullary branches descend in the pyramids, forming in them bundles of straight twigs (Arteriolæ rectæ).

The **veins** correspond in general to the arteries. In the superficial part of the cortex the veins form star-like figures (Venæ stellatæ) by the convergence of several small radicles to a common trunk.

Lymph Vessels.—These may be divided into two sets, capsular or superficial, and parenchymatous or deep.

Nerve-supply.—The nerves are derived from the renal plexus of the sympathetic, and form a plexus around the vessels.

THE URETERS

The **ureters** are the narrow part of the excretory ducts of the kidneys. Each begins at the renal pelvis and terminates at the bladder. It is about $\frac{1}{3}$ to $\frac{1}{4}$ inch (ca. 6 to 8 mm.) in diameter, and its average length is about 28 inches (ca. 70 cm.). The **abdominal part** (Pars abdominalis) of each ureter emerges ventrally from the hilus of the kidney, and curves backward and inward toward the lateral face of the posterior vena cava (right side) or the posterior aorta (left side). They then pass almost straight backward in the subperitoneal tissue on the surface of the psoas minor, cross the external iliac vessels, and enter the pelvic cavity. The **pelvic part** (Pars pelvina) passes backward and a little downward on the lateral wall of the pelvic cavity, turns inward, and pierces the dorsal wall of the bladder near the neck.

In the male the pelvic part enters the urogenital fold and crosses the vas deferens. In the female the ureter is situated in the greater part of its course in the dorsal part of the broad ligament of the uterus.

The wall of the ureter is composed of three coats. The outer **fibrous coat** (Tunica adventitia) is composed of loose fibrous tissue. The **muscular coat** (Tunica muscularis) consists of inner and outer layers of longitudinal fibers, with a stratum of circular fibers between them. The **mucous membrane** (Tunica mucosa) is covered with transitional epithelium; glands (Glandulæ mucosæ ureteris) resembling those of the renal pelvis occur in the first three or four inches of the ureter.

THE URINARY BLADDER

The **urinary bladder** (Vesica urinaria) (Figs. 270, 271, 272) differs in form, size, and position according to the amount of its contents. When empty and contracted it is a dense, pyriform mass, about the size of a fist, lies on the ventral wall of the pelvic cavity, and does not reach to the inlet. When moderately filled, it is ovoid in form, and extends a variable distance along the ventral abdominal wall. Its physiological capacity varies greatly, but may be estimated approximately at about three or four quarts.

The anterior rounded blind end is termed the vertex;[1] on its middle is a mass of cicatricial tissue (Centrum verticis), a vestige of the urachus, which in the fœtus forms a tubular connection between the bladder and the allantois. The body or middle part (Corpus vesicæ) is rounded, and is somewhat flattened dorso-ventrally, except when distended. It presents two surfaces, dorsal and ventral, the former being the more strongly convex, especially in its posterior part in front of the entrance of the ureters.[2] The posterior narrow extremity, the neck (Collum vesicæ), joins the urethra.

The relations of the bladder vary according to the degree of fullness of the organ, and also differ in important respects in the two sexes. The ventral surface lies on the ventral wall of the pelvis, and extends forward on the abdominal wall as the bladder fills. The dorsal surface in the male is related to the rectum, the urogenital fold, the terminal parts of the vasa deferentia, the vesiculæ seminales, and the prostate; in the female it is in contact, instead, with the body of the uterus and the vagina. The vertex of the full bladder is related to coils of the small intestine and small colon, and to the pelvic flexure of the large colon.

Fixation.—Displacement of the bladder is limited chiefly by three peritoneal folds, termed the middle and lateral ligaments (Figs. 257, 272). The middle ligament (Plica umbilicalis media) is a median triangular fold, formed by the reflection of the peritoneum from the ventral surface of the bladder on to the ventral wall of the pelvis and abdomen. In the new-born animal it is extensive and reaches to the umbilicus; in the adult it is usually much reduced in length relatively. It contains elastic and muscular fibers in its posterior part. The lateral ligaments (Plicæ umbilicales laterales) stretch from the lateral aspects of the bladder to the lateral pelvic walls. Each contains in its free edge a round, firm band, the round or umbilical ligament (Lig. umbilicale s. teres); this is the remnant of the large fœtal umbilical artery, the lumen of which in the adult is very small. The retroperitoneal part of the bladder is attached to the surrounding parts by loose connective tissue, in which there is a quantity of fat. It is evident that the posterior part of the bladder has a definite fixed position, while its anterior part is movable.

Structure.—The wall of the bladder consists of a partial peritoneal investment, the muscular coat, and the mucous lining.

The serous coat (Tunica serosa) covers the greater part of the dorsal surface, from which it is reflected in the male to form the urogenital fold; in the female it passes on to the vagina, forming the vesico-genital pouch. Ventrally the peritoneum covers only the anterior half or less of the bladder, and is reflected posteriorly on to the pelvic floor.

The muscular coat (Tunica muscularis) is relatively thin when the bladder is full. It is unstriped, pale, and not clearly divided into layers, but has rather a plexiform arrangement. Longitudinal fibers occur on the dorsal and ventral surfaces, but laterally they become oblique and decussate with each other. A distinctly circular arrangement is found at the neck, where the fibers form a sphincter (Annulus urethralis).

The mucous coat (Tunica mucosa) is pale and thin. It is in general attached by a highly elastic submucosa to the muscular coat, and forms numerous folds when the organ is empty and contracted. It is modified dorsally in the vicinity of the neck over a triangular area, termed the trigonum vesicæ; the angles of this space lie at the orifices of the two ureters and the urethra, which are close together.

[1] This is commonly termed the fundus by veterinarians, but is not the homologue of the fundus of the human bladder.

[2] This would correspond to the fundus vesicæ of man.

Here the mucous membrane is closely attached and does not form folds. From each **ureteral orifice** (Orificium ureteris) a fold of mucous membrane (Plica ureterica) passes backward and inward, uniting with its fellow to form a median crest (Crista urethralis) in the first part of the urethra. The ureteral orifices are a little more than one inch (ca. 3 cm.) apart. The terminal part of the ureter, after piercing the muscular coat of the bladder, passes for a distance of about an inch (ca. 2 to 3 cm.) between the muscular and mucous coats before piercing the latter; this arrangement constitutes a valve which prevents absolutely the return of the urine from the bladder into the ureter. The **internal urethral orifice** (Orificium urethræ internum) lies at the apex of the trigonum, and is about an inch and a half (ca. 4 cm.) behind the ureteral orifices. The mucous membrane is covered with transitional epithelium like that of the ureter and renal pelvis. It contains lymph nodules.

Blood-supply.—This is derived chiefly from the vesico-prostatic branch of the internal pudic artery. It is also supplied by small twigs from the obturator and umbilical arteries. The veins terminate chiefly in the internal pudic veins. They form plexuses posteriorly.

Lymph Vessels.—These form plexuses on both surfaces of the muscular coat. They go to the internal iliac and lumbar glands.

Nerves.—The nerves are derived from the pelvic plexus (sympathetic and ventral branches of third and fourth sacral nerves). They form a plexus in the submucosa which presents microscopic ganglia.

In the fœtus and new-born animal the bladder is situated chiefly in the abdomen. It is long, narrow, and fusiform. Its abdominal end lies at the umbilicus, through which it is continued by the urachus to the extra-embryonic part of the allantois. As the pelvis increases in size and the large intestine grows, the bladder retracts into the pelvis and changes its form.

The urethra will be described with the genital organs.

THE ADRENAL BODIES

The **adrenal bodies** or **suprarenal glands** (Glandulæ suprarenales)[1] are two small, flattened organs, which lie in contact with the anterior part of the inner border of the kidneys (Figs. 376, 377). They are ductless.

In the horse they are red-brown in color, about three and a half to four inches (ca. 9 to 10 cm.) long, one to one and a half inches (ca. 3 to 4 cm.) wide, and about half an inch or more (ca. 1 to 5 cm.) in thickness. The weight varies from one to two ounces (ca. 28 to 56 gm.).

The **right adrenal** is related internally to the posterior vena cava, to which it is adherent. Its anterior part curves dorsally around the inner border of the right kidney. Its posterior part is flattened and is related ventrally to the pancreas and cæcum, dorsally, to the right renal vessels. The anterior extremity is concealed in the renal impression of the liver; the posterior is related to the ureter.

The **left adrenal** is a little shorter than the right one, and its extremities are rounded; it is usually curved, so that its internal border partly embraces the anterior mesenteric artery. Its dorsal surface is related to the kidney, the renal artery, the aorta, and the left cœliaco-mesenteric ganglion. The ventral surface is in relation with the left extremity of the pancreas and the root of the great mesentery. The posterior extremity often curves inward behind the anterior mesenteric artery; it is related behind to the left renal vein.

When hardened *in situ* the adrenals present several features not evident in the soft organs. The anterior part of the right adrenal is twisted upward and outward over the inner margin of the kidney, so that this part is prismatic and has three surfaces; of these, the concave outer one is applied to the kidney, the dorsal one is related to the right crus of the diaphragm and the liver,

[1] From the standpoint of comparative anatomy the term "adrenal" seems decidedly preferable to "suprarenal."

and the inner one is in contact with the posterior vena cava. The anterior mesenteric artery is nearly always more or less enlarged as a result of verminous arteritis, and the form and degree of curvature of the left adrenal seem to vary in conformity with the condition of the artery.

Structure.—The fibrous **capsule** adheres intimately to the surface of the organ. It contains elastic fibers, and in its deep part unstriped muscle-fibers. From it trabeculæ pass radially into the substance, blending with the fine supporting reticulum. The **parenchyma** consists of a cortical and a medullary portion. The **cortical substance** (Substantia corticalis) is red-brown in color, and is clearly distinguishable from the yellow **medullary substance** (Substantia medullaris). A large **central vein** (Vena centralis) is visible on cross-sections.

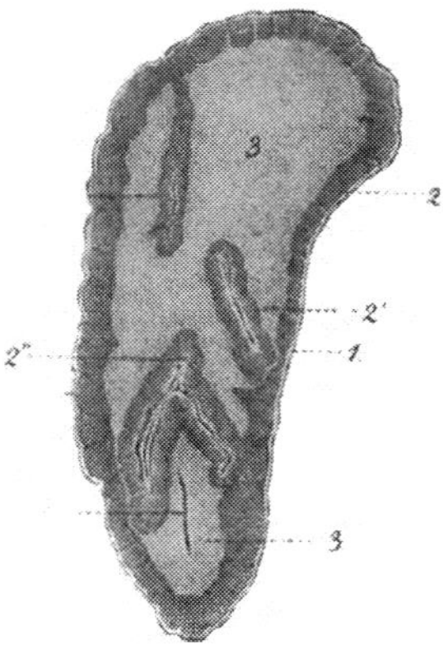

FIG. 381.—ADRENAL BODY OF HORSE; HORIZONTAL SECTION, REDUCED.

1, Capsule; *2*, *2'*, cortical substance; *3*, medullary substance; *4*, blood-vessel in section. (From Leisering's Atlas, reduced.)

The cells of the cortex are arranged in chains of one or two rows. In the peripheral portion the cells are of high cylindrical shape, and the chains form connecting loops; Günther has proposed the name zona arcuata for this part, instead of the usual term zona glomerularis. More deeply the chains are distinctly palisade-like, and this region is called the zona fasciculata. Next to the medulla is the zona reticularis, in which the chains form a network. The cells in these two zones are polygonal and contain a brown pigment.

The cells of the medulla are arranged in irregular groups or form sheaths around the veins. They react to chromic salts by assuming a yellow or yellow-brown color, and are termed chromaffin cells; they share this peculiarity with certain cells of the sympathetic ganglia and paraganglia, with which they are probably related genetically. The alkaloid adrenalin appears to be formed in the medullary cells.

Vessels and Nerves.—The adrenals receive a relatively large blood-supply through the **adrenal arteries** (Aa. suprarenales), which arise from the renal arteries or from the aorta directly. The **veins** terminate in the posterior vena cava and the left renal vein. The **lymph vessels** go to the renal lymph glands. The numerous **nerves** are derived from the sympathetic system through the solar and renal plexuses. The fibers form a rich interlacement, especially in the medullary substance. Ganglion cells are found chiefly in the medulla, but also occur in the deeper part of the cortex.

URINARY ORGANS OF THE OX

The **kidneys** are superficially divided into polygonal lobes by fissures of variable depth. The lobes vary in size, and are commonly about twenty to twenty-five in number. The fissures are filled with fat.

The right **kidney** has an elongated elliptical outline, and is flattened dorso ventrally. It lies ventral to the last rib and the first two or three lumbar transverse processes. The dorsal surface is rounded, and is in contact chiefly with the sublumbar muscles. The ventral surface is less convex, and is related to the liver, pancreas, duodenum, and terminal part of the colon. The hilus is situated on the anterior part of this surface near the inner border. The internal border is nearly straight, and lies parallel with the posterior vena cava. The external border is convex. The anterior extremity occupies the renal impression of the liver, and is capped by the adrenal body.

The left **kidney** occupies a remarkable position, and when hardened *in situ*, differs strongly in form from the right one. When the rumen is full, it pushes the kidney backward and across the median plane, so that it is situated on the right side, behind and at a lower level than the right kidney. It then lies usually under the third, fourth, and fifth lumbar vertebræ. When the rumen is not full, the left kidney may lie partly to the left of the median plane. It has three surfaces. The dorsal surface is convex, and presents on its antero-external part the hilus, which opens outward. The ventral surface is related to the intestine. The third face

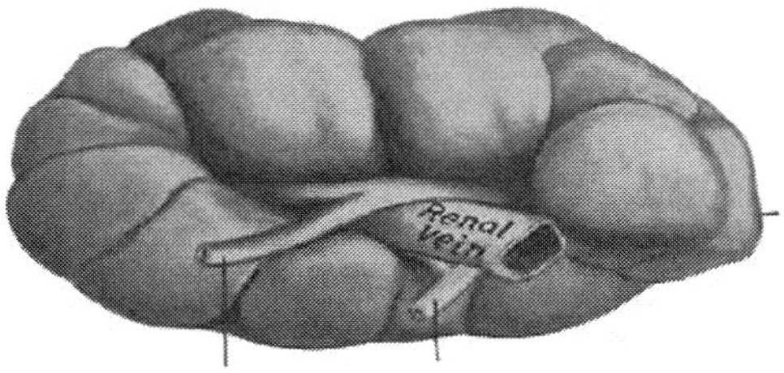

Fig. 382.—Right Kidney of Ox, Ventral Face.
Organ hardened *in situ*. Fat has been removed from fissures between lobes.

is often more or less flattened by contact with the rumen, and may be termed the ruminal surface. The anterior extremity is small, the posterior large and rounded.

The preceding statements refer to the adult subject, and are based on investigations made on living subjects, and studies of frozen sections and material hardened *in situ*. In the young calf the kidneys are almost symmetrically placed, but as the rumen grows it pushes the left kidney to the right and backward *pari passu*. It also usually causes a rotation of the kidney, so that the primary dorsal surface comes to lie almost in a sagittal plane. Further, the gland is bent so that the hilus is largely closed up and faces outward (to the right). In very fat subjects the three-sided appearance of the kidney may be absent, and about one-third or more may remain to the left of the median plane, even where the rumen is pretty well filled.

The kidneys are embedded in a large amount of perirenal fat. The weight

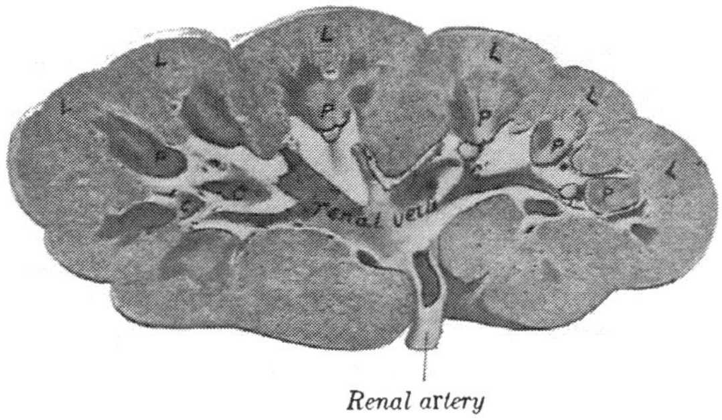

Fig. 383.—Frontal Section of Kidney of Ox.
L Lobes of cortex; *P*, papillæ; *C*, calyx major; *c'*, calyces minores.

of a kidney is about 20 to 25 ounces (ca. 570 to 700 gm.), the left one being usually an ounce or more the heavier. The two form about ¼ per cent. of the body-weight.

The right kidney measures about 8 to 10 inches (ca. 20 to 25 cm.) in length, 4 to 5 inches (ca. 10 to 12 cm.) in width, and 2½ to 3 inches (ca. 7 cm.) in thickness. The left kidney is one or two inches (ca. 2 to 5 cm.) shorter, but its posterior part is much thicker than the right one.

Structure.—The hilus is equivalent to the hilus and sinus of the kidney of the horse; in the right kidney it is an extensive elliptical cavity, in the left, a deep fissure. The pelvis is absent. The ureter begins at the junction of two wide, thin-walled tubes, the **calyces majores**; the anterior calyx is usually the larger. Each calyx major gives off a number of branches, and these divide into several funnel-shaped **calyces minores,** each of which embraces a renal papilla. The space not occupied by the calyces and vessels is filled with fat.

On section through the kidney the **renal pyramids** are easily made out. The blunt apex of each pyramid, the **papilla renalis,** projects into a calyx minor. On each papilla are small orifices (Foramina papillaria) by which the terminal renal tubules (Ductus papillares) open into the calyx. The renal columns are much more distinct than in the horse.

At the hilus the renal artery is dorsal, the vein in the middle, and the ureter ventral; a quantity of fat surrounds these structures in the hilus.

The kidneys of the **sheep** are bean-shaped and smooth, without any superficial lobation. The soft organ is regularly elliptical in form, with convex dorsal and ventral surfaces and rounded extremities; its length is about 2½ to 3 inches (ca. 5 to 8 cm.), its width about 1½ to 2 inches (ca. 4 to 5 cm.), and its thickness a little

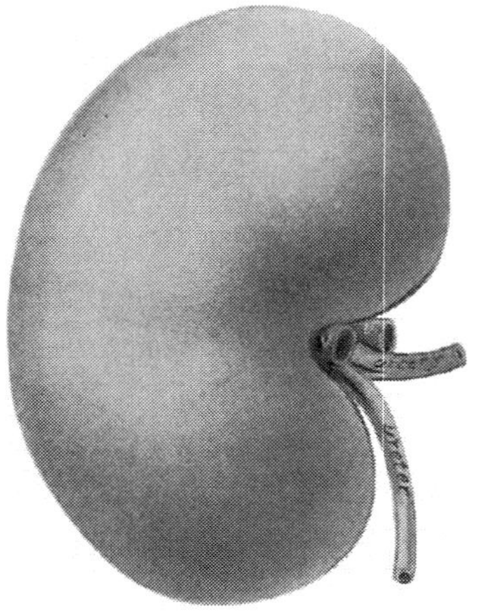

FIG. 384.—KIDNEY OF SHEEP, VENTRAL VIEW. *V.V.*, Branches of renal vein.

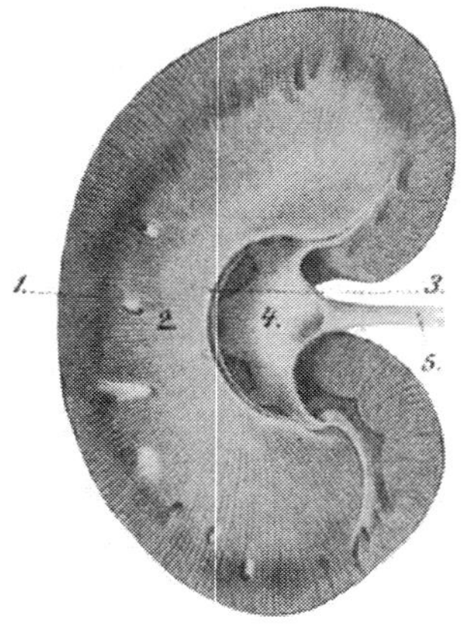

FIG. 385.—KIDNEY OF SHEEP, HORIZONTAL SECTION. *1*, Cortical substance; *2*, medullary substance; *3*, renal crest; *4*, renal pelvis; *5*, ureter. (From Leisering's Atlas, reduced.)

more than 1 inch (ca. 3 cm.). In position they resemble those of the ox, except that the right one is usually a little further back, and lies under the first three lumbar transverse processes. The average weight of each is about four ounces. The hilus is in the middle of the inner border. There is a renal crest or common papilla formed by the fusion of twelve to sixteen pyramids.

When the rumen is full, the left kidney (which is attached by a short mesentery) usually lies entirely to the right of the median plane, under the third, fourth, and fifth lumbar transverse processes. The primitive dorsal surface has become ventro-medial, and is somewhat flattened by contact with the rumen.

The **ureters** are, in general, like those of the horse, except in regard to the first part of the left one, which has a peculiar course, in conformity with the remarkable position of the kidney. It begins at the ventral part of the hilus (which faces toward the right), curves upward and inward over the outer aspect of the kidney to its dorsal surface, crosses the median plane, and runs backward on the left side.

The bladder is longer and narrower than that of the horse, and extends further forward on the abdominal floor. The peritoneal coat extends backward further than in the horse.

THE ADRENAL BODIES

The **right adrenal** lies against the inner part of the anterior pole of the right kidney. When hardened *in situ* it is pyramidal in form. Its inner surface is flattened and is in contact with the right crus of the diaphragm. The outer surface is convex and lies in the renal impression of the liver. The ventral surface is grooved for the posterior vena cava; on this surface a relatively large vein emerges near the apex. The base is concave and rests obliquely against the anterior pole of the kidney. The apex fits into the angle between the posterior vena cava and the dorsal border of the liver.

The **left adrenal** lies on the inner face of the posterior vena cava just behind the anterior mesenteric artery, and is therefore practically median in position. It is flattened, and irregularly triangular or heart-shaped in outline. Its left face

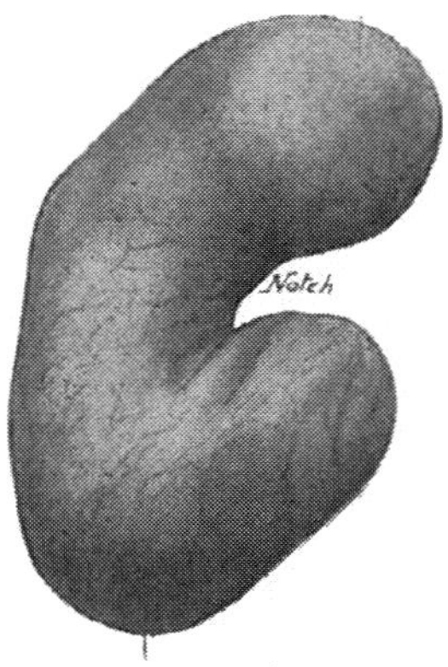

Fig. 386.—Left Adrenal of Ox, Ventral View: Hardened *in situ*.

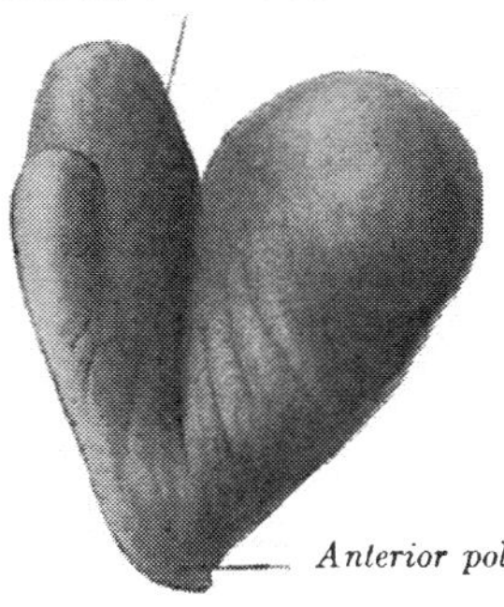

Fig. 387.—Right Adrenal of Ox, Ventral View: Hardened *in situ*.

is related to the dorsal sac of the rumen. Its right face is related to the vena cava, and presents a large emergent vein. The posterior border or base is deeply notched.

It is interesting to note that the left adrenal does not migrate with the kidney, but retains its primitive position; it lies usually about two inches (ca. 5 cm.) in front of a transverse plane through the anterior pole of the left kidney.

The adrenals of the **sheep** are both bean-shaped. The right one lies along the anterior part of the inner border of the kidney, at the angle of the junction of the right renal vein and the posterior vena cava. It is a little over an inch (ca. 3 cm.) long, and about an inch (ca. 12 to 15 mm.) wide. The left adrenal is longer, flatter, and somewhat bent. It lies across the left renal vein, to which it is attached, but is not in contact with the kidney.

URINARY ORGANS OF THE PIG

The **kidneys** are smooth and bean-shaped; they are more flattened dorsoventrally, more elongated, and smaller at the extremities than those of the dog. The length is about twice the width. They are usually almost symmetrically placed

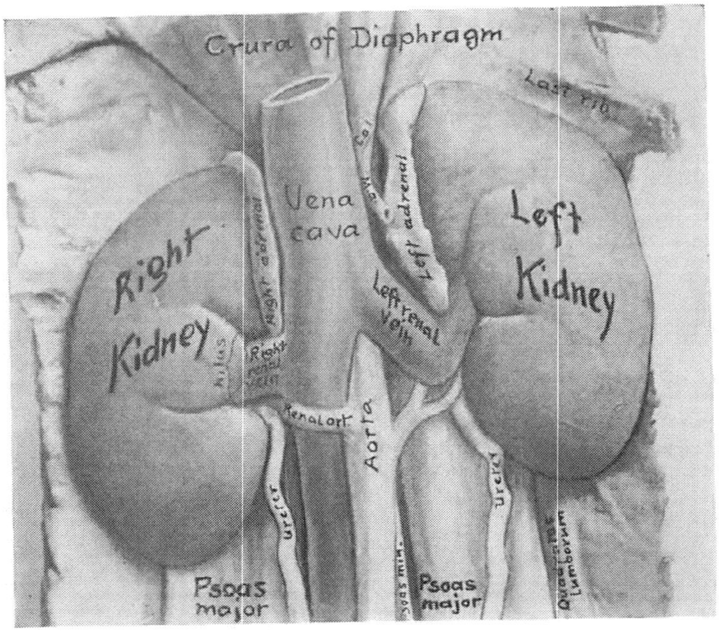

FIG. 388.—KIDNEYS OF PIG *in situ*, VENTRAL VIEW.
C.a., Hepatic artery; *M.a.*, gastro-splenic artery.

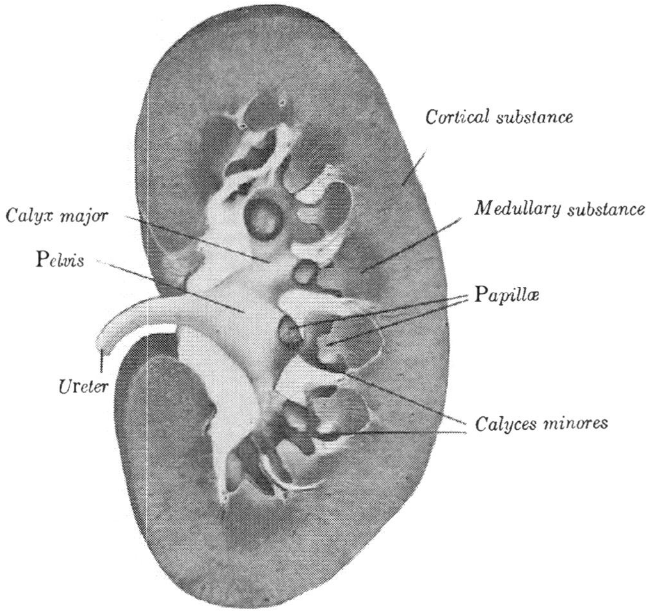

FIG. 389.—FRONTAL SECTION OF KIDNEY OF PIG.

on either side of the first four lumbar vertebræ. (Variations in position are not rare, and involve the left kidney oftener than the right. The former has been found near the pelvic inlet.) The external border lies against the flank parallel with the edge of the longissimus muscle. The posterior extremity usually lies about midway between the last rib and the external angle of the ilium. The anterior extremity of the right kidney usually extends as far forward as the last rib, but has no contact with the liver.

The weight of the kidney of a medium-sized pig is about seven to nine ounces (200 to 250 grams). The ratio of their combined weight to that of the body is about 1 : 150–200.

Structure.—The hilus is about in the middle of the inner border. The pelvis is funnel-shaped, and divides into two calyces majores, which pass in a curve forward and backward respectively, and give off some eight to twelve short calyces minores; each of the latter contains a papilla Some papillæ are narrow and conical, and correspond to a single pyramid; others are wide and flattened, and result from the fusion of two or more pyramids; some project directly through the wall of the pelvis without the formation of a calyx. The renal pyramids are distinct, but it is apparent that some are compound, *i. e.*, formed by fusion of primitively separate pyramids. The renal artery enters the ventral part of the hilus, and the ureter leaves it dorsally.

The only special feature in regard to the ureter is that it is at first relatively wide and gradually diminishes in caliber.

The **bladder** is relatively very large; when full, it lies chiefly in the abdominal cavity. It is almost completely covered with peritoneum.

URINARY ORGANS OF THE DOG

The **kidneys** are relatively large, forming about $\frac{1}{150}$ to $\frac{1}{200}$ of the body-weight; the weight of the kidney of a medium-sized dog is about two ounces (ca. 50 to 60 grams). They are both bean-shaped, thick dorso-ventrally, with a rounded ventral surface and a less convex dorsal surface; the surfaces are smooth.

The **right kidney** (Fig. 343) is not subject to much variation in position; it is situated usually under the last rib and the first three lumbar transverse processes. Its anterior part lies in the deep renal impression of the liver; its posterior part is related to the sublumbar muscles dorsally, and the pancreas and duodenum ventrally.

The **left kidney** (Fig. 342) is subject to some variation in position; this is due to the fact that it is loosely attached by the peritoneum, and is affected by the degree of fullness of the stomach. When the stomach is nearly empty, the kidney usually lies under the transverse processes of the second, third, and fourth lumbar vertebræ, so that its anterior pole is opposite to the hilus of the right kidney. As the stomach fills it pushes the left kidney backward, so that the anterior pole of the latter may be opposite the posterior pole of the right kidney. The dorsal surface is related to the sublumbar muscles. The ventral surface is in contact with the terminal part of the colon (Colon descendens). The external border is related to the spleen and the flank. The anterior extremity touches the stomach and the left extremity of the pancreas.

The external border of the left kidney has considerable contact with the flank, and hence it may be palpated more or less distinctly in the living animal about half-way between the last rib and the crest of the ilium.

Structure.—The hilus is in the middle of the inner border and is, relatively wide. Cortex, limiting zone, and medulla are clearly defined. On frontal sections it is seen that the medullary substance forms a horizontal renal crest like that of the horse, but with the important difference that curved ridges proceed dorsally and ventrally from the crest somewhat like buttresses. Sections above or below the renal crest often cut these ridges in such a manner as to give the appearance of conical papillæ, and thus tend strongly to produce a false impression. The pelvis is adapted to this arrangement of the medullary substance. It incloses a central cavity into which the renal crest projects, and is prolonged outward between the ridges, forming cavities for the latter, thus simulating the appearance of calyces which do not exist.

The **ureters** present no special features.

The **bladder** is abdominal in position, the neck lying at the anterior border of the pubic bones. It is relatively large, and when full, the vertex may reach to the umbilicus. It has a practically complete peritoneal coat.

THE ADRENALS

The right **adrenal** lies between the anterior part of the inner border of the kidney and the posterior vena cava. It is somewhat prismatic, and is pointed at either end.

The left **adrenal** lies along the posterior aorta, from the renal vein forward, but is not in contact with the kidney. It is elongated and flattened dorso-ventrally. (There is a furrow on the ventral surface for the vein which crosses it; the part in front of this furrow is discoid, and may be taken for the entire organ in a fat subject.)

The cortex is pale yellow in color, the medulla dark brown.

THE MALE GENITAL ORGANS

The **male genital organs** (Organa genitalia masculina) are: (1) The two **testicles,** the essential reproductive glands, with their coverings and appendages; (2) the **vasa deferentia,** the ducts of the testicles; (3) the **vesiculæ seminales;** (4) the **prostate,** a musculo-glandular organ; (5) the two **bulbo-urethral** (or Cowper's) **glands;** (6) the male **urethra,** a canal which transmits the generative and urinary secretions; (7) the **penis,** the male copulatory organ. The vesiculæ seminales, the prostate, and the bulbo-urethral glands discharge their secretions into the urethra, where they mix with the seminal fluid secreted by the testicles; hence they are often termed the accessory sexual glands.

MALE GENITAL ORGANS OF THE HORSE

THE TESTICLES

The **testicles** (Testes) are situated in the inguinal region, inclosed in a diverticulum of the abdomen termed the scrotum. Their long axes are nearly longitudinal. They are ovoid in form, but considerably compressed from side to side. Each presents two surfaces, two borders, and two extremities. The **internal** and **external surfaces** (Facies medialis, lateralis) are convex and smooth. The **free** or ventral **border** (Margo liber) is convex in both directions. The **attached** or dorsal **border** (Margo epididymidis) is nearly straight, and is the one by which the gland is suspended in the scrotum by the spermatic cord; the epididymis is attached to this border and overlies it externally. The **anterior** and **posterior extremities** (Extremitas capitata, caudalis) are rounded.

At the anterior extremity there is often a sessile or pedunculated sac which contains a clear fluid; this is the **appendix** testis or hydatid of Morgagni, from which a thread-like process extends backward toward the vas deferens. It is regarded as a remnant of the Müllerian duct of the embryo.

A testicle of average size of an adult stallion is about four or five inches (ca. 10 to 12 cm.) long, two and a half inches (ca. 6 to 7 cm.) high, and one and a half to two inches (ca. 4 to 5 cm.) wide; it weighs about ten and one half ounces (ca. 300 grams). They vary much in size in different subjects, and are commonly of unequal size, the left one being more often the larger.

The **epididymis** is adherent to the attached border of the testicle, and overlaps somewhat the external surface. Its anterior enlarged end is termed the **head** or globus major (Caput epididymidis), and its posterior, slightly enlarged end is the **tail** or globus minor (Cauda epididymidis); while the intermediate narrow part is the **body** (Corpus epididymidis). The head is closely connected with the testicle by the efferent ducts of the latter, by connective tissue, and by the serous membrane. The body is less closely attached by the serous covering, which forms externally a pocket beneath the epididymis termed the **digital fossa** (Sinus epididymidis). The tail is firmly attached to the posterior extremity of the testicle by a short ligament (Lig. epididymidis), formed by a thick fold of the tunica vaginalis, which contains smooth muscle-fibers; it is continued by the vas deferens.

Structure of the Testicle and Epididymis.—The greater part of the surface of the testicle is covered by a serous membrane, the **tunica vaginalis propria,** which is the visceral layer of the serous envelop of the cord and testicle; this is reflected from the attached border of the gland, leaving an uncovered area at which the vessels and nerves in the spermatic cord reach the testicle. Beneath this serous covering is the **tunica albuginea,** a strong capsule composed of dense white inelastic fibrous tissue and unstriped muscle-fibers. From the deep surface of this tunic delicate membranous **septa** (Septula testis) pass into the gland, dividing it into pyramidal spaces, the bases of which are peripheral. At the anterior part of the attached border of the testicle connective tissue and smooth muscle-fibers pass into the substance of the gland, forming the **mediastinum testis**; from this the septa radiate. The mediastinum contains a network of fine canals, the **rete testis**;

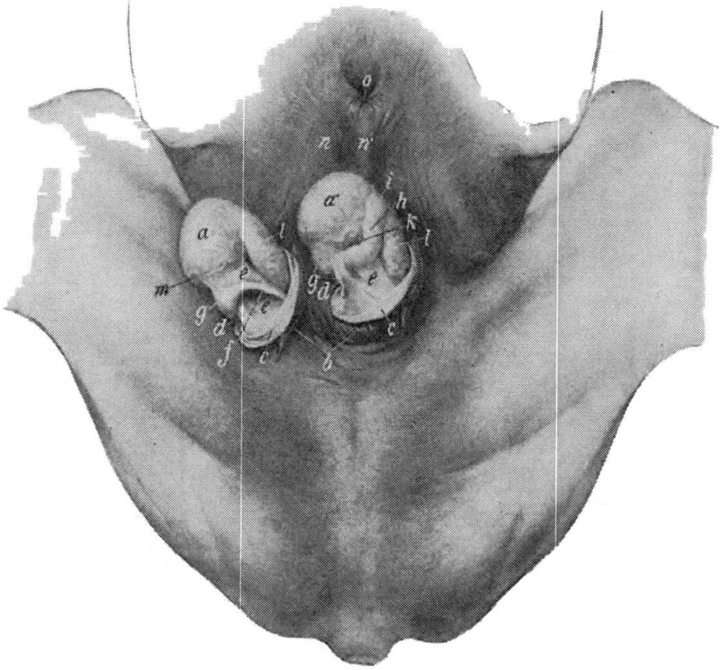

FIG. 390.—INGUINAL REGION OF STALLION, WITH TESTICLES EXPOSED.

a, a', Testicles; *b*, scrotum, opened and reflected; *c*, tunica vaginalis communis, opened and reflected; *d*, ligament of epididymis; *e*, tunica vaginalis propria (mesorchium); *f*, vas deferens; *g, g'*, tail of epididymis; *h*, body of same; *i*, head of same; k, digital fossa or sinus epididymidis; *l*, spermatic vessels showing through tunica vaginalis propria; *m*, spermatic artery; *n*, prepuce; *n'*, raphé; *o*, preputial orifice. (After Ellenberger-Baum, Top. Anat. d. Pferdes.)

it is traversed by blood-vessels, which radiate on the septa to the deep face of the tunica albuginea, forming a delicate network—the so-called tunica vasculosa. The spaces imperfectly marked off by the septa contain the **parenchyma testis,** which consists of **seminiferous tubules** (Tubuli seminiferi), supported by loose intertubular connective tissue. The tubules are collected into small masses or lobules (Lobuli testis). They are at first very tortuous (Tubuli contorti); toward the apex of the lobule they unite with other tubules, forming larger straight tubules (Tubuli recti); these pass into the mediastinum testis, where they form the **rete testis.** From the latter a number (ca. 15 to 20) of larger **efferent tubules** (Vasa efferentia) pierce the albuginea and enter the head of the epididymis.

The **epididymis** is covered by the tunica vaginalis propria and a thin albuginea.

Its head consists of lobules (Lobuli epididymidis), each of which consists of a coiled tubule or **conus vasculosus,** which succeeds a vas efferens. By the union of these tubules is formed a single tube, the **duct of the epididymis** (Ductus epididymidis), which, by its complex coils, forms the body and tail of the epididymis and terminates in the vas deferens. The tubules and the coils of the duct of the epididymis are held together by connective tissue and unstriped muscle-fibers. The tubules and duct are lined with ciliated epithelium, and the duct has a muscular coat which consists of longitudinal and circular fibers.

Vessels and Nerves.—The testicle is richly supplied with blood by the **spermatic artery,** a branch of the posterior aorta. The artery descends in the anterior part of the spermatic cord, and is very tortuous near the testicle; on reaching the attached border of the gland it passes backward in a flexuous manner, giving branches to the testicle and epididymis, turns around the posterior extremity,

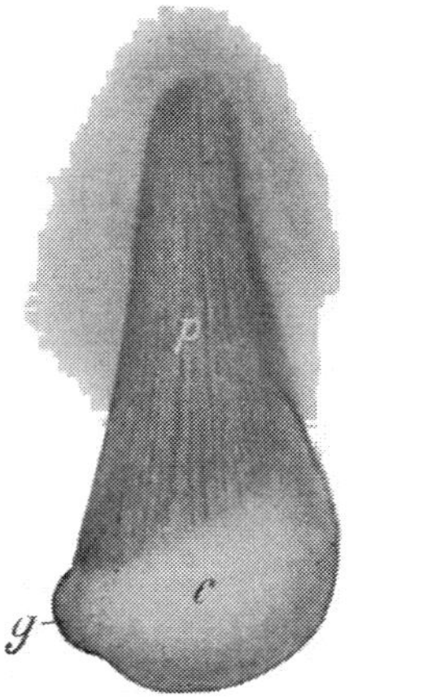

Fig. 391.—Right Testicle and Spermatic Cord of Horse, Inclosed in Tunica Vaginalis.

c, Tunica vaginalis communis; *g*, prominence caused by tail of epididymis; *p*, cremaster externus muscle. (After Ellenberger-Baum, Top. Anat. d. Pferdes.)

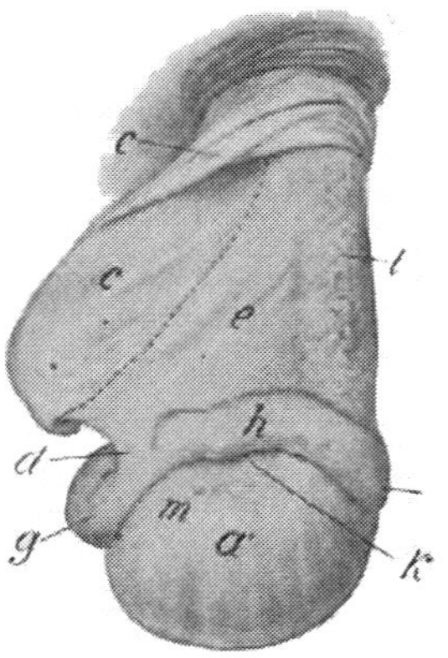

Fig. 392.—Right Testicle and Spermatic Cord of Horse, Exposed.

a', External surface of testicle; *c*, tunica vaginalis, cut and reflected; *d*, ligament of epididymis; *e*, mesorchium; *g*, tail, *h*, body, *i*, head of epididymis; *k*, digital fossa or sinus epididymidis; *l*, spermatic vessels showing through tunica vaginalis propria; *m*, end of spermatic artery. Dotted line indicates position of vas deferens on other side of mesorchium. (After Ellenberger-Baum, Top. Anat. d. Pferdes.)

and runs forward on the free border to the anterior extremity. It is partially embedded in the tunica albuginea, and detaches lateral branches which ascend in a tortuous fashion on each surface of the testicle; these give off small branches which enter the gland on the septa.

The **spermatic veins** on leaving the testicle, form the **pampiniform plexus** around the artery in the spermatic cord. The vein which issues from this plexus usually joins the posterior vena cava on the right side, the left renal vein on the left side.

The **nerves,** derived from the renal and posterior mesenteric plexuses, form the **spermatic plexus** around the vessels.

THE SCROTUM

The **scrotum,** in which the testicles and the lower parts of the spermatic cords are situated, is somewhat globular in form, but is commonly asymmetrical, since one testicle—more often the left—is the larger and more dependent. It varies in form and appearance in the same subject, according to the condition of its subcutaneous muscular tissue. The latter contracts on exposure to cold, so that the scrotum is drawn up and becomes thicker and wrinkled; when relaxed under the influence of heat or fatigue, or from debility, it becomes smooth and pendulous, with a constriction or neck superiorly. It consists of layers which correspond with those of the abdominal wall; considered from without inward these are:

(1) The **skin,** which is thin, elastic, usually black in color, and smooth and oily to the touch. It presents scattered short fine hairs, and is abundantly supplied with very large sebaceous and sweat glands. It is marked centrally by a longitudinal furrow, in which is a line, the **raphe scroti**; this is continued forward on the prepuce and behind on the perineum.

(2) The **dartos** (Tunica dartos) is reddish in color and is closely adherent to the skin except superiorly. It consists of fibro-elastic tissue and unstriped muscle. Along the raphe it forms a median partition, the **septum scroti,** which divides the scrotum into two pouches. Dorsally the septum divides into two layers which diverge on either side of the penis to join the abdominal tunic. At the bottom of the scrotum fibers connect the dartos closely with the tunica vaginalis and the tail of the epididymis, constituting the **scrotal ligament.**[1] Elsewhere the dartos is loosely connected with the underlying tunic by areolar tissue which contains no fat.

(3) The scrotal **fascia,** which is apparently derived from the oblique abdominal muscles.

It has been customary to describe three layers of fascia, in conformity with the accounts given in text-books of human anatomy. These are: (1) the intercolumnar or spermatic fascia, derived from the margin of the external inguinal ring; (2) the cremasteric fascia, derived from the internal oblique muscle; (3) the infundibuliform fascia, derived from the fascia transversalis. The first two cannot be distinguished by dissection and the third is (in the scrotum) fused with the parietal peritoneum of the tunica vaginalis.

(4) **The parietal** layer of **the tunica vaginalis.**—This is a fibro-serous sac which is continuous with the parietal peritoneum of the abdomen at the internal inguinal ring. It is thin above, but is thick in its scrotal part, where it is strengthened by fibrous tissue (Lamina fibrosa) derived from the transversalis fascia. It will be described further under the caption tunica vaginalis.[2]

THE VAS DEFERENS

This tube (Ductus deferens) extends from the tail of the epididymis to the ejaculatory duct. It passes upward in the inguinal canal, inclosed in a fold detached from the inner surface of the mesorchium, near the posterior (attached) border of the latter. At the vaginal ring it separates from the other constituents of the spermatic cord, and turns backward and inward into the pelvic cavity (Fig. 272). For some distance it lies in the free edge of the urogenital fold, by which it is attached to the lower part of the lateral wall of the pelvis. In its further course (over the dorsal surface of the bladder) it leaves the edge of the fold and inclines inward between its layers, coming in contact with the inner face of the vesicula seminalis. Over the neck of the bladder the two vasa lie very close together, flanked laterally by the necks of the vesiculæ seminales, and having the uterus masculinus between them. They then disappear under the isthmus of the prostate, and are continued through the wall of the urethra by the ejaculatory ducts. The latter are formed in the urethral wall by the union of the

[1] This is a remnant of the gubernaculum testis of the fœtus.

[2] The tunica vaginalis is not a part of the scrotum in the strict or narrow sense of that term, but is included here on practical grounds.

vas deferens with the duct (or neck) of the corresponding vesicula seminalis; they are thin-walled tubes, about 2 to 3 mm. long and 6 to 7 mm. wide, which open into the urethra on either side of the colliculus seminalis. In about 15 per cent. of subjects the vas deferens and duct of the seminal vesicle do not unite, but open side by side into the urethra. From its origin until it reaches the dorsal surface of the bladder the vas deferens has a uniform diameter of about a quarter of an inch (ca. 6 mm.). It then forms a fusiform dilatation, the **ampulla ductus deferentis** (Fig. 394); this part is about six to eight inches (ca. 15 to 20 cm.) long, and in its largest part nearly an inch (ca. 2 cm.) in diameter in the stallion; in geldings the dilatation is usually not very pronounced. Beyond the ampulla the duct abruptly contracts.

Structure.—The wall of the vas deferens is thick and the lumen relatively small, so that the tube has a firm and cord-like character. It is covered with peritoneum, except in the last few inches of its course. The loose **adventitia** contains numerous vessels and nerves. The thick **muscular coat** consists of longitudinal and circular layers. The **mucous membrane** has an epithelium of short columnar cells. In the posterior part of the tube, and especially in the ampulla, there are numerous tubulo-alveolar glands.

Blood-supply.—Spermatic and umbilical arteries.

Nerve-supply.—Spermatic and pelvic plexuses.

THE SPERMATIC CORD

The **spermatic cord** (Funiculus spermaticus) consists of the structures carried down by the testicle in its migration through the inguinal canal from the abdominal cavity to the scrotum. It begins at the internal inguinal ring, where its constituent parts come together, extends obliquely downward through the inguinal canal, passes over the side of the penis, and ends at the attached border of the testicle. It consists of the following structures:

(1) The **spermatic artery.**

(2) The **spermatic veins,** which form the pampiniform plexus around the artery.

(3) The **lymphatics,** which accompany the veins.

(4) Sympathetic **nerves,** which run with the artery.

(5) The **vas deferens.**

(6) The **internal cremaster muscle,** which consists of bundles of unstriped muscular tissue.

(7) The **visceral** layer of the **tunica vaginalis** or **mesorchium.**

The first four of these constituents are gathered into a rounded mass which forms the anterior part of the cord; they are united by connective tissue, interspersed with which are bundles of the cremaster internus. The vas deferens is situated posteriorly, inclosed in a special fold detached from the inner surface of the mesorchium; hence it is not visible externally.

The term spermatic cord is to a certain extent misleading as applied to most animals, while in man the structure is distinctly cord-like. In the horse, when the tunica vaginalis is slit open and the "cord" stretched out, the latter is seen to have the form of a wide sheet, the mesorchium, which has a thick, rounded anterior edge, the so-called "vascular part" of the cord. The posterior edge of the mesorchium is continuous with the parietal layer of the tunic; its inner surface presents posteriorly the deferential fold (Plica ductus deferentis). Between the two layers of the mesorchium are bundles of unstriped muscle (cremaster internus) and small vessels.

THE TUNICA VAGINALIS

The **tunica vaginalis** is a somewhat pyriform serous sac which extends from the internal inguinal ring through the inguinal canal to the bottom of the scrotum.

Like the abdominal peritoneum, of which it is an evagination, it consists of two layers—parietal and visceral. The **parietal layer,** or **tunica vaginalis communis** (s. reflexa), lines the scrotum below; its narrow, tubular part lies in the inguinal canal and is directly continuous with the parietal peritoneum of the abdomen at the internal inguinal ring. The **cavity** of the tunica vaginalis (Cavum vaginale) is a diverticulum of the general peritoneal cavity, with which it communicates through the **vaginal ring** (Annulus vaginalis). It contains normally a small quantity of serous fluid. The parietal layer is reflected from the posterior wall of the inguinal canal around the structures of the cord, forming the **mesorchium,** a fold analogous to the mesentery of the intestine. The **visceral layer,** or **tunica vaginalis propria,** covers the spermatic cord, testicle, and epididymis.

The **external cremaster muscle** (M. cremaster externus) lies on the outer and posterior part of the tunic, to the scrotal part of which it is attached.

Confusion has arisen from the use of the term internal abdominal or inguinal ring in two senses. The term is used to designate the upper or abdominal opening of the inguinal canal, but it is also applied to the upper opening of the cavity of the tunica vaginalis. It should only be applied to the abdominal opening of the canal, the **subperitoneal ring.** The **peritoneal ring** at which the cavity of the tunica vaginalis opens into the general peritoneal sac is distinguished by the name **vaginal ring.** It is placed about four or five inches (ca. 10 to 12 cm.) from the linea alba, and about two or three inches (ca. 6 to 8 cm.) in front of the ilio-pectineal eminence. In stallions it will usually admit the end of the finger readily, but it may be abnormally large and allow a loop of bowel to enter the cavity of the tunica vaginalis. In the gelding it is smaller and sometimes partially occluded. In man the cavity is almost always obliterated early, except in its scrotal portion, thus abolishing the vaginal ring.

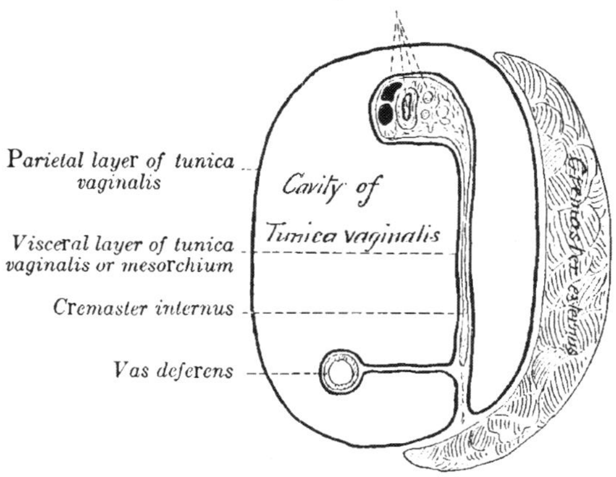

FIG. 393.—DIAGRAM OF CROSS-SECTION OF SPERMATIC CORD AND TUNICA VAGINALIS; LATTER REPRESENTED AS DISTENDED.

DESCENT OF THE TESTICLES

During early fœtal life the testicle is situated against the dorsal wall of the abdominal cavity, in contact with the ventral surface of the corresponding kidney. As growth proceeds it gradually migrates from this primitive position, and finally passes down the inguinal canal into the scrotum. Previous to its descent through the abdominal wall the testicle is suspended by a fold of peritoneum, termed the **mesorchium.** This fold contains the vessels and nerves of the testicle in its anterior border. In its posterior edge is the elongated tail of the epididymis, and two cords of fibrous tissue and unstriped muscle. One of these cords is short and connects the tail of the epididymis with the testicle; later it becomes shorter, and is termed the ligament of the epididymis. The other cord, the **gubernaculum testis**, extends from the tail of the epididymis to the subperitoneal tissue in the vicinity of the future vaginal ring. The **deferential fold** (Plica ductus deferentis) is given off from the inner face of the mesorchium, and joins the urogenital fold posteriorly. The body of the epididymis at this time lies in the edge of an oblique fold formed by the outer layer of the mesorchium. After the middle of fœtal life, a pouch or diverticulum of the peritoneum, the **processus vaginalis**, grows downward through the inguinal canal, carrying with it cremaster fibers derived from the internal oblique muscle and a layer from the transversalis fascia. It is aecompanied by an inguinal extension of the gubernaculum testis. The latter blends below with the subcutaneous tissue which later becomes the dartos. The tail of the epididymis first enters the processus vaginalis, followed by the testicle with its mesorchium, which descends within this diverticulum of the peritoneum until it reaches the scrotum. The vas deferens and its fold descend synchronously with the epididymis and testicle.

The mechanical factors concerned in the migration of the testicle are matters on which much uncertainty still exists. That the gubernaculum exerts sufficient traction to guide the epididymis and testicle to the inguinal canal seems plausible. The internal inguinal ring may constitute a locus minoris resistentiæ in the abdominal wall, especially after the descent of the processus vaginalis. Progressive shortening of the gubernaculum was formerly considered to be the chief cause of the descent through the abdominal wall. Increase in the intra-abdominal pressure is probably an important factor.

In the foal the descent of the testicles is often complete at birth, but it frequently happens that one testicle or both may be retained in the inguinal canal or in the abdomen for some months. In other cases the testicle may return into the canal or abdomen, since in the young foal the vaginal ring is large and the testicle small and soft, and not yet closely anchored by the scrotal ligament. In rare cases the descent may be completed as late as the fourth year (personal observation).

Indefinite retention of one testicle or both in the abdominal cavity or inguinal canal is not rare in horses; this condition is termed **cryptorchism**. Abdominal retention is the more usual form of cryptorchism in adult horses, inguinal retention being usually temporary. The retained testicle is usually, but not always, small, thin, soft, and flabby, and is non-spermiogenic. The processus vaginalis and the inguinal part of the gubernaculum are usually present, but may be rudimentary. The ligament of the epididymis and the corresponding part of the mesorchium are often so long that the tail of the epididymis may be several inches distant from the testicle. The abdominal part of the gubernaculum may be 8 to 10 inches (ca. 20 to 25 cm.) long, and the ligament of the epididymis much elongated (10 to 15 cm. in length according to Vennerholm); thus the testicle may have a wide range. The vaginal ring is sometimes closed.

In many mammals the testicles normally remain in the abdominal cavity; such animals are termed testiconda, and include the elephant, some insectivora, hyrax, sloths, ant-eaters, armadillos, and cetacea. In others the testicles descend periodically during the period of œstrum, and then return into the abdomen, or they may be extruded and retracted voluntarily; this is true of most rodents, many insectivora (moles, shrews, hedgehog), and bats.

THE VESICULAE SEMINALES

The **vesiculæ seminales** (Fig. 394) are two elongated and somewhat pyriform sacs, which lie on either side of the posterior part of the dorsal surface of the bladder. They are partly inclosed in the urogenital fold, and are related to the rectum dorsally. Their long axes are parallel with the vas deferentia and converge posteriorly. Each consists of a rounded blind end, the **fundus**, a middle, slightly narrower part, the body, and a posterior constricted part, the **neck** or duct.

In the stallion they are about six to eight inches (ca. 15 to 20 cm.) long, and their greatest diameter is about two inches (ca. 5 cm.); in the gelding they are usually much smaller.[1]

[1] Sometimes one vesicula or both are very large in the gelding. The writer has seen four cases in the dissecting room, three of which were bilateral, the other unilateral. The vesicula resembled the urinary bladder in appearance and contained about a quart of thick, amber-colored secretion.

The vesiculæ are, for the most part, retroperitoneal, but the fundus extends forward into the urogenital fold and hence has a serous covering. The **neck** or **duct** (Ductus excretorius) dips under the prostate, and usually unites with the end of the vas deferens to form the ejaculatory duct.

Structure.—The wall, exclusive of the partial serous coat, consists of a fibrous

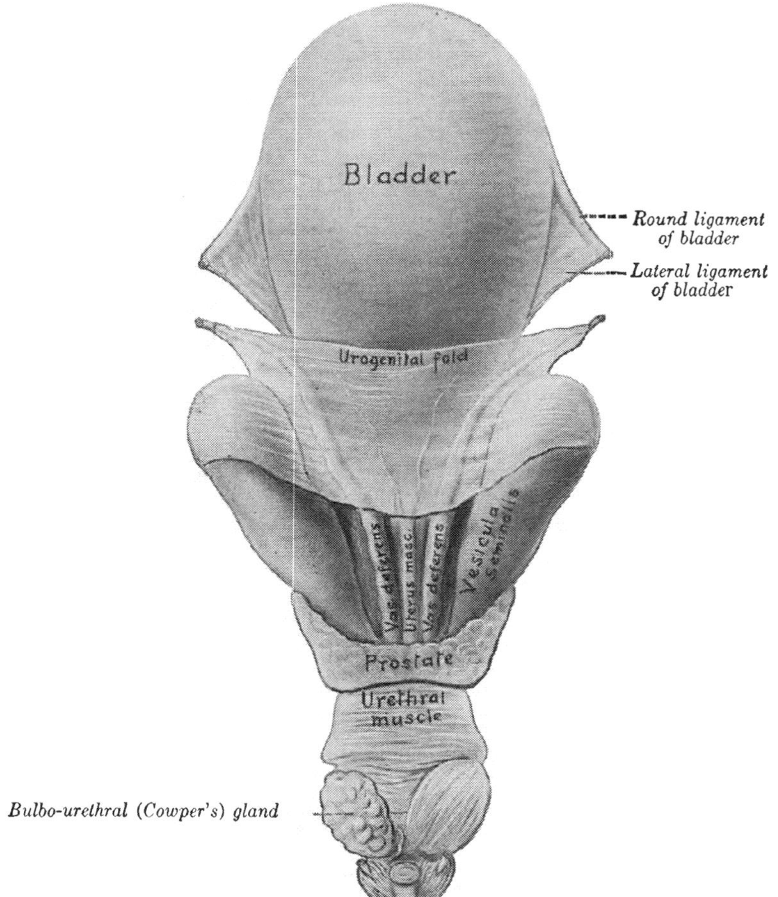

Fig. 394.—Internal Genital Organs of Stallion, Dorsal View.
On left side urethral muscle has been removed over bulbo-urethral gland. Cornua of uterus masculinus are indicated in urogenital fold.

adventitia, a middle muscular coat, and a mucous lining. The muscular coat is thickest at the fundus, and consists of two planes of longitudinal fibers with a circular layer between them. The mucous membrane is thin, and is arranged in numerous folds which form a network; the spaces so inclosed present the openings of tubulo-alveolar glands. The epithelium is columnar. The blood-supply is derived from the internal pudic artery.

THE PROSTATE

The **prostate** (Prostata) is a musculo-glandular organ which lies on the neck of the bladder and the beginning of the urethra, beneath the rectum. It consists of two lateral lobes and a connecting isthmus.

The **lateral** lobes, right and left (Lobus dexter et sinister), are somewhat prismatic in form, and are directed forward, outward, and somewhat upward. The antero-internal surface of each lobe is concave and partly embraces the corresponding vesicula seminalis. The dorsal surface is concave and is in relation with the rectum. The ventral surface is convex and lies on the obturator internus muscle and fat. The apex is pointed and lies near the posterior end of the superior ischiatic spine.

The **isthmus** is a thin, transverse band, about four-fifths of an inch (ca. 2 cm.) wide. It lies over the junction of the bladder with the urethra, the uterus masculinus, the terminal parts of the vasa deferentia, and the necks of the vesiculæ seminales. Dorsally it is partly covered by transverse fibers of the urethral (Wilson's) muscle.

Structure.—The prostate is inclosed in a fibro-muscular **capsule,** which sends thick, somewhat radially arranged **trabeculæ** into the gland substance, dividing it into spheroidal or ovoid **lobules.** The lobules contain a central space in which the prostatic secretion (Succus prostaticus) collects. The walls of these spaces are pouched out to form tubular diverticula, and the latter present saccular dilatations. These cavities are all lined by cubical epithelium. There are 15 to 20 **prostatic ducts** (Ductus prostatici) on either side, which perforate the urethra and open lateral to the colliculus seminalis. The **blood-supply** is derived from the **internal pudic artery.**

The surface of the prostate is commonly tuberculate in old subjects, and amyloid bodies and calcareous concretions may be found in it.

THE UTERUS MASCULINUS

The **uterus masculinus** or **prostatic utricle** is a rudimentary structure of variable size and form, situated centrally on the posterior part of the dorsal surface of the bladder. When well developed, it consists of a median flattened tube, some three or four inches (ca. 7.5 to 10 cm.) long, and about half an inch (ca. 1 to 1.5 cm.) wide, the anterior part of which lies in the urogenital fold and gives off two slender processes or cornua; the latter curve forward and outward in the fold a variable distance, being sometimes traceable as far as the anterior end of the ampulla of the vas deferens. The posterior extremity of the tube passes under the isthmus of the prostate, and opens into the urethra on the summit of the colliculus or joins an ejaculatory duct. It has a muscular coat and a mucous lining. In many cases it consists merely of a very small central tubule with a blind anterior end, or a band, not at all sharply marked off from the adjacent tissue; in other cases it cannot be recognized. It is interesting chiefly as being a remnant of the ducts of Müller and the homologue of the uterus and vagina.

THE BULBO-URETHRAL GLANDS

The **bulbo-urethral** (or Cowper's) **glands** (Glandulæ bulbourethrales) are two in number, and are situated on either side of the pelvic part of the urethra close to the ischial arch (Fig. 452). They are covered by the urethral (Wilson's) muscle. They are ovoid in form, somewhat depressed dorso-ventrally, and their long axes are directed obliquely forward and outward. In the stallion they may measure about two inches (ca. 5 cm.) in length, and an inch or more (ca. 3 cm.) in width. In the gelding they are about the size of an average hazel nut.

Structure.—They resemble the prostate in general structure, but the interstitial tissue is much less abundant, especially in regard to its muscular elements. In the peripheral part there are striped muscle-fibers. Each gland has six to eight **excretory ducts** (Ductus excretorii) which open into the urethra on a series of small papillæ behind the prostatic ducts and close to the median plane. The **blood-supply** comes from the **internal pudic** artery

THE PENIS

The **penis,** the male organ of copulation, is composed essentially of erectile tissue, and incloses the extrapelvic part of the urethra. It extends from the ischial arch forward between the thighs on to the umbilical region of the abdominal wall. It is supported by the fascia penis and the skin, and its prescrotal portion is situated

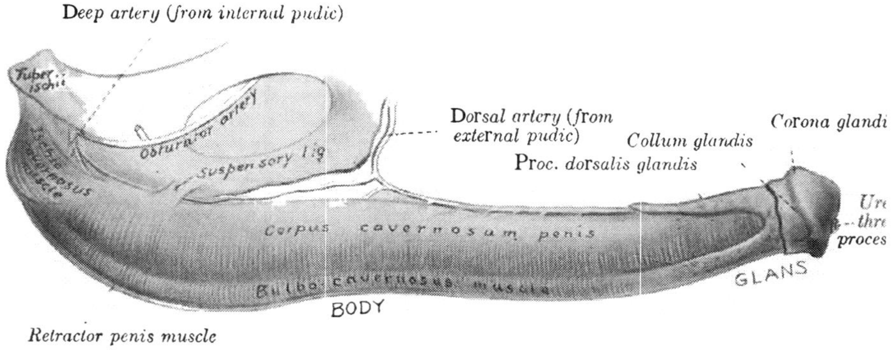

Fig. 395.—Penis of Horse, Lateral View.

in a cutaneous pouch, the prepuce or sheath. It is cylindrical in form, but much compressed laterally in the greater part of its extent.

In the quiescent state it is about 20 inches (ca. 50 cm.) long; of this, about 6 to 8 inches (ca. 15 to 20 cm.) is free in the prepuce. In erection it increases 50 per cent. or more in length.

It may be divided into a root, a body, and a terminal enlargement, the glans.

The root (Radix penis) is attached to the lateral parts of the ischial arch by two **crura,** which converge and unite below the arch (Fig. 452). The urethra passes over the ischial arch between the crura, and curves forward to become incorporated with the penis.

The **body** (Corpus penis) begins at the junction of the crura and constitutes the bulk of the organ. At its origin it is attached to the symphysis ischii by two strong flat bands, the **suspensory ligaments** of the penis (Ligamenta suspensoria penis), which blend with the tendon of origin of the graciles muscles (Figs. 451, 456). This part of the penis is flattened laterally for the most part, but becomes rounded and smaller anteriorly. It presents four surfaces. The dorsal **surface** or **dorsum penis,** is narrow and rounded; on it are the dorsal arteries and nerves of the penis and a rich venous plexus. The **ventral** or urethral **surface** (Facies urethralis) is rounded, and along it runs the urethra, embedded in the deep **urethral groove** of the corpus cavernosum. The **lateral surfaces** are high and flattened, except anteriorly, where they are lower and rounded.

The **glans penis** is the enlarged free end of the organ. It is marked off from the body by a faintly marked **neck** (Collum glandis). In front of this is a prominent circular ridge, the **corona glandis,** which is notched below. The base of the glans is rounded and extends further backward dorsally than ventrally; it is marked in its lower part by a deep depression, the **fossa glandis,** in which the urethra protrudes for about an inch (ca. 2.5 cm.) as a free tube, the **urethral process** (Processus urethræ), covered by a thin integument. The urethra is thus surrounded by a circular fossa, which opens superiorly into the **urethral sinus,** a bilocular diverticulum lined by thin black skin. This diverticulum is filled sometimes with a caseous mass of sebaceous matter and epithelial débris.

Structure.—The penis consists essentially of two erectile bodies, the corpus cavernosum penis and the corpus spongiosum.

The **corpus cavernosum penis** forms the greater part of the bulk of the penis except at its free extremity. It arises from each side of the ischial arch by a **crus,** which is embedded in the ischio-cavernosus muscle. Below the ischial arch the crura fuse completely to form the laterally compressed body of the corpus cavernosum; this presents ventrally the **urethral groove** (Sulcus urethralis), which contains the urethra and corpus spongiosum. Anteriorly, the corpus cavernosum divides into three processes, a long central one, which is capped by the glans penis, and two short blunt lateral ones. The corpus cavernosum is inclosed by the **tunica albuginea,** a thick capsule of fibrous tissue which contains many elastic fibers and some unstriped muscle. Externally the fibers are chiefly longitudinal; internally they are mainly circular and are looser in arrangement. Numerous **trabeculæ** pass inward from the tunic and form a sponge-like framework in the interior of the corpus cavernosum, which is thus divided into numerous spaces (Cavernæ). These spaces may be regarded as greatly enlarged capillaries; they contain blood, are lined with flat endothelial cells, and are directly continuous with the veins of the penis. Their walls are composed very largely of unstriped muscle. Erection is produced by distention of these spaces with blood; at other times the spaces are mere slits.

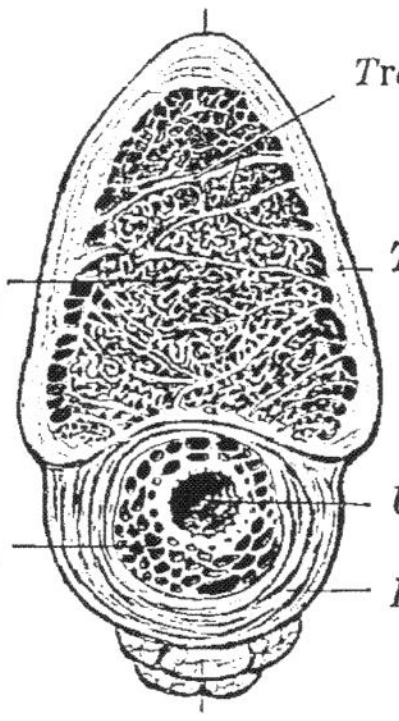

Fig. 396.—Cross-section of Body of Penis of Horse.

In man there are two distinct corpora cavernosa, separated by a complete septum penis, except in the middle part of the organ, where the septum is composed of vertical trabeculæ, between which are slit-like intervals; through the latter the blood-spaces of the two corpora cavernosa communicate. In the horse no distinct septum exists except near the root, but in the proximal and distal parts of the corpus cavernosum there are vertical trabeculæ.

The **corpus spongiosum** or **corpus cavernosum urethræ** forms a tube around the urethra, and is much enlarged at its free end to form the bulk of the glans penis; throughout the remainder of its course it is practically uniform in size, and does not form any very distinct bulb (Bulbus urethræ) at its origin, as in man and many animals. The glans has been described in part; it should be noted that the corpus spongiosum extends backward dorsally a distance of about four inches (ca. 10 cm.) on the middle process of the corpus cavernosum penis, forming the processus dorsalis glandis. The urethral process is covered by a thin layer of corpus spongiosum.

In structure the corpus spongiosum has a general resemblance to the corpus cavernosum, but the trabeculæ are finer and more elastic. In the glans the trabeculæ are highly elastic, and the spaces are large and very extensible; the latter are continuous at the extremity of the processus dorsalis with large veins on the dorsum penis. There is a partial septum glandis. The skin covering the glans is thin, destitute of glands, and richly supplied with nerves and special nerve-endings.

Vessels and Nerves.—The penis is supplied with blood by three **arteries**, viz., the **internal pudic**, **obturator**, and **external pudic**. The **veins** form a rich plexus on the dorsum and sides of the penis, which is drained by the **external pudic** and **obturator veins**; from the root the blood is carried by the **internal pudic veins**. The **lymphatics** run with the veins and go to the inguinal and lumbar glands. The **nerves** are derived chiefly from the **pudic nerves** and the **pelvic plexus** of the sympathetic.

MUSCLES OF THE PENIS (Figs. 183, 451, 452, 456)

1. The **ischio-cavernosus** (or erector penis) is a short but strong paired muscle, which arises from the tuber ischii and the adjacent part of the sacro-sciatic ligament, and is inserted on the crus and adjacent part of the body of the penis. It is somewhat fusiform, incloses the crus as in a sheath, and is situated in a deep depression in the semimembranosus muscle. It pulls the penis against the pelvis, and assists in producing and maintaining erection by compressing the dorsal veins of the penis. Its blood-supply is derived from the obturator artery, and the nerve-supply from the pudic nerve.

2. The **retractor penis** is an unstriped muscle which arises on the ventral surface of the first two or three coccygeal vertebræ. It divides into two flat bands, half an inch or more (ca. 1.5 cm.) in width, which pass downward over the sides of the rectum to meet below the anus. Here there is a decussation of fibers, thus forming a sort of suspensory apparatus for the posterior part of the rectum and the anus. From the decussation the muscle passes for a short distance between superficial and deep layers of the bulbo-cavernosus, and then along the ventral surface of the penis, to which it is loosely attached. Near the glans penis it splits up into bundles which pass through the bulbo-cavernosus and are attached to the tunica albuginea. Below the anus the muscle is attached to the sphincter ani externus. On the penis the two muscles are intimately united to each other. Their action is to withdraw the penis into the sheath after erection or protrusion. The proximal part would draw the anus upward and forward and support it during defecation.

THE PREPUCE

The **prepuce** (Præputium), popularly called the "sheath," is a double invagination of the skin which contains and covers the free or prescrotal portion of the penis when not erect. It consists of two parts, external and internal. The external part or sheath extends from the scrotum forward close to the umbilicus, where the external layer is reflected ventrally and laterally, forming the thick margin of the **preputial orifice** (Ostium præputiale); dorsally it is directly continuous with the integument of the abdominal wall. It is marked by a median **raphe præputii**, a continuation of the scrotal raphé. At the lower margin of the preputial orifice there are often in the stallion two papillæ, which are rudimentary teats or nipples. The internal layer passes backward from the preputial orifice a distance of about six to eight inches (ca. 15 to 20 cm.), lining the cavity of the external prepuce, and is then reflected forward until it approaches the orifice, where it is again reflected backward. It thus forms within the cavity of the sheath a secondary tubular invagination, the prepuce proper, in which the anterior part of the penis lies. This tubular cavity is closed behind by the reflection of the internal layer on to the penis to form the penile layer of the prepuce. Its orifice is surrounded by a thick margin, the **preputial ring** (Annulus præputialis), which is connected ventrally with the outer part of the sheath by the **preputial frenum** (Frenulum præputii).

The arrangement differs from that found in man in the fact that the inner part of the prepuce as described above is equivalent to the entire human prepuce. This part, the prepuce proper, is well seen on sagittal sections, and can be demonstrated by pulling the penis, inclosed in this prepuce, out of the cavity of the sheath; the arrangement of the free part of the penis and prepuce is then like that in man. (In paraphimosis the penis is strangulated by the preputial ring.)

Structure.—The **external skin** of the prepuce resembles that of the scrotum. The **inner** layers of skin are hairless, variable in color, and often irregularly pigmented; they form irregular folds, and are supplied with numerous large sebaceous glands and coil glands, which reach their greatest size at the preputial ring. Be-

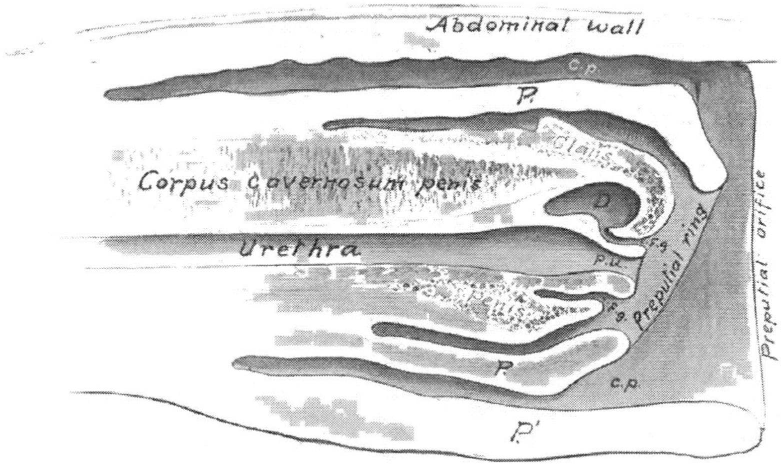

Fig. 397.—Sagittal Section of Prepuce and Part of Penis of Horse.
P, Internal part of prepuce or prepuce proper; *P'*, external part of prepuce or sheath; *c.p.*, preputial cavity; *F.g.*, fossa glandis; *D*, diverticulum of fossa glandis; *p.u.*, processus urethræ.

yond this the glands are absent, and the skin resembles a non-glandular mucous membrane. The secretion of the **preputial glands** (Glandulæ præputiales), together with desquamated epithelial cells, forms the fatty **smegma præputii**, which has a strong unpleasant odor, and often accumulates in considerable amount. Beneath the skin is a large amount of loose connective tissue, except over the glans penis, where the skin is closely attached to the tunic of the corpus spongiosum. The external part of the prepuce is strengthened by a layer of elastic tissue, derived from the abdominal tunic, and termed the suspensory ligament.

Vessels and Nerves.—The **arteries** are branches of the **external pudic artery**, and the **veins** go chiefly to the **external pudic vein**. The **lymphatics** go to the superficial inguinal and lumbar lymph glands. The **nerves** are derived from the **pudic**, **ilio-hypogastric**, and **ilio-inguinal** nerves.

THE MALE URETHRA

The **urethra** of the male (Urethra masculina) is the long mucous tube which extends from the bladder to the glans penis. It passes backward on the floor of the pelvis, turns around the ischial arch, forming an acute angle, and passes forward inclosed in the corpus spongiosum. It may, therefore, be divided into two segments, pelvic and extrapelvic.

The **pelvic part** (Pars pelvina) is four or five inches (ca. 10 to 12 cm.) long. At its origin it is not distinguishable from the neck of the bladder in size or structure; in fact no line of demarcation exists between the two. Behind the prostate the tube dilates to a potential width of two inches or more (ca. 5 to 6 cm.). Near the ischial arch, between the bulbo-urethral (Cowper's) glands, it contracts again, forming the **isthmus urethræ**. It is related dorsally to the rectum and the prostate, ventrally to the internal obturator muscles, and laterally to the bulbo-urethral

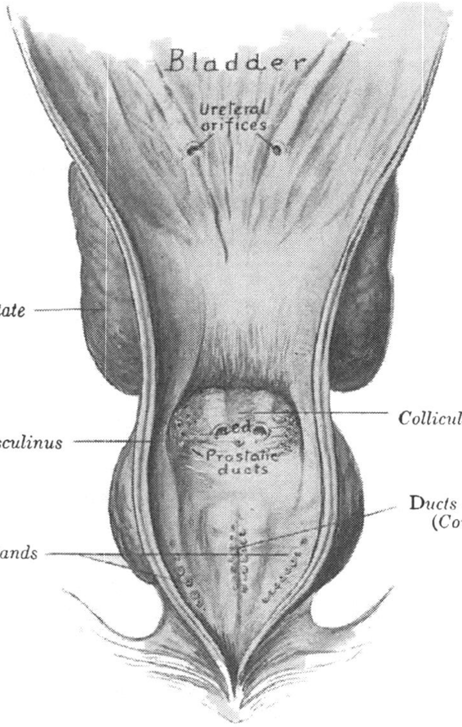

Fig. 398.—Pelvic Urethra and Posterior Part of Bladder of Horse Slit Ventrally and Laid Open. *e.d.*, Ejaculatory ducts.

glands. It is inclosed, except at its origin, by the urethral (Wilson's) muscle. Beneath this is a rich venous plexus, forming a sort of erectile tissue.[1]

The **extrapelvic part** (Pars cavernosa) passes between the two crura of the penis and runs along the groove on the ventral surface of the corpus cavernosum penis, inclosed by the corpus spongiosum and the bulbo-cavernosus muscle. It passes through the glans penis and projects forward about an inch in the fossa glandis as a free tube, the **processus urethræ**; this part is covered by a delicate integument, under which there is a thin layer of erectile tissue.

[1] It has been customary to divide the pelvic part of the urethra into prostatic and membranous parts. These terms apply well in human anatomy, but have no special value in comparative anatomy. In the horse a prostatic part hardly exists, unless we assume that it and the neck of the bladder together are only about an inch in length. There is no membranous part in the sense in which that term is used in regard to man.

The lumen of the tube is largely obliterated in the inactive condition of the parts. When moderately distended its dimensions in a horse of medium size are as follows: At its origin the diameter is about half an inch (1 to 1.5 cm.). The pelvic dilatation at its widest part measures one and a half to two inches (ca. 3.5 to 5 cm.) transversely, and about an inch (2 to 3 cm.) vertically; it is elliptical in cross-section when fully distended. The isthmus at the ischial arch is a little smaller than the initial part. Beyond this the lumen is about one-half to three-fourths of an inch (ca. 1.5 cm.) in diameter, and is fairly uniform to the glans penis. Here there is a slight fusiform dilatation (Fossa navicularis), beyond which the tube contracts.

The opening from the bladder into the urethra is termed the **internal urethral orifice** (Orificium urethræ internum); it is closed except during urination. The terminal opening is the **external urethral orifice** (Orificium urethræ externum) or meatus urinarius. The two orifices of the **ejaculatory ducts** are situated dorsally on either side of the colliculus seminalis, about two inches (ca. 5 cm.) behind the internal urethral orifice; they are slit-like and close together. The small orifice of the uterus masculinus is placed centrally on the colliculus; it is inconstant. The orifices of the **prostatic ducts** are on two groups of small papillæ, placed lateral to the openings of the ejaculatory ducts. The **ducts** of the **bulbo-urethral** (Cowper's) **glands** open on two lateral series of small papillæ, about an inch (ca. 2.5 cm.) further back and close to the median line. The small orifices of the **urethral glands** are situated laterally in the wide pelvic portion.

Structure.—The **mucous membrane** contains an unusually large amount of fine elastic fibers, and in its pelvic part there are alveolar **glands** (Glandulæ urethrales). The epithelium is at first like that of the bladder, then becomes cylindrical, and in the terminal part is stratified squamous. In the dorsal wall the membrane forms a median ridge, the **urethral crest** (Crista urethralis); this terminates about two inches from the internal urethral orifice in a rounded elevation, the **colliculus seminalis,** on the sides of which the ejaculatory ducts open.

At the origin of the urethra there is a layer of circular **unstriped muscle-fibers** outside of the mucous coat. Beyond this the latter is inclosed by a layer of **erectile tissue,** composed of plexuses of veins supported by trabeculæ of elastic and smooth muscular tissue. This is continued by the corpus spongiosum. Outside of the erectile tissue there is a continuation of the intrinsic unstriped muscular coat, consisting of external and internal longitudinal strata, with a layer of circular fibers between them.

Except at its origin and termination the urethra is provided with a continuous layer of striped muscle, placed outside of the erectile tissue. This is described as consisting of two parts or muscles.

(1) The **urethral** (or Wilson's) **muscle** (M. urethralis) consists of dorsal and ventral layers of transverse fibers on the wide pelvic part of the urethra, and covers the bulbo-urethral (Cowper's) glands. It is a compressor of the pelvic part of the urethra and the bulbo-urethral glands. By its forcible contraction it plays an important rôle in the ejaculation of the seminal fluid, and also in evacuating the last of the urine in micturition.[1]

(2) The **bulbo-cavernosus muscle** (or accelerator urinæ) is the continuation of the urethral muscle on the extrapelvic part of the urethra; it extends from the ischial arch to the glans penis. At the root of the penis it is the thickest, and forms a complete layer of circular fibers which inclose the corpus spongiosum and the urethra. Beyond this it diminishes very gradually in thickness, and consists of fibers which arise on a median ventral raphé and curve around the corpus spongiosum to end on the tunica albuginea of the corpus cavernosum. Its action is to empty the extrapelvic part of the urethra.

The **ischio-urethral muscles** (Fig. 452) are small bands which arise on the ischial arch and crura of the penis and pass forward to become lost on the ventral layer of the urethral muscle. They may assist in erection of the penis by exerting pressure on the dorsal veins.

[1] The statement often made that it acts as a sphincter of the bladder is a hypothesis of doubtful plausibility. In material hardened *in situ*, in which the internal urethral orifice is tightly closed, the urethral muscle apparently takes no part in the closure.

MALE GENITAL ORGANS OF THE OX

The **scrotum** is situated somewhat further forward than in the horse. It is long, pendulous, and has a well-marked neck. The skin here is usually flesh-colored, but in some breeds is more or less pigmented; it is sparsely covered with short hairs. Just in front of it are four (sometimes only two) rudimentary teats.

The **testicles** are relatively larger than those of the horse, and have an elongated, oval outline. The long axis is vertical. The inner surface is somewhat flattened.

A testicle of an adult bull measures on the average about four or five inches (10 to 12 cm.) in length, exclusive of the epididymis; with the latter the length is about six inches (15 cm.). The

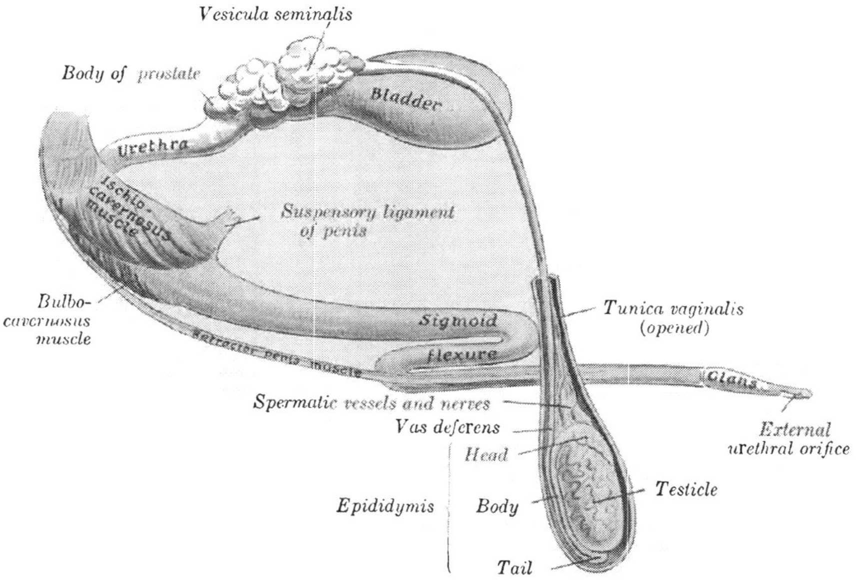

FIG. 399.—GENERAL VIEW OF GENITAL ORGANS OF BULL.

width is about two and a half to three inches (ca. 6 to 8 cm.), and the antero-posterior diameter about the same. The weight is about nine or ten ounces (ca. 250 to 300 grams).

The tunica albuginea is thin. The parenchyma is yellowish in color. The mediastinum testis descends from the anterior part of the upper extremity deeply into the gland as an axial strand about 5 mm. in thickness. The vasa efferentia leave at the upper end of the mediastinum.

The **epididymis** is very closely attached to the testicle. The head is long; it curves over the upper extremity and nearly half way down the anterior border of the testicle. The body is very narrow, and lies along the outer part of the posterior border of the testicle, to which it is attached by a narrow peritoneal fold. The tail is large and is closely attached to the lower extremity of the testicle.

The **spermatic cord** and the **tunica vaginalis** are much longer than in the horse; the extra-inguinal part of the cord is about eight to ten inches (20 to 25 cm.) in length. The **cremaster externus** is well developed, and almost completely incloses the tunic to the neck of the scrotum; it does not extend so far down as in the horse, but is inserted about at the level of the upper pole of the testicle. The **vaginal ring** is relatively very small, and is about four inches (ca. 10 cm.) from the linea alba. The cremaster internus is feeble.

The spermatic cords emerge through the outer angles of the external inguinal rings, and curve downward and inward to the neck of the scrotum. The external rings are about four inches (ca. 10 cm.) long, and are two and a half to three inches (6 to 8 cm.) apart. In animals in good condition there is a large mass of fat above the neck of the scrotum, between the spermatic

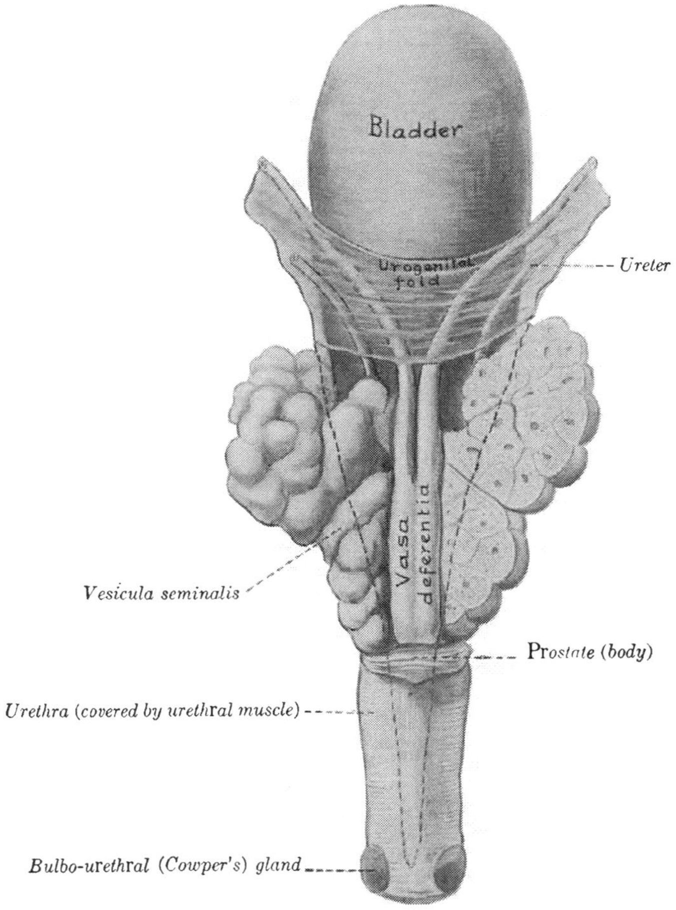

FIG. 400.—INTERNAL GENITAL ORGANS OF BULL; DORSAL VIEW.
The right vesicula is sectioned frontally. The dotted line indicates the backward extension of the peritoneum.

cords. The mesorchium extends to the bottom of the tunica vaginalis, forming a narrow fold (ca. 1 cm. wide) which attaches the epididymis to the posterior part of the tunic.

The inguinal canal presents several special features in the bull. The internal ring is very long. Its anterior border, formed by the edge of the internal oblique, is decidedly concave and is tendinous in its inner part. The long axis of the external ring is directed outward, forward, and downward. The spermatic cord lies in its outer part, the external pudic vessels in its middle. A muscular band about an inch wide, detached from the internal oblique muscle, crosses the outer side of the vaginal ring.

The **vas deferens** is small in caliber. The urogenital fold is narrow, so that the vasa are closer together in it than in the horse. On reaching the posterior part of the bladder they are in apposition for a distance of about four inches

(10 cm.), flanked and overlapped by the vesiculæ seminales. They form ampullæ about four or five inches (10 to 12 cm.) long and half an inch (1.2 to 1.5 cm.) wide, the mucous lining of which is plicated. They then pass under the body of the prostate and unite with the ducts of the vesiculæ seminales to form the ejaculatory ducts. The latter have slit-like openings on either side of the colliculus seminalis

The **vesiculæ seminales** are not bladder-like sacs, as in the horse, but are compact glandular organs with a lobulated surface. In the adult they measure about four or five inches (ca. 10 to 12 cm.) in length, two inches (5 cm.) in width in their largest part, and an inch or more (ca. 3 cm.) in thickness. The dorsal surface of each faces upward and inward and is partially covered with peritoneum. The ventral surface faces in the opposite direction and is non-peritoneal. Each may be regarded as consisting of a very thick-walled, sacculated tube, bent on itself in a tortuous manner. This tube, if straightened out, would be about ten inches (25 cm.) in length. They are commonly unsymmetrical in size and shape. Short branches are often given off from the chief tube.

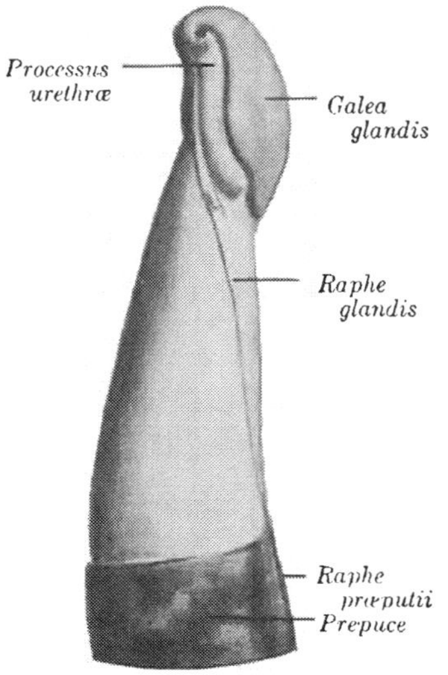

FIG. 401.—ANTERIOR EXTREMITY OF PENIS OF BULL, LEFT VIEW. (After Böhm.)

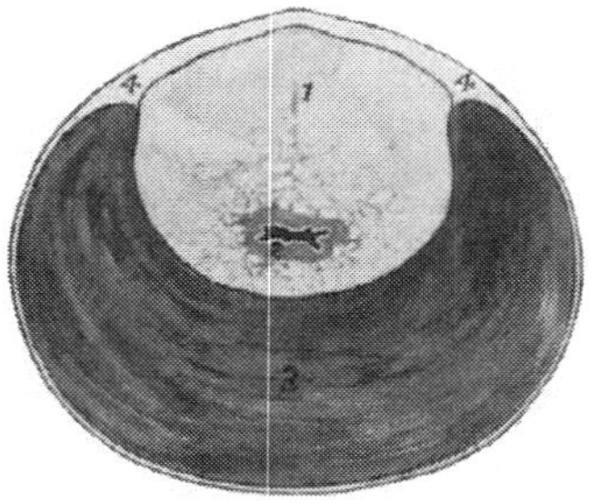

FIG. 402.—CROSS-SECTION OF PELVIC URETHRA OF BULL.

1, Prostate gland (pars disseminata); *2*, urethra; *3*, urethral muscle; *4*, aponeurosis. The lumen of the urethra is black.

The excretory duct or neck joins the outer side of the vas deferens at an acute angle to form the ejaculatory duct.

The structure of the vesicula is masked by a thick capsule of fibrous tissue and unstriped muscle, which maintains it in its bent condition and also sends trabeculæ between the alveoli. There is a central canal into which the secretion formed in the alveoli passes. The cavities (central canal and alveoli) are lined with columnar epithelium. On account of this structure the term glandulæ vesiculares is preferred by some anatomists.

The **prostate** is pale yellow in color, and consists of two parts. The **body** (Corpus prostatæ) is a mass which stretches across the dorsal surface of the neck of the bladder and the origin of the urethra. It measures about an inch and a half (ca. 3.5 to 4 cm.) transversely, and about half an inch (ca. 1 to 1.5 cm.) in width and thickness. The **pars disseminata** surrounds the pelvic part of the urethra; dorsally it forms a layer about half an inch (ca. 10 to 12 mm.) thick, but ventrally it is quite thin. It is concealed by the urethral (Wilson's) muscle; hence it often escapes notice, but is very evident on cross-section (Fig. 402). The **prostatic ducts** open into the urethra in rows between two folds of the mucous membrane which proceed backward from the colliculus seminalis.

The **uterus masculinus** appears to be absent frequently. Ellenberger states that it opens between the ejaculatory ducts, while Martin says that it usually has two orifices at the colliculus, but that it often unites with the vasa deferentia.

The **bulbo-urethral** (Cowper's) **glands** are somewhat smaller than in the stallion. They are liable to escape notice, since they are covered by a thick layer of dense fibrous tissue and also partially by the bulbo-cavernosus muscle. Each has a single duct which opens into the urethra under cover of a fold of the mucous membrane.

The **penis** is cylindrical, and is longer and of very much smaller diameter than in the horse. Just behind the scrotum it forms an S-shaped curve, the **sigmoid flexure;** thus about one foot is folded up when the penis is fully retracted. The flexure is effaced during erection. The **glans penis** is about three inches (ca. 8 cm.) in length. It is flattened dorso-ventrally, and its extremity is pointed and twisted. The **external urethral orifice** is situated at the end of a groove formed by this twist; it is only large enough to admit a probe of medium size. Even in the non-erect state the penis is remarkably dense and firm. The **tunica albuginea** is very thick, and incloses the urethra. In the first part, as far as the first curve, there is a thick median **septum penis.** Beyond this there is a central axial rod of dense fibrous tissue from which numerous strong trabeculæ radiate. The erectile tissue is small in amount, so that the organ undergoes very little enlargement in erection.

The length of the penis in the adult is about three feet (ca. 90 cm.). The crura are flattened laterally. The suspensory ligaments are attached to the ventral ridge on the symphysis. The body is somewhat flattened dorso-ventrally beyond the first curve. The extremity of the glans is unsymmetrical, the urethral orifice being situated ventro-laterally. The glans contains little erectile tissue, and hence undergoes little enlargement in erection.

The **bulbo-cavernosus muscle** presents several remarkable features. It is for the greater part an inch or more (ca. 3 cm.) in thickness, but its length is only six to eight inches (15 to 20 cm.). It is covered by a strong aponeurosis, and is divided by a median raphé into two lateral halves except at its origin. It diminishes in size from behind forward, and its anterior extremity is pointed.

The **ischio-cavernosus muscle** resembles in general that of the horse, but is flattened laterally. It is covered by a close aponeurosis.

The **retractor penis** muscle resembles that of the horse in origin. Its two parts are about an inch (ca. 2 to 5 cm.) apart on the root of the penis, where they lie in a groove on either side of the bulbo-cavernosus. They then come close together and pass on either side of the ventral curve of the sigmoid flexure. Further forward they lie along the ventral aspect of the penis, and end about five or six inches (ca. 12 to 15 cm.) behind the glans.

The **prepuce** is very long and narrow. Its orifice is about two inches (ca. 5 cm.) behind the umbilicus; it is only large enough to admit a finger readily, and is surrounded by long hairs. The cavity of the sheath is about fifteen inches (35 to 40 cm.) long, and a little over an inch (ca. 3 cm.) in diameter. The lining membrane forms longitudinal folds; it is covered with squamous stratified epithelium, and has coiled tubular glands. The penile layer is glandless, and is reddish in color. It presents lymph nodules in its posterior part.

There are two pairs of **preputial muscles** which are derivatives of the panniculus carnosus. The anterior pair, the **protractors** of the prepuce (Mm. præputiales craniales), are two flat bands, two inches or more (5 to 6 cm.) in width, which arise close together in the xiphoid region, about eight inches (20 cm.) in front of the preputial orifice. Traced backward they diverge, leaving the umbilicus and an area about one and a half inches wide free, and then unite behind the preputial orifice. They draw the prepuce forward. The posterior pair, the **retractors** of the prepuce (Mm. præputiales caudales), arise in the inguinal region and converge on the anterior part of the prepuce. They draw the prepuce backward.

These muscles are subject to a good deal of variation. The retractor may be absent. Many fibers come in from the panniculus on either side, dip under the protractor, and are inserted into the skin just behind the preputial opening. The homologue of the protractor is present in the cow.

The urethra in its pelvic part is about five inches (12 cm.) long, and is of relatively small and uniform caliber. The urethral (Wilson's) muscle incloses the tube ventrally and laterally; it is very thick, crescentic in cross-section, and is covered by an aponeurosis. Dorsally, the aponeurosis is thick and the muscle absent. Inside of these the pars disseminata of the prostate surrounds the urethra as far back as the bulbo-urethral glands. The colliculus seminalis is short, but prominent; from it the urethral crest extends forward to the trigonum vesicæ. The extrapelvic part has an enlargement, the bulb, at its origin; it then gradually

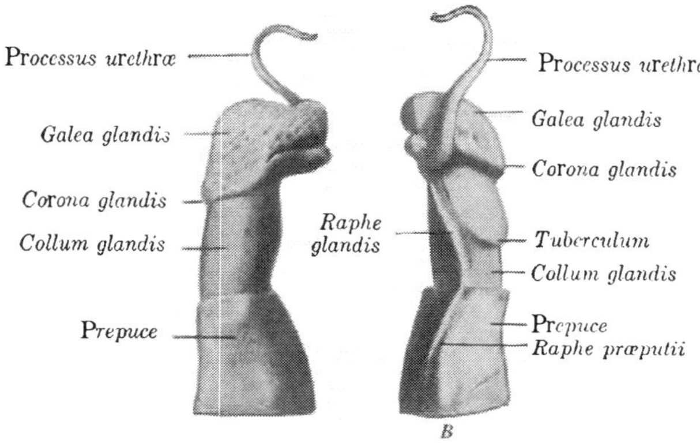

FIG. 403.—ANTERIOR PART OF PENIS OF RAM.
A, Right side; *B*, left side. (After Böhm.)

diminishes in diameter, and is relatively very small at its termination. Other features have been mentioned in preceding paragraphs.

In the ram the urethra lies in a groove on the ventral surface of the corpus cavernosum. Its terminal part projects commonly 3 to 4 cm. beyond the glans penis, forming a twisted processus urethræ.

MALE GENITAL ORGANS OF THE PIG

The **scrotum** is situated a short distance from the anus, and is not so sharply defined from the surrounding parts as in the other animals.

The **testicles** are very large and are soft in texture. Their long axis is almost vertical, the free border being posterior and the tail of the epididymis dorsal. The mediastinum testis is well developed. The epididymis is closely attached to the testicle and the tunica vaginalis; the tail is specially large.

The **spermatic cord** is necessarily very long (20 to 25 cm. in a boar of medium size). The **vas deferens** in its testicular part is flexuous, and is closely attached to the tunica vaginalis; it forms no ampullæ. The **cremaster externus** is well developed, and extends to about the middle of the scrotal part of the tunic.

The vesiculæ **seminales** are exceedingly large, and extend into the abdominal cavity. They are three-sided pyramidal masses, are in apposition with each other medially, and cover the posterior part of the bladder and the ureters, the vasa deferentia, the body of the prostate, and the anterior part of the urethra. They are pale pink in color, distinctly lobulated and glandular in structure, and contain large alveoli, but no central cavity. There are two excretory ducts which open into the urethra close to the vasa deferentia; the two ducts frequently unite.

In the adult boar the vesiculæ are about five to six inches (ca. 12 to 15 cm.) long, two to three inches (ca. 5 to 8 cm.) wide, and one and a half to two inches (ca. 4 to 5 cm.) thick; they weigh about 6 to 8 ounces each.

The **prostate** consists of two parts, as in the ox. The body is about an inch (2.5 cm.) wide, and embraces the neck of the bladder and the urethra at their junction dorsally and laterally. It is concealed by the vesiculæ seminales. The **pars disseminata** forms a layer which surrounds the pelvic part of the urethra, and is covered by the urethral muscle.

The uterus **masculinus** is small.

The bulbo-urethral (Cowper's) **glands** are very large and dense. They are somewhat cylindrical, and lie on either side of and upon the posterior two-thirds of the pelvic urethra. In a large boar they are about five inches (ca. 12 cm.) in length and an inch or more (ca. 2.5 to 3 cm.) in diameter. They are partially covered with a layer of striated muscle (M. ischio-glandularis), and have a lobulated surface. Each gland has a large excretory duct which leaves at the posterior extremity, perforates the dorsal wall of the urethra at the ischial arch, and opens in a cul-de-sac covered by a fold of mucous membrane.

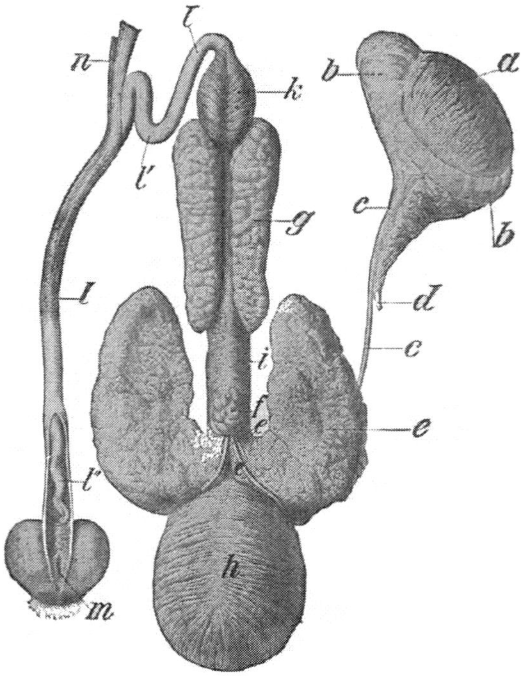

FIG. 404.—GENITAL ORGANS OF BOAR.

a, Testicle; *b*, epididymis; *c*, vas deferens; *d*, spermatic artery; *e*, vesicula seminalis reflected to show the body of the prostate. *f*; *e'*, excretory ducts of vesiculæ; *g*, bulbo-urethral (Cowper's) gland; *h*, urinary bladder; *i*, urethral muscle; k, bulbo-cavernosus muscle; *l*, penis; *l'*, sigmoid flexure of penis; *l''*, spiral anterior part of penis, exposed by slitting open prepuce; *m*, orifice of preputial pouch; *n*, retractor penis muscle. (Ellenberger-Baum, Anat. d. Haustiere.)

It is to be noted that these accessory glands are very small in animals which have been castrated early.

The **penis** resembles in general that of the ox. The sigmoid flexure is, however, prescrotal. The anterior portion has no glans, and is spirally twisted, especially in erection. The **urethral orifice** is slit-like and is situated ventrolaterally, close to the pointed extremity. The penis in the adult boar measures about 18 to 20 inches (ca. 45 to 50 cm.) in length. Its muscles resemble those of the bull; the bulbo-cavernosus is very strong but short.

The **prepuce** has a narrow orifice, around which there are a number of stiff hairs. The cavity is partially divided by a circular fold into a posterior narrow portion and a much wider anterior portion. The lining membrane of the posterior part is papillated, and is in close contact with the penis. In the dorsal wall of the wide part there is a circular opening which leads into a cul-de-sac, the **preputial diverticulum.** This pouch is ovoid in form (when distended), and varies greatly in size in different subjects. It extends for the most part backward over the narrow part of the prepuce. Its cavity is partially divided by a narrow median septum. It contains usually decomposing urine and macerated epithelium, which have a characteristic and very unpleasant odor. Concrements have been found in it.

Oehmke found that a cast of the pouch in a Yorkshire boar weighing about 500 pounds measured 9 cm. in length, 12½ cm. in breadth, and 6 cm. in height. The opening into the prepuce will admit two fingers in the adult, but is ordinarily closed by folds of the lining membrane. The sac is much smaller in animals which were castrated young, and the opening is vertical and further back; in them it is often empty or contains only a little clear urine. The pouch is covered by a layer of striped muscle which is mainly derived from the homologue of the protractor of the prepuce of ruminants.

The **urethra** has a very long pelvic portion (ca. 15 to 18 cm. long in the adult); it is inclosed (with the pars disseminata of the prostate) by a thick **urethral muscle.** There is a distinct **bulb** at the root of the penis. The penile part is of small caliber, and is surrounded by erectile tissue which, however, does not extend to the extremity of the penis.

MALE GENITAL ORGANS OF THE DOG

The **scrotum** is situated about half way between the inguinal region and the anus. The skin covering it is pigmented and is covered sparsely with fine hairs. The raphé is not very distinct.

The **testicles** are relatively small, and have a round-oval form. The long axis is oblique, and is directed upward and backward. The mediastinum testis is central and is well developed. The epididymis is large, and is closely attached along the outer part of the dorsal border of the testicle.

The **spermatic cord** and the **tunica vaginalis** are long; they cross the side of the penis very obliquely. The upper end of the tunic is sometimes closed, so that there is then no vaginal ring. The vasa deferentia have very narrow ampullæ.

The **vesiculæ seminales** are absent; hence there are no ejaculatory ducts.

The **prostate** is relatively large; it is yellowish in color, dense in structure, and lies at the anterior border of the pubis. It is globular, and surrounds the neck of the bladder and the urethra at their junction. A faint median furrow indicates a division into two lateral lobes. The capsule and stroma contain a large amount of unstriped muscle. The ducts are numerous. Lobules of prostatic tissue (pars disseminata) are also found on the urethra further back. The gland is subject to much variation in size, and is often enlarged, especially in old subjects.

The **uterus masculinus** is a very small saccule (Utriculus prostaticus), often difficult to find.

The **bulbo-urethral** (Cowper's) **glands** are absent.

The **penis** presents several special features. In its posterior part there are two distinct corpora cavernosa, separated by a median septum penis. In its anterior part there is a bone, the **os penis,** which in large dogs reaches a length of four inches (ca. 10 cm.) or more. It is regarded as a continuation forward of the corpus cavernosum. Ventrally it is grooved for the urethra; dorsally it is convex, and anteriorly it becomes smaller and has a curved fibrous prolongation. The **glans penis** is very long, extending over the entire length of the os penis; posteriorly it forms a rounded enlargement, the **bulbus glandis**; anteriorly it is cylindrical, smaller, and pointed at the extremity. Just in front of the bulbus glandis there is a thick circular layer of glands, forming the **annulus glandularis** (Schmaltz). The two dorsal veins arise from the bulbus glandis, pass backward on the dorsum penis, and unite at the ischial arch. A small muscle (M. compressor venæ dorsalis penis) arises from the tuber ischii on either side; the two converge on the dorsum penis near the bulbus glandis. They compress the dorsal veins, and may also tend to elevate the penis and thus assist in copulation. The other muscles offer no features worthy of special description.

The **prepuce** forms a complete sheath around the anterior part of the penis. The outer layer is ordinary integument. The inner layer has the character of a

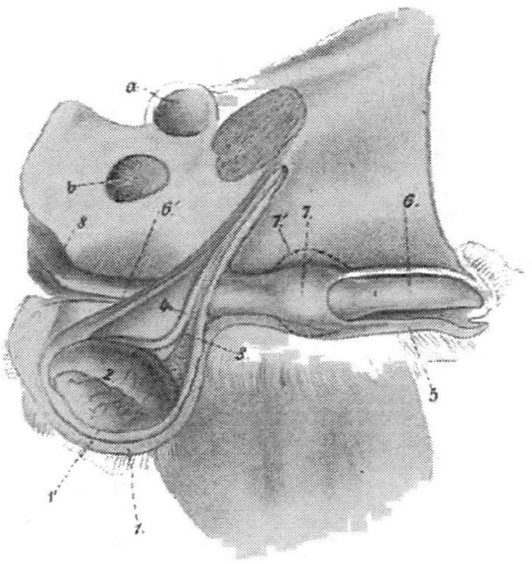

FIG. 405.—EXTERNAL GENITAL ORGANS OF MALE DOG, VENTRO-LATERAL VIEW OF PREPARATION.

1, Scrotum; *1'*, tunica vaginalis; *2*, epididymis; *3*, vascular part of spermatic cord; *4*, vas deferens; *5*, prepuce; *6*, glans penis; *6'*, corpus cavernosum penis; 7, bulbus glandis; *7'*, contour of bulbus in erection; *8*, ischio-cavernosus muscle: *a*, acetabulum; *b*, obturator foramen. (After Ellenberger, in Leisering's Atlas.)

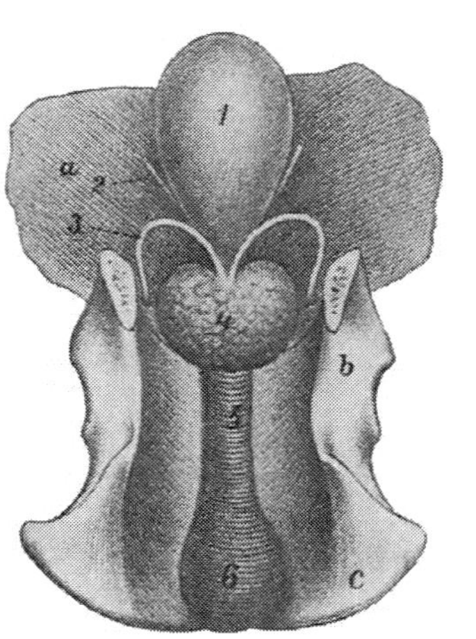

FIG. 406.—INTERNAL GENITAL ORGANS OF MALE DOG.

1, Urinary bladder; *2*, ureter; *3*, vas deferens; *4*, prostate; *5*, urethral muscle; *6*, bulb of urethra: *a*, abdominal wall; *b*, ilium; *c*, ischium. (After Ellenberger, in Leisering's Atlas.)

glandular mucous membrane; it is thin and reddish in color. The penile layer is glandless. In the fundus of the præputial cavity there are numerous lymph follicles. The protractor muscles arise in the xiphoid region and decussate posteriorly around the extremity of the penis.

The pelvic part of the **urethra** is relatively long. Its first part is inclosed in the prostate.[1] At the ischial arch the urethra has a well-developed bilobed bulb, formed by an enlargement here of the corpus spongiosum. It is covered by the strong but short bulbo-cavernosus muscle. The other erectile bodies have been described.

The **urethral** (Wilson's) **muscle** is very strong; it encircler the urethra and has a median raphé dorsally.

[1] This is clinically important, since enlargement of the prostate may interfere with micturition.

THE FEMALE GENITAL ORGANS

The **female genital organs** (Organa genitalia feminina) are: (1) The two **ovaries,** the essential reproductive glands, in which the ova are produced; (2) the **uterine** or **Fallopian tubes,** which convey the ova to the uterus; (3) the **uterus,** in which the ovum develops; (4) the **vagina,** a dilatable passage through which the fœtus is expelled from the uterus; (5) the **vulva,** the terminal segment of the genital tract, which serves also for the expulsion of the urine; (6) the **mammary glands,** which are glands of the skin, but are so closely associated functionally with the generative organs proper as to be described with them.

GENITAL ORGANS OF THE MARE

THE OVARIES

The **ovaries** (Ovaria) of the mare are bean-shaped, and are much smaller than the testicles. Their size varies much in different subjects, and they are

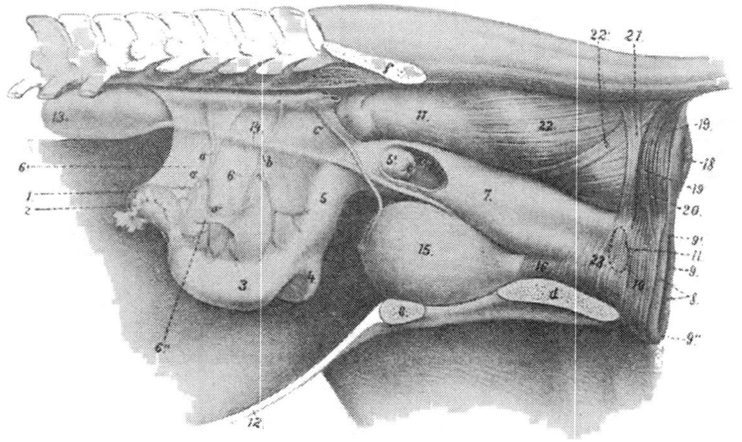

FIG. 407.—LATERAL VIEW OF GENITAL ORGANS AND ADJACENT STRUCTURES OF MARE.

The removal of the other abdominal viscera has allowed the ovaries and uterus to sink down, whereas they are normally in contact with the roof of the cavity in the non-pregnant subject. *1*, Left ovary; *2*, Fallopian tube; *3*, left cornu uteri; *4*, right cornu uteri; *5*, corpus uteri; *5'*, portio vaginalis uteri, and *5"*, os uteri, seen through window cut in vagina; *6*, broad ligament of uterus; *6"*, round ligament; *7*, vagina; *8*, labia vulvæ; *9*, rima vulvæ; *9'*, superior commissure, and *9"*, inferior commissure of vulva; *10*, constrictor vulvæ; *11*, position of vestibular bulb; *12*, ventral wall of abdomen; *13*, left kidney; *14*, left ureter; *15*, urinary bladder; *16*, urethra; *17*, rectum; *18*, anus; *19*, *19'*, unpaired and paired parts of sphincter ani externus; *20*, retractor ani cut at disappearance under sphincter; *21*, suspensory ligament of anus; *22*, longitudinal muscular layer of rectum; *22'*, recto-coccygeus; *23*, constrictor vaginæ; *a*, utero-ovarian artery, with ovarian (*a'*) and uterine (*a"*) branches; *b*, uterine artery; *c*, umbilical artery; *d*, ischium; *e*, pubis; *f*, ilium. (After Ellenberger, in Leisering's Atlas.)

normally larger in young than in old animals; one ovary is often larger than the other. They are about three inches (ca. 7 to 8 cm.) long and an inch to an inch and a half (ca. 3 to 4 cm.) thick. The weight is about two and a half to three ounces (ca. 70 to 80 grams).

Each presents for description two surfaces, two borders, and two extremities or poles. The **surfaces** are termed internal and external (Facies medialis, lateralis); they are both smooth and rounded.[1] The **attached** or **mesovarial** border (Margo mesovaricus) is convex. It is inclosed in a part of the broad ligament termed the mesovarium; the vessels and nerves reach the gland at this border. The **free border** (Margo liber) is marked by a notch which leads into a depression, the **ovulation fossa.** The **tubal** or **anterior extremity** (Extremitas tubaria) is rounded, and is related to the fimbriated end of the uterine or Fallopian tube. The **uterine** or **posterior extremity** (Extremitas uterina) is also round, and is connected with the horn of the uterus by the ovarian ligament.

The ovaries are situated in the sublumbar region of the abdominal cavity, about a handbreadth behind the corresponding kidney. They are in contact with the lumbar wall of the abdomen, and are commonly about two or three inches (ca. 5 to 7.5 cm.) from the median plane. The distance from the ovaries to the vulvar orifice is about twenty inches (ca. 50 cm.) in a mare of medium size. The attached (mesovarial) border is commonly directed toward the median plane, the free border laterally and somewhat ventrally.

The position of the ovaries is not constant, but is subject to less variation than might be expected from their mode of attachment. The normal variations in the non-pregnant state are chiefly in a transverse direction, and do not usually exceed two or three inches (ca. 5 to 7 cm.). It is not at all rare to find the ovary deflected medially, so that the external surface faces ventrally. In the longitudinal direction little variation appears to occur. The right ovary is usually about four or five inches (ca. 10 to 12 cm.), and the left one about three or four inches (ca. 8 to 10 cm.), behind the corresponding kidney. Thus they lie about in a transverse plane tangent to the external angles of the ilia, *i. e.*, through the fifth lumbar vertebra. They may be about two inches (ca. 5 cm.) from the extremity of the corresponding cornu of the uterus or in contact with it. The right ovary commonly lies a little (ca. 2.5 cm.) further forward than the left one. Except during pregnancy, they are normally in contact with the lumbar abdominal wall, and do not hang down among the adjacent viscera.

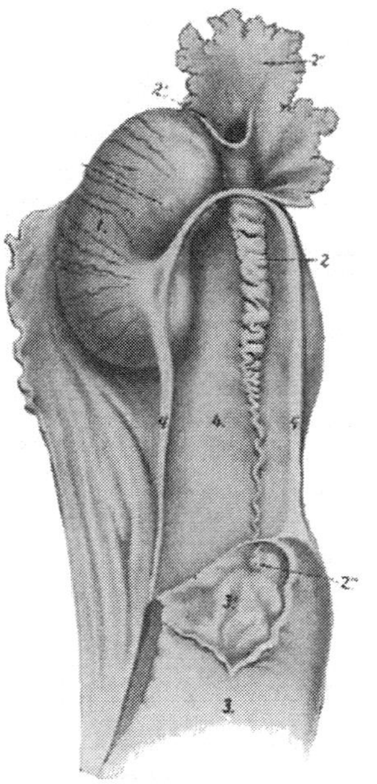

FIG. 408.—RIGHT OVARY OF MARE, WITH ADJACENT STRUCTURES.

The extremity of the cornu uteri is opened. *1*, Ovary; *2*, Fallopian tube, with its ostium abdominale (*2'*), fimbriæ (*2''*), and ostium uterinum (*2'''*); *3*, cornu uteri, with its mucous lining (*3'*); *4*, ovarian ligament; *4'*, mesosalpinx. (After Ellenberger, in Leisering's Atlas, reduced.)

The ovary is attached to the sublumbar region by the anterior part of the broad ligament; this part of the ligament, the **mesovarium,** is about three or four inches (ca. 8 to 10 cm.) wide, measured from the ovary directly to the parietal attachment. The uterine or posterior extremity of the ovary is connected with the extremity of the cornu of the uterus by the **ovarian ligament** (Ligamentum ovarii proprium); this is a band of unstriped muscle inclosed between the layers of the broad ligament.

Structure.—The greater part of the surface of the ovary has a covering of peritoneum. The peritoneal investment is absent at the attached border where

[1] These terms apply properly only when the adjacent viscera are removed and the ovaries are actually "suspended" by the broad ligaments. When the ovary is in its natural position, the surfaces are dorsal and ventral, the former corresponding to the "external" surface if the free border is directed outward, to the "internal" if the free edge is medial.

the vessels and nerves enter; this area is termed the **hilus.** The ovulation fossa is covered by a layer of columnar cells, a remnant of the primitive **germinal epithelium.** The **stroma** of the ovary (Stroma ovarii) is a network of connective tissue and unstriped muscular fibers. In the deeper or medullary portion of the stroma (Zona vasculosa) the meshes are largely occupied by the numerous blood-vessels. In the peripheral or cortical portion (Zona parenchymatosa) are numerous **ova** (Ovula) in various stages of development. The immature ova are surrounded by follicle cells; those more advanced in development are inclosed also by a condensation of the stroma termed the **theca folliculi;** within the theca is a quantity of fluid, the **liquor folliculi.** These constitute the **Graafian follicles** (Folliculi oöphori), which enlarge as they mature, becoming visible to the naked eye as vesicles with a diameter of a centimeter or more. When fully developed, the follicles are superficially situated, and often project slightly from the surface of the ovary. At intervals follicles rupture and their contents escape. This process, which sets free the ovum, is termed **ovulation;** it takes place in the mare only at the ovulation fossa, and occurs during the periods of œstrum.

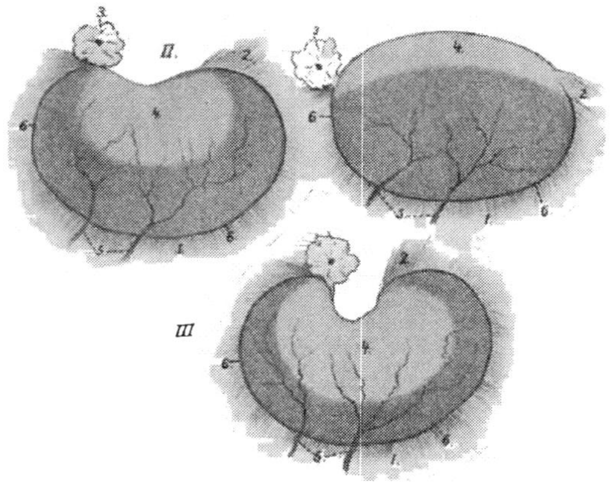

FIG. 409.—SCHEMATIC REPRESENTATION OF CHANGES IN OVARY OF MARE FROM FŒTAL TO ADULT STATE. (After Born.)

The changes affect chiefly the free border (upper in figure) and the extent and form of the area covered by germinal epithelium (*4*). *1*, Peritoneum (broad ligament); *2*, ligament of ovary; *3*, fimbria of Fallopian tube; *4*, germinal epithelium; *5*, vessels, which reach the ovary at the attached border (*6*). The latter represents the hilus, while the deep depression at the free border is the ovulation fossa. (Ellenberger, in Leisering's Atlas.)

After rupture of a follicle its cavity is partly occupied by a blood-clot, constituting what may be termed a **corpus rubrum.** By proliferation and enlargement and fatty changes, the follicle cells are transformed into lutein cells, forming a yellow mass known as a **corpus luteum.** If impregnation takes place, the accompanying increase in vascularity of the organs may cause the corpus luteum to reach a large size; if impregnation does not occur, it is much smaller, and is sooner replaced by scar tissue, the **corpus albicans.**

In the young foal the ovaries are large and oval in form. The free border is convex and is covered by germinal epithelium, which extends over part of the surfaces also. This area is distinguishable by its dull gray appearance from the peritoneal surface, which has the usual smooth glistening character. As growth proceeds the ovary gradually becomes bent until it assumes its definitive curved shape. The germinal epithelium is then limited to the ovulation fossa. The ovary migrates somewhat during development from its primitive position, which is the same as that of the testicle.

In old animals the ovaries commonly consist largely of fibrous tissue, in which there are often cysts of various sizes. The ova, present in enormous number at birth, have then been extruded, or destroyed by phagocytic action or degeneration.

Vessels and Nerves.—The **arteries** of the ovary are derived from the **ovarian artery.** The artery is relatively large and is flexuous; it reaches the attached border of the ovary by passing between the layers of the mesovarium. The **veins** are large and numerous. They form a plexus somewhat like that of the spermatic cord. The **lymph vessels** pass to the lumbar glands. The **nerves** are derived from the sympathetic system through the renal and aortic plexuses. They accompany the arterial branches.

THE UTERINE OR FALLOPIAN TUBES

The uterine or Fallopian tubes (Tubæ uterinæ) act as excretory ducts of the ovaries, since they convey the ova from the reproductive glands to the uterus. They are not, however, in direct continuity with the glands, but rather partly in contiguity with, and partly attached to, them.[1] They are two flexuous tubes, about ten to twelve inches (ca. 25 to 30 cm.) long, which extend from the extremities of the uterine cornua to the ovaries. Each is inclosed in a peritoneal fold, derived from the external layer of the broad ligament, and termed the **mesosalpinx.** This largely covers the outer aspect of the ovary, and forms with it and the broad ligament a pouch called the **bursa ovarica.** The **uterine extremity** of the tube communicates with the cavity of the cornu by a minute orifice, the **ostium uterinum.** The **ovarian** or **fimbriated extremity** is expanded into a funnel-shaped **infundibulum.** The margin of the latter is slit into irregular processes or **fimbriæ,** some of which, the **fimbriæ ovaricæ,** are attached in the ovulation fossa. In the center of the fimbriated extremity is a small opening, the **ostium abdominale,** by which the tube communicates with the peritoneal cavity. The tube appears normally to be applied to the ovary, so that the extruded ova pass into it and are conveyed to the uterus.[2]

Pedunculated cysts, the **hydatids of Morgagni,** are often found on one or more of the fimbriæ. In the mesosalpinx are blind flexuous tubules, which constitute the **paroöphoron,** a remnant of the Wolffian body. They are most evident in the young adult, and tend to disappear with increasing age. Not uncommonly they give rise to cysts.

Structure.—The tube is covered externally by a **serous coat** formed by the mesosalpinx. The serous membrane is continued on the fimbriæ, and meets the mucous lining on them. The **fibrous coat** or adventitia is continuous with the fibrous lamina of the broad ligament. The **muscular coat** consists chiefly of circular fibers, although longitudinal fibers occur externally. The **mucous coat** is thin and is much plicated. The folds (Plicæ tubariæ) are chiefly longitudinal, but in the wide part of the tube (Ampullæ tubæ) they are very complex, so that on cross-sections the spaces between the folds may be mistaken for branched tubular glands. The folds are continued on to the fimbriæ. The **epithelium** is a single layer of columnar ciliated cells, the cilia producing a current directed toward the uterus. At the fimbriated extremity this epithelium passes gradually into the squamous type of the serous coat.

Vessels and Nerves.—The **arteries** are derived from the utero-ovarian **artery.** The **veins** are satellites of the arteries. The **lymphatics** pass with the ovarian vessels to the lumbar glands. The nerves have a similar origin to those of the ovary.

THE UTERUS

The **uterus** is a hollow muscular organ, which receives the Fallopian tubes anteriorly and opens into the vagina posteriorly. It is situated chiefly in the abdominal cavity, but extends a short distance into the pelvic cavity. It is attached to the lumbar wall of the abdomen and the lateral walls of the pelvic cavity by two folds of peritoneum termed the broad ligaments. It consists of two cornua or horns, the body, and the neck.

The **cornua** or **horns** of the uterus (Cornua uteri) are situated entirely in the abdomen. They appear to vary considerably in position; commonly they

[1] The Fallopian tubes may be regarded, both in structure and morphology, as prolongations of the uterus (McMurrich).

[2] The arrangement is the only exception to the general rule that the serous cavities are closed. In this case the mucous membrane of the fimbriated extremity is continuous with the adjacent peritoneum, a persistence of the embryonic relations of the Müllerian duct.

are pressed up against the sublumbar muscles by the intestine (left portions of large colon, small colon, and small intestine). They are cylindrical, and are about ten inches (ca. 25 cm.) in length. The anterior extremity of each forms a blunt point which receives the Fallopian tube. Posteriorly they increase somewhat in caliber, converge, and unite with the body. The **dorsal** (or attached) **border** is slightly concave and is attached to the broad ligament. The **ventral** border is convex and free.

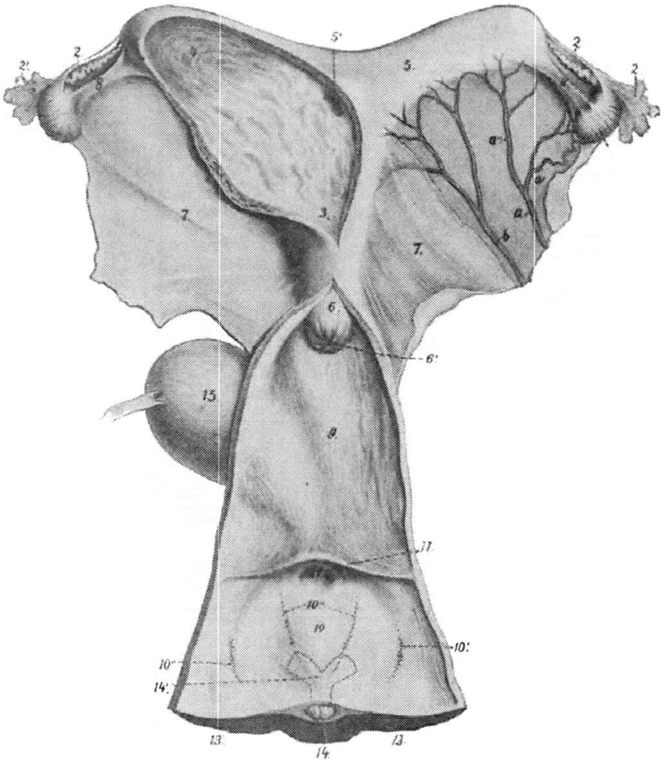

FIG. 410.—GENITAL ORGANS OF MARE, DORSAL VIEW.

The left cornu and adjacent part of the body of the uterus and the vagina and vulva are opened up. *1*, Ovary; *2*, Fallopian tube, with *2'*, its fimbriated end; *3*, cavity of corpus uteri; *4*, cavity of left cornu; *5*, right cornu, with *5'*, its communication with the body; *6*, portio vaginalis uteri; *6'*, os uteri; *7*, broad ligament of uterus; *8*, ligament of ovary; *9*, vagina; *10*, vulva; *10'*, glandulæ vestibulares majores; *10''*, glandulæ vestibulares minores; *11*, transverse fold; *12*, external urethral opening; *13*, *13'*, labia vulvæ; *14*, glans clitoridis; *14'*, junction of crura to form corpus clitoridis indicated by dotted lines; *15*, urinary bladder; *a*, utero-ovarian artery with ovarian (*a'*) and uterine (*a''*) branches; *b*, uterine artery. (After Ellenberger, in Leisering's Atlas.)

When a soft uterus is distended, the cornua are strongly curved, but this does not represent the natural form. When fixed *in situ* the horns are either slightly curved or nearly straight. The two horns are commonly unsymmetrical in length and diameter in mares which have borne young.

The body of the uterus (Corpus uteri) is situated partly in the abdomen, partly in the pelvic cavity. It is cylindrical, but considerably flattened dorso-ventrally, so that in cross-section it is elliptical. Its average length is about six inches (15 cm.), and its diameter, when moderately distended, about four inches (10 cm.). Its dorsal surface (Facies rectalis) is related to the small colon and rec-turn. Its **ventral surface** (Facies vesicalis) is in contact with the bladder, and has inconstant relations with various parts of the intestine. The term **fundus uteri** is applied to the anterior wide part from which the cornua diverge.

The position of the body of the uterus is variable, especially in regard to its anterior part. It is often pressed up against the rectum, and may be deflected to either side—most frequently to the left—by the pelvic flexure of the colon or coils of the small colon.

The **cervix** or **neck** of the uterus (Cervix uteri) is the constricted posterior part which joins the vagina. Part of it (Portio vaginalis uteri) projects into the cavity of the vagina; it is therefore not visible externally, but may be felt through the vaginal wall. It is about two inches (5 cm.) in length, and an inch and a half (3.5 to 4 cm.) in diameter.

Attachments.—The body and cornua are attached to the abdominal and pelvic walls by two extensive peritoneal folds, the **broad ligaments** (Ligamenta lata). These extend on either side from the sublumbar region and the lateral pelvic walls to the dorsal border of the cornua and the lateral margins of the body of the uterus. They contain the vessels and nerves of the uterus and ovaries, connective tissue, and unstriped muscular fibers. The ureters are situated along their parietal margins. The outer layer of each forms a fold, the **round ligament** of the uterus (Ligamentum teres uteri), which blends with the parietal peritoneum over the internal inguinal ring; its anterior extremity is situated above the extremity of the cornu and is rounded and free. It contains muscular tissue, vessels, and nerves, and is the homologue of the gubernaculum testis. The anterior part of the neck is continuous with the vagina, and thus has a more fixed position than the rest of the organ.

The **cavity** of the uterus (Cavum uteri) is largely obliterated in the non-pregnant state by the contraction of the wall and by folds of the mucous lining. At the extremity of each cornu it communicates by a minute opening with the Fallopian tube. The cavity of the neck is termed the **cervical canal** (Canalis cervicis); it is closed ordinarily by mucous folds and a plug of mucus. It opens into the vagina by the **os uteri externum**, and into the body by the **os uteri internum.**

Structure.—The wall of the uterus consists of three coats—an external serous, a middle muscular, and an internal mucous. The **serous coat** (Perimetrium) is, for the most part, closely adherent to the muscular coat. It is continuous with the broad ligaments. The **muscular coat** consists essentially of two layers, a thin external stratum of longitudinal fibers, and a thick layer of circular fibers. Between these is a very vascular layer (Stratum vasculare) of connective tissue with circular and oblique muscular fibers in it. The circular coat is very thick in the neck, where it forms a **sphincter** half an inch or more (ca. 1.5 cm.) in thickness. The **mucous membrane** rests directly on the muscular coat. It is thick, and is covered by columnar epithelium. It contains numerous long tubular **uterine glands** (Glandulæ uterinæ). It is brownish-red in color, except in the neck, where it is pale.

Vessels and Nerves.—The chief **arteries** are the **uterine** and the **uterine branch** of the **utero-ovarian,** which have a flexuous course in the broad ligaments; there is also a branch from the **internal pudic** artery. The veins form pampiniform plexuses and accompany the arteries. The **lymphatics** are numerous and go to the internal iliac and lumbar glands. The **nerves** are derived from the sympathetic through the uterine and pelvic plexuses.

The foregoing statements refer to the non-gravid uterus. In the pregnant state it undergoes important changes in size, position, and structure. The increase in size affects chiefly the gravid cornu (except in the case of twins) and the body. The cornu attains a length of about two and a half to three feet (ca. 80 to 90 cm.), and a corresponding diameter; in this process it extends much beyond the ovary, and the broad ligament. The gravid uterus is entirely abdominal in position, and extends along the ventral wall, chiefly to the left of the median plane. It weighs about nine pounds (ca. 4 kg.), according to Ellenberger. The broad ligaments increase greatly in size and contain more muscular tissue. The vessels are greatly enlarged and form new branches. The muscular coat, in spite of the increase in size and number of the fibers, is somewhat thinner, except in the neck. The mucous membrane is thicker and more vascular; the epithelium becomes non-ciliated and stratified.

THE VAGINA

The **vagina** is the passage which extends horizontally through the pelvic cavity from the neck of the uterus to the vulva. It is tubular, is about six to eight inches (ca. 15 to 20 cm.) in length, and, when slightly distended, about four or five inches (ca. 10 to 12 cm.) in diameter. Its dilatability appears to be limited only by the pelvic wall. There is no external line of demarcation between the vagina and the uterus or the vulva.

It is related dorsally to the rectum, ventrally to the bladder and urethra, and laterally to the pelvic wall. The recto-genital pouch of the peritoneum extends between the vagina and rectum for a distance of about two inches (5 cm.), and ventrally the vesico-genital pouch passes backward somewhat less between the vagina and bladder. Thus most of the vagina is retroperitoneal and is surrounded by a quantity of loose connective tissue, a venous plexus, and a variable amount of fat.

Structure.—With the exception of the short peritoneal part, as indicated above, the proper wall of the vagina is composed of muscular and mucous coats. The **muscular coat** is composed of a thin layer of longitudinal fibers, and a thicker layer of circular fibers; it contains also many elastic fibers. The **mucous coat** is highly elastic, and is covered with a stratified epithelium. It has no glands.

Under usual conditions the cavity is practically obliterated by apposition of the walls, so that the lumen is a transverse slit; this condition is pronounced when the ampulla of the rectum is full. The anterior end of the vagina is largely occupied by the intravaginal part of the neck of the uterus, so that the cavity is here reduced to an annular recess termed the **fornix vaginæ**. The posterior part is directly continuous with the vulva without any line of demarcation except the valvular fold, which covers the external urethral orifice; in very young subjects this fold is continued on either side, forming the **hymen,** which narrows the entrance to the vagina (Introitus vaginæ).[1]

Vessels and Nerves.—The blood-supply is derived from the branches of the **internal pudic arteries.** The **veins** form a plexus which is drained by the **internal pudic veins.** The **lymphatics** pass to the internal iliac lymph glands. The **nerves** are derived from the sympathetic through the pelvic plexus.

THE VULVA

The **vulva** or **urogenital sinus** is the terminal part of the genital tract.[2] It is continuous in front with the vagina, and opens externally at the vulvar cleft below the anus. There is no external line of demarcation between the vagina and vulva. The tube is about five inches (ca. 12 cm.) in length, measured from the external urethral orifice to the inferior commissure; dorsally it is considerably shorter. It is related dorsally to the rectum and anus, ventrally to the pelvic floor, and laterally to the sacro-sciatic ligament, the semimembranosus muscle, and the internal pudic artery. The external orifice or **vulvar cleft** (Rima vulvæ) has the form of a vertical slit, about four to six inches (ca. 10 to 15 cm.) high, and is margined

[1] In formalin-hardened subjects there is frequently a pronounced ring-like constriction at the beginning of the vulva.

[2] The term vulva is used here in the sense in which it is understood generally by English and French veterinarians. In the German works it is applied only to the labia and other structures around the external orifice of the urogenital sinus, while the sinus itself is termed the vestibule of the vagina (Vestibulum vaginæ).

by two prominent rounded folds, the labia. The **labia** of the vulva (Labia vulvæ) meet above at an acute angle, forming the **superior commissure** (Commissura dorsalis), which is about two inches (ca. 5 cm.) below the anus. Below they unite to form the thick rounded **inferior commissure** (Commissura ventralis), which lies about two inches (ca. 5 cm.) behind and below the ischial arch. When the labia are drawn apart, a rounded body, about an inch (ca. 2.5 cm.) wide, is seen in the inferior commissure; this is the **glans clitoridis,** the homologue of the glans penis. Overlying it is a thin fold, the **prepuce** of the clitoris (Præputium clitoridis). At the anterior extremity of the ventral wall of the vulva, *i. e.*, about four or five inches (ca. 10 to 12 cm.) from the inferior commissure, is the **external urethral orifice** or meatus urinarius (Orificium urethræ externum). It readily admits the finger and is very dilatable. It is covered by a fold of mucous membrane, the free edge of which is directed backward.

Structure.—The labia are covered by thin, pigmented, smooth skin, which is richly supplied with sebaceous and sweat glands. This is continuous at a distance of about half an inch (ca. 1 to 1.5 cm.) from the free edge with a thin glandless mucous membrane. Between these is a layer of striped muscle, the **constrictor vulvæ;** this fuses above with the sphincter ani, and embraces the clitoris below, spreading out laterally at the inferior commissure. It constricts the vulvar orifice and elevates the clitoris. The **constrictor vestibuli** muscle embraces the vulva in front of the preceding; it is joined on either side by a band of unstriped muscle which arises from the first and second coccygeal vertebræ, and is homologous with the proximal part of the retractor penis. It constricts the vulva. Under this muscle in the lateral wall is a flattened, oval body, the **bulbus vestibuli** (Fig. 453); this is an erectile structure, homologous with the corpus spongiosum urethræ of the male. It is about two and a half to three inches (ca. 6 to 8 cm.) long, and an inch or more (ca. 3 cm.) wide. It consists of a venous network inclosed in a fibrous capsule, and is supplied with blood by a large branch of the internal pudic artery. The **mucous membrane** of the vulva is reddish in color, and forms longitudinal and transverse folds. It presents ventrally two linear series of small papillæ which converge toward the inferior commissure; these mark the orifices of the ducts of the **glandulæ vestibulares minores.** On either side of the dorsal wall is a group of eight to ten larger prominences on which the ducts of the **glandulæ vestibulares majores** (of Bartholin) open.

Quite exceptionally there may be found on either side of the urethral orifice the opening of the canals of Gartner (Ductus epoöphori longitudinales).

The **clitoris** is the homologue of the penis. It arises from the ischial arch by two **crura,** which unite to form a body as large as one's little finger. This projects backward into the inferior commissure of the vulva, capped by a small rounded **glans.** The organ is composed of erectile tissue similar to the corpus cavernosum penis. The **ischio-cavernosus** (or erector clitoridis) is a very feeble muscle which depresses the clitoris. The veins of the clitoris communicate by an intermediate plexus on either side with the bulbus vestibuli.

THE FEMALE URETHRA

The female **urethra** (Urethra feminina) represents only that part of the canal of the male which lies between the internal urethral orifice and the openings of the ejaculatory ducts. Its length is about two inches (5 cm.), and its lumen is sufficient to admit of the introduction of the finger; it is, however, capable of remarkable dilatation if sufficient care and patience are exercised in the process. It lies centrally on the pelvic floor, and is related and attached dorsally to the vagina.

Structure.—The intrinsic **muscular coat** consists of longitudinal and circular layers of unstriped fibers. Between these is a layer of areolar tissue which contains a rich **venous plexus**. The **mucous membrane** is thrown into longitudinal folds when the canal is closed; it is highly elastic, and is covered with stratified epithelium.

The urethral **muscle** (M. compressor urethræ) embraces the urethra and is continued backward for some distance under the constrictor vestibuli. It is covered by a fibro-elastic membrane.

THE MAMMARY GLANDS

The **mammary glands** (Glandulæ lactiferæ) are modified cutaneous glands which are so closely associated functionally with the genital organs as to be considered accessory to them.

In the mare they are two in number, and are placed on either side of the median plane in the inguinal region. Each gland has the form of a short cone, much compressed transversely, and having a flat inner surface. It consists of the glandular mass or body of the gland (Corpus mammæ) and the **teat** or **nipple** (Papilla mammæ). The base is related to the abdominal wall, to which it is attached by areolar tissue, which contains a venous plexus, the superficial inguinal lymph glands, and a variable amount of fat. The apex is constituted by the teat, which is also flattened transversely and varies in length from one to two inches (ca. 2.5 to 5 cm.). Between the bases of the teats is the intermammary groove. On the apex of each teat two or three small orifices are placed close together; these are the openings of the lactiferous ducts.

Structure.—The **skin** over the glands is thin, pigmented, chiefly hairless, and supplied with numerous large sebaceous and sweat glands. Under this are two layers of **fascia** except on the teats. The superficial fascia presents no special features. The deep fascia consists of two laminæ detached from the abdominal tunic which descend on either side of the median plane, forming a **septum** between the two glands, and constituting their ligamentum suspensorium.

These laminæ are separated by a layer of areolar tissue, so that it is possible to remove one gland if diseased by careful dissection between the layers of the septum.

The **gland substance** or **parenchyma** is pinkish gray in color, and of firmer consistence than the fat which is found around and within the gland. It is inclosed by a fibro-elastic capsule which sends inward numerous trabeculæ; these form the **interstitial tissue,** and divide the gland into **lobes** and **lobules.** In the latter are the secretory **tubules** and **alveoli,** which unite to form the larger **ducts.** Each lobe has a duct, which opens at the base of the teat into a space called the **lactiferous sinus** (Sinus lactiferus); this is lined with mucous membrane, and from it two (or three) **lactiferous ducts** (Ductus lactiferi) pass through the extremity of the nipple. These ducts are lined with a non-glandular mucous membrane, which is covered with stratified squamous epithelium. They are surrounded by unstriped muscular tissue, the bulk of the fibers being arranged in a circular manner to form a **sphincter.**

The size and form of the mammary glands are subject to much variation. In the young subject, before pregnancy, they are small and contain little gland tissue. During the latter part of gestation, and especially during lactation, they increase greatly in size, and the gland tissue is highly developed. After lactation the secretory structures undergo marked involution, and the gland is much reduced in size. The relative amounts of gland substance and interstitial tissue vary greatly; in some cases a gland of considerable size contains little secretory tissue and is consequently functionally deficient.

Vessels and Nerves.—The **arteries** are derived from the **external pudic artery,** which enters the gland at the posterior part of its base. The **veins** form **a**

plexus on either side of the base of the gland, which is drained by the **external pudic vein** chiefly. The **lymphatics** are numerous and pass chiefly to the superficial inguinal (or supramammary) lymph glands. The **nerves** are derived from the **inguinal nerves** and the posterior **mesenteric plexus** of the sympathetic system.

GENITAL ORGANS OF THE COW

The **ovaries** of the cow are much smaller than those of the mare, measuring usually about one to one and a half inches (ca. 3 to 4 cm.) in length, and a little less than an inch (ca. 2 cm.) in thickness in their largest part. They are oval in form, pointed at the uterine end, and have no ovulation fossa. They are situated usually a little above the middle of the lateral margin of the pelvic inlet in the non-pregnant subject, but may be found a little further forward. They are thus about 16 to 18 inches (ca. 40 to 45 cm.) from the vulva in a cow of medium size.

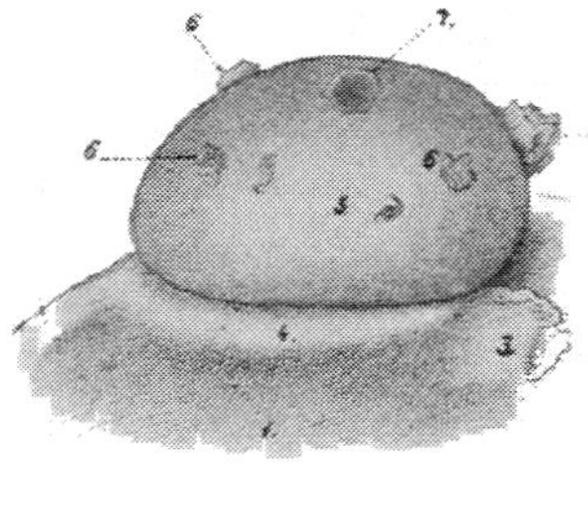

FIG. 411.—OVARY OF COW.

1, Broad ligament of uterus; *2*, ligament of ovary; *3*, fimbria ovarica; *4*, attachment of broad ligament; *5*, surface of ovary covered with germinal epithelium; *6*, corpora lutea; *7*, Graafian follicle. (From Leisering's Atlas.)

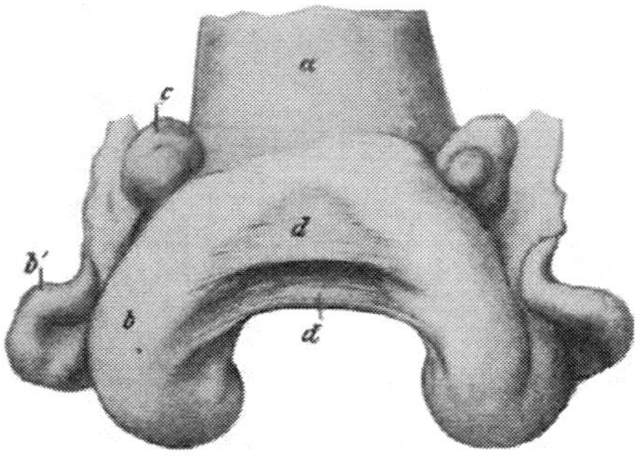

FIG. 412.—UTERUS OF COW, CONTRACTED, DORSAL VIEW.

a, Body of uterus; *b*, *b'*, horn of uterus; *c*, ovary; *d*, *d'*, triangular folds connecting horns of uterus (Lig. intercornualia). (After Zieger.)

The greater part of the surface of the gland is covered with germinal epithelium, the peritoneal epithelium being limited to a narrow zone along the attached border. Follicles of various sizes are often seen projecting from the surface, as well as corpora lutea; a corpus luteum verum has a pronounced yellow color, and may reach a width of half an inch or more (ca. 1 to 1.5 cm.).

The **Fallopian** or **uterine** tubes are long and less flexuous than in the mare. The junction with the cornu of the uterus is not so abrupt as in the mare, since the extremities of the horns are pointed. The uterine orifice of the tube is rather large and funnel-shaped. The fimbriæ are not so extensive as in the mare.

The **uterus** lies almost entirely within the abdominal cavity in the adult. The **body** is only about one inch (ca. 2 to 3 cm.) in length, although externally it appears to be much longer. This false impression is due to the fact that the posterior parts of the cornua are united by connective and muscular tissue and have a common peritoneal covering. The **cornua** are, therefore, really longer than they appear externally. They taper gradually toward the free end, so that the junction with the Fallopian tubes is not abrupt, as in the mare. The free part of the horn curves at first downward, forward, and outward, and then turns upward, forming a spiral coil. The **cervix** is about four or five inches (ca. 8 to 10 cm.) long;

its wall is remarkably dense, and may be nearly an inch (ca. 2 cm.) in thickness. Its lumen, the **cervical canal,** is spiral, and is ordinarily tightly closed and very difficult to dilate. The **muscular coat** of the uterus is thicker than in the mare. It consists of an external longitudinal layer and two circular strata. The inner circular layer is about a fourth of an inch (ca. 6 mm.) thick in the cervix. The other layers are continued in the vagina. The **mucous membrane** of the horns and body presents as a characteristic feature the **uterine cotyledons** (Cotyledones uterinæ). These are oval prominences, about a hundred in number, which are either irregularly scattered over the surface or arranged in rows of about a dozen.

In the non-gravid uterus they average about ½ to ¾ inch (ca. 15 to 18 mm.) in length, ⅓ inch (ca. 8 mm.) in width, and ⅛ inch (ca. 2 to 4 mm.) in thickness. During pregnancy they become greatly enlarged and pedunculated. The larger ones then measure about 4 to 5 inches (10 to 12 cm.) in length, 1 to 1½ inches (3 to 4 cm.) in width, and 1 inch (2 to 2.5 cm.) in thickness. The deep face has a hilus at which the vessels enter. The rest of the surface has a spongy appearance, due to numerous crypts which receive the villi of the chorion.

The **uterine glands** are long and branched. The mucous membrane of the cervix is pale and forms numerous folds. The latter are arranged in several series which obliterate the lumen. At the external orifice (os uteri) the folds (Plicæ palmatæ) form rounded prominences arranged circularly, which project into the cavity of the vagina. There are no glands in the cervix, but a thick mucus is secreted by goblet cells.

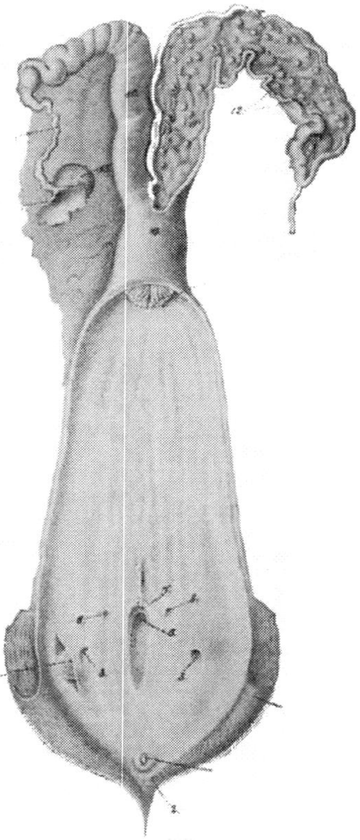

FIG. 414.—GENITAL ORGANS OF COW, DORSAL VIEW.

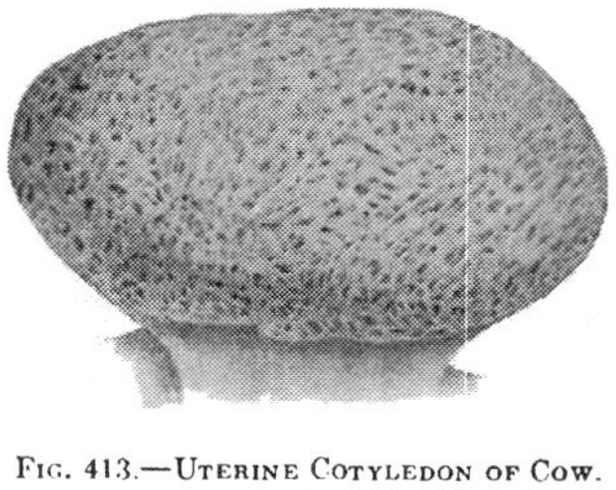

FIG. 413.—UTERINE COTYLEDON OF COW.
The figure represents a cotyledon of medium size. (After Ellenberger, in Leisering's Atlas.)

The **broad ligaments** are not attached in the sublumbar region as in the mare, but to the upper part of the flanks, about a handbreadth below the level of the external angle of the ilium. They contain a conspicuous amount of unstriped muscle. The **round ligaments** are well developed, and can be traced distinctly to the vicinity of the internal inguinal ring.

The **vagina** is somewhat longer and more roomy than that of the mare; its wall is also thicker. Its average length in the non-pregnant animal is about eight inches (ca. 20 cm.); but in the pregnant cow the length increases to twelve inches (30 cm.) or more. The recto-genital pouch of peritoneum extends backward about five inches (ca. 12 cm.) on the dorsal surface, while ventrally the serous coat only extends backward about two inches (ca. 5 cm.).

This gives ample space dorsally for the incision of the fornix vaginæ in oöphorectomy.

In the ventral wall of the vagina, between the muscular and mucous coats, there are frequently present the two **canals** of **Gartner** (Ductus epoöphori longitudinales). When well developed they may attain the diameter of a goose quill, and may be traced forward to the anterior part of the vagina or even further. They open posteriorly near the external urethral orifice.

These tubes are remnants of the Wolffian ducts, and, like other fœtal vestiges, are very variable. Röder states that the right canal was absent in over 52 per cent., the left in only 22 per cent., of the cows examined by him. In some cases they may be traced in the broad ligaments for a variable distance toward the ovary. They are of clinical interest in that cysts frequently form along their course.

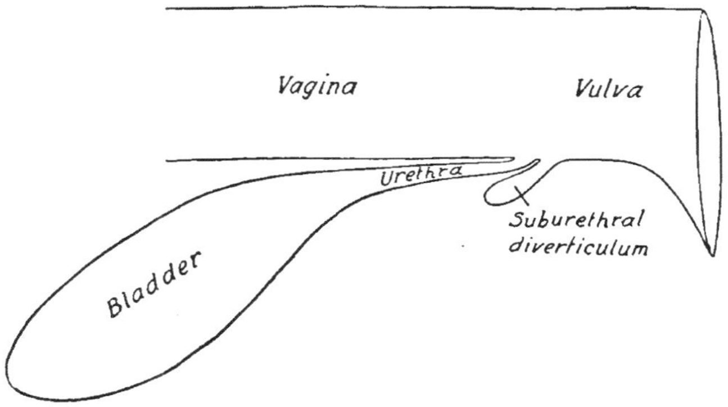

FIG. 415.—DIAGRAMMATIC SAGITTAL SECTION OF PART OF UROGENITAL TRACT OF COW, SHOWING SUBURETHRAL DIVERTICULUM.

The **vulva** has thick wrinkled labia, and both commissures are acute; the lower one is pointed, and has on it a number of long hairs; it lies about two inches (5 cm.) behind, and about the same distance below, the level of the ischial arch. The **glans clitoridis** is small; the **crura** are about four inches (ca. 10 cm.) long and are flexuous. The **external urethral orifice** or meatus urinarius is four or five inches (10 to 12 cm.) from the ventral commissure. Beneath it is a blind pouch, the **suburethral diverticulum,** which is more than an inch (ca. 3 to 4 cm.) long, and readily admits the end of a finger.

The form and position of this pouch should be carefully noted on account of the difficulty it causes in catheterizing the bladder. If the catheter is passed along the ventral wall of the vulva (as in the mare), it will always enter the pouch instead of the urethra.

The **glandulæ vestibulares majores** (or glands of Bartholin) are situated on the lateral walls of the vulva, under the constrictor vulvæ. They are little over an inch (ca. 3 cm.) long and about half an inch (ca. 1.5 cm.) in width. Each has a single duct which opens about an inch and a half (ca. 3 to 4 cm.) lateral to and behind the external urethral orifice.

The **urethra** of the cow is about four inches (10 cm.) in length; it is narrower and much less dilatable than that of the mare. It is fused dorsally with the wall of the vagina, while laterally and ventrally it is covered by the constrictor vaginæ muscle.

The **mammary glands,** normally two in number, are popularly termed the udder. They are very much larger than in the mare, and the body of each is somewhat ellipsoidal in form, but flattened transversely. The base (or dorsal surface) of each gland is slightly concave and slopes obliquely downward and forward in adaptation to the abdominal wall, to which it is adherent; posteriorly it is in relation to the large supramammary lymph glands and a quantity of fat. The inner surface is flat, and is separated from the other gland by a well-developed double septum. The outer surface is convex. Four well-developed teats are present; they average about three inches (ca. 7 to 8 cm.) in length. It is customary

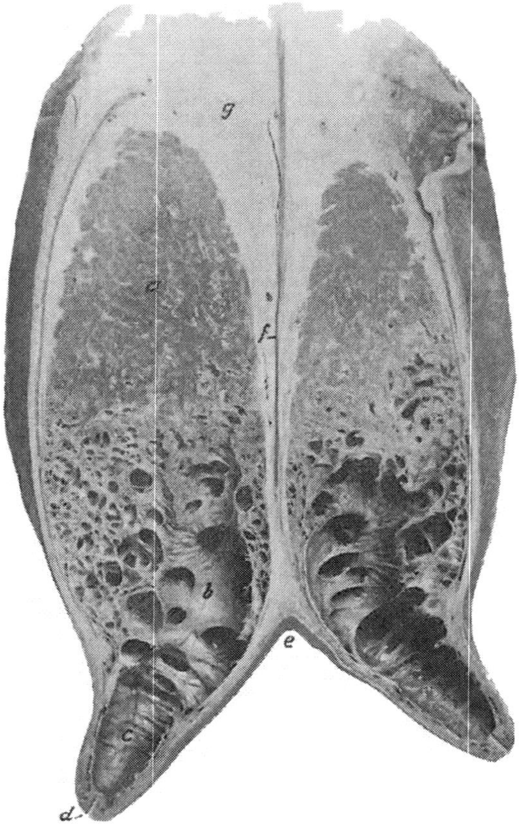

FIG. 416.—CROSS-SECTION OF MAMMARY GLANDS OF COW.
a Body of gland; *b*, lactiferous sinus; *c*, cavity of teat; *d*, duct of teat; *e*, intermammary groove; *f*, septum between glands; *g*, supramammary fat.

to consider the udder to consist of four "quarters." There is no septum nor visible division between the two quarters of the same side, but, on the other hand, injections of fluids of different colors into the two teats of the gland demonstrate that the cavities drained by them do not communicate.

The size and form of the glands vary greatly; in the highly specialized dairy breeds (*e. g.*, Holsteins) they often attain enormous dimensions. The size of the udder is not a certain index of its productivity, since some so-called "fleshy" udders contain a very large amount of interstitial tissue and relatively little parenchyma. Small accessory teats often occur posteriorly; commonly these are rudimentary and imperforate (polythelia), but sometimes they drain a small amount of gland substance (polymastia). Sanson described a case in which there were seven teats, all giving milk.

Each teat has a single duct which widens superiorly and opens freely into a roomy lactiferous sinus or milk cistern (Sinus lactiferus). The lactiferous duct or teat canal is lined by a glandless mucous membrane which is covered with stratified squamous epithelium; the lower part (ca. 1 cm.) of the canal is narrow, and is closed by a sphincter of unstriped muscle. The mucous membrane of the sinus forms numerous folds which render the cavity multilocular.

Vessels and Nerves.—The blood-supply is derived from the external pudic arteries. The veins form a circle at the base of the udder, from which the blood is drained by three trunks, viz., the very large subcutaneous abdominal ("milk vein"), the external pudic, and the perineal vein. The lymphatics are numerous, and pass to the supramammary glands chiefly. The nerves are derived from the inguinal nerves and the posterior mesenteric plexus of the sympathetic.

GENITAL ORGANS OF THE SOW

The ovaries are concealed in the bursa ovarii, owing to the large extent of the mesosalpinx. They are more rounded than in the bitch, and have a distinct hilus.

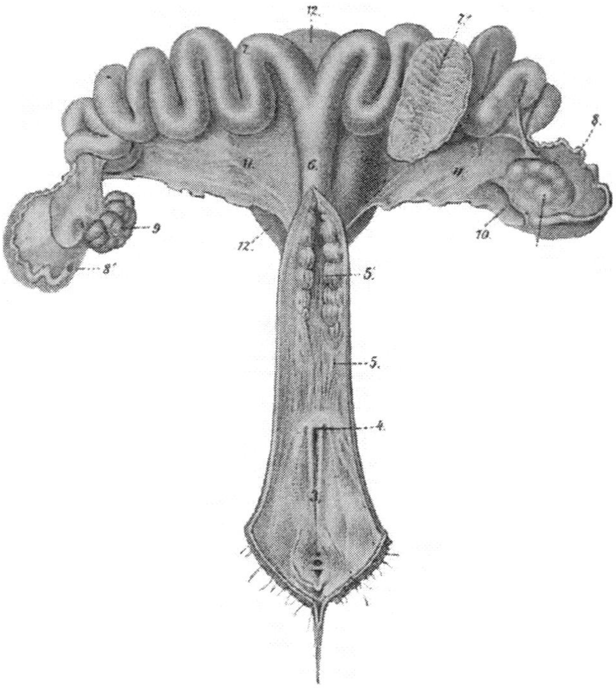

Fig. 417.—Genital Organs of Sow Dorsal View. The Vagina and Cervix Uteri are Slit Open.

1, Labia vulvæ; *2*, glans clitoridis; *3*, vulva; *4*, external urethral orifice; *5*, vagina; *5'*, cervix uteri; *6*, corpus uteri; *7*, cornua uteri, one of which is opened at *7'* to show folds of mucous membrane; *8*, Fallopian tube; *8'*, abdominal opening of tube; *9*, ovaries; *10*, ovarian bursa; *11*, broad ligaments of uterus; *12*, urinary bladder. (From Leisering's Atlas.)

They are situated usually as in the cow, but their position is quite variable in animals which have borne young. The surface commonly presents rounded prominences, so that sometimes the gland has an irregular, mulberry-like aspect; this is due to the fact that there is very little stroma and the larger Graafian follicles project from the surface.

The **Fallopian** or **uterine tubes** are long (ca. 15 to 30 cm.), and less flexuous than in the mare. The fimbriated extremity forms an ampulla and has a large abdominal opening. The uterine end shades insensibly into the small extremity of the cornu of the uterus.

The **uterus** presents several striking features. The **body** is only about two inches (ca. 5 cm.) long. The **horns** are extremely long and flexuous, and are freely movable, on account of the large extent of the broad ligaments. The extremities of the horns taper to about the diameter of the Fallopian tubes.[1] The **neck** is remarkable for its length (ca. 15 to 20 cm.) and the fact that it is directly continued by the vagina without forming any intravaginal projection (os uteri). It can be distinguished by the transverse folds of its mucous membrane and the thickness of its wall.

The changes in form and position of the uterus during pregnancy are similar to those mentioned later in the case of the bitch.

The **vagina** is about four or five inches (ca. 10 to 12 cm.) long in a sow of medium size. It is small in caliber, and has a thick muscular coat which consists mainly of circular fibers. The mucous membrane is plicated, and is intimately united with the muscular coat.

The **vulva** is relatively long. The inferior commissure is pointed and dependent. The mucous lining is plicated. There is a small **suburethral diverticulum.** The vestibular glands are small and variable in number. The vestibular bulbs are little developed. The canals of Gartner may sometimes be traced as far as the ovary, but are often difficult to find.

The **clitoris** is long, flexuous, and pointed; beneath it is a cul-de-sac.

The **urethra** is very long; its vulvar orifice is not concealed by a valvular fold.

The **mammary glands** are usually ten or twelve in number, and are arranged in two rows, as in the bitch. Each teat has commonly two excretory ducts.

GENITAL ORGANS OF THE BITCH

The **ovaries** (Fig. 336) are small, elongated-oval in outline, and flattened. Each ovary is situated close to or in contact with the posterior pole of the corresponding kidney, and thus lies ventral to the third or fourth lumbar vertebræ, or about half way between the last rib and the crest of the ilium. Each is concealed in a peritoneal pouch, the **bursa ovarii,** which has a slit-like opening ventrally. The two folds which form this pouch contain a quantity of fat and unstriped muscle. They are continued to the cornu of the uterus, constituting the **mesosalpinx** and the **ovarian ligament.** The surface of the ovary presents prominences caused by projecting Graafian follicles. There is no distinct hilus.

The **Fallopian** or **uterine tubes** are small and average two or three inches (ca. 5 to 8 cm.) in length. Each passes at first forward and then turns backward, having a straight or only slightly flexuous course. The fimbriated extremity lies in the bursa ovarii, and has a rather large opening. The uterine orifice is very small.

The **uterus** has a very short body and two long narrow horns. In a bitch of medium size the body is about an inch (ca. 2 to 3 cm.) and the cornua five or six

[1] Lesbre states that the cornua may attain a length of 45 to 50 cm.

inches (ca. 12 to 15 cm.) long. The horns are of uniform diameter, are nearly straight, and lie entirely within the abdomen. They diverge from the body in the form of a V toward each kidney. Their posterior parts are united by the peritoneum. The neck is very short and is fused dorsally with the vagina. It has a thick muscular coat. The mucous membrane of the uterus has long uterine glands and also short tubular crypts.

The **broad ligaments** contain fat and unstriped muscle. They are much longer in the middle than at either end. The posterior part is attached to the anterior part of the vagina. The **round ligaments** are very long, extending through the inguinal canals, and traceable almost to the vulva.

The horns of the gravid uterus present dilatations or **ampullæ,** which contain the fœtuses, and are separated by constrictions. The gravid uterus lies on the ventral abdominal wall, and toward the end of gestation extends forward to the stomach and liver.

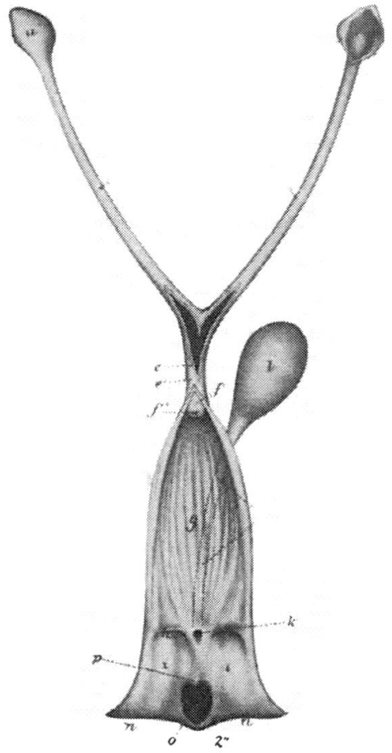

FIG. 418.—GENITAL ORGANS OF BITCH.

Vulva, vagina, and uterus (in part) are slit open. *a*, Ovarian bursa; *b*, same opened to show the right ovary, *c*; *d*, *d*, horns of uterus; *e*, *e'*, body of uterus; *f*, neck of uterus; *f'*, os uteri; *g*, vagina; *h*, hymen; *i*, vulva; k, external urethral orifice; *l*, urinary bladder; *m*, urethra; *n*, *n*, labia vulvæ; *o*, fossa clitoridis; *p*, clitoris. (After Ellenberger, in Leisering's Atlas.)

The **vagina** is relatively long. It is narrow anteriorly, and has no distinct fornix. The muscular coat is thick and consists chiefly of circular fibers. The mucous membrane forms longitudinal folds. The canals of Gartner are usually absent.

The **vulva** has thick labia which form a pointed inferior commissure. The mucous lining is smooth. On either side of the urethral orifice there is a small depression. The glandulæ vestibulares majores are absent, but the smaller glands are present, and their ducts open ventrally on either side of a median ridge. The vestibular bulbs are relatively large and join dorsally. The clitoris has a small pointed glans, beneath which is a diverticulum. The corpus cavernosum is a little more than an inch (ca. 3 to 4 cm.) long in a subject of medium size, and is infiltrated with fat.

The **mammary** glands are usually ten in number, and are arranged in two series extending from the posterior part of the pectoral region to the inguinal region; they are, therefore, designated according to location as **pectoral, abdominal,** and **inguinal.** The teats are short, and present on their apices six to twelve small orifices of the excretory ducts.

ANGIOLOGY: THE VASCULAR SYSTEM

Angiology is the description of the organs of circulation of the blood and lymph—the heart and vessels. The **heart** is the central hollow muscular organ which functions as a suction and force pump; the differences in pressure caused by its contraction and relaxation determine the circulation of the blood and lymph. It is situated in the middle mediastinal space of the thorax, between the two lungs, and is inclosed in a fibro-serous sac—the pericardium. The vessels are tubular and run through almost all parts of the body. They are designated according to their contents as blood- and lymph-vessels.

The **blood-vascular system** consists of: (1) the **arteries**, which convey blood from the heart to the tissues; (2) the **capillaries**, microscopic tubes in the tissues which permit of the necessary interchange between the blood and the tissues; (3) the **veins**, which convey the blood back to the heart.

The blood-vessels are divided into the **pulmonary** and the **systemic**. The **pulmonary artery** conveys the blood from the right ventricle of the heart to the lungs, where it is arterialized, and is returned by the **pulmonary veins** to the left atrium of the heart, and passes into the left ventricle. The **systemic arteries** convey the blood from the left ventricle all over the body, whence it is returned by the **venæ cavæ** to the right atrium, and passes into the right ventricle.

It should be noted, however, that the lungs receive arterial blood through the systemic bronchial arteries. This blood is returned in part by the bronchial veins to the right atrium (indirectly), in part by the pulmonary veins to the left atrium.

The term **portal system** is often applied to the portal vein and its tributaries which come from the stomach, intestine, pancreas, and spleen. The vein enters the liver, where it branches like an artery, so that the blood in this subsidiary system passes through a second set of capillaries before being conveyed to the heart by the hepatic veins and the posterior vena cava.

The **arteries** (Arteriæ), as a rule, divide at an acute angle, giving off finer and finer branches. In some cases branches come off at a right angle, and others are recurrent, *i. e.*, run in a direction opposite to that of the parent stem. The intercommunication of branches of adjacent arteries is termed **anastomosis.** Most commonly the connections are made by a network of numerous fine branches (Plexus vasculosus). Relatively large communicating branches (Rami communicantes) occur in certain places; they may be transverse or in the form of arches. Wide-meshed networks of vessels are termed **Retia vasculosa. Terminal** or **end arteries** are such as form isolated networks, *i. e.*, do not anastomose with adjacent arteries. A **rete mirabile** is a network intercalated in the course of an artery. A **collateral vessel** (Vas collaterale) is one which pursues a course near and similar to that of a larger vessel.

The **veins** (Venæ) are in general arranged like the arteries, but are usually of greater caliber. When a vein accompanies an artery, it is termed a **vena comitans** or **satellite vein**; in many places two veins accompany a single artery. The primitive venous trunks do not run with the arteries, and most of the superficial veins (Venæ cutaneæ) pursue independent courses. They anastomose even more freely than the arteries, and large communicating branches are very common. The veins form very rich plexuses (Plexus venosi) in many places. Some veins which are without independent walls and are inclosed by dense membranes and run usually in bony grooves are termed (venous) **sinuses**; examples of this are the sinuses of the dura mater of the brain.

Structure of Arteries.—The wall consists of three coats. The **external coat** (Tunica externa) consists chiefly of fibrous connective tissue. In the deeper part are some elastic fibers, and in some arteries there are also longitudinal unstriped muscle-fibers. The **middle coat** (Tunica media) is composed of unstriped muscle and elastic tissue in medium-sized arteries. In small vessels there is only the muscular tissue, and in the largest trunks only elastic tissue. The **internal coat** or **intima** (Tunica intima) consists of a layer of endothelial cells, resting on an elastic membrane. The **sheath** (Vagina vasis) is a condensation of the surrounding connective tissue, and is attached more or less closely to the external coat.

Structure of Veins.—The walls of veins are similar in structure to those of the arteries, but are very much thinner, so that veins collapse more or less completely when empty, while arteries do not. The **middle coat** is very thin and consists to a large extent of ordinary connective tissue. The **intima** is also less elastic than in the arteries. In many veins this coat forms semilunar **valves**, the free edges of which are directed toward the heart. They are most numerous in the veins of the skin and the deep veins of the extremities (except the foot), while in most veins of the body cavities and viscera they are absent or occur only where the veins open into larger ones or where two veins join.

The walls of the vessels are supplied with blood by numerous small arteries, called **vasa vasorum.** These arise from branches of the artery which they supply or from adjacent arteries, ramify in the external coat, and enter the middle coat also.

The **nerves** of the vessels consist of both medullated and non-medullated fibers. They form plexuses around the vessels, from which fibers pass mainly to the muscular tissue of the middle coat.

BLOOD-VASCULAR SYSTEM OF THE HORSE

THE PERICARDIUM[1]

The **pericardium** is the fibro-serous sac which surrounds the heart, and also the great vessels in connection with it to a greater or less extent. Its form is in general similar to that of the heart. The **fibrous layer** is relatively thin, but strong and inelastic. It is attached dorsally to the large vessels at the base of the heart, and is continued in part up to the longus colli muscle. Ventrally it is firmly attached to the middle of the posterior half of the thoracic surface of the sternum. The **serous layer** is a closed sac, surrounded by the fibrous pericardium, and invaginated by the heart. It is smooth and glistening, and contains a small amount of clear serous fluid, the **liquor pericardii.** Like other serous membranes, it may be regarded as consisting of two parts, parietal and visceral. The **parietal part** lines the fibrous layer, to which it is closely attached. The **visceral layer** covers the heart and parts of the great vessels, and is therefore also termed the **epicardium.** The serous pericardium is composed of a connective-tissue membrane, rich in elastic fibers, and covered on its free surface by a layer of flat endothelial cells.

The pericardium is covered by the mediastinal pleura (Pleura pericardica) and is crossed laterally by the phrenic nerves. Its lateral surfaces are related chiefly to the lungs, but the lower part is in partial contact with the chest-wall. On the left side the area of contact is from the third to the fifth intercostal space inclusive. On the right side the contact is smaller and is at the third and fourth

[1] The pericardium is described before the heart since it must be examined first in the laboratory.

ribs. The anterior border of the base is opposite to the second intercostal space, and the posterior border is opposite to the sixth rib or space. The base is related to the great vessels, the trachea and its bifurcation, the bronchial lymph glands, the œsophagus, and the vagus, left recurrent, and cardiac nerves.

The two parts of the serous pericardium are, of course, continuous with each other at the line of reflection on to the great vessels. The latter are covered in varying degree by the visceral layer. The aorta and pulmonary artery are inclosed in a complete common sheath as far as the bifurcation of the latter. A pouch passes inward between the pulmonary artery and the left auricle, and is connected with another pouch which passes backward between the right auricle and the aorta, thus forming the great transverse sinus of the pericardium. The posterior vena cava is covered on the right and below for a distance of an inch or a little more (ca. 3 cm.). The pulmonary veins receive practically no serous covering. The epicardium is closely adherent to the muscular tissue of the heart, but is attached to the vessels by loose tissue and fat, and hence is easily dissected off them.

THE HEART

The heart (Cor) occupies the greater part of the middle mediastinal space. Its shape is that of an irregular and somewhat flattened cone. It is attached at

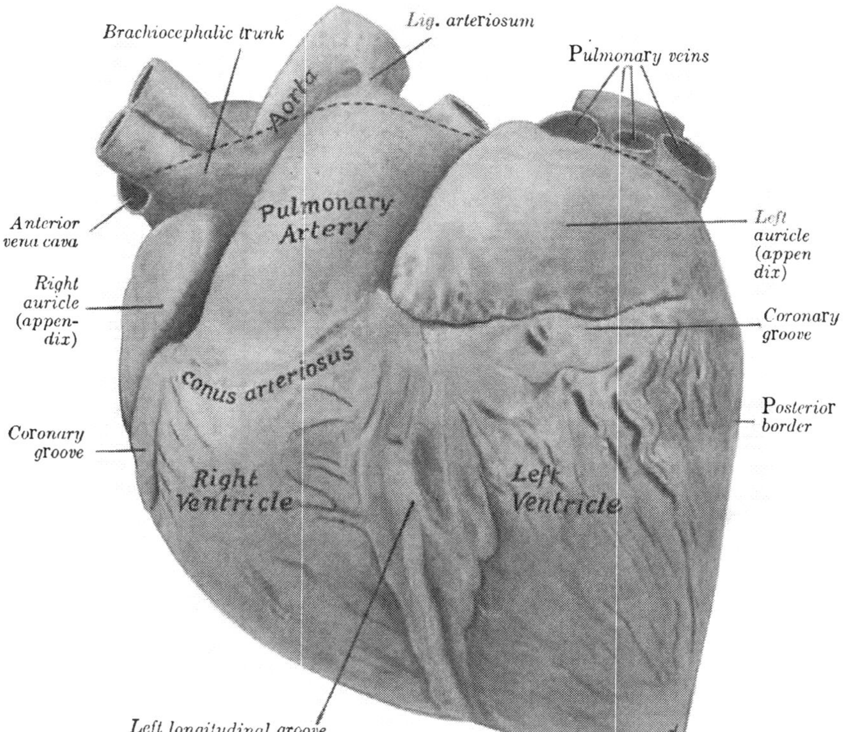

FIG. 419.—HEART OF HORSE, LEFT VIEW. HARDENED *in situ.*
The dotted line indicates the line of reflection of the serous pericardium. The epicardium and subepicardial fat have not been removed from the heart.

its base by the great vessels, but is otherwise entirely free in the pericardium. It presents two surfaces, two borders, a base, and an apex for description.

In position the heart is decidedly asymmetrical, about two-fifths being to the right of the median plane and three-fifths to the left. The long axis (from the middle of the base to the apex) is directed downward, backward, and somewhat to the left. The **base** (Basis cordis) is directed dorsally and lies a little above the middle of the dorso-ventral diameter of the thorax. It is opposite to the ribs from the third to the sixth inclusive. The **apex** (Apex cordis) lies above the last segment of the sternum, and is separated by a very short interval from the sternal part of the diaphragm. The **anterior** border (Margo cranialis) is strongly convex and is directed obliquely downward and backward; its lower part is parallel with the sternum. The **posterior border** (Margo caudalis) is much shorter, nearly vertical,

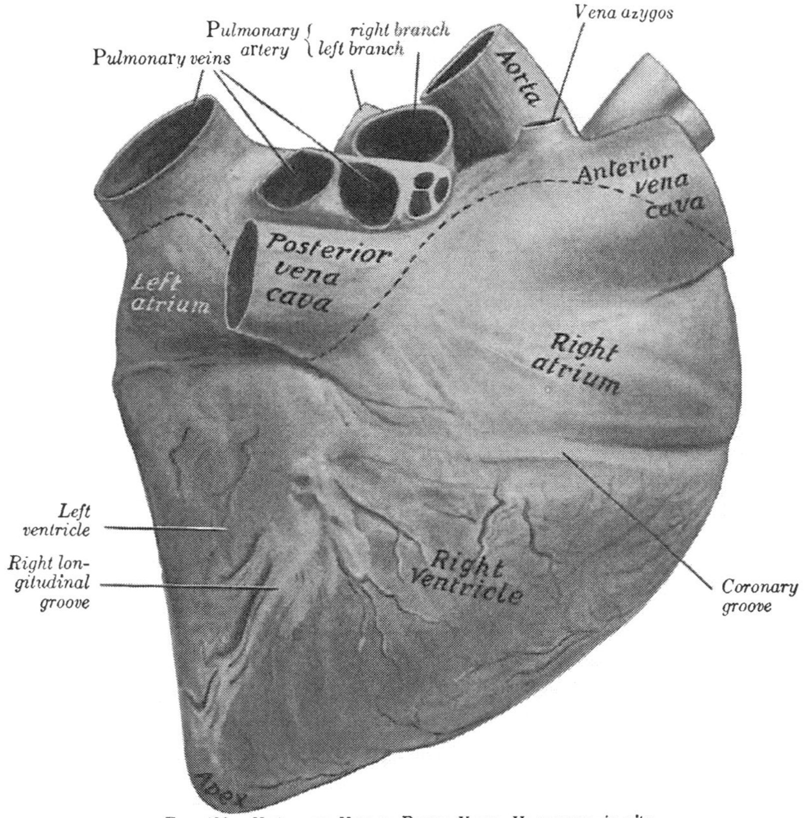

FIG. 420.—HEART OF HORSE, RIGHT VIEW. HARDENED *in situ*.
Line of reflection of serous pericardium dotted. Epicardium and subepicardial fat have not been removed from heart. Left ventricle is considerably contracted.

and is opposite to the sixth rib or intercostal space. The **surfaces**, right and left (Facies dextra, sinistra), are convex and are marked by grooves which indicate the division of the heart into four chambers, the two atria above and two ventricles below. The left surface (covered by the pericardium) is in contact with the lower third of the chest-wall from the third to the fifth intercostal space. On the right side the cardiac notch of the lung is smaller and further forward, so that the area of contact is at the third and fourth ribs.

The **coronary** or **atrio-ventricular groove** (Sulcus coronarius) indicates the division between the atria and the ventricles. It almost completely encircles the heart, but is interrupted by the origin of the pulmonary artery. The **longitudinal** or **interventricular grooves,** right and left (Sulci longitudinales sinister et dexter), correspond to the septum between the ventricles. The left groove is left-anterior in position. It begins at the coronary groove behind the origin of the pulmonary artery, and passes downward almost parallel to the posterior border, but does not reach the apex. The right groove is right-posterior in position. It begins at the coronary groove below the termination of the posterior vena cava and passes downward and a little backward, ending about an inch and a half (ca. 3 to 4 cm.)

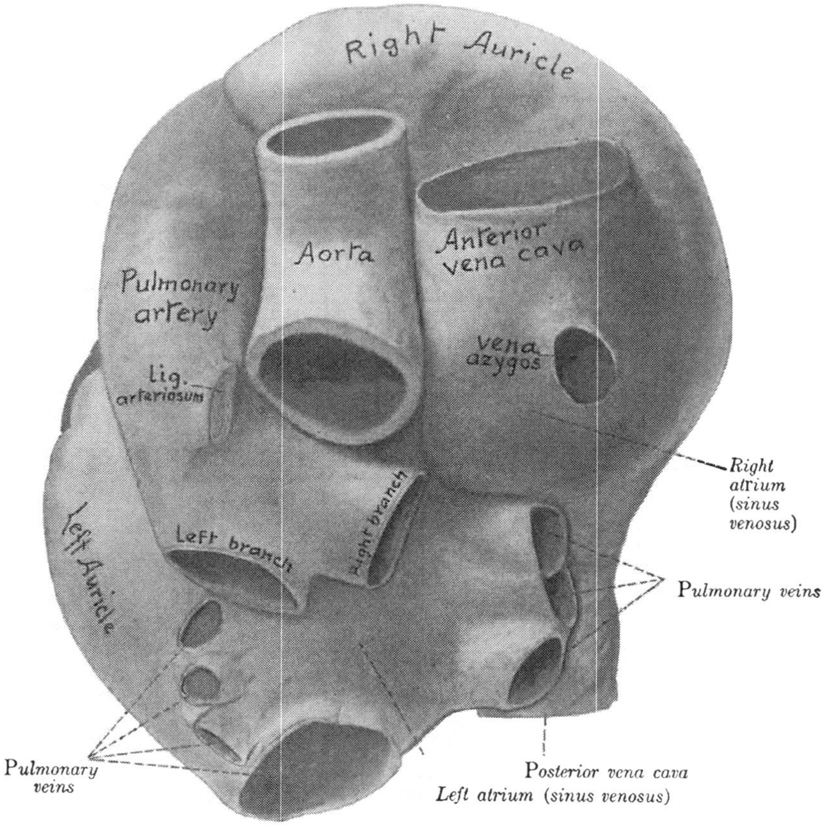

FIG. 421.—BASE OF HEART OF HORSE WITH LARGE VESSELS, DORSAL VIEW. SPECIMEN HARDENED *in situ.*

above the apex. The grooves are occupied by the coronary vessel and a variable quantity of fat.

Size and Weight.—In horses of medium size the heart usually weighs about seven or eight pounds (ca. 3.5 kg.), or about 0.7 per cent. of the body-weight. There is, however, great range of variation in apparently normal specimens.

The following measurements were obtained in medium-sized hearts in diastole:

Sagittal diameter of base	25 cm.
Greatest width of base	18 to 20 cm.
Circumference at coronary groove	65 to 70 cm.
Distance between origin of pulmonary artery and apex	25 cm.
Distance between termination of posterior vena cava and apex	18 to 20 cm.

THE RIGHT ATRIUM

The right **atrium** (Atrium dextrum) or auricle forms the right-anterior part of the base of the heart, and lies above the right ventricle. It consists of a **sinus venosus**, into which the veins open, and an **auricle** or auricular appendix. The latter is a conical diverticulum which curves around the right and anterior surfaces

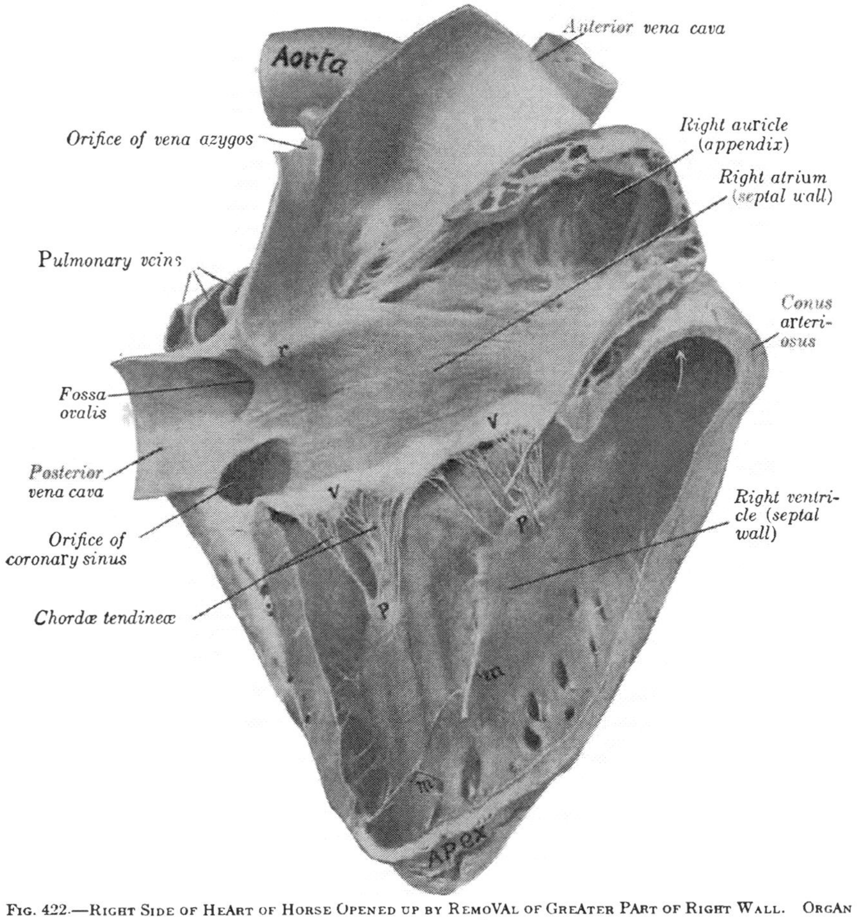

FIG. 422.—RIGHT SIDE OF HEART OF HORSE OPENED UP BY REMOVAL OF GREATER PART OF RIGHT WALL. ORGAN HARDENED *in situ*.

The right ventricle was in diastole. *r*, intervenous crest; *v*, *v*, tricuspid valve; *p*, *p*, papillary muscles; *m*, *m*, moderator bands. Arrow points into origin of pulmonary artery.

of the aorta, its blind end appearing on the left side in front of the origin of the pulmonary artery.

There are five chief openings in the right atrium. The **opening of the anterior vena cava** (Ostium venæ cavæ cranialis) is in the upper and fore part. The **opening of the posterior vena cava** (Ostium venæ cavæ caudalis) is at the lower posterior part. Between the two the wall pouches upward somewhat, forming what is sometimes termed the sinus venosus or sac of Lower. In the anterior part of this the **vena azygos** opens. The **coronary sinus** opens immediately below the posterior vena cava; the orifice is provided with a small semilunar valve or valve of Thebesius (Valvula sinus coronarii). The middle coronary vein has a separate opening in some cases close to that of the coronary sinus. The **atrio-ventricular opening** is in the lower part, and leads into the right ventricle. In addition to the foregoing there are several small orifices of the venæ cordis parvæ; these are concealed in the depressions between the musculi pectinati.

The atrium is lined with a glistening membrane, the **endocardium.** Its walls are smooth except on the right and in the auricle (or appendix), where it is crossed in various directions by muscular ridges, the **musculi pectinati.** Small bands extend across some of the spaces inclosed by the musculi pectinati. The latter terminate above on a curved crest, the **crista terminales,** which indicates the junction of the primitive sinus venosus of the embryo with the atrium proper, and corresponds with the sulcus terminalis externally. The openings of the venæ cavæ are without valves. A ridge, the intervenous crest,[1] projects downward and forward from the roof just in front of the opening of the posterior vena cava; it tends to direct the flow of blood from the anterior vena cava to the atrio-ventricular opening. The **fossa ovalis** is an oval depression in the septal wall at the point of entrance of the posterior vena cava, bounded internally by a thick margin (Limbus fossæ ovalis). The fossa is the remains of an opening, the **foramen ovale,** through which the two atria communicate in the fœtus.

The Left Atrium

The left **atrium** (Atrium sinistrum) or auricle forms the posterior part of the base of the heart. It lies behind the pulmonary artery and the aorta and above the left ventricle. The auricle (or appendix) extends outward and forward on the left side, and its blind end is behind the origin of the pulmonary artery. The **pulmonary veins,** usually seven or eight in number, open into the atrium behind and on the right side. The cavity of the atrium is smooth, with the exception of the auricle (or appendix), in which the musculi pectinati are present. In some cases there is a depression on the septal wall opposite the fossa ovalis, bounded above by a fold which is the remnant of the valve of the foramen ovale of the fœtus. The **atrio-ventricular opening** is situated below and in front; it usually appears smaller than the right one on account of the contraction of the left ventricle in the dead subject. The apertures of small veins of the heart are found in the spaces inclosed by the musculi pectinati.

The number and the arrangement of the pulmonary veins are variable. They may be five to nine in number. The largest orifice is posterior. Usually three veins of considerable size enter close together on the right above the posterior vena cava, and three or four open clos to the ridge which projects from the roof at the base of the auricle (appendix).

The Right Ventricle

The **right ventricle** (Ventriculus dexter) constitutes the right-anterior part of the ventricular mass. It forms almost all of the anterior border of the heart, but does not reach the apex, which is formed entirely by the left ventricle. It extends from the third rib to the fourth intercostal space on the left side, to the fifth rib and space on the right side. It is somewhat triangular in outline, and is semilunar in cross-section. Its base faces upward and a little to the right and is connected largely with the right atrium, with which it communicates through the atrio-ventricular orifice; but its left part projects higher and forms the **conus arteriosus,** from which the pulmonary artery arises. Its apex is two inches or more (ca. 5 to 6 cm.) above the apex of the heart. On opening the cavity it is seen that the two openings are separated by a thick rounded ridge (Crista supraventricularis).

[1] This is termed the tubercle of Lower in human anatomy and the tuberculum intervenosum by German veterinary anatomists.

The axis of the cavity, taken from this ridge to the apex forms a spiral curve downward and to the right. The septal wall is convex and faces obliquely forward and to the right.

The **right atrio-ventricular orifice** (Ostium venosum dextrum) is oval and is situated opposite to the lower parts of the third and fourth ribs. It is guarded by a **tricuspid valve** (Valvula tricuspidalis); of the three large cusps of this valve, one is between the atrio-ventricular opening and the conus arteriosus, one is septal, and the third is on the right margin. Small intermediate cusps intervene between the large ones. The peripheral edges of the cusps are attached to the fibrous ring at the atrio-ventricular opening. The central edges are irregular and hang down

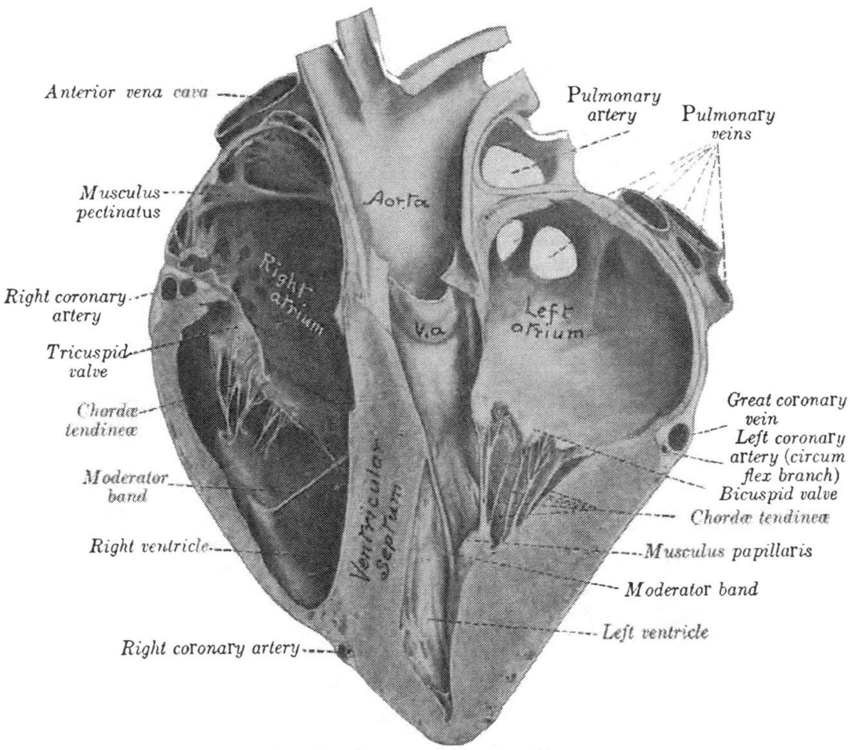

FIG. 423.—SECTION OF HEART OF HORSE.
Specimen hardened *in situ* and cut nearly at right angles to the ventricular septum. The left ventricle is contracted but not *ad maximum*. *V. a.*, Segment of aortic valve.

into the ventricle; they give attachment to chordæ tendineæ. The auricular surfaces are smooth. The ventricular surfaces are rough and furnish attachment to interlacing branches of the chordæ tendineæ. The valves are folds of the endocardium, strengthened by fibrous tissue and at the periphery by muscular fibers also. The **chordæ tendineæ** are attached below to the three **musculi papillares,** which project from the ventricular wall; superiorly they divide into branches which are inserted into the ventricular surfaces and the free edges of the valves. Each segment of the valve receives chordæ tendineæ from two papillary muscles. Of the latter, two are on the septum and the third and largest springs from the anterior wall.

The **pulmonary orifice** (Ostium arteriæ pulmonalis) is circular and is situated at the summit of the conus arteriosus, opposite to the lower part of the third intercostal space. It is guarded by the **pulmonary valve,** composed of three semilunar cusps (Valvulæ semilunares arteriæ pulmonalis); of these, one is internal, one external, and the third posterior. The convex peripheral border of each cusp is attached to the fibrous ring at the junction of the pulmonary artery and the conus arteriosus. The central border is free and slightly concave. Each cusp consists of a layer of endocardium on its ventricular surface, a continuation of the inner coat of the artery on its arterial surface, and an intermediate layer of fibrous tissue. The upper edge of the conus arteriosus forms three arches with intermediate projecting angles or horns, to all of which the cusps are attached; and the

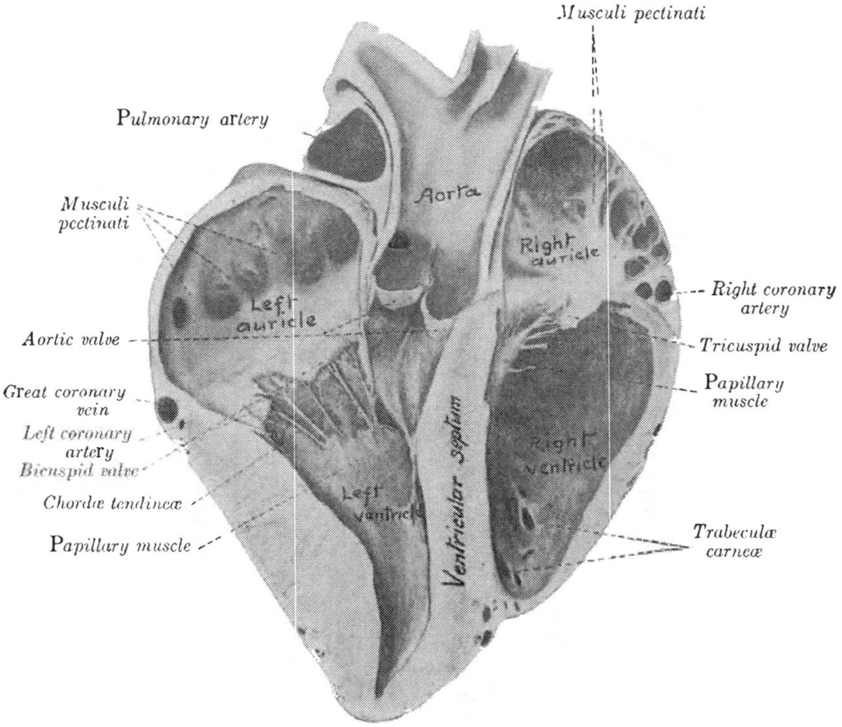

FIG. 424.—SECTION OF HEART OF HORSE. SPECIMEN HARDENED *in situ.*
The section is cut nearly at right angles to the ventricular septum, and is viewed from the right and posteriorly.

artery forms opposite each cusp a pouch, the sinus of the pulmonary artery (or of Valsalva).

The walls of the ventricle (except in the conus arteriosus) bear muscular ridges and bands, termed **trabeculæ carneæ.** These are of three kinds, viz., (1) ridges or columns in relief; (2) musculi papillares, somewhat conical flattened projections, continuous at the base with the wall and giving off the chordæ tendineæ to the tricuspid valve; (3) moderator bands (Musculi transversi cordis) which extend from the septum to the opposite wall. The latter are partly muscular, partly tendinous, and vary in different subjects. The strongest one is usually about midway between the base and apex and extends from the septum to the base of the anterior musculus papillaris. It is considered that they tend to prevent overdistention.

THE LEFT VENTRICLE

The **left ventricle** (Ventriculus sinister) forms the left posterior part of the ventricular mass. It is more regularly conical than the right ventricle and its wall is much thicker except at the apex. It forms all of the posterior border of the ventricular part and the apex of the heart. Its base is largely continuous with the left atrium, with which it communicates through the left atrio-ventricular opening, but in front it opens into the aorta. The cavity usually appears smaller than that of the right ventricle in the dead subject, on account of the greater contraction of its wall. It is almost circular in cross-section.

The **left atrio-ventricular orifice** (Ostium venosum sinistrum) is opposite to the fifth rib and intercostal space. It is almost circular and is guarded by the

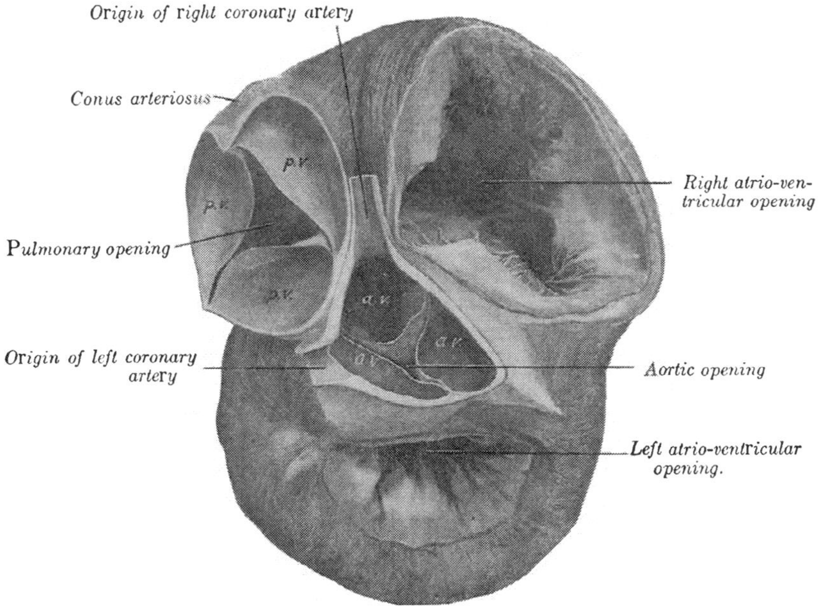

FIG. 425.—THE BASES OF THE VENTRICLES OF THE HEART OF THE HORSE.
The atria have been removed and the aorta and pulmonary artery cut off short. The left ventricle is contracted. *p.v.*, Pulmonary valve; *a.v.*, aortic valve.

bicuspid or **mitral valve** (Valvula bicuspidalis). The two segments of this valve are larger and thicker than those of the right side of the heart. One is placed in front and separates the atrio-ventricular and aortic openings. The other is placed behind and laterally and is usually divided into two or three flaps.

The **aortic orifice** (Ostium aorticum) is directed upward and slightly forward. It is situated opposite to the fourth rib. It is guarded by the **aortic valve,** composed of three semilunar cusps (Valvulæ semilunares aortæ); one cusp is anterior, the others right and left posterior. They are similar to those of the pulmonary valve, but are much stronger. The free edge of each contains a central nodule of fibrous tissue, the corpus Arantii (Nodulus valvulæ semilunaris).

The **chordæ tendineæ** are fewer but larger than those of the right ventricle.

There are two large **musculi papillares,** one on each side; they are usually compound. The moderator bands are variable. Commonly two or three larger ones (which are often branched) extend from the musculi papillares to the septum. Smaller ones may be found in various places, especially at the apex. The other trabeculæ are fewer and less prominent than in the right ventricle.

The **interventricular septum** (Septum ventriculorum) is the musculo-membranous partition which separates the cavities of the two ventricles. It is placed obliquely. One surface is convex, faces forward and to the right, and bulges into the right ventricle. The other surface, which faces into the left ventricle, is concave and looks backward and to the left. The greater part of the septum is thick and muscular (Septum musculare), but the upper part is thin and membranous (Septum membranaceum). The latter intervenes between the left ventricle, on the one hand, and the right ventricle and atrium on the other.

Structure of the Heart

The heart-wall consists mainly of peculiar striped muscle, the myocardium, which is covered externally by the visceral part of the serous pericardium or epicardium, and is lined by the endocardium.

The **epicardium** is in general closely attached to the muscular wall, but is loosely attached over the coronary vessels and the associated subepicardial fat. It consists of a layer of flat polygonal cells, resting on a membrane of white and elastic fibers.

The **myocardium** consists of planes of fibers arranged in a somewhat complicated manner. The muscular tissue of the atria is almost completely separated from that of the ventricles by the fibrous rings around the atrio-ventricular orifices.

In the atria the muscle bands fall naturally into two groups—superficial and deep. The former are common to both atria, the latter special to each. The **superficial** or **common fibers** for the most part begin and end at the atrio-ventricular rings, but some enter the interatrial septum. The **deep** or **special bundles** also form two sets. Looped fibers pass over the atria from ring to ring, while annular or spiral fibers surround the ends of the veins which open into the atria, the auricles, and the fossa ovalis.

The muscular wall of the ventricles is much stronger than that of the atria. That of the left ventricle is in general about three times as thick as that of the right one, but is thin at the apex. The **superficial fibers** are attached above to the atrio-ventricular fibrous rings and pass in a spiral toward the apex. Here they bend upon themselves and pass deeply upward to terminate in a papillary muscle of the ventricle opposite to that in which they arose. The loops so formed at the apex constitute a whorl, the **vortex cordis.** The **deep fibers,** although they appear to be proper to each ventricle, have been shown by MacCallum to be in reality almost all common to both. Their arrangement is scroll-like. They begin on one side, curve around in the wall of that ventricle, then pass in the septum to the opposite side, and curve around the other ventricle. There is a layer of deep fibers which is confined to the basal part of the left ventricle; it is attached to the left atrio-ventricular ring.

Four **fibrous rings** (Annuli fibrosi) surround the orifices at the bases of the ventricles. The atrio-ventricular rings separate the musculature of the atria from that of the ventricles. Those which surround the origins of the pulmonary artery and aorta are festooned in conformity with the attached borders of the valves. The aortic ring contains on the right side a plate of cartilage (Cartilago cordis), which frequently becomes more or less calcified in old animals. Sometimes a smaller plate is present on the left side.

The **endocardium** lines the cavities of the heart and is continuous with the internal coat of the vessels which enter and leave the organ. Its free surface is smooth and glistening and is formed by a layer of endothelial cells. The latter rest on a thin layer of connective tissue, which is connected with the myocardium by a subendocardial elastic tissue containing vessels and nerves.

Vessels and Nerves.—The heart receives its blood-supply through the two **coronary arteries** which arise from the aorta opposite to the anterior and left cusps of the aortic valve. Most of the blood is returned by the **coronary veins,** which open into the right atrium by the coronary sinus.[1] A few small veins open directly into the right atrium, and others are said to open into the left atrium and the ventricles. The **lymph-vessels** form a subepicardial network which communicates through stomata with the cavity of the pericardium. There is a less distinct subendocardial network. The vessels converge usually to two trunks which accompany the blood-vessels in the atrio-ventricular grooves and enter the glands at the bifurcation of the trachea. The **nerves** are derived from the **vagus** and **sympathetic** through the cardiac plexus.

THE ARTERIES

THE PULMONARY ARTERY

The **pulmonary artery** (A. pulmonalis) springs from the conus arteriosus at the left side of the base of the right ventricle. It curves upward, backward, and inward, and divides behind the arch of the aorta into right and left branches. It is related in front to the right auricle (appendix), behind to the left auricle (appendix), and internally to the aorta. It is enveloped with the latter in a common sheath of the visceral layer of the serous pericardium. Near the bifurcation it is connected with the arch of the aorta by a fibrous band about half an inch (ca. 1.2 cm.) in width; this is the **ligamentum arteriosum,** a remnant of the large **ductus arteriosus,** which conducts most of the blood from the pulmonary artery to the aorta in the fœtus. The artery is bulbous at its origin, and forms three **sinuses** or pouches, which correspond to the cusps of the semilunar valve. Beyond this it gradually diminishes in caliber.

In a horse of medium size the artery is about seven inches (ca. 17 to 18 cm.) long. At the origin it is about two and a half inches (ca. 6 to 6.5 cm.) in width; at the bifurcation its caliber is about one and a half inches (ca. 3.5 to 4 cm.). The wall is relatively thin, especially at the origin.

The **right branch** (Ramus dexter) of the pulmonary artery is a little longer and wider than the left one. It passes over the fore part of the left atrium and below the bifurcation of the trachea to the hilus of the right lung, and enters the latter below the right bronchus. In the lung it passes to the outer and lower side of the stem-bronchus and accompanies it to the base of the organ. The branches correspond to the ramification of the bronchi. The **left branch** (Ramus sinister) is very short. It passes backward and enters the lung below the left bronchus. Its branches within the lung are arranged like that of the right one.

THE SYSTEMIC ARTERIES

The **aorta** is the main systemic arterial trunk. It begins at the base of the left ventricle and is practically median at its origin. It passes upward and slightly forward between the pulmonary artery on the left and right atrium on the right. It then curves sharply backward and upward and inclines somewhat to the left, forming the **arch of the aorta** (Arcus aortæ), and reaches the ventral surface of the spine at the eighth or ninth thoracic vertebra. After passing backward along the ventral aspect of the bodies of the vertebræ between the lungs it traverses the hiatus

[1] These vessels will be described later in their systematic order.

aorticus and enters the abdominal cavity, where it lies below the vertebral bodies and the psoas minor, just to the left of the median plane. It divides under the fifth lumbar vertebra into the two internal iliac or hypogastric arteries.

From the bifurcation a small vessel, the middle sacral artery (A. sacralis media), sometimes passes backward on the pelvic surface of the sacrum. It becomes lost in the periosteum or joins the coccygeal artery, or in exceptional cases is traceable to the sphincter ani externus.

The caliber of the aorta is greatest at its origin, which is termed the bulbus aortæ. Here it forms three pouch-like dilatations, the sinuses of the aorta (or of Valsalva). These correspond to the cusps of the aortic valve, and the coronary arteries arise from the left posterior and anterior sinuses. At the arch the

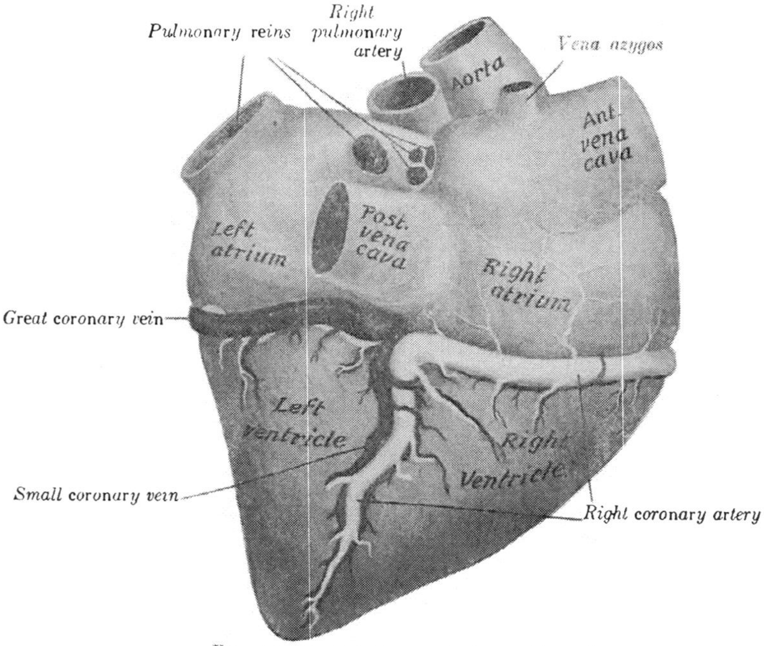

FIG. 426.—CARDIAC VESSELS OF HORSE, RIGHT SIDE.
Veins are black, arteries white.

diameter is about two inches (ca. 5 cm.), and beyond this it diminishes gradually in width.

It is convenient to divide the aorta into thoracic and abdominal parts. The thoracic aorta (Aorta thoracica) lies within the pericardium to the point of attachment of the ligamentum arteriosum, and is inclosed with the pulmonary artery in a prolongation of the epicardium. Beyond this it is between the two pleural sacs. It is crossed on the right by the œsophagus and trachea, on the left by the left vagus nerve. The left recurrent nerve winds around the concavity of the arch from left to right, and the vena azygos and thoracic duct lie along the dorsal part of its right face. The trachea causes it to deviate to the left; but beyond this it becomes median. The abdominal aorta (Aorta abdominalis) (Fig. 450) is related above to the lumbar vertebræ, the inferior common ligament, and the left psoas minor muscle; in the hiatus aorticus it is related to the cisterna chyli. On its right is the posterior vena cava, and on its left the left kidney and ureter.

BRANCHES OF THE THORACIC AORTA

1. CORONARY ARTERIES

The two coronary arteries, right and left, are distributed almost entirely to the heart, but send some small twigs to the origins of the great vessels.

The **right coronary artery** (A. coronaria dextra) arises from the anterior sinus of the aorta. It passes forward between the conus arteriosus and the right auricle (appendix) to the coronary groove, in which it curves around to the right and backward. It then descends in the right ventricular groove almost to the apex of the heart.

The **left coronary artery** (A. coronaria sinistra) arises from the left posterior

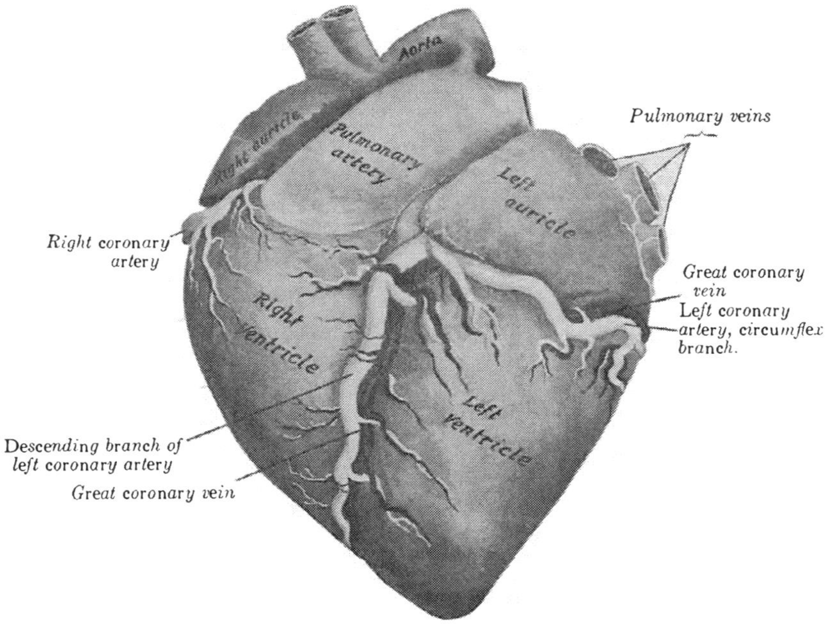

FIG. 427.—CARDIAC VESSELS OF HORSE, LEFT SIDE.
The dotted lines indicate part of the left coronary artery which is concealed by the left auricle.

sinus of the aorta, passes to the left behind the origin of the pulmonary artery, and divides into two branches. The **descending branch** (Ramus descendens) passes down the left ventricular groove toward the apex. The **circumflex branch** (Ramus circumflexus) runs backward in the coronary groove, in which it winds around to the right side.

2. COMMON BRACHIOCEPHALIC TRUNK OR ANTERIOR AORTA

The **common brachiocephalic trunk** or **anterior aorta** (Truncus brachiocephalicus communis) is a very large vessel which arises from the convexity of the arch of the aorta within the pericardium. It is directed forward and upward. Its length in horses of medium size is usually about two inches (ca. 5 to 6 cm.), but it is sometimes only half an inch or less (ca. 1 cm.). It is crossed on the left by the left vagus and cardiac nerves, and the left recurrent nerve runs between it and the trachea. It divides opposite to the second intercostal space or third rib into the brachiocephalic and left brachial arteries.

The brachiocephalic artery (A. brachiocephalica) is directed forward and a little upward in the anterior mediastinum, beneath the trachea. Opposite the first rib it gives off the bicarotid trunk and is continued as the right brachial artery. The latter (A. subclavia dextra) turns downward and bends around the anterior border of the first rib and the insertion of the scalenus muscle above the brachial vein. Its course and branches beyond this point will be described with the vessels of the thoracic limb.

The left brachial artery (A. subclavia sinistra) is longer than the right one and rises to a higher level. It forms an almost semicircular curve, the concavity being

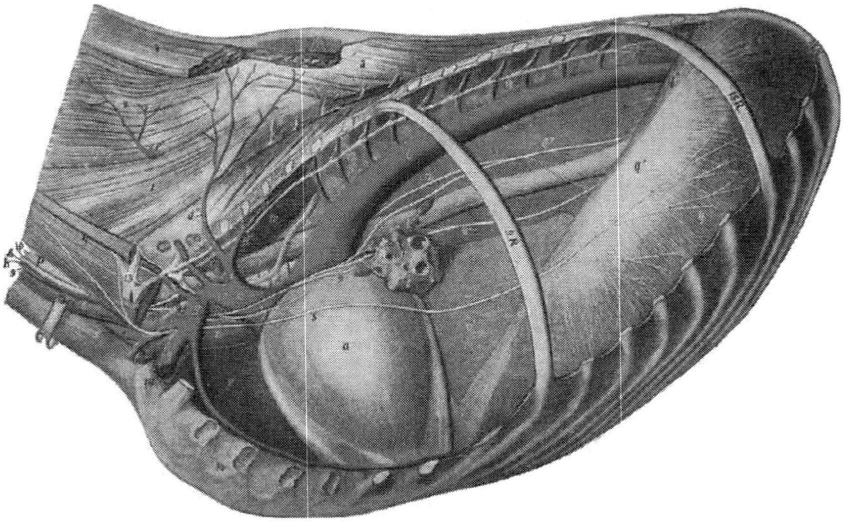

FIG. 428.—TOPOGRAPHY OF THORACIC CAVITY OF HORSE, LEFT SIDE, AFTER REMOVAL OF LEFT LUNG.

The ninth, fifteenth, and eighteenth ribs are retained. *a*, Pericardium; *b*, thoracic aorta; *c*, brachiocephalic trunk; *d*, *d″*, dorsal artery; *d′*, subcostal artery; *e*, *e′*, superior or deep cervical artery; *f*, vertebral artery; *g*, *g′*, left brachial artery; *h*, inferior cervical artery; *i*, internal thoracic artery; *k*, common carotid artery; *l*, jugular vein; *m*, brachial vein; *m′*, inferior cervical vein; *n*, anterior vena cava; *o*, thoracic duct; *p*, œsophagus; *q*, costal part of diaphragm; *q′*, tendinous center of same; *q″*, left crus of same; r, anterior mediastinal lymph-glands; *s*, trachea; *t*, bronchial lymph-glands; *u*, root of left lung; *v*, anterior mediastinum; *v′*, posterior mediastinum; *w*, longus colli; *x*, sterno-cephalicus; *y*, scalenus; *z*, transversalis costarum; *1*, longissimus; *2*, splenius; *3*, spinalis et semispinalis; *4*, *4′*, rhomboideus; *5*, left phrenic nerve; *6*, left vagus; *6′*, *6″*, œsophageal continuations of vagi; *7*, dorsal branch of right vagus; *8*, cardiac nerve; *9*, left recurrent nerve; *10*, cervical trunk of sympathetic; *11*, first thoracic ganglion of sympathetic; *12*, thoracic trunk of sympathetic; *13*, brachial plexus. (After Ellenberger-Baum, Top. Anat. d. Pferdes.)

ventral. It is related internally to the œsophagus, trachea, and thoracic duct and the left vagus, phrenic, and cardiac nerves cross under its origin. It emerges from the thorax like the artery of the right side. There is thus a difference at first between the trunks of opposite sides, but beyond this their course and distribution are similar.

The brachial and brachiocephalic arteries within the thorax give off the dorsal, superior cervical, vertebral, and internal thoracic arteries. At the first rib they give off the external thoracic and inferior cervical arteries.

1. The left dorsal or dorso-intercostal artery (A. costo-cervicalis) passes dorsally across the left face of the trachea and œsophagus toward the second intercostal space. The right artery arises usually by a common trunk with the

superior cervical, crosses the right face of the trachea and has no contact with the œsophagus. Both detach small branches to the trachea, lymph glands, and pleura, and divide on reaching the longus colli into two branches. Of these the **subcostal artery** (A. intercostalis suprema) is the smaller. It passes backward under the costo-vertebral joints with the sympathetic trunk. It gives off the second, third, and fourth intercostal arteries, and ends at the fifth space, where it anastomoses with the first aortic intercostal artery, or constitutes the fifth intercostal artery, or dips into the longissimus muscle. It also gives off spinal branches and twigs to the longus colli and the pleura. The other branch (A. transversa colli) is the direct continuation of the trunk. It emerges through the upper end of

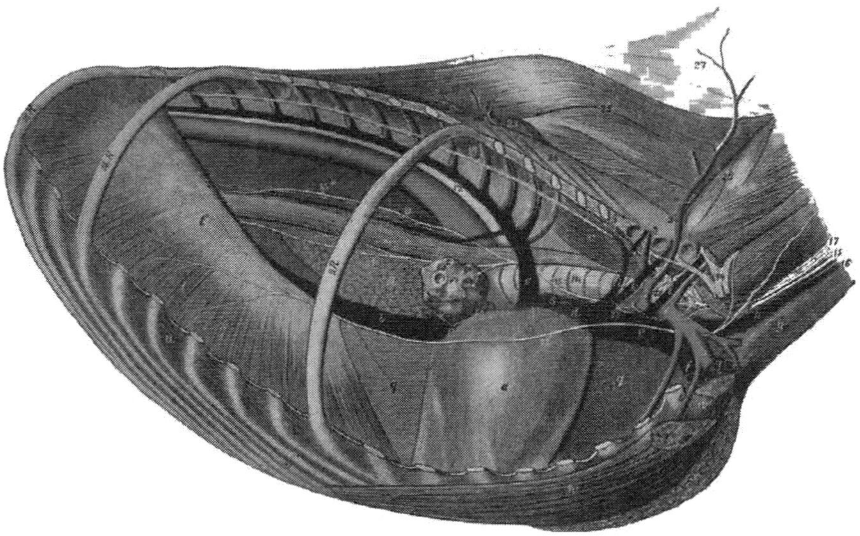

FIG. 429.—TOPOGRAPHY OF THORACIC CAVITY OF HORSE, RIGHT VIEW.

The ninth, fifteenth, and eighteenth ribs are retained. *a*, Pericardium; *b*, posterior vena cava; *c*, vena azygos; *c'*, œsophageal vein; *d*, *e*, anterior vena cava; *f*, brachial vein; *g*, inferior cervical vein; *h*, jugular vein; *i*, vertebral vein; *k*, superior cervical vein; *l*, dorsal vein; *m*, trachea; *n*, root of right lung; *o*, œsophagus; *p*, mediastinal lobe of right lung; *q*, mediastinum; *r*, bronchial lymph glands; *s*, mediastinal lymph glands; *t*, costal part of diaphragm; *t'*, tendinous center of same; *u*, intercostal muscle; *v*, longus colli; *w*, posterior deep pectoral muscle; *w'*, anterior deep pectoral muscle; *x*, superficial pectoral muscle; *y*, sterno-cephalicus; *z*, scalenus; *1*, *5*, right brachial artery; *2*, dorso-cervical trunk; *2'*, superior or deep cervical artery; *3*, dorsal artery (cut); *3'*, subcostal artery; *4*, internal thoracic artery; *6*, external thoracic artery; *7*, inferior cervical artery; *8*, bicarotid trunk; *10*, aorta; *11*, œsophageal artery; *12*, thoracic duct; *13*, right phrenic nerve; *14*, brachial plexus; *15*, right vagus; *15'*, *15''*, œsophageal continuations of vagi; *16*, right recurrent nerve; *17*, cervical trunk of sympathetic; *18*, thoracic trunk of sympathetic; *20*, inferior cervical ganglion; *21*, first thoracic ganglion of sympathetic; *22*, right cardiac nerve; *23*, longissimus; *24*, transversalis costarum; *25*, spinalis; *26*, multifidus; *27*, ligamentum nuchæ. (After Ellenberger-Baum, Top. Anat. d. Pferdes.)

the second intercostal space, passes across the transversalis costarum and longissimus toward the withers, and divides into several diverging branches. An anterior branch passes upward and forward between the splenius and complexus and anastomoses with branches of the superior cervical artery; the others are directed upward under the serratus magnus and rhomboideus to the withers, supplying the muscles and skin of this region.

The left dorsal artery sometimes arises with the superior cervical by a common trunk. On the right side there may be a common stem for the dorsal, superior cervical, and vertebral arteries. Occasionally the artery arises from the anterior aorta. Sometimes it emerges through the third space. The subcostal may arise independently behind the dorsal or from the superior cervical artery.

2. The superior or **deep cervical artery** (A. cervicalis profunda) arises in front of the dorsal or by a common trunk with it. It crosses the œsophgaus (left side), the trachea (right side), and the longus colli, and emerges from the thoracic cavity by passing through the space behind the first costo-transverse articulation. In the thorax it gives off a small branch (A. mediastini cranialis) to the mediastinum and the pericardium; also the first intercostal artery (A. intercostalis prima), a very small vessel which passes down in the first intercostal space. After leaving the thorax the artery passes upward and forward on the spinalis muscle and the lamellar part of the ligamentum nuchæ, covered by the complexus. Its terminal branches anastomose with branches of the occipital and vertebral arteries in the region of the axis. Numerous collateral branches are detached to the extensor muscles of the head and neck, the ligamentum nuchæ, and the skin, and anastomoses occur with the dorsal artery above and the vertebral artery below.

The artery sometimes emerges through the second intercostal space.

3. The **vertebral artery** (A. vertebralis) arises from the brachial (or brachiocephalic) opposite the first intercostal space and passes upward and forward. On the left side it crosses the œsophagus, on the right the trachea. Emerging from the thorax it passes between the longus colli internally and the scalenus externally, under the transverse process of the seventh cervical vertebra, and continues along

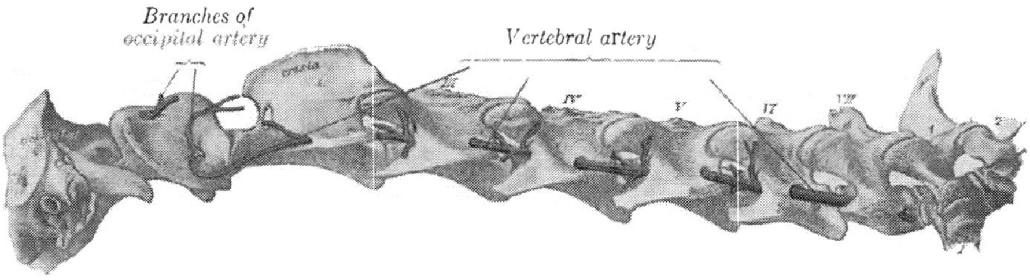

FIG. 430.—VERTEBRAL ARTERY OF HORSE. (After Schmaltz, Atlas d. Anat. d. Pferdes.)

the neck through the series of foramina transversaria, between which it is covered by the intertransversales colli. Emerging from the foramen of the axis, it crosses the capsule of the atlanto-axial joint, and joins the retrograde branch of the occipital artery under cover of the great oblique muscle of the head. At each intervertebral foramen a **spinal branch** (Ramus spinalis) is given off which enters the vertebral canal and reinforces the ventral spinal artery. It also gives off series of dorsal and ventral **muscular branches** (Rami musculares). The dorsal branches are the larger; they supply the deep extensor muscles of the head and neck, and anastomose with the deep cervical and occipital arteries. The ventral branches supply chiefly the scalenus, longus colli, intertransversales, and rectus capitis anterior major. The artery is accompanied by the vertebral vein and a sympathetic nerve trunk.

In some cases the last cervical transverse process has a foramen transversarium, through which the artery passes.

4. The **internal thoracic artery** (A. thoracica s. mammaria interna) is a large vessel which arises from the ventral side of the brachial opposite the first rib. It curves downward and backward, being at first on the inner surface of the rib, and then crosses the lower part of the first intercostal space and passes under the transversus thoracis muscle. It runs backward under cover of that muscle over the chondro-sternal joints to the eighth costal cartilage, where it divides into asternal and anterior abdominal branches. At each intercostal space two collateral

branches are detached. The **intercostal branches** (Rami intercostales) pass upward in the intercostal spaces and anastomose with homonymous descending arteries. The lower branches detach small twigs to the transversus thoracis, pleura, and pericardium, and pass out between the costal cartilages as **perforating branches** (Rami perforantes) to supply the pectoral muscles and skin, anastomosing with the external thoracic artery. A very small pericardiaco-phrenic artery ascends in the mediastinum on the left side, in the caval fold of pleura on the right side; it supplies fine twigs to the pericardium and pleura and accompanies the phrenic nerve to the diaphragm. In the young subject it gives small branches (Aa. thymicæ) to the thymus gland. The **asternal artery** (A. musculophrenica) passes along the ninth costal cartilage and continues along the costal attachment of the transversus abdominis (Fig. 185). It gives off intercostal branches which anastomose with those descending from the thoracic aorta, and twigs to the diaphragm and transversus abdominis. The **anterior abdominal artery** (A. epigastrica cranialis) is the direct continuation of the internal thoracic. It passes between the ninth costal cartilage and the xiphoid cartilage, runs backward on the abdominal surface of the rectus abdominis and then becomes embedded in it (Fig. 466). It supplies the ventral wall of the abdomen and anastomoses with the posterior abdominal artery.

5. The **external thoracic artery** (A. thoracica externa) is given off from the ventral aspect of the brachial, usually at the inner surface or anterior border of the first rib. It turns around the first rib below or behind the brachial vein (when given off within the thorax) and passes backward under the deep pectoral muscle; it is continued as a small vessel in the panniculus carnosus, where it accompanies the external thoracic ("spur") vein. It sends branches to the pectoral muscles and the axillary lymph glands.

This artery varies in origin and size. Not rarely it arises from the internal thoracic or from the brachial outside of the thorax. In other cases it arises by a common trunk with the inferior cervical. It may be very small or even absent, in which case the perforating branches of the internal thoracic compensate.

6. The **inferior cervical artery** (Truncus omo-cervicalis) arises usually from the dorsal surface of the brachial opposite the first rib or where that vessel winds around the rib. It is directed downward and a little forward across the external surface of the jugular vein and the deep face of the scalenus among the lymph glands at the thoracic inlet, and divides into ascending and descending branches. The **ascending branch** (A. cervicalis ascendens) passes upward and forward along the external surface of the jugular vein, then turns sharply backward and runs upward along the anterior border of the anterior deep pectoral muscle, between the omo-hyoideus and mastoido-humeralis and in relation to the prescapular lymph-glands; it gives branches to these muscles and the prepectoral and prescapular lymph glands. The **descending branch** (A. transversa scapulæ) passes downward and outward across the surface of the anterior deep pectoral and then runs in the groove between that muscle and the mastoido-humeralis in company with the cephalic vein. It supplies branches to these muscles and the skin of the breast.

THE COMMON CAROTID ARTERY

These two vessels (Arteriæ carotides communes) arise from the brachio cephalic artery by a common trunk. This stem, the **truncus bicaroticus** or **cephalic artery**, is detached from the inner face of the brachiocephalic opposite the first rib and passes forward in the median plane beneath the trachea. It is related ventrally to the prepectoral lymph glands, the terminal parts of the jugular veins, and the anterior vena cava, and laterally to the vagus and recurrent nerves. It is commonly two or three inches (ca. 5 to 7 cm.) in length, but it may vary between one and eight inches (ca. 2.5 to 20 cm.).

The **right common carotid** artery passes obliquely from the ventral face of the trachea to its right side. In this position it runs upward and forward and divides at the crico-pharyngeus muscle and under the submaxillary gland into external carotid, internal carotid, and occipital arteries. It is inclosed in a fibrous sheath, and is accompanied dorsally by the vagus and sympathetic

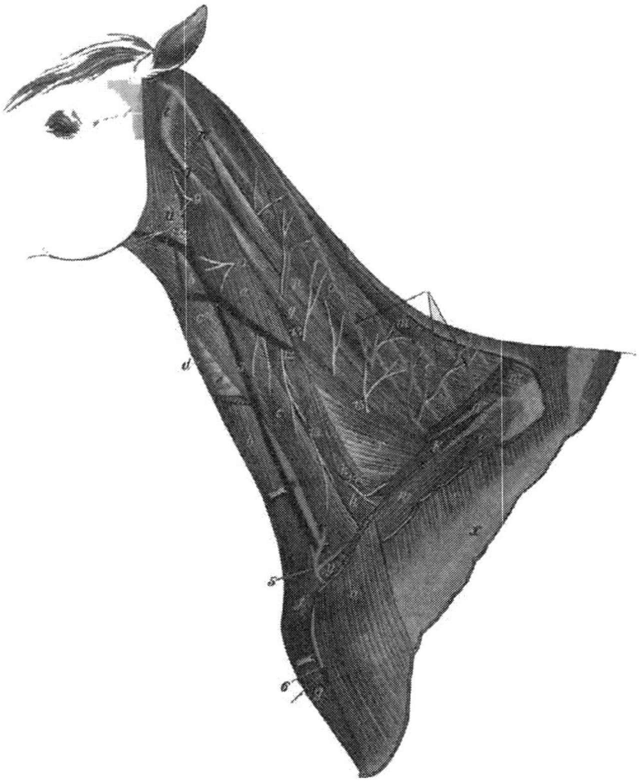

FIG. 431.—VESSELS AND NERVES OF NECK OF HORSE.

a, Mastoido-humeralis; *b*, sterno-cephalicus; *c*, omo-hyoideus; *d*, sterno-thyro-hyoideus; *e*, trachea; *f*, position of cariniform cartilage; *g*, anterior superficial pectoral muscle; *h*, scalenus; *i*, intertransversales; k, insertion of serratus cervicis; *l*, origin of trapezius; *m*, rhomboideus; *n*, splenius; *o*, complexus; *p*, q, trachelo-mastoideus; *p'*, *q'*, tendons of same; *r*, longissimus; *s*, obliquus capitis posterior; *t*, wing of atlas; *u*, parotid gland; *v*, supraspinatus; *w*, anterior deep pectoral; *x*, spine of scapula; *y*, prescapular lymph glands; *1*, external maxillary vein; *2*, *3*, jugular vein; *4*, carotid artery, exposed by drawing jugular vein aside; *5*, *6*, ascending and descending branches of inferior cervical artery; *7*, cephalic vein; *8*, branches of superior or deep cervical artery; *9–14*, ventral branches of second to seventh cervical nerves; *15*, branches of dorsal divisions of cervical nerves. (Ellenberger-Baum, Top. Anat. d. Pferdes.)

nerves, ventrally by the recurrent nerve. At the last two cervical vertebræ it is in contact superficially with the jugular vein, but further forward the omo-hyoideus muscle intervenes between the artery and vein. Near its termination the artery becomes more deeply placed and is related externally to the submaxillary and parotid glands, internally to the œsophagus. In some cases it is in contact ventrally with the thyroid gland, especially when the latter is larger than usual.

The left **common carotid artery** differs from the right one in that it is related deeply to the œsophagus, which separates it from the trachea in the greater part of its course.

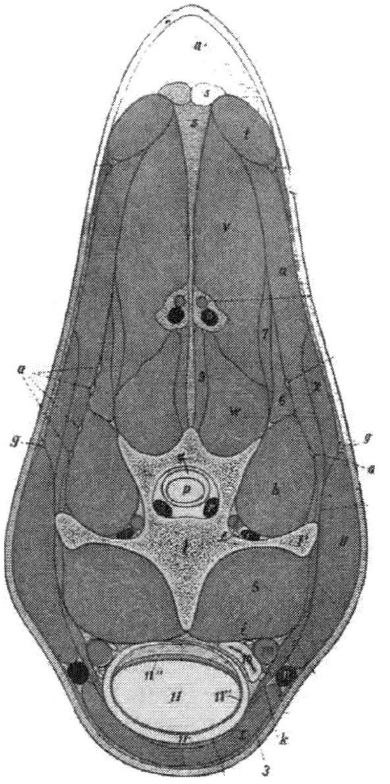

Fig. 432.—Cross-section of Neck of Horse, Passing through Fifth Cervical Vertebra; Anterior View.

a, Branches of cervical nerves; *a′*, nuchal fat; *b*, intertransversalis muscle; *c*, longissimus muscle; *d*, vertebral artery; *e*, vertebral vein; *f*, vertebral nerve; *g*, spinal accessory nerve (upper division); *h*, recurrent nerve; *i*, vago-sympathetic trunk; *k*, tracheal lymph duct; *l*, body of fifth cervical vertebra; *l′*, transverse process of same; *m*, carotid artery; *n*, jugular vein; *o*, superior cervical artery; *o′*, satellite vein of *o*; *p*, spinal cord; *q*, dura mater; *r*, spinal vein; *s*, ligamentum nuchæ; *t*, rhomboideus muscle; *u*, splenius; *v*, complexus; *w*, multifidus; *x*, serratus cervicis; *y*, mastoido-humeralis; *z*, sterno-cephalicus; *1*, rectus capitis ant. major; *2*, omo-hyoideus; *3*, panniculus; *4*, sterno-thyro-hyoideus; *5*, longus colli; *6*, *7*, trachelo-mastoideus; *8*, trapezius; *9*, spinalis; *10*, œsophagus; *11*, trachea, with cartilaginous ring (*11′*), mucous membrane (*11″*), and muscular layer (*11‴*). (After Ellenberger, in Leisering's Atlas.)

The collateral branches of the common carotids are in the main small. They comprise:

1. **Muscular branches** (Rami musculares) of variable size, which go to the ventral muscles of the neck and the skin.

2. **Œsophageal** and **tracheal branches** (Rami œsophagei et tracheales). Small twigs go to the cervical lymph glands also.

3. The **parotid artery**. This comes off near the termination and enters the ventral part of the parotid gland. It also supplies the subparotid lymph glands, and sometimes sends a branch to the submaxillary gland. It is inconstant.

4. The **thyro-laryngeal artery** (A. thyreoidea cranialis). This, the largest collateral branch of the carotid, arises from the latter two or three inches before it divides. It curves over the anterior end of the thyroid gland, into which it sends several branches. It gives off a **laryngeal branch** (A. laryngea), which sends twigs to the external muscles of the larynx and the constrictors of the pharynx, passes between the cricoid and thyroid cartilages, and supplies the internal muscles and the mucous membrane of the larynx. A small **pharyngeal branch** (A. pharyngea ascendens) runs upward and forward to the crico-pharyngeus, and supplies twigs to the posterior part of the pharynx and the origin of the œsophagus. Small innominate twigs are given off to the trachea, the œsophagus, and the sterno-thyro-hyoideus and omohyoideus muscles.

In some cases the thyroid and laryngeal arteries arise from the carotid separately or by a short common stem. A laryngeal branch is often detached from the carotid in front of the thyro-laryngeal and enters the larynx with the superior laryngeal nerve. The pharyngeal branch frequently comes directly from the carotid.

5. The **accessory thyroid artery** (A. thyreoidea caudalis) is an inconstant vessel which arises from the carotid at a variable distance behind the thyro-laryngeal—sometimes from the latter or from the parotid artery. It sends branches into the posterior part of the thyroid gland and detaches small tracheal and muscular twigs. In some cases it is distributed chiefly or entirely to the adjacent muscles.

THE OCCIPITAL ARTERY

The occipital artery (A. occipitalis) is the second in size of the terminals of the carotid. It arises usually just in front of the internal carotid, but in some cases

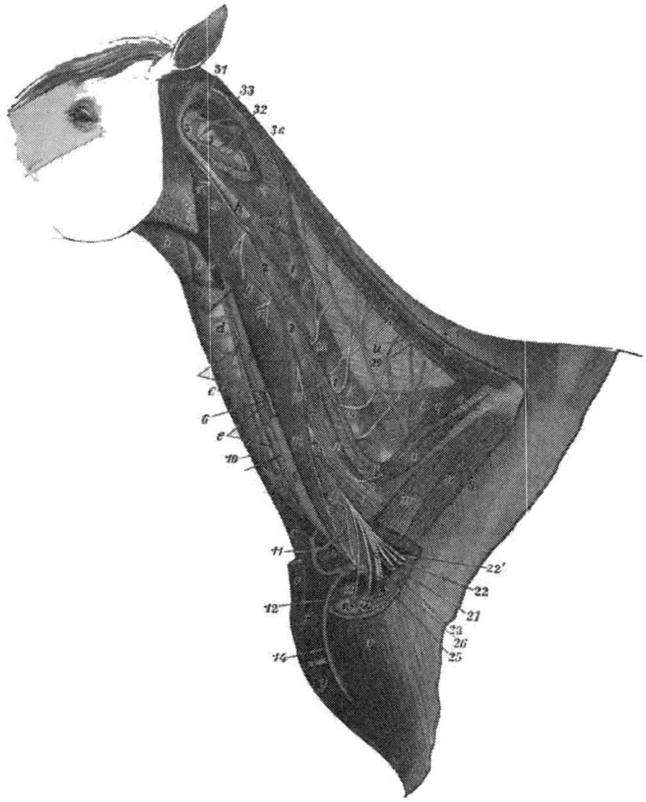

FIG. 433.—DEEP DISSECTION OF NECK OF HORSE.

a, a, Ends of sterno-cephalicus; *b,* anterior part of omo-hyoideus; *c,* sterno-thyro-hyoideus; *d,* trachea; *e,* œsophagus; *f,* cariniform cartilage; *g,* rectus cap. ant. major; *h,* stump of trachelo-mastoideus; *i,* intertransversales; *k,* multifidus; l, *m,* scalenus; *n,* serratus cervicis; *o, o,* stumps of splenius, *p,* longissimus, *q,* complexus (most of which is removed); *r,* rhomboideus; *s,* trapezius; *t,* spinalis et semispinalis; *u,* lamellar part of lig. nuchæ; *v,* mastoido-humeralis; *w,* anterior deep pectoral; *x,* supraspinatus; *y,* anterior superficial pectoral; *z,* scapular tuberosity; *1, 1,* articular processes of cervical vertebræ; *2, 2,* transverse processes of same; *3,* atlas; *3',* axis; *4, 4,* jugular vein (remainder removed); *5,* common carotid artery, from which a piece is removed to show the accompanying nerves; *6,* vago-sympathetic trunk; *7, 7,* tracheal and muscular branches of carotid artery; *8,* recurrent nerve; *10,* left tracheal lymph-duct; *11, 12,* ascending and descending branches of inferior cervical artery (*13*); *14,* cephalic vein; *15–20,* ventral branches of second to seventh cervical nerves; *21,* roots of phrenic nerve; *22,* thoracic or pectoral nerves; *22',* nerve to serratus magnus; *23,* musculo-cutaneous nerve; *24,* median nerve; *25,* ulnar nerve; *26,* radial nerve; *27,* axillary nerve; *28,* dorsal branches of cervical nerves; *28',* accessory nerve (cut); *29,* superior or deep cervical artery; *30,* muscular branch of vertebral artery; *31,* posterior (anastomotic) branch of occipital artery; *32,* vertebral artery; *33,* muscular branches of occipital artery; *34,* obliquus capitis post.; *35,* obl. cap. ant.; *36,* twig from dorsal branch of third cervical nerve. (After Ellenberger-Baum, Top. Anat. des Pferdes.)

with that artery by a common trunk of variable length. It pursues a somewhat flexuous course to the fossa atlantis, where it divides into anterior and posterior branches. It is related superficially to the submaxillary gland and the mastoido-humeralis, and deeply to the guttural pouch and the rectus capitis anterior major.[1] The internal carotid artery, the inferior cerebral vein, and the accessory, vagus, and sympathetic nerves cross its deep face. It gives twigs to the sub maxillary gland, the anterior straight muscles, the guttural pouch and the adjacent lymph glands, and two named collateral branches. The condyloid or **prevertebral artery** (A. condyloidea) is a small vessel which passes upward and forward on the guttural pouch, and divides into muscular and meningeal branches. The latter enter the cranium through the foramen lacerum and hypoglossal foramen and are distributed to the dura mater. This artery is very variable in its origin. The posterior **meningeal** or **mastoid artery** (A. meningea caudalis) is a much larger vessel which runs upward and forward between the small oblique muscle and the paramastoid process, passes through the mastoid foramen into the parieto-temporal canal, enters the cranial cavity, and is distributed to the dura mater.

The posterior or **retrograde branch** (Ramus descendens) of the occipital passes up through the foramen transversarium of the atlas and joins the vertebral artery. It gives branches to the great oblique muscle of the head, which covers it.

The **anterior** or **occipital branch** (Ramus occipitalis) passes through the alar (antero-external) foramen of the atlas and supplies the muscles and skin of the poll, anastomosing with the deep cervical artery and its fellow of the opposite side. In the alar furrow it gives off the cerebro**spinal artery,** which enters the spinal canal through the intervertebral (antero-internal) foramen of the atlas, perforates the dura mater, and divides into cerebral and spinal branches. The **cerebral branch** unites with that of the opposite side to form the **basilar**

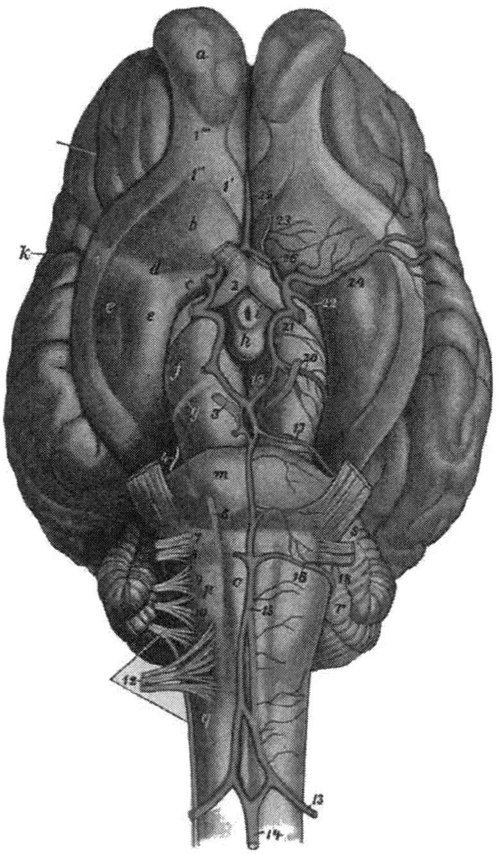

FIG. 434.—VESSELS AND NERVES OF BASE OF BRAIN OF HORSE.

13, Cerebro-spinal artery; *14*, middle spinal artery; *15*, basilar artery; *16*, posterior cerebellar artery; *17*, anterior cerebellar artery; *18*, internal auditory artery; *19*, posterior cerebral artery; *20*, deep cerebral artery; *21*, stump of internal carotid artery; *22*, anterior choroid artery; *23*, anterior meningeal artery; *24*, middle cerebral artery; *25*, artery of corpus callosum; *26*, anterior communicating artery; *1*, *1'*, *1''*, olfactory tracts; *1'''*, olfactory peduncle; *2-12*, cranial nerves; *a*, olfactory bulb; *b*, trigonum olfactorium; *c*, lamina perforata anterior; *d*, fossa transversa; *e*, pyriform lobe; *f*, cerebral peduncle; *g*, tractus transversus; *h*, corpus mammillare; *i*, tuber cinereum; *k*, lateral fissure (of Sylvius); *l*, presylvian fissure; *m*, pons; *o*, pyramid; p, facial eminence; *q*, corpus restiforme; r, cerebellum; *s*, middle peduncle of cerebellum. (After Ellenberger Baum, Top. Anat. d. Pferdes.)

[1] The relation to the guttural pouch is not constant. In some cases—especially when the head and neck are extended—the artery lies behind the pouch. The backward extension of the latter is variable.

artery, and the **spinal branch** similarly forms by union with its fellow the **middle spinal artery.**

The **basilar artery** (A. basilaris cerebri) passes forward in the median groove on the ventral surface of the medulla and pons and divides into the two posterior cerebral arteries. The collateral branches of the basilar are:

1. Medullary branches (Rami medullares), ten or twelve in number, distributed to the medulla oblongata.

2. Posterior cerebellar arteries (Aa. cerebelli caudales) which pass outward around the medulla behind the pons to the cerebellum, to which they are distributed after giving twigs to the medulla and pons.

3. The small auditory artery (A. auditiva interna) accompanies the eighth nerve to the internal ear. It often arises from the posterior cerebellar.

4. Anterior cerebellar arteries (Aa. cerebelli nasales). These are very variable in number and origin. There are often two or three on either side and they frequently arise from the posterior cerebrals. They pass outward in front of the pons and supply the anterior part of the cerebellum.

The **posterior cerebral arteries** (Aa. communicantes caudales) diverge at an acute angle and join the posterior communicating branches of the internal carotid arteries on the inferior surface of the cerebral peduncles. They are connected by a transverse branch and by a network of fine twigs which form often a rete mirabile.

THE INTERNAL CAROTID ARTERY (Figs. 434, 436, 437)

This artery (A. carotis interna) is somewhat smaller than the occipital. It usually arises just behind that artery, crosses its deep face, and runs upward and forward on the guttural pouch to the foramen lacerum. It is closely related to the vagus nerve and the superior cervical ganglion of the sympathetic nerve, fibers from which accompany it. It is crossed externally by the ninth and twelfth cranial nerves and the pharyngeal branch of the vagus. It passes through the inferior petrosal sinus and enters the cavernous sinus, within which it forms an S-shaped curve. It is connected with the opposite artery by a transverse branch (A. intercarotica), which lies behind the pituitary body in the intercavernous sinus. A branch (A. caroticobasilaris) sometimes connects it with the basilar artery. It then perforates the dura mater, gives off the posterior communicating branch, and passes forward and divides at the side of the optic chiasma into anterior and middle cerebral arteries.

The **posterior communicating artery** (A. communicans posterior) turns backward and joins the posterior cerebral. It gives off the **deep cerebral artery** (A. cerebri profunda) which winds around the cerebral peduncle and is distributed chiefly to the mid-brain. A smaller collateral branch is the anterior choroid artery (A. chorioidea nasalis) which passes along the optic tract and is distributed in the choroid plexus of the lateral ventricle.

The **anterior cerebral artery** (A. cerebri anterior) unites with the corresponding branch of the opposite artery above the optic chiasma. From this junction proceeds the **artery of the corpus callosum** (A. corporis callosi), which turns around the genu of the corpus callosum, enters the great longitudinal fissure, divides into two branches, and is distributed to the inner aspect of the cerebral hemispheres. A small anterior meningeal branch (A. meningea nasalis) of the anterior cerebral is distributed to the anterior part of the dura, and assists in forming a network in the ethmoidal fossa (Rete ethmoidale), anastomosing with the ethmoidal branch of the ophthalmic artery.

The **middle cerebral artery** (A. cerebri media) passes outward in the lateral fissure (of Sylvius) and divides into branches on the outer surface of the hemisphere.

The **arterial circle of Willis** (Circulus arteriosus) (Fig. 434) is formed at the interpeduncular space of the base of the brain by the union of the anterior cerebral arteries in front, by the diverging posterior cerebral arteries behind, and is completed laterally by the junction of the latter with the posterior communicating arteries and by the internal carotid. It is irregularly polygonal in outline.

The cerebral arteries are very variable in arrangement, and the foregoing account is a brief statement of the more usual disposition of the larger vessels. The internal carotid artery often arises with the occipital by a common trunk of variable length.

THE EXTERNAL CAROTID ARTERY (Figs. 436, 437)

This artery (A. carotis externa) by its size and direction constitutes the continuation of the common carotid. It passes forward on the lateral wall of the pharynx at the lower border of the guttural pouch, covered by the submaxillary gland and the stylo-maxillaris, digastricus, and stylo-hyoideus muscles. It then emerges between the stylo-hyoideus and the great cornu of the hyoid bone, passes upward on the latter parallel with the posterior border of the lower jaw, and terminates about two inches (ca. 5 cm.) below the temporo-maxillary articulation by dividing into superficial temporal and internal maxillary branches. It is crossed deeply near its origin by the superior laryngeal and pharyngeal branches of the vagus nerve. Just before its emergence its superficial face is crossed by the hypoglossal nerve, and the glosso-pharyngeal nerve passes over its inner surface at the ventral border of the great cornu. The chief collateral branches are the masseteric, external maxillary, and posterior auricular. It also furnishes variable branches to the submaxillary and parotid glands, the guttural pouch, and the pharyngeal lymph glands, as well as twigs to some adjacent muscles.

1. The **inferior masseteric** or maxillo-muscular artery (A. masseterica inferior) is given off from the external carotid at its emergence from beneath the stylo-hyoideus. It passes downward and slightly forward under cover of the parotid gland and over the tendon of insertion of the sterno-cephalicus to the posterior border of the mandible and appears on the masseter muscle, into which it plunges after a short course on its surface. It gives branches also to the internal pterygoid and stylo-maxillaris muscles and the parotid gland.

2. The **external maxillary, facial,** or **submaxillary artery** (A. maxillaris externa)[1] arises from the external carotid on the inner surface of the posterior belly of the digastricus (Fig. 436). It runs downward and forward on the lateral wall of the pharynx across the deep face of the stylo-hyoideus toward the great cornu of the hyoid bone, accompanied by the glosso-pharyngeal nerve in front and the hypoglossal nerve behind. After giving off the lingual artery at the posterior border of the great cornu, it inclines more ventrally on the inner surface of the internal pterygoid muscle, crosses over the hyo-glossus muscle, the hypoglossal nerve, the submaxillary duct, and the intermediate tendon of the digastricus, and turns forward in the submaxillary space. Here it lies on the lower part of the internal pterygoid muscle, and is related internally to the submaxillary lymph glands, above to the anterior belly of the digastricus, and below to the homonymous vein. At the anterior border of the masseter it turns around the lower border of the jaw and runs upward on the face in front of that muscle.[2] At the turn the artery is in front, the vein in the middle, and the parotid duct posterior. The artery and vein pass upward along the anterior border of the masseter, under cover of the facial panniculus and the zygomaticus, and are crossed superficially by branches

[1] By some authors the term facial is applied to the artery only after it turns around the lower border of the jaw.

[2] The artery is conveniently placed at its inflection for taking the pulse, since it is superficial and lies directly on the bone.

of the facial nerve and deeply by the parotid duct. The artery terminates over the levtaor labii superioris proprius by dividing into the dorsal nasal and the angular artery of the eye. The chief branches of the external maxillary are as follows:

(1) The pharyngeal artery (A. palatina ascendens) arises usually behind the stylo-pharyngeus, passes between that muscle and the great cornu, and runs forward on the lateral wall of the pharynx under the elastic pharyngeal fascia. It is distributed to the soft palate, pharynx, and tonsil.

(2) The lingual artery (A. lingualis) is a large branch which diverges from the parent trunk at an acute angle, runs along the ventral border of the great cornu of the hyoid bone, and dips under the hyo-glossus muscle. It then passes across

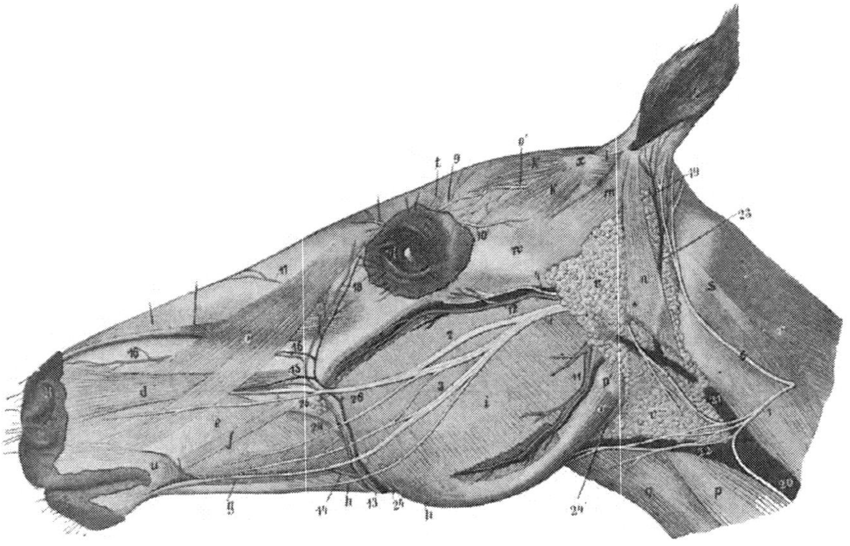

FIG. 435.—SUPERFICIAL DISSECTION OF HEAD OF HORSE. MOST OF THE PANNICULUS IS REMOVED.

a, Dilatator naris superior; *b*, levator labii superioris proprius; *c*, levator naso-labialis; d, dilatator naris lateralis; *e*, buccinator; *f*, zygomaticus; *g*, depressor labii inferioris; *h*, stump of retractor anguli oris; *i*, masseter; *k*, *k*, scutularis; *l*, scutulo-auriculares superficiales; *m*, zygomatico-auricularis; *n*, parotido-auricularis; *o*, stylo-maxillaris; *p*, sterno-cephalicus; *p′*, tendon of *p*; *q*, omo-hyoideus; *r*, splenius; *s*, tendon of splenius and trachelo-mastoideus; *t*, corrugator supercilii; *u*, orbicularis oris; *v*, parotid gland; *w*, zygomatic arch; *x*, scutiform cartilage; *y*, upper commissure of nostril; *1*, facial nerve; *2*, superior buccal nerve; *3*, inferior buccal nerve; *4*, transverse facial nerve; *5*, cervical branch of facial nerve; *6*, posterior auricular branch of second cervical nerve; *7*, cutaneous cervical branch of same; *8*, infratrochlear nerve; *9*, frontal nerve; *10*, lacrimal nerve; *10′*, end of auriculo-palpebral nerve; *11*, inferior masseteric artery and vein; *12*, transverse facial artery and vein; *13*, facial artery; *14*, inferior labial artery; *15*, superior labial artery; *16*, lateral nasal artery; *17*, dorsal nasal artery; *18*, angular artery of the eye; *19*, posterior auricular artery; *20*, *21*, jugular vein; *22*, external maxillary vein; *23*, great auricular vein; *24*, parotid duct; *24′*, origin of same. (After Ellenberger-Baum, Top. Anat. d. Pferdes.)

the kerato-hyoideus, turns inward under the intercornual joint of the hyoid bone, and runs forward in the tongue between the hyo-glossus and genio-glossus. This part (A. profunda linguæ) is flexuous and is accompanied by branches of the hypoglossal and lingual nerves. It is the chief artery of the tongue, and anastomoses with the opposite artery and the sublingual.

(3) The sublingual artery (A. sublingualis) is a smaller vessel which arises at the anterior extremity of the submaxillary gland (Fig. 436). It passes forward on the anterior belly of the digastricus between the ramus of the mandible and the mylohyoideus, perforates the latter, runs along the lower border of the sublingual gland, and ramifies in the mucous membrane of the anterior part of the floor of the mouth.

It detaches branches to the muscles and skin in the submaxillary space, the submaxillary lymph glands, and the sublingual gland. It also gives off the small **submental artery,** which runs forward superficially toward the lower lip, supplying twigs to the skin and the mylo-hyoideus.

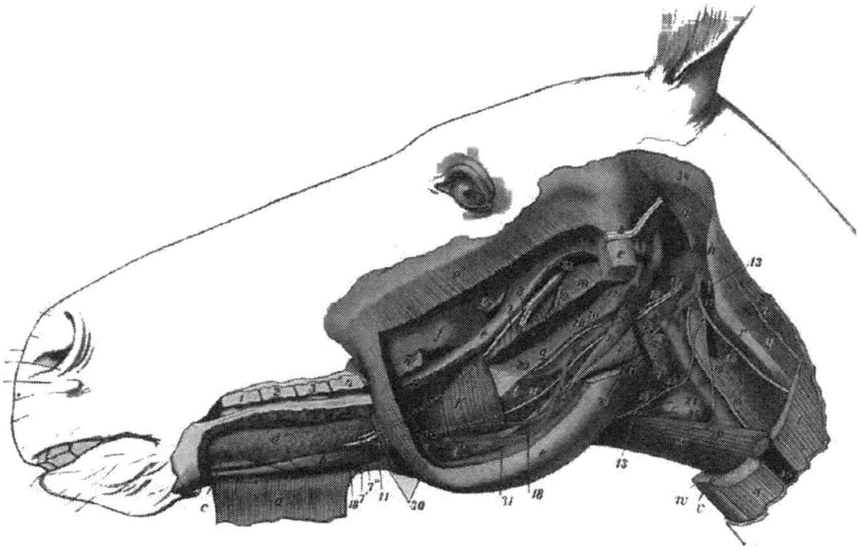

FIG. 436.—PAROTID, MASSETERIC, AND LINGUAL REGIONS OF HORSE: DEEP DISSECTION, THIRD LAYER.

a, Mylo-hyoideus, anterior part, reflected; *b*, genio-hyoideus; *c*, genio-glossus; *d*, sublingual gland; *e*, ramus of mandible, the greater part of which is removed; *e'*, stump of masseter; *f*, maxillary tuberosity; *g*, great cornu of hyoid bone; *h*, wing of atlas; *i*, intermediate tendon of digastricus; *i'*, anterior belly, *i''*, posterior belly of digastricus; k, posterior part of mylo-hyoideus; *l*, hyo-glossus; *m*, pterygoideus internus (cut); *n*, stylo-hyoideus; *o*, stylo-maxillaris (cut); *p*, crico-pharyngeus; q, obliquus capitis ant.; *r*, tendon of trachelo-mastoideus; *s*, rectus cap. ant. major; *t*, mastoido-humeralis (cut); *u*, sterno-cephalicus (cut); *v*, sterno-thyroideus (cut); *w*, sterno-hyoideus (cut); *x*, omo-hyoideus; *y*, obliquus cap. post.; *z*, splenius (cut); *1–4*, upper cheek teeth; *4'*, last cheek tooth; *5*, stump of facial nerve; *6*, stump of buccinator nerve; *7*, lingual nerve; *7'*, superficial branch, *7''*, deep branch of lingual nerve; *8*, stumps of inferior alveolar artery, vein and nerve; *9*, mylo-hyoid nerve (cut); *10*, glosso-pharyngeal nerve; *11*, hypoglossal nerve; *12*, superior laryngeal nerve; *13*, ventral branch of first cervical nerve; *14*, vagus and sympathetic; *15*, dorsal branch of spinal accessory nerve; *16*, ventral branch of same; *17*, inferior cerebral vein; *18*, submaxillary duct; *19*, common carotid artery; *20*, parotid branch; *21*, thyro-laryngeal artery; *22*, pharyngeal artery; *23*, laryngeal artery; *24*, internal carotid artery; *25*, occipital artery; *26*, external carotid artery; *27–31*, external maxillary artery; *28*, posterior palatine artery; *29*, lingual artery; *30*, sublingual artery; *32*, internal maxillary artery; *33*, internal maxillary vein (origin); *34*, remnant of parotid gland; *35*, thyroid gland; *36*, jugular vein; *37*, pharyngeal lymph glands. (After Ellenberger-Baum, Top. Anat. d. Pferdes.)

In some cases the sublingual artery arises from the lingual and the submental from the external maxillary. Sometimes the sublingual remains on the external face of the mylo-hyoideus —thus resembling the submental of man—and the sublingual gland is supplied by a special branch of the lingual.

Not uncommonly a considerable branch, given off in the submaxillary space, turns round the lower border of the jaw and enters the middle of the lower part of the masseter muscle. In some cases this artery is of large size and its pulsation can be felt. It is accompanied by a vein.

(4) The **inferior labial artery** (A. labialis inferior) arises from the facial a little before it reaches the depressor labii inferioris (Fig. 435). It passes forward, dips under the depressor muscle, and continues to the lower lip. It supplies branches to the muscles and skin in this region, to the inferior buccal glands, the mucous membrane of the cheek, and the lower lip, anastomosing with the mental artery and the corresponding vessels of the opposite side. It detaches a branch (A. anguli oris) to the angle of the mouth, which anastomoses with the superior labial.

(5) The **superior labial artery** (A. labialis superior) arises from the facial in front of the facial crest (Fig. 435). It passes forward under the dilatator naris lateralis and levator nasolabialis to the upper lip, gives twigs to the upper part of the cheek and the lateral nasal region, and ramifies in the upper lip, anastomosing with the opposite artery and the palato-labial.

(6) The **lateral nasal artery** (A. lateralis nasi) arises usually a little above the preceding one, and runs forward parallel with it and under the levator nasolabialis to the nostril (Fig. 435). It supplies branches to the lateral nasal region and the nostril.

The vessel is often double. It may arise from the superior labial at the point of bifurcation of the facial or with the dorsal nasal from the infraorbital artery (as in the ox). In some cases it gives off a dorsal nasal branch.

(7) The **dorsal nasal artery** (A. dorsalis nasi) arises on the levator labii superioris proprius and passes forward under the levator nasolabialis to the dorsum nasi (Fig. 435).

(8) The **angular artery of the eye** (A. angularis oculi) runs toward the internal canthus of the eye, where it anastomoses with the orbital branch (Ramus malaris) of the infraorbital artery (Fig. 435).

In addition to the preceding, unnamed branches are supplied to the submaxillary salivary gland and the submaxillary lymph glands.

3. The **posterior auricular artery** (A. auricularis posterior) arises at an acute angle from the external carotid just above the origin of the masseteric. It passes upward under cover of the parotid gland, to which it gives branches, and divides into several branches which supply the skin and muscles of the external ear (Fig. 435). The **posterior branch** passes to the posterior part of the base of the ear, where it divides into two branches; of these, one (Ramus intermedius) passes up the convex surface of the external ear to the apex, while the other (Ramus medialis) winds around to the anterior (inner) border, and forms an arch with the intermediate branch. The **external branch** (Ramus lateralis) passes up the posterior (external) border of the ear and forms an arch with the intermediate branch. The **deep branch** (A. auricularis profunda) enters the interval between the external auditory canal and mastoid process, and passes through an opening into the interior of the external ear and ramifies in the skin which lines it. It gives off the **stylomastoid artery**, which passes through the stylomastoid foramen into the tympanum, forms an arch around the membrana tympani, and supplies the middle ear and its muscles.

THE SUPERFICIAL TEMPORAL ARTERY

This artery (A. temporalis superficialis) is much the smaller of the two terminal branches of the external carotid. It passes upward behind the posterior border of the ramus of the mandible under cover of the parotid gland, and divides below the level of the condyle into the anterior auricular and transverse facial arteries. It is crossed superficially by the facial nerve.

The **anterior auricular artery** (A. auricularis anterior) passes upward behind the temporo-mandibular articulation under cover of the parotid gland, crosses the zygomatic arch, and reaches the temporalis muscle. It is crossed deeply at its origin by the superficial temporal nerve and is accompanied by a satellite vein and the auriculo-palpebral branch of the facial nerve. It is distributed to the skin and the temporal and anterior auricular muscles, and sends a branch through the conchal cartilage to the skin which lines it. Collateral twigs are detached to the parotid gland, and an anterior branch anastomoses with the supraorbital artery. A branch sometimes passes into the parieto-temporal canal and anastomoses with the posterior meningeal (mastoid) artery.

The **transverse facial artery** (A. transversa faciei) is larger than the preceding.

It turns around the neck below the condyle of the mandible and emerges from beneath the parotid gland (Fig. 435). It then passes forward a short distance on the masseter about half an inch below the zygomatic arch and plunges into the muscle, in which it commonly divides into two chief branches. It is accompanied by a vein and a branch of the superficial temporal nerve. It supplies the

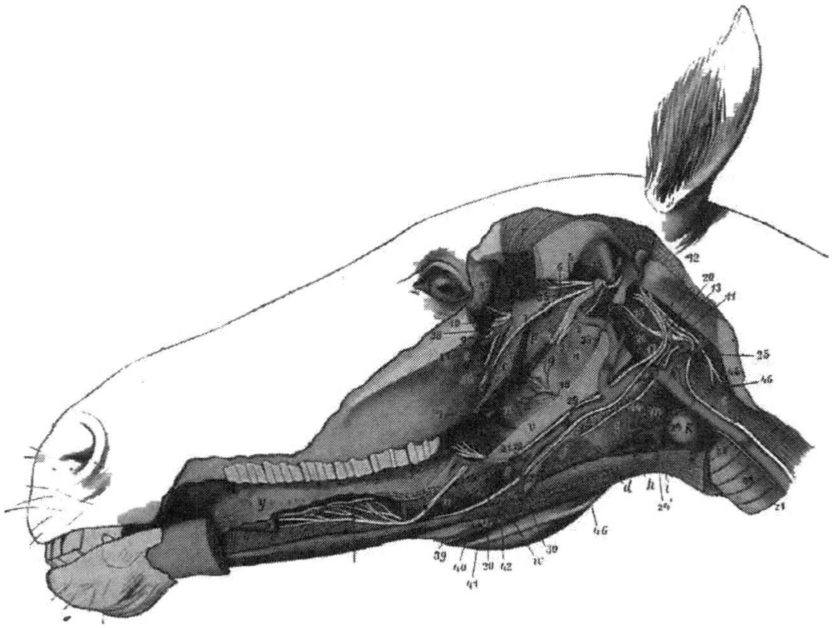

FIG. 437.—DEEP DISSECTION OF HEAD OF HORSE.

The left ramus of the mandible and structures connected with it have been removed. *a, a*, Stumps of styloglossus; *b*, genio-glossus; *c*, genio-hyoideus; *d*, omo-hyoideus; *e*, kerato-hyoideus; *f*, thyro-hyoideus; *g*, thyro-pharyngeus; *h*, crico-thyroideus; *i*, sterno-thyroideus; k, thyroid gland; *m*, crico-pharyngeus; *n*, palatinus and palato-pharyngeus; *o*, pterygoideus externus; *p*, tensor palati; q, levator palati; *r*, temporalis; *s*, rectus cap. ant. major; *t*, obliquus cap. ant.; *u*, guttural pouch; *v*, great cornu of hyoid bone, posterior extremity of which is removed and indicated by dotted line; *w*, position of small cornu, dotted line; *x*, thyroid cornu; *y*, tongue; *z*, anterior pillar of soft palate; *1*, superficial temporal nerve; *2*, chorda tympani; *3*, stump of inferior alveolar nerve; *4*. *4*, lingual nerve, intermediate part removed; *5*, deep temporal nerve; *6*, masseteric nerve; *7*, buccinator nerve; *8*, great palatine nerve; *9*, infraorbital nerve; *10*, sphenopalatine and posterior nasal nerves; *11*, spinal accessory nerve; *12*, vagus; *13*, pharyngeal branch of vagus; *14*, superior laryngeal nerve; *15*, vago-sympathetic trunk; *16*, sympathetic, with superior cervical ganglion a little further back; *17*, glosso-pharyngeal nerve; *18*, pharyngeal and *19*, lingual branches of glosso-pharyngeal; *20*, hypoglossal nerve; *21*, left recurrent nerve; *22*, common carotid artery; *23*, parotid branch; *24*, thyro-laryngeal artery; *24'*, laryngeal artery; *25*, occipital artery; *26*, internal carotid artery; *27*, external carotid artery; *28–30*, external maxillary artery; *29*, pharyngeal artery; *31*, lingual artery; *32*, internal maxillary artery; *33*, stump of inferior alveolar artery; *34*, middle meningeal artery; *35*, deep temporal artery; *36*, buccinator artery; *37*, palatine artery; *38*, end of internal maxillary artery; *39*, right external maxillary artery; *40*, satellite vein of *39*; *41*, right parotid duct; *42*, submaxillary lymph glands; *43*, pharyngeal lymph glands; *44*, trachea; *45*, wing of atlas; *46*, dotted line indicating outline of submaxillary gland; *47*, lacrimal gland. (After Ellenberger-Baum, Top. Anat. d. Pferdes.)

masseter and the skin of this region, and anastomoses with the external maxillary and posterior deep temporal arteries.

The pulse may usually be felt in this artery as it passes below the articulation of the jaw.

THE INTERNAL MAXILLARY ARTERY (Figs. 437, 438, 439)

This artery (A. maxillaris interna) is much the larger of the two terminal branches of the external carotid. It begins at the inner side of the posterior border of the mandible about two inches (ca. 5 cm.) below the articulation of the jaw and ends in the anterior part of the pterygo-palatine fossa. On account of its complex course and the large number of branches given off it is convenient to divide it into three parts.

The first **part** is much the longest, forms an S-shaped curve, and is in great part in contact with the guttural pouch. It passes upward and forward on the inner surface of the mandible a distance of about an inch (ca. 2 to 3 cm.) and is related here to the vein, which is ventral. It then turns inward below the external pterygoid muscle and the inferior maxillary nerve, passes between that muscle and the tensor palati, and runs forward to enter the alar (pterygoid) foramen. This part gives off the following branches:

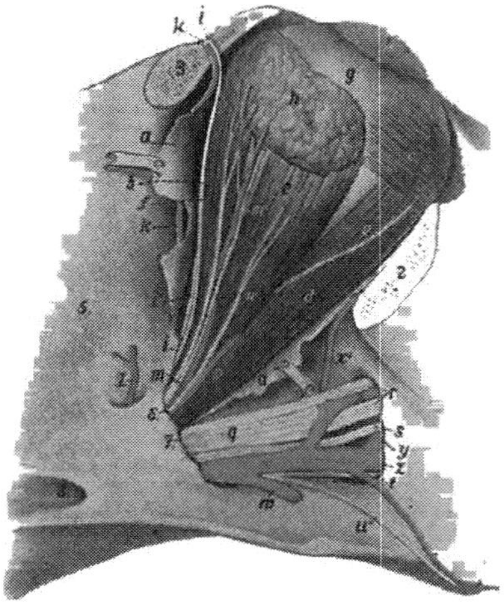

FIG. 438.—RIGHT EYE OF HORSE.

a, Remnants of periorbita; *b*, levator palpebræ superioris; *c*, obliquus oculi inferior; *d*, rectus oculi inferior; *e*, rectus oculi externus; *f*, rectus oculi superior; *g*, sclera; *g*.' cornea; *h*, lacrimal gland; *i*, frontal nerve; k, frontal artery; *l*, branch of lacrimal nerve to gland; *m*, lacrimal artery; *n*, zygomatic nerve; *o*, branch of ophthalmic artery; *p*, branch of oculomotor nerve to obliquus oculi inferior; *q*, maxillary nerve; *r*, infraorbital nerve; *s*, posterior nasal nerve; *t*, great palatine nerve; *u*, small palatine nerve; *v*, internal maxillary artery; *w*, buccinator artery (cut); *x*, infraorbital artery; *x'*, malar artery; *y*, sphenopalatine artery; *z*, great palatine artery; *z'*, small palatine (or staphyline) artery; *1*, posterior deep temporal artery; *2*, *3*, stumps of orbital margin; *4*, facial crest; *5*, temporal fossa; *6*, foramen lacerum orbitale; *7*, anterior end of alar canal; *8*, posterior opening of same. (After Ellenberger, in Leisering's Atlas.)

1. The **inferior alveolar** or **dental artery** (A. alveolaris mandibulæ s. inferior) passes downward and forward with the homonymous vein and nerve, being at first between the external and internal pterygoid muscles, then between the latter and the ramus of the mandible. It enters the mandibular foramen, passes downward and forward in the mandibular canal, and terminates at the mental foramen by dividing into mental and incisor branches. The **mental branch** (A. mentalis) emerges through the mental foramen and anastomoses in the lower lip with the opposite artery and the inferior labial. The **incisor branch** continues forward in the bone, supplies twigs to the canine and incisor teeth, and anastomoses with its fellow of the opposite side. Collateral branches are detached to the pterygoid and mylo-hyoid muscles, and within the bone to the teeth, alveolar periosteum, the gums, and the spongy substance of the mandible.

2. The **pterygoid arteries,** two or three in number, are distributed to the pterygoid and tensor and levator palati muscles.

3. The **tympanic artery** is a very small vessel which passes along the Eustachian tube to the petro-tympanic fissure (of Glaser) and enters the middle ear.

4. The **middle meningeal artery** (A. meningea media) arises beneath the buccinator nerve where the internal maxillary turns forward. It passes backward across the temporal wing of the sphenoid to the antero-external part (foramen spinosum) of the foramen lacerum. Entering the cranium, it divides into branches which course in the grooves on the temporal and parietal bones and supply the dura mater. It anastomoses with the posterior meningeal.

The size of this artery is variable, and is in inverse ratio to that of the posterior meningeal.

5. The **posterior deep temporal artery** (A. temporalis profunda aboralis)

arises from the internal maxillary just before the latter enters the canal of the pterygoid process. It passes upward and backward in the temporal fossa on the deep face of the temporalis muscle, in which it ramifies. It sends a branch outward to the masseter, and anastomoses with the superficial temporal and middle meningeal arteries.

In some cases the tympanic and middle meningeal arise from this artery.

The **second part** lies in the alar canal and is about an inch (ca. 2 to 3 cm.) in length. It gives off two branches—the anterior deep temporal and the ophthalmic.

1. The **anterior deep temporal artery** (A. temporalis profunda oralis) emerges from the canal through the temporal or small alar foramen, and passes upward in the anterior part of the temporal fossa on the deep face of the temporalis muscle,

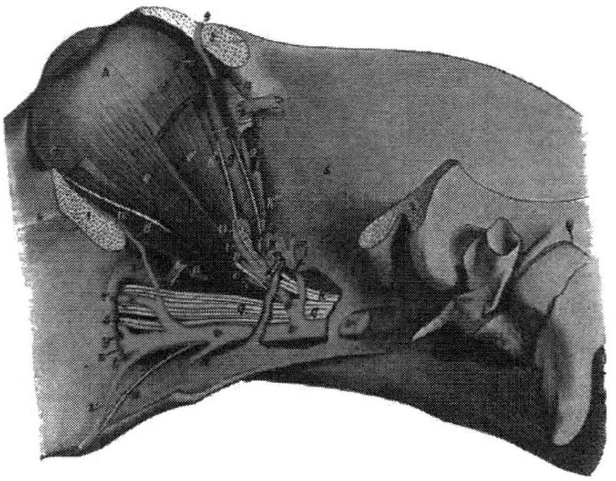

FIG. 439.—LEFT EYE OF HORSE, DEEPER DISSECTION.

The outer plate of bone has been removed behind the pterygoid crest to expose the vessels and nerves. *a, a*, Remnants of periorbita; *b*, stump of rectus oculi superior; *c*, obliquus oculi inferior; *d*, rectus oculi inferior; *e*, rectus oculi lateralis; *e'*, retractor oculi; *f*, rectus oculi internus; *g, g*, obliquus oculi superior; *h*, eyeball; *i*, trochlear nerve; *k*, ophthalmic nerve; *k'*, nasal nerve; *k''*, infratrochlear nerve; *k'''*, ethmoidal nerve; *l*, optic nerve; *m*, frontal nerve; *n*, lacrimal nerve; *o*, zygomatic nerve; *p*, nerve to obliquus inferior (from oculomotor); *q*, maxillary nerve; *r*, infraorbital nerve; *s*, sphenopalatine nerve; *t*, great palatine nerve; *u*, small palatine nerve; *v*, internal maxillary artery; *w*, buccinator artery (cut off); *x*, infraorbital artery; *x'*, malar artery; *y*, sphenopalatine artery; *z*, great palatine artery; *z'*, small palatine (or staphyline) artery; *1, 2*, stumps of zygomatic arch; *3*, stump of supraorbital process; *4*, facial crest; *5*, temporal fossa; *6*, ophthalmic artery; *7*, muscular branch of *6*; *8*, lacrimal artery (cut); *9*, frontal artery; *10*, anterior deep temporal artery; *11*, ethmoidal artery. (After Ellenberger-Baum, Top. Anat. d. Pferdes.)

in which it is chiefly distributed. It gives twigs to the orbital fat and the skin of the frontal region.

2. The **ophthalmic artery** (A. ophthalmica externa) emerges from the anterior opening of the alar canal, and enters the apex of the periorbita or ocular sheath. Within this it forms a semicircular bend under the rectus oculi superior and is continued by the ethmoidal artery. Its branches are as follows:

(*a*) The **supraorbital** or **frontal artery** (A. supraorbitalis)[1] is a small vessel which often arises from the anterior deep temporal or the internal maxillary. It passes along the inner wall of the orbit in company with the nerve of the same name to the supraorbital foramen, through which it emerges. It is distributed to the orbicularis oculi, the corrugator supercilii, and the skin of the supraorbital region.

(*b*) The **lacrimal artery** (A. lacrimalis) runs upward and forward within the

[1] This vessel appears to represent both the supraorbital and frontal of man.

periorbita along the outer edge of the levator palpebræ superioris to the lacrimal gland, in which it is chiefly distributed. It also sends twigs to the upper eyelid.

(*c*) **Muscular branches** (Rami musculares) supply the orbital muscles, the periorbita, the third eyelid, and the conjunctiva.

(*d*) **Ciliary branches** (Aa. ciliares), two sets of very slender arteries, arise from the ophthalmic direct and from the muscular branches. The anterior ciliary arteries (Aa. ciliaries anteriores) pierce the sclera in front of the equator and ramify chiefly in the ciliary body and the iris. The posterior ciliary arteries (Aa. ciliares posteriores) pierce the posterior part of the sclera; most of them ramify in the choroid coat as the short ciliary arteries, but two of larger size, the long ciliary

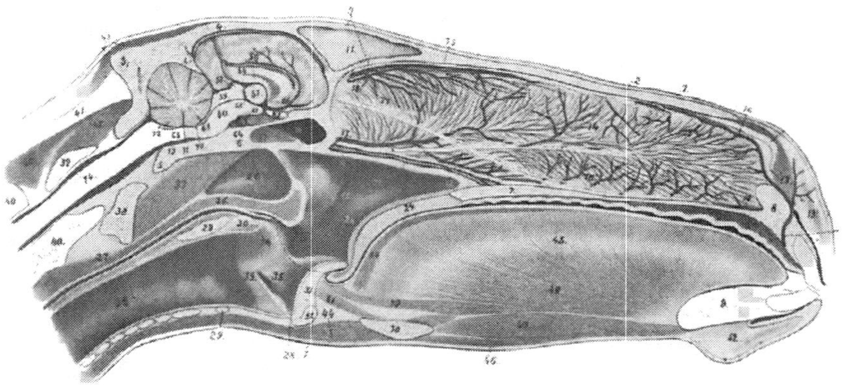

FIG. 440.—SAGITTAL SECTION OF HEAD OF HORSE, CUT A LITTLE TO THE RIGHT OF THE MEDIAN PLANE.

1, Skin; *2*, nasal bone; *3*, frontal bone; *4*, parietal bone; *4'*, tentorium osseum; *5*, occipital bone; *6*, sphenoid bone; *7*, hard palate; *8*, premaxilla; *9*, mandible; *10*, hyoid bone; *11*, septum between frontal sinuses; *12*, alar cartilage; *13*, dilatator naris transversus; *14*, septum nasi with venous plexuses; *15*, palato-labial artery; *16*, *16'*, upper and lower septal branches of *15*; *17*, septal branch of sphenopalatine artery and satellite vein; *18*, septal branch of ethmoidal artery; *19*, sphenoidal sinus; *20*, guttural pouch; *21*, pharynx; *22*, pharyngeal orifice of Eustachian tube; *23*, posterior naris; *24*, soft palate; *25*, palatinus muscle; *26*, pharyngeal muscles; *27*, œsophagus; *28*, dotted line indicating position of posterior pillar of soft palate; *29*, lamina; *29'*, arch of cricoid cartilage; *30*, arytenoideus transversus muscle; *31*, epiglottis; *32*, body of thyroid cartilage; *33*, vocal process and cord; *34*, arytenoid cartilage; *35*, lateral ventricle of larynx; *36*, trachea; *37*, ventral straight muscles of head; *38*, longus colli; *39*, atlas; *40*, axis; *41*, lig. nuchæ; *42*, dorsal spinal muscles; *43*, muscles of external ear; *44*, omo- and sterno-hyoideus; *45*, tongue; *46*, mylo-hyoideus; *47*, genio-hyoideus; *48*, genio-glossus; *49*, longitudinalis inferior; *50*, longitud. superior; *51*, hyo-epiglotticus; *52*, chin and mentalis muscle; *53*, venous plexus of hard palate; *54*, corpus callosum; *55*, septum pellucidum; *56*, fornix; *57*, thalamus; *58*, pineal body; *59*, corpora quadrigemina; *60*, cerebral peduncle; *61*, corpus mammillare; *62*, pituitary body; *63*, chiasma opticum; *64*, intercarotid artery; *65*, medulla oblongata; *66*, interventricular foramen; *67*, infundibulum; *68*, third ventricle; *69*, cerebral aqueduct; *70*, anterior medullary velum; *71*, fourth ventricle; *72*, posterior medullary velum; *73*, basilar artery; *74*, spinal cord; *75*, ethmoidal nerve; *76*, septal branch of posterior nasal nerve; *76'*, branch of same to organ of Jacobson; *77*, olfactory nerve to organ of Jacobson; *78*, nasal branches of palatine artery. (After Ellenberger, in Leisering's Atlas.)

arteries, run forward, one on each side, between the sclera and choroid to the periphery of the iris. Here they divide into branches which anastomose and form a circle (Circulus iridis major). From this secondary branches are detached which form a second circle around the pupil (Circulus iridis minor).

(*e*) The **central artery of the retina** (Arteria centralis retinæ) is a small vessel which arises from the ophthalmic or from a posterior ciliary artery. It pierces the optic nerve a short distance behind the sclera and runs in its center to the lamina cribrosa, where it breaks up in thirty to forty fine branches. These appear in the fundus of the eye at the margin of the optic papilla and radiate in the posterior part of the retina.

(*f*) The **ethmoidal artery** (A. ethmoidalis) is the continuation of the ophthalmic. It enters the cranial cavity through the ethmoidal foramen, passes inward on the cribriform plate, and divides into meningeal and nasal branches. The former ramify in the anterior part of the dura mater and anastomose with branches of the artery of the corpus callosum. The nasal branch passes through the cribriform plate, gives branches to the mucous membrane of the lateral mass of the ethmoid and the adjacent part of the septum nasi, and runs forward on the superior turbinal.

The **third part** passes forward in the pterygo-palatine fossa, accompanied by branches of the maxillary nerve. On reaching the posterior palatine foramen it is continued by the palatine artery. Its branches are as follows:

(1) The **buccinator artery** (A. buccinatoria) arises from the lower aspect of the internal maxillary shortly after its emergence (Fig. 437). It turns around the maxillary tuberosity, accompanied by the buccinator nerve, and under the masseter muscle, enters the cheek, and runs forward in it. It supplies branches to the cheek, the superior buccal glands, and the masseter and pterygoid muscles. Near its origin it gives off a branch to the orbital fat behind the periorbita.

(2) The **infraorbital** or **superior dental artery** (A. infraorbitalis) arises from the upper aspect of the internal maxillary a little in front of the preceding vessel. It passes upward and forward to the maxillary foramen, runs in the infraorbital canal in company with the nerve of the same name, and is continued forward within the jaw to the incisor teeth. It gives branches to the teeth and gums, and detaches a branch through the infraorbital foramen which anastomoses with the lateral nasal and superior labial. About midway between its origin and the maxillary foramen it gives off the **malar** or **orbital branch** (Ramus malaris), which passes along the floor of the orbit to end in the lower lid and anastomose with the angularis oculi. It gives twigs to the inferior oblique muscle and the lacrimal sac.

The infraorbital artery is usually small at its emergence upon the face, but in some cases it is rather large and may partially replace the superior labial and lateral nasal arteries.

(3) The **staphyline** or **small palatine artery** (A. palatina minor) is a small vessel which passes forward in the groove at the inner side of the maxillary tuberosity to the soft palate. In the groove it is accompanied by the nerve of the same name and the palatine vein.

(4) The **sphenopalatine artery** (A. sphenopalatina) arises in the extreme anterior part of the pterygo-palatine fossa and passes into the nasal cavity, where it divides into internal and external branches. The internal branch is distributed to the mucous membrane of the septum nasi; the external one goes to the inferior turbinal, the inferior meatus, the posterior nares, and the maxillary and frontal sinuses. It may arise from the infraorbital.

(5) The **palatine** or **palato-labial artery** (A. palatina major) is the direct continuation of the internal maxillary. It passes through the palatine canal to the roof of the mouth, accompanied by the palatine nerve, and runs forward in the palatine groove, where it is joined by the vein. A little behind the plane of the corner incisor teeth it curves inward over a bar of cartilage to the foramen incisivum, where it unites with its fellow of the opposite side. The single artery thus formed passes up through the foramen and divides under the transverse dilator of the nostril into two branches. These ramify in the upper lip and anastomose with the lateral nasal and superior labial arteries. In its course in the roof of the mouth the palatine artery gives off branches to the hard and soft palate and the gums, and others which pass through the accessory palatine foramina to be distributed in the mucous membrane of the lower part of the nasal cavity. Commonly two branches, right and left, are detached from the convexity of the arch formed by the union of the two arteries; these run forward in the anterior part of the hard palate.

ARTERIES OF THE THORACIC LIMB

THE BRACHIAL ARTERY

The **brachial artery,** after turning around the lower border of the scalenus at the first rib, passes backward and a little downward across the origin of the coraco-brachialis and the insertion of the subscapularis muscle at the inner side of the shoulder joint. At the posterior border of the subscapularis it gives off the subscapular artery, and turns downward on the inner surface of the arm. In its course in the arm it inclines a little forward, crosses the humerus very obliquely, and divides at the antero-internal aspect of the distal third of the shaft of the bone into the anterior and posterior radial arteries.[1]

It is related internally to the serratus magnus and the posterior deep pectoral muscles, and the cubital lymph glands. Externally it lies on the subscapularis, the brachialis, the insertion of the teres major and latissimus dorsi, and the inner head of the triceps. The coraco-brachialis muscle lies along the front of the artery, which, however, overlaps the muscle distally. The vein crosses the inner face of the artery and runs down behind it, accompanied part way by the ulnar and radial nerves. The musculo-cutaneous and median nerves form a loop around the artery close to its origin, and the latter nerve then passes down in front of the artery. The chief branches are as follows

1. The **suprascapular artery** (A. thoracico-acromialis) is a small and somewhat flexuous vessel, which arises near the anterior border of the subscapularis, runs upward, and dips in between that muscle and the supraspinatus. It gives branches to these muscles, the anterior deep pectoral, and the mastoido-humeralis. A branch passes in front of the coraco-brachialis to the shoulder joint and the proximal end of the humerus.

This vessel may be double, or be represented by one or more branches of the inferior cervical artery.

2. The **subscapular artery** (A. subscapularis) is a very large vessel which arises at the posterior border of the subscapularis muscle. It passes upward in the interstice between that muscle and the teres major on the inner surface of the long head of the triceps, turns around the posterior border of the scapula below the posterior angle, and ends in the infraspinatus and deltoid. Besides collaterals (Rami musculares) to the subscapularis, teres major, triceps, and tensor fasciæ antibrachii it gives off the following named branches:

(*a*) The **thoracico-dorsal** (A. thoracicodorsalis) is a long artery which is usually given off about an inch from the origin of the subscapular, crosses the inner face of the teres major, and runs upward and backward on the latissimus dorsi. It gives branches to these muscles, the abdominal panniculus and the axillary lymph glands.

(*b*) The **posterior circumflex artery** (A. circumflexa humeri posterior) arises a little above the preceding vessel and passes outward behind the shoulder joint between the long and external heads of the triceps with the axillary (or circumflex) nerve. It gives branches to these muscles, the joint capsule, and the muscles and skin of the outer side of the shoulder, anastomosing with the anterior circumflex artery.

(*c*) The **circumflex artery of the scapula** (A. circumflexa scapulæ) arises about two or three inches (ca. 5 to 7.5 cm.) above the shoulder joint, passes forward to the posterior border of the scapula, and divides into two branches. The outer one runs forward on the external surface of the scapula below the spine and gives branches to the supraspinatus, infraspinatus, and teres minor. The inner branch passes forward in a similar fashion on the costal surface of the scapula and supplies branches to the subscapularis.

[1] The term axillary is often applied to the artery from the first rib to the point of origin of the subscapular branch.

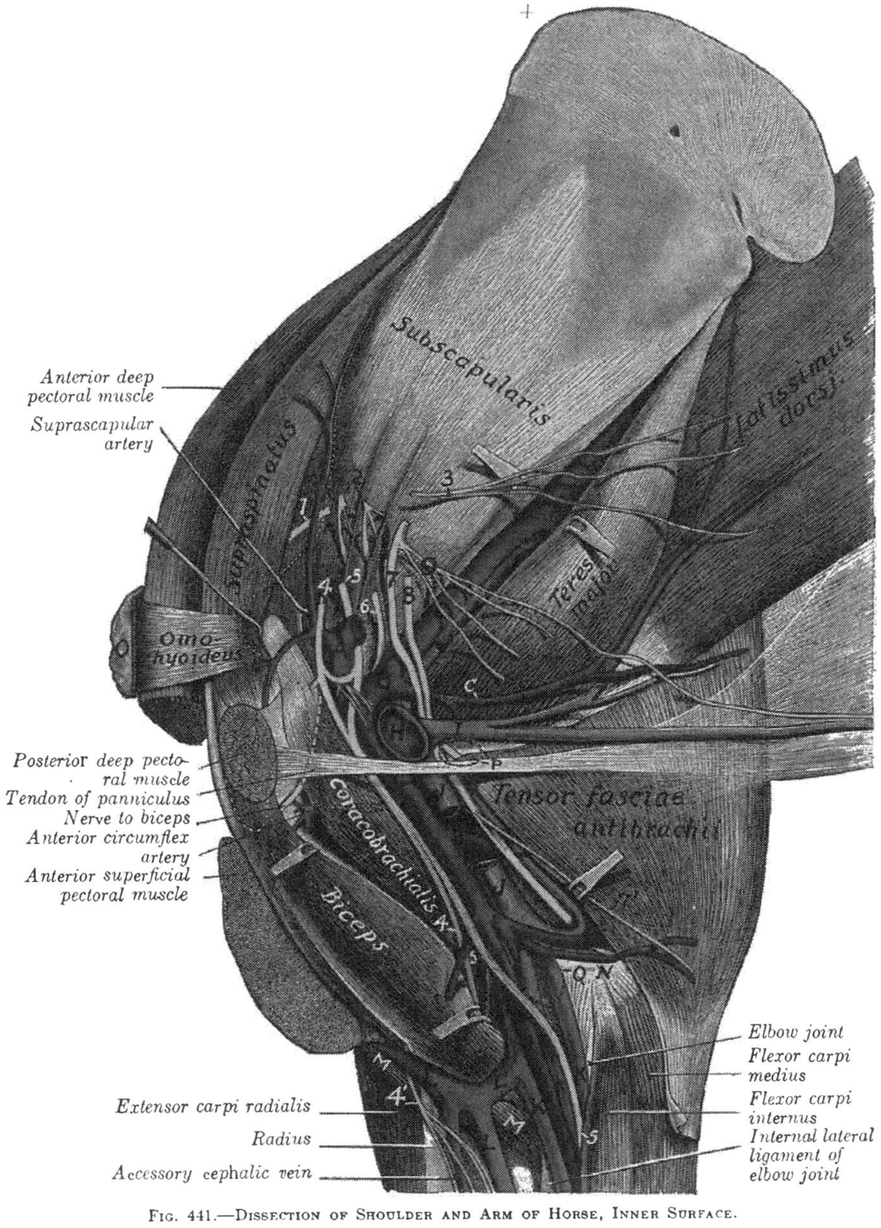

FIG. 441.—DISSECTION OF SHOULDER AND ARM OF HORSE, INNER SURFACE.

A, Brachial artery; *B*, subscapular artery; C, thoracico-dorsal artery; *D*, deep brachial artery; *E*, ulnar artery; *F*, anterior radial artery; *G*, posterior radial (or median) artery; *H*, brachial vein; *I*, external thoracic (or "spur") vein; *J*, brachial vein; *K*, *K*, *K*, posterior radial veins; *L*, cephalic vein; *L'*, communicating vein; *M*, brachialis muscle; *N*, internal epicondyle of humerus; *O*, prescapular lymph glands; *P*, position of axillary lymph glands; *Q*, position of cubital lymph glands; *1*, suprascapular nerve; *2*, subscapular nerves; *3*, thoraco-dorsal nerve; *4*, musculo-cutaneous nerve; *4'*, cutaneous branch of musculo-cutaneous nerve; *5*, median nerve; *6*, axillary nerve; *7*, ulnar nerve; *8*, radial nerve; *9*, thoracic nerves. (After Schmaltz, Atlas d. Anat. d. Pferdes.)

3. The **anterior circumflex** (or prehumeral) **artery** (A. circumflexa humeri anterior) arises usually at the upper border of the teres major. It passes forward and outward between the two parts of the coraco-brachialis or between the latter

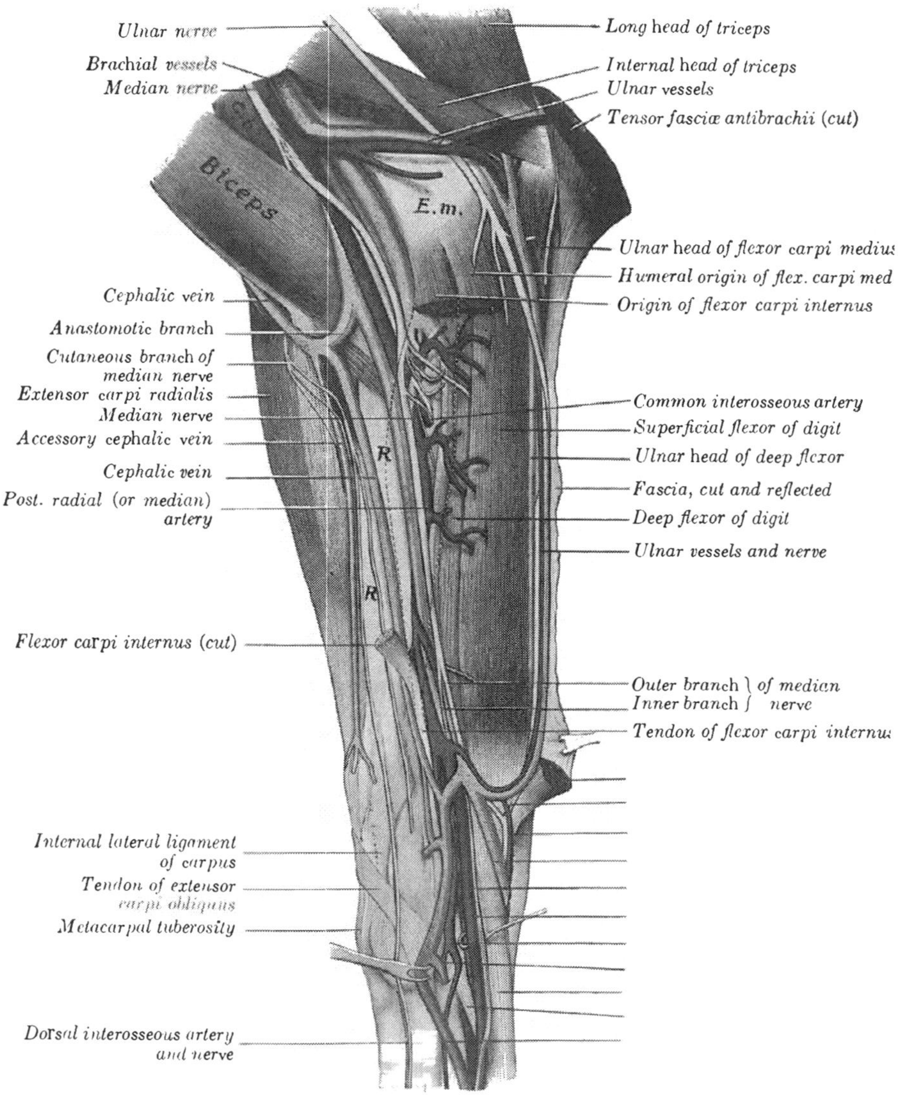

FIG. 442.—DISSECTION OF RIGHT FOREARM AND CARPUS OF HORSE, INTERNAL SURFACE.
C.b., Coraco-brachialis muscle; *E.m.*, internal epicondyle of humerus; *R*, subcutaneous surface of radius. (After Schmaltz, Atlas d. Anat. d. Pferdes.)

and the humerus. It gives branches to the coraco-brachialis and deep pectoral and ends in the upper part of the biceps and in the mastoido-humeralis. It anastomoses with the posterior circumflex.

Not rarely it arises below the middle of the humerus and passes upward between the biceps and coraco-brachialis. In these cases a small branch for the coraco-brachialis is usually given off at the usual point of origin of the anterior circumflex.

4. The **deep brachial artery** (A. profunda brachii) is a large but short trunk which arises usually about the middle of the humerus. It passes backward and divides into several branches which supply the triceps, tensor fasciæ antibrachii, anconeus, and brachialis. A branch runs in the musculo-spiral groove with the radial nerve to the front of the elbow joint and anastomoses with the anterior radial. A slender branch passes down along the external border of the extensor carpi and supplies cutaneous twigs. Anastomoses occur with the ulnar and recurrent interosseous arteries.

The point of origin is inconstant and it is not uncommon to find two arteries instead. Often a large branch for the posterior deep pectoral muscle is detached close to the origin or arises from the brachial directly.

5. **Muscular branches** (Rami musculares) are distributed to the teres major, deep pectoral, coraco-brachialis, and biceps. The largest and least variable of these supplies the lower part of the biceps.

6. The **ulnar artery** (A. collateralis ulnaris superior) arises a little below the nutrient foramen of the humerus and passes downward and backward along the lower edge of the internal head of the triceps under cover of the brachial vein and the tensor fascia antibrachii. It gives branches to these muscles, the posterior superficial pectoral, the cubital lymph glands, panniculus, and skin. At the internal epicondyle of the humerus it is joined by the ulnar nerve and turns downward under the ulnar head of the flexor carpi medius. It continues with the vein and nerve under the deep fascia of the forearm between the ulnar and humeral heads of the perforans, and in the distal half of the region between the external and middle flexors of the carpus. It unites just above the carpus (under cover of the flexor carpi externus) with a branch of the radial artery, with which it forms the supracarpal arch. It detaches small collaterals to the muscles along which it passes and terminal twigs to the outer surface of the carpus.

7. The **nutrient artery of the humerus** (A. nutritia humeri) is a short vessel which enters the nutrient foramen of the humerus. It often arises from the ulnar.

8. The **anterior radial artery** (A. collateralis radialis inferior) passes downward and a little outward on the anterior face of the humerus under cover of the biceps and brachialis to the front of the elbow joint, where it is joined by the radial nerve. It then descends on the anterior surface of the radius under cover of the anterior extensor of the digit to the carpus, where it concurs in the formation of the rete carpi dorsale, anastomosing with the posterior radial and interosseous arteries. It supplies branches to the elbow joint, the biceps, brachialis, and the extensors of the carpus and digit. A cutaneous branch emerges between the distal end of the biceps and the brachialis.

THE POSTERIOR RADIAL ARTERY

The **posterior radial** or **median artery** (A. mediana) is the direct continuation of the brachial. It passes downward and slightly backward, at first on the inner surface of the humerus, and then over the capsule and internal lateral ligament of the elbow joint, under cover of the posterior superficial pectoral muscle.[1] Below the elbow it dips under the flexor carpi internus and passes down the inner part of the posterior surface of the radius. In the distal part of the forearm it inclines backward and is separated from the radius by the reinforcing band (Caput tendineum) of the superficial flexor of the digit and is continued by the large metacarpal artery.

[1] The pulse can be taken where the artery lies on the lateral ligament, since the pectoral muscle is thin here.

It is accompanied by the median nerve, which lies in front of the artery at its origin, then crosses over it obliquely at the elbow joint and becomes posterior. In the arm the brachial vein lies behind and partly upon the artery; lower down there

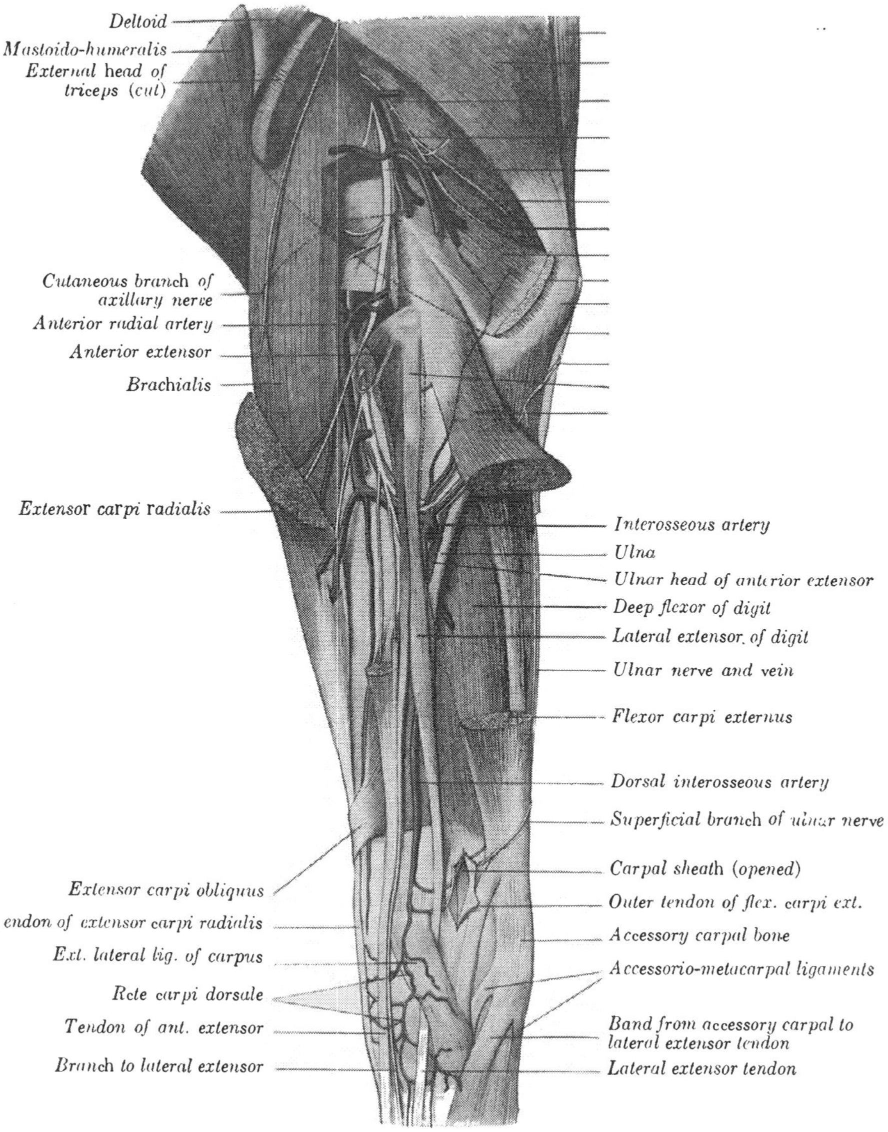

FIG. 443.—DISSECTION OF LEFT FOREARM OF HORSE, EXTERNAL SURFACE. (After Schmaltz, Atlas d. Anat. d. Pferdes.)

are usually two satellite veins, anterior and posterior. The chief collateral branches are as follows:

1. Articular branches for the elbow joint.

2. **Muscular branches** to the flexors of the carpus and digit. The largest of these arise at the proximal third of the forearm.

3. The **common interosseous artery** (A. interossea communis) is a vessel of

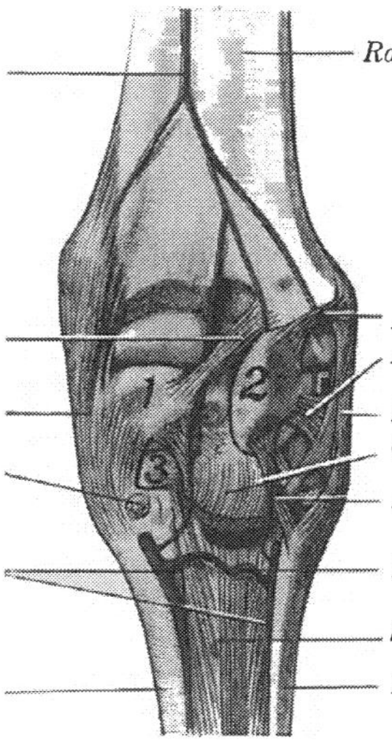

FIG. 444.—DEEP DISSECTION OF RIGHT CARPUS OF HORSE, POSTERIOR VIEW.
1, Radial carpal bone; *2*, accessory carpal bone; *3*, second carpal bone. (After Schmaltz, Atlas d. Anat. d. Pferdes.)

considerable size which arises at the level of the interosseous space, through which it passes. Before entering the space it gives off a small branch, the volar interosseous (A. interossea volaris), which descends to the radial head of the perforans. In the space it supplies the nutrient arteries of the radius and ulna. Emerging

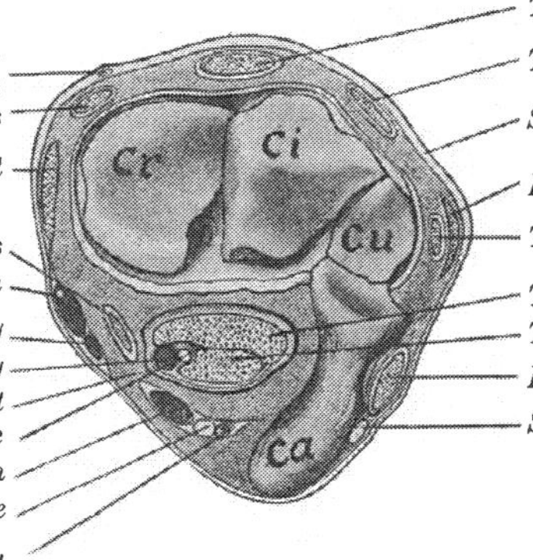

FIG. 445.—CROSS-SECTION OF RIGHT CARPUS OF HORSE.
The soft structures are cut at the level of the radio-carpal articulation, exposing the proximal row of carpal bones. *Cr*, Radial carpal bone; *Ci*, intermediate carpal bone; *Cu*, ulnar carpal bone; *Ca*, accessory carpal bone. (After Schmaltz, Atlas d. Anat. d. Pferdes.)

from the space it gives off branches to the flexor carpi externus, a small **recurrent branch** (A. interossea recurrens) which passes upward on the outer surface of the ulna and anastomoses with the deep brachial and ulnar arteries, and is continued as the **dorsal interosseous artery.** This vessel (A. interossea dorsalis) passes down between the anterior and lateral extensors of the digit and concurs with the anterior radial in forming a network on the anterior surface of the carpus, the **rete carpi dorsale.** From the latter arise two small vessels, the **internal** and **external dorsal metacarpal arteries** (A. metacarpea dorsalis medialis, lateralis), which run distally in the grooves between the large and small metacarpal bones and anastomose with the volar metacarpal arteries.

4. The **artery of the rete carpi volare** (A. retis carpi volaris) is a small vessel which arises at the distal third of the forearm and passes downward to the posterior surface of the carpus, where it concurs with branches of the volar metacarpal arteries in forming the rete carpi volare.

5. The **external volar metacarpal artery** (A. metacarpea volaris lateralis) is a small vessel which arises just above the carpus under cover of the flexor carpi medius and anastomoses with the ulnar artery, forming the supracarpal arch. From the latter a branch descends with the outer branch of the median nerve, inclines outward toward the posterior border of the accessory carpal bone, and arrives at the head of the external metacarpal bone. Here it is connected with the internal volar metacarpal artery, usually by two transverse branches, thus forming the **deep** volar or **subcarpal arch** (Arcus volaris profundus). One of these branches lies between the subcarpal check ligament and the suspensory ligament; the other (not always present) lies beneath the latter on the large metacarpal bone. A small branch descends to the fetlock with the external metacarpal nerve. Below the arch the artery pursues a flexuous course downward on the posterior face of the large metacarpal bone alongside of the external small metacarpal and under cover of the suspensory ligament. At the distal third of the metacarpus it commonly unites with the corresponding vessel of the inner side to form a short trunk which passes backward through the angle of divergence of the branches of the suspensory ligament and joins the external digital or the common digital artery.

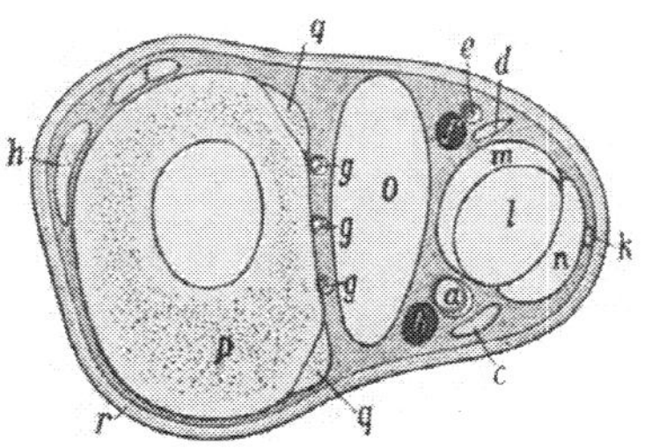

FIG. 446.—CROSS-SECTION OF MIDDLE OF RIGHT METACARPUS OF HORSE.

a, Common digital (or large metacarpal) artery; *b*, internal metacarpal vein; c, internal metacarpal nerve; *d*, external metacarpal nerve; *e*, branch of external volar metacarpal artery; *f*, external metacarpal vein; *g*, *g*, *g*, deep volar or interosseous metacarpal arteries; *h*, tendon of anterior extensor; *i*, tendon of lateral extensor; *k*, anastomotic branch connecting metacarpal nerves; *l*, deep flexor tendon; *m*, check ligament; *n*, superficial flexor tendon; *o*, suspensory ligament; p, large metacarpal bone; *q*, *q*, small metacarpal bones; *r*, skin. (After Ellenberger, in Leisering's Atlas.)

6. The internal volar or **small metacarpal artery** (A. metacarpea volaris medialis) is given off from the posterior radial at an acute angle, usually a little above the external one or by a common trunk with it. It passes down the inner side of the carpus behind the tendon of the flexor carpi internus and embedded in the posterior annular ligament. Arriving at the proximal end of the inner metacarpal bone it becomes more deeply placed and is connected with the external volar artery by one or two transverse branches as stated above. It then pursues a flexuous course downward alongside of the inner small metacarpal bone, like the corresponding external artery, with which it commonly unites as described above. It is larger than the external artery and supplies the nutrient artery to the large metacarpal bone.

The foregoing account describes the most common arrangement of the dorsal and volar metacarpal arteries. Variations in their origin and connections are common, but have no great surgical importance. Collateral branches are omitted for the same reason. In some cases the internal volar metacarpal is connected with the common digital or large metacarpal artery a little below the carpus by a branch passing obliquely across the inner border of the deep flexor tendon; this forms a superficial volar arch.

THE COMMON DIGITAL ARTERY

The **common digital** or **large metacarpal artery**[1] is the direct continuation of the posterior radial. It descends in the carpal canal along the inner side of

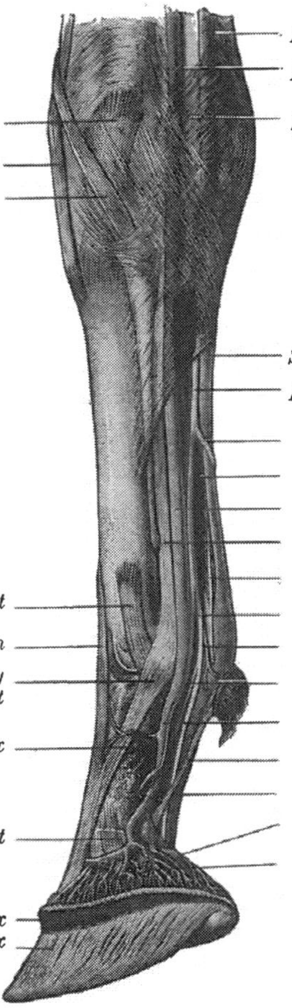

FIG. 447.—DISSECTION OF RIGHT CARPUS, METACARPUS, AND DIGIT OF HORSE, INNER VIEW. (After Schmaltz Atlas d. Anat. d. Pferdes.)

the flexor tendons in company with the inner branch of the median nerve and a satellite vein. Continuing down the limb it preserves this relation to the tendons to the distal third of the metacarpus, where it inclines toward the middle line of the limb behind the suspensory ligament, and divides into the internal and external digital arteries. In the metacarpus the artery is related to the vein in front and the artery behind, and is covered by the fascia and skin. It furnishes collateral branches to the suspensory ligament, the flexor tendons, and the skin.

[1] This vessel is also termed the A. metacarpea volaris superficialis or the palmar metacarpal artery.

THE DIGITAL ARTERIES

The internal and external digital arteries (A. digitalis medialis, lateralis) are formed by the bifurcation of the common digital at the distal third of the meta carpus. They diverge, pass down over the outer surface of the corresponding sesamoid at the fetlock, and descend parallel with the borders of the deep flexor tendon to the volar grooves and foramina of the third phalanx. Entering the latter the two arteries unite in the semilunar canal and form the terminal arch (Arcus terminalis), from which numerous branches pass through the bone to the wall surface and ramify in the matrix of the wall and sole of the hoof. A number of branches emerge through the foramina at the lower border, where they anastomose with each other in arciform fashion. These branches were named by Spooner the inferior communicating arteries, and the anastomotic arch formed by them is termed the circumflex artery of the third phalanx (Chauveau) or the artery of the lower border of the third phalanx (Leisering).

Each artery is accompanied by a vein and by the digital nerves. Above the fetlock the artery is most deeply placed and is covered by the vein; the nerve is behind the vein. At the fetlock the artery has become superficial and is related to the vein in front and the posterior branch of the nerve behind. The anterior branch of the nerve crosses over the artery obliquely to the lateral aspect of the first phalanx. The vessels and nerves are crossed obliquely by a small tendinous band, the ligament of the ergot, which begins in the fibrous basis of the ergot at the back of the fetlock and extends downward and forward to end in the fascia at the side of the pastern joint.

In addition to branches to the joints, tendons and synovial sheath, ergot, and skin, the digital arteries give off:

1. The artery of **the first** phalanx or perpendicular artery (A. phalangis primæ), a short trunk which arises at a right angle about the middle of the first phalanx, and divides into dorsal and volar branches (Rami dorsales et volares) The dorsal (anterior) branch passes between the first phalanx and the extensor tendon and ramifies on the front of the digit, anastomosing with its fellow. The volar (posterior) branch dips in between the flexor tendons and the inferior sesamoidean ligaments and anastomoses with the opposite artery.

2. The artery of the plantar cushion (A. toricæ phalangis tertiæ) arises at the proximal border of the lateral cartilage and passes backward and downward to ramify in the plantar cushion and the matrix of the heels and frog.

3. The dorsal artery of the second phalanx (Ramus dorsalis phalangis secundæ) arises a little above the navicular bone, and passes forward under cover of the lateral cartilage and the extensor tendon to the front of the second phalanx, where it anastomoses with the opposite vessel. It gives branches to the skin, the tendon, the coffin joint, and the coronary matrix of the hoof.

4. The volar artery of the second phalanx (Ramus volaris phalangis secundæ) is smaller than the preceding, opposite to which it arises. It passes above the proximal border of the third sesamoid and unites with the opposite artery.

The arteries of the second phalanx form what is termed by Chauveau the **coronary circle.** The dorsal (anterior) part of the circle gives off commonly an artery (A. coronalis phalangis tertiæ) near either side of the extensor tendon, which divides into two branches. The central branch unites with that of the opposite side, while the other joins a branch of the artery of the plantar cushion. In this way is formed the **circumflex artery of the coronary cushion,** an anastomotic arch which lies on the extensor tendon at the coronet. In some cases descending branches of the arteries of the first phalanx concur in the formation of the arch.

5. The dorsal artery of the **third** phalanx or preplantar artery (A. dorsalis phalangis tertiæ) arises at the deep face of the wing of the third phalanx, passes outward through the notch or foramen there, and runs forward in the groove on the wall surface. It gives off ascending and descending branches, which ramify in the matrix

of the wall of the hoof, anastomosing above with the circumflex artery of the coronary cushion and below with the circumflex artery of the third phalanx. Before passing through the wing it detaches a retrograde branch to the plantar cushion, and after emerging one which ramifies on the outer aspect of the lateral cartilage.

The terminal part of the digital artery after giving off the preceding vessel is sometimes termed the plantar.

BRANCHES OF THE THORACIC AORTA

In addition to the coronary arteries and the common brachiocephalic trunk (which have been described), the thoracic part of the aorta gives off branches to the thoracic walls and viscera and to the spinal cord and its membranes. The visceral **branches** (Rami viscerales) are the bronchial and œsophageal, which arise by a broncho-œsophageal trunk. The **parietal branches** (Rami parietales) are the intercostal and phrenic arteries.

1. The **broncho-œsophageal** (Truncus broncho-œsophageus) is a short, usually bulbous, trunk which arises at the sixth thoracic vertebra from the aorta or in common with the first aortic intercostal arteries. It passes (under cover of the vena azygos) down the right face of the aorta toward the bifurcation of the trachea and divides into bronchial and œsophageal branches.

(*a*) The **bronchial artery** (A. bronchialis) crosses the left face of the œsophagus to the bifurcation of the trachea, where it divides into right and left branches. Each enters the hilus of the corresponding lung above the bronchus, which it accompanies in its ramification. It supplies the lung tissue and also detaches twigs to the bronchial lymph glands and the mediastinum.

(*b*) The **œsophageal artery** (A. œsophagea) (Fig. 429) is a small vessel which passes backward above the œsophagus in the posterior mediastinum and anastomoses with the œsophageal branch of the gastric artery. It detaches twigs to the œsophagus and the mediastinal lymph glands and pleura, and also gives off two branches which pass between the layers of the ligaments of the lungs and ramify in the subpleural tissue. Very commonly there is another artery which runs backward ventral to the œsophagus.

In some cases there is no broncho-œsophageal trunk, the bronchial and œsophageal arising separately. In other cases the second aortic intercostal arises in common with them also.

2. The **intercostal arteries** (Aa. intercostales) (Figs. 428, 429) number eighteen pairs. The first arises from the deep cervical artery, the next three from the subcostal branch of the dorsal artery, and the remainder from the aorta. The aortic intercostals arise from the dorsal face of the aorta in pairs close together; the fifth and sixth usually spring from a common stem. Each passes across the body of a vertebra to the corresponding intercostal space, detaches twigs to the vertebræ and the pleura, and divides into dorsal and ventral branches. The **dorsal branch** (Ramus dorsalis) gives off a spinal branch (Ramus spinalis) which passes through the inter vertebral foramen, gives twigs to the membranes of the spinal cord, perforates the dura, and reinforces the ventral spinal artery. A muscular branch passes to the muscles and skin of the back. The **ventral branch** (Ramus ventralis) is much the larger. It passes downward, at first almost in the middle of the intercostal space between the intercostal muscles, then gains the posterior border of the rib and is subpleural. Each is accompanied by a vein and nerve, the artery being in the middle and the vein in front. At the lower part of the space it unites with a ventral intercostal branch of the internal thoracic or the asternal artery. It supplies the intercostal muscles, the ribs and the pleura, and gives off perforating branches which pass out to the serratus magnus, the abdominal muscles, and the skin.

3. The **phrenic arteries** (Aa. phrenicæ) are two or three small vessels which arise at the hiatus aorticus from the ventral aspect of the aorta, often by a common

trunk. They supply the crura of the diaphragm. In some cases they arise in common with an intercostal artery.

BRANCHES OF THE ABDOMINAL AORTA

The collateral branches of the abdominal part of the aorta are distributed chiefly to the walls and contents of the abdominal cavity, but some branches are supplied to the spinal cord and its membranes, and others extend into the pelvis and to the scrotum. The **visceral branches** are the cœliac, anterior mesenteric, renal, posterior mesenteric, and the spermatic or utero-ovarian. The **parietal branches** are the lumbar arteries.

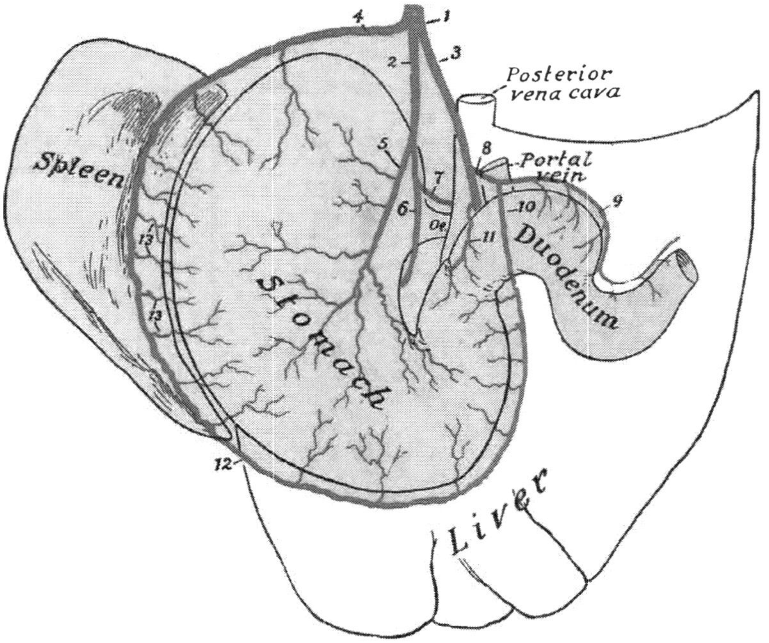

FIG. 448.—PLAN OF BRANCHES OF CŒLIAC ARTERY OF HORSE.
1, Cœliac artery; *2*, gastric artery; *3*, hepatic artery; *4*, splenic artery; *5*, posterior gastric artery; *6*, anterior gastric artery; *7*, œsophageal branch; *8*, gastro-duodenal artery; *9*, pancreatico-duodenal artery; *10*, right gastro-epiploic artery; *11*, pyloric artery; *12*, left gastro-epiploic artery; *13*, short gastric branches of splenic.

I. The **cœliac artery** or **axis** (A. cœliaca) is an unpaired vessel, usually half an inch or less (ca. 1 cm.) in length, which arises from the ventral aspect of the aorta at its emergence from the hiatus aorticus. It divides on the dorsal surface of the pancreas into three branches—the gastric, hepatic, and splenic.

1. The **gastric artery** (A. gastrica sinistra) passes downward and forward in the gastro-phrenic ligament, gives off œsophageal and pancreatic branches, and divides above and behind the cardia into anterior and posterior branches.

(*a*) The anterior branch (Ramus cranialis) crosses the lesser curvature just to the right of the cardia and ramifies on the parietal surface of the stomach. The branches pursue a flexuous course toward the greater curvature and anastomose with the short gastric arteries and the gastric branch of the hepatic artery.

(*b*) The **posterior** branch (Ramus caudalis) is distributed in a similar fashion on the visceral surface.

(c) The **œsophageal branch** (Ramus œsophageus) passes through the hiatus œsophageus into the thoracic cavity above the œsophagus and anastomoses with the œsophageal branch of the broncho-œsophageal artery.

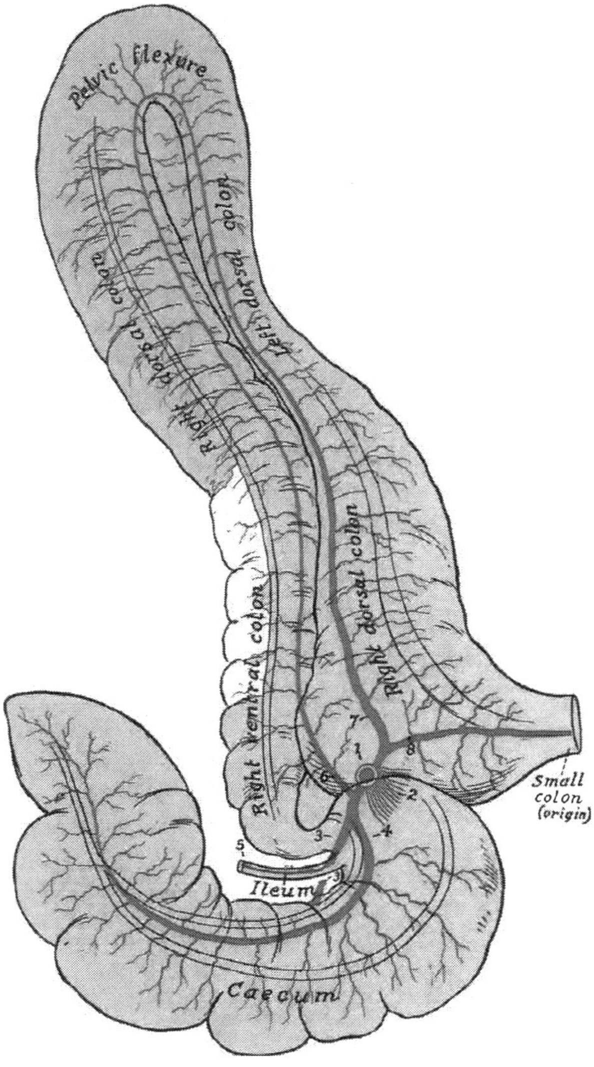

Fig. 449.—Plan of Chief Branches of Anterior Mesenteric Artery of Horse.

1, Stump of anterior mesenteric artery; *2*, stumps of arteries of small intestine; *3*, external cæcal artery; *4*, internal cæcal artery; *5*, ileal artery; *6*, ventral colic artery; *7*, dorsal colic artery; *8*, middle colic or first artery of small colon.

The gastric artery often arises by a common trunk with the splenic. The two terminal branches may arise separately, or the anterior from the splenic and the posterior from the hepatic. The œsophageal branch often arises from the splenic or the posterior gastric.

2. The **hepatic artery** (A. hepatica) is larger than the gastric. It passes forward to the right and ventrally on the dorsal surface of the pancreas, covered by

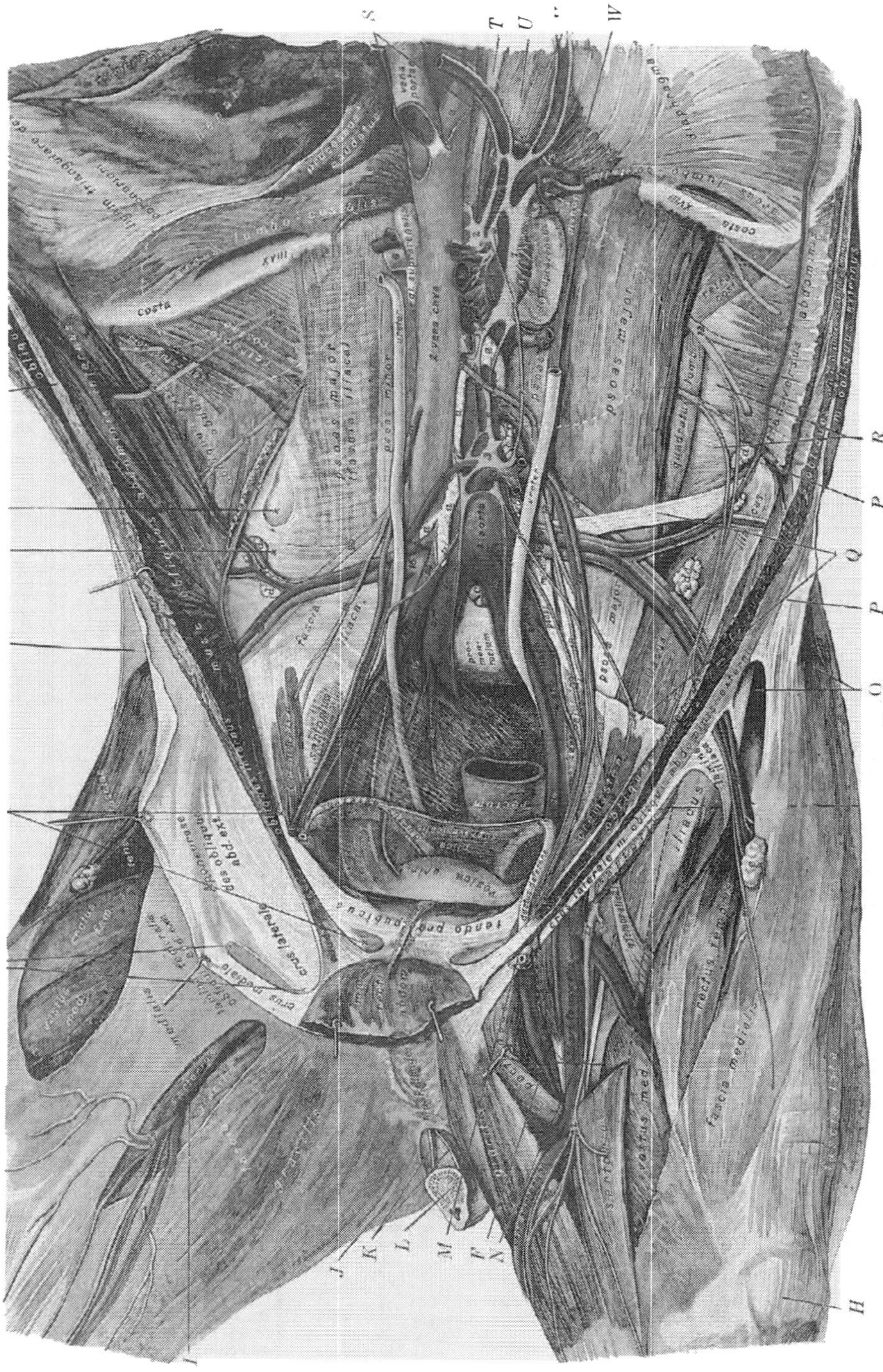

Fig.

FIG. 450.—DISSECTION OF SUBLUMBAR REGION, PELVIC INLET, AND INNER SURFACE OF THIGH OF HORSE.

Bl od-vessels: *1*, Aorta; *2*, posterior v ea ax; *3*, hepatic; *4*, gastric; *5*, splenic; *6*, *7*, renal; *8*, an erior mesenteric; *9*, arteries of sall intestine; *10*, ile co-colic; *1* dorsal coli; *12*, artery of sall colon; *13*, posterior mesenteric; *14*, external iliac; *15*, internal iliac; *16*, circumflex iliac; *17*, *9*, anterior and posterior branches of *16*; *18*, anastomosis wi h inter-da; *20*, spermatic; *21*, cremasteric; *22*, lateral sacral; *23*, internal pudic; *24*, umbilical; *25*, femoral; *26*, deep femoral; *27*, anterior femoral; *28*, b a ch to gracilis; *29*, sps.

Lymph-vessels and glands: *a*, Lymph-vessels; *b*, lumbar glands; *c*, in tal iliac glands; *d*, external iliac glands; *e*, precrural glands; *f*, deep inguinal glands (position indicated by d tal line).

Nerves and ganglia: *1*, *2*, left and right cœliaco-mesenteric ganglia; *3*, posterior mesenteric ganglion; *4*, connection between *1* and *2*; *5*, connection be en hepatic and splenic nerves; *6*, *7*, connections b een anterior and posterior mesenteric ganglia; *8*, splanchnic nerve; *9*, lumbar trunk of sympathetic; *10*, pelvic branches of pos eor mesenteric ganglion; *11*, internal spermatic nerve; *12*, last thoracic nerve; *13*, ilio-hypogastric nerve; *14*, anastomosis tween *13* and ilio-inguinal nerve; *16*, *17*, cutaneous and muscular branches of *15*; *18*, *9*, muscular and scrotal branches of external spermatic nerve; *20*, external cutaneous nerve of thigh; *21*, em ral r; *22*, saphenous re; *23*, branch of *22* to sartorius.

A, Cut surface of obliquus abdominis externus; *B*, ut surface of obliquus abdominis internus; *C*, depression due to disappearance of fat in interval dn ur border of psoas major and iliacus; *D*, thick part of iliac fascia which xals fm dn of psoas minor to external angle of ilium; *E*, super cial a of flk; *F*, internal inguinal ring; *G*, external nguinal ring; *H*, patella; *I*, femoral canal; *J*, semimembranosus; *K*, suspensory ligaments of penis; *L*, cross-section of penis; *M*, stump of spe matic cord; *N*, il-psoas; *O*, tensor asciæ latæ; *P*, *P*, extremities of sternal angle of ilium; *Q*, remains of iliac fascia; *R*, ilio-lumbar ligament or deep l r of h- odsal fcia; *S*, line of tachment of gastro-pancreatic old; *T*, endon of right crus of diaphragm; *U*, right cs; *V*, aorta at hiatus aorticus; *W*, left cs of diaphragm. The posi on of the kidneys is indi ated by dotted lines. (After Schma tz, Atlas d. Anat. d. Pferdes.)

the gas
under t
border o
or four
of the li
portal v
following

(*a*)
re give
in which

(*b*)
arises ab
descends
first par
anastom
epiploic
duodena

(*c*)
duodena
duodenu
epiploic
right ga
dextra)
duodenu
which
greater

(*d*) The left gastro-epiploic **artery** (A. gastroepiploica sinistra) is the continuation of the splenic artery. It passes to the right in the great omentum, parallel with the greater curvature of the stomach, and anastomoses with the right gastro-epiploic. It gives off branches to the greater curvature of the stomach, and twigs to the omentum.

II. The anterior or **great** mesenteric **artery** (A. mesenterica cranialis) arises from the ventral face of the aorta at the first lumbar vertebra. It is a large unpaired trunk, about an inch (ca. 2 to 3 cm.) in length, which passes ventrally between the vena cava and the left adrenal into the root of the great mesentery, when it divides into three branches—left, right, and anterior.[1]

1. The left **branch** gives off at once about fifteen to twenty **arteries** of **the small** intestine (Aa. intestinales).[2] These come off close together and pass in divergent fashion between the layers of the great mesentery, each dividing into two branches which anastomose with adjacent branches to form a series of arches. In the anterior part of the series secondary arches are formed by the union of branches given off from the primary set of arches. From the convex side of these arches terminal branches pass to the wall of the small intestine, in which they ramify and form a vascular network. They are accompanied by satellite veins and by nerves and lymph-vessels. The first artery anastomoses with the pancreatico-duodenal, and the last with the ileal branch of the great mesenteric artery. Branches are supplied to the mesenteric lymph glands.

2. The **right branch** (A. ileo-cæco-colica) might be regarded as the continuation of the trunk. It runs downward and a little forward and to the right and gives off the ileal, the two cæcal, and the ventral colic arteries.

(1) The **ileal** or **ileo-cæcal** artery (A. ilea) passes in retrograde fashion along the terminal part of the ileum and unites with the last branch of the left division.

(2) The **external** or **inferior cæcal artery** (Ramus cæcalis lateralis) passes between the cæcum and the origin of the colon and runs on the external muscular band of the cæcum to the apex, where it anastomoses with the internal artery. Besides numerous collaterals to the cæcum, it gives off the artery of the arch, which passes along the lesser curvature of the base of the cæcum and runs on the outer face of the origin of the great colon.

(3) The **internal** or **superior cæcal artery** (Ramus cæcalis medialis) passes along the inner band to the apex of the cæcum, where it anastomoses with the external cæcal artery.

(4) The **ventral**, right, or **direct colic artery** (A. colica ventralis) runs along the opposed surfaces of the ventral (first and second) parts of the great colon to the pelvic flexure, where it unites with the dorsal colic artery. It supplies the ventral parts of the great colon and sends a branch to the base of the cæcum.

3. The **anterior branch** divides after a very short course into the dorsal and middle colic arteries.

(1) The **dorsal, left,** or **retrograde** colic **artery** (A. colica dorsalis) is a large vessel which passes along the dorsal (fourth and third) parts of the great colon to the pelvic flexure, where it joins the ventral colic artery.

(2) The **middle** colic **artery** or **first artery** of **the small** colon (A. colica media) is a much smaller vessel which passes to the origin of the small colon, enters the colic mesentery, and forms an arch by joining the first branch of the posterior mesenteric artery close to the lesser curvature of the bowel. It sends an anasto motic branch to the dorsal colic artery.

[1] In the great majority of subjects this vessel and some of its branches are the seat of more or less extensive verminous aneurysm, produced by the Sclerostomum armatum. In the author's experience an entirely normal specimen is quite exceptional in adult horses.

[2] The left branch is a descriptive convention rather than a reality, since the arteries of the small intestines spring from the mesenteric trunk either directly or by short common stems with an adjacent vessel.

III. The **renal arteries** (Aa. renales), right and left, are relatively large vessels which arise from the aorta near the anterior mesenteric. The right **artery** is the longer of the two. It crosses over the dorsal surface of the vena cava to the right and somewhat forward. At the hilus it divides into several (five to eight) branches; some of these enter the gland at the hilus, while others pass to the ventral surface and enter there. The left **artery** is short and usually arises a little further back: it passes directly outward to the kidney and is then disposed like the right one. Small collateral branches are supplied to the ureters and the adrenals. The latter also receive small vessels directly from the aorta. The distribution within the kidney has been described.

Variations in the renal arteries are frequent. Two or more arteries may occur on one or both sides. Accessory arteries are more common on the left side and usually enter the posterior pole of the gland. They may arise from the aorta, the external iliac, or the circumflex iliac artery.

IV. The **posterior** or **small mesenteric artery** (A. mesenterica caudalis) is an unpaired vessel which arises from the ventral face of the aorta at the fourth lumbar vertebra, *i. e.*, about five or six inches (ca. 12 to 15 cm.) behind the origin of the anterior mesenteric artery. It is much smaller than the latter and supplies the greater part of the small colon and rectum. It descends in the colic mesentery and divides into two branches. The anterior branch (A. colica sinistra) gives off three or four arteries which divide and form anastomotic arches close to the bowel. The first arch is formed by union with the middle colic branch of the anterior mesenteric. The posterior branch or anterior hæmorrhoidal artery (A. hæmorrhoidalis cranialis) passes backward in the upper part of the mesentery and the mesorectum and terminates near the anus by anastomosing with the internal pudic artery. Three or four of its anterior collateral branches form arches.

V. The **spermatic arteries** (Aa. spermaticæ internæ), right and left, are long slender arteries which arise from the aorta near the posterior mesenteric and supply the testicle and epididymis. Each passes backward in a narrow fold of peritoneum (Plica vasculosa) to the internal inguinal ring and descends through the inguinal canal to the scrotum. In the canal and scrotum it pursues a very flexuous course in the anterior border of the spermatic cord, surrounded by the pampiniform plexus of veins, and associated closely with the spermatic nerves and lymphatics and unstriped muscle-fibers. It passes between the epididymis and testicle, runs in flexuous fashion along the attached border of the latter, turns around the posterior pole, and runs forward on the free border to the anterior pole. The largest branches arise from its ventral part, pass tortuously up either side of the gland embedded in the tunica albuginea, and give off fine branches to the gland substance. Small collateral branches are detached to the ureter and the spermatic cord.

The **utero-ovarian arteries** in the female correspond to the preceding vessels, but are much shorter. Each is placed in the anterior part of the broad ligament of the uterus and divides into ovarian and uterine branches. The **ovarian branch** (A. ovarica) pursues a flexuous course to the ovary, which it supplies. The **uterine branch** (A. uterina cranialis) passes to the concave border of the cornu of the uterus, which it supplies, anastomosing with the uterine artery.

VI. The **lumbar arteries** (Aa. lumbales) are in series with the intercostal arteries and have a similar origin and distribution. There are usually six pairs of lumbar arteries, of which five arise from the aorta and the sixth from the internal iliac or the lateral sacral at the junction of the last lumbar vertebra and the sacrum. Each passes across the body of a lumbar vertebra to the intertransverse space, gives branches to the sublumbar muscles, and divides into dorsal and ventral branches. The **dorsal branch** (Ramus dorsalis), the larger of the two, passes upward to ramify in the extensor muscles of the spine and the skin of the loins; it gives off a **spinal branch** (Ramus spinalis) which comports itself like the corresponding branch of an aortic intercostal artery. The **ventral branch** (Ramus

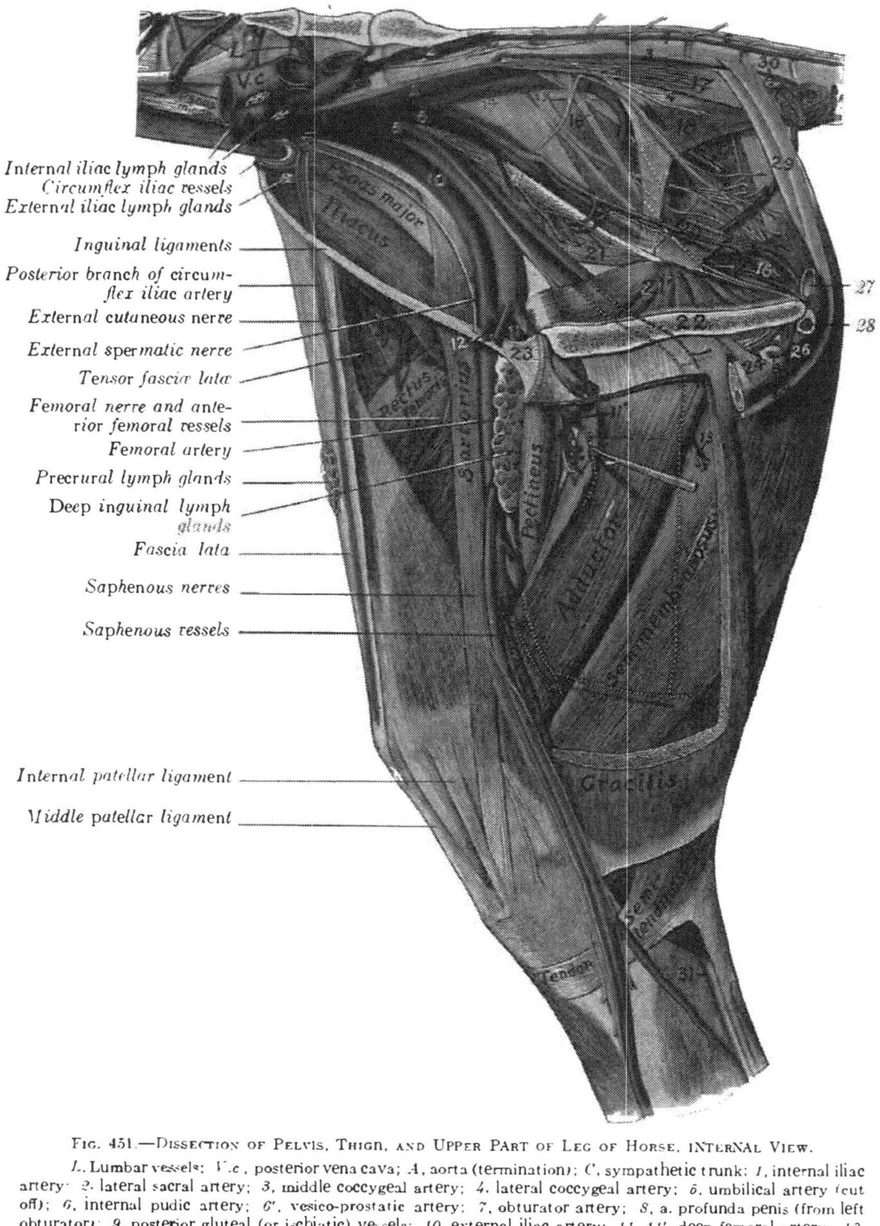

FIG. 451.—DISSECTION OF PELVIS, THIGH, AND UPPER PART OF LEG OF HORSE, INTERNAL VIEW.

L, Lumbar vessels; *V.c*, posterior vena cava; *A*, aorta (termination); *C*, sympathetic trunk; *1*, internal iliac artery; *2*, lateral sacral artery; *3*, middle coccygeal artery; *4*, lateral coccygeal artery; *5*, umbilical artery (cut off); *6*, internal pudic artery; *6'*, vesico-prostatic artery; *7*, obturator artery; *8*, a. profunda penis (from left obturator); *9*, posterior gluteal (or ischiatic) vessels; *10*, external iliac artery; *11*, *11'*, deep femoral artery; *12*, prepubic artery; *13*, branch of deep femoral artery; *14*, great sciatic nerve; *15*, posterior gluteal nerve; *16* (above), internal pudic nerve; *16* (below near pelvic outlet), suburethral venous plexus; *17*, sacro-coccygeus inferior; *18*, coccygeus; *19*, recto-coccygeus; *20*, retractor ani; *21*, *21'*, two heads of obturator internus; *22*, symphysis pelvis; *23*, prepubic tendon; *24* suspensory ligament of penis; *25*, retractor penis muscle; *26*, bulbo-cavernosus muscle; *27*, urethra (cross-section); *28*, crus penis (cross-section); *29*, suspensory ligaments of anus (= upper part of retractor penis muscle); *30*, anal lymph glands; *31*, tibial nerve. (After Schmaltz, Atlas d. Anat. d. Pferdes.)

ventralis) runs outward in the intertransverse space, passes between the transversus and obliquus internus abdominis, gives branches to these muscles, and ends in the obliquus externus, the panniculus, and the skin of the flank.

THE INTERNAL ILIAC ARTERY

The **internal iliac** or **hypogastric arteries** (Aa. hypogastricæ) result from the bifurcation of the aorta under the fifth or sixth lumbar vertebra. They diverge at an angle of about 60 degrees, and each passes backward under the wing of the

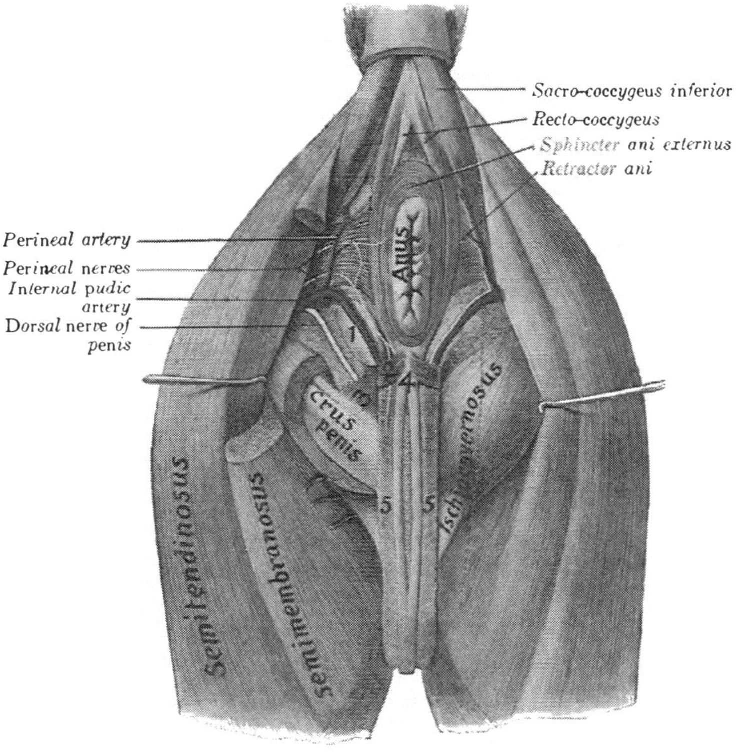

FIG. 452.—DISSECTION OF PERINEUM OF HORSE (MALE).

1 Bulbo-urethral (Cowper's) gland; *2*, transversus perinei muscle (?); *3*, ischio-urethral muscle: retractor penis muscle; *5*, bulbo-cavernosus muscle. (After Schmaltz, Atlas d. Anat. d. Pferdes.)

sacrum, then inclines downward on the pelvic surface of the shaft of the ilium, and divides a little above the psoas tubercle into iliaco-femoral and obturator arteries. The chief branches are as follows:

1. The last pair of **lumbar arteries** pass up through the foramina at the junction of the last lumbar vertebra and the sacrum.

2. The **internal pudic artery** (A. pudenda interna) arises near the origin of the internal iliac. It passes backward and somewhat downward, at first along the iliac head of the obturator internus, then above the superior ischiatic spine on the inner surface of the sacro-sciatic ligament, perforates the latter and runs for a variable distance in its substance or on its external face. It then re-enters the pelvic cavity, passes backward on the retractor ani to the ischial arch, and divides

into the perineal and the artery of the bulb in the male, perineal and artery of the clitoris in the female. It is accompanied by the internal pudic nerve. Its chief branches are as follows:

(1) The **umbilical** artery is given off from the internal pudic about an inch (ca. 2 to 3 cm.) from the origin of that vessel. It is a very large artery in the fœtus, in which it curves downward and forward at the side of the bladder in the edge of the umbilical fold of peritoneum, passes through the umbilical opening, becomes a component of the umbilical cord and ramifies in the fœtal placenta. After birth it extends only to the vertex of the bladder and is much reduced. Its lumen is almost obliterated and its wall is very thick, giving the vessel a cord-like character, hence it is commonly termed the round ligament of the bladder.[1] It

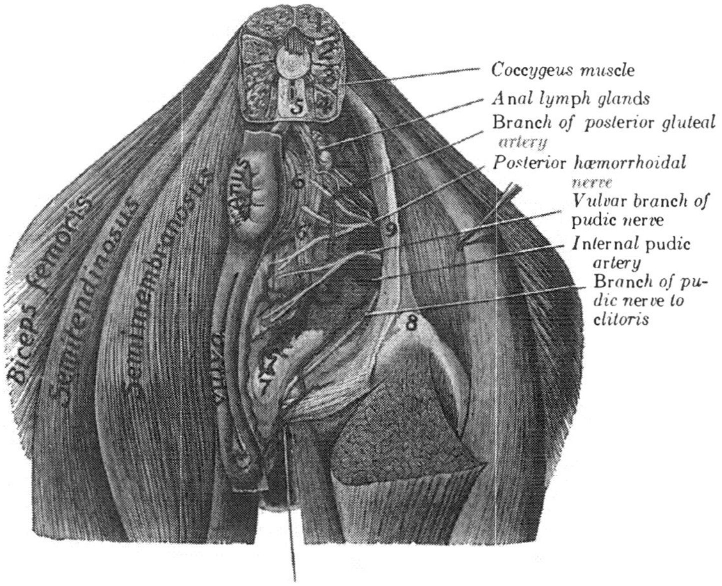

Fig. 453.—Dissection of Perineum of Mare.

1 Sacro-coccygeus superior; 2, sacro-coccygeus lateralis; 3, intertransversales; 4, sacro-coccygeus inferior; 5 recto-coccygeus; 6, sphincter ani externus; 6′, branch connecting sphincter ani with constrictor vulvæ; 7, vestibular bulb; 8, tuber ischii; 9, sacro-sciatic ligament. (After Schmaltz, Atlas d. Anat. d. Pferdes.)

gives off small vesical **branches** (Aa. vesicales craniales) to the bladder, and twigs to the prostate and vasa deferens in the male. In the mare a small branch runs forward along the ureter into the broad ligament of the uterus.

(2) The middle **hæmorrhoidal** or vesico-**prostatic artery** (A. hæmorrhoidalis media) in the male arises usually near the prostate and runs backward lateral to the rectum. It supplies branches to the rectum, bladder, urethra, and accessory genital glands. In the female the homologous vessel is much larger and gives off the posterior uterine **artery** (A. uterina caudalis). This runs forward on the side of the vagina, to which it gives branches, and ramifies on the body of the uterus, anastomosing with the anterior and middle uterine arteries. (In some cases this artery arises from the internal iliac or the umbilical.)

(3) The perineal artery (A. perinei) is relatively small in the male. It passes

[1] The obliteration in the adult extends a variable distance from the vesical end toward the origin, but usually involves only a small part.

upward at the side of the anus, which it supplies, and gives twigs to the bulbo-cavernosus muscle and the skin of the perineum. In the female it is large and is distributed to the anus and vulva, and gives a large branch to the vestibular bulb.

(4) The **artery of the bulb** (A. bulbi urethræ) may be regarded as the direct continuation of the internal pudic in the male. It lies at the side of the urethra above the ischial arch, dips under the bulbo-cavernosus muscle, and ramifies in the corpus spongiosum. Before doing so it gives off a small branch which turns around the ischial arch to reach the dorsum penis, and anastomoses with the deep branch of the obturator.

(4*a*) The **artery of the clitoris** (A. clitoridis) is the homologue in the female of the preceding vessel, but is much smaller. It passes to the ventral surface of the vulva with the internal pudic nerve, supplies the clitoris, and gives twigs to the vulva.

3. The **lateral sacral artery** (A. sacralis lateralis) arises at the lumbo-sacral

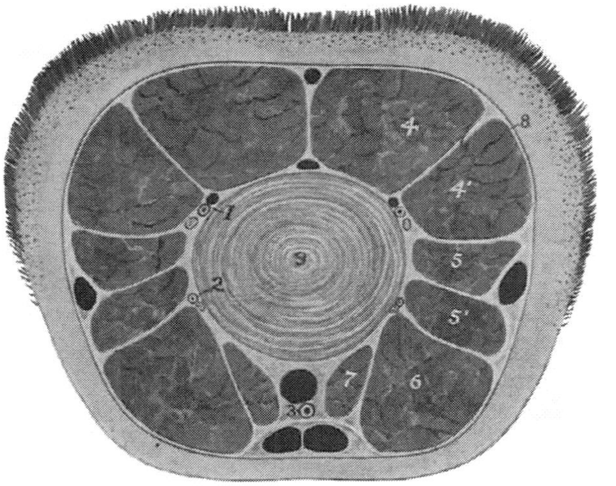

FIG. 454.—CROSS-SECTION OF TAIL OF HORSE.

1, Dorso-lateral coccygeal vessels and nerve; *2*, ventro-lateral coccygeal artery and nerve; *3*, middle coccygeal artery; *4*, sacro-coccygeus superior; *4'*, sacro-coccygeus lateralis; *5*, *5'*, intertransversales; *6*, sacro-coccygeus inferior; *7*, recto-coccygeus; *8*, coccygeal fascia; *9*, fibro-cartilage between fourth and fifth coccygeal vertebræ. The veins are black.

articulation (Fig. 451). It passes backward under the wing of the sacrum, then along the pelvic surface of the bone below the inferior sacral foramina and the nerves emerging from them, and is continued by the lateral coccygeal artery. The branches are as follows:

(1) **Spinal branches** (Rami spinales) enter the vertebral canal through the foramen between the last lumbar vertebra and the sacrum and through the ventral sacral foramina. They give off branches to the spinal cord and its membranes which reinforce the ventral spinal artery, and others which emerge through the dorsal sacral foramina and supply the muscles and skin of the croup.

(2) The **middle coccygeal artery** (A. coccygea) is an unpaired vessel which arises from the right or left lateral sacral or from a lateral coccygeal artery. It passes backward on the pelvic surface of the sacrum to the median line and continues in that position along the tail between the depressor muscles, supplying these and the skin.

(3) The **posterior gluteal or ischiatic artery** (A. glutea caudalis) emerges

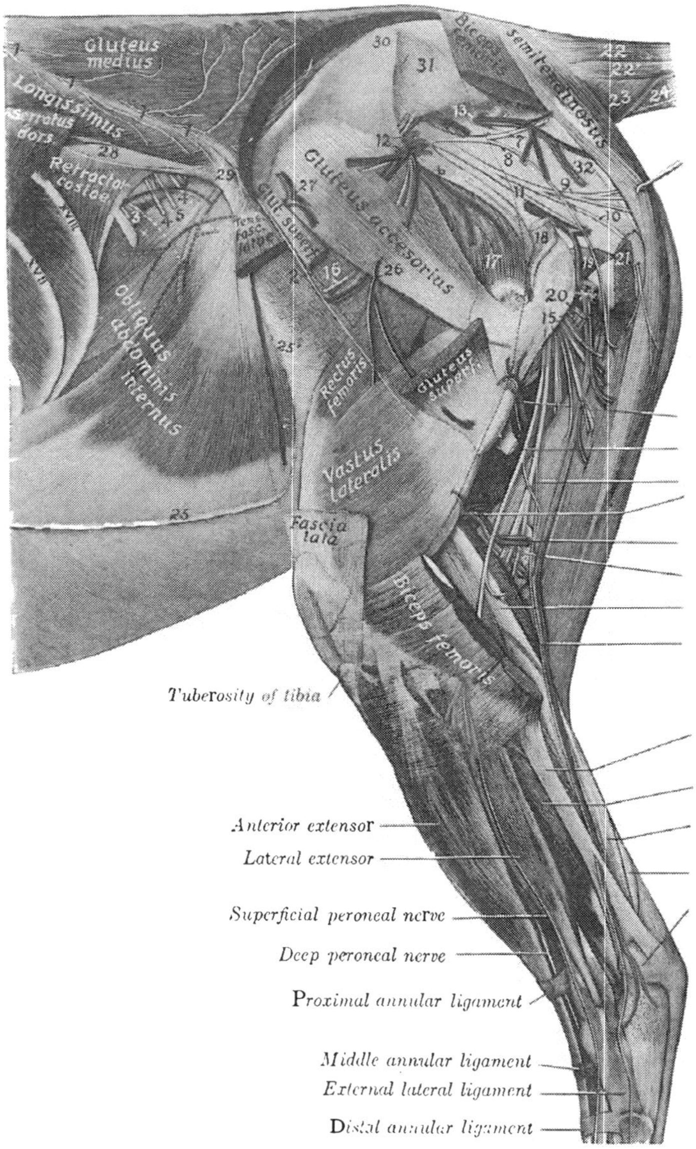

FIG. 455.—DISSECTION OF PELVIS, THIGH, AND LEG OF HORSE, EXTERNAL VIEW.

1, Dorsal branches of last intercostal and first three lumbar nerves; *2*, cutaneous branch of fourth lumbar nerve; *3*, ventral branches of last intercostal nerve; *4*, branches of ilio-hypogastric nerve; *5*, superficial branch of ilio-inguinal nerve; *6*, great sciatic nerve; *7*, *8*, nerves to biceps femoris (from posterior gluteal nerve); *9*, nerve to semitendinosus (from same); *10*, posterior cutaneous nerve of thigh; *11*, internal pudic nerve; *12*, anterior gluteal vessels and nerves; *13*, posterior gluteal (or ischiatic) vessels; *14*, branches of obturator vessels; *15*, proximal muscular branches of great sciatic nerve to biceps femoris, semitendinosus, and semimembranosus; *16*, nerve to tensor fasciæ latæ (from anterior gluteal nerve); *17*, gluteus profundus; *18*, stump of gluteus medius; *19*, gemellus; *20*, trochanter major; *21*, stump of biceps femoris; *22*, sacro-coccygeus superior; *22'*, sacro-coccygeus lateralis; *23*, coccygeus; *24*, sacro-coccygeus inferior; *25*, line of fusion of aponeuroses of internal and external oblique muscles of abdomen; *25'*, aponeurosis of external oblique muscle (lamina iliaca); *26*, branches of iliaco-femoral vessels; *27*, ilio-lumbar vessels; *28*, ilio-lumbar ligament or deep layer of lumbo-dorsal fascia; *29*, external angle of ilium; *30*, internal angle of ilium; *31*, lateral sacro-iliac ligament; *32*, sacro-sciatic ligament. (After Schmaltz, Atlas d. Anat. d. Pferdes.)

through the upper part of the sacro-sciatic ligament and runs backward and downward on the latter under cover of the biceps femoris (Fig. 455). It gives branches to that muscle and to the semitendinosus and semimembranosus, and anastomoses with the obturator, deep femoral, and posterior femoral arteries.

(4) The **lateral coccygeal artery** (A. caudalis lateralis ventralis) continues the direction of the lateral sacral, but is much smaller than the preceding vessel. It passes back between the depressor and intertransversales muscles of the tail and divides into two branches which supply twigs to the muscles and skin.

4. The **ilio-lumbar artery** (A. iliolumbalis) arises at a right angle from the internal iliac and runs outward behind the sacro-iliac joint, crossing the ventral surface of the ilium under cover of the iliacus muscle. It gives branches to the iliopsoas and longissimus, and terminates by turning around the external border of the

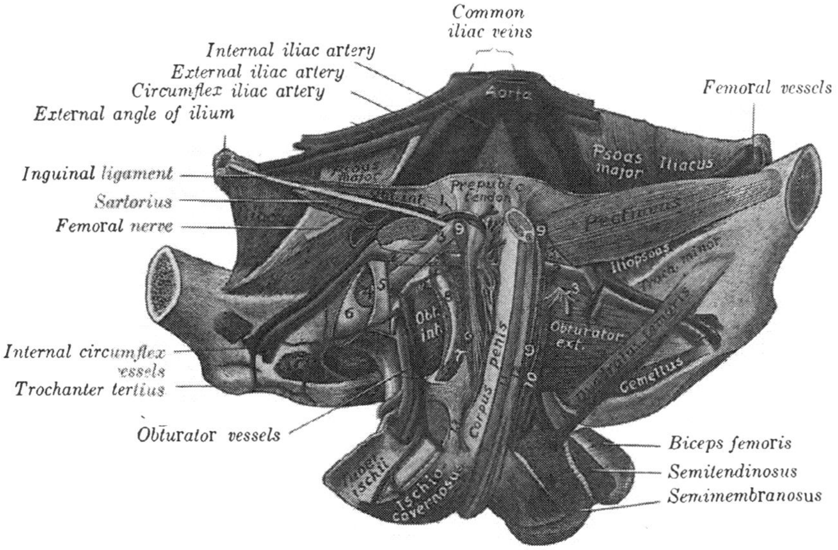

FIG. 456.—DEEP DISSECTION OF VENTRAL WALL OF PELVIS OF HORSE (MALE).

1, External pudic artery and small satellite vein; *2*, anastomosis between external pudic and internal circumflex veins; *3*, accessory ligament; *4*, round ligament; *5*, transverse ligament; *6*, head of femur; *7*, obturator externus (stumps); *8*, inner margin of obturator foramen; *9*, origin of gracilis; *10*, origin of adductor; *11*, bulbocavernosus; *12*, retractor penis; *13*, suspensory ligament of penis. (After Schmaltz, Atlas d. Anat. d. Pferdes.)

ilium a little behind the external angle, giving branches to the gluteus medius and tensor fasciæ latæ (Fig. 455).

5. The **anterior gluteal artery** (A. glutea cranialis) is the largest branch of the internal iliac. It arises usually opposite to the preceding vessel and passes outward through the great sacro-sciatic foramen, dividing into several branches as it emerges; these enter the gluteal muscles (Fig. 455).

6. The **iliaco-femoral** or **external circumflex artery** (A. circumflexa femoris lateralis) passes downward and outward across and beneath the shaft of the ilium, under cover of the iliacus muscle, and dips in between the rectus femoris and vastus externus. It is accompanied by two satellite veins. It gives collateral branches to the iliopsoas, the glutei, and the tensor fasciæ latæ, supplies the nutrient artery of the ilium, and terminates in the quadriceps femoris (Fig. 455).

7. The **obturator artery** (A. obturatoria), the inner terminal branch of the internal iliac, passes downward and backward on the pelvic surface of the shaft of

the ilium along the ventral border of the iliac head of the obturator internus, accompanied by the satellite vein and nerve, which lie in front of the artery (Fig. 451). On reaching the anterior border of the obturator foramen it dips under the obturator internus and passes obliquely through the foramen. In this part of its course it gives off a vesical branch and twigs to the obturator internus and the hip-joint. After its emergence from the pelvic cavity it runs backward on the ventral face of the ischium, passes through the semimembranosus and, in the male, enters the crus penis, forming the arteria profunda penis. It anastomoses with the internal pudic, and usually with the external pudic by a branch which runs forward on the dorsum penis. Large collateral branches are detached to the adductors of the thigh, the biceps femoris and semitendinosus, forming anastomoses with the deep femoral and posterior femoral arteries. In the female the terminal part is small and enters the root of the clitoris.

ARTERIES OF THE PELVIC LIMB

The main arterial trunk of each pelvic limb descends as far as the lower border of the popliteus muscle, where it divides into the anterior and posterior tibial arteries. The different parts of the trunk receive special names which correspond to the several regions through which it passes. In the abdomen it is termed the **external iliac artery,** in the proximal two-thirds of the thigh it is called the **femoral artery,** while below this it is termed the **popliteal artery.**

THE EXTERNAL ILIAC ARTERY (Figs. 450, 451)

The **external iliac artery** (A. iliaca externa) arises from the aorta under the fifth lumbar vertebra, usually just in front of the origin of the internal iliac. It descends at the side of the pelvic inlet along the tendon of the psoas minor, crosses the insertion of that muscle, and reaches the level of the anterior border of the pubis, where it becomes the femoral artery. It is covered by the peritoneum and fascia, and is related behind to the corresponding vein. Its branches are as follows:

1. The **circumflex iliac artery** (A. circumflexa ilium profunda) arises from the external iliac at its origin or from the aorta directly. It passes across the iliac fascia toward the external angle of the ilium, near which it divides into two branches. The artery lies between the fascia and the peritoneum and is accompanied by two veins and the external cutaneous nerve of the thigh. The **anterior branch** gives twigs to the iliacus and psoas muscles, and passes downward and forward in the flank between the obliquus internus and transversus abdominis, in which it ramifies. The **posterior branch** perforates the abdominal wall and runs downward on the inner face of the tensor fasciæ latæ to the fold of the flank, supplying branches to that muscle, the panniculus, the precrural lymph-glands, and the skin.

2. The **cremasteric artery** (A. spermatica externa) is a very small vessel which arises in a variable manner. It springs most often from the external iliac near its origin, but may come from the circumflex iliac, the aorta between the external and internal iliac, or the latter vessel. It accompanies the cremaster muscle to the inguinal canal, supplies twigs to that muscle, the tunica vaginalis, and other constituents of the spermatic cord (Fig. 450).

2*a*. The **middle uterine artery** (A. uterina media) of the female is regarded as the homologue of the preceding vessel. It has a similar origin, but is a much larger artery, which passes between the layers of the broad ligament and reaches the horn of the uterus close to its junction with the body. It is distributed to both, and anastomoses with the anterior and posterior uterine arteries.

THE FEMORAL ARTERY (Figs. 450, 451)

The **femoral artery** is the main arterial trunk of the thigh. It begins at the level of the anterior border of the pubis, from which it is separated by the femoral vein. It descends almost vertically in the femoral canal behind the sartorius muscle, covered at first by the internal femoral fascia and lower down by the gracilis. After passing over the insertion of the pectineus, it perforates the adductor muscle, crosses in the vascular groove of the posterior surface of the femur and is continued between the two heads of the gastrocnemius as the popliteal artery.

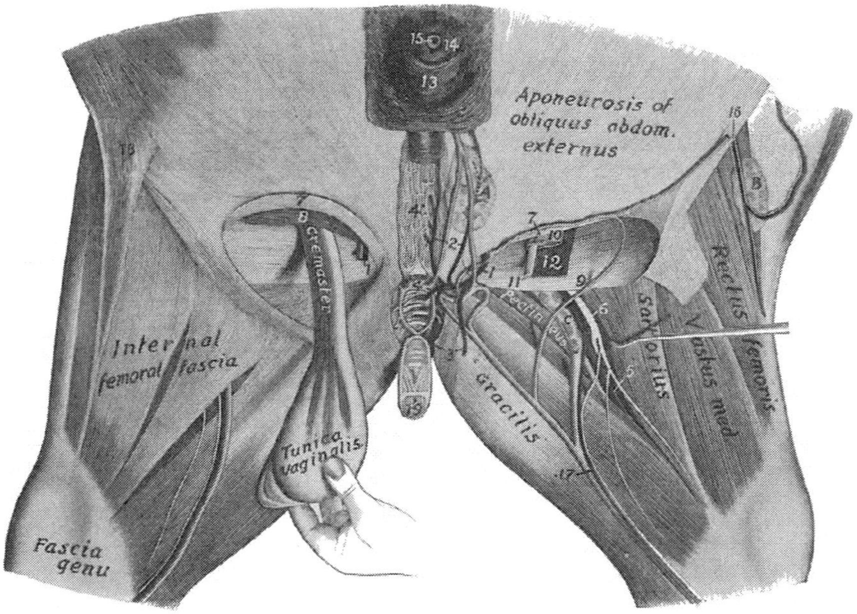

FIG. 457.—DISSECTION OF INGUINAL REGION AND INNER SURFACE OF THIGH OF HORSE.

1, External pudic artery; *2*, anterior branches of *1*; *3*, posterior branches of *1*; *4*, transverse anastomosis between external pudic veins; *4'*, venous plexus of dorsum penis; *5*, femoral artery; *6*, saphenous nerve; *7*, anterior border of external inguinal ring; *8*, obliquus abdominis internus; *9*, posterior border of external inguinal ring; *10*, tunica vaginalis; *11*, vas deferens; *12*, cremaster muscle; *13*, prepuce; *14*, glans penis; *15*, external urethral orifice; *16*, posterior branches of circumflex iliac vessels; *17*, saphenous vessels; *18*, fold of flank; *19*, penis (cut); *A*, superficial inguinal lymph glands; *B*, precrural lymph glands; *C*, deep inguinal lymph glands. (After Schmaltz, Atlas d. Anat. d. Pferdes.)

It is related at its origin to the sartorius in front, the femoral vein behind (which separates it from the pectineus), and the iliacus externally. Lower down it is related superficially to the deep inguinal lymph glands, and deeply to the vastus internus, while the saphenous nerve is in front of it, and the vein passes to its external face. The chief branches are as follows:

1. The **prepubic artery** (Truncus pudendo-epigastricus) arises from the femoral artery at its origin, usually by a common trunk with the deep femoral. It passes forward and a little inward and downward across the edge of the inguinal ligament, and then runs on the abdominal surface of the ligament to the inner part of the internal inguinal ring, where it divides over the upper border of the internal oblique muscle into the posterior abdominal and external pudic arteries.

(1) The **posterior abdominal artery** (A. epigastrica caudalis) passes along the

external border of the rectus abdominis and anastomoses in the umbilical region with the anterior abdominal artery (Figs. 272). It supplies branches to the rectus and obliquus internus muscles.

(2) The **external pudic artery** (A. pudenda externa) descends on the inguinal ligament through the inner part of the inguinal canal and emerges at the inner angle of the external ring. In the male it divides into the **subcutaneous abdominal artery** and the **dorsal artery of the penis.** The former runs forward a short distance from the linea alba, and gives branches to the superficial inguinal lymph glands, the sheath, and the scrotum. The latter passes to the dorsum penis and ends at the glans as the arteria glandis. It gives off collateral branches (Rami profundi penis) to the corpus cavernosum, one of which usually passes backward and anastomoses with a branch of the obturator artery. Branches are also supplied to the superficial inguinal lymph glands, the prepuce, and the scrotum. In the female the **mammary artery** takes the place of the dorsal artery of the penis; it plunges into the base of the mammary gland.

2. The **deep femoral artery** (A. profunda femoris) arises either by a common trunk with the prepubic or a little distal to it (Fig. 451). It passes backward and downward across the inner face of the femoral vein, then below the pubis in the space between the hip joint and the pectineus muscle. On reaching the obturator externus it inclines more ventrally and outward, passes out between the internal border of the femur and the quadratus femoris, and ramifies in the biceps femoris and semitendinosus. It supplies large collateral branches to the adductor muscles and twigs to the deep inguinal lymph glands and the hip joint.

3. The **anterior femoral artery** (A. femoralis cranialis) arises a little distal to the preceding vessel from the opposite side of the femoral trunk. It passes forward, outward, and a little downward across the deep face of the sartorius, and dips in between the rectus femoris and vastus internus (Fig. 451). It is related externally to the ilio-psoas and the femoral nerve.

In some cases this artery is replaced by a large branch of the external circumflex, which passes between the ilio-psoas and rectus femoris and enters the interstice between the latter muscle and the vastus internus.

4. Innominate **muscular branches** (Rami musculares) of variable size and arrangement are given off to the muscles of this vicinity.

5. The **saphenous artery** (A. saphena) is a small vessel which arises from the femoral about its middle or from a muscular branch, and emerges between the sartorius and gracilis or through the latter to the inner surface of the thigh (Fig. 457). It is joined by the large saphenous vein and the saphenous nerve and passes down superficially on the fore part of the gracilis, continues on the deep fascia of the leg, and divides above the hock into two branches, which accompany the radicles of the vein. It gives off cutaneous twigs and anastomoses with the recurrent tibial artery.

In some cases this anastomosis does not occur. The artery may be larger and directly continuous with the internal tarsal artery.

6. The **articular branch** (A. genu suprema) is a slender artery which arises from the femoral just before it passes through the adductor. It descends along the posterior border of the vastus internus to the inner surface of the stifle joint, where it ramifies.

7. The **nutrient artery of the femur** (A. nutritia femoris) is given off at the middle of the femur and enters the nutrient foramen.

8. The **posterior femoral** or **femoro-popliteal artery** (A. femoris caudalis) is a large vessel which arises from the posterior face of the femoral just before the trunk passes between the two heads of the gastrocnemius (Fig. 455). It is very short and divides into two branches. The ascending branch passes upward and outward

between the adductor (in front) and the semimembranosus (behind), and enters the biceps femoris, in which it ramifies. The descending branch passes downward and backward on the external head of the gastrocnemius, then curves upward between the biceps femoris and semitendinosus (crossed externally by the tibial nerve) and divides into branches to these muscles. A branch is detached from the convexity of the curve which passes down between the heads of the gastrocnemius, gives branches to that muscle and the flexor perforans, and is continued by a slender artery which accompanies the tibial nerve and unites with the recurrent tibial artery. A branch ascends alongside of the sciatic nerve between the biceps and semitendinosus and anastomoses with a descending branch of the obturator.

The Popliteal Artery

This artery (A. poplitea) is the direct continuation of the femoral. It lies between the two heads of the gastrocnemius, at first on the posterior face of the femur, then on the femoro-tibial joint capsule. It then passes down through the popliteal notch under cover of the popliteus, inclines outward, and divides near the upper part of the interosseous space into anterior and posterior tibial arteries. The satellite vein lies along its inner side. Collateral branches are supplied to the stifle joint and the gastrocnemius and popliteus.

POSTERIOR TIBIAL ARTERY

The **posterior tibial artery** (A. tibialis posterior) is much the smaller of the two terminals of the popliteal. It lies at first between the tibia and the popliteus, then between that muscle and the deep and inner heads of the deep flexor. Lower down it descends along the tendon of the inner head, becomes superficial in the distal third of the leg, and passes behind the tendon. At the level of the tuber calcis it forms an ᔕ-shaped curve, runs downward along the deep flexor tendon accompanied by the plantar nerves, and divides at the lower part of the hock into internal and external plantar arteries. The collateral branches are as follows:

1. The **nutrient artery of the tibia** (A. nutritia tibiæ).
2. **Muscular branches** (Rami musculares) to the popliteus and deep flexor.
3. The **external tarsal artery** (A. tarsea lateralis) arises at the distal end of the leg and is distributed to the outer surface of the hock. It gives off a small recurrent branch which ascends along the external border of the gastrocnemius tendon and anastomoses with a branch of the posterior femoral artery.
4. The **recurrent tibial artery** (A. tibialis recurrens) is given off from the second part of the curve, ascends in relation to the tibial nerve, and anastomoses with the descending branch of the posterior femoral and with the saphenous artery.
5. Small branches (internal calcaneal) to the inner aspect of the hock.
6. The **plantar arteries,** internal and external (A. plantaris medialis, lateralis), are the small terminals of the posterior tibial. They descend along the sides of the tarsal sheath of the deep flexor with the plantar nerves to the proximal part of the metatarsus, where they unite with the perforating tarsal artery to form the **plantar arch** (Arcus plantaris). Four **plantar metatarsal arteries** proceed from this arch. The two slender **superficial plantar metatarsal arteries** (A. metatarsea plantaris superficialis medialis, lateralis) descend on either side of the deep flexor tendon with the plantar nerves and unite with the great metatarsal or with the corresponding digital artery. The two **deep** or **interosseous plantar metatarsal arteries** (A. metatarsea plantaris profundus medialis, lateralis) descend between the suspensory ligament and the corresponding small metatarsal bone and unite near the fetlock with the great metatarsal. The inner artery is the larger of the

two and usually appears to be the continuation of the perforating tarsal. It supplies the nutrient artery of the large metatarsal bone. In other cases it is

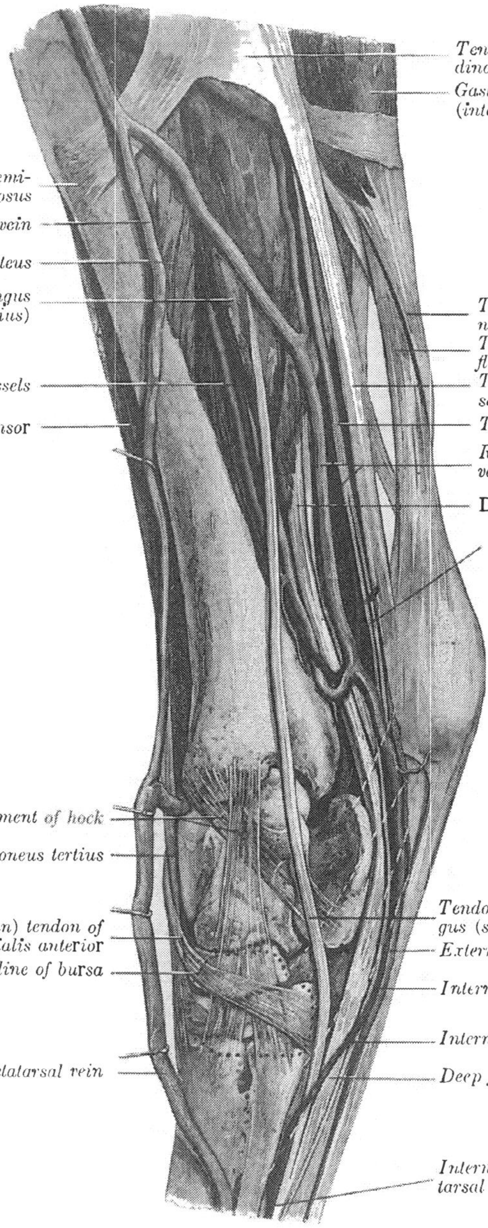

Fig. 458.—Dissection of Leg and Hock of Horse, inner View. (After Schmaltz, Atlas d. Anat. d. Pferdes.)

the direct continuation of the internal plantar artery, the external artery only uniting with the perforating tarsal.

ANTERIOR TIBIAL ARTERY

The anterior tibial artery (A. tibialis anterior) is much the larger of the two terminal branches of the popliteal. It passes forward through the upper part of

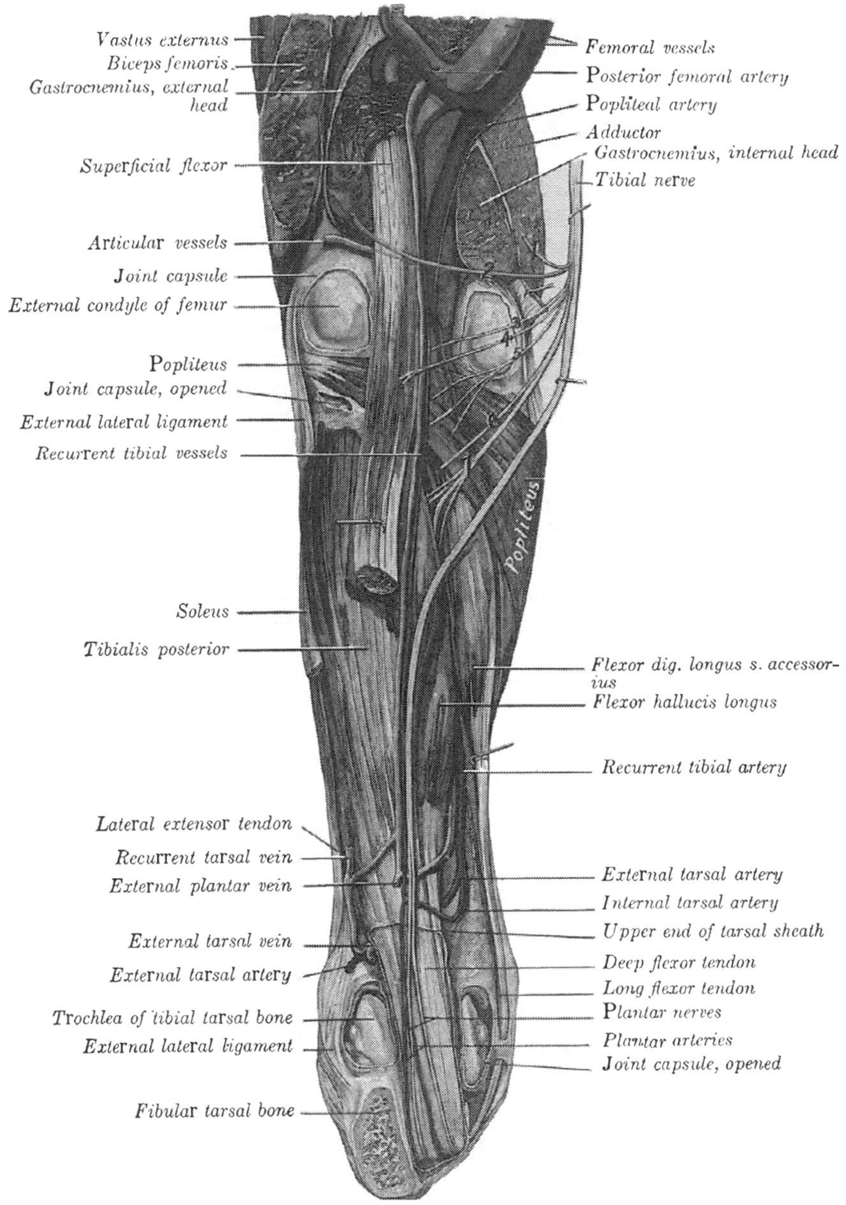

Fig. 459.—Deep Dissection of Right Stifle, Leg, and Hock of Horse, Posterior View.

The hock is flexed at a right angle, and the tuber calcis is sawn off. The tibial nerve is drawn inward to show its muscular branches. Branches of tibial nerve: *1*, *2*, to gastrocnemius; *3*, *4*, to superficial flexor; *5*, to popliteus; *6*, to flexor longus or accessorius; *7*, to deep flexor. (After Schmaltz, Atlas d. Anat. d. Pferdes.)

the interosseous space and descends with two satellite veins on the outer part of the front of the tibia, under cover of the tibialis anterior. At the lower part of the

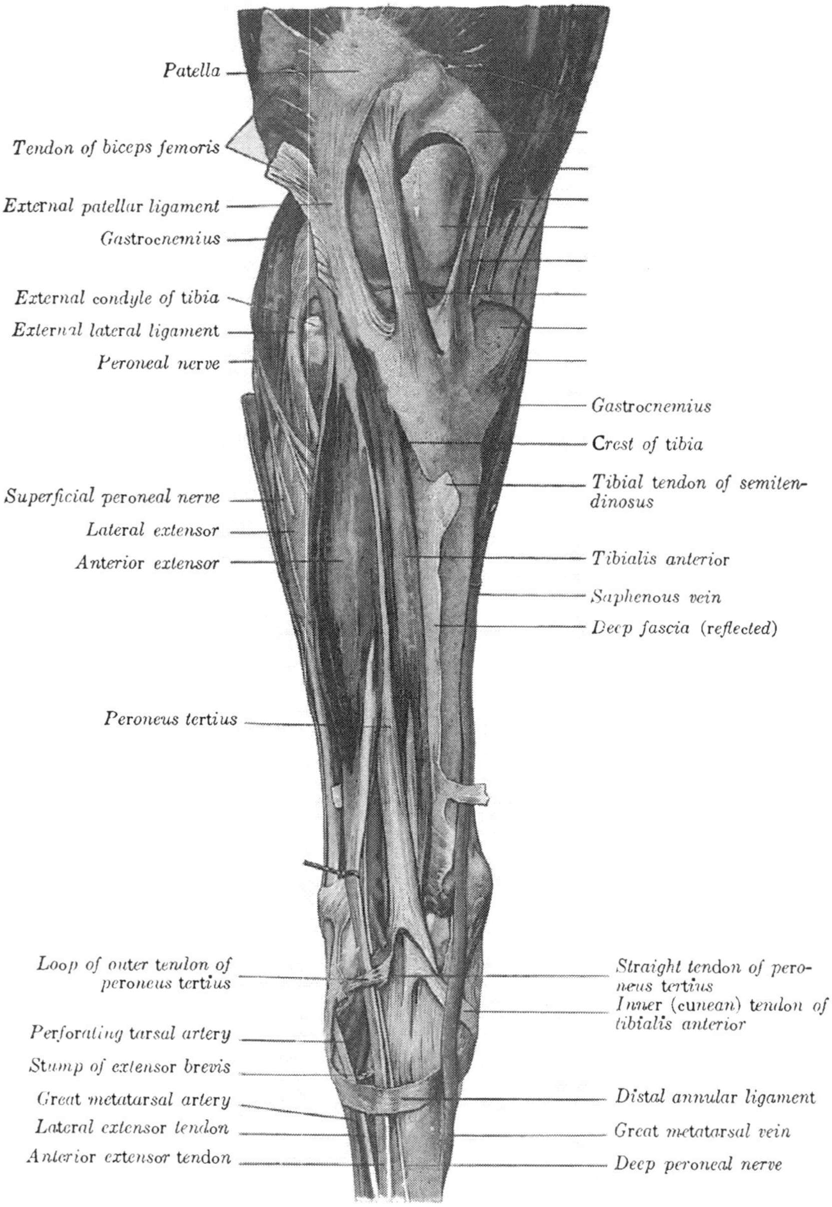

Fig. 460.—Superficial Dissection of Right Stifle, Leg, and Hock of Horse, Front View. (After Schmaltz, Atlas d. Anat. d. Pferdes.)

leg it deviates to the outer border of the tendon of this muscle, passes on to the capsule of the hock joint, gives off the perforating tarsal artery, and is continued as the great metatarsal artery. It gives off muscular branches to the dorso-lateral group of muscles of the leg and articular branches to the hock. The peroneal branch (A. peronea) is a variable vessel which descends along the fibula under the lateral extensor; it gives off muscular branches and one which perforates the fascia and divides into ascending and descending cutaneous twigs.

The perforating tarsal artery (A. tarsea perforans) is given off under cover of the outer tendon of the peroneus tertius. It passes backward through the vascular canal of the tarsus with a satellite vein and unites on the upper part of the suspensory ligament with the plantar arteries (or only with the external plantar) to form the plantar arch.

In well-injected specimens it is seen that there is a fine arterial network (Rete tarsi dorsale) on the flexor surface of the hock, which is formed by twigs from the anterior tibial and lateral tarsal arteries. From it proceed two very slender dorsal metatarsal arteries. The inner one descends in the furrow between the inner small and large metatarsal bones, and anastomoses usually in the proximal part of the metatarsus with the internal superficial plantar metatarsal, uniting sometimes with the deep plantar metatarsal. The external vessel passes down under the periosteum on the anterior face of the large metatarsal bone and becomes lost or joins the large metatarsal artery.

Sometimes the anterior tibial artery passes undivided through the tarsus, gives off the internal deep plantar metatarsal, and is continued as a very large internal superficial plantar metatarsal along the deep flexor tendon, thus resembling the arrangement in the fore limb.

In a few cases the perforating tarsal is a large vessel, directly continuing the anterior tibial, and is continued by a large internal deep plantar metatarsal. The great metatarsal is then small. Other variations are common.

THE GREAT METATARSAL ARTERY

This artery (A. metatarsea dorsalis lateralis) is the direct continuation of the anterior tibial. It passes downward and outward under the extensor brevis and the tendon of the lateral extensor, at first on the joint capsule and then in the oblique vascular groove on the upper part of the large metatarsal bone. It then descends in the groove formed by the apposition of the large and external small metatarsals, inclines inward between the two, and divides on the lower part of the posterior face of the large metatarsal bone into the internal and external digital arteries. It is not usually accompanied by a vein. Beyond this the arterial arrangement is the same as in the thoracic limb.

THE VEINS[1]

PULMONARY VEINS

The terminal pulmonary veins (Vv. pulmonales), usually seven or eight in number, return the aërated blood from the lungs and open into the left atrium of the heart. They are destitute of valves. Their tributaries arise in the capillary plexuses in the lobules of the lungs, and unite to form larger and larger trunks which accompany the branches of the bronchi and pulmonary arteries. A very large vein is formed by the union at an acute angle of a trunk from each lung, where the latter are adherent to each other.

SYSTEMIC VEINS

The Veins of the Heart (Figs. 426, 427)

The coronary sinus (Sinus coronarius) is a very short bulbous trunk which receives most of the blood from the wall of the heart. It is situated just

[1] Most of the veins are depicted in the illustrations of the section on the arteries, to which reference is to be made.

below the termination of the posterior vena cava and is covered in part by a thin layer of ventricular muscle-fibers. It opens into the right atrium just below the posterior vena cava. It is formed by the union of two tributaries. The **great cardiac or left coronary vein** (V. cordis magna) begins at the left side of the apex of the heart, ascends in the left longitudinal groove and turns backward in the coronary groove, in which it winds around the posterior border of the heart to the right side and joins the coronary sinus. The **middle cardiac or right coronary vein** (V. cordis media) begins on the right side of the apex, ascends in the right longitudinal groove and joins the coronary sinus, or opens separately into the atrium just in front of the orifice of the left vein, so that a common trunk (coronary sinus) does not then exist.

The **small cardiac veins** (Vv. cordis minores), three to five in number, are small vessels which return some blood from the right ventricle and atrium; they open into the latter near the coronary groove in spaces between the musculi pectinati.

THE ANTERIOR VENA CAVA (Fig. 429)

The anterior vena cava (V. cava cranialis) returns to the heart the blood from the head, neck, thoracic limbs, and the greater part of the thoracic wall. It is formed at the ventral part of the thoracic inlet by the confluence of the two jugular and two brachial veins. Its origin is attached to the first pair of ribs. It passes backward in the anterior mediastinum, at first median and ventral to the common carotid trunk, then deviates to the right of the anterior aorta, and opens into the right atrium opposite to the third rib. The demarcation between vein and atrium is not very distinct. It contains no valves except at the mouths of its radicles. Its length is about five to six inches (ca. 12 to 15 cm.) and its caliber about two inches (ca. 5 cm.) in a subject of medium size. Its right face is crossed by the right phrenic nerve, and on the left it is related to the anterior aorta and brachiocephalic artery. It receives, in addition to small pericardial and mediastinal veins, the following tributaries:

1. The **internal thoracic vein** (V. thoracica interna) is a satellite of the artery of that name. It opens into the anterior vena cava at the first rib.

2. The **vertebral vein** (V. vertebralis) corresponds to the homonymous artery. On the right side it terminates either in front of the deep cervical vein or by a short common trunk with it. On the left side it almost always unites with the deep cervical and vertebral vein to form a common trunk.

3. The **deep or superior cervical vein** (V. cervicalis profunda) corresponds to the artery. On the right side it leaves the artery at the first intercostal space, crosses the right face of the trachea and opens into the vena cava; it may form a common trunk with the dorsal or vertebral. On the left side there is nearly always a common trunk for all three.

4. The **dorsal vein** (V. costo-cervicalis) corresponds to the artery. On the right side it leaves the artery on entering the thorax, crosses the right face of the trachea, and opens into the vena cava in front of the deep cervical or by a common trunk with it. On the left side it almost always joins the deep cervical and vertebral to form a short common trunk which crosses the left face of the intrathoracic part of the brachial artery opposite the second rib and opens into the anterior vena cava.

The Vena Azygos

The vena azygos (Fig. 429) is an unpaired vessel which arises at the level of the first lumbar vertebra by radicles coming from the psoas and the crura of the diaphragm; it is connected with the first lumbar vein. It passes forward along the right side of the bodies of the thoracic vertebræ, in contact usually with the thoracic duct, which separates the vein from the aorta. At the seventh vertebra it leaves the spine, curves downward and forward over the right side of the thoracic duct, trachea, and œsophagus, and opens into the right atrium opposite the third intercostal space. Its tributaries are:

1. The last fourteen **intercostal veins** (Vv. intercostales) of the right side. On the left side the last four to seven intercostal veins usually empty into the vena **hemiazygos**. This vessel runs on the left side of the aorta from the fourteenth to the eleventh thoracic vertebra, passes between the aorta and the spine, and joins the vena azygos. In its absence its tributaries join the vena azygos.

2. The **œsophageal vein** (V. œsophagea), satellite of the œsophageal artery, joins the vena azygos as it inclines downward.

3. The **bronchial vein** (Vena bronchialis) unites with the preceding to form a short common trunk (Ellenberger-Baum), or empties into the great coronary vein (Chauveau).[1]

VEINS OF THE HEAD AND NECK

Jugular Veins

The **jugular veins** (Vv. jugulares), right and left (Fig. 431), arise behind the posterior border of the lower jaw about two and a half inches (ca. 6 to 7 cm.) below the temporo-maxillary articulation by the union of the superficial temporal and internal maxillary veins. Each passes downward and backward, at first embedded more or less in the parotid gland, and continues in the jugular furrow to the thoracic inlet, where it unites with its fellow and the two brachial veins to form the anterior vena cava. In the neck it is covered by the skin, fascia, and panniculus, and is superficial to the carotid artery, from which it is separated in the anterior two-thirds of the region by the omo-hyoideus muscle.[2] It contains valves at the mouths of its tributaries and has several pairs of semilunar valves variably disposed along its course. Its tributaries are as follows:

1. The **internal maxillary vein** (V. maxillaris interna) is larger than the external maxillary. It may be considered to begin as the continuation backward of the buccinator vein where the vessel crosses the alveolar border of the mandible (about two inches (ca. 5 cm.) behind the last molar tooth). It runs backward on the inner surface of the ramus below the external pterygoid and covered by the internal pterygoid muscle for a distance of about three inches (ca. 7 to 8 cm.), then inclines a little downward and runs ventral to the artery for about an inch (ca. 2 to 3 cm.). It crosses the external face of the artery at the posterior border of the jaw, and is joined by the superficial temporal vein to form the jugular. Its principal radicles are:

(1) The **dorsal lingual vein** (V. dorsalis linguæ), which is a satellite of the lingual nerve.

(2) The **inferior alveolar** or **dental vein** (V. alveolaris mandibulæ), a satellite of the corresponding artery. It often unites with the preceding.

(3) **Pterygoid veins** (Rami pterygoidei).

(4) The **deep temporal vein** (V. temporalis profunda) is a large vessel which receives tributaries from the temporalis muscle and emissaries from the parieto-temporal canal. It is connected with the anterior cerebral vein and usually with

[1] Chauveau says "the bronchial veins, which ramify on the bronchi like the arteries of which they are satellites, open into the great coronary vein very near its mouth, after having united to form a single vessel, which sometimes opens directly into the atrium." Ellenberger and Baum state that the bronchial and œsophageal veins open into the vena azygos separately or by a common trunk. Martin describes a short broncho-œsophageal trunk, but the vein which he figures as the bronchial does not come from the lungs, but is a small mediastinal vessel. The author finds such a vessel entering the terminal part of the œsophageal vein, but no distinct bronchial vein in the horse.

[2] M'Fadyean records a case in which the vein lay on the deep face of the omo-hyoideus with the carotid artery.

the meningeal veins by its frontal branch. The latter drains chiefly the lacrimal gland and passes behind the supraorbital process.

2. The superficial temporal vein (V. temporalis superficialis) is a satellite of the corresponding artery. It is formed by the confluence of the anterior auricular and transverse facial veins. The former receives the superior cerebral vein (V. cerebralis dorsalis), which is the emissary of the transverse sinus of the dura mater; it emerges from the parieto-temporal canal behind the postglenoid process. The transverse facial vein (V. transversa faciei) runs at first above the artery of like name, then plunges deeply into the masseter and unites in front with the facial vein. It is connected with the vena reflexa.

3. The inferior masseteric or maxillo-muscular vein (V. masseterica) joins the jugular at the upper border of the sterno-cephalicus tendon. It is a short trunk formed by the confluence at the posterior border of the jaw of masseteric and

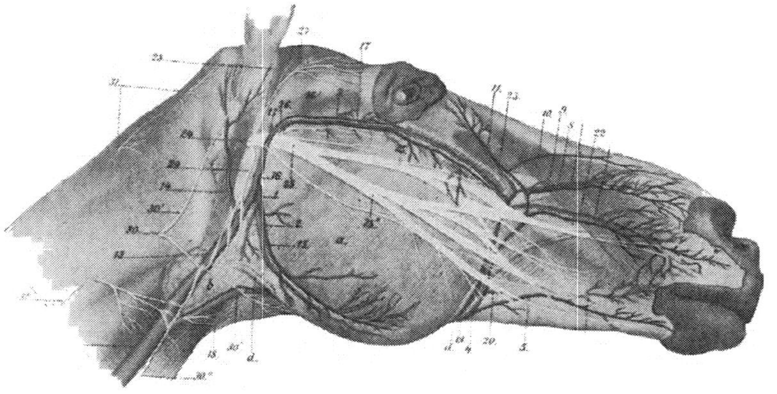

Fig. 461.—Superficial Vessels and Nerves of Head and Anterior Part of Neck of Horse.

a, Masseter; *b*, parotid gland; *c*, parotido-auricularis; *1*, masseteric artery; *2*, parotid branch; *3*, transverse facial artery; *4*, facial artery; *5*, *6*, inferior labial artery; *7*, superior labial artery; *8*, lateral nasal artery; *9*, infraorbital artery; *10* dorsal nasal artery; *11*, angular artery of eye; *12*, *13*, jugular vein; *14*, great auricular vein; *15*, masseteric vein; *16*, superficial temporal vein; *17*, transverse facial vein; *17'*, deep temporal vein; *18*, external maxillary vein; *19*, facial vein; *20*, labial vein; *21*, dorsal nasal vein; *22*, lateral nasal vein; *23*, angular vein of eye; *24*, *25*, facial nerve; *25'*, *25''*, superior and inferior buccal nerves; *26*, transverse facial nerve; *27*, auriculo-palpebral nerve; *28*, anterior auricular nerve; *29*, cervical branch of facial nerve; *30*, ventral branch of second cervical nerve; *30'*, *30''*, *30'''*, auricular and cutaneous branches of *30*; *31*, branches of dorsal division of first and second cervical nerves; *32*, dorsal branch of spinal accessory nerve. (After Leisering's Atlas.)

pterygoid veins. The former is usually connected by a large branch with the buccinator vein.

4. The great auricular vein (V. auricularis magna) is a satellite of the posterior auricular artery above, but joins the jugular a variable distance below and behind the point of origin of the artery.

5. The inferior cerebral vein (V. cerebralis ventralis) is an emissary of the cavernous sinus of the dura. It is a satellite of the internal carotid artery, receives the condyloid vein, and joins the jugular near the occipital vein or by a common trunk with it.

6. The occipital vein (V. occipitalis) arises in the fossa atlantis by the union of muscular and cerebrospinal branches. The former comes from the muscles of the poll and passes through the foramen transversarium. The latter is connected with the occipital sinus of the dura mater and emerges from the spinal canal by the intervertebral foramen.

7. The external maxillary or facial vein (V. maxillaris externa) arises by radicles which correspond in general to the branches of the artery of like name. It passes

down over the cheek along the anterior border of the masseter muscle behind the artery, crossing over the parotid duct, which lies behind the vein lower down. Thus on the ramus and as they turn around its lower border the artery is in front, the vein in the middle, and the duct posterior. In the submaxillary space the vein is ventral to the artery for some distance, then parts company with the artery, runs straight backward along the lower border of the parotid gland, and opens into the jugular vein at the posterior angle of the gland.[1] The chief differences in the tributaries of the vein as compared with the branches of the corresponding artery are as follows:

The **labial veins** (Vv. labiales) form a plexus in the submucous tissue of the cheek from which two veins emerge. The upper one passes back and joins the buccinator vein. The lower one (V. labialis communis) joins the external maxillary vein.

Three veins connect with the external maxillary at the anterior border of the masseter.

The upper one is the **transverse facial,** which unites close to the end of the facial crest.

A little lower is the large valveless **vena reflexa** or **alveolar vein.** This passes back under the upper part of the masseter on the maxilla, turns around the tuber maxillare, perforates the periorbita, and joins the ophthalmic vein. It is relatively small at each end, but presents one or two large fusiform dilatations. It receives the following tributaries: (*a*) The **palatine vein** (V. palatina major), which separates from the palatine artery at the anterior palatine foramen and passes in the groove between the tuber maxillare and the palate bone. The palatine veins form a very rich plexus of valveless vessels in the submucosa of the hard palate, which consists of several layers anteriorly. (*b*) The **sphenopalatine vein** (V. spheno-palatina) forms a rich plexus of valveless vessels on the turbinal bones and the septum nasi. It is usually joined by the **infraorbital vein** (V. infraorbitalis) to form a short common trunk.

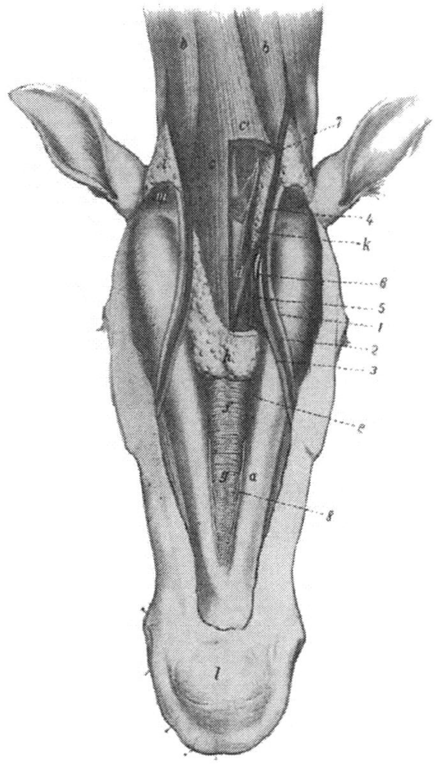

Fig. 462.—Dissection of Submaxillary Space and Adjacent Part of Neck of Horse.

a, Ramus of mandible; *b*, sterno-cephalicus muscle; *c*, *c'*, omo-hyoidei and sterno-hyoidei (portion removed on right side); *d*, hyoid bone; *e*, anterior belly of digastricus; *f*, *g*, mylo-hyoideus; *h*, submaxillary lymph glands (portion removed on right side); *i*, parotid gland; *k*, submaxillary gland; *l*, chin; *m*, stylo-maxillaris; *1*, parotid duct; *2*, facial vein; *3*, facial artery; *4*, external maxillary vein; *5*, sublingual vein; *6*, sublingual artery; *7*, ventral branch of first cervical nerve; *8*, mylo-hyoid nerve. (After Ellenberger, in Leisering's Atlas.)

The venous plexuses are remarkably developed in certain parts of the nasal mucosa. On the septum a little below its middle and on the turbinals the veins are in several layers. The olfactory region does not share in this arrangement and the veins here are small and join the ethmoidal vein.

[1] The venous angle formed by this junction indicates the position of the thyroid gland.

(*c*) The **ophthalmic vein** (V. ophthalmica) is a short trunk, connected in front with the vena reflexa and behind with the cavernous sinus through the foramen lacerum orbitale. It receives veins which correspond to the arterial branches.

The **buccinator vein** (V. buccinatoria) extends backward from the external maxillary along the lower border of the depressor labii inferioris and buccinator under cover of the masseter, passes between the ramus of the mandible and the tuber maxillare and is continued as the internal maxillary vein. It has a large fusiform dilatation and is valveless. It receives a large common labial vein from the labial plexus, and is usually connected with the masseteric vein.

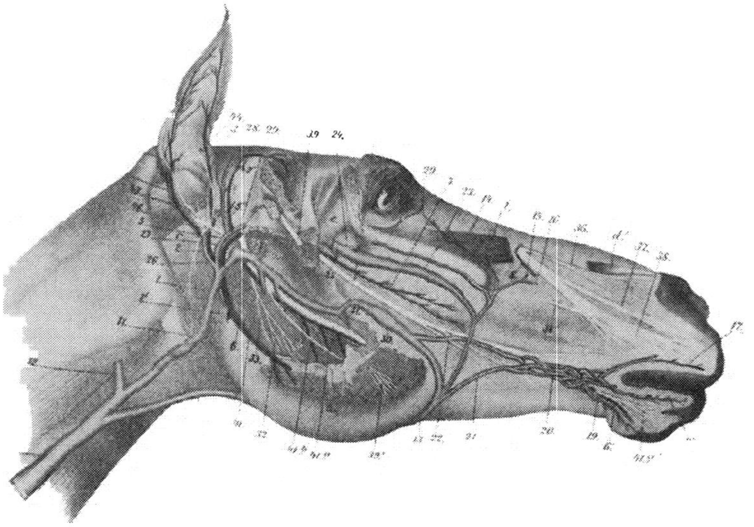

FIG. 463.—DEEPER VESSELS AND NERVES OF HEAD OF HORSE.

The parotid gland, most of the masseter muscle, and a portion of the ramus of the mandible are removed. *a* Remnant of masseter muscle; *b*, internal pterygoid muscle; *c*, stylo-mandibularis; *d*, *d'*, levator labii superioris proprius (portion removed); *e*, periorbita; *1*, masseteric artery; *1'*, parotid branch; *2*, trunk for anterior (*3*) and posterior (*4*) auricular arteries; *5*, *5'*, superficial temporal artery; *5''*, transverse facial artery; *6*, inferior alveolar (or dental) artery; *6'*, mental continuation of *6*; *7*, buccinator artery; *8*, infraorbital artery; *9*, *11*, jugular vein; *10*, external maxillary vein; *12*, inferior cerebral vein; *13*, facial vein; *14*, angular vein of eye; *15*, dorsal nasal vein; *16*, lateral nasal vein; *17*, superior labial vein; *18*, *19*, inferior labial veins; *20*, labial plexus; *21*, *22*, emergent veins of plexus; *23*, vena reflexa; *24*, trunk of sphenopalatine and infraorbital veins; *25*, palatine vein; *26*, great auricular vein; *27*, *28*, superficial temporal vein; *29*, transverse facial vein; *30*, buccinator vein; *31*, dorsal lingual vein; *32*, inferior alveolar or dental vein; *33*, pterygoid vein; *34*, deep temporal vein; *35*, superior cerebral vein; *36*, external nasal nerve; *37*, anterior nasal nerve; *38*, superior labial nerve; *39*, masseteric nerve; *39'*, end branches of *39*; *40*, buccinator nerve; *41*, pterygoid nerve; *41a*, inferior alveolar or dental nerve; *41b*, mylo-hyoid nerve; *42*, posterior auricular nerve; *43*, auricular branch of vagus; *44*, internal auricular nerve; *45*, auriculo-palpebral nerve (cut); *46*, digastric nerve. (After Leisering's Atlas.)

The **lingual vein** (V. lingualis) is not a satellite of the artery. It is formed at the side of the lingual process of the hyoid bone by the confluence of several veins which come from the substance of the tongue. One or two considerable vessels run partly in the substance of the hyo-glossus, and another in the genio-hyoideus. The vein is at first covered by the mylo-hyoideus, perforates that muscle, runs back along the omo-hyoideus in relation to the submaxillary lymph glands, and joins the external maxillary near the posterior border of the jaw. Near its termination it receives the **sublingual vein**, or the latter may open into the external maxillary directly.

8. The **thyroid vein** (V. thyreoidea) is a large vessel which joins the jugular near the external maxillary vein. It receives anterior thyroid, laryngeal, and pharyngeal radicles, and sometimes a posterior thyroid vein.

9. **Muscular, tracheal, and œsophageal veins.**

10. The **cephalic vein** (Vena cephalica) enters the jugular near its termination. It will be described with the veins of the thoracic limb.

11. The **inferior cervical vein** (V. cervicalis ascendens) accompanies the artery. It may open into the brachial vein.

The Sinuses of the Dura Mater

These (Sinus duræ matris) are blood-spaces between the meningeal and periosteal layers of the dura mater and are lined with endothelium. In many places the lumen is crossed by fibrous strands. They receive the veins of the brain, communicate with the meningeal and diploic veins, and with veins outside of the cranium; their connections with the latter are by means of small **emissary veins** (Emissaria). They convey the blood directly or indirectly to the jugular veins. Some are paired, others unpaired. They may be divided into dorsal and basilar systems. The **dorsal system** comprises the following:

The **superior longitudinal** or **sagittal sinus** (S. sagittalis superior) is situated in the upper border of the falx cerebri along the internal sagittal crest. It begins at the crista galli and ends at the tentorium osseum by dividing into two transverse sinuses. It receives the superior cerebral veins. Along each side are small pouches

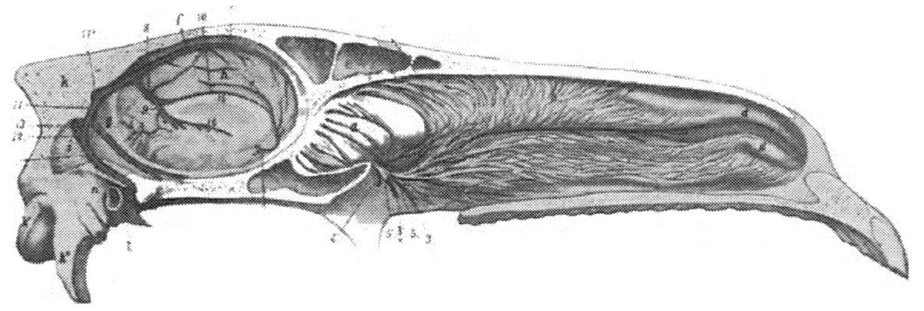

Fig. 464.—Median Section of Head of Horse, Upper Part with Septum Nasi Removed.

a, Lateral mass of ethmoid bone; *b*, superior turbinal; *c*, inferior turbinal; *d*, *d'*, turbinal folds; *e*, frontal sinus; *f*, falx cerebri; *g*, tentorium cerebelli; *h*, medial surface of hemisphere; *i*, cerebellum; k, occipital bone; k', occipital condyle; k'', paramastoid process; *l*, external auditory meatus; *m*, temporal condyle; *n*, parieto-temporal canal; *1*, branches of ethmoidal artery; *2*, *2'*, branches of sphenopalatine artery; *3*, *3'*, branches of sphenopalatine vein; *4*, branches of ethmoidal nerve; *5*, *5'*, branches of sphenopalatine nerve; *6*, artery of corpus callosum; *7*, superior sagittal sinus; *8*, straight sinus; *9*, vena magna cerebri; *10*, inferior sagittal sinus; *11*, *11'*, transverse sinuses; *12*, superior petrosal sinus; *13*, superior occipital sinus; *14*, superior cerebral vein; *15*, corpus callosum; *16*, fornix. (After Ellenberger, in Leisering's Atlas.)

(Lacunæ laterales) into which the veins open. The lumen of the sinus is traversed by fibrous bands and is partially divided by a longitudinal septum.

The **transverse sinuses** (S. transversi), right and left, pass outward in the transverse grooves of the parietal bones, enter the parieto-temporal canals, and are continued by the superior cerebral veins to the superficial temporal veins. The two sinuses are connected by the sinus communicans.

The **inferior longitudinal** or **sagittal sinus** (S. sagittalis inferior) runs backward on the upper surface of the corpus callosum along the concave edge of the falx cerebri and joins the great cerebral vein (of Galen) to form the straight sinus.

The **straight sinus** (S. rectus) passes upward and backward between the cerebral hemispheres and in the tentorium cerebelli and joins the superior sagittal sinus. The point of meeting is the confluence of the sinuses (Confluens sinuum).

The **occipital sinuses** (S. occipitales) lie on either side of the vermis cerebelli. They empty anteriorly into the sinus communicans and communicate behind with the spinal veins.

The **superior petrosal sinuses** (S. petrosi superiores) pass in the tentorium cerebelli to end in the transverse sinuses.

The **basilar system** consists of the following:

The **cavernous sinuses** (S. cavernosi) lie in the inner grooves of the root of the temporal wings of the sphenoid bone at either side of the sella turcica. The two are connected by a wide traverse branch (Sinus intercavernosus) behind and below the posterior part of the pituitary body. Each is continuous in front with the ophthalmic vein and below with the inferior petrosal sinus. The third, sixth, and the ophthalmic and maxillary divisions of the fifth nerve lie along the outer wall of the sinus. The internal carotid artery traverses the sinus and is connected with its fellow by a transverse branch which lies in the corresponding part of the sinus. An oval opening in the floor communicates with the inferior petrosal sinus and transmits the internal carotid artery.

The sinus is not subdivided by strands of fibrous tissue as in man, but a few delicate bands attach the artery to its wall.

The **inferior petrosal sinuses** (S. petrosi inferiores)[1] lie along the borders of the basilar part of the occipital bone, inclosed in the thick dura which closes the foramen lacerum. The anterior part extends about half an inch (ca. 12 mm.) under the temporal wing of the sphenoid. Here communications exist with veins in the pterygo-palatine fossa. The posterior end is bulbous and lies in the condyloid fossa; it communicates with the condyloid vein issuing from the hypoglossal foramen and is drained by the inferior cerebral vein; it also receives an emissary vein from the parieto-temporal canal. The roof of the sinus is perforated by an oval opening at the carotid notch which opens into the cavernous sinus and transmits the internal carotid artery; the latter forms the first bend of its **S**-shaped curve in the petrosal and the second in the cavernous sinus.

The **basilar plexus** (Plexus basilaris) is a venous plexus situated on the upper surface of the basilar part of the occipital bone. It is connected through the hypoglossal foramen with the inferior petrosal sinus and communicates behind with the spinal veins.

The Veins of the Cranium

The **veins of the brain** (Venæ cerebri) do not in general accompany the cerebral arteries. They have very thin walls, no muscular coat, and no valves. They are arranged in two sets, superficial or cortical and deep or central. The superficial veins are more numerous and larger than the arteries. They lie on the surface of the brain in the pia mater and the subarachnoid space.

The **superior cerebral veins** drain the upper and outer part of the cerebral cortex. They receive veins from the medial surfaces of the hemispheres and open into the superior sagittal sinus. Their terminal parts are bulbous and their openings are directed obliquely forward, *i. e.*, contrary to the direction of the bloodstream in the sinus.

The **inferior cerebral veins** lie on the inferior and external aspect of the hemispheres. They open into the inferior system of sinuses. The **middle cerebral vein** runs in the lateral fissure (of Sylvius) and opens into the cavernous sinus.

The **deep cerebral veins** issue from the central or ganglionic parts of the brain at the transverse fissure. They converge to form the **great cerebral vein** (of Galen) (V. magna cerebri). This passes upward and backward behind the splenium of the corpus callosum and is continued as the straight sinus to join the sagittal sinus.

The **superior cerebellar veins** ramify on the upper surface of the cerebellum. They open into the superior system of sinuses and the great cerebral vein. The **inferior cerebellar veins** are larger and go chiefly to the basilar plexus. The veins of the medulla and pons end in the inferior system of sinuses.

The **meningeal veins** (Venæ meningeæ) arise in capillary plexuses in the superficial and deep faces of the dura mater. Some end in the sinuses of the dura, others accompany the meningeal arteries.

[1] These are termed by Chauveau and M'Fadyean the subsphenoidal confluents.

The **diploic veins** (Venæ diploicæ) are anastomosing channels in the spongy substance of the cranial bones. Their walls are thin, consisting in many places only of the endothelium, and they have no valves. Some open inward into venous sinuses, others into extracranial veins.

Spinal Veins

Two **longitudinal spinal veins** or **sinuses** (Sinus columnæ vertebralis) extend along the floor of the vertebral canal, one on either side of the superior common ligament. They are continuous in front with the basilar plexus. They lie in the grooves on the bodies of the vertebræ and are connected by a series of transverse anastomoses which pass between the central part of the bodies of the vertebræ and the superior common ligament or in channels in the bone. They receive veins from the spinal cord, the dura mater, and the bodies of the vertebræ (Venæ basis vertebræ). Through the intervertebral foramina efferent vessels connect with the vertebral, intercostal, lumbar, and lateral sacral veins.

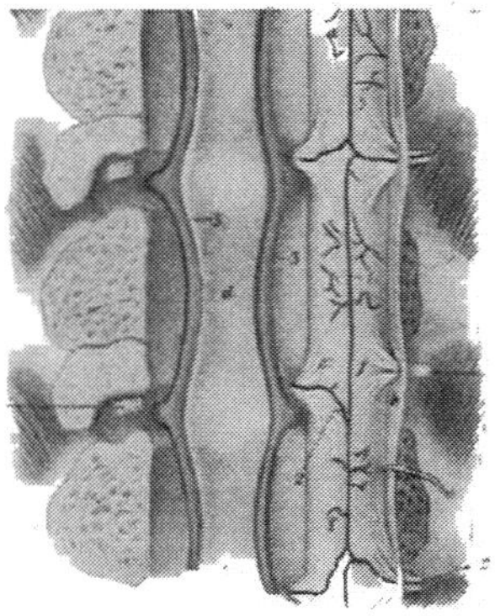

Fig. 465.—Spinal Vessels of Horse.
The vertebral canal has been opened by sawing off the arches. The nerve-roots are cut on one side and the spinal cord turned over to right. *1*, Ventral or middle spinal artery; *2*, reinforcing branches from vertebral, intercostal, or lumbar arteries (according to region); *3*, longitudinal vertebral sinuses; *a*, ventral surface of spinal cord; *b*, dura mater (cut); *c*, nerve-roots; *d*, superior common ligament. (After Ellenberger, in Leisering's Atlas.)

VEINS OF THE THORACIC LIMB

The **brachial vein** (V. brachialis) is a satellite of the extrathoracic part of the brachial artery. It arises at the inner side of the distal end of the shaft of the humerus and passes upward in the arm behind the artery under cover of a layer of fascia and the posterior superficial pectoral muscle. At the shoulder it is ventral to the artery, crosses the anterior border of the first rib, and concurs with its fellow and the two jugulars in the formation of the anterior vena cava. The roots of the vein are somewhat variable, but most often four radial veins in addition to a large oblique branch from the cephalic unite in its formation. Its tributaries correspond in general to the branches of the artery, but a few differences are worthy of notice. The **thoracico-dorsal vein** joins the brachial directly or opens into the deep brachial. The **external thoracic** or **"spur" vein** (V. thoracica externa) is a large vessel which arises in the ventral wall of the abdomen, passes forward (embedded more or less in the panniculus) along the outer border of the posterior deep pectoral muscle, and joins the brachial vein near the first rib. It often communicates with the subscapular vein.

The **cephalic vein** (V. cephalica) arises at the inner side of the carpus as the continuation of the internal superficial metacarpal vein. It runs upward on the deep fascia of the forearm at first in the furrow between the flexor carpi internus and the radius. Toward the middle of the forearm it inclines gradually forward on the inner surface of the radius, accompanied by a cutaneous branch of the median nerve, and arrives at the insertion of the biceps. Here it detaches a large branch (Ramus communicans) which passes upward and backward over the inner insertion of the biceps, the posterior radial artery, and the median nerve, and joins the brachial vein. The vein to this point is often termed the internal subcutaneous vein of the forearm (V. cephalica antebrachii). It is continued (as the V. cephalica humeri) in the furrow between the mastoido-humeralis and the anterior superficial pectoral with a branch of the inferior cervical artery, crosses the deep face of the cervical panniculus, and opens into the terminal part of the jugular or the brachial vein. It receives an **accessory cephalic vein** (V. cephalica accessoria), which arises from the carpal network, runs upward along the inner border of the extensor carpi,

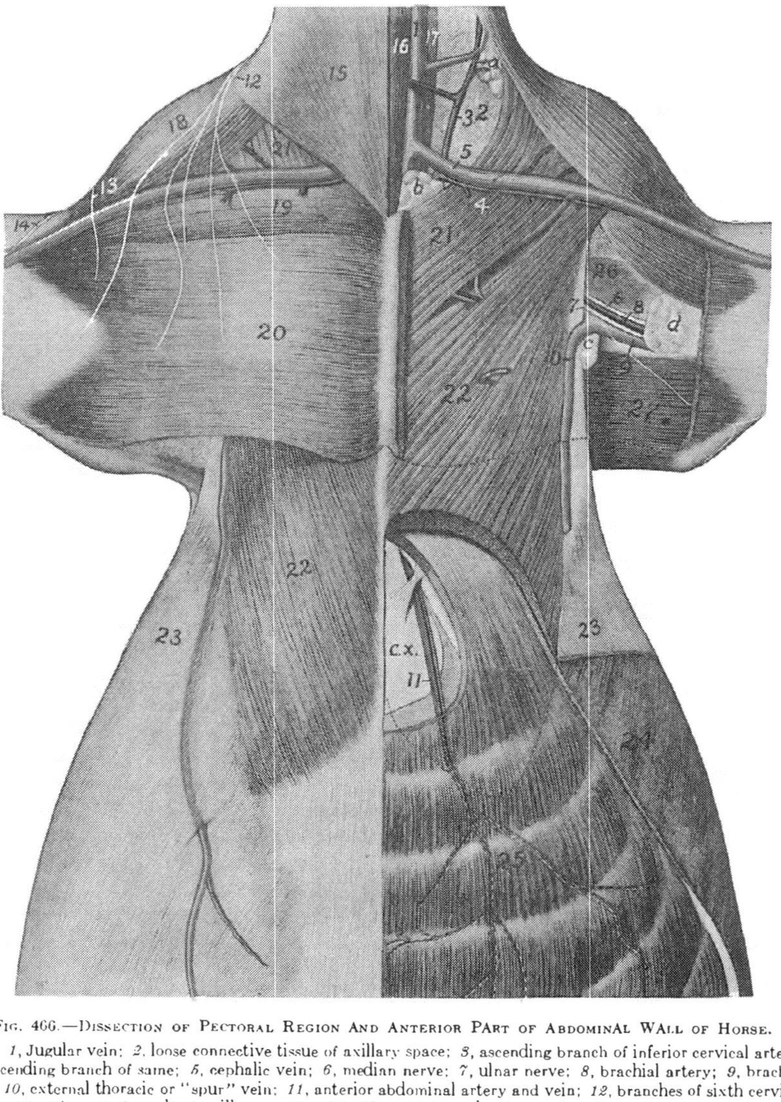

Fig. 466.—Dissection of Pectoral Region and Anterior Part of Abdominal Wall of Horse.

1, Jugular vein; *2*, loose connective tissue of axillary space; *3*, ascending branch of inferior cervical artery; *4*, descending branch of same; *5*, cephalic vein; *6*, median nerve; *7*, ulnar nerve; *8*, brachial artery; *9*, brachial vein; *10*, external thoracic or "spur" vein; *11*, anterior abdominal artery and vein; *12*, branches of sixth cervical nerve; *13*, cutaneous branch of axillary nerve; *14*, cutaneous branch of musculo-cutaneous nerve; *15*, cervical panniculus; *16*, sterno-cephalicus; *17*, scalenus; *18*, mastoido-humeralis; *19*, anterior superficial pectoral; *20*, posterior superficial pectoral; *21*, anterior deep pectoral; *22*, posterior deep pectoral; *23*, abdominal panniculus; *24*, obliquus abdominis externus; *25*, rectus abdominis; *26*, coraco-brachialis; *27*, tensor fasciæ antibrachii; *a*, prescapular lymph glands; *b*, prepectoral lymph glands; *c*, axillary lymph glands; *d*, cubital lymph glands; *c.x.*, xiphoid cartilage. (After Schmaltz, Atlas d. Anat. d. Pferdes.)

turns along the lower border of the brachialis, passes under the superficial tendon of the biceps and joins the cephalic.

The deep veins of the forearm are variable. Commonly two **posterior radial veins** (Venæ medianoradiales) accompany the artery of like name, one in front and one behind. A third vein arises by radicles emerging from the proximal part of the deep flexor; it joins the posterior satellite of the posterior radial artery or forms one of the roots of the brachial vein. The **common interosseous vein** joins the posterior satellite. The **anterior radial vein** (V. collateralis radialis) is a satellite of the artery. The **ulnar vein** is usually double at its proximal part, and communicates with the deep brachial vein.

There are three chief **metacarpal veins.** The **internal metacarpal vein** (V. metacarpea volaris superficialis medialis) arises from the volar venous arch above the fetlock. It is the largest vein of the region and lies in front of the large metacarpal artery. It separates from the artery at the proximal end of the metacarpus, passes upward on the inner part of the posterior surface of the carpus, under cover of the superficial layer of the posterior annular ligament, and is continued as the cephalic vein. It communicates at its proximal part with the origin of the posterior radial veins by a short but relatively large branch. The **external metacarpal vein** (V. metacarpea volaris superficialis lateralis) arises from the venous arch above the fetlock and passes upward behind the external border of the suspensory ligament in front of the external branch of the median nerve and accompanied by a small artery. At the proximal end of the metacarpus it is connected with the deep metacarpal vein by two transverse anastomoses which pass across the suspensory ligament. It then passes upward as a satellite of the external volar metacarpal artery and concurs in the origin of the ulnar and posterior radial veins. The **deep metacarpal vein** (V. metacarpea volaris profunda medialis) arises from the venous arch, passes forward between the two branches of the suspensory ligament, and ascends on the posterior surface of the large metacarpal bone. At the proximal end of the latter it communicates with the other metacarpal veins, ascends with the small metacarpal artery, and concurs in forming the radial veins.

The **venous arch** (Arcus venosus volaris), from which the metacarpal veins arise, is situated above the sesamoids of the fetlock between the suspensory ligament and the deep flexor tendon. It is formed by the junction of the two digital veins.

The **digital veins,** internal and external (V. digitalis medialis, lateralis), drain the venous plexuses of the foot. They arise at the upper edge of the lateral cartilages and ascend in front of the corresponding arteries.

It is convenient to recognize the following venous plexuses of the foot, which, however, communicate very freely:

1. The **coronary plexus** encircles the upper part of the foot. It is attached to the terminal part of the extensor tendon, the lateral cartilages, and the bulbs of the plantar cushion.
2. The **dorsal** (or laminal) **plexus** covers the dorsal or wall surface of the third phalanx in the deep layer of the matrix of the wall of the hoof. It forms the circumflex vein of the third phalanx or vein of the distal border of the third phalanx, which corresponds to the artery of like name.
3. The **volar plexus** is in the deep layer of the matrix of the sole of the hoof and on the deep surface of the lateral cartilages. It communicates around the inferior border of the third phalanx with the dorsal plexus and through the lateral cartilages with the coronary plexus.

The deep vein of the third phalanx accompanies the terminal part of the digital artery. It drains the **intraosseous plexus.**

THE POSTERIOR VENA CAVA (Figs. 270, 450)

The **posterior vena cava** (V. cava caudalis) returns almost all of the blood from the abdomen, pelvis, and pelvic limbs. It is formed by the confluence of the right and left common iliac veins at the fifth lumbar vertebra, above the terminal part of the aorta and chiefly to the right of the median plane.

The mode of origin is variable. In some cases there is a common trunk formed by the union of the two internal iliac veins so that the arrangement resembles the termination of the aorta. In other cases the internal iliac vein does not exist.

It passes forward on the ventral face of the psoas minor to the right of the abdominal aorta. At the last thoracic vertebra it separates from the aorta and runs forward between the right crus of the diaphragm and the pancreas till it reaches the liver. Here it inclines downward along the inner border of the right lobe and the parietal surface of the liver, largely embedded in the gland substance, and passes through the foramen venæ cavæ of the diaphragm. It then runs forward and somewhat downward between the mediastinal lobe and the main mass of the right lung at the upper margin of a special fold of the right pleura, accompanied by the right phrenic nerve, and opens into the posterior part of the right atrium. It receives the following tributaries:

1. The **lumbar veins** (Vv. lumbales) correspond to the arteries. Five pairs usually empty into the vena cava. Sometimes the corresponding veins of opposite sides unite to form a common trunk. The first communicate with the vena azygos.

2. The **spermatic veins** (Vv. spermaticæ internæ) (Fig. 450) accompany the arteries of like name. In the spermatic cord they form the pampiniform plexus about the artery and nerves. Their termination is variable. The right one commouly joins the vena cava near the renal vein, often by a common trunk with the left one. Frequently the left vein joins the left renal, and sometimes the right one ends similarly.

2*a*. The **utero-ovarian veins** are much larger than the preceding and are satellites of the arteries in the broad ligaments. The ovarian branch is plexiform near the ovary. The uterine branches form a rich plexus in the wall of the uterus. The trunk is very short.

3. The **renal veins** (Vv. renales), satellites of the arteries, are of large caliber and thin-walled. The right vein passes inward and backward on the ventral face of the kidney between the artery in front and the ureter behind. It joins the vena cava above the right adrenal. The left vein is somewhat longer. It passes inward at first like the right one, then bends around the posterior end of the adrenal, crosses the origin of the renal artery and opens into the vena cava a little further back than the right one. They receive veins from the adrenals, but some adrenal veins open directly into the vena cava.

4. The **hepatic veins** (Vv. hepaticæ) return the blood from the liver, and open into the vena cava as it lies in the groove in the liver. Three or four large vessels open into the vena cava just before it leaves the liver, and numerous small ones discharge into its embedded part.

5. The **phrenic veins** (Vv. phrenicæ), two or three in number, return the blood from the diaphragm. They are very large in comparison with the arteries, and join the vena cava as it lies in the caval opening.

In some cases there is a small middle sacral vein (V. sacralis media), a satellite of the artery. It opens into the angle of junction of the common iliac veins or into one of the latter.

THE PORTAL VEIN

The **portal vein** (V. portæ) is a large trunk which returns the blood carried to the viscera by the gastric, splenic, and mesenteric arteries. Its peripheral tributaries correspond closely with the branches of the arteries, but the terminal trunks do not. The vein is formed behind the pancreas and below the posterior vena cava by the confluence of the **anterior** and **posterior mesenteric** and **splenic veins**. It passes forward, traverses the posterior part of the pancreas very obliquely, inclines ventrally and a little to the right, and reaches the portal fissure of the liver. Here it divides into three branches which enter the liver and ramify in the substance of the gland like an artery, terminating in the lobular capillaries. From the lobules the blood passes into the hepatic veins and through these to the posterior vena cava. Thus the blood which is distributed to the stomach, nearly the entire intestinal tract, the pancreas, and the spleen, passes through two sets of capillaries prior to its return to the heart, viz., the capillaries of these viscera and of the liver.

1. The **anterior mesenteric vein** (V. mesenterica cranialis) is the largest of the portal radicles. It is situated to the right of the artery of like name, and its tributaries correspond in general to the branches of the artery. Usually a single colic vein corresponds to the two arteries of the right portions of the colon.

2. The **posterior mesenteric vein** (V. mesenterica caudalis) is the smallest of the radicles of the portal. It accompanies the artery in the colic mesentery and its rectal branches anastomose with those of the internal pudic vein.

3. The **splenic vein** (V. lienalis) is the very large satellite of the splenic artery. It is formed by the union of two radicles at the base of the spleen. On leaving the hilus of the spleen it passes inward between the anterior pole of the left kidney and the saccus cæcus of the stomach and above the left end of the pancreas, receives commonly the **posterior gastric vein** (V. gastrica caudalis), and unites with the anterior mesenteric at the posterior border of the pancreas.

The collateral tributaries of the portal veins are as follows:

(1) **Pancreatic veins** (Rami pancreatici).

(2) The **gastro-duodenal vein** (V. gastroduodenalis) corresponds mainly to the extrahepatic branches of the hepatic artery.

(3) The **anterior gastric vein** (V. gastrica cranialis) joins the portal at the portal fissure.

THE COMMON ILIAC VEINS (Fig. 456)

These (V. iliacæ communes) are two very large but short trunks which result from the union of the internal and external iliac veins of each side at the sacro-iliac articulation. The left one is the longer and crosses obliquely over the terminal part of the aorta. The chief tributaries of each are as follows:

1. The last **lumbar vein**.

2. The **circumflex iliac veins** (Vv. circumflexæ ilium profundæ) are the two satellites of each corresponding artery, on either side of which they are placed. They may open directly into the posterior vena cava or into the external iliac vein.

3. The **ilio-lumbar vein** (V. iliolumbalis) may open into the common iliac, the external iliac, or the internal iliac vein.

THE INTERNAL ILIAC VEINS

The **internal iliac** or **hypogastric veins** (Vv. hypogastricæ), right and left, are usually formed by the confluence of lateral sacral, gluteal, and internal pudic veins. The obturator vein may open into them also. They are short trunks and are smaller than the external iliac veins. The tributaries correspond in general to the branches of the three arteries of like names. The internal pudic veins receive affluents from the venous plexuses of the prepuce and penis in the male; of the mammary gland, vulva, vagina, and vestibular bulb in the female.

THE VEINS OF THE PELVIC LIMB

The **external iliac vein** (V. iliaca externa) (Figs. 450, 451) lies behind the corresponding artery at the brim of the pelvis. It is the upward continuation of the femoral vein, and unites at the sacro-iliac joint with the internal iliac to form the common iliac vein. Its tributaries are as follows:

1. The **obturator vein** (V. obturatoria) is a satellite of the artery and usually opens into the external iliac at the insertion of the psoas minor. Its radicles anastomose with those of the internal and external pudic veins (Figs. 451, 455).

2. The **iliaco-femoral** or **external circumflex veins** (Vv. circumflexæ femoris laterales) are the two satellites of the homonymous artery. They open a little higher than the obturator.

The **femoral vein** (Figs. 450, 451) lies behind the artery in the upper part of the thigh, external to it lower down. Its chief tributaries are:

1. A very large but short trunk formed by the union of the deep femoral and the external pudic vein. The **deep femoral vein** (V. profunda femoris) corresponds otherwise to the artery. The **external pudic vein** (V. pudenda externa) arises chiefly from a rich plexus of large veins situated above and along the sides of the penis and prepuce in the male, the mammary glands in the female. It passes through a foramen in the anterior part of the tendon of origin of the gracilis and runs outward in the subpubic groove behind the pectineus to unite with the deep femoral vein. The right and left veins are connected by a large transverse anastomosis and each has a large connection with the obturator vein. Each receives the **posterior abdominal** vein (V. epigastrica caudalis) which accompanies the artery of like name. The **subcutaneous abdominal vein** (V. abdominalis subcutanea) arises in the skin and panniculus of the ventral abdominal wall, anastomoses with the internal and external thoracic and deep abdominal veins, and joins the external pudic or posterior abdominal vein.

A small vein accompanies the external pudic artery in the inguinal canal.

2. The **anterior femoral vein** (V. femoris cranialis) accompanies the artery.

3. The **saphenous vein** (V. saphena) (Figs. 451, 458, 460) arises at the inner side of the flexion surface of the tarsus as the upward continuation of the internal metatarsal vein. Its course is distinctly visible. It ascends on the subcutaneous surface of the tibia and the popliteus muscle, inclosed between layers of the deep fascia, inclines a little backward to the proximal part of the leg, then deviates slightly forward, runs upward on the gracilis, passes between that muscle and the sartorius, and joins the femoral or the external pudic vein.[1] On the upper part of the capsule of the hock joint it forms an arch with the anterior tibial vein. The vein has numerous valves. The satellite artery is relatively small and lies in front of the vein as far as the junction with the recurrent tibial vein, which it accompanies on the leg. It receives the **recurrent tibial vein** (V. recurrens tibialis)[2] at the proximal fourth of the leg. This vessel arises at the inner surface of the tarsus and forms an arch with the posterior tibial vein at the level of the tuber calcis. It ascends in the furrow in front of the gastrocnemius tendon, inclines forward at the proximal third of the leg, and joins the saphenous vein at an acute angle. It has numerous valves. A smaller vein from the anterior face of the metatarsus joins the saphenous at the hock.

4. **Muscular branches** which correspond to the arteries.

5. The **posterior femoral** or **femoro-popliteal** vein (V. femoris caudalis) is a satellite of the artery. It receives the **recurrent tarsal** or **external saphenous vein** (V. tarsea recurrens), which arises at the outer side of the hock, ascends on the deep fascia of the external surface of the leg in front of the tendo Achillis, passes between the biceps femoris and semitendinosus, and joins the posterior femoral vein. It is connected with the recurrent tibial vein by a large anastomotic branch which crosses in front of the tuber calcis. Usually a branch from it ascends along the great sciatic nerve and anastomoses with the obturator vein.

[1] The place and mode of termination is quite variable. It may disappear from the surface of the thigh at any point above the distal third. In some cases it passes through the anterior part of the gracilis instead of dipping in between that muscle and the sartorius.

[2] This often joins the posterior femoral or the popliteal vein.

The **popliteal vein** (V. poplitea) lies along the inner side of the artery (Fig. 459). It is formed by the confluence of anterior and posterior tibial veins.

Two **anterior tibial veins** (Vv. tibiales anteriores) usually accompany the artery of like name; the outer vein is much the larger. In other cases there is a single large vein in the proximal part of the leg, two lower down. They arise from a number of anastomosing radicles on the front of the capsule of the hock joint, chiefly as the continuation of the perforating tarsal vein. The origin of the chief vein is connected with the saphenous by a large anastomotic branch.

The **posterior tibial vein** (V. tibialis posterior) is commonly double (Fig. 458). It arises at the level of the tuber calcis, where it has a communication with the recurrent tibial vein. It is a satellite of the artery

The **internal** or **great metatarsal vein** (V. metatarsea dorsalis medialis) (Figs. 458, 460) arises from the venous arch above the sesamoids at the fetlock, but is practically the upward continuation of the internal digital vein. It ascends along the inner border of the deep flexor tendon, then in the groove on the inner aspect of the proximal part of the large metatarsal bone to the capsule of the hock joint, and is continued by the saphenous vein.

The **external metatarsal vein** (V. metatarsea plantaris lateralis) arises from the venous arch above the fetlock, but appears to be the upward continuation of the external digital vein. It ascends along the outer border of the deep flexor tendon in front of the plantar nerve, and is connected with the deep metatarsal vein at the proximal part of the metatarsus by a transverse branch. It then passes upward along the deep flexor tendon in relation to the plantar nerves and the inner tarsal artery and is continued by the recurrent tibial vein.

The **deep metatarsal vein** (V. metatarsea plantaris medialis) arises from the plantar venous arch, passes forward between the branches of the suspensory ligament, and ascends on the posterior face of the large metatarsal bone. At the proximal end of the metatarsus it is connected with the external metatarsal vein by a transverse branch. It then passes (as the perforating tarsal vein) through the vascular canal of the tarsus and forms the chief radicle of the anterior tibial vein.

The **plantar venous arch** (Arcus venosus plantaris) and the digital veins are arranged like those of the thoracic limb.

THE LYMPHATIC SYSTEM

The **lymphatic system** (Systema lymphaticum) is subsidiary to the venous part of the circulatory system, from which it arises in the embryo. It consists of the lymph vessels and glands.

The **lymph vessels** (Vasa lymphatica) contain a colorless fluid, the lymph, which contains numerous lymphocytes.[1] They resemble the veins in structure but have thinner walls and are provided with more numerous valves. The vessels are sacculated opposite the segments of the valves and have a characteristic beaded appearance when distended. The collecting lymph vessels do not usually form rich plexuses, as veins often do, their branching is more limited and less tree-like than that of the blood-vessels, and their caliber therefore increases less from the periphery toward their termination. All of the lymph is ultimately carried into the venous system by two trunks, the **thoracic duct** and the **right lymphatic duct**. Almost all of the lymph passes through at least one group of lymph glands before entering the blood-vascular system.

The **lymph glands** or **nodes** (Lymphoglandulæ) are intercalated in the course of the lymph vessels. They vary widely in size, some being microscopic, others

[1] The term chyle is often applied to the lymph carried by the efferent vessels of the intestine when it contains products of digestion, and these vessels may be designated as lacteals or chyle vessels.

several inches in length. In form they may be globular, ovoid and flattened, elongated, or irregular. In certain situations they are aggregated into groups, and a knowledge of the position of these and the territory drained into them is important. It is convenient, when possible, to indicate their position with regard to arteries on the course of which they are placed. In color they are usually gray or yellowish-brown in the dead subject, pink or reddish-brown during life, but this varies according to their position and functional state. The bronchial glands are often blackened by infiltration with carbon. The mesenteric glands are creamy or white while the chyle is passing through, but pink at other times. Vessels which carry lymph to a gland are called **afferent**; the **efferent** vessels which convey it away are larger and fewer. Each gland has a depression, the **hilus,** at which the blood-vessels enter and the efferent lymph vessels emerge.

Lymph nodules or **follicles** (Noduli lymphatici) are minute masses of lymphoid tissue which occur in certain mucous membranes. They may be solitary, as in the solitary glands of the intestine, or aggregated into masses or patches, as in the tonsils and the so-called Peyer's patches.

The lymph nodule or follicle is the unit of structure of the lymph gland. It consists essentially of an artery surrounded by a reticulum of connective tissue, the meshes of which contain numerous lymphocytes. Surrounding this is a rich plexus of lymph vessels, forming the so-called sinus, inclosed in some cases by a fibrous capsule. The gland consists of a mass of follicles, inclosed in a fibrous **capsule,** from which **trabeculæ** pass in and unite the follicles. Beneath the capsule is the **peripheral sinus,** which consists of a very rich plexus of lymph vessels; to this the afferent vessels pass at various points of the surface. In the **cortical substance** the cells are in rounded masses, the cortical nodules, while in the **medullary substance** they lie around the arteries, forming the so-called medullary cords. The medulla is redder than the cortex, since it is more vascular; it contains the **central lymph sinuses,** which have a similar structure to the peripheral sinus.

The **hæmolymph glands** differ from the lymph glands in color and structure. They are of a deep red color, which is due to the high vascularity of the cortical substance. The peripheral sinuses especially are greatly developed and contain numerous red blood-cells. There is no clear division into cortical and medullary substance, and the trabeculæ contain smooth muscle-cells. Some have afferent and efferent lymph vessels and others do not. They resemble the spleen in some respects, but their significance is not yet clear. They are numerous in the ox and sheep, much fewer in the dog, and apparently are absent in the horse. They occur along the course of the aorta, in the perineal fat, at the portal fissure, and with the gastric and mesenteric lymph glands. In the ox they are also found under the trapezius muscle, under the skin of the upper part of the flank, and in other places less constantly.

The **tissue** or **lymph spaces** are interstices of varying size between cells or in the meshes of connective tissue. They contain a fluid derived from the blood-plasma, which is usually called **lymph.** They are drained by the veins and lymph vessels. The large serous sacs are often included in this category.

The exact relationship between the lymphatic capillaries and the tissue spaces is still a matter of controversy. It is held by some that the lymph-vessels are in direct communication with the tissue spaces, while others maintain that the lymphatics are complete closed tubes. Communication between the spaces and vessels is in general very free. Mall has shown that granules injected into the hepatic artery are returned by the lymphatics as well as by the veins, and intramuscular injections will enter the lymph-vessels of the tendon in spite of the absence of lymphatics in muscle.

LYMPHATIC SYSTEM OF THE HORSE

THE THORACIC DUCT (Figs. 428, 429)

The **thoracic duct** (Ductus thoracicus) is the chief collecting trunk of the lymphatic system. It begins as an elongated irregular dilatation, the **cisterna** or **receptaculum chyli,** which is situated between the right side of the aorta and the right crus of the diaphragm at the first and second lumbar vertebræ. The duct enters the thorax through the hiatus aorticus and runs forward on the right of the median plane between the vena azygos and the aorta, covered by the pleura. At the sixth or seventh thoracic vertebra it inclines somewhat ventrally, crosses obliquely over the left face of the œsophagus, and passes forward on the left side of the trachea to the inlet of the thorax. The extrathoracic terminal part passes downward and forward a variable distance (3 to 4 cm.) on the deep face of the left scalenus muscle, bends inward and backward under the bicarotid trunk, and opens into the upper part of the origin of the anterior vena cava just behind the angle of junction of the jugular veins. The terminal bend is ampullate and sometimes divides into two very short branches which open close together.

Since the duct develops from a plexus of ducts in the embryo, considerable variation from the more usual course occurs. There is often a left duct which arises at the cisterna or at a variable point from the right duct, runs across the left intercostal arteries parallel to the latter, and unites with it over the base of the heart or further forward. The two are connected by cross-branches. In some cases the left duct is the larger, and there may indeed be none on the right side. Other variations are common.

The chief tributaries of the thoracic duct are as follows:

1. The two **lumbar trunks** (Trunci lumbales) are formed by the confluence of the efferent ducts of the lumbar glands, and commonly unite with each other and with the posterior intestinal trunk before opening into the cistern.

2. The **intestinal trunks** (Trunci intestinales), two or three in number, receive the efferents of the lymph glands of the intestine, stomach, liver, and spleen.[1]

In its course through the thorax the thoracic duct receives efferents from the intercostal, mediastinal, and bronchial glands. At the thoracic inlet it is joined by ducts from the prepectoral and right axillary glands, and by the left tracheal duct. The duct is provided with several pairs of valves; the best developed are at its termination.

THE RIGHT LYMPHATIC DUCT

This vessel (Ductus lymphaticus dexter)—when present—collects the lymph from the right side of the head, neck, and thorax, and from the right thoracic limb. It is most frequently absent, being represented by a number of short ducts which terminate in the thoracic duct, the right jugulo-brachial junction, or the origin of the anterior vena cava. When present in its typical form, it results from the confluence of efferent ducts from the right axillary and prepectoral lymph glands with the right tracheal duct. It lies on the deep face of the scalenus muscle above the terminal part of the right jugular vein. It is more or less ampullate and usually opens into the anterior vena cava to the right of the thoracic duct. It may be connected with the latter by considerable anastomoses and may join it.

The duct is very variable in form and in regard to its afferents. Often it is a very short, irregular, and bulbous trunk; in some cases it is about an inch and a half (ca. 3 to 4 cm.) in length and receives the tracheal duct at its terminal bend. The lymphatico-venous connections here need further study.

THE LYMPH GLANDS AND VESSELS OF THE HEAD AND NECK

1. The **submaxillary lymph glands** (Lg. submaxillares) (Figs. 437, 462) are arranged in two elongated groups in the submaxillary space along each side of the omo-hyoid muscles. The two groups are in apposition in front of the insertion of these muscles and diverge posteriorly in the form of a V, extending backward about four or five inches (ca. 10 to 12 cm.). They are covered by the skin and a

[1] The lymph vessels of these organs appear to vary considerably in their mode of termination, and the arrangement needs further study. Some ducts from the stomach, liver, and spleen open directly into the cistern.

thin layer of fascia and panniculus, and are therefore palpable. Anteriorly they are firmly attached to the mylo-hyoidei, but otherwise they are rather movable in the normal state. Each group is related externally to the external maxillary artery and the anterior belly of the digastricus, below to the external maxillary vein, and above to the lingual and sublingual veins.

They receive **afferent** vessels from the lips, nostrils, nasal region, cheeks, the anterior part of the tongue, the jaws, the floor of the mouth, and the greater part of the hard palate and nasal cavity. The **efferent** vessels pass to the anterior cervical and pharyngeal glands.

The superficial lymph vessels of the face converge to twelve to fifteen trunks which turn around the lower border of the jaw with the facial vessels. Those of the lips form plexuses at the commissures. The nasal mucous membrane is richly supplied with lymph vessels which accompany the veins; posteriorly they communicate with the subdural and subarachnoid spaces and send efferents to the pharyngeal and anterior cervical glands.

2. The **pharyngeal lymph glands** (Figs. 436, 437, 569) may consist of two groups. One lies on the lateral surface of the pharynx along the course of the external carotid artery. These glands are related externally to the stylo-maxillaris and digastricus and often to the submaxillary gland also, above to the guttural pouch. Other glands (Lg. retropharyngeales) are commonly found on the guttural pouch along the course of the internal carotid artery. They lie below the artery and are covered by the aponeurosis of the mastoido-humeralis and the cervical end of the submaxillary gland.

They receive afferent vessels from the cranium, the posterior part of the tongue, the soft palate, pharynx, guttural pouch, larynx, posterior part of the nasal cavity, and efferents from the submaxillary glands.

3. The **anterior cervical lymph glands** (Lg. cervicales craniales) are situated chiefly along the course of the common carotid artery in the vicinity of the thyroid gland, under cover of the cervical angle of the parotid gland. Some occur between the thyroid and the submaxillary salivary gland, others above and partly upon the thyroid. They are related deeply to the posterior part of the larynx, the trachea, the thyroid gland, and the œsophagus; below to the external maxillary vein and the outer border of the omo-hyoideus.[1]

These glands are variable. Often there are none in front of the thyroid and the group may extend back a considerable distance along the course of the carotid artery.

Their afferents are deep lymph vessels from the head, the pharynx, larynx, guttural pouch, and thyroid gland, and efferents from the submaxillary and pharyngeal glands. Their efferent vessels go to the middle and posterior cervical glands.

4. The **middle cervical lymph glands** (Lg. cervicales mediæ) form an inconstant group situated a little in front of the middle of the neck on the trachea below the carotid artery. The group is usually small and in some cases is absent, being replaced by a number of glands occurring at intervals along the course of the carotid artery. In other subjects the group consists of several glands of considerable size. They are intercalated in the course of the tracheal lymph ducts.

5. The **posterior cervical** or **prepectoral lymph glands** (Lg. cervicales caudales) form a large group below the trachea at the entrance to the thorax (Fig. 466). They occupy the interstices between the vessels and muscles and extend forward a variable distance on the ventral aspect of the trachea. They are covered by the panniculus and sterno-cephalicus. Their afferent vessels come from the head, neck, thorax, and thoracic limb. They receive efferent ducts of the anterior and middle cervical, prescapular, and axillary glands. Their efferents go to the thoracic duct on the left, to the right lymphatic duct on the right, or open directly into the vena cava.

6. The **prescapular** or **superficial cervical lymph glands** (Lg. cervicales

[1] Abscess here can be reached readily by an incision between the vein and the omo-hyoideus.

superficiales) lie on the anterior border of the anterior deep pectoral muscle, in relation to the omo-hyoideus internally and the mastoido-humeralis externally (Figs. 431, 441, 466). They are on the course of the ascending branch of the inferior cervical artery. They receive afferents from the neck, breast, shoulder, and arm. Their efferents pass to the prepectoral glands.

The **tracheal ducts,** right and left (Ductus trachealis dexter, sinister), are colleeting trunks for the lymph of the head and neck. They lie on the trachea in relation to the carotid arteries. The right one goes to the prepectoral glands or to the right lymphatic duct, the left one to the terminal part of the thoracic duct.

THE LYMPH GLANDS AND VESSELS OF THE THORAX

1. The **intercostal lymph glands** (Lg. intercostales) are small and are situated at the sides of the bodies of the thoracic vertebræ, in series corresponding to the intercostal spaces. They receive afferents from the vertebral canal, the spinal muscles, the diaphragm, intercostal muscles, and pleura. The efferent vessels go to the thoracic duct.

In the young subject these glands are more numerous than in the adult, and there are also glands along the dorsal face of the thoracic aorta which seem to disappear later.

2. The **anterior mediastinal lymph glands** (Lg. mediastinales craniales) (Fig. 428) are numerous. Some are situated on the course of the brachial arteries and their branches; on the right side they are related deeply to the trachea, on the left to the œsophagus also. They are variable in size and disposition and are continuous in front with the prepectoral glands. Other glands lie along the ventral face of the trachea on the anterior vena cava and the right atrium of the heart; these are continuous behind with the bronchial glands. A few glands usually occur along the dorsal surface of the trachea, and there is often one at the angle of divergence of the brachiocephalic trunk. The afferent vessels come chiefly from the pleura, the pericardium, the heart, the thymus or its remains, the trachea, and the œsophagus. Their efferent vessels pass to the prepectoral glands and the thoracic duct.

The glands along the ventral face of the trachea are frequently enlarged and usually pigmented in dissecting-room subjects. The left recurrent nerve lies above them on the ventral face of the trachea.

3. The **bronchial lymph glands** (Lg. bronchiales) are grouped around the terminal part of the trachea and the bronchi. One group lies on the upper surface of the bifurcation of the trachea and is continued a short distance backward under the œsophagus (Fig. 428). Others lie below the trachea and bronchi and also occupy the angle between the aortic arch and the pulmonary artery, concealing the left recurrent nerve and often covering the vagus in this part of its course. Small glands occur along the chief bronchi in the substance of the lungs (Lg. pulmonales). They receive the deep and most of the superficial lymph vessels of the lungs, and the efferents from the posterior mediastinal glands. Their efferent vessels go to the thoracic duct and the anterior mediastinal glands. The deep lymph vessels of the lung arise in plexuses which surround the terminal bronchi and accompany the bronchi to the root of the lung. The superficial vessels form a rich network under the pleura; most of them pass to the bronchial glands.

The bronchial glands are commonly pigmented except in young subjects and are often enlarged and indurated.

4. The **posterior mediastinal lymph glands** (Lg. mediastinales caudales) are usually small and are scattered along the posterior mediastinum above the œsophagus. They receive afferent vessels from the œsophagus, mediastinum, diaphragm, and liver. The efferents go to the bronchial and anterior mediastinal lymph glands, partly to the thoracic duct directly.

Sometimes one or two small glands are situated in the acute angle between the posterior vena cava and the diaphragm.

THE LYMPH GLANDS AND VESSELS OF THE ABDOMEN AND PELVIS

The **lymph glands of the abdomen** consist of two main groups, parietal and visceral. The **parietal glands** lie in the subperitoneal or subcutaneous tissue; they receive the lymph vessels from the abdominal and pelvic walls, from parts of the viscera, and from the proximal lymph glands of the pelvic limbs. The **visceral glands** lie on the walls of the viscera or in the peritoneal folds which connect the organs with the wall or with adjacent viscera. They receive all or most of the lymph vessels from the organs with which they are connected.

The **parietal glands** comprise the following:

1. The **lumbar lymph glands** (Lg. lumbales) lie along the course of the abdominal aorta and posterior vena cava (Fig. 450). Some are placed along the lower surface and sides of the vessels, others above. A few small glands may be found above the sublumbar muscles. The small nodes which are situated at the hilus of the kidneys are often termed the renal lymph glands. They receive afferent vessels from the lumbar wall of the abdomen and the paired viscera (kidneys, adrenals, genital organs), also the inguinal vessels and the efferents of the iliac glands. Their efferents go to the thoracic duct, constituting the lumbar trunks of origin of that vessel.

2. The **internal iliac lymph glands** (Lg. iliacæ internæ) are grouped about the terminal part of the aorta and the origins of the iliac arteries (Fig. 450). Their afferent vessels come chiefly from the pelvis, pelvic viscera, and tail, and they receive efferent vessels of the external iliac and deep inguinal glands.

3. The **external iliac lymph glands** (Lg. iliacæ externæ) form a group on either side on the iliac fascia at the bifurcation of the circumflex iliac artery (Fig. 450). Their afferent vessels come from the flank and abdominal floor, the outer surface of the thigh, and the precrural glands. The efferent vessels go to the lumbar and internal iliac glands.

4. The **sacral lymph glands** (Lg. sacrales) are small nodes situated along the borders of the sacrum and on its pelvic surface. They receive afferents from the roof of the pelvis and from the tail, and their efferent vessels pass to the internal iliac glands.

5. The **superficial inguinal lymph glands** (Lg. inguinales superficiales) lie on the abdominal tunic in front of the external inguinal ring (Fig. 457). They form an elongated group along the course of the subcutaneous abdominal artery, on either side of the penis in the male, above the mammary glands in the female; in the latter they are often termed **mammary**. Their afferents come from the inner surface of the thigh, the abdominal floor, the sheath and scrotum in the male, and the mammary glands in the female. The efferent vessels ascend through the inguinal canal and go to the deep inguinal and lumbar glands.

6. The **ischiatic lymph gland** (Lg. ischiadica) is a small node which may be found at the lesser sciatic notch. It receives lymph from the adjacent parts and from the popliteal glands, and sends efferents to the sacral and internal iliac glands.

The **visceral glands** include the following:

1. The **gastric lymph glands** (Lg. gastricæ) are situated along the course of the gastric arteries. Several occur along the attachment of the gastro-phrenic ligament. A group lies at the lesser curvature a short distance below the cardia. There is another small group on the visceral surface where the posterior gastric artery divides into its primary branches. Two or three small nodes are usually found on the ventral aspect of the pylorus. Other small glands are scattered

along the course of the gastro-epiploic and short gastric arteries in the great and gastro-splenic omenta. The efferent vessels pass largely to the cœliac radicle of the thoracic duct, but along the left part of the great curvature they go to the splenic glands.

2. The **hepatic lymph glands** (Lg. hepaticæ) lie along the portal vein and hepatic artery and in the lesser omentum. Their efferent vessels go to the cœliac radicle of the cisterna chyli.

Many of the lymph vessels from the parietal surface of the liver pass in the falciform and lateral ligaments to the diaphragm and anastomose with its lymphatics. Some pass through the diaphragm with the vena cava and go to the mediastinal glands.

The **pancreatic lymph vessels** follow the course of the blood-vessels which supply the gland; most of them go to the splenic and hepatic glands.

3. The **splenic lymph glands** (Lg. lienales) lie along the course of the splenic blood-vessels. Their afferent vessels come from the subscapular network of the spleen, from the greater curvature of the stomach, and from the left part of the pancreas. The efferents pass to the cœliac radicle of the thoracic duct.

4. The **mesenteric lymph glands** (Lg. mesentericæ) are situated in the great mesentery near its root. They are numerous and hence lie close together. They receive a very large number of afferent vessels (400 to 500) from the small intestine. They have several considerable efferents which concur in the formation of the intestinal radicles of the cisterna chyli.

The lymph vessels of the intestine form three sets of capillary plexuses, viz., in the subserosa, submucosa, and mucosa. The lymph follicles, solitary and aggregate, lie in the zone of the plexus of the mucosa. The collecting vessels arise from the subserous plexus.

5. The **lymph glands of the cæcum** are numerous and are distributed along the course of the cæcal blood-vessels. Their efferents enter into the formation of an intestinal radicle of the cisterna chyli.

6. The **lymph glands of the great colon** are extremely numerous and are placed close together along the colic blood-vessels. Their efferent vessels are large and numerous. They converge to two large trunks which concur with those of the cæcum and small intestine to form an intestinal radicle of the cisterna chyli.

The intestinal radicles of the cisterna chyli are formed by the confluence of efferents from the intestinal lymph glands. The anterior trunk lies on the left side of the anterior mesenteric artery, passes between that vessel and the cœliac artery, turns sharply backward across the right renal vessels and opens into the cisterna. It is formed by the union of the cœliac trunk with efferents from the glands of the small intestine, cæcum and colon. It is about four inches (ca. 10 cm.) in length and is ampullate. The posterior trunk receives vessels from the small intestine and small colon. It usually opens into a trunk formed by the union of the right and left lumbar ducts. It is usually ampullate at its termination (Franck). The arrangement of these collecting trunks is, however, very variable.

7. The **lymph glands of the small colon** are situated in part on the wall of the bowel along the attachment of the mesentery, in part between the layers of the latter along the course of the blood-vessels. The efferent vessels go to the lumbar glands and to the posterior intestinal radicle of the thoracic duct.

The **lymph vessels of the rectum** pass chiefly to the lumbar and internal iliac glands.

8. The **anal lymph glands** (Lg. anales) form a small group on either side of the sphincter ani externus (Figs. 451, 453). They receive afferents from the anus, perineum, and tail. Their efferents go to the internal iliac glands.

THE LYMPH GLANDS AND VESSELS OF THE THORACIC LIMB

1. The **axillary lymph glands** (Lg. axillares), some ten to twelve in number, are grouped on the inner face of the distal part of the teres major and the tendon of the latissimus dorsi at the angle of junction of the external thoracic and subscapular

veins with the brachial (Fig. 466). Their efferents include most of the lymph vessels of the limb, which come directly or as efferents from the cubital glands. They receive also lymph vessels from the thoracic wall. The efferents accompany the brachial blood-vessels and end in the prepectoral glands and the thoracic and right lymphatic ducts.

2. The **cubital lymph glands** (Lg. cubitales), usually eight to ten in number, form a discoid oval group at the inner side of the distal part of the shaft of the humerus (Figs. 441, 446). They lie behind the biceps muscle on the brachial vessels and median nerve and are covered by the deep fascia and the posterior superficial pectoral muscle. They receive as afferents most of the vessels from the limb below this point. Their efferents pass chiefly to the axillary glands, but in part to the prescapular glands also.

A number of superficial lymph vessels ascend with or near the subcutaneous veins (cephalic and accessory cephalic) and join the prescapular and prepectoral glands. Superficial vessels from the chest-wall and shoulder run across the latter to the prescapular glands. The superficial lymphatics of the pectoral region form a plexus which drains into the prepectoral and prescapular glands by a number of vessels which accompany the cephalic vein. The deep lymph vessels of the pectoral region run with the external thoracic vein to the axillary glands.

THE LYMPH GLANDS AND VESSELS OF THE PELVIC LIMB

1. The **precrural** or **subiliac lymph** glands (Lg. subiliacæ) are situated in the fold of the groin on the anterior border of the tensor fasciæ latæ, about midway between the point of the hip and the patella (Figs. 450, 451, 457). They lie on the course of the posterior branch of the circumflex iliac artery, and number usually about a dozen. They receive superficial lymph vessels from the hip, thigh, and flank. Their efferent vessels ascend with the posterior circumflex iliac vein, enter the abdomen near the external angle of the ilium, and join the external iliac lymph glands.

2. The **deep inguinal lymph glands** (Lg. inguinales profundæ) form a large group situated in the upper part of the femoral canal between the pectineus and sartorius muscles (Figs. 451, 457). They cover the femoral vessels and are related superficially to the inguinal ligament. They receive nearly all of the lymph vessels of the limb below them. Their efferent vessels ascend to the internal iliac glands.

3. The **popliteal lymph glands** (Lg. popliteæ), usually four to six in number, lie behind the origin of the gastrocnemius and between the biceps femoris and semitendinosus at the division of the posterior femoral artery into its primary branches (Fig. 455). They receive the deep lymph vessels of the distal part of the limb. Their efferent vessels chiefly follow the course of the femoral vessels to the deep inguinal glands, but one or two ascend in company with a vein along the great sciatic nerve and may enter a gland at the lesser sciatic notch. From this a vessel accompanies the internal pudic vein and joins the internal iliac glands.

Several superficial lymph vessels ascend with or near the internal metatarsal and saphenous veins, enter the femoral canal, and end in the deep inguinal glands.

THE FŒTAL CIRCULATION

The blood of the fœtus is oxygenated, receives nutrient matter, and gives off waste matter by close contiguity with the maternal blood in the placenta. The chief differences in the blood-vascular system as compared with that which obtains after birth are correlated with this interchange.

The **umbilical arteries**, right and left, are large vessels which arise from the internal iliac arteries and pass downward and forward in the umbilical folds of peritoneum on either side of the bladder to the umbilicus. Here they are incorporated with the umbilical vein and the urachus in the umbilical cord, ramify in the allantois, and end as the capillaries of the fœtal placenta. They conduct the impure blood to the placenta. After birth these vessels retract with the bladder to the pelvic cavity; their lumen becomes greatly reduced and the wall thickened so that they are cord-like and are termed the round ligaments of the bladder.

The **umbilical vein** receives the oxygenated blood from the placenta. Its radicles converge to form in the horse a single large trunk which separates from the other constituents of the umbilical cord on entering the abdomen and passes forward along the abdominal floor in the free border of the falciform ligament of the liver. It enters the latter at the umbilical fissure and joins the portal vein, so that the blood conveyed by it passes through the capillaries of the liver before entering the posterior vena cava.

In the ox and dog some of the blood in the umbilical vein is conveyed directly to the vena cava by the **ductus venosus** (Arantii). This vessel is given off within the liver from a venous sinus formed by the confluence of the portal and umbilical veins and passes directly to the posterior vena cava.

The **foramen ovale** is an opening in the septum between the atria, by which the latter communicate with each other. It is guarded by a valve (Valvula foraminis ovalis) which prevents the blood from passing from the left atrium to the right. After birth the foramen soon closes, but this part of the septum remains membranous, and there is a deep **fossa ovalis** in the right atrium which indicates the position of the former opening. In some cases the foramen persists to a variable extent in the adult without apparent disturbance of the circulation.

The **pulmonary circulation** is very limited in the fœtus, and most of the blood which enters the pulmonary artery passes through the **ductus arteriosus** to the aorta. This vessel is larger than the divisions of the pulmonary which go to the lungs and joins the left side of the aortic arch. After birth the pulmonary circulation undergoes promptly an enormous increase and the ductus is rapidly transformed into a fibrous cord—the **ligamentum arteriosum.**

The only arterial blood in the fœtus is that carried by the umbilical vein. This blood is mixed in the liver with the venous blood of the portal vein, and after passing through the capillaries of the liver is carried by the hepatic veins to the posterior vena cava. The latter receives also the venous blood from the posterior part of the trunk and the pelvic limbs. It is generally believed that the blood carried into the right atrium by the posterior vena cava passes largely, if not entirely, through the foramen ovale into the left atrium, while the blood flowing into it through the anterior vena cava passes into the right ventricle. On this basis the blood received by the left atrium consists chiefly of mixed blood from the posterior vena cava, since the small amount of blood conveyed by the pulmonary veins is venous. This mixed blood passes into the left ventricle and is forced into the systemic arteries. The venous blood from the anterior part of the body and the thoracic limbs is conveyed by the anterior vena cava to the right atrium, passes into the right ventricle, and is forced into the pulmonary artery. A small amount is carried to the lungs, but the bulk of it passes by the ductus arteriosus into the aorta behind the point of origin of the brachiocephalic trunk (anterior aorta), and is carried to the posterior part of the body, a large part passing by the umbilical arteries to the placenta.

THE BLOOD-VASCULAR SYSTEM OF THE OX

The Pericardium and Heart

The **pericardium** is attached by two fibrous bands (Ligamenta sterno-pericardiaca) to the sternum opposite the facets for the sixth costal cartilages; these ligaments, right and left, are embedded in the mass of fat which separates the apex of the pericardium from the floor of the thorax.

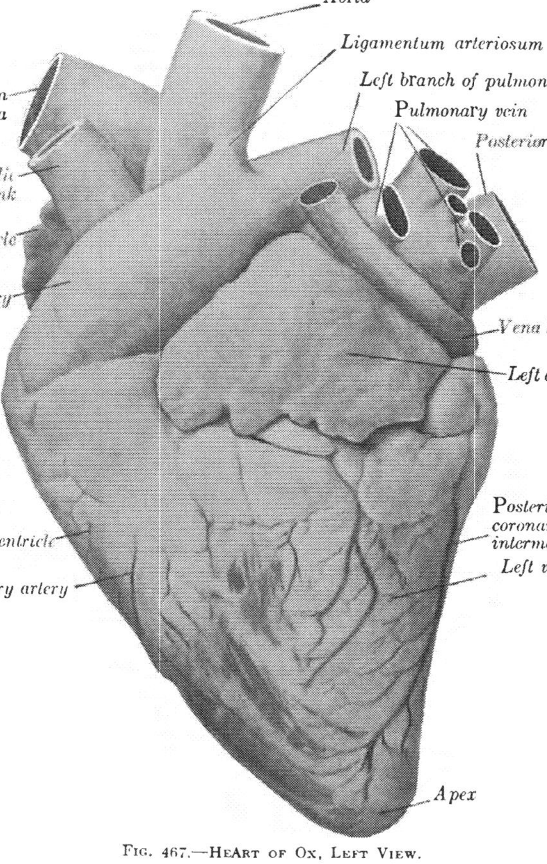

Fig. 467.—Heart of Ox, Left View.

The **heart** of the adult ox has an average weight of about 5½ to 6 pounds (ca. 2.5 to 2.7 kg.) or about 0.4 to 0.5 per cent. of the body-weight. Its length from base to apex is relatively longer than that of the horse and the base is smaller in both its diameters.

A shallow **intermediate groove** (Sulcus intermedius) extends from the coronary groove down the left side of the posterior border, but does not reach the apex. The amount of fat in and near the grooves is much greater than in the horse.

The heart is situated more to the left of the median plane than in the horse and is opposite to the third, fourth, and fifth ribs when it is contracted. It has extensive contact with the lateral wall of the thorax on the left side, but none on the right side, where a considerable thickness of lung covers the pericardium.[1]

Two bones, the **ossa cordis**, develop in the aortic fibrous ring. The right one is in apposition with the atrio-ventricular rings and is irregularly triangular in form. Its left face is concave and gives attachment to the right posterior cusp of the aortic valve. The right surface is convex from before backward. The base is superior. The posterior border bears two projections separated by a notch. It is usually a little more than an inch (ca. 4 cm.) in length. The left bone is smaller and is inconstant. Its concave right border gives attachment to the left posterior cusp of the aortic valve. There is a large fleshy moderator band in the right ventricle.

THE ARTERIES[2]

The great arterial trunks in the thorax resemble those of the horse in general disposition.

The left **coronary artery** is much larger than the right one; it gives off a branch which descends in the intermediate groove, and terminates by running downward in the right longitudinal groove. The **right artery,** after emerging from the interval between the right auricle and the pulmonary artery, divides into branches which are distributed to the wall of the right ventricle.

The **brachiocephalic trunk** (anterior aorta) is usually four or five inches (ca. 10 to 12 cm.) in length.

The **brachial arteries** give off in the thorax the following branches:

1. A common trunk for the subcostal, dorsal, superior or deep cervical, and vertebral arteries.

(1) The **subcostal artery** commonly arises separately, but may be given off as in the horse. It supplies the first three intercostal arteries.

(2) The **dorsal artery** is relatively small. It usually ascends in front of the first costo-vertebral joint and is distributed as in the horse.

(3) The **superior** or **deep cervical artery** may arise from a common stem (Truncus vertebro-cervicalis) with the vertebral, or may constitute a branch of that artery. It passes up between the first thoracic and last cervical vertebræ or between the sixth and seventh cervical and is distributed as in the horse.

(4) The **vertebral artery** passes along the neck as in the horse to the intervertebral foramen between the second and third cervical vertebræ, gives off a muscular branch, and enters the vertebral canal (Fig. 469). It runs forward on the floor of the canal—connected with its fellow by two or three transverse anastomoses—and divides in the atlas into two branches. The smaller internal division (cerebrospinal artery) passes forward to the floor of the cranium and concurs with the condyloid artery and branches of the internal maxillary in the formation of a large **rete mirabile.** The large external branch emerges through the intervertebral foramen of the atlas and ramifies in the muscles of the neck in that region, compensating for the smallness of the branches of the occipital artery. It also sends a branch to the rete mirabile. The collateral branches detached to the cervical muscles are large and compensate for the small size of the deep cervical artery. The collateral spinal branches of the vertebrals pass through the intervertebral foramina, divide into anterior and posterior branches, and form two longitudinal trunks which are connected by cross-branches so as to form irregular polygonal figures.

2. The **internal thoracic artery.**

[1] It is, of course, only the pericardium which comes in contact with the wall, but it is customary as a matter of convenience to speak of the relation of the heart as though it were direct.

[2] Only the most important differential features of the arrangement of the vessels as compared with those of the horse will be considered.

3. The **inferior cervical** artery corresponds usually to the ascending branch of that vessel in the horse.

4. The **external thoracic** artery is large and usually gives off a branch which is equivalent to the descending branch of the inferior cervical artery of the horse.

THE COMMON CAROTID ARTERY

The **carotid arteries** usually arise from a common trunk about two inches (ca. 5 cm.) in length, but in exceptional cases are given off separately from the brachio-

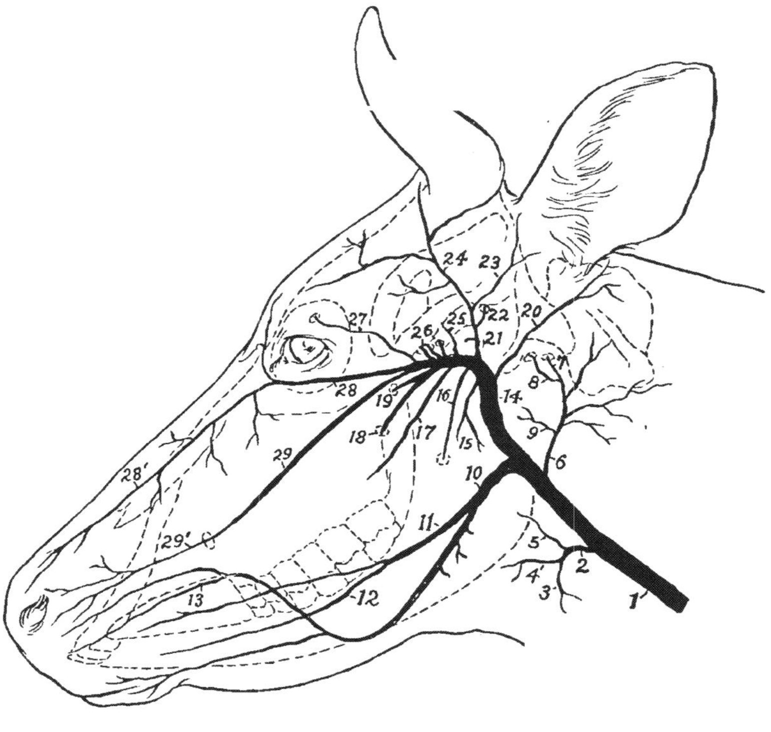

FIG. 468.—SCHEMA OF CHIEF ARTERIES OF HEAD OF COW.
1, Common carotid artery; *2*, thyro-laryngeal; *3*, thyroid; *4*, laryngeal; *5*, pharyngeal; *6*, occipital; *7*, condyloid; *8*, middle meningeal; *9*, pharyngeal; *10*, external maxillary; *11*, lingual; *12*, sublingual; *13*, superior labial; *14*, internal maxillary; *15*, masseteric; *16*, inferior alveolar; *17*, buccinator; *18*, great palatine; *19*, sphenopalatine; *20*, posterior auricular; *21*, superficial temporal; *22*, posterior meningeal; *23*, anterior auricular; *24*, artery to matrix of horn; *25*, deep temporal; *26*, arteries to rete mirabile; *27*, frontal; *28*, malar; *28'*, dorsal nasal continuation of malar; *29*, infraorbital; *29'*, lateral nasal continuation of *29*.

cephalic. Each pursues a course similar to that of the horse and is accompanied by the small internal jugular vein, but is separated from the external jugular vein by the omo-hyoid and sterno-mastoid muscles. It divides at the digastricus into occipital, external maxillary, and external carotid arteries. In addition to tracheal, œsophageal, and muscular branches, it gives off the thyroid and laryngeal arteries. The **thyroid artery** (A. thyreoidea cranialis) bends around the anterior end of the thyroid gland, in which it ramifies. The accessory thyroid artery is usually absent. The **laryngeal artery** may arise with the thyroid.

1. The **occipital artery** is relatively small. It gives off:

(1) The **pharyngeal artery**, which, however, may arise from the external carotid.

(2) Several branches to the muscles (chiefly the flexors) and to the atlanto-occipital joint.

(3) The **condyloid artery** passes into the cranium through the anterior foramen in the condyloid fossa, and joins the vertebral in the formation of the rete mirabile about the pituitary gland. Before entering the cranium it gives off a branch to the pharyngeal lymph glands, and the middle meningeal artery; the latter passes through the foramen lacerum. Another branch enters the temporal canal and gives twigs to the temporalis muscle and the mucous membrane of the frontal sinus. A muscular branch emerges from the intervertebral foramen of the atlas. A diploic branch goes into the occipital condyle and squama, and emits twigs to the occipital muscles.

2. The **external maxillary** artery is smaller than that of the horse, but pursues

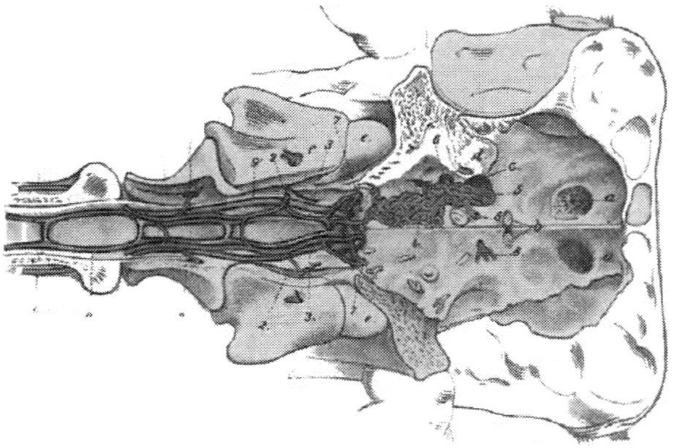

FIG. 469.—FLOOR OF CRANIUM AND ANTERIOR PART OF VERTEBRAL CANAL OF OX.

1, Vertebral artery; *2*, muscular branches of *1*; *3*, branches of *1* to the rete mirabile, *4*; *5*, branches of internal maxillary artery to rete; *6*, branch of internal maxillary artery entering cranium through foramen ovale; *7*, condyloid artery; *8*, emergent artery from rete, distributed like internal carotid artery of horse; *9*, *9'*, longitudinal vertebral sinuses; *a*, cribriform plate; *b*, optic foramina; *c*, for. lacerum orbitale + rotundum; *d*, foramen ovale; *e*, occipital condyle; *f*, *g*, *h*, first, second, and third cervical vertebræ. (After Leisering's Atlas.)

a similar course. The **lingual artery** is large, and often arises separately from the common carotid; it gives off a branch to the submaxillary gland, and the **sublingual artery**. After turning around the jaw the facial gives off the two **labial arteries.** The **superior labial** is large; it usually gives off a branch which runs forward almost parallel with the lateral nasal. The **angular artery** is absent or rudimentary, and the **lateral** and **dorsal nasal arteries** spring from branches of the internal maxillary.

3. The **external carotid artery** passes upward between the stylo-hyoideus and the great cornu of the hyoid bone, turns forward across the external face of the latter, and divides into superficial temporal and internal maxillary arteries. It gives off the following collateral branches:

(1) Branches to the parotid and submaxillary glands.

(2) The **pharyngeal artery**, which, however, often arises from the occipital.

(3) The **posterior auricular**, which resembles that of the horse and sends a stylo-mastoid branch into the tympanum. It may arise from the superficial temporal.

(4) The masseteric artery resembles that of the horse, but is smaller.

The superficial temporal artery is large and presents the following special features: (1) Its transverse facial branch passes into the central part of the masseter. (2) It gives off a branch which corresponds to the posterior meningeal artery of the horse, enters the temporal canal, and ramifies in the dura mater, giving off twigs to the external ear, the temporal muscle, and the frontal sinus. (3) It usually gives off the anterior auricular artery. (4) Branches are supplied to the frontalis muscle and the eyelids. (5) A large branch passes around the outer side of the base of the horn-core, supplies the matrix of the horn, and anastomoses across the back of the frontal eminence with the artery of the opposite side.

The internal maxillary artery is less curved than in the horse and is entirely extraosseous, since the alar canal is absent. The principal differential features in its branching are as follows:

(1) The ophthalmic artery forms a rete mirabile within the periorbita. Its frontal branch enters the supraorbital canal and ramifies chiefly in the frontal sinus.

(2) Several branches take the place of the internal carotid artery. One of these enters the cranial cavity through the foramen ovale and several small ones pass through the foramen which represents the foramen rotundum and foramen lacerum orbitale of the horse. They concur with the vertebral and condyloid arteries in the formation of an extensive rete mirabile on the cranial floor around the sella turcica. From each side of the rete an artery arises which is distributed in general like the internal carotid of the horse.

(3) The malar artery is large; it arises by a common trunk with the infraorbital and gives off the dorsal nasal and the angular artery of the eye.

(4) The infraorbital artery is large and emerges from the infraorbital foramen to form the lateral nasal artery.

(5) The palatine artery is smaller than in the horse and usually arises by a common trunk with the sphenopalatine. It passes through the palatine canal and along the palatine groove, enters the nasal cavity through the incisive fissure, and does not go to the upper lip. It forms a rete mirabile about the nasopalatine canal and terminates in the mucous membrane of the anterior part of the nasal cavity.

ARTERIES OF THE THORACIC LIMB

The brachial artery pursues the same course in the arm as that of the horse. At the elbow it becomes the median.[1] The chief differential features in its branches are as follows:

1. The subscapular artery is almost as large as the continuation of the brachial. The posterior circumflex artery sends branches backward and downward into the triceps, taking the place in part of the deep brachial artery. The thoracico-dorsal artery supplies branches to the pectoral muscles and the triceps as well as the teres major and latissimus dorsi; it may arise directly from the brachial.
2. The deep brachial artery is small.
3. The superior collateral ulnar artery is often double, and does not extend to the carpus.

The median artery (posterior radial artery) descends along the inner part of the posterior surface of the radius and divides near the middle of the forearm into the radial and ulnar arteries. It gives off at the upper third of the forearm the common interosseous artery, a large vessel which anastomoses with the deep brachial, passes through the proximal interosseous space, and descends (as the dorsal interosseous) in the groove between the radius and ulna, and concurs in the formation of the rete carpi dorsale. At the distal end of the forearm it sends a branch

[1] The homologies of the vessels of the lower parts of the limbs are still uncertain. The account given here is mainly based on the views of Sussdorf and Baum.

through the distal interosseous space, which passes downward, assists in forming the rete carpi volare, and is continued in the metacarpus as the external deep volar metacarpal artery. This is a small vessel which passes down under the outer border of the suspensory ligament and assists in forming the deep volar arch near the fetlock.

The **radial artery** is smaller than the ulnar. It descends on the flexor carpi internus, passes over the postero-internal surface of the carpus, and is continued as the internal deep volar metacarpal. At the distal end of the forearm and at the carpus it furnishes branches to the retia carpi. Another branch (A. met. perforans

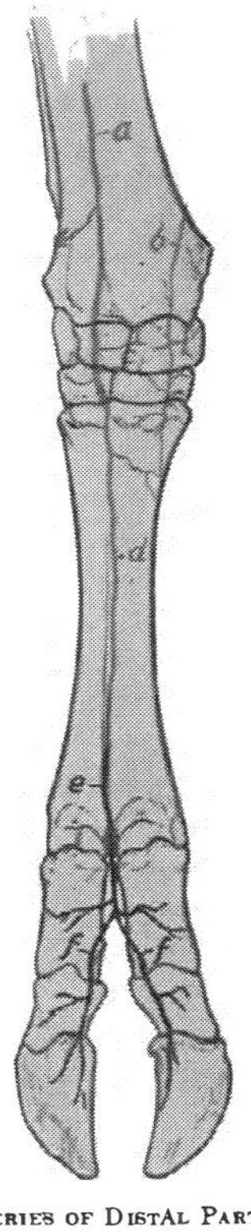

Fig. 470.—Arteries of Distal Part of Right Fore Limb of Ox, Anterior View.

a, Interosseous artery; *b*, dorsal branch of radial artery; *c*, rete carpi dorsale; *d*, dorsal metacarpal artery; *e*, dorsal common digital artery; *f*, *f*, dorsal proper digital arteries.

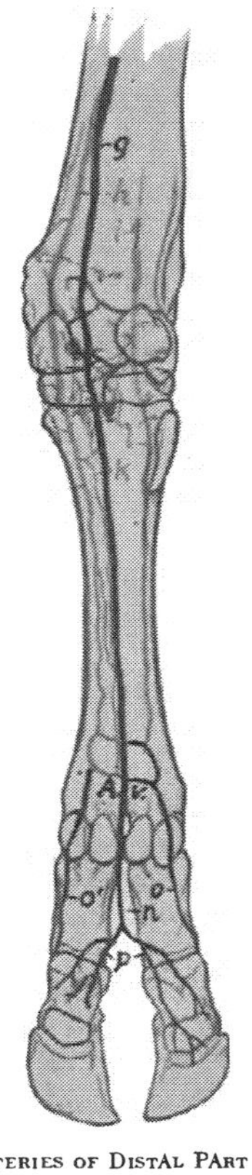

Fig. 471.—Arteries of Distal Part of Right Fore Limb of Ox, Posterior View.

g, Ulnar artery; *h*, radial artery; *i*, volar branch of common interosseous artery; *k*, *l*, *m*, deep volar metacarpal arteries; *A.v.*, volar arches; *n*, volar common digital artery; *o*, *o'*, *p*, volar proper digital arteries.

proximalis) runs outward between the suspensory ligament and the large metacarpal bone, passes through the proximal foramen of the bone, and unites with the interosseous artery; before passing through the foramen it detaches the middle deep volar metacarpal artery (A. met. volaris prof. III.), which descends on the posterior face of the metacarpal bone, receives an anastomotic branch from the internal deep artery, and concurs in the formation of the deep volar arch above the fetlock.

The **ulnar artery**, the larger of the two divisions of the median, descends under cover of the flexor carpi internus without giving off any large branches in the forearm. It passes through the carpal canal and continues along the inner side of the deep flexor tendon as the volar **common digital artery.** At the distal third of the metacarpus this vessel is joined by a branch from the internal deep volar metacarpal artery, forming the superficial volar arch. Near this another branch of the common digital (or of the internal digital) passes around the outer border of the flexor tendons to the posterior face of the metacarpal bone and concurs with the deep volar metacarpal arteries in the formation of the deep volar arch. A branch from the arch passes forward through the inferior foramen of the metacarpal bone and joins the dorsal metacarpal artery which descends from the rete carpi dorsale in the anterior metacarpal groove.

The volar **common digital artery** (A. metacarpea volaris superficialis III.) passes into the interdigital space and divides into two **volar proper digital arteries,** which descend along the interdigital surfaces of the chief digits and pass through the foramina at the upper part of the interdigital surfaces of the third phalanges, enter the cavities in these bones, and ramify in a manner similar to the corresponding vessels in the horse. The volar common digital detaches a branch (A. interdigitalis perforans) which passes forward through the upper part of the interdigital space and anastomoses with the dorsal metacarpal artery.

The volar proper digital arteries (or the common digital) give off, in addition to other collaterals, branches which correspond to the arteries of the plantar cushion of the horse. These pass to the bulbs of the claws and anastomose with each other and with the inner and outer digital arteries, forming an arch from which numerous branches are distributed to the matrix of the hoofs.

The dorsal **metacarpal artery** (A. met. dorsalis III.) is a small vessel which arises from the rete carpi dorsale, descends in the groove on the anterior face of the metacarpal bone, and is joined by the inferior perforating metacarpal artery from the deep volar arch to constitute the dorsal common digital artery. This vessel (A. digitalis communis dorsalis III.) divides into two **dorsal proper digital arteries.**

The **internal digital artery** (A. digiti III. medialis) is the continuation of the internal deep volar metacarpal artery. It descends on the inner side of the inner digit and terminates at the bulb of the claw by anastomosing with the corresponding volar proper digital artery. It gives off a branch to the rudimentary digit and forms a transverse anastomosis behind the first phalanx with the volar common digital or its inner division.

The **external digital artery** (A. digiti IV. lateralis) arises from the deep volar arch, passes down on the outer side of the external digit and is distributed like the inner one.

BRANCHES OF THE THORACIC AORTA

The **bronchial** and **œsophageal** arteries often arise separately.

Ten pairs of **intercostal arteries** usually arise from the aorta. The other three come from the subcostal artery.

The two **phrenic arteries** are very variable in origin. They may come from the aorta, the cœliac, left ruminal, or an intercostal or lumbar artery.

BRANCHES OF THE ABDOMINAL AORTA

The **cœliac artery** is about four to five inches (ca. 10 to 12 cm.) in length. It passes downward and curves forward between the rumen and pancreas on the left and the right crus of the diaphragm and the posterior vena cava on the right. It gives off five chief branches.

1. The **hepatic artery** arises from the convex side of the curve of the cœliac artery as it crosses the posterior vena cava. It passes downward, forward, and to

the right above the portal vein to the portal fissure, and gives off the following branches:

(1) Pancreatic branches.

(2) Dorsal and ventral branches to the liver. The ventral branch is the larger; it gives off the right gastric artery, which runs in the lesser omentum to supply the origin of the duodenum and the pylorus, anastomosing with the dorsal branch of the omaso-abomasal artery.

(3) The cystic artery supplies the gall-bladder.

(4) The gastro-duodenal artery divides into right gastro-epiploic and pancreatico-duodenal branches. The right gastro-epiploic artery anastomoses with the left gastro-epiploic. The pancreatico-duodenal artery anastomoses with the first intestinal branch of the anterior mesenteric artery.

2. The **right ruminal artery** (A. ruminalis dextra) is the largest branch, and usually arises by a short common trunk with the splenic. It runs downward and backward on the right face of the dorsal sac of the rumen to the posterior transverse fissure, in which it turns around to the left and anastomoses with branches of the left ruminal artery. It gives off a pancreatic branch, dorsal and ventral coronary arteries, branches to the great omentum, and ramifies on both surfaces of the rumen.

3. The **left ruminal artery** (A. ruminalis sinistra) runs downward on the anterior part of the right face of the rumen, enters the anterior furrow, in which it runs from right to left, and continues backward in the left longitudinal groove, anastomosing with branches of the right artery. It supplies chiefly the left face of the rumen, but not its posterior part. It usually gives off near its origin the **reticular artery** (A. reticularis); this rather small vessel passes forward on the dorsal curvature of the rumen and turns downward in the rumino-reticular groove, in the bottom of which it runs around ventrally to the right side. It gives off a branch which passes to the left of the cardia and along the lesser curvature of the reticulum to the neck of the omasum. The reticular branches anastomose with the omaso-abomasal and left ruminal arteries.

4. The **omaso-abomasal artery** (A. gastrica sinistra) appears as the continuation of the cœliac. It passes forward and downward to the greater curvature of the omasum and divides after a course of four or five inches into two branches. The **dorsal branch** curves sharply backward on the dorsal surface of the omasum, continues along the lesser curvature of the abomasum, and anastomoses with the hepatic artery. It supplies branches to the omasum and to the lesser curvature and pyloric part of the abomasum. The **ventral branch** (A. gastro-epiploica sinistra) runs forward and downward over the anterior extremity of the omasum, passes backward in the great omentum close to the ventral curvature of the abomasum, and anastomoses with the right gastro-epiploic. A considerable branch from it curves around in front of the neck of the omasum to communicate with the reticular artery. Another branch runs back across the left side of the omaso-abomasal junction, and a third goes to the lesser (ventral) curvature of the omasum.

5. The **splenic artery** usually arises by a common trunk with the right ruminal artery. It passes forward and to the left across the dorsal curvature of the rumen and enters the hilus of the spleen.

The **anterior mesenteric artery** arises from the aorta just behind the cœliac, and has about the same caliber as the latter. It passes downward and a little to the right, and crosses the colon as it emerges from the spiral to run backward. After detaching twigs to the pancreas it gives off in succession the following branches:

1. A branch (A. colica media) passes to the colon as it emerges from the spiral arrangement. This artery is comparable to the middle colic or artery of the small colon of the horse; it runs backward along the terminal part of the colon, which it supplies.

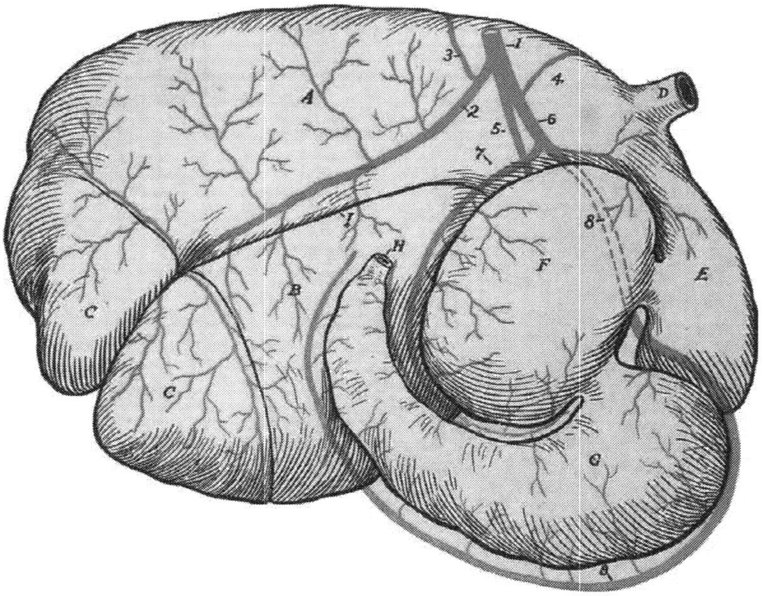

FIG. 472.—GASTRIC ARTERIES OF OX, RIGHT VIEW (PARTLY SCHEMATIC).

1, Cœliac artery; *2*, right ruminal; *3*, splenic; *4*, reticular; *5*, left ruminal; *6*, omaso-abomasal; *7*, dorsal branch of *6*; *8*, ventral branch of *6* (= left gastro-epiploic); *A*, dorsal sac of rumen; *B*, ventral sac of rumen; *C*, *C*, posterior blind sacs; *D*, œsophagus; *E*, reticulum; *F*, omasum; *G*, abomasum; *H*, duodenum; *I*, right longitudinal furrow of rumen. By an oversight the reticular artery is shown as arising from the omaso-abomasal.

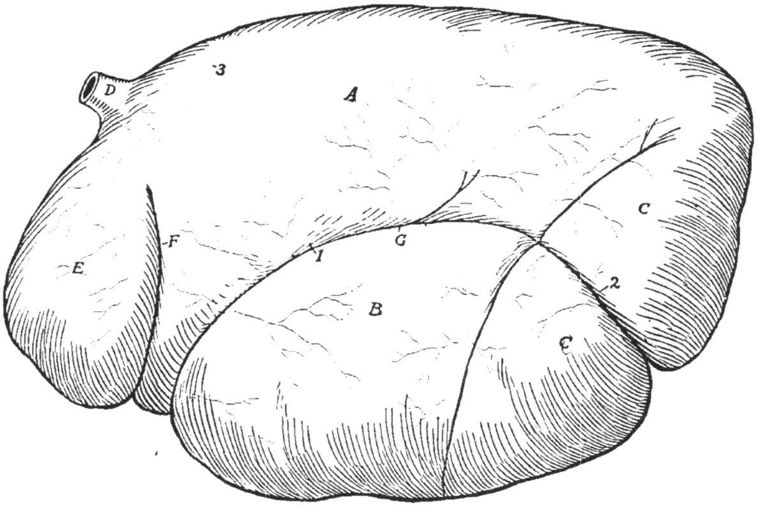

FIG. 473.—GASTRIC ARTERIES OF OX, LEFT VIEW (PARTLY SCHEMATIC).

1, Left ruminal artery; *2*, continuation of right ruminal artery; *3*, reticular artery, which disappears into rumino-reticular groove; *A*, dorsal sac of rumen; *B*, ventral sac of rumen; *C*, *C*, posterior blind sacs; *D*, œsophagus; *E*, reticulum; *F*, rumino-reticular groove; *G*, left longitudinal furrow of rumen.

2. The ileo-cæco-colic artery ramifies on the right face of the spiral part of the colon. It gives off the ileo-cæcal artery, which divides into ileal and cæcal arteries.

3. An artery (Ramus collateralis) runs in the mesentery in a curve along the ventral border of the coils of the colon. (This vessel is absent in the sheep.)

4. An artery which constitutes the direct continuation of the anterior mesenteric pursues a course in the mesentery corresponding to the series of mesenteric lymph glands.

The two preceding vessels are essentially the arteries of the small intestine,

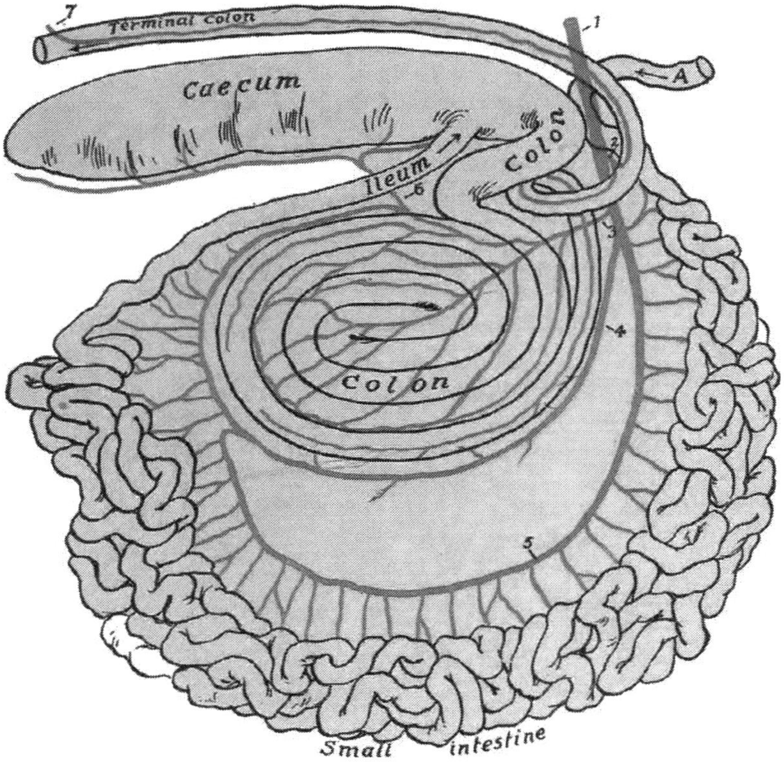

FIG. 474.—PLAN OF BRANCHES OF ANTERIOR MESENTERIC ARTERY OF OX.

1, Anterior mesenteric artery; *2*, middle colic artery; *3*, ileo-cæco-colic artery; *4*, ramus collateralis; *5*, continuation of anterior mesenteric artery, giving off branches to small intestine; *6*, cæcal artery; *7*, colic branch of posterior mesenteric artery; *A*, termination of duodenum.

which they supply with the exception of its initial and terminal parts. The first gives off no considerable branches in its course along the ventral border of the coils of the colon, but on curving upward along the latter it anastomoses with the second artery and detaches numerous branches to the small intestine which form series of superposed anastomotic arches. It supplies, roughly speaking, about one-third of the small intestine and terminates by joining the ileal artery. The second artery gives off numerous branches which also form arches and supply about the first two-thirds of the small intestine, exclusive of the small part supplied by branches of the cœliac artery. Both arteries give branches to the lymph glands.[1]

[1] It is difficult to make the arrangement of these vessels clear in a brief textual description, but a reference to the schematic figure will explain the main facts.

The **posterior mesenteric artery** arises from the aorta near its termination. It is small and supplies branches to the terminal part of the colon and to the rectum.

The **renal arteries** arise from the aorta close together. The right one passes outward and forward across the dorsal face of the posterior vena cava to the hilus of the kidney. The left one runs backward, but necessarily varies in direction in conformity with the position of the kidney (*q. v.*)

The **spermatic arteries** resemble those of the horse.

The **utero-ovarian arteries** are small.

The five pairs of **lumbar arteries** derived from the aorta are distributed much as in the horse. The sixth usually comes from the internal iliac artery.

The **middle sacral artery** is a vessel about 5 mm. in diameter which continues

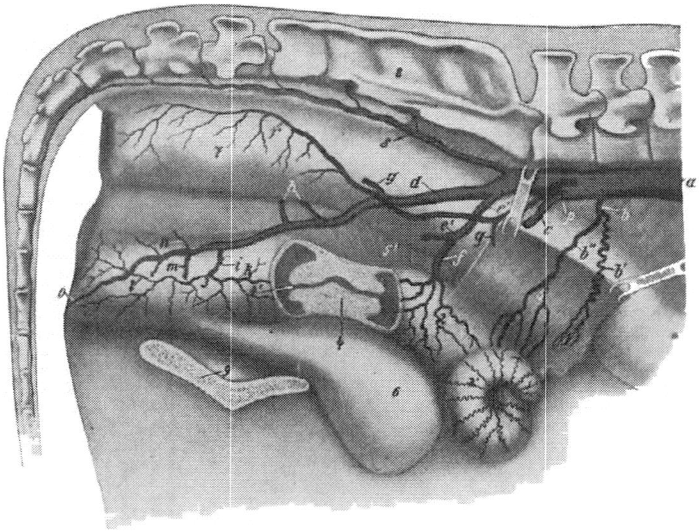

FIG. 475.—PELVIC ARTERIES OF COW.

Part of the right wall of the uterus and vagina is removed and the cervix uteri is shown in sagittal section. *a*, Aorta; *b*, utero-ovarian artery; *b'*, ovarian, and *b''*, uterine branch of *b*; *c*, external iliac artery; *d*, right internal iliac artery; *e*, common trunk of umbilical artery (*e'*) and middle uterine artery (*f*); *g*, ilio-lumbar artery; *h*, anterior gluteal arteries; *i*, middle hæmorrhoidal artery; k, posterior uterine artery; *l*, perineal artery; *m*, posterior gluteal artery; *n*, obturator arteries; *o*, artery of clitoris; *p*, posterior mesenteric artery; *r*, anterior hæmorrhoidal artery; *s*, middle sacral artery; *1*, ovary; *2*, apparent body of uterus, really apposed horns; *2'*, cornu; *3*, vagina; *4*, cervix uteri; *4'*, vaginal part of uterus (os uteri); *5*, *5'*, broad ligaments, large part of right one removed; *6*, urinary bladder; *7*, rectum; *8*, sacrum; *9*, symphysis pelvis. (After Zieger.)

the aorta. It arises from the dorsal face of the aorta at the angle of divergence of the internal iliacs, runs backward on the pelvic surface of the sacrum a little to the left of the median line, and is continued as the middle coccygeal artery. It gives off small collateral branches to the spinal cord and the muscles of the tail and the **lateral coccygeal arteries.** The latter may have a common trunk of origin, and each divides into dorsal and ventral branches. The **middle coccygeal artery** runs through the ventral (hæmal) arches of the coccygeal vertebræ. The coccygeal arteries are connected at pretty regular intervals by segmental anastomoses.

The **internal iliac arteries** are much longer than in the horse. Each passes backward on the sacro-sciatic ligament and divides about the middle of the pelvic wall into posterior gluteal and internal pudic branches. The chief differences in its distribution are : (1) A large trunk gives origin to the umbilical and middle uterine arteries. The **umbilical artery** is usually largely obliterated and its terminal branches receive their blood through anastomoses with the internal pudic. It gives off near its origin two small vessels, the ureteral artery (A. ureterica) and the deferential artery (A. deferentialis), which accompany the ureter and the vas deferens respectively. The **middle uterine artery** (A. uterina media) is very large. It is distributed chiefly to the cornu of the uterus, and compensates for the small size of the utero-ovarian artery. (2) The **ilio-lumbar** artery is relatively small and is distributed chiefly to the sublumbar muscles. It is sometimes replaced by branches of the circumflex iliac and gluteal arteries. (3) The **anterior gluteal artery** is commonly represented by several vessels. (4) The **obturator** artery is represented by several small branches which supply the obturator and adductor muscles. (5) The **iliaco-femoral** and **lateral sacral arteries** are absent. The absence of the latter is compensated by the middle sacral and gluteal arteries. (6) The **posterior gluteal** (or ischiatic) artery is large. It emerges through the lesser sciatic notch and ramifies in the biceps femoris and adjacent muscles. (7) The **internal pudic** artery (A. urethro-genitalis) is the direct continuation of the internal iliac. It gives off branches to the rectum, bladder, urethra, and genital organs. In the male it supplies the accessory genital glands and divides into dorsal and deep arteries of the penis; the a. dorsalis penis runs along the dorsum penis to the glans and gives twigs to the prepuce; the a. profunda penis gives off a perineal branch and enters the corpus cavernosum penis. In the female it gives off a large posterior uterine artery, which supplies the posterior part of the uterus and gives branches to the vagina and bladder. It ends as the a. clitoridis, which supplies the clitoris and adjacent parts.

ARTERIES OF THE PELVIC LIMB

The **external iliac artery** has the same course as in the horse. The circumflex iliac artery is large. A branch from it emerges between the abdominal and lumbar muscles near the external angle of the ilium and ramifies like the terminals of the ilio-lumbar artery of the horse.

The **femoral** and **popliteal arteries** pursue a similar course to those of the horse. The chief differences in their branches are as follows:

1. The **external pudic artery** is distributed chiefly to the scrotum in the male. In the cow it is usually termed the **mammary** and is very large, especially during lactation. Each divides at the base of the mammary gland into two branches which are distributed to the anterior and posterior parts ("quarters") of the gland. A small branch accompanies the subcutaneous abdominal vein to the xiphoid region.

2. The **deep femoral artery** gives off an obturator branch which passes up through the obturator foramen to supply the obturator internus and compensates otherwise for the absence of the obturator artery.

3. The **anterior femoral artery** is large. It often gives off the **external circumflex artery** of the thigh, which perforates the proximal end of the quadriceps, gives branches to that muscle, the iliacus, glutei, and tensor fasciæ latæ.

4. The **saphenous artery** is large. It descends in front of the homonymous vein to the postero-internal surface of the hock, where it divides into two plantar branches. The **internal plantar artery** (A. plantaris medialis) is the direct continuation of the saphenous. It descends at first along the inner border of the superficial flexor tendon and is continued as the **internal superficial plantar metatarsal artery** along the inner side of the deep flexor tendon with the internal plantar nerve. It anastomoses at the proximal end of the metatarsus with the perforating metatarsal artery, assisting in the formation of the proximal plantar arch. Near the fetlock it concurs with the perforating branch of the dorsal metatarsal artery in the formation of the distal plantar arch. Below this it is continued as the **internal**

digital artery. The external plantar artery (A. plantaris lateralis) is small. It descends along the outer border of the deep flexor tendon with the external plantar nerve, concurs with the perforating tarsal and the internal plantar arteries in the formation of the proximal plantar arch, and gives branches to the rete tarsi dorsale. Continuing downward along the deep flexor tendon as the external

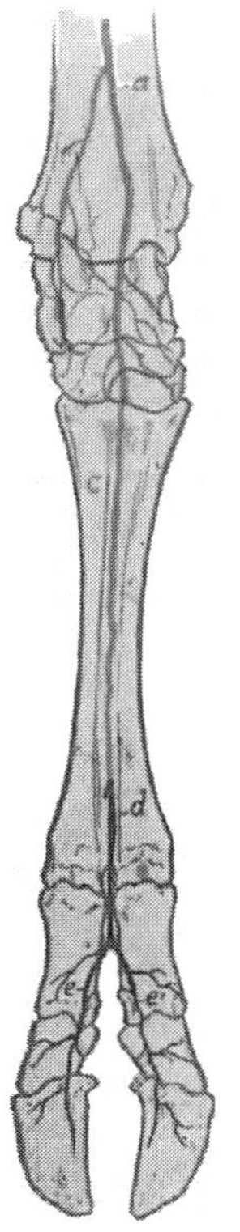

FIG. 476.—ARTERIES OF DISTAL PART OF RIGHT HIND LIMB OF OX ANTERIOR VIEW.

a, Anterior tibial artery; *b*, proximal perforating metatarsal artery; *c*, dorsal metatarsal artery; *d*, dorsal common digital artery; *e*, *e'*, dorsal proper digital arteries.

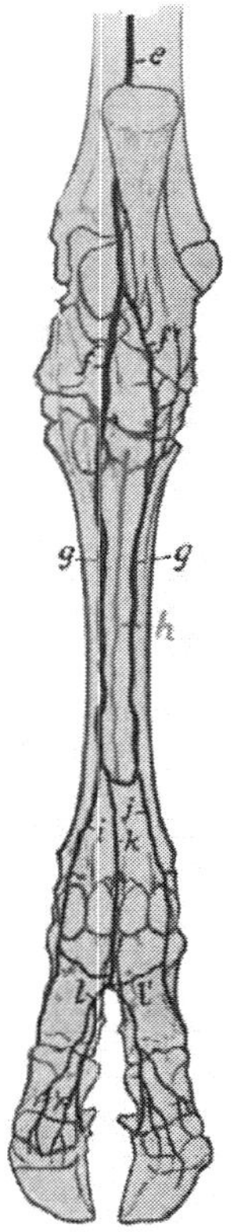

FIG. 477.—ARTERIES OF DISTAL PART OF RIGHT HIND LIMB OF OX, POSTERIOR VIEW.

e, Saphenous artery; *f*, *f'*, internal and external plantar arteries; *g*, *g'*, internal and external superficial plantar metatarsal arteries; *h*, deep plantar metatarsal artery; *i*, *j*, internal and external plantar digital arteries; *k*, plantar common digital artery; *l*, *l'*, internal and external plantar digital arteries.

superficial plantar metatarsal artery, it assists in forming the distal plantar arch and becomes the external digital artery.

The posterior tibial artery is relatively small and is distributed chiefly to the muscles on the posterior surface of the tibia. Lower down it is replaced by the saphenous artery as described above.

The anterior tibial artery has the same course as in the horse. It is continued down the groove on the front of the metatarsal bone as the dorsal metatarsal artery. This is the chief artery of the region and is accompanied by two veins. It detaches the proximal perforating metatarsal artery, which passes through the proximal foramen of the metatarsal bone and concurs with the superficial plantar arteries in forming the proximal plantar arch. Near the distal end of the metatarsal bone it gives off the distal perforating metatarsal artery which passes back through the distal metatarsal foramen and assists in forming the distal plantar arch. The two arches are connected by the small **deep plantar metatarsal artery** which lies in the groove on the posterior face of the large metatarsal bone.

The **dorsal common digital artery** is the direct continuation of the dorsal metatarsal. It divides into two branches which unite in the interdigital space with the corresponding branches of the plantar common digital to form the proper digital arteries.

The **plantar common digital artery** descends from the distal plantar arch, anastomoses in the interdigital space with the internal and external digitals, and divides into two branches which join those of the dorsal common digital artery as before mentioned.

The foregoing is a brief statement of the more common arrangement of the vessels in the distal part of the limb, but minor variations are very common.

THE VEINS [1]

The **vena hemiazygos** usually takes the place of the vena azygos. It lies along the left side of the aorta and the bodies of the thoracic vertebræ, turns down across the left face of the aorta and left pulmonary artery, runs back over the left auricle and opens into the great coronary vein or the right atrium. It receives the intercostal veins.

Two **jugular veins** occur on either side. The **internal jugular vein** (V. jugularis interna) is a relatively small vessel which accompanies the carotid artery. It arises by occipital, laryngeal, and thyroid radicles, receives tracheal, œsophageal, and muscular branches, and joins the external jugular near its termination. It is sometimes absent, but in some cases it appears, on the other hand, to be large enough to interfere with venesection practised on the external jugular. The **external jugular vein** (V. jugularis externa) is very large and corresponds to the single jugular of the horse. It is separated from the carotid artery in the greater part of its course by the sternocephalicus and omo-hyoideus muscles.

The **inferior cerebral vein** usually does not unite with the occipital; the latter is continued by the internal jugular vein.

The **orbital veins** form a network between the periorbita and the muscles of the eyeball. This plexus communicates with the cavernous sinus and with the superior cerebral vein. It is also drained by the frontal vein which runs in the supraorbital canal and groove and joins the angular vein of the eye.

The **dorsal nasal vein** is usually double.

The **superior labial vein** usually joins the infraorbital.

The **vena reflexa** is absent and the radicles which are received by it in the horse go to the internal maxillary vein.

The **sublingual vein** is very large.

The **veins of the thoracic limb** differ chiefly in the distal part; the special features are as follows:

The **dorsal digital veins** ascend on the front of the digits and are connected with the other digital veins by transverse branches. They unite near the fetlock to form the **dorsal metacarpal vein.** This runs upward on the anterior face of the metacarpus and carpus, inclines to the inner surface of the radius, and joins the accessory cephalic or the cephalic vein.

The **volar digital veins** are larger than the dorsal. They lie on the interdigital

[1] Most of the differences in the veins of the ox are correlated with those of the arteries of which they are satellites and will not be described. The account here given consists chiefly of those differential features which could not be deduced from a knowledge of the arteries.

surfaces of the digits and unite in the interdigital space to form a trunk which is a satellite of the volar common digital artery.

The **internal** and **external digital veins** lie in front of the corresponding arteries. They are connected with the volar digital vein by a large branch which passes between the flexor tendons and the first phalanx. At the distal end of the metacarpus each inclines forward and anastomoses with the volar common digital vein to form the volar venous arch. The inner vein is continued as the internal volar metacarpal vein along the inner border of the suspensory ligament, and becomes a satellite of the radial artery in the forearm, while the outer one is continued on the posterior face of the metacarpal bone by two irregular veins, the external and middle volar metacarpals. The latter anastomose freely with each other and with the inner vein. They unite below the carpus or join the volar common digital vein.

The **accessory cephalic vein** is the upward continuation of the dorsal metacarpal vein and is much larger than in the horse.

The posterior vena cava is partially embedded in the medial border of the liver. Its abdominal part has a thicker wall than in the horse. Its affluents correspond to the arteries of which they are satellites. The **renal veins** are large and thick-walled; they run obliquely forward and join the vena cava at an acute angle. The left one is much the longer.

Two **middle sacral veins** usually accompany the artery.

The **veins of the mammary glands** deserve special notice. They converge to a venous circle at the base of the udder, which is drained chiefly by two pairs of veins. The **subcutaneous abdominal vein** (anterior mammary or "milk" vein) is very large in animals of the dairy breeds and its course along the ventral wall of the abdomen is easily followed. It is usually flexuous. It emerges at the anterior border of the udder about two or three inches (ca. 5 to 8 cm.) from the linea alba, runs forward (deviating a little outward), dips under the panniculus, passes through a foramen in the abdominal wall about a handbreadth from the median plane, and joins the internal thoracic vein. The **external pudic vein** (middle mammary vein) is also of considerable size. It ascends in the inguinal canal as a satellite of the artery and joins the external iliac vein. The right and left veins are connected at the posterior border of the base of the udder by a large transverse branch. From the latter arises the **perineal vein** (posterior mammary vein), which runs medially upward and backward to the perineum, turns around the ischial arch, and joins the internal pudic vein. In the male these veins are relatively small.

The deep veins of the thigh and leg resemble those of the horse, but there is no recurrent tibial vein.

The saphenous vein is much smaller than in the horse.

The **recurrent tarsal vein** (external saphenous) is large. It is the upward continuation of the external plantar metatarsal vein and anastomoses with the anterior tibial and saphenous veins. It arises on the outer face of the hock, ascends at first in front of the tendo Achillis, then crosses the latter externally, passes up between the biceps femoris and semitendinosus, and joins the posterior femoral vein.

There are three chief metatarsal veins. The great **dorsal metatarsal vein** arises at the distal part of the metatarsus by the union of the dorsal digital vein and a large branch from the venous arch above the sesamoids. It ascends superficially between the long and lateral extensor tendons and becomes the chief radicle of the anterior tibial vein. The **internal plantar metatarsal vein** arises from the venous arch above the fetlock, ascends along the inner border of the suspensory ligament, passes through the vascular canal of the metatarsus and centro-tarsal (as the perforating tarsal) and joins the anterior tibial vein. The **external plantar**

metatarsal vein is larger than the preceding. It passes superficially over the outer face of the hock and is continued by the recurrent tarsal vein.

The **digital veins** differ from those of the fore limb chiefly in that the dorsal vein is large and the plantar absent or small.

The **portal vein** is formed usually by the confluence of two radicles, gastric and mesenteric. It receives the right gastro-epiploic vein and veins of the pancreas. The gastric vein is the largest affluent. It is formed by the junction of three veins, the left of which receives the splenic vein. The anterior mesenteric vein is also formed by the confluence of three radicles; it usually receives the small posterior mesenteric vein. The portal tributaries are in general satellites of the corresponding arteries.

The Lymph Vessels and Glands

The **thoracic duct** arises from a small cisterna chyli and is very variable. It is exceptional to find a single trunk throughout, as is often the case in the horse. The duct is largely covered by fat and small lymph glands. There are often two ducts, one on either side of the aorta, which may join at a variable point or terminate close together at the junctions of the jugular and brachial veins. In other cases the duct is single for a variable distance, then bifurcates or divides into three or four branches, which are often connected by plexiform anastomoses.

The efferent vessels from the intestine converge to a large trunk which accompanies the anterior mesenteric artery and vein. It passes below the pancreas and receives usually a large duct which is formed by efferent vessels from the stomach, liver, and spleen; this duct sometimes opens directly into the cisterna. The gastro-intestinal trunk receives the collecting duct (truncus lumbalis) of the lumbar lymph vessels, forms a bend around the right renal vessels, and joins the cisterna.

The **lymph glands** in the ox are in general less numerous but larger than those of the horse, and in some situations a single large gland occurs instead of a group of smaller ones, as found in the latter animal.

The **submaxillary lymph glands** are usually two in number, right and left; each is situated under the external maxillary vein between the submaxillary salivary gland and the sterno-cephalicus muscle. Usually one or two hæmolymph glands are near it. There is generally a small gland on the deep face of the anterior part of the submaxillary salivary gland, and small nodes may be found further forward in the submaxillary space.

A large **subparotid lymph gland** lies on the postero-superior part of the masseter muscle, partly under cover of the upper end of the parotid gland. Several hæmolymph glands lie on its deep face.

The **pharyngeal lymph glands** number two or three on each side. Of these, two large **suprapharyngeal glands** (Lg. retropharyngeales) are situated about an inch apart between the dorsal wall of the pharynx and the ventral straight muscles (Figs. 281, 365). These are two to three inches long. Enlargement of them is likely to cause difficulty in swallowing and in respiration. Behind these are several hæmolymph glands. An **atlantal gland** is situated below the wing of the atlas on the spinal accessory nerve. It is discoid, oval in outline, and may be an inch and a half or more in length. It is partly covered by the upper end of the submaxillary salivary gland.

A smaller lymph gland (parapharyngeal) is usually found along the lower border of the carotid artery (*i. e.*, ventral to the atlantal gland) on the lateral wall of the pharynx and under cover of the submaxillary salivary gland or at its posterior border.

Two or three small **anterior cervical lymph glands** commonly lie along the carotid artery a little further back.

The middle cervical lymph glands comprise a series of small nodes along the dorsal face of the trachea.

In the sheep and goat there is a lymph gland at the middle of the neck, in the angle between the spinalis and complexus, covered by the splenius. It receives vessels from the atlantal gland and sends efferents to the prescapular gland.

The prescapular or superficial cervical lymph gland is situated at the anterior border of the supraspinatus under cover of the mastoido-humeralis and omo-transversarius. It is elongated and may be an inch or more in width and four or five inches long. Two occur in exceptional cases.

A chain of hæmolymph glands lies along the front of the shoulder, covered above by the trapezius. Others are frequently found (in the calf especially) on the surface of the omo-transversarius at the point where it passes under the mastoido-humeralis (Forgeot).

The posterior cervical or prepectoral lymph glands number commonly three or four on each side. One or two are placed on the brachial vessels, one below the

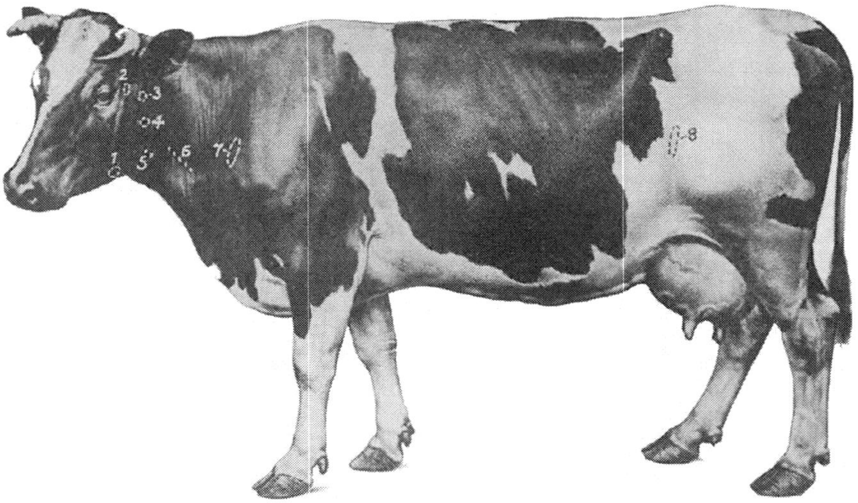

Fig. 478.—Superficial Lymph Glands of Cow Projected on Surface of Body.
1 Submaxillary; *2*, subparotid; *3*, atlantal; *4*, parapharyngeal; *5*, anterior cervical; *6*, middle cervical; *7*, prescapular; *8*, precrural. (With use of fig. in Ellenberger-Baum, Anat. f. Künstler.)

brachial vein at the first rib, and one at the junction of the common trunk of the external and subcutaneous thoracic veins with the brachial.

The intercostal lymph glands are situated, as in the horse, at the upper parts of the intercostal spaces. Associated with them are hæmolymph glands.

The sternal lymph glands are situated along the course of the internal thoracic artery at the lower part of the intercostal spaces. The largest is close to the thoracic inlet. Several glands occur in the fat about the apex of the pericardium.

4. Several anterior mediastinal lymph glands are placed along the œsophagus and the trachea.[1] Hæmolymph glands occur here also.

Usually three large bronchial lymph glands are present (Fig. 289). One is situated at the origin of each chief bronchus and the third is under the trachea at the origin of the special bronchus of the apical lobe of the right lung. Another

[1] The upper series is continuous with the posterior mediastinal (œsophageal) glands and the lower or tracheal glands with the bronchial. Hence we might well designate the mediastinal glands as œsophageal (anterior and posterior) and tracheo-bronchial.

may lie between the aorta and the left branch of the pulmonary artery. These glands are often pigmented. Other small nodes are situated on the bronchi within the lungs.

The **posterior mediastinal lymph glands** comprise two or three of large size placed along the dorsal wall of the œsophagus. There may be a single gland about eight inches (ca. 20 cm.) long, the anterior half of which lies on the œsophagus (Fig. 289).[1] A small gland is situated in the acute angle formed by the posterior vena cava and the diaphragm.

A single **axillary lymph gland** is situated on the distal part of the teres major on the course of the vein from the latissimus dorsi.

The **lumbar lymph glands** form an irregular series scattered along the abdominal aorta and posterior vena. A bean-shaped **renal lymph gland** occurs at the hilus of each kidney. **Hæmolymph glands** occur along the course of the aorta.

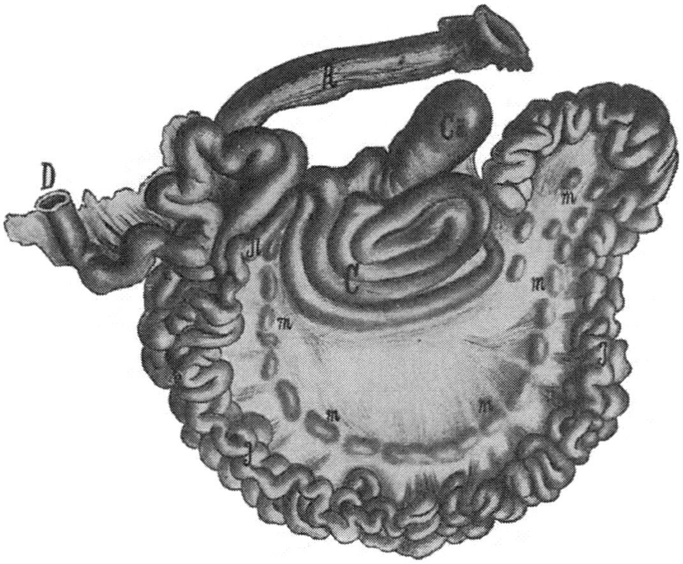

Fig. 479.—Intestine of Ox, Spread Out.
Ca Cæcum; C, colon; *D*, duodenum; *Il*, ileum; *J*, jejunum; *R*, rectum; *m*, mesenteric lymph glands. (After Edelmann.)

The **internal iliac lymph glands** comprise a group of five or six at the termination of the aorta and the origin of the vena cava. A discoid gland, two inches or more in diameter, occurs near the side of the pelvic inlet at the angle of divergence of the circumflex iliac artery from the external iliac. A small gland is sometimes found at the origin of the prepubic artery.

The **external iliac lymph glands** number commonly two on either side, and are situated near the point of the hip in front of the anterior branch of the circumflex iliac artery.

The superficial **inguinal lymph glands** are situated centrally below the prepubic tendon and in the narrow space between the origins of the graciles. In the male there are usually two or three on either side of the penis behind the sigmoid flexure. In the cow they are supramammary, *i. e.*, are situated above the posterior margin

[1] When enlarged, as is often the case in tuberculosis, this gland frequently causes difficulty in swallowing and in rumination and produces chronic or recurrent bloating.

of the base of the udder; two large glands which are in apposition with each other medially are constant, and above these there are often two smaller glands.

An **ischiatic lymph gland**, which is discoid and usually about an inch in diameter, is situated on the lower part of the sacro-sciatic ligament near the lesser sciatic notch under cover of the biceps femoris.

An **anal lymph gland** is situated on the retractor ani on either side.

The **gastric lymph glands** are numerous and comprise: (1) a chain along the course of the right ruminal artery and two or three in the left groove of the rumen; (2) several on the reticulum above and below the junction with the omasum; (3) a series along the course of the superior omasal vessels and the lesser curvature of the abomasum; (4) an extensive chain along the ventral face of the omasum and the great curvature of the abomasum at the attachment of the great omentum.

Two or three large hepatic or **portal lymph glands** are found at the upper part of the portal fissure of the liver.

No lymph glands occur at the hilus of the spleen. The efferent vessels from the spleen appear to go to glands along the course of the cœliac artery.

A large discoid **cœliac lymph gland** lies on the pancreas and the cœliac artery, covering the latter as it gives off its primary branches.

The **mesenteric lymph glands** are large and numerous. They form a chain in the lower part of the mesentery along the course of the great mesenteric artery. They are chiefly elongated and narrow, and some have a length of six to eight inches (15 to 20 cm.) or more. Sometimes several unite and form a narrow band about two feet in length. A large gland occurs at the origin of the spiral part of the colon, a group is found near the anterior mesenteric trunk, and others are scattered along the coils of the colon, which are best seen on the right side. A chain of small lymph glands extends along the terminal part of the colon and the dorsal face of the rectum.

The **precrural lymph gland** is situated on the aponeurosis of the external oblique at the anterior border of the tensor fasciæ latæ a short distance above the stifle. It is elongated like the prescapular gland and may be six inches (ca. 15 cm.) long. Several subcutaneous hæmolymph glands occur in this vicinity; others are situated further forward on the flank not far from the last rib. There is usually a round, flattened lymph gland about an inch in diameter on the upper part of the quadriceps femoris under cover of the tensor fasciæ latæ, and one or more small ones occur on the surface of the latter muscle.

No **deep inguinal lymph glands** are present.

A single **popliteal lymph gland** an inch or more in length is situated somewhat lower down on the gastrocnemius than in the horse, behind the tibial and peroneal nerves.

CIRCULATORY SYSTEM OF THE PIG

THE HEART

The pericardium is attached to the sternum from a point opposite to the third rib as far as the xiphoid cartilage, and also to the sternal part of the diaphragm.

The heart is small in proportion to the body-weight, especially in fat animals. It is relatively short and wide. The apex is blunt and is marked by a notch (Incisura apicis). Its long axis is more oblique, but it is less asymmetrical with regard to the median plane, than in the horse or ox. The lower border of the left auricle (appendix) is marked by several notches and is situated at a lower level than the right one. The right longitudinal groove is placed far back and there is no posterior sulcus.

THE ARTERIES

The **pulmonary vessels** present no remarkable features.

The aorta resembles that of the horse and ox in its course and relations, but the arch is more strongly curved. There is no common brachiocephalic trunk (anterior aorta).

The **brachiocephalic artery** arises first from the aortic arch and passes forward below the trachea to the first rib. Here it gives off the common **carotid arteries**, and is continued around the first rib as the right brachial.

The **superior cervical, vertebral,** and **dorsal arteries** usually arise by a common trunk.

The **inferior cervical artery** is large; its ascending branch gives off the **posterior thyroid artery** and **parotid branches.**

The **internal** and **external thoracic arteries** give branches to the pectoral mammary glands; the external may be absent.

The left **brachial artery** arises from the aortic arch just above the brachiocephalic. It curves forward and downward and turns around the anterior border of the first rib. Its superior cervical, vertebral, and dorsal branches usually arise separately.

The **carotid arteries** arise from the brachiocephalic close together or by a very short common trunk. They terminate in occipital and internal and external carotid divisions.

The **occipital artery** resembles that of the horse.

The **internal carotid artery** usually arises by a common trunk with the occipital. After giving off a large meningeal branch it passes through the foramen lacerum and forms with the opposite artery a rete mirabile which resembles that of the ox, but is smaller and is not connected with the vertebral and condyloid arteries.

The **external carotid artery** has the same course and termination as in the horse. Its branches present the following special features: (1) The **lingual artery** is relatively large and supplies the pharyngeal artery, the sublingual, muscular branches, and branches to the soft palate, submaxillary gland, and larynx. (2) The **external maxillary artery** is small and is distributed chiefly to the submaxillary gland, the pharyngeal lymph glands, the masseter and the panniculus. It does not extend upon the lateral surface of the face. (3) The **posterior auricular artery** is long and relatively large; it gives off the posterior meningeal.

The **internal maxillary artery** pursues a flexuous course between the ramus of the mandible and the pterygoid muscles. Its branches offer the following special features: (1) The **inferior alveolar** (or dental) is large; branches from it emerge through four or five mental foramina and take the place of the inferior labial. (2) The **buccinator artery** is also large and extends to the lips. (3) The **infraorbital artery** extends to the snout and replaces the superior labial largely and the lateral nasal in part. The malar branch compensates largely for the absence of the lateral and dorsal nasal. (4) The **palatine artery** is small.

The **intercostal arteries** number fourteen to sixteen in either side; of these ten to twelve arise from the aorta, usually by short common trunks. Frequently an intercostal artery is given off from that of an adjacent space.

The **bronchial** and **œsophageal arteries** usually arise separately.

The **cœliac artery** is half an inch to an inch long. It supplies a branch to the left crus of the diaphragm and divides into two primary branches, gastro-hepatic and splenic. The gastro-hepatic artery is the larger. It gives off pancreatic branches, the anterior gastric artery, branches to the lesser curvature of the stomach, pyloric and gastro-duodenal arteries. The latter divides into pancreatico-duodenal and right gastro-epiploic. The anterior gastric usually supplies the œsophageal artery. The continuing trunk (A. hepatica propria) gives off a cystic branch and divides in the portal fissure into four branches which supply the liver. The splenic artery gives off the posterior gastric (usually), branches to the stomach above the cardia, twigs to the pancreas, short gastric arteries to the left part of the great curvature, and splenic branches, and is continued as the left gastro-epiploic artery.

The posterior gastric may arise from the gastro-hepatic or in the angle of divergence of the two primary divisions of the cœliac. The œsophageal branch may come from the splenic.

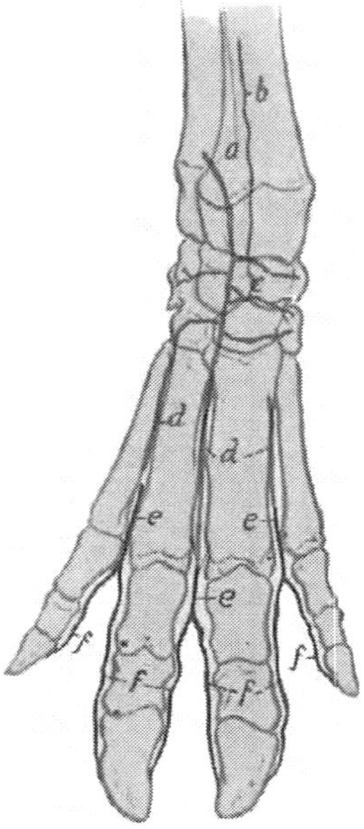

Fig. 480.—Arteries of Distal Part of Right Fore Limb of Pig, Anterior View.

a, Terminal part of volar interosseous artery; *b*, dorsal interosseous artery; *c*, rete carpi dorsale; *d*, dorsal metacarpal arteries; *e*, dorsal common digital arteries; *f*, dorsal proper digital arteries.

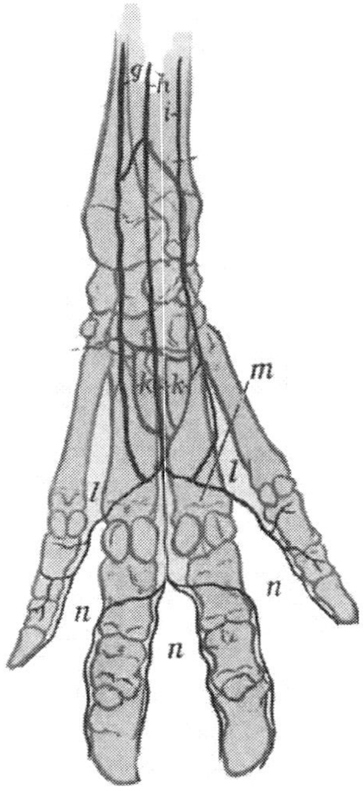

Fig. 481.—Arteries of Distal Part of Right Fore Limb of Pig, Posterior View.

g, Ulnar artery; *h*, superficial branch of radial artery; *i*, collateral ulnar artery; *j*, volar interosseous artery; *h*, deep branch of radial artery; *k*, deep volar metacarpal arteries; *l*, superficial volar metacarpal arteries; *m*, volar common digital artery; *n*, volar proper digital arteries.

The anterior mesenteric artery is long like that of the ox. It gives twigs to the pancreas, the ilio-cæcal and two colic arteries, and is continued in the mesentery as the artery of the small intestine. This gives off numerous branches which form a series of arches along the mesenteric lymph glands. From these is formed a rich network which gives off innumerable fine branches placed close together. The colic arteries enter the axis of the spiral coil of the colon and anastomose at its apex. Their branches also form rich networks.

A phrenico-abdominal artery arises on either side a little in front of the renals. It divides into branches which go to the costal part of the diaphragm and the abdominal muscles.

The renal and spermatic arteries present no special characters.

The posterior mesenteric artery arises near the termination of the aorta. It is small and is distributed like that of the ox.

Six pairs of lumbar arteries arise from the aorta. The seventh comes from the middle sacral.

The terminal branches of the aorta resemble those of the ox.

The arteries of the shoulder, arm, and forearm resemble in general those of the ox.

The main facts as to the metacarpal and digital arteries are as follows: The rete carpi dorsale is formed essentially by the terminals of the interosseous artery of the forearm. It gives rise to three dorsal metacarpal arteries which descend in

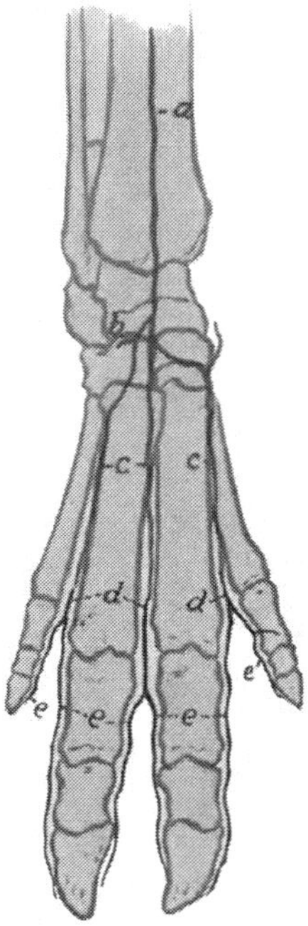

FIG. 482.—ARTERIES OF DISTAL PART OF RIGHT HIND LIMB OF PIG ANTERIOR VIEW.

a, Anterior tibial artery, continued on tarsus as the dorsalis pedis; *b*, perforating tarsal artery; *c*, dorsal metatarsal arteries; *d*, common digital arteries; *e*, proper digital arteries.

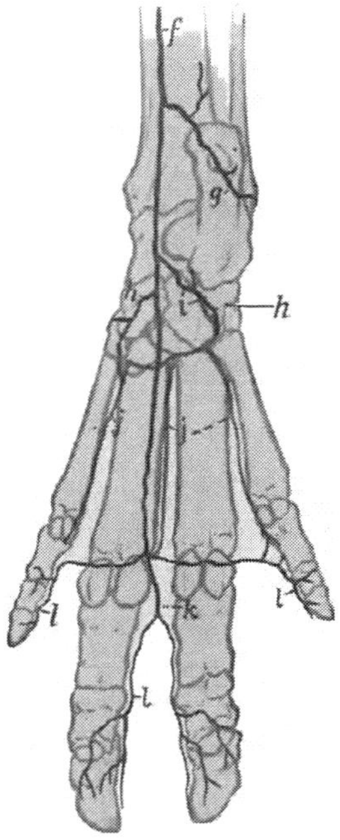

FIG. 483.—ARTERIES OF DISTAL PART OF RIGHT HIND LIMB OF PIG, POSTERIOR VIEW.

f, Saphenous artery, continued as internal tarsal artery; *g*, external tarsal artery; *h*, internal plantar artery; *h'*, external plantar artery; *i*, perforating tarsal artery; *j*, deep plantar metatarsal arteries; *k*, common digital artery; *l*, proper digital arteries.

the corresponding interosseous spaces and unite with branches of the volar metacarpals to form three common digital arteries. Each of these divides into two proper digital arteries, which descend along the interdigital surfaces of the digits. On the volar surface are two volar arches, superficial and deep, from which three superficial and three deep volar metacarpal arteries arise. The deep arteries unite near the distal end of the space between the principal metacarpal bones to form a stem which unites with the middle (third) superficial artery. The superficial arteries unite to form an arch from which proper digital arteries are given off to the axial aspect of the small digits, and a common digital which supplies two volar proper digital arteries to each of the chief digits.

The arteries of the hip, thigh, and leg are arranged much as in the ox. A few special features may be noted.

The **ilio-lumbar artery** gives off a branch to the quadriceps femoris. It may also supply the posterior abdominal artery, which otherwise arises from the deep femoral.

The **deep femoral artery** is given off above the level of the pubis. The posterior abdominal and external pudic arteries may arise from it by a short common trunk or separately. The **external pudic** gives branches to the prepuce but not to the penis. The **popliteal artery** gives off the peroneal.

The **femoral artery** gives off a short trunk which divides into anterior femoral and external circumflex arteries, the latter being much the larger.

The **saphenous artery** is large. It descends on the inner surface of the leg and hock and concurs with the perforating tarsal artery in forming the proximal plantar arch.

The **posterior tibial artery** is small, being replaced distally by the saphenous. It gives branches to the muscles on the posterior face of the tibia and supplies the nutrient artery of that bone.

The **anterior tibial artery** is continued as the dorsalis pedis on the flexion surface of the tarsus. This gives off the **perforating tarsal artery**, which passes back through the vascular canal of the tarsus and unites with the terminal branches of the saphenous to form the proximal plantar arch.

The **metatarsal** and **digital arteries** resemble in arrangement the corresponding vessels of the fore limb.

THE VEINS

The **veins** resemble in general those of the ox. Thus there is a hemiazygos vein and two jugular veins, the internal one being relatively larger than in the ox. A few differential features may be noted.

The **buccinator vein** resembles that of the horse, and unites with the **vena reflexa** to form a short common trunk which joins the facial.

The **facial vein** resembles in general that of the horse. The **dorsal nasal vein** is large, receives the veins from the snout, runs backward in the groove of the nasal bone and joins the frontal vein; it is connected with its fellow by a transverse branch, and anastomoses freely with the malar and facial.

The veins of the distal parts of the limbs naturally present differences which are correlated with those of the arteries.

THE LYMPH VESSELS AND GLANDS

The **thoracic duct** often divides near its termination into two branches which unite to form an ampulla. The latter suddenly contracts and opens into the terminal part of the left jugular vein.

The **submaxillary lymph glands** are situated in the space between the omohyoid and internal pterygoid muscles in relation to the lower part of the anterior border of the submaxillary salivary gland. There are commonly two on each side, one large, the other small.

The **parotid lymph glands** (Fig. 309) are reddish-brown in color. There are usually four of considerable size on either side. One is situated at the upper part of the posterior border of the masseter, partly covered by the parotid gland. Another large subparotid gland lies below the base of the ear. Ventral to this are two smaller glands, one above and one below the external jugular vein.

The **pharyngeal** (or retropharyngeal) **lymph glands** (Fig. 310) are situated on the dorsal wall of the pharynx above the external carotid artery and below and behind the paramastoid process. There are usually two of considerable size on either side.

The **middle cervical lymph glands** form a group on the mastoido-humeralis on the course of the external jugular vein.

The **prescapular lymph glands** are situated at the anterior border of the anterior deep pectoral muscle under cover of the trapezius and omo-transversarius.

The **prepectoral lymph glands** are reddish in color and usually three in number. The largest is placed centrally under the trachea; the others are situated on the brachial vessels as they turn around the first rib.

The **axillary lymph glands** are usually absent, but very small nodes may be found near the insertion of the latissimus dorsi. Cubital glands are not present.

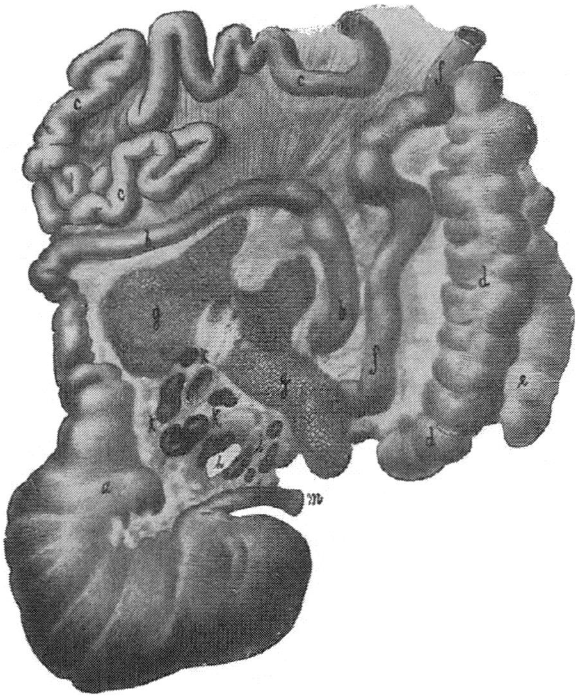

FIG. 484.—STOMACH AND PART OF INTESTINE OF PIG, SPREAD OUT.
a, Pyloric portion of stomach; *b*, duodenum; *c*, jejunum; *d*, cæcum; *e*, *f*, colon; *g*, pancreas; *h*, epiploic foramen (of Winslow); *i*, portal vein; k, hepatic lymph glands; *l*, gastric lymph glands; *m*, œsophagus. (After Edelmann.)

The **thoracic lymph glands** comprise: (1) a gland of considerable size on the first segment of the sternum; (2) about half a dozen reddish glands along the upper face of the thoracic aorta; (3) several glands along the lower face of the trachea; (4) the **bronchial lymph glands;** one of these lies on the bifurcation of the trachea and another at the apical bronchus of the right lung (Fig. 371).

The **lumbar lymph glands** are scattered along the abdominal aorta and the vena cava. Those placed near the hilus of the kidney are often designated **renal.**

The **internal iliac lymph glands** are rounded and relatively large. They comprise: (1) three or four glands situated on and between the origin of the circumflex iliac and the external and internal iliac arteries; (2) a gland in the angle of divergence of the internal iliac arteries.

The **external iliac lymph** glands are small, two or three in number, and lie in front of the circumflex iliac vessels near the point of the hip.

The visceral lymph glands of the abdomen comprise:

1. **Gastric** lymph **glands** on the lesser curvature of the stomach.
2. Several small **hepatic** lymph **glands** along the portal vein.
3. An elongated **splenic** lymph **gland** on the splenic vessels near the dorsal end of the spleen.
4. A series of **mesenteric** lymph **glands** situated along the anastomotic arches formed by the vessels of the small intestine.
5. Several **cæcal** lymph **glands** situated along the first part of the cæcal vessels.
6. Two series of **colic** lymph **glands** which accompany the arteries of the spiral part of the colon, and are exposed by separating the coils of the bowel. Small glands are placed in the colic mesentery and above the rectum.
7. The **anal** lymph **glands** are situated on either side on the retractor ani.

A small **ischiatic** lymph **gland** is found on the sacro-sciatic ligament near the lesser sciatic notch.

The **precrural** lymph **glands** are situated on the aponeurosis of the external oblique below the external angle of the ilium.

The **superficial inguinal** lymph **glands** are situated behind the external inguinal ring. No deep inguinal lymph glands are present.

The **popliteal** lymph **glands** are small normally and may escape notice.

A few nodules occur in front of the distal part of the tendo Achillis.

CIRCULATORY SYSTEM OF THE DOG

THE PERICARDIUM AND HEART

The **pericardium** is attached to the sternal part of the diaphragm by a fibrous band, and is connected with the sternum only by the mediastinal pleura.

The **heart** is almost globular in form, the apex being much blunter than in the other animals, and marked by a notch. Its long axis is almost parallel with the sternum and the apex (covered by the pericardium) is directed against the sternal part of the diaphragm. Its weight averages about 0.8 to 1 per cent. of the body-weight.[1]

The base extends forward to a transverse plane through the lower ends of the third pair of ribs. The apex lies opposite the sixth costal cartilage in expiration. On the right side the pericardium is in direct contact with the chest-wall over a narrow triangular area (base anterior) from the fourth to the sixth intercostal space inclusive. On the left side the area of contact is smaller and is at the fourth, fifth, and sixth cartilages.

The two coronary arteries may arise by a common trunk. Each divides into circumflex and descending branches. The left artery is twice as large as the right one.

The great coronary vein ascends in the left longitudinal groove to the coronary groove, in which it winds around the posterior face of the heart to the right side and opens into the right atrium below the posterior vena cava. Near its termination it receives one or two veins which ascend along the right longitudinal furrow. Several small veins from the wall of the right ventricle open into the right atrium separately or by a common trunk.

[1] The relative weight is subject to wide variation. It is large in hunting dogs and such as are trained for speed or worked.

THE ARTERIES

There is no common brachiocephalic trunk (anterior aorta). Two large vessels arise from the convexity of the aortic arch; these are the **brachiocephalic** and **left brachial arteries.** The **brachiocephalic** gives off the two **carotid arteries,** no common trunk being present. It frequently also supplies the posterior thyroid artery. The intrathoracic branches of the brachial arteries are as follows:

A common trunk gives off the **dorsal, subcostal,** and **superior cervical arteries.** The dorsal artery passes out in front of the first rib, and the superior cervical through the first intercostal space. The latter is relatively small.

The **vertebral artery** may arise either in front of or behind the trunk above mentioned; in the latter case it crosses the inner face of the trunk. It passes along

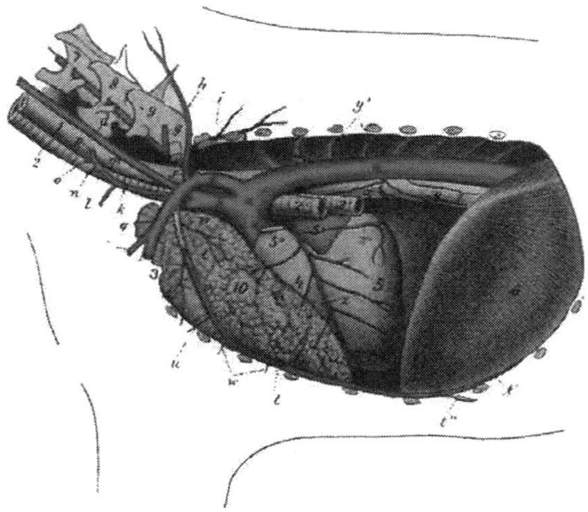

FIG. 485.—ARTERIES OF THORACIC CAVITY AND PART OF NECK OF DOG.

a, Aortic arch; *a'*, thoracic aorta; *b*, brachiocephalic artery; *c*, left brachial artery; *d*, *d*, common carotid arteries; *e*, vertebral artery; *f*, dorsal artery; *g*, deep or superior cervical artery (usually given off from a common trunk with *f*); *h*, extrathoracic part of *f*; *i*, subcostal artery; *k*, inferior cervical artery; *l*, descending branch of *k*; *m*, ascending branch of *k*; *n*, internal scapular; *o*, acromial; *p*, superficial cervical; *q*, *s*, extrathoracic part of left brachial; *r*, external thoracic; *t*, internal thoracic; *t'*, asternal; *t''*, anterior abdominal; *u*, perforating branch of *t*; *v*, anterior mediastinal (thymic); *w*, ventral intercostals; *x*, bronchial; *y*, œsophageal; *y'*, dorsal intercostals; *z*, descending branch of left coronary artery; *z'*, circumflex branch of same; *1*, œsophagus; *2*, trachea; *2'*, bronchi; *3*, first rib (sawn off); *4*, right ventricle; *5*, left ventricle; *5'*, left auricle; *5''*, pulmonary artery (cut off); *6*, diaphragm; *7*, *8*, *9*, last three cervical vertebræ; *10*, thymus. (After Ellenberger, in Leisering's Atlas.)

the neck in typical fashion to the third cervical vertebra and divides into three branches. The largest of these supplies the muscles in this region, compensating for the absence of branches of the superior cervical artery. The second passes between the second and third cervical vertebræ into the vertebral canal and unites with the opposite artery and a branch of the occipital artery to form the basilar. The third branch is the small continuation of the parent trunk; it passes to the wing of the atlas and anastomoses with the occipital.

The **inferior cervical artery** gives off the superficial cervical which ascends in front of the supraspinatus.

The **internal thoracic artery** is large and sends perforating branches to the pectoral mammary glands.

The **external thoracic artery** arises outside of the thorax and sends branches to the mammary glands.

The **common carotid arteries,** left and right, arise in that order from the brachiocephalic. In the neck the right one lies on the trachea, the left on the œsophagus. Collateral branches are the posterior thyroid (which may, however, arise from the right or left brachial or the inferior cervical), pharyngeal, thryo-laryngeal, muscular, tracheal, and glandular (to the submaxillary gland). Each carotid divides under the wing of the atlas into occipital and internal and external carotid branches.

The **occipital artery** is small. It gives off **condyloid** and **posterior meningeal** branches, passes up through the notch on the anterior margin of the wing of the atlas, and is distributed to the muscles of this region. Its **cerebrospinal** branch

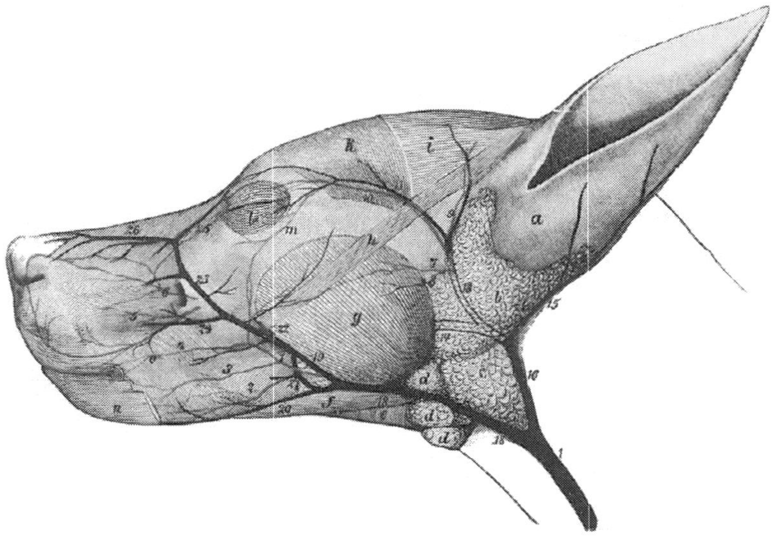

FIG. 486.—SUPERFICIAL VESSELS OF HEAD OF DOG.

1, Facial artery; *2*, inferior labial artery; *3*, artery of angle of mouth; *4*, superior labial artery; *5*, lateral nasal artery; *6*, dorsal nasal artery; *7*, superficial temporal artery; *8*, transverse facial artery; *9*, anterior auricular artery; *10*, zygomatico-orbital artery; *11*, satellite vein of *10*; *12*, ant. auricular vein; *13*, superficial temporal vein; *14*, internal maxillary vein; *15*, post. auricular vein; *16*, *17*, external jugular vein; *18*, external maxillary vein; *19*, *23*, facial vein; *20*, inf. labial vein; *21*, buccinator vein; *22*, vena reflexa; *24*, superior labial vein; *25*, vena angularis oculi; *26*, dorsal nasal vein; *a*, concha; *b*, parotid gland; *c*, submaxillary gland; *d*, submaxillary lymph glands; *e*, mylo-hyoideus; *f*, digastricus; *g*, masseter; *h*, zygomaticus; *i*, scutularis; k, temporalis; *l*, orbicularis oculi; *m*, zygomatic arch; *n*, retractor anguli oris; *o*, buccinator. (Ellenberger-Baum, Anat. d. Hundes.)

passes through the intervertebral foramen, and unites in the vertebral canal with its fellow and a branch from the vertebral artery to form the basilar. A retrograde branch anastomoses with the vertebral as in the horse.

The **internal carotid artery,** also small, passes to the foramen lacerum posterius, enters the carotid canal and forms a bend before entering the cranium through the carotid foramen. It forms a plexus which is connected by branches with the middle meningeal and ophthalmic arteries. It then perforates the dura mater and enters into the formation of the arterial circle (of Willis).

The **external carotid artery** is the direct continuation of the common carotid. It passes along the lateral wall of the pharynx, emerges from beneath the digastricus, and divides into superficial temporal and internal maxillary arteries. It gives off the large flexuous **lingual artery** which has a course similar to that of the horse.

The **external maxillary**, smaller than the lingual, passes along the upper border of the digastricus, gives off the sublingual, gains the anterior border of the masseter, and divides into superior and inferior labial and the angularis oris. The last-named vessel passes forward on the cheek between the labials to the angle of the mouth. The **sublingual artery** passes at first along the upper border of the digastricus and continues between the mylo-hyoideus and the ramus of the mandible. The **posterior auricular artery** arises at the anterior border of the digastricus, gives branches to the salivary glands and the adjacent muscles, and ascends on the convex face of the concha. It divides into two branches which return along the borders of the external ear.

The **superficial temporal artery**, after giving off the **anterior auricular artery** and a small **transverse facial artery**, turns forward under the temporal fascia toward the eye, and divides into upper and lower branches which supply the frontal region and the eyelids. It also supplies branches to the parotid gland and the masseter and temporalis muscles.

The **internal maxillary artery** pursues a course similar to that of the horse. The mental branches of the **inferior alveolar** (or dental) **artery** are of considerable size and are distributed in the lower lip and gums. Two or three **deep temporal arteries** are present. The anterior one may arise from the buccinator; it gives off the middle meningeal, which sends a branch to the carotid plexus. The **ophthalmic artery** gives off a branch which enters the cranium through the foramen lacerum orbitale and connects with the internal carotid; this is termed the internal ophthalmic and gives off the arteria centralis retinæ. The superficial branches of the **infraorbital artery** replace the dorsal and lateral nasal arteries, and compensate for the small size of the superior labial.

The **brachial artery** in its course in the arm presents no special features. At the elbow it passes between the biceps and the pronator teres, descends (as the median) under the flexor carpi radialis about a third of the way down the forearm, and divides into radial and ulnar arteries. Among its collateral branches are: (1) The **subscapular artery**, which passes up between the subscapularis and teres major, turns around the posterior angle of the scapula and terminates in the supraspinatus, deltoid, trapezius, and mastoido-humeralis. In about half the cases it gives off the **anterior circumflex**, which often arises with the **posterior circumflex**. Its other branches resemble those of the horse. (2) The **anterior circumflex artery** (in about half the cases). (3) The **deep brachial** arises about a third of the way down the arm. (4) The **bicipital artery** (for the biceps) is given off at the lower part of the arm. (5) The **proximal collateral radial artery** (not present in the horse) arises at the lower fourth of the arm, crosses over the terminal part of the biceps, descends on the extensor carpi radialis, and concurs with a branch of the volar interosseous in forming the rete carpi dorsale. It often supplies the bicipital artery. (6) The **anterior radial artery** (A. collateralis radialis distalis) is very small. (7) The **common interosseous artery** is given off a little below the elbow. It supplies branches to the flexor muscles and the **dorsal interosseous artery**, which passes through the interosseous space, gives branches to the extensor muscles, and by its terminal twigs concurs in the formation of the rete carpi dorsale. The direct continuation of the trunk is the **volar interosseous artery**, which descends under cover of the pronator quadratus, gives off a branch to the rete carpi dorsale and the **fifth volar metacarpal artery**, and terminates by joining the volar branch of the radial artery to form the deep volar arch. (8) The **volar antibrachial artery** (Ramus volaris antibrachii) arises below the interosseous and descends at first under the flexor carpi radialis, then between the heads of the deep flexor, and divides into ascending and descending branches.

The **radial artery**, the smaller terminal of the brachial, descends along the inner border of the radius, and divides near the carpus into dorsal and volar branches.

The dorsal branch assists in forming the rete carpi dorsale. The larger volar branch descends behind the inner border of the carpus and joins the end of the volar interosseous in forming the deep volar arch. From this arch three deep volar

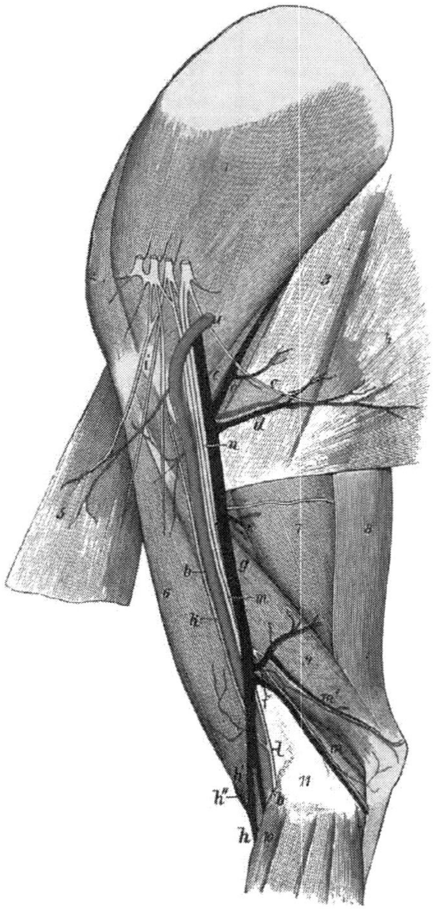

FIG. 487.—VESSELS AND NERVES OF INNER SURFACE OF SHOULDER AND ARM OF DOG.

a, *b*, Brachial artery; *c*, subscapular vessels; *d*, thoracico-dorsal vessels; *e*, deep brachial vessels; *f*, superior collateral ulnar vessels; *g*, brachial vein; *h*, *h''*, cephalic vein; *h'*, mediano-radial vein; *i*, anterior thoracic nerves; k, musculo-cutaneous nerve; *l*, median nerve; *m*, ulnar nerve; *n*, radial nerve; *o*, thoracico-dorsal nerve; *1*, subscapularis muscle; *2*, supraspinatus muscle; *3*, teres major, *4*, latissimus dorsi; *5*, deep pectoral muscle; *6*, biceps brachii; *7*, long head of triceps; *8*, tensor fasciæ antibrachii; *9*, internal head of triceps; *10*, pronator teres. (Ellenberger-Baum, Anat. d. Hundes.)

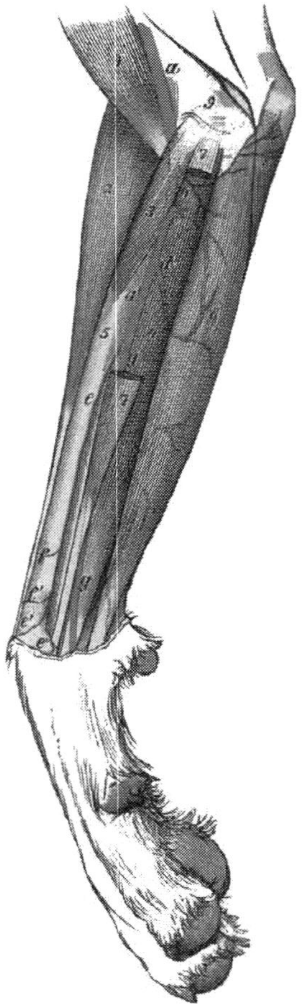

‥, *2*,

metacarpal arteries descend in the second, third, and fourth intermetacarpal spaces and concur with the corresponding superficial volar and the dorsal arteries to form the common digitals.

The **ulnar artery** descends on the deep flexor of the digit, and sends a connecting branch to the radial above the carpus. Near the middle of the metacarpus it gives off the **first volar metacarpal artery** and divides into the **second, third,** and **fourth superficial volar metacarpal arteries.** The first volar artery unites with the corresponding dorsal artery to form the **first common digital artery,** which supplies proper digital arteries for the opposed surfaces of the first and second digits. The superficial volar arteries descend in the spaces between the other metacarpal bones, unite near the metacarpo-phalangeal joints with the corresponding deep volar and dorsal metacarpal arteries to form three **common digital arteries.** Each of the latter

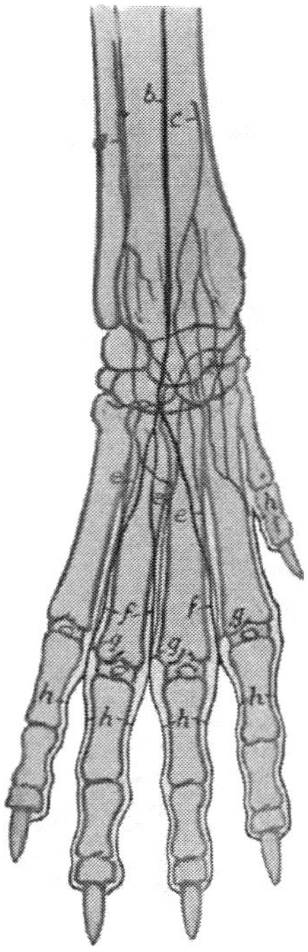

Fig. 489.—Arteries of Distal Part of Right Fore Limb of Dog, Anterior View.

a, Branch of volar interosseous artery; *b*, proximal collateral radial artery (external branch); *c*, radial artery (dorsal branch); *d*, rete carpi dorsale; *e*, deep dorsal metacarpal arteries; *f*, superficial dorsal metacarpal arteries; *g*, common digital arteries; *h*, proper digital arteries.

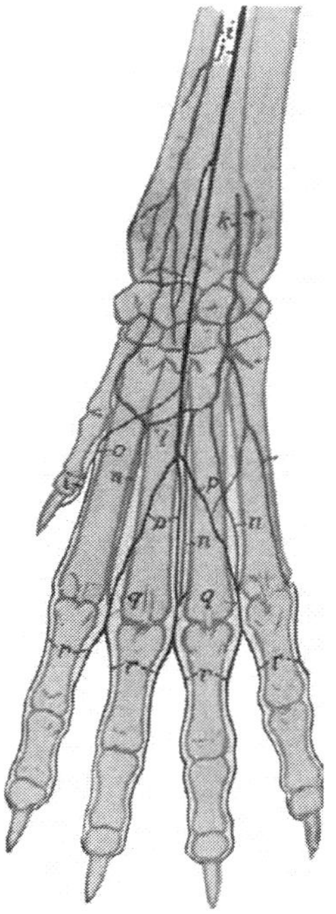

Fig. 490.

i, Radial artery; *j*, ulnar artery; *k*, volar interosseous artery; *l*, deep volar arch; *m*, external (fifth) volar metacarpal artery; *n*, deep volar metacarpal arteries; *p*, superficial volar metacarpal arteries; *o*, *q*, common digital arteries; *r*, proper digital arteries.

divides after a short course into two **proper digital arteries,** which run along the opposed surfaces of the second to the fifth digits. The external digital artery of the fifth digit comes from the **superficial volar arch** formed by the union of a branch of the volar interosseous with the fourth superficial volar metacarpal artery.

The rete carpi dorsale gives off four **dorsal metacarpal arteries** which descend in the intermetacarpal spaces and unite near the metacarpo-phalangeal joints with the volar arteries to form the common digitals.

The **thoracic aorta** supplies the last nine or ten pairs of intercostal arteries, but no anterior phrenic arteries. It gives off two or more œsophageal branches, in addition to the broncho-œsophageal, which arises close to or with the sixth intercostal and ramifies in the usual manner.

The **abdominal aorta,** after giving off the external iliac arteries, continues about half an inch to an inch (ca. 1 to 3 cm.) under the last lumbar vertebræ, gives off the internal iliacs, and is continued by the middle sacral artery. This small vessel runs backward under the sacrum and coccygeal vertebræ and gives off branches in segmental fashion.

The **cœliac artery** gives off the hepatic artery and forms a short **gastro-splenic trunk.** The **hepatic artery** gives off several hepatic branches, and the pyloric or right gastric artery, which passes along the lesser curvature of the stomach, anastomoses with the (left) gastric artery, and is continued by the gastro-duodenal. This

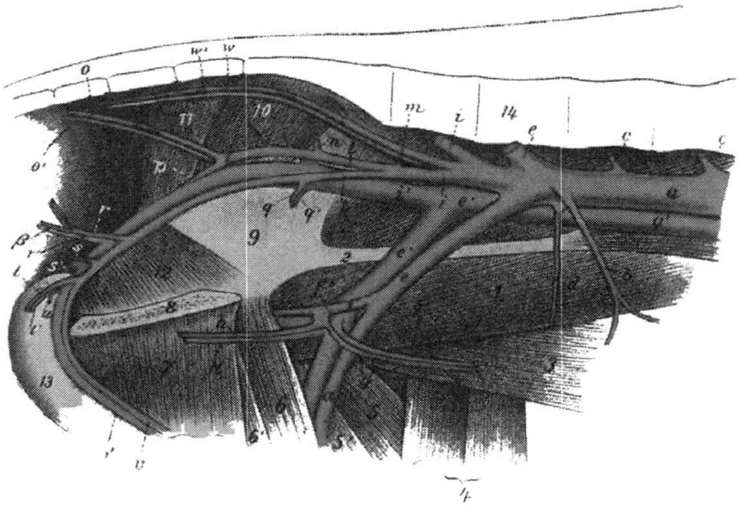

FIG. 491.—END BRANCHES OF AORTA AND RADICLES OF POSTERIOR VENA CAVA OF DOG.

a, Abdominal aorta; *b*, posterior mesenteric artery; *c*, lumbar arteries; *d*, circumflex iliac artery; *e*, external iliac artery; *f*, deep femoral artery; *g*, posterior abdominal artery; *h*, external pudic artery; *a*, femoral artery; *i*, *i*, internal iliac arteries; *k*, visceral branch of *i*; *l*, parietal branch of *i*; *m*, ilio-lumbar artery; *n*, anterior gluteal artery; *o*, lateral coccygeal artery; *p*, posterior gluteal artery; q, umbilical artery; *r*, middle hæmorrhoidal artery; *β*, posterior hæmorrhoidal artery; *s*, perineal artery; *t*, art. profunda penis; *n*, art. bulbi urethræ; *v*, art. dorsalis penis; *w*, middle sacral artery; *a′*, posterior vena cava; other veins are satellites of arteries and correspondingly named; *1*, ilio-psoas muscle; *2*, tendon of psoas minor; *3*, abdominal muscles; *4*, sartorius; *5*, rectus femoris; *5′*, vastus internus; *6*, pectineus; *6′*, adductor; *7*, gracilis; *8*, symphysis pelvis; *9*, ilium; *10*, pyriformis; *11*, gluteus superficialis; *12*, obturator internus; *13*, penis; *14*, lumbar vertebræ. (After Ellenberger, in Leisering's Atlas.)

divides near the pylorus into right gastro-epiploic and pancreatico-duodenal. The (left) **gastric artery** passes to the lesser curvature of the stomach and ramifies chiefly on the left part of the stomach, giving off a branch which anastomoses with the pyloric branch of the hepatic. The **splenic artery** gives off pancreatic branches, and reaches the lower part of the spleen. It gives off the left gastro-epiploic, and a branch which passes to the dorsal end of the spleen, which it supplies, besides giving off twigs to the left extremity of the stomach.

The **anterior mesenteric artery** arises close behind the cœliac. It gives off a common trunk for two colic arteries and the ileo-cæeo-colic. The former supply the transverse and the anterior part of the left or descending colon, while the latter divides into branches for the ileum, cæcum, and first part of the colon. The trunk is continued as the artery of the small intestine, giving off fourteen to sixteen branches (Aa. jejunales), which form a series of anastomotic arches in the mesentery near the bowel.

Two **phrenico-abdominal arteries** (Aa. phrenicæ caudales) come off from the aorta behind the anterior mesenteric, and divide into phrenic and abdominal branches. Each phrenic artery diverges from its fellow in descending on the abdominal surface of the corresponding crus of the diaphragm to the sternal part. The inner branches anastomose with those of the opposite artery, the outer branches with intercostal arteries chiefly. The abdominal arteries give branches to the lumbar muscles, the renal fat and capsules, and ramify in the oblique abdominal muscles.

The **renal** and **spermatic arteries** offer no special features.

The **utero-ovarian artery** divides near the ovary into three or four branches which supply the ovary and uterus, anastomosing with the uterine artery.

The **posterior mesenteric** artery is small. It divides into two branches which supply the terminal part of the colon and the anterior part of the rectum.

The **circumflex iliac artery** usually arises from the terminal part of the aorta.

The **external iliac** artery usually gives off no collateral branches.

The **femoral artery** has the usual course. The deep femoral gives off the posterior abdominal and external pudic arteries by a very short common trunk or separately. In the female the external pudic divides into anterior and posterior branches; the former runs forward, supplies branches to the inguinal lymph glands, the mammary glands and skin, and anastomoses with the mammary branch of the internal thoracic artery; the posterior branch pursues a flexuous course between the thighs to the vulva, where its terminal branches anastomose with the internal pudic artery. The anterior femoral may arise by a short common trunk with the external circumflex. The former, accompanied by the anterior branch of the

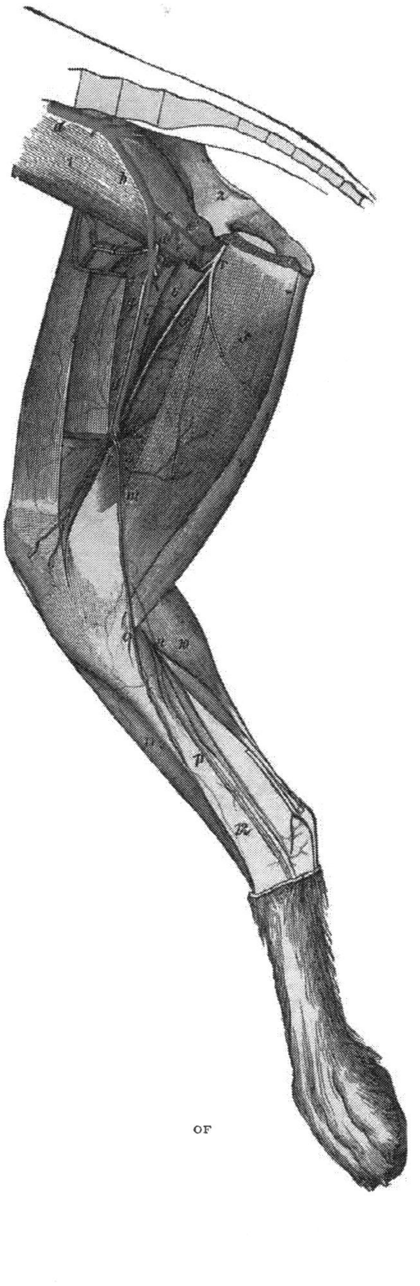

femoral nerve, dips in between the rectus femoris and vastus internus. The external circumflex artery passes forward between the sartorius internally and the rectus femoris and tensor fasciæ latæ externally and supplies branches to these muscles and the glutei. In addition to muscular branches of considerable size, an articular branch (A. genu suprema) arises a little below the middle of the thigh and runs downward and forward to the inner face of the stifle joint. The **saphenous artery** is large. It arises from the inner surface of the femoral a little below the middle of the femur, descends superficially to the upper part of the leg and divides into two branches. The smaller **anterior branch** (Ramus dorsalis) passes obliquely

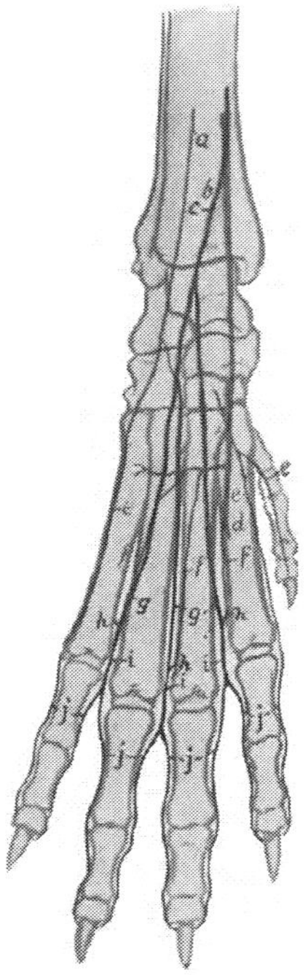

FIG. 493.—ARTERIES OF DISTAL PART OF RIGHT HIND LIMB OF DOG, ANTERIOR VIEW.

a, External branch of anterior tibial artery; *b*, anterior tibial artery; *c*, saphenous artery (anterior branch); *d*, perforating metatarsal artery; *e*, dorsal metatarsal arteries; *f*, deep dorsal metatarsal arteries; *g*, superficial dorsal metatarsal arteries; *h*, anastomoses between dorsal and plantar arteries; *i*, common digital arteries; *j*, proper digital arteries.

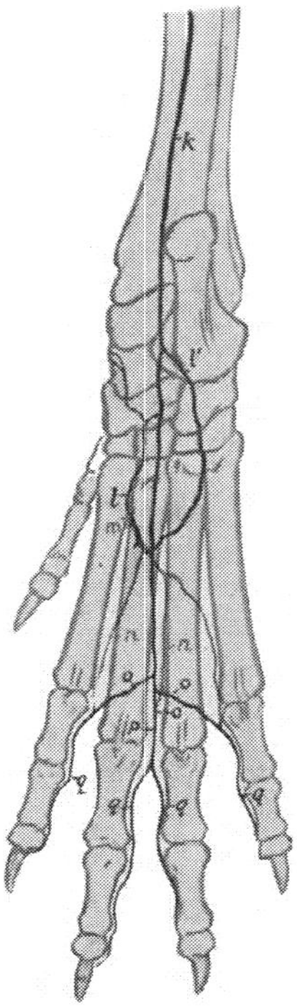

FIG. 494.—ARTERIES OF DISTAL PART OF RIGHT HIND LIMB OF DOG, POSTERIOR VIEW.

k, Saphenous artery (posterior branch); *l*, *l'* internal and external plantar arteries; *m*, perforating metatarsal artery; *n*, deep plantar metatarsal arteries; *o*, superficial plantar metatarsal arteries; *p*, common digital artery; q, proper digital arteries.

downward and forward across the inner surface of the tibia to the flexion surface of the hock and terminates in three **superficial dorsal metatarsal arteries.** The posterior branch (Ramus plantaris) passes down on the inner face of the gastrocnemius and the long digital flexor. It gives off a branch (A. tarsea lateralis) which descends obliquely to the external surface of the tarsus, and at the posterior face of the tarsus detaches the **internal** and **external plantar arteries;** these descend on either side of the deep flexor tendon and unite with the perforating metatarsal artery to form the proximal plantar arch. The artery continues down the middle of the plantar surface of the metatarsus and divides near the metacarpo-phalangeal joints into three **superficial plantar metatarsal arteries.** These vessels unite with three deep **plantar metatarsal** arteries which descend from the proximal plantar arch and with branches from the dorsal metatarsal arteries. From these anastomoses four digital arteries result; of these, the central two have a common digital trunk.

The **popliteal** and **posterior femoral arteries** present nothing of special interest.

The **posterior tibial artery** is small, being replaced largely by the saphenous. It supplies twigs to the flexor muscles at the upper part of the leg.

The **anterior tibial artery** descends on the anterior face of the tibia and tarsus and is continued as the perforating metatarsal artery, which passes through the upper part of the space between the second and third metatarsal bones and concurs with the plantar branches of the saphenous in the formation of the plantar arch. Besides muscular and articular branches, the anterior tibial supplies the external or fifth dorsal metatarsal artery for the outer side of the fifth digit. At the proximal part of the metatarsus it gives off three **deep dorsal metatarsal arteries** which descend in the intervals between the metatarsal bones and concur with the superficial dorsal and the plantar arteries in the formation of the **digital arteries.** The latter resemble in general arrangement the corresponding arteries of the thoracic limb.

The **internal iliac artery** (Fig. 491) runs backward and a little outward across the ilio-psoas, and on reaching the ilium divides into parietal and visceral branches. The **parietal** branch is the larger. It runs backward on the lateral wall of the pelvis, passes out through the lesser sciatic notch, and breaks up into branches which supply the muscles in this region like the posterior gluteal (or ischiatic) artery of the horse. It gives off the following branches: (1) The **ilio-lumbar artery** passes outward between the ilio-psoas and the shaft of the ilium and ramifies in the gluteus medius, giving branches to the ilio-psoas and tensor fasciæ latæ; it may arise from the internal iliac. (2) The **anterior gluteal artery** passes out behind the posterior superior spine of the ilium and supplies branches to the glutei. (3) **Muscular branches** go to the obturator internus, coccygeus, and retractor ani. (4) The **lateral coccygeal artery** (A. caudalis lateralis superficialis) passes back at first on the outer face of the coccygeus and continues beneath the skin along the side of the tail. The **visceral branch** or **internal pudic artery** passes back below the parietal branch on the lateral face of the rectum, retractor ani, and coccygeus. Its chief collateral branches are: (1) The **umbilical artery,** which pursues a flexuous course and supplies twigs to the bladder, ureter, and vas deferens. In the bitch it gives off a large **uterine artery** which ramifies chiefly in the body and neck of the uterus and the vagina and anastomoses with the utero-ovarian. (2) The **middle hæmorrhoidal artery** arises near the ischial arch, passes upward and forward on the lateral surface of the rectum, gains its dorsal surface and anastomoses with the posterior mesenteric; it supplies the rectum and the anus, together with its muscles and glands. (3) A small **perineal artery** is detached to the perineum. In the male the trunk turns around the ischial arch as the **artery of the penis** (A. penis). This vessel, after giving off the **deep artery of the penis** (A. profunda penis), which supplies the **artery of the bulb** (A. bulbi urethræ) and enters the corpus cavernosum, is continued as the **dorsal artery of the penis** (A. dorsalis penis) along the dorsum penis. In the female the terminal branches of the trunk go to the vulva, vestibular bulb, and clitoris.

THE VEINS

The arrangement of the veins is, of course, correlated in general with the arterial system, but a few special features are worthy of mention.

The **anterior vena cava** is formed by the junction of short right and left **brachiocephalic** (or subclavian) **veins,** and each of the latter results from the confluence of jugular and **brachial veins.**

The **vena azygos** resembles that of the horse, and receives at the ninth or tenth thoracic vertebra a **vena hemiazygos.**

Two **jugular veins** are present on each side. The **external jugular vein** is formed by the union of external and internal maxillary veins at the posterior border of the submaxillary gland. The two external jugulars are commonly united by a transverse branch below the cricoid cartilage. Each passes along the neck on the sterno-cephalicus, covered only by the skin and panniculus, dips under the cleido-cervicalis, and joins the internal jugular.

The **external maxillary vein** arises on the lateral nasal region by the junction of the dorsal nasal vein with the angularis oculi. Near the infraorbital foramen it receives the lateral nasal vein, and a little lower the superior labial. In its course along the anterior border of the masseter it receives the vena reflexa, which arises in the pterygo-palatine fossa by the junction of infraorbital, sphenopalatine, and palatine radicles, together with a branch from the cavernous sinus. At the lower border of the mandible it is joined by the inferior labial vein, which receives the buccinator vein. The lingual vein is connected with its fellow by a superficial transverse branch at the insertion of the sterno-hyoidei. The sublingual and submental veins terminate in a variable manner, but often form a common trunk which joins the lingual.

The **internal maxillary vein** arises from the pterygoid plexus, formed chiefly by dorsal lingual, inferior alveolar, deep temporal, pterygoid, and meningeal tributaries. It receives the superior cerebral, auricular, superficial temporal, transverse facial, and masseteric veins, and often a trunk formed by the union of the inferior cerebral and occipital veins.

The **internal jugular vein** results usually from the junction of laryngeal and thyroid veins, but in some cases it is formed by the confluence of the inferior cerebral and occipital veins.

The **brachial** and **radial veins** are satellites of the arteries.

The **ulnar vein** is usually double. It unites below the carpus with a branch of the interosseous vein to form the superficial venous arch.

The **cephalic vein** accompanies the ulnar artery in the forearm and joins the superficial venous arch below.

The **accessory cephalic vein** arises from the union of three dorsal metatarsal veins. It joins the cephalic about the middle of the forearm.

There are three short volar **metacarpal veins** which open into the superficial venous arch. They are formed above the metacarpo-phalangeal joints by the junction of the volar digital **veins,** of which there are two for each of the chief digits. The volar vein of the first digit joins the superficial venous arch.

Each of the chief digits has two dorsal **digital veins,** while the first digit has one.

The **posterior vena cava,** its collateral affluents, and common iliac radicles present no special features of importance.

The **internal iliac vein** corresponds in regard to its tributaries with the branches of the artery, except that it is not divided into dorsal and ventral branches.

The **external iliac, femoral,** and **popliteal veins** with their collateral tributaries are satellites of the arteries.

The **anterior tibial vein** is usually double, and the **posterior tibial vein** is very small.

The **internal saphenous vein** is the upward continuation of the internal plantar metatarsal vein. It communicates by a large branch with the dorsal metatarsal vein, and ascends the leg as a satellite of the saphenous artery and its plantar (posterior) branch. The **recurrent tarsal** or **external saphenous vein** is larger. It is formed at the lower part of the leg by the union of dorsal and external plantar metatarsal veins, crosses the outer surface of the leg obliquely upward and backward, ascends behind the gastrocnemius and joins the posterior femoral vein.

The **metatarsal** and **digital veins** resemble in general the corresponding vessels of the fore limb.

The Lymph Vessels and Glands

The **cisterna chyli** is large and fusiform. The **thoracic duct** may be single throughout, but often divides anteriorly into two branches, which may then unite and form a dilatation which receives the left tracheal duct and the vessels from the fore limb. The primitive plexiform arrangement persists in varying degree. The duct terminates in the left brachiocephalic vein.

The **tracheal ducts** accompany the internal jugular veins. The right duct opens into the right brachiocephalic vein.

The **submaxillary lymph glands** (Fig. 486) are commonly three in number on each side. They are situated in the angle between the masseter and the submaxillary salivary gland, in relation to the external maxillary vein and covered only by the skin and panniculus. The number may be reduced to two or one with a corresponding increase in size.

A small round **parotid** or **auricular lymph gland** is situated superficially between the upper part of the posterior border of the masseter and the parotid gland.

The **pharyngeal** (or retropharyngeal) **lymph glands,** one or two in number on each side, lie on the pharynx chiefly under cover of the submaxillary salivary gland.

The **prescapular** or **superficial cervical lymph glands** lie on the serratus magnus at the anterior border of the supraspinatus, embedded in a mass of fat. Usually two or three are present on each side, but there may be only one. They are oval and are about an inch long in a dog of medium size when two are present.

The **axillary lymph gland** lies in a mass of fat on the inner face of the lower part of the teres major. It is discoid.

The **cubital lymph gland** is inconstant. It is situated on the deep face of the long head of the triceps or on the latissimus dorsi.

The **mediastinal lymph glands** are small and quite variable in arrangement. Usually one or two glands are found on the course of the internal thoracic vessels at the second segment of the sternum.

The **bronchial lymph glands** are commonly four in number. The largest is situated in the angle of divergence of the chief bronchi, two lie on the origin of the right apical bronchus, and the fourth is between the aortic arch and the anterior face of the left bronchus. They are commonly pigmented.

The **lumbar lymph glands** are small.

The **mesenteric lymph glands** are represented chiefly by a long flattened mass (formerly known as the pancreas Aselli) which lies in the mesentery along the course of the anterior mesenteric artery and vein. It is succeeded by three or four glands which lie along the portal vein and appear to receive vessels from the stomach, spleen, liver, pancreas, and great omentum. A few very small nodes occur along the colon.

The **iliac lymph glands** are relatively large and are situated at the termination of the aorta and the origin of the iliac arteries. Commonly four are present. Of these, the two largest lie on the psoas minor on each side in relation to the aorta and vena cava respectively. The other two are in the angle of divergence of the internal iliac arteries.

The **superficial inguinal lymph glands** are situated in the subcutaneous fat behind the external inguinal ring. They are relatively large, especially when there is only one on each side; two smaller ones may be found instead.

The **popliteal lymph gland**—usually unique, but sometimes double—lies in a pad of fat on the upper part of the gastrocnemius between the biceps femoris and semitendinosus. It may project back so as to be superficial and palpable.

NEUROLOGY

THE NERVOUS SYSTEM

The nervous system is a complex mechanism by which the organism is brought into functional relation with its environment, and its various parts are coördinated. For purposes of gross description it is divided primarily into two parts, central and peripheral.

The **central nervous system** (Systema nervorum centrale) comprises (*a*) the **spinal cord** (Medulla spinalis), and (*b*) the **brain** (Encephalon).

The **peripheral nervous system** (Systema nervorum periphericum) includes (*a*) the **cerebral** and **spinal nerves** with their **ganglia**, and (*b*) the **sympathetic nervous system.**

The division into central and peripheral parts is quite arbitrary and is employed purely as a matter of convenience of description. The fibers of which the nerves are composed either arise or end within the central system, and therefore constitute an integral part of the latter. The structural and functional unit of the nervous system is the **neurone,** which consists of the **cell-body,** usually termed the **nerve-cell,** and all its **processes.** The processes arise as outgrowths from the cell-body and conduct impulses to or from the cell. They vary greatly in length, some being less than a millimeter long, while others extend from a cell in the spinal cord to the distal end of a limb. A nerve is composed of such processes, usually inclosed in a protecting and insulating sheath, and united into bundles by connective tissue. The neurones are embedded in a peculiar supporting tissue termed **neuroglia.** This consists of a very intricate feltwork of glia-fibers, many of which are connected with the small glia-cells or astrocytes. In addition the nervous tissue is invested closely by a vascular layer of connective tissue, the pia mater, from which ingrowths extend into the nervous substance proper.[1]

To the naked eye the central nervous system appears to be composed chiefly of two kinds of substance, white and gray. The **white matter** (Substantia alba) is dead white in color and is soft in the natural state. It consists largely of medullated nerve-fibers, packed closely together and arranged more or less clearly in large or small bundles or tracts (Funiculi, fasciculi). The **gray matter** (Substantia grisea) is usually brownish-gray in color, often with a tinge of pink. It is softer than the white substance and much more vascular. It is composed chiefly of cell-bodies and non-medullated processes. In some situations it is modified to form the **gelatinous substance** (Substantia gelatinosa), which is pale yellowish-gray and jelly-like.

Ganglia are gray masses found on the dorsal roots of the spinal nerves and on the course of many nerves. They are commonly ovoid in form and are inclosed in a fibrous capsule. They are composed largely of the cell-bodies of neurones, but have connected with and passing through them nerve-fibers (processes) which extend peripherally and centrally. In origin and function the spinal ganglia belong properly to the central system, but it is customary to include them with the peripheral part in gross anatomical descriptions.

Nerves are conducting trunks composed of bundles of parallel nerve-fibers. They are enveloped in a fibro-elastic sheath, the epineurium, which contains the blood and lymph vessels. They are classified according to their central connections as **cranial** or **cerebral, spinal,** and **sympathetic.** The groups of cells of which the nerve-fibers are processes are termed the **nuclei of origin** or **termination** of the nerves, according as the latter conduct impulses in a peripheral or central direction. On the same basis the nerve-fibers are designated **efferent** and **afferent**

[1] Limitations of space and the purpose of this work preclude consideration of the finer structure of the nervous system, for which ample literature is available.

respectively. A bundle of fibers which passes from one nerve-trunk to another is called an **anastomotic branch** (Ramus anastomoticus). In some situations the exchange of branches between adjacent nerves is so free as to constitute a **nerve-plexus** (Plexus nervorum). The term **ramus communicans** is properly restricted to branches which connect the ventral divisions of the spinal nerves with adjacent ganglia or nerves of the sympathetic system. The terminal twigs of the nerves are designated according to their distribution as **muscular branches** (Rami musculares), **cutaneous nerves** (Nervi cutanei), and **articular nerves** (Nervi articulares). The muscular branches are motor in function, the cutaneous and articular sensory, but all contain vasomotor fibers which control the caliber of the blood-vessels.

THE MENINGES

The central organs of the nervous system are inclosed in three meninges or membranes. From without inward these are: (1) the dura mater, (2) the arachnoidea, and (3) the pia mater.

THE DURA MATER

The **dura mater** is a dense resistant membrane of white fibrous tissue; in the fresh state it is bluish-white in color. On account of the difference in its arrangement within the cranium from that in the spinal canal it is customary to describe it as consisting of two parts, cerebral and spinal; these portions are continuous with each other at the foramen magnum.

The **cerebral dura mater** (Dura mater encephali) is adherent to the interior of the cranium, and may be regarded as forming an internal periosteum for the bones here as well as being an envelope of the brain. Its outer surface is connected with the bony wall of the cranial cavity by numerous fine fibrous strands and by blood-vessels; hence it appears rough in many places when separated from the wall. The degree of adhesion varies greatly at different points. It is most firmly attached at the various projections, *e. g.*, the internal sagittal crest, the tentorium osseum, the petrosal crest; also at the base and the foramen magnum. Before the sutures are closed the dura is connected with the sutural ligaments and through them is continuous with the external periosteum. The cranial nerves receive sheaths from the dura, which is thus continuous without the cranium with the epineurium and periosteum. Along the roof and sides (except as noted above) the adhesion is relatively slight, and lymph-spaces are said to exist between the dura and the bone. The internal surface of the dura is smooth and glistening, since it is lined by endothelium and is moistened by a fluid resembling lymph; it forms the outer boundary of the subdural space. In accordance with its double function the dura is composed of two layers, which are, however, intimately adherent to each other in most places in the adult. The venous sinuses are channels between the two layers and are lined by endothelium. They have been described with the other vessels.

Several folds or septa are given off from the inner surface of the dura; these project into the cavity between the gross subdivisions of the brain. These septa are: (1) the falx cerebri; (2) the tentorium cerebelli; and (3) the diaphragma sellæ.

The **falx cerebri** is a sickle-shaped median partition which projects downward in the great longitudinal fissure between the cerebral hemispheres. It is attached above to the internal sagittal crest, in front to the crista galli, and behind to the tentorium osseum. Its superior border is convex and separates into two layers which inclose the superior longitudinal sinus. Its lower border is concave and lies over the corpus callosum. The falx is thick above, but much thinner below, and in some places cribriform.

In the horse the posterior part of the falx cerebri does not extend to the corpus callosum, and hence the hemispheres are here in contact and adherent to each other over a small area. In the ox and pig the falx does not descend so far as in the horse, while in the dog it completely separates the hemispheres.

The **tentorium cerebelli** is a crescentic transverse fold which separates the cerebellum from the posterior poles of the cerebral hemispheres. It is attached above to the tentorium osseum and laterally to the petrosal crests. Its lower border is thin, concave, and free; it forms the upper and lateral boundaries of an opening (Incisura tentorii) which incloses the mid-brain.

The **diaphragma sellæ** is a small circular fold which roofs over the sella turcica and the pituitary body. It is perforated centrally by an opening (Foramen diaphragmatis) for the infundibulum.

The falx cerebelli, a sickle-shaped fold which projects into the median notch between the cerebellar hemispheres in man, is not present in the domesticated animals. There is instead merely a slight thickening of the dura.

The **spinal dura mater** (Dura mater spinalis) forms a tube around the spinal cord from the foramen magnum to the second or third segment of the sacrum. It is separated from the periosteum of the spinal canal by a considerable **epidural space** (Cavum epidurale) which is occupied by fatty connective tissue and veins. It is held in position chiefly by the sheaths which it furnishes to the roots of the spinal nerves, and in its anterior part by two ligaments; the latter connect it with the inferior atlanto-occipital membrane and with the odontoid process. It is large in proportion to its contents, but its diameter is not uniform. It is largest in the atlas, small in the thoracic region, and becomes very small in its terminal part, where it incloses the delicate filum terminale of the spinal cord.

The **subdural space** (Cavum subdurale) is the cavity between the inner surface of the dura mater and the arachnoidea. It is a mere capillary space which contains just sufficient fluid to moisten its surfaces; this fluid is usually regarded as lymph, which is replenished by filtration through the walls of the blood-vessels. The space is in communication with the lymph-paths of the nerve-sheaths.

THE ARACHNOIDEA

The **arachnoidea** is a very delicate and transparent membrane situated between the dura and pia mater. Its outer surface forms the inner wall of the subdural space and is covered by a layer of endothelium continuous with that of the opposed surface of the dura mater. Between it and the pia mater is the **subarachnoid space** (Cavum subarachnoideale) which contains the cerebrospinal fluid. An inner surface can scarcely be said to exist, since deeply the membrane becomes a reticulum of fine fibers which traverse the subarachnoid space and are attached to the pia mater. The arachnoidea furnishes sheaths to the cerebral nerves from their superficial origins to a variable but usually short distance beyond the emergence from the dursal sac. In the case of the optic nerve this sheath extends to the eyeball.

The **arachnoidea of the brain** (Arachnoidea encephali), except in the case of the great longitudinal and transverse fissures, does not dip into the sulci on the surface of the brain. On the summits of the gyri it is so closely attached to the pia mater that the two form practically a single membrane. Its outer part bridges over the sulci, and here the subarachnoid space is partially divided up by the loose arachnoid tissue into intercommunicating cavities. In certain situations the arachnoidea is separated from the pia by spaces of considerable depth and extent. These enlargements of the subarachnoid space are termed **subarachnoid cisterns** (Cisternæ subarachnoidales). In them the subarachnoid tissue does not form a close network, but consists of a relatively small number of long, thread-like strands which traverse the cavity.

The chief cisternæ are: (1) the cisterna magna, which is at the angle formed between the posterior face of the cerebellum and the upper surface of the medulla oblongata. It communicates with the fourth ventricle through the foramen of Magendie (in man); and behind with the wide subarachnoid space of the spinal cord; (2) the cisterna pontis on the ventral surface of the pons; (3) the cisterna basalis, which lies at the base of the cerebrum and is divided by the optic chiasma into two parts (cisterna chiasmatis, cisterna interpeduncularis); (4) the cisterna fossæ lateralis, situated at the lower part of the lateral fissure (of Sylvius), and continuous with the cisterna basalis.

Along the upper border of the falx cerebri the arachnoidea bears bulbous excrescences, the **arachnoid granulations** or **Pacchionian bodies.** These are inclosed in thin evaginations of the dura mater and project into the sagittal sinus or the parasinoidal sinuses along either side of it. In some cases they are sufficiently large to exert pressure on the bone and produce in it depressions of variable depth.

The **spinal arachnoidea** (Arachnoidea spinalis) is directly continuous with that of the brain at the foramen magnum. It forms a relatively wide tube around the spinal cord, so that the latter (inclosed in the pia) is surrounded by a very considerable quantity of cerebrospinal fluid. The spinal subarachnoid space is traversed by fewer arachnoid trabeculæ than is the case in the cranium. It is partially subdivided by three imperfect septa. One of these, the septum dorsale, is median and dorsal. The other two, the ligamenta denticulata, are lateral and will be described with the pia mater.

PIA MATER

The **pia mater** is a delicate and very vascular membrane which invests closely the surface of the brain and spinal cord and sends processes into their substance. It also furnishes sheaths to the nerves, which blend outside of the dural sac with the epineurium.

The **pia mater** of **the brain** (Pia mater encephali) follows accurately all the inequalities of the surface, dipping into all the fissures and sulci of the cerebrum, and into the larger fissures of the cerebellum. Its external surface, which forms the inner boundary of the subarachnoid space, is covered by a layer of endothelium. From its deep face numerous trabeculæ are given off which penetrate into the substance of the brain and cord, forming a path for the blood-vessels, and concurring with the neuroglia in forming the supporting tissue of the nervous-substance proper. The larger blood-vessels of the brain lie within the subarachnoid space, but the smaller vessels ramify in the pia, forming rich plexuses. The twigs which penetrate into the gray matter are inclosed in pial sheaths. They are end-arteries, *i. e.*, constitute the entire supply of the district which they enter and do not anastomose with adjacent vessels.

Two important folds of the pia extend into the two great transverse fissures of the brain; these processes overlie the third and fourth ventricles and are known as the **telæ chorioideæ** of these cavities. They constitute paths for the deeper vessels and their edges contain vascular convolutions which are known as chorioid plexuses. They will receive further consideration more appropriately later.

The **spinal pia mater** (Pia mater spinalis) is thicker and denser than that of the brain. It has a strong outer layer of fibrous tissue, most of the fibers of which are longitudinal. The inner layer is vascular and adheres closely to the surface of the cord because it sends numerous processes into it. It sends a fold into the median ventral fissure and also helps to form the median dorsal septum of the cord. Along the median ventral line it forms a band-like thickening, the linea splendens, along which the ventral spinal artery runs. On each side the pia mater gives off a strong longitudinal band, the **ligamentum denticulatum,** which is connected externally with the dura mater. The inner or pial border extends in a line between the dorsal and ventral roots of the nerves. The outer or dural border is denticulated and to a large extent free. The denticulations are attached to the dura between the nerve-roots.

NERVOUS SYSTEM OF THE HORSE

THE SPINAL CORD

The **spinal cord** (Medulla spinalis) is the part of the central nervous system which is situated in the vertebral canal. It extends from the foramen magnum to about the middle of the sacrum.

In the horse its average length is about 76 to 78 inches (ca. 190 to 195 cm.), and its weight about 8½ to 9 ounces (ca. 240 to 255 grams).

It is approximately cylindrical, but more or less flattened dorso-ventrally. There is no line of demarcation between it and the medulla oblongata, but for practical purposes the division is usually assumed to be at the posterior border of the foramen magnum. Its posterior part tapers rapidly to a point, forming the **conus medullaris.** This is prolonged for a short distance by the slender **filum terminale.**

Forty-two pairs of spinal nerves are connected with the sides of the spinal cord. They are classified as eight cervical, eighteen thoracic, six lumbar, five sacral, and five coccygeal. According to the attachments of these series of nerves the spinal cord is divided into **cervical, thoracic, lumbar,** and **sacral** parts.

In a horse about 16½ hands high these parts measured 65 cm. (ca. 26 in.), 86 cm. (ca. 34.4 in.), 27 cm. (ca. 10.8 in.), and 15 cm. (ca. 6 in.) respectively (Dexler).

In the embryo these divisions correspond primitively to the regions of the vertebral column, but later, through unequal growth of the cord and spine, the correspondence between the two is not at all exact in the anterior regions and is lost in the last two. The lumbar part of the cord in the horse ends at the junction of the fifth and sixth lumbar vertebræ, so that the roots of the last lumbar nerve must run backward the length of the last lumbar vertebra to reach the intervertebral foramen through which it emerges. The conus medullaris reaches only to the anterior part of the sacral canal, so that the roots of the sacral and coccygeal nerves extend backward in the spinal canal for a considerable distance, forming a leash of bundles, in the center of which lie the conus medullaris and the filum terminale. This arrangement is expressively designated the **cauda equina.**

Each pair of spinal nerves is attached by its root-fibers to a certain length of the cord, and the latter is, therefore, regarded as consisting of as many **segments** as there are nerves. It is to be noted, however, that there is no line of demarcation between the segments other than the intervals between the root-fibers of adjacent nerves.

The segments are of different lengths; the longest are the third to the sixth cervical, which measure 11, 10, 10, and 8.5 cm. respectively. The spinal nerves are in general designated according to the vertebræ behind which they emerge from the vertebral canal. In the neck, however, there are eight pairs of nerves and only seven vertebræ; here the first nerve emerges through the intervertebral foramen of the atlas and the eighth between the last cervical and the first thoracic vertebra.

In the greater part of the thoracic region the spinal cord is fairly uniform in size, but there are two conspicuous wide enlargements which involve the segments with which the nerves of the limbs are connected. The **cervical enlargement** (Intumescentia cervicalis) begins gradually in the fifth cervical vertebra and subsides in the second thoracic. Its maximum transverse diameter is about an inch (ca. 25 mm.) and its dorso-ventral nearly half an inch (ca. 12 mm.). The **lumbar enlargement** (Intumescentia lumbalis) is situated in the fourth and fifth lumbar vertebræ. It is a little narrower than the cervical enlargement, and its dorso-ventral diameter is also slightly smaller. Behind this the cord tapers rapidly to form the **conus medullaris.** The tip of the latter is continued by a delicate glistening strand, the **filum terminale,** which is composed largely of fibrous tissue continued from the pia mater, covered by arachnoid.

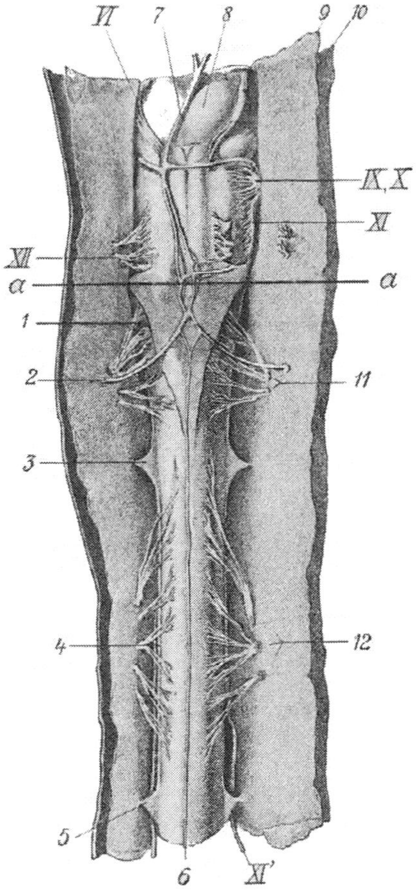

FIG. 495.—VENTRAL VIEW OF MEDULLA OBLONGATA AND FIRST AND SECOND SEGMENTS OF SPINAL CORD OF HORSE; THE MEMBRANES ARE CUT AND REFLECTED.

1, Lig. suspensorium arachnoideale; *2*, right cerebrospinal artery; *3*, *5*, digitations of lig. denticulatum; *4*, free border of lig. denticulatum; *6*, middle spinal artery; *7*, basilar artery; *8*, pons; *9*, arachnoidea; *10*, dura mater; *11*, *12*, ventral root-bundles of first and second segments of spinal cord; *VI.*, N. abducens; *IX*, *X*, glosso-pharyngeus and vagus; *XI*, accessory, medullary part; *XI'*, accessory, spinal part; *a*, line between medulla oblongata and spinal cord. (Dexler, in Ellenberger-Baum, Anat. d. Haustiere.)

The surface of the spinal cord is divided into two similar halves by a **dorsal median groove** (Sulcus medianus dorsalis) and a **ventral median fissure** (Fissura mediana ventralis). On either side of the former is the **dorso-lateral groove** (Sulcus dorsalis lateralis) at which the fibers of the dorsal nerve-roots enter the cord; it is faint except at the enlargements, and is represented by two grooves in the first cervical segment. The ventral root-fibers as they emerge from the cord do not form a continuous series, but arise from a zone (Area radicularis ventralis) 3 to 5 mm. in width a little lateral to the ventral median fissure, and no groove is found here. In the greater part of the cervical region and the anterior part of the thoracic region there is a shallow **dorsal paramedian groove** (Sulcus intermedius dorsalis) a short distance lateral to the median

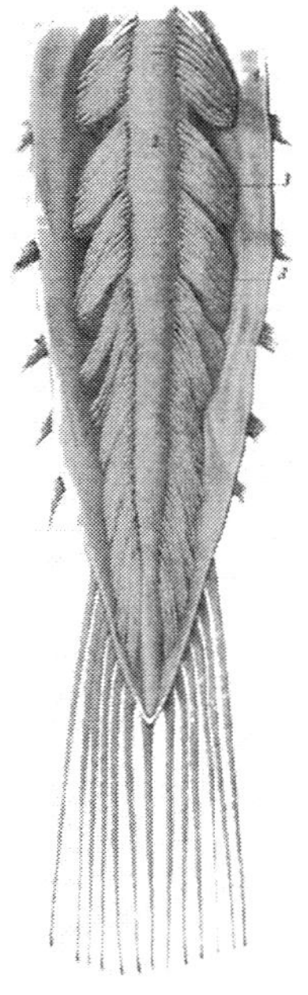

FIG. 496.—CAUDA EQUINA.

1, Dura and arachnoidea divided and reflected; *2*, spinal cord; *3*, nerve-roots. (From Leisering's Atlas, reduced.)

groove. These grooves indicate the division of the white matter of the cord into columns to be described later.

Examination of cross-sections of the spinal cord shows that it is a bilaterally symmetrical structure, incompletely divided into right and left halves by a ventral fissure and a dorsal septum. The **ventral median fissure** (Fissura mediana ventralis) is narrow and penetrates nearly to the middle of the dorso-ventral diameter of the cord. It is occupied by a fold of pia mater. The **dorsal median septum** (Septum medianum dorsale) is a partition which descends from the posterior median groove to about the middle of the cord. It apparently consists of condensed neuroglia with an admixture of pial tissue. The two halves of the cord are connected by commissures of gray and white matter. The **gray commissure** (Commissura grisea) is a transverse band of gray matter at the ventral end of the dorsal septum. It is divided into dorsal and ventral parts by the central canal of the cord. The

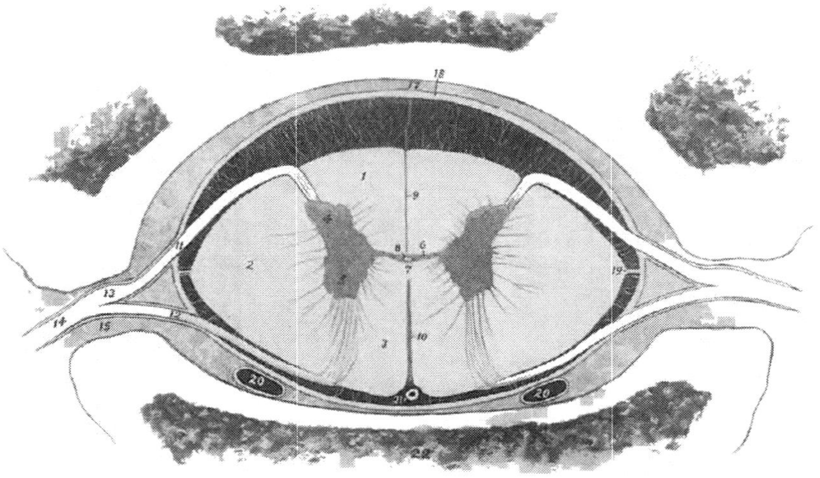

FIG. 497.—CROSS-SECTION OF SPINAL CORD *in situ*, IN PART SCHEMATIC.

1, Dorsal column; *2*, lateral column; *3*, ventral column; *4*, dorsal horn; *5*, ventral horn; *6*, gray commissure; *7*, white commissure; *8*, central canal; *9*, dorsal septum; *10*, ventral fissure; *11*, dorsal nerve-root; *12*, ventral nerve-root; *13*, spinal ganglion; *14*, nerve; *15*, intervertebral foramen; *16*, arch of vertebra; *17*, epidural space; *18*, dura mater (represented a little too thick); *19*, ligamentum denticulatum; *20*, *20*, longitudinal venous sinuses; *21*, middle spinal artery. The subdural and subarachnoid spaces (black) are traversed by delicate trabeculæ. The outer part of the arachnoid and the pia mater are not shown.

white commissure (Commissura alba) is a bridge of white matter which connects the ventral columns of the cord over the dorsal end of the ventral median fissure, and constitutes a conducting path from one side to the other.

The **central canal** of the cord (Canalis centralis), the spinal vestige of the lumen of the embryonal neural tube, is a minute passage which tunnels the gray commissure. It opens at its anterior end into the posterior part of the fourth ventricle of the brain, and its terminal part in the conus medullaris forms a slight dilatation, the ventriculus terminalis. It is lined by epithelium and is surrounded by a layer of modified neuroglia (Substantia grisea centralis).

The **gray matter** of the spinal cord as seen in cross-sections resembles roughly a capital H, the cross-bar of the letter being formed by the gray commissure. Each lateral part is considered as consisting of dorsal and **ventral gray columns or horns** (Columna grisea dorsalis, ventralis). In the greater part of the cord the dorsal column or horn is elongated and narrow and tapers to a point which extends almost to the surface of the cord at the attachment of the dorsal root-fibers of the spinal nerves. Its apex or tip consists of gray matter which is lighter in color and less opaque than that of the rest of the horn and is termed the **substantia gelatinosa** (Rolandi). The ventral column or horn is short, thick and rounded, and is separated from the surface of the cord by a thick layer of white matter, through which the fibers of the ventral roots of the spinal nerves pass. From the middle of the cervical region to the lumbar region there is a medial projection of gray matter on the lower part of the dorsal column; this is the **nucleus dorsalis** or Clarke's column. In the anterior part of the cord there is an outward projection of the gray matter at the base of the ventral horn; this is termed the **lateral column** or **horn.** The demarcation between the gray and white matter is in many places indistinct; this is especially the case laterally, where processes of gray matter extend into the white substance, producing what is known as the **formatio reticularis.**

Cross-sections of the spinal cord present the following gross regional characters: (1) The cervical cord near the medulla is compressed dorso-ventrally. Its width is about 18 mm. and its greatest thickness about 8 mm. It has dorsally a deep median sulcus and a distinct dorso-lateral sulcus. Lateral grooves are also present. The dorsal cornua are strongly everted. Each has an expanded head, which comes very close to the surface of the cord, and has an extensive cap of substantia gelatinosa. The neck is distinct. The ventral cornua are short and blunt and diverge very little. The gray commissure is about in the middle of the section and 2.5 mm. in length. According to Dexler the column between the median and lateral grooves dorsally is the funiculus cuneatus, the funiculus gracilis being very small and not showing on the surface in this region. In the middle of the cervical region the diameters are about 16 mm. and 10 mm. respectively. The ventral surface is somewhat flattened. The dorsal cornua have pointed ends and turn decidedly outward. The ventral cornua are short and thick and are directed very slightly outward; their ends are about 4 mm. from the ventral surface. The gray commissure is just above the middle of the section and is about 2 mm. long. The cervical enlargement measures about 25 mm. transversely and 12 mm. vertically. The dorsal cornua are smaller than the ventral and have a large cap of substantia gelatinosa. The ventral cornua are short and thick, curve strongly outward, and are about 4 mm. from the ventral surface. Each bears a prominence on its inner side near the base. The gray commissure is considerably above the middle of the section and is about 4 mm. long. (2) In the middle of the thoracic region the cross-section is biconvex, the ventral surface being the more strongly curved. The transverse diameter is about 15 mm. and the dorso-ventral about 10 mm. The gray columns are close together, the gray commissure being only about 1 mm. in length, and lying considerably above the middle of the section. The dorsal cornua are short and have slightly enlarged ends. The ventral cornua have a uniform diameter, turn very little outward, and end about 3 mm. from the ventral surface. (3) The lumbar enlargement is much flattened, especially dorsally. The transverse diameter is about 22 mm. and the dorso-ventral 9 to 10 mm. The cornua are very large. The ventral cornua are thick and rounded and turn sharply outward; they end about 2 mm. from the ventral surface. The dorsal cornua are smaller and shorter and do not diverge so strongly. The gray commissure is about in the middle of the section and is about 3 mm. long. In the third lumbar vertebra the cord is about 3 mm. narrower and thicker, and both surfaces are about equally convex. The dorsal cornua are smaller, considerably everted, and constricted in the middle. The ventral cornua are very short and do not turn outward. (4) In the first sacral vertebra the cord is almost round and is 5 to 6 mm. in diameter; the cornua are relatively very large and the commissure has the form of a high intermediate mass.

The ventral horn contains large cells, the axones of which emerge as the fibers of the ventral nerve-roots (Fila radicularia). The axones of many cells cross to the opposite side in the white commissure and pass out in a ventral root of that side, or enter the white matter and pass forward and backward, associating various segments of the cord. Some pass to the ventral horn of the opposite side at the same or at different levels. Others pass to the periphery of the cord, join the cerebellospinal fasciculus, and extend to the cerebellum. Scattered through the gray matter are many smaller cells with axones which pursue a short course and serve to connect different parts of the gray matter.

The **white matter** of the spinal cord is divided into three pairs of **columns.** The **dorsal columns** (Funiculi dorsales) lie on either side of the dorsal median septum and extend outward to the dorso-lateral groove and the dorsal gray column. The **ventral columns** (Funiculi ventrales) are situated on either side between the median fissure and the ventral gray columns. They are connected above the fissure by the white commissure. The **lateral columns** (Funiculi laterales) lie external to the gray columns on either side; their limits are indicated superficially by the dorso-lateral groove and the emergence of the ventral root-fibers. The paramedian groove (where present) indicates a subdivision of the dorsal column into two fasciculi or tracts; the inner of these is the **fasciculus gracilis** (Goll's column); the outer, the **fasciculus cuneatus** (Burdach's column).

The amounts of gray and white matter vary greatly in different parts of the cord both absolutely and relatively. In cross-section the absolute areas of both are greatest in the enlargements. The relative area of gray matter is smallest in the thoracic region (except at its anterior end), and increases from the lumbar enlargement backward.

Investigations have shown that in man the columns of white matter are subdivided into fasciculi or tracts, which constitute definite conducting paths of greater or less length. Our knowledge of the tracts in the domesticated animals is very limited, and it is quite unsafe to make inferences from the arrangement in man. As evidence of this it may be noted that the ventral cerebrospinal or direct pyramidal tract of man cannot be recognized as such.

The dorsal white columns consist essentially of two sets of axones. The afferent or sensory axones which come from the cells of the spinal ganglia enter as the dorsal roots of the spinal nerves and divide into two branches in the vicinity of the dorsal gray column. The anterior (ascending) branches form the direct sensory path to the brain and extend in the fasciculus cuneatus and fasciculus gracilis or corresponding tracts to nuclei in the medulla oblongata. The posterior (descending) branches extend backward for varying distances and give off numerous collaterals to cells of the gray column, thus forming part of the mechanism for the mediation of reflex action. Some collaterals cross in the white commissure to the opposite side. Many of these fibers are collected in the comma-shaped tract between the fasciculus gracilis and cuneatus. The second set of axones arises from the smaller cells of the gray column. They enter the white matter, divide into anterior and posterior branches, forming the fasciculi proprii or ground bundles of the cord. Some branches cross to the opposite side. The function of this set of axones is chiefly to associate various levels of the cord.

The lateral columns contain some axones of the dorsal nerve-roots, which (in man) are grouped in the marginal tract of Lissauer, situated just dorsal to the apex of the dorsal horn. The cerebellospinal fasciculus (direct cerebellar tract of Flechsig) extends along the periphery of the lateral column. It contains the axones of the cells of the nucleus dorsalis (Clarke's column), which proceed to the medulla oblongata and enter the cerebellum by the restiform body. The rubrospinal tract of Monakow appears to take the place of the lateral cerebrospinal fasciculus or crossed pyramidal tract of man. It lies at the inner side of the cerebellospinal fasciculus. Its fibers arise in the nucleus ruber of the mid-brain, cross the median plane (decussation of Forel), and pass backward in the tegmentum and medulla oblongata to the lateral column of the cord. It is a path for motor impulses coming from the cerebral cortex and the cerebellum. The lateral fasciculus proprius or ground-bundle is deeply situated at the side of the gray columns. The bulk of its fibers are axones of cells of the posterior cornu which divide into anterior and posterior branches. They are intersegmental paths which associate different levels of the gray matter of the cord. The significance of the remaining fibers is not yet known.

The ventral white columns do not contain a ventral cerebrospinal or direct pyramidal tract, as in man. There is a small tract (Fasciculus intracommissuralis ventralis) above the white commissure, which separates it from the rest of the ventral column. It extends to the middle of the thoracic region. It consists of intersegmental fibers, and contains in the anterior part of the cervical cord in the sheep and goat both crossed and direct pyramidal fibers. The descending cerebellospinal fasciculus extends from the cerebellum to the lumbar region. In the cervical region it occupies a semilunar area which reaches almost to the surface ventro-laterally. Scattered fibers belonging to it lie also in the medial part of the ventral column. Posteriorly it diminishes in size and comes to occupy a position next to the ventral median fissure, corresponding to the sulco-marginal fasciculus of man (Dexler).

THE BRAIN

The **brain** or **encephalon** is the part of the central nervous system that is situated in the cranial cavity. It is the enlarged and highly modified cephalic part of the primitive neural tube. It conforms rather closely in size and shape to the cavity in which it lies.

Its average weight without the dura mater is about 23 ounces (ca. 650 gm.), and forms about $\frac{1}{7}$ of 1 per cent. of the body-weight.

It is desirable to examine the general external configuration of the brain before studying its various parts in detail.[1]

When divested of its membranes and vessels (Figs. 499, 500), its ventral

[1] The description given here is intended to present the chief facts in regard to the brain as they may be studied in the dissecting room. The vessels and membranes which must be examined first have been described.

surface or base presents the median **brain stem,** which is continuous with the spinal cord without any natural line of demarcation; it divides in front into two branches, the cerebral peduncles, each of which disappears into the mass of the corresponding cerebral hemisphere. The brain stem consists of three parts. The **medulla oblongata** is the posterior part which extends forward as the direct continuation of the spinal cord. The **pons** (Varolii) is a transversely elongated mass which appears to turn up on either side into the cerebellum. The **cerebral peduncles** extend forward from the pons and diverge to plunge into the ventral part of the cerebral hemispheres. The area between them is the **interpeduncular** space. It is largely covered by the **pituitary body** or **hypophysis,** a yellowish-brown, discoid structure, which is connected with the base of the cerebrum by a delicate tube called the **infundibulum.**[1] On drawing the pituitary body gently aside, the infundibulum is seen to be attached to a slight gray eminence, the tuber **cinereum.** Behind this is the **mammillary body,** a well-marked round prominence. The posterior part of the space is perforated by numerous openings for the passage of small arteries, and hence is termed the **locus perforatus posticus.** Two large bands of white matter, the **optic tracts,** cross the anterior ends of the cerebral peduncles and unite at the **optic chiasm** or **commissure,** forming the anterior boundary of the interpeduncular space. Above and in front of the chiasm the hemispheres are separated by the median **longitudinal fissure.** In contact with the anterior extremity of each hemisphere is the **olfactory bulb,** an oval enlargement adapted to the ethmoidal fossa of the cranium. This appears as a gray swelling on a wide flat band, the **olfactory peduncle,** which is continued behind by two divergent bands, the **olfactory tracts** or **striæ.** The **internal tract** disappears after a very short course on to the inner surface of the hemisphere. The **external tract** is larger and longer; it runs backward, inclines at first outward and then curves inward and disappears on the concealed or tentorial surface of the hemispheres. It is separated from the lateral cerebral gyri by a distinct groove (Sulcus rhinalis). Along the inner side of the stria are two eminences. The anterior of these is the **trigonum olfactorium,** a gray elevation situated in the angle of divergence of the inner and outer striæ. Behind this is a depression, the **fossa transversa,**[2] which is continued across the external stria and sharply limits the second and much larger eminence, the **pyriform lobe.**

The superficial origins of most of the cranial nerves are visible on the base of the brain.

The olfactory **nerve-fibers** join the convex surface of the olfactory lobe and give it a shaggy appearance in specimens which have been removed intact—a difficult proceeding.

The **second** or **optic nerves** converge to the optic chiasm.

The **third** or oculomotor **nerve** arises from the inner part of the cerebral peduncle.

The fourth or **trochlear nerve** may be seen emerging between the pons and the hemisphere, but its connection with the brain is not visible.

The **fifth** or **trigeminal nerve** is connected with the lateral part of the pons.

The **sixth** or **abducent nerve** arises just behind the pons and lateral to the pyramid of the medulla.

The **seventh** or **facial** and the **eighth** or **auditory nerves** arise close together just behind the pons proper on the extremity of the corpus trapezoideum.

The **ninth** or **glosso-pharyngeal,** the **tenth** or **vagus,** and the **eleventh** or **spinal**

[1] Unless care is used in removing the brain the infundibulum is likely to be torn and the pituitary body left in the cranium. In this case there is a small opening which communicates with the third ventricle.

[2] The fossa corresponds in position to the locus perforatus anticus of the human brain, but is not pierced by numerous openings for vessels in the horse.

accessory nerves are connected by a linear series of roots with the lateral aspect of the ventral surface of the medulla. The spinal part of the accessory nerve comes forward along the edge of the medulla to join its medullary root.

The twelfth or **hypoglossal nerve** arises from the posterior part of the medulla along the lateral edge of the pyramid.

The parts that are visible when the brain is viewed from above are the cerebral hemispheres, the cerebellum, and part of the medulla oblongata. The **cerebral**

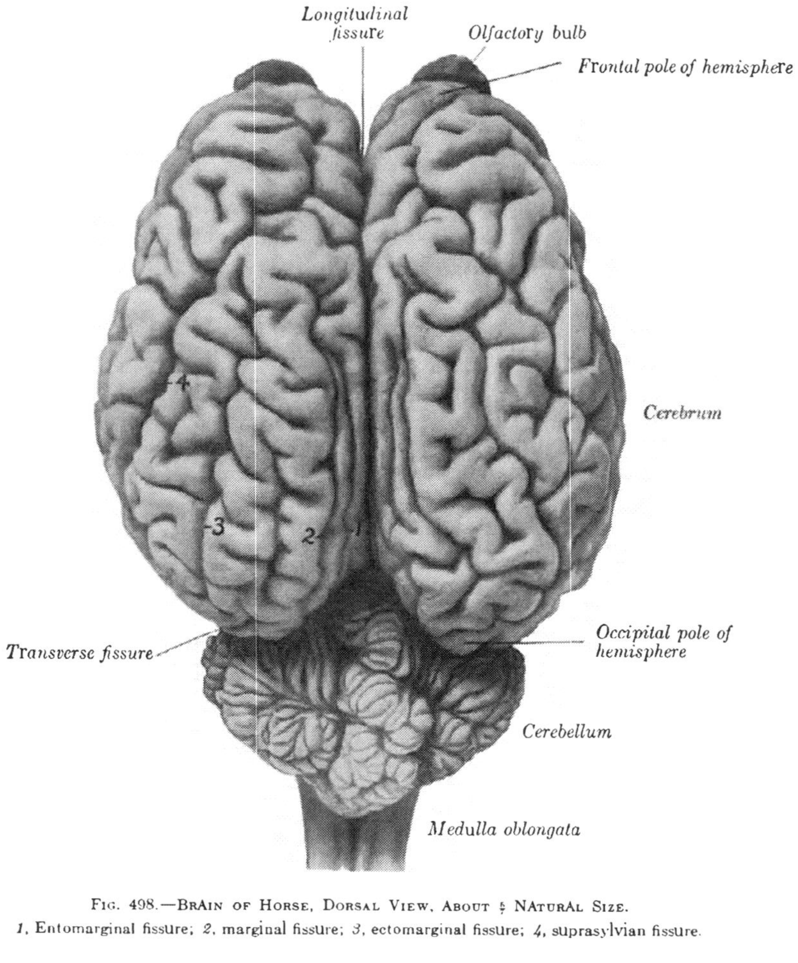

FIG. 498.—BRAIN OF HORSE, DORSAL VIEW, ABOUT $\frac{5}{7}$ NATURAL SIZE.
1, Entomarginal fissure; *2*, marginal fissure; *3*, ectomarginal fissure; *4*, suprasylvian fissure.

hemispheres form an ovoid mass, and are separated from each other by the median **longitudinal fissure,** in which the falx cerebri is situated. Their surfaces are marked by thick folds, the **gyri cerebri,** separated by **sulci.** The upturned ends of the **olfactory** bulbs are seen in front of the frontal poles of the hemispheres. The occipital poles of the hemispheres overlie the anterior part of the cerebellum, from which they are separated by the **transverse fissure** and the tentorium cerebelli contained in it. The **cerebellum** is a much smaller rounded mass which conceals the greater part of the medulla oblongata. Its surface is divided into a middle lobe, the **vermis,** and two lateral **hemispheres.** It is marked by numerous gyri and narrow sulci which have in general a transverse direction. The posterior third of the **medulla** oblongata is not covered by the cerebellum.

The brain is developed from the expanded cephalic part of the neural tube of the embryo. The process comprises a series of thickenings, flexures, and unequal growth and expansion of various parts of the tube. In the higher animals the result is that the tubular character of the brain is not very evident, since the lumen comes to consist of four irregular cavities, the ventricles, which are connected by narrow passages. The tube is first subdivided by two constrictions into three brain vesicles, termed respectively the hind-brain or rhombencephalon, the mid-brain or mesencephalon, and the fore-brain or prosencephalon. The hind-brain gives rise to three secondary segments and the fore-brain to two. The annexed table indicates the origin of the principal structures of the fully developed brain from the primitive vesicles. It has become customary to describe the brain with reference to its embryological relations.

TABLE INDICATING THE DERIVATION OF THE PRINCIPAL PARTS OF THE BRAIN

Primary Segments.	Secondary Segments.	Derivatives.	Cavities.
Rhombencephalon (posterior vesicle)	Myelencephalon	Medulla oblongata	Fourth ventricle
	Metencephalon	Pons Cerebellum	
	Isthmus rhombencephali	Anterior cerebellar peduncles Anterior medullary velum	
Mesencephalon (middle vesicle)	Mesencephalon	Corpora quadrigemina Cerebral peduncles	Cerebral aqueduct
Prosencephalon (anterior vesicle)	Diencephalon	Optic thalami Subthalamic tegmenta Pineal body	Posterior part of third ventricle
	Telencephalon	Pituitary body Optic nerves and retinæ Cerebral hemispheres Olfactory tracts and bulb	Anterior part of third ventricle. Lateral ventricles and olfactory continuations.

THE RHOMBENCEPHALON

The Medulla Oblongata

The **medulla oblongata** lies on the basilar part of the occipital bone. It is quadrilateral in outline, but much wider in front than behind, and compressed dorso-ventrally. Its length, measured from the root of the first cervical nerve to the pons, is about two inches (ca. 5 cm.).

Its **ventral surface** is convex in the transverse direction. It is marked by a **median fissure** (Fissura mediana ventralis) which is continuous behind with the similar fissure of the spinal cord. The posterior part of the fissure is faintly marked, but in front it becomes deeper and ends in a small depression (Foramen cæcum) behind the central part of a transverse band, the **corpus trapezoideum.** On either side of the fissure is a rounded tract, the **pyramid** (Pyramis), which is bounded externally by a faint lateral groove (Sulcus intermedius ventralis). The pyramids join the pons in front; behind they become narrower and disappear into the substance of the medulla, in which their fibers intercross, forming the **decussation of the pyramids** (Decussatio pyramidum).[1]

The superficial origin of the **sixth cranial nerve** (N. oculomotorius) is just lateral to the anterior end of the pyramid. The **corpus trapezoideum** is a transverse band which extends across the surface immediately behind the pons. It is crossed by the pyramids, which cut off a small central part. The lateral part extends out to the roots of the seventh and eighth nerves on either side. Behind the outer part of the corpus trapezoideum there is a variably developed rounded eminence, the **tuberculum faciale.** The root-fibers of the twelfth or hypoglossal nerve form an oblique linear series lateral to the posterior part of the pyramid.

The **dorsal surface** is largely concealed by the cerebellum and forms the greater part of the floor of the fourth ventricle. The **dorsal median fissure** (Fissura mediana dorsalis), the direct continuation of the corresponding groove of the spinal

[1] The decussation varies superficially in different specimens. In some there is a distinct superficial crossing of fibers so that the median fissure is practically effaced at this point.

cord, extends forward to about the middle of the surface. Here the **restiform bodies,** which constitute the lips of the fissure, diverge to form the lateral boundaries of a triangular depression; this is the posterior part of the rhomboid fossa or floor of the fourth ventricle of the brain. The dorso-lateral fissure winds outward

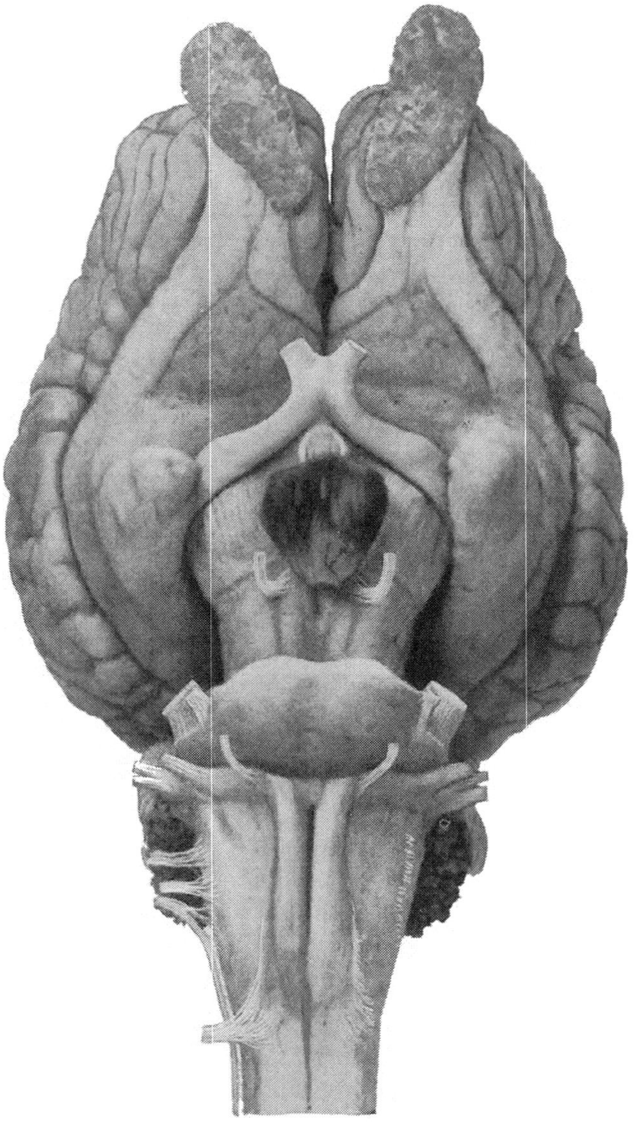

FIG. 499.—BASE OF BRAIN OF HORSE NATURAL SIZE.

and forward to the lateral aspect of the medulla, where it presents the roots of the **ninth, tenth,** and **eleventh cranial nerves.** External to it is a distinct oval eminence on the anterior part of the lateral column, termed the **tuberculum cinereum.** The central canal of the cord is continued in the posterior part of the medulla, inclines dorsally, and opens in the posterior angle of the fourth ventricle. Hence it is customary to distinguish a closed and an open part of the medulla. The dorsal aspect of the latter, which is concealed at present, will be considered later in the description of the fourth ventricle.

The lateral surface is narrow behind, wider and rounded in front. From it the root-fibers of the ninth, tenth, and eleventh cranial nerves arise in a linear series, and alongside of it the spinal part of the eleventh nerve passes forward to join the medullary root. Close inspection reveals the presence of striæ which curve obliquely downward and backward from the surface of the restiform body

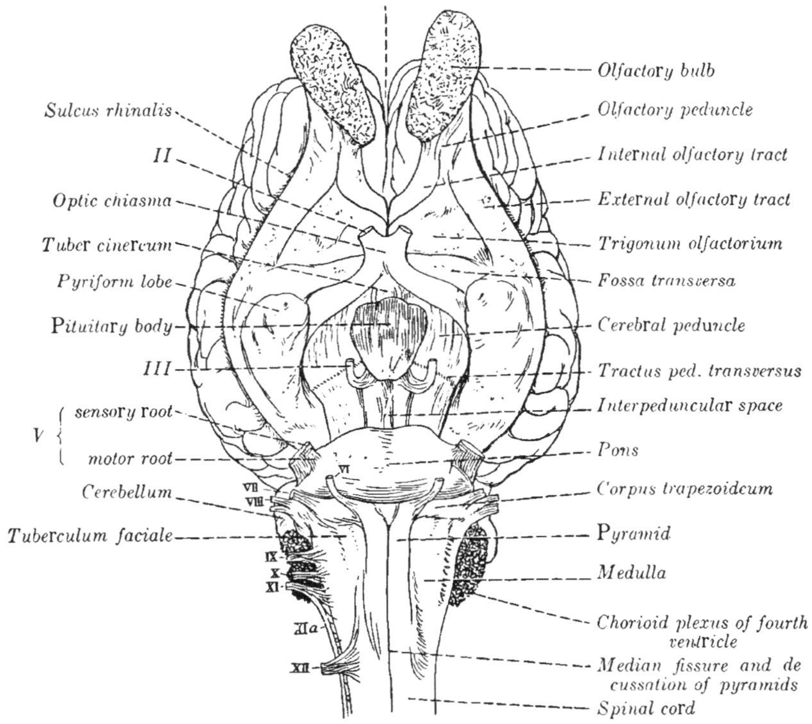

FIG. 500.—LINE DRAWING OF BASE OF BRAIN OF HORSE. (KEY TO FIG. 499.)

toward the hypoglossal root-fibers; these are the **external arcuate fibers** (Fibræ arcuatæ externæ). The recess between the lateral aspect of the medulla and the cerebellum is occupied by an irregular mass of villous projections of the pia mater, containing tufts of vessels; this is the **chorioid plexus of the fourth ventricle,** and is the lateral edge of the **tela chorioidea** of the ventricle. On raising the chorioid plexus it is seen that the tela chorioidea is attached to the dorsal aspect of the medulla, and reinforces here the wall of the fourth ventricle; also that the restiform body terminates in front by entering the base of the cerebellum, forming its posterior peduncle.

In the medulla the fiber tracts of the spinal cord either terminate in the nuclei of the gray matter or undergo changes in their relative position, and new tracts appear. The gray matter is highly modified and forms masses which have no homologues in the cord. The central canal of the closed part of the medulla is surrounded by a thicker layer of gray matter than is the case in the spinal cord. As the medulla opens out this gray matter is naturally spread in the floor of the fourth ventricle. The dorsal horns of gray matter become wide, spread apart, and are broken up to a great extent in the formatio reticularis. Two elongated masses of cells appear above the central gray matter; these are the **nucleus gracilis** and **nucleus cuneatus**, and in them the fasciculi of like name gradually end. In front of these are the **terminal nuclei** of the afferent or sensory cranial nerves and of the sensory portions of the mixed nerves. The ventral horns are succeeded by the **nuclei of origin** of the efferent or motor cranial nerves and the motor root-fibers of the mixed nerves. Of the twelve pairs of cranial nerves, the last eight are connected with nuclei in the medulla and pons. The **posterior olivary nucleus** (Nucleus olivaris caudalis) is a conspicuous gray mass which lies above the pyramid on each side. On cross-sections it appears as a wavy layer of gray matter which is folded on itself so as to inclose a mass of white matter. It is about 2 cm. long in the horse, but is smaller in circumference than in man and hence does not cause any very distinct external enlargement (olivary eminence), as in the latter. It is connected with the opposite side of the cerebellum by the cerebello-olivary fibers. At its inner side are two small accessory olivary nuclei. The **pyramidal tracts**, which are small in ungulates, send most of their fibers across to the opposite side in the posterior part of the medulla, forming the **pyramidal decussation.** Some fibers, however, continue in the ventral column of the same side of the cord, and others are connected with the nuclei of the motor nerve-roots. From the nucleus gracilis and nucleus cuneatus fibers arise which are traceable forward to the thalamus.

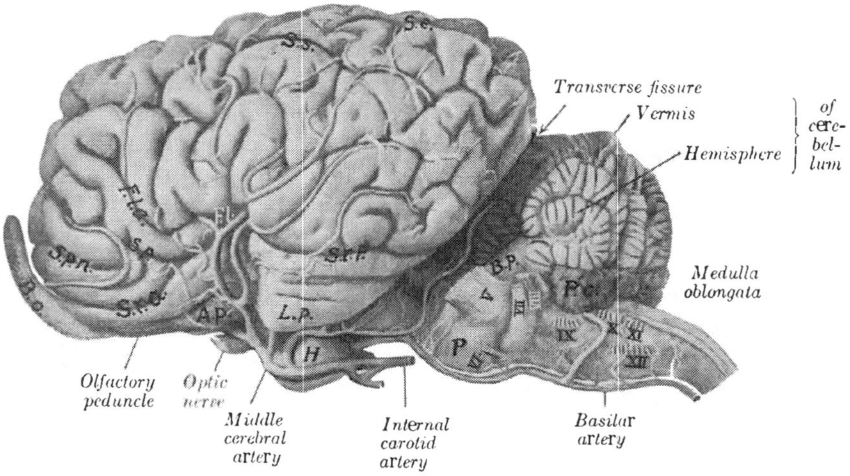

FIG. 501.—BRAIN OF HORSE, LEFT LATERAL VIEW.

The larger arteries are shown. The nerve-roots are indicated by Roman numerals. *P.c.*, Chorioid plexus of fourth ventricle; *B.p.*, middle peduncle of cerebellum; *P*, pons; *H*, pituitary body; *L.p.*, pyriform lobe; *A.p.*, trigonum olfactorium; *B.o*, olfactory bulb; *S.r.a.*, sulcus rhinalis anterior; *S.r.p.*, sulcus rhinalis posterior; *F.l.*, lateral fissure (of Sylvius); *F.l.a.*, anterior branch of lateral fissure; *S.p.*, presylvian fissure; *S.p.n.*, anterior presylvian fissure; *S.s.*, suprasylvian fissure; *S.e.*, ectomarginal fissure.

These are the **internal arcuate fibers** (Fibræ arcuatæ internæ), which curve across the median plane below the central gray matter and form with those of the opposite side the **decussation of the fillet** (Decussatio lemniscorum). Beyond the decussation the fibers form an important longitudinal tract which extends forward in the mid-brain. This is the **fillet** or **lemniscus**, the chief continuation of the sensory conducting path from the dorsal roots of the spinal nerves. The **external arcuate fibers**, some of which were seen on the lateral aspect of the medulla, have a similar origin. Part of them (Fibræ dorsales) pass directly to the dorsal aspect of the restiform body of the same side; others (Fibræ ventrales) cross to the opposite side, descend close to the ventral fissure, and then curve upward and forward to the restiform body. The decussation of the arcuate fibers forms the distinct median raphe seen on cross-sections of the medulla anterior to the pyramidal decussation. The restiform body, situated dorso-laterally, contains, in addition to the arcuate fibers, the **cerebello-olivary fasciculus** before mentioned, and the **cerebello-spinal fasciculus** or direct cerebellar tract. The **dorsal longitudinal fasciculus** corresponds to the ventral ground-bundle of the spinal cord, displaced dorsally by the decussation of the pyramids and fillet. In the posterior part of the medulla it is not marked off from the fillet, along the dorsal edge of which it lies. From the level of the hypoglossal nucleus forward it is distinct and can be traced as a conspicuous tract in the ventral margin of the gray matter of the floor of the fourth ventricle and of the central gray matter of the mid-brain. Below the restiform body and related externally to the external arcuate fibers, there is a considerable bundle of longitudinal fibers, the **spinal root** (Tractus spinalis) **of the fifth nerve**; internal to it is the terminal nucleus of the sensory root of the nerve.

THE PONS

The **pons** (Varolii) is that part of the brain stem which lies between the medulla and the cerebral peduncles; it is marked off from these ventrally by anterior and

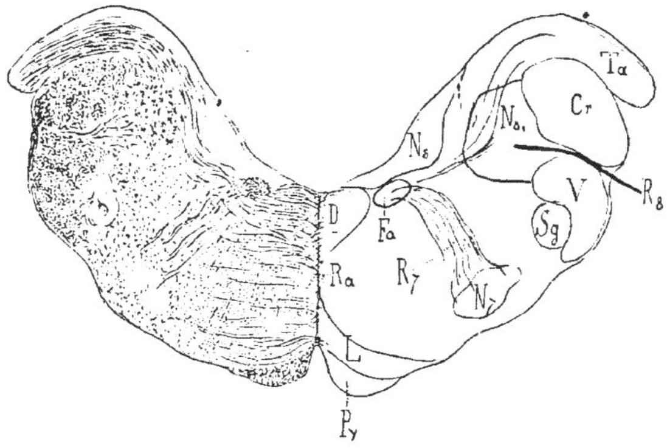

FIG. 502.—CROSS-SECTION OF MEDULLA OBLONGATA OF HORSE, PASSING THROUGH FACIAL NUCLEUS.

Cr, Corpus restiforme; *D*, dorsal longitudinal fasciculus; *Fa*, ascending part of facial nerve; *L*, fillet; *N7*, nucleus of facial nerve; *N8*, triangular nucleus of vestibular root of eighth nerve; *N8'*, spinal root of eighth nerve; *Py*, pyramid; *Ra*, raphe; *R7*, radicular part of facial nerve; *R8*, vestibular root of eighth nerve; *Sg*, substantia gelatinosa; *Ta*, posterior end of tuberculum acusticum; *V*, spinal root of trigeminus. (Ellenberger-Baum, Anat. d. Haustiere.)

posterior grooves. Viewed from below it is elongated transversely, convex in both directions, and presents a wide shallow median groove (Sulcus basilaris), which

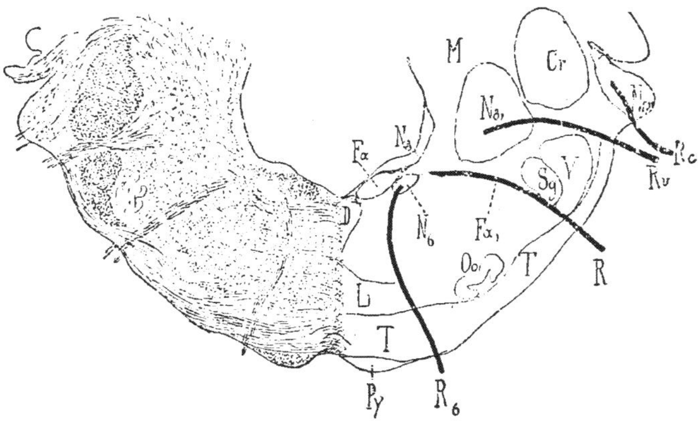

FIG. 503.—CROSS-SECTION OF MEDULLA OBLONGATA OF HORSE; SECTION PASSES THROUGH MIDDLE OF CORPUS TRAPEZOIDEUM.

Cr, Corpus restiforme; *D*, dorsal longitudinal bundle; *Fa*, ascending part of facial nerve; *Fa'*, emergent or descending part of facial nerve; *R7*, root of facial nerve; *L*, fillet; *M*, central white matter of cerebellum; *N6*, abducens nucleus; *N8*, triangular nucleus; *N8'*, nucleus of Deiters; *N8''*, tuberculum acusticum; *Oo*, anterior olive; *Py*, pyramid; *R6*, root of abducens nerve; *R7*, root of facial nerve; *Rc*, cochlear nerve; *Rv*, vestibular nerve; *Sg*, substantia gelatinosa; *T*, corpus trapezoideum; *V*, spinal root of trigeminus. (Ellenberger-Baum, Anat. d. Haustiere.)

lodges the basilar artery. Laterally a large part of its mass curves upward and backward into the base of the cerebellum, forming the **middle cerebellar peduncle** (Brachium pontis). The superficial origin of the trigeminal (fifth) nerve is at the lateral limit of the ventral surface. Transverse striations indicate the course of its superficial (ventral) fibers which connect the two sides of the cerebellum. The dorsal surface is blended on either side with the overlying anterior peduncles of the cerebellum; the central free portion forms the anterior part of the floor of the fourth ventricle, and will be considered in the account of that cavity.

On cross-section the pons is seen to be composed of dorsal and ventral parts. The **dorsal part** (Pars dorsalis pontis) consists superficially of a layer of gray matter covered by the ependyma of the fourth ventricle. Beneath this the median raphe of the medulla is continued into the pons, dividing it into similar halves. In the anterior part of the pons the fillet divides into an inner and outer part, the **medial and lateral fillets** (Lemniscus medialis, lateralis); the latter arches outward to reach the outer side of the anterior cerebellar peduncle. The **dorsal longitudinal fasciculus** becomes sharply defined into a round bundle which lies close to the raphé under the gray matter of the floor of the fourth ventricle. In cross-section the **formatio reticularis** forms a large area below the superficial gray matter and the longitudinal bundles. Dorso-laterally is the large rounded section of the **anterior cerebellar peduncle**. Lower down is a large bundle, the **sensory root of the fifth nerve**. In front of this is the **motor nucleus** of the same nerve, external to which is its **motor root**. The **ventral part** of the pons (Pars basilaris pontis) is composed of transverse and longitudinal fibers, and a large amount of gray matter which is broken up into small masses (Nuclei pontis) by the intersection of the fibers. The **transverse fibers** are gathered laterally into a compact mass which turns upward and backward and enters the central white matter of the cerebellum, forming the **middle cerebellar peduncle**. Centrally the fibers are arranged in bundles which intercross. The transverse fibers are chiefly of two kinds. Some arise from the Purkinje cells of the cerebellar cortex and pass either to the opposite side of the cerebellum or turn at the raphé and run forward and backward in the brain-stem. Others are axones of cells of the nuclei pontis, and pass to the hemispheres of the cerebellum. The corpus trapezoideum is mainly the central continuation of the cochlear division of the auditory nerve. Above it is the small **anterior olivary nucleus** (Nucleus olivaris nasalis). The longitudinal fibers of the ventral part of the pons consist chiefly of the **cerebrospinal** or **pyramidal fasciculi.** These come from the ventral part (pes) of the cerebral peduncles and are situated laterally, interspersed among the deep transverse fibers in the anterior part of the pons. Toward the posterior part the bundles incline toward the median plane and become collected into a compact mass which appears superficially at the posterior border. Many fibers come from the cerebral cortex and terminate in the nuclei of the gray matter of the pons; they may be designated **corticopontile fibers.**

THE CEREBELLUM

The **cerebellum** is situated in the posterior fossa of the cranium, and is separated from the cerebral hemispheres by the transverse fissure and the tentorium cerebelli which occupies it. It overlies the pons and the greater part of the medulla, from which it is separated by the fourth ventricle. Its average weight is about two ounces (ca. 60 gm.) or about 9 per cent. of the weight of the entire brain. Its shape is approximately globular but very irregular. It is somewhat compressed dorso-ventrally and its transverse diameter is the greatest.

The **anterior surface** faces upward and forward and is covered partially by the tentorium cerebelli. The **posterior surface** is almost vertical. The **ventral surface** or base lies over the fourth ventricle, and is connected bv three pairs of peduncles with the medulla, pons, and mid-brain.

It is customary to recognize three gross divisions of the cerebellum, viz., the median vermis and two lateral hemispheres. The **vermis** (cerebelli) is curved in a circular manner so that its two extremities are close together or even in contact on the ventral surface. The anterior extremity is termed the **lingula;** it lies between the cerebellar peduncles and gives attachment to the **anterior medullary velum,** a thin lamina which forms the anterior part of the roof of the fourth ventriele. The posterior extremity, the **nodulus,** gives attachment to the **posterior medullary velum** which covers the posterior recess of the fourth ventricle. The **hemisoheres** (Hemisphæria cerebelli) are clearly separated from the vermis by two deep paramedian fissures. They lie in the lateral depressions of the cerebellar compartment of the cranium.

In tracing the fissures from behind forward it will be noticed that they are nearly sagittal as far as the anterior surface, where they diverge widely, so that the vermis forms all of the fore part of the cerebellum.

The surface of the cerebellum is further cut up into numerous **gyri** or **folia** by narrow and relatively deep **sulci**, many of which approach a transverse direction. Certain of the sulci are more pronounced than the others, and by means of them it is possible to define groups of gyri. Such groups are termed **lobes**, and have received specific names, derived chiefly from the systematic descriptions of the human cerebellum.

The lobes of the vermis are readily distinguished on a median section. Enumerated from the anterior to the posterior extremity they are: (1) lingula, (2) lobus centralis, (3) lobus ascendens, (4) lobus culminis, (5) lobus clivi, (6) tuber vermis, (7) pyramis, (8) uvula, (9) nodulus. Each hemisphere is cut into laterally by two sulci which mark off two sagittal discoid masses, termed by Ziehen tabulations. The external tabulation consists of four or five lobules, the lowest of which is regarded as the flocculus. The inner part of the hemisphere is divided into three or four lobes. In the absence of a satisfactory morphological basis it seems undesirable to deal with the lobation of the cerebellum in further detail.

The **cerebellar peduncles**, three on each side, join the central white matter of the cerebellum at the base. The **posterior peduncle** is the restiform body of the medulla, a large rounded tract derived from the lateral and ventral columns of the cord. Near the middle of the medulla it inclines outward, forms the lateral wall of the fourth ventricle, and ends by entering the central white matter of the cerebellum. The **middle peduncle** is formed, as previously seen, by the brachium pontis. The **anterior peduncles** (Brachia conjunctiva) pass forward on either side on the dorsal surface of the pons, forming the lateral boundary of the fore part of the fourth ventricle. They disappear under the corpora quadrigemina into the substance of the mid-brain. At the point of disappearance the **trochlear** (fourth) **nerve** emerges from the mid-brain. In some cases two or three bundles of fibers (Fila lateralia pontis) arise in the angle between the middle and anterior peduncle, curve obliquely forward and downward over the outer aspect of the latter, and spread out on the ventral face of the cerebral peduncle just in front of the pons.

On sagittal section the cerebellum is seen to consist of a layer of **cortical gray matter** (Substantia corticalis) and the **medullary white matter**. The white matter consists of a large basal mass (Corpus medullare), which is joined by the peduncles, and gives off primary laminæ to the lobules; from these secondary and tertiary laminæ arise, the latter entering the gyri. The arrangement on sagittal section is tree-like, hence the classical term "arbor vitæ" which is applied to it. The central gray matter consists of groups of cells which form small **nuclei** embedded in the central white substance.

As noted above the central gray matter does not form a large nucleus, the corpus dentatum, which is so conspicuous an object on sagittal sections of the cerebellar hemisphere in man.

The principal connections established by the peduncular fibers of the cerebellum are as follows: The posterior peduncle (Corpus restiforme) is composed of afferent and efferent fibers which connect the cerebellum with the medulla and spinal cord. The **cerebello-spinal fasciculus** or **direct cerebellar tract**, which arises from the cells of the nucleus dorsalis (Clarke's column) of the cord, ends in the cortex of the vermis; many of its fibers cross to the opposite side. Numerous **arcuate fibers** from the nucleus gracilis and nucleus cuneatus of the same and opposite sides establish connections with cells of the cerebellar cortex. **Clivo-cerebellar** fibers (chiefly afferent) connect with the olivary nucleus of the same and of the opposite side of the medulla oblongata. The **nucleo-cerebellar fasciculus** comprises fibers derived from the nuclei of the fifth, eighth, and tenth cranial nerves (Edinger). The **descending cerebello-spinal fasciculus** consists of fibers which terminate in relation with cells of the ventral horns of the spinal cord. The chief facts concerning the middle peduncle have been mentioned in the description of the pons. The anterior peduncle is essentially an efferent tract, the fibers of which pass forward to the tegmentum of the cerebral peduncle, the subthalamic region, and the thalamus. After the peduncles disappear under the corpora quadrigemina, they converge and many of their fibers intercross, forming the **decussation of the superior peduncle**. A considerable number of fibers end in the nucleus ruber. Thence impulses are transmitted in two directions: first, by **thalamo-cortical fibers** to the cerebral cortex; second, by the **rubro-spinal tract** through the brain-stem and lateral columns of the cord to the ventral horn cells. The ventro-lateral cerebellospinal fasciculus (Gowers' tract) is an ill-defined tract which connects the spinal cord with the cerebellum. Its fibers appear to be axones of cells of the posterior horns of the cord; they pass in the lateral column of the cord, become scattered in passing through the reticular formation of the medulla and pons, and enter the cerebellum by way of the anterior medullary velum.

The Fourth Ventricle

The fourth ventricle (Ventriculus quartus) is the cavity of the rhombencephalon; it communicates with the central canal of the spinal cord behind, and through the aqueduct with the third ventricle in front. It is somewhat rhomboid in outline, elongated from before backward and narrowest behind. It is lined completely by an epithelium (Ependyma) and contains a small amount of fluid.

Its **floor** (Fossa rhomboidea) is formed by the **medulla** and **pons** and is marked by three longitudinal furrows which converge behind. It is widest and deepest a little in front of its middle. The posterior part narrows to a point at the opening of the central canal, and on account of its appearance in man it has been termed the

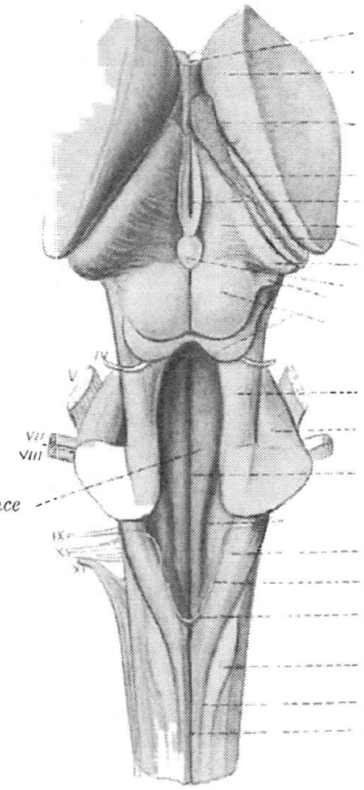

Fig. 504.—Brain Stem and Basal Ganglia of Horse, Dorsal View.
The cranial nerve-roots are designated by Roman numerals.

calamus scriptorius. The **median sulcus** (Sulcus medianus) extends the entire length of the floor and is deepest toward the ends. The **limiting** sulci (Sulci limitantes) begin on either side of the opening of the central canal and extend forward as the lateral limits of the rhomboid fossa. Just beyond the middle of the fossa they expand into a shallow depression, the **anterior fovea** (Fovea nasalis). On either side of the median sulcus and margined by the limiting sulcus is a slightly rounded column, the **eminentia medialis.** Opposite the fovea this presents an elongated prominence, the **colliculus facialis,** so named because it overlies the bend formed by the fibers of origin of the facial nerve. External to the limiting sulcus is a long fusiform elevation, the **area acustica,** from which a band of fibers (Striæ acusticæ) winds over the anterior end of the restiform body to the superficial origin of the cochlear nerve.

The **lateral wall** is formed by the restiform body and the anterior peduncle of the cerebellum.

The roof is formed in its middle part by the vermis of the cerebellum, covered by the epithelium before mentioned. There is commonly a dorsal recess (Recessus tecti s. fastigium) between the extremities of the vermis. The anterior part of the roof is formed by a thin lamina of white substance, the **anterior medullary velum** (or valve of Vieussens), which extends backward from the corpora quadrigemina, and is attached on either side to the anterior peduncles of the cerebellum. Its anterior part is relatively thick and contains the decussation of the fibers of the trochlear nerves. Posteriorly it blends with the white matter of the cerebellum. A thin lamina of white matter, the **posterior medullary velum,** backed by pia mater, completes the roof posteriorly. After removal of the cerebellum the line of attachment (Tænia ventriculi quarti) to the medulla is seen; it begins centrally over the opening of the central canal, runs forward on the inner face of the restiform body, and turns outward behind the brachium pontis. The thick part which stretches over the posterior angle of the ventricle is termed the **obex.** The posterior part of the ventricle forms three recesses, of which two are lateral and the third median and posterior. The **lateral recesses** communicate with the sub

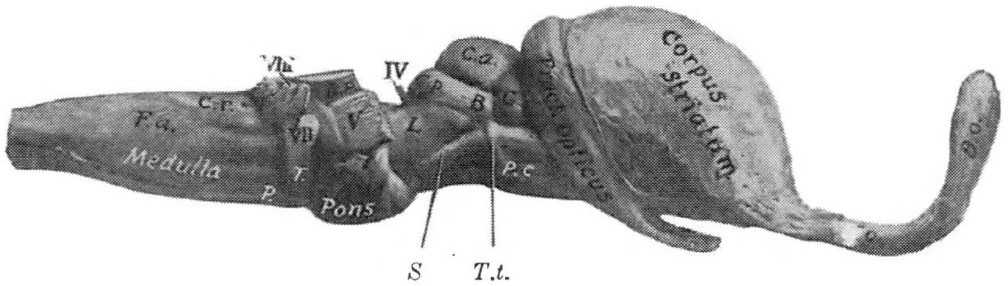

Fig. 505.—Brain Stem and Basal Ganglia of Horse, Right View.

F.a., External arcuate fibers; *C.r.*, corpus restiforme; *P*, pyramid; *T*, corpus trapezoideum; *B.p.*, middle peduncle of cerebellum; *P.c.*, cerebral peduncle; *S*, sulcus lateralis; *T.t.*, tractus transversus; *L*, trigonum lemnisci; *C.a.*, corpus quad. ant.; *C.p.*, corpus quad. post.; *B*, commissure of *C.p.*; *G*, corpus geniculatum internum; *T.o.*, olfactory peduncle; *B.o.*, olfactory bulb.

arachnoid space by distinct openings (Aperturæ laterales). The layer of pia which strengthens the roof here is named the **tela chorioidea** of the fourth ventricle. It is triangular in outline and closely adherent to the velum. It forms three fringed masses which contain vascular convolutions and are designated the **median** and **lateral chorioid plexuses** of the fourth ventricle. They appear to lie within the ventricle, but are really excluded from the cavity by the epithelial lining, which they invaginate.

THE MESENCEPHALON

The **mesencephalon** or **mid-brain** connects the rhombencephalon with the fore-brain. In the undissected brain it is covered dorsally by the cerebral hemispheres. It consists of a dorsal part, the corpora quadrigemina, and a larger ventral part, the cerebral peduncles, which are visible on the base of the brain. It is traversed longitudinally by a narrow canal, the cerebral aqueduct, which connects the fourth ventricle with the third.

The **corpora quadrigemina**[1] are four rounded eminences which lie under the posterior part of the cerebral hemispheres. They consist of two pairs, separated by a transverse groove. The **anterior pair** (Colliculi nasales) are larger and much

[1] In the new nomenclature the term lamina quadrigemina is applied to the dorsal mass of the mid-brain, and the four eminences which it bears are the corpora quadrigemina.

higher than the posterior pair. They are gray in color, almost hemispherical, and are separated by a narrow furrow which leads forward to the subpineal fovea. A wide groove intervenes between them and the optic thalami. The **posterior pair** (Colliculi caudales) are relatively small and are paler than the anterior pair. They are marked by a wide median depression, and are limited below by a transverse furrow (Sulcus postquadrigeminus), at either side of which the **trochlear** (fourth) **nerve** emerges. Laterally each is prolonged to the inner geniculate body by a band of white matter termed the inferior brachium.[1]

The **cerebral peduncles** or crura cerebri (Pedunculi cerebri) appear on the base of the brain as two large rope-like stalks which emerge from the pons close together and diverge as they extend forward to enter the cerebrum. At the point of disappearance the **optic tract** winds obliquely across the peduncle. About half an inch further back a small tract (Tractus peduncularis transversus) curves across the peduncles, and behind this near the median line is the superficial origin of the **oculomotor** (third) **nerve.** The triangular depression between the diverging peduncles is the **interpeduncular space** (Fossa interpeduncularis). It is covered to a large extent by the **pituitary** body, a discoid brown mass which is connected with the base of the brain by a hollow stalk, the **infundibulum.** The posterior part of the space is pierced by numerous minute openings which transmit blood-vessels, and is therefore termed the **locus perforatus posticus.** The objects in the space belong to the diencephalon, and will be described later. The lateral aspect of the peduncle is marked by a groove (Sulcus lateralis mesencephali) which indicates the division into a dorsal part, the **tegmentum,** and a ventral part the **basis pedunculi**; these are separated by a layer of dark gray matter, the **substantia nigra.** The triangular area (Trigonum lemnisci) above the lateral groove is faintly marked by fibers passing obliquely upward and backward to the anterior cerebellar peduncle; these belong to the fillet or lemniscus, an important tract that connects the thalamus and corpora quadrigemina with the sensory reception nuclei of the opposite side of the medulla.

The **aqueduct of the cerebrum** or of Sylvius (Aquæductus cerebri) is the canal which extends through the mid-brain from the fourth to the third ventricle. It is surrounded by a layer of gray matter (Stratum griseum centrale), in the ventral part of which are the nuclei of origin of the oculomotor and trochlear nerves, and laterally nuclei of the mesencephalic roots of the trigeminal nerves.

THE DIENCEPHALON

The diencephalon or **inter-brain** comprises the thalamus and a number of other structures grouped about the third ventricle, the cavity of this division of the brain.[2] To expose its dorsal aspect, the greater part of the cerebral hemispheres, the corpus callosum, the fornix, the hippocampus, and the tela chorioidea of the third ventricle must be removed.

The **thalamus** (or optic thalamus) is the principal body in this part of the brain. It is a large ovoid gray mass placed obliquely across the dorsal face of each cerebral peduncle, so that the long axes of the two thalami would meet in front about at a right angle. Medially they are fused to a large extent, and around the area of adhesion they are separated by a sagittal circular space, the third ventricle. The dorsal surface is convex in both directions, and is separated from the overlying hippocampus by the tela chorioidea (or velum interpositum). Laterally it is sep-

[1] In man a distinct superior brachium connects the superior pair with the lateral geniculate body, but in the domesticated animals the union with the optic thalamus is too direct to allow of any definite arm being recognized.

[2] On a strictly embryological basis the optic part of the hypothalamus, comprising the anterior part of the third ventricle and the structures associated with it, belong to the telencephalon, but will be considered here as a matter of convenience.

arated from the nucleus caudatus by an oblique groove in which there is a band of white matter termed the **stria terminalis** or tænia semicircularis. Internally it is bounded by a narrow band, the **stria medullaris,** on which is a delicate ridge of ependyma termed the **tænia thalami**. The striæ unite posteriorly and blend with the stalk of the pituitary body. Near this point they present a small enlargement caused by the nucleus habenulæ. Anteriorly there is a small eminence, the **anterior tubercle.** The posterior part of the thalamus has the form of a rounded ridge which is continuous laterally with the optic tract.[1] Behind the point of origin of the tract, in the angle between the thalamus and the cerebral peduncle, is the **internal geniculate** body (Corpus geniculatum mediale), a well-defined oval prominence.

The outer surface is separated from the lenticular nucleus by the **internal capsule**, an important mass of white matter composed of fibers passing to and from the cerebral cortex. These fibers go to form a large part of the ventral portion (basis) of the cerebral peduncle. From the entire external surface of the thalamus fibers pass into the internal capsule and radiate to reach the cerebral cortex; similarly fibers coming from the cortex converge in the internal capsule to enter the thalamus. This arrangement is termed the thalamic radiation. Ventral to the thalamus proper is the **subthalamic tegmental region.** This is the continuation of the tegmental part of the cerebral peduncle into the diencephalon. It contains the **red nucleus** (Nucleus ruber) an important ganglion on the course of the motor tracts. It receives numerous fibers from the cerebral cortex and the corpus striatum. From it fibers proceed to the thalamus and to the spinal cord; the fibers to the cord (Tractus rubro-spinalis of Monakow) cross to the opposite side and extend back in the tegmentum to the lateral columns of the cord. Lateral to the red nucleus a conspicuous lenticular area of dark gray matter is visible on cross-sections of the subthalamic region; this is the **subthalamic nucleus** (Nucleus hypothalamicus s. corpus Luysi), which consists of pigmented nerve-cells scattered through a dense network of fine medullated fibers, and is richly supplied with capillary blood-vessels. The two nuclei are connected by a transverse commissure (Commissura hypothalamica), which crosses the floor of the third ventricle above the mammillary body.

The **pineal body** or **epiphysis** is a small ovoid or fusiform red brown mass situated in a deep central depression between the thalami and corpora quadrigemina. It is variable in size, but is commonly about 10 to 12 mm. long and 6 mm. wide. It is attached at the postero-superior quadrant of the third ventricle by a short stalk, in which is a small recess of that cavity. Its base blends in front with the junction of the striæ medullares of the thalamus. Immediately under the posterior part of the stalk is a short transverse band of white matter, the **posterior commissure.**

The pineal body is inclosed in a fibrous capsule from which numerous trabeculæ pass inward, dividing the organ into spaces occupied by round epithelial cells of the same origin as the ependyma of the ventricle.

The **mammillary** body (Corpus mammillare) is a white round elevation a little larger than a pea which projects ventrally at the anterior end of the median furrow of the interpeduncular space. While it is a single body in external form in the horse, sections show that it is double in structure and contains a nucleus of gray matter on either side.

Three sets of fibers are connected with the mammillary body. The anterior pillar of the fornix curves down in the lateral wall of the third ventricle to the body and many of the fornix fibers end in it. A bundle (Fasciculus thalamo-mammillaris) passes upward and backward from it into the anterior part of the thalamus, and a tract (Fasciculus pedunculo-mammillaris) extends back in the floor of the third ventricle to the tegmentum of the mid-brain.

The **pituitary** body or **hypophysis** was mentioned as covering part of the interpeduncular space. It is oval in outline, flattened dorso-ventrally, and nearly an inch (ca. 2 cm.) in width. It is attached by a delicate tubular stalk, the **infundibulum,** to the tuber **cinereum,** a small gray prominence situated between the optic chiasm in front and the mammillary body behind.

The pituitary body consists of two parts which can be distinguished readily on sections by their color. The glandular (or anterior) lobe is brown in color and is inclosed in a fibrous capsule.

[1] This backward projection of the thalamus is equivalent to the pulvinar and lateral geniculate body of man, which are not superficially divided in the domestic animals.

It is glandular in character and there is good ground for the view that it is an organ of internal secretion. Besides the chief cells which stain lightly, it contains large deeply staining chromophile cells. It arises as an outgrowth from the primitive mouth cavity. The cerebral (or posterior) lobe is pale and is connected with the infundibulum so as to form a rather flask-shaped arrangement. It is almost entirely inclosed by the glandular part. It arises as an outgrowth from the primitive diencephalon, but loses most of its earlier nervous character.

The optic chiasm and tracts form the anterior boundary of the interpeduncular space. The **optic chiasm** or **commissure** (Chiasma opticum) is formed by the convergence of the optic nerves and the crossing of the major part of the fibers of the nerve of one side to the tract of the opposite side. From the chiasm each **optic tract** (Tractus opticus) curves over the cerebral peduncle outward, back-

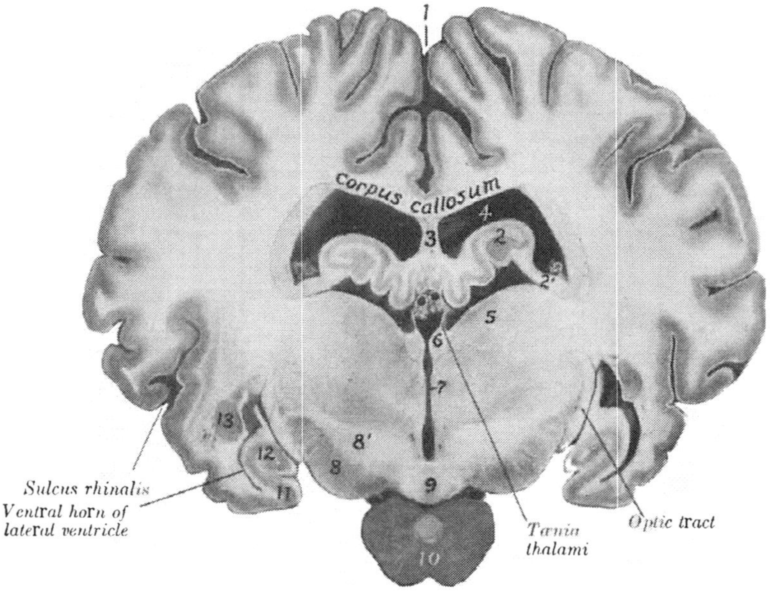

FIG. 506.—CROSS-SECTION OF BRAIN OF HORSE, NATURAL SIZE.

Section passes through posterior part of third ventricle and is viewed from behind. *1*, Longitudinal fissure; *2*, hippocampus; *2'*, fimbria; *3*, septum pellucidum; *4*, lateral ventricle; *5*, thalamus; *6*, habenula; *7*, third ventricle; *8*, cerebral peduncle; *8'*, hypothalamus; *9*, mammillary body; *10*, pituitary body; *11*, pyriform lobe; *12*, ventral end of hippocampus; *13*, amygdaloid nucleus. Between the upper parts of the tæniæ thalami is the chorioid plexus of the third ventricle, and above this are the internal cerebral veins.

ward, and upward to the posterior part of the thalamus and the internal geniculate body; some fibers reach the anterior quadrigeminal body.

All the fibers in the chiasm are not derived from the optic nerves. The posterior part contains fibers which pass from one tract to the other and are connected with the internal geniculate bodies; this bundle is called Gudden's commissure (Commissura inferior). Above it is Meynert's commissure (Commissura superior), the fibers of which enter the subthalamic body.

The **third ventricle** (Ventriculus tertius) is the narrow annular space between the thalami. It communicates by means of the aqueduct with the fourth ventriele behind, and in front it is continuous with the lateral ventricle on each side through the interventricular foramen. Its floor is formed by the structures of the interpeduncular space and to a small extent by the tegmentum of the cerebral peduncles. The roof is formed in the strict sense only by the ependyma, above which is a fold of pia mater, termed the **tela chorioidea** of the third ventricle or **velum interpositum.** The roof is invaginated by two delicate **chorioid plexuses** which appear to lie within the ventricle, although they are excluded from the cavity by the epithelium. When the tela is removed, the delicate ependyma of the roof is torn away with it, leaving the line of attachment to the stria medullaris to constitute the tænia thalami. The **anterior** wall is formed by the **lamina terminalis** (s. cinerea), a thin layer of gray matter which extends upward from the optic chiasm to the corpus callosum. A distinct rounded band of white matter extends across its posterior face, bulging into the ventricle. This is the **anterior commissure** (Commissura nasalis) of the cerebrum; its fibers extend to the olfactory bulb and to the pyriform lobe. A similar but more slender **posterior commissure** (Commissura caudalis) crosses the posterior wall above the entrance to the aqueduct; the connections of its fibers are not yet clearly known. The **interventricular foramen** (of Monroe) is situated on either side of the anterior part of the ventricle and leads outward and slightly upward between the anterior pillar of the fornix and the anterior tubercle of the thalamus. The cavity presents three **recesses** or diverticula, of which two are ventral and the third is supero-posterior. The **optic recess** (Recessus opticus) lies above the optic chiasm. Just behind it is the **infundibular recess** (Recessus infundibuli) which extends through the infundibulum to the pituitary body. The **pineal recess** (Recessus pinealis) is in the stalk of the pineal body.

THE TELENCEPHALON

The **telencephalon** or **end-brain** comprises two principal parts, the cerebral hemispheres and the optic part of the hypothalamus. The latter has been considered as a matter of convenience in the description of the diencephalon.

The Cerebral Hemispheres

The **cerebral hemispheres** (Hemisphæria) form the greater part of the fully developed brain. Viewed from above (Fig. 498) they form an ovoid mass, of which the broader end is posterior, and the greatest transverse diameter is a little behind the middle. The two hemispheres are separated by a deep median cleft, the **longitudinal fissure** of the cerebrum, which is occupied by a sickle-shaped fold of dura mater, the falx cerebri. In front the separation is complete, and it appears to be behind also, but here the two hemispheres are attached to each other over a small area by the pia mater. When the hemispheres are gently drawn apart, it is seen that the fissure is interrupted in its middle part at a depth of a little more than an inch (ca. 3 cm.) by a white commissural mass, the **corpus callosum**; this connects the hemispheres for about half of their length. The **transverse fissure** separates the hemispheres from the cerebellum, and contains the tentorium cerebelli.

The **convex** or **dorso-lateral surface**[1] conforms closely to the cranial wall. The **medial** or **internal surface** is flat and sagittal and bounds the longitudinal fissure; to a large extent it is in contact with the falx cerebri, but behind the great cerebral vein the two hemispheres are in contact and are attached to each other over a small area as noted above. In well hardened specimens there is usually an impression for the vein in front of the area of adhesion. The **base** or **ventral surface** (Fig. 499) is irregular. Its anterior two-thirds is adapted to the cerebral fossa of the cranial floor. Crossing this area in front of the optic tract is a depression, the **transverse fossa** (vallecula or fossa of Sylvius), which leads outward to the **lateral fissure** (fissure of Sylvius), and lodges the middle cerebral artery. In front of the fossa there is a considerable rounded elevation known as the **trigonum olfactorium.** The trigonum and the inner part of the fossa are pierced

[1] In order to study the configuration of the hemisphere it should be separated from its fellow by median section and from the brain stem by cutting across the mid-brain. Material for this purpose should be hardened *in situ*.

by numerous openings for the passage of small blood-vessels and are equivalent to the locus perforatus anticus of man. Behind the outer part of the fossa is the rounded anterior end of the **pyriform lobe.** Traced backward the lobe curves upward and inward over the optic tract and the thalamus to the tentorial aspect of the hemisphere; its continuation, the hippocampus, forms part of the floor of the lateral ventricle, and will be examined later.

The posterior part or **tentorial area** is flattened, faces inward and backward as well as downward, and rests largely on the tentorium cerebelli; on its anterior part there is a shallow depression adapted to the corpora quadrigemina and the pineal body.

The **frontal pole** or anterior extremity (exclusive of the olfactory bulb) is compressed laterally, and the **occipital pole** or posterior extremity forms a blunt point.

The hemisphere comprises: (1) the **pallium** or **mantle,** which consists of an outer layer of gray matter, the **cortex** (Substantia corticalis), covering a large mass

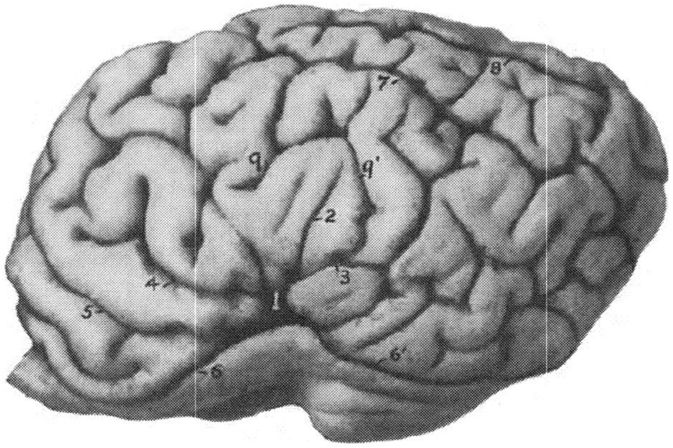

FIG. 507.—LEFT CEREBRAL HEMISPHERE OF HORSE, LATERAL VIEW. THE OLFACTORY BULB IS CUT OFF.

1, Lateral fissure (of Sylvius); *2, 3, 4*, middle, posterior, and anterior branches of *1*; *5*, presylvian fissure; *6 6,'* sulcus rhinalis, anterior et posterior; *7*, suprasylvian fissure; *8*, ectomarginal fissure; *9, 9'*, ectosylvian fissure.

of white matter (Centrum semiovale); (2) the **rhinencephalon** or olfactory portion of the brain; (3) the **corpus callosum** and **fornix,** the great commissural white masses; (4) the **lateral ventricle** and certain important structures associated therewith.

The **pallium** is thrown into numerous folds, the **gyri cerebri,** which are separated by **sulci** or **fissures** of varying depth. The general pattern of the gyri and sulci is similar in normal brains of the same species, but the details are very variable and are never alike on the two hemispheres of the same brain. In the horse the arrangement is complicated by the existence of numerous short accessory fissures which cut into the gyri at right angles and tend to confuse the observer. The principal fissures and sulci of the convex surface (Figs. 497, 507) are as follows:

1. The **lateral fissure** (Fissura lateralis Sylvii) ascends on the lateral surface of the hemisphere as the continuation of the fossa transversa in front of the pyriform lobe. After crossing the external olfactory tract it divides into three branches; of these one passes upward, one runs obliquely forward and upward, and the third is directed upward and backward.

2. The **suprasylvian fissure** (F. suprasylvia)[1] is long and divides a large part

[1] Termed by Lesbre the parietal fissure and by M'Fadyean the great oblique fissure.

of the convex surface of the hemisphere into dorsal and lateral portions. It begins on the dorso-medial border near its anterior end and, inclining gradually downward, passes back to end on reaching the tentorial surface. It is continuous internally with the transverse fissure usually and in front with the presylvian fissure.

3. The **presylvian fissure** (F. præsylvia) is the continuation forward of the preceding. It passes forward, outward, and downward almost to the frontal pole, and then inclines backward to end at the groove which marks the upper limit of the rhinencephalon (Sulcus rhinalis).

4. The **marginal** fissure (F. marginalis) extends along the dorso-medial border. It begins a little in front of the middle of the border and turns around the occipital pole to end on its tentorial aspect.

5. The **entomarginal fissure** (F. entomarginalis) lies internal to the dorso-medial border. It does not extend quite as far forward as the marginal fissure, from which it is separated by a narrow gyrus.

6. The **ectomarginal fissure** (F. ectomarginalis) lies about midway between the marginal fissure and the posterior part of the suprasylvian fissure.

7. The **sulcus rhinalis** is a very distinct furrow on the lower part of the lateral surface which marks off the olfactory part of the brain (rhinencephalon) from the rest of the hemisphere. It is undulating and is highest where it is crossed by the lateral fissure (of Sylvius).[1]

On the medial surface (Fig. 508) the main fissures and sulci are as follows:

1. The **calloso-marginal fissure** (F. calloso-marginalis) is extensive and well-defined. It is approximately parallel to the dorso-medial border of the hemisphere, from which it is about half an inch distant. It begins in front a short distance below and in front of the anterior bend (genu) of the corpus callosum and forms a C-shaped curve, its posterior part extending on the tentorial surface to a point behind the depression for the corpora quadrigemina. It separates the marginal gyri above from the gyrus fornicatus, which extends down to the corpus callosum.

2. The **transverse** fissure (F. transversa) begins a little behind the middle of the calloso-marginal fissure, passes obliquely upward and forward to the dorso-medial border—into which it cuts deeply—and usually joins the suprasylvian fissure.[2]

3. The **sublimbic fissure** (F. sublimbica) curves over the gyrus fornicatus a short distance above the corpus callosum. Its middle part is commonly indistinct, and it is often divided into anterior and posterior parts.

4. The **callosal sulcus** (Sulcus corporis callosi) separates the corpus callosum from the gyrus fornicatus.

The **hippocampus** (or cornu Ammonis) is a gyrus which curves from the deep face of the pyriform lobe around the thalamus and forms the posterior part of the floor of the lateral ventricle. It can be displayed by cutting away the brain-stem up to the optic tract and the interventricular foramen. Viewed from below the hippocampal gyrus is seen to form a semicircular curve from the apex of the pyriform lobe to the angle of divergence of the posterior pillars of the fornix, *i. e.*, to a point under the central part of the corpus callosum. It is separated deeply by the hippocampal fissure from the **gyrus dentatus.** Along the concave margin of the latter is a band of white matter, termed the **fimbria,** which is the prolongation of the greater part of the posterior pillar of the fornix into this region. The ventricular surface of the hippocampus (Fig. 511) is covered with a thin layer of white matter, the **alveus,** which is also derived from the posterior pillar of the fornix, and

[1] Just above this point is a lobe which is homologous with the insula of man. When the overhanging gyri which partly conceal it—forming the operculum—are removed, there are disclosed several short, deeply placed gyri (Gyri breves).

[2] By some authors this is regarded as the homologue of the cruciate fissure of the dog, but it seems likely that the latter is represented by a short and inconstant sulcus situated further forward.

is therefore continuous with the fimbria. The two hippocampi are connected at their highest parts by transverse fibers which constitute the **hippocampal commissure.**

The interval between the hippocampus and fimbria on the one hand and the brain-stem on the other is a lateral continuation of the great transverse fissure of the brain, and is termed the **chorioid fissure.** It is occupied by a fold of pia mater, the **tela chorioidea** of the third ventricle, or **velum interpositum.** This fold i triangular in outline and its apex reaches to the interventricular foramen. Its base is continuous at the transverse fissure with the pia which covers the surface of the brain. Its middle part lies over the epithelial roof of the third ventricle, as has

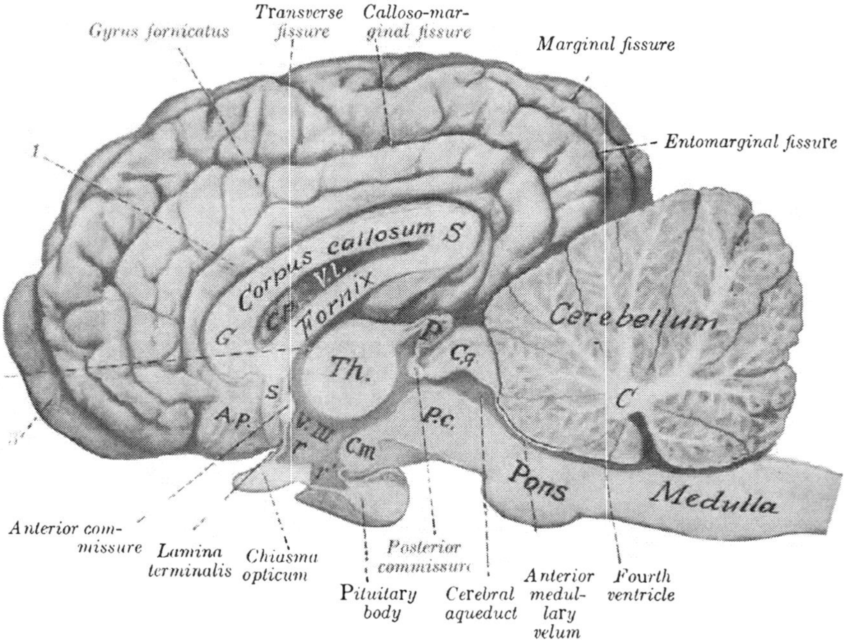

FIG. 508.—MEDIAN SECTION OF BRAIN OF HORSE.

The membranes and vessels are removed. *C*, Central white matter (corpus medullare) of cerebellum· *P.c.*, cerebral peduncle; *C.q.*, corpora quadrigemina; *P*, pineal body; *Th.*, thalamus; *V.III.*, third ventricle; *r*, optic recess; *r'*, infundibular recess; *C.m.*, mammillary body; *s*, subcallosal gyrus; *A.p.*, area parolfactoria· *G*, genu of corpus callosum; *S*, splenium of same; *1*, callosal sulcus; *2*, interventricular foramen; *3*, olfactory bulb. The cerebral lobe of the pituitary body is distinguished by its lighter color.

been seen (Fig. 506). The lateral borders will be seen on the floor of the lateral ventricles, where they form thick rounded bands containing convolutions of blood-vessels, known as the **chorioid plexuses** of the lateral ventricles (Fig. 511).

When the tela is pulled out one may easily get the impression that the lateral ventricle communicates with the exterior by means of the chorioid fissure. Such is not the case, since the chorioid plexus is covered by the epithelial lining of the ventricle, which has been torn away.

The **rhinencephalon** or olfactory part of the brain comprises the olfactory bulb, peduncle and tracts or roots, the trigonum olfactorium, the area parolfactoria, and the pyriform lobe.[1]

[1] From the morphological point of view other structures should be included, but in descriptive anatomy it is usual to limit the application of the term to the parts enumerated above.

The **olfactory bulb** (Bulbus olfactorius) is an oval enlargement which curves upward in front of the frontal pole of the hemisphere. Its convex superficial face fits into the ethmoidal fossa and receives numerous olfactory nerve-fibers through the cribriform plate; hence it is very difficult to remove the bulb intact. It contains a considerable **cavity** (Ventriculus bulbi olfactorii) which is connected with the lateral ventricle by a small canal in the middle olfactory tract. The deep face is largely in contact with the frontal pole of the hemisphere and is connected with the olfactory peduncle.

The gray matter of the bulb is external and is thickest on the convex anterior surface. The posterior surface consists to a large extent of fibers which are the axones of the mitral cells of the deep layer of the gray substance and go to form the peduncle and striæ.

The **olfactory peduncle** (Tractus olfactorius) is a very short but wide band of white substance which arises in the olfactory bulb and extends back to be continued by the olfactory tracts.

The **olfactory tracts** or **striæ** (Striæ olfactorii) are three in number. The

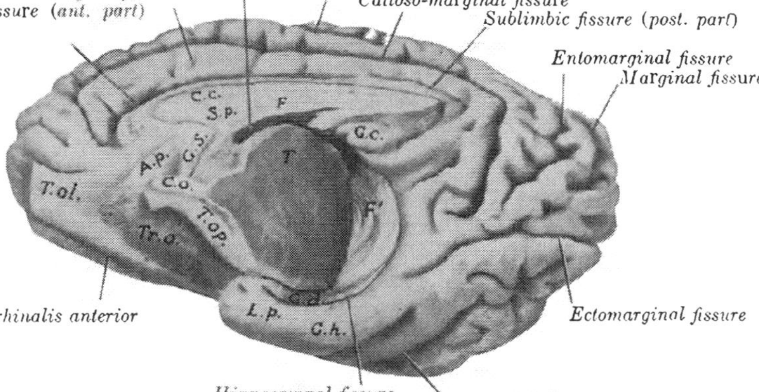

FIG. 509.—MEDIO-VENTRAL ASPECT OF RIGHT CEREBRAL HEMISPHERE OF HORSE.

The olfactory bulb is cut off. *T.ol.*, Olfactory peduncle; *A.p.*, area parolfactoria; *Tr.O.*, trigonum olfactorium; *T.op.*, optic tract; *C.o.*, chiasma opticum; *G.s.*, subcallosal gyrus; *C.c.*, corpus callosum; *S.p.*, septum pellucidum; *F*, fornix; *G.c.*, callosal gyrus; *T*, cut surface of thalamus; *F'*, fimbria; *G.d.*, gyrus dentatus; *L p.*, pyriform lobe; *G.h.*, hippocampal gyrus.

external tract (Stria lateralis) is much the largest and most distinct. It passes backward, upward, and outward, widens out and joins the pyriform lobe. It is clearly defined dorsally by the sulcus rhinalis and is marked off from the trigonum olfactorium by the sulcus arcuatus. The **intermediate tract** (Stria intermedia) is short, ill defined, and flat; it contains the canal which opens into the anterior horn of the lateral ventricle. The **internal tract** (Stria medialis) is small, short, and not well defined; it bends over to the parolfactory area (of Broca) on the inner face of the hemisphere below the genu of the corpus callosum.

The **trigonum olfactorium** is the prominent gray area situated in the angle of divergence of the internal and external olfactory striæ. It is bounded externally by the external olfactory stria, from which it is defined by the arcuate sulcus. It is continuous with the **area parolfactoria** on the medial surface; behind the latter a band descends from the rostrum of the corpus callosum and is continuous below with the anterior perforated space; it is termed the **subcallosal gyrus** or peduncle of the corpus callosum.

The **pyriform lobe** (Lobus piriformis) is the well-marked prominence on the base lateral to the optic tract and cerebral peduncle, from which it is separated by a deep fissure. Its nipple-like apex lies behind the fossa transversa and covers the optic tract. The external surface is marked by one or two sulci (lobi piriformis). The lobe contains a cavity, the ventral horn of the lateral ventricle.

The fibers of the olfactory tracts go to the pyriform lobe and hippocampus, the trigonum olfactorium, the area parolfactoria, the subcallosal gyrus, and part of the gyrus fornicatus. The central connections of the olfactory apparatus are complex and are not yet fully understood. The anterior cerebral commissure contains fibers which pass from the olfactory bulb of one side by way of the inner tracts to the bulb of the opposite side; also fibers which cross in it from the inner tract of one side to the pyriform lobe of the opposite side. Many fibers pass by way of the septum pellucidum, fornix, and fimbria to the hippocampus. Other fibers pass in the anterior pillar of the fornix to the mammillary body and thence to the thalamus by the thalamo-mammillary bundle.

The **corpus callosum** is the great transverse commissure which connects the two cerebral hemispheres through about half of their length. On median section (Fig. 508) it is seen to be arched from before backward, white in color, and com-

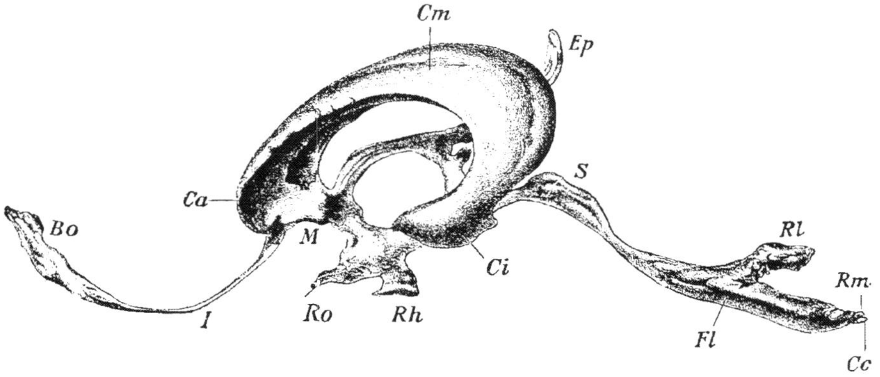

Fig. 510.—Lateral View of Cast of Cavities of Brain of Horse.

Bo, Cavity of olfactory, which communicates through the canal *I* with a lateral ventricle; *Ca*, anterior horn, *Cm*, body, *Ci*, ventral horn of lateral ventricle; *M*, isthmus which connects lateral and third ventricles *Ep*, suprapineal recess, below which is the small infrapineal recess; *Ro*, optic recess; *Rh*, infundibular and pituitary recess; *S*, aqueduct; *Fl*, ridge corresponding to sulcus limitans; *Rl*, lateral recess, *Rm*, posterior recess, of fourth ventricle; *Cc*, beginning of central canal of spinal cord. (Dexler.)

posed substantially of transverse fibers. The middle part or **truncus** (Truncus corporis callosi) slopes downward and forward and is thinner than the ends. The anterior thickened end, the **genu**, bends downward and backward and thins out to form the **rostrum**; the latter is continuous with the lamina terminalis. The posterior end, the **splenium**, also thick, lies at a considerably higher level than the genu. The **upper surface** is convex in its length, concave transversely. Its central part forms the floor of the longitudinal fissure. It is covered by a thin layer of gray matter (Induseum griseum), in which are strands of longitudinal fibers (Striæ longitudinales); the latter are arranged in median and lateral bundles (Stria medialis, striæ laterales).[1] The **lower surface** has the reverse configuration, and forms the roof of the lateral ventricles. Along the median line the septum pellucidum is attached to it. The fibers of the corpus callosum (with the exception of the longitudinal striæ) run transversely and spread out laterally in all directions in the central white matter of the hemispheres to the cortex, forming the **radiation of the corpus callosum** (Radiatio corporis callosi).

[1] It is generally believed that these constitute an olfactory path.

The **fornix** is a bilateral structure composed of white fibers which arch chiefly over the thalamus and the third ventricle. It is described as consisting of a body and two pairs of pillars. The body (Corpus fornicis) is formed by the fusion of the two arches of which the fornix is composed. It is triangular and overlies the anterior parts of the thalami and the third ventricle. The upper surface gives attachment to the septum pellucidum and on either side forms part of the floor of the lateral ventricle. The lateral border is related to the chorioid plexus of the lateral ventricle and forms the inner boundary of the interventricular foramen. The **anterior pillars** or **columns** (Columnæ fornicis) (Fig. 512) are two slender round bundles which emerge from the body in front of the interventricular foramen

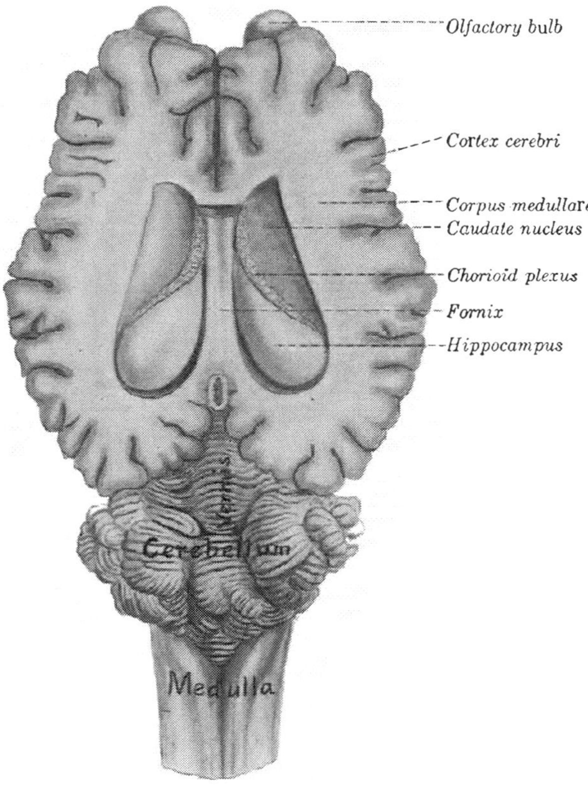

Fig. 511.—Brain of Horse, with Lateral Ventricles Opened by Removal of Upper Part of Cerebral Hemispheres.

and diverge slightly as they curve downward and backward to the mammillary body.

From the mammillary body the greater part of these fornix fibers are continued to the thalamus by the thalamo-mammillary fasciculus (or bundle of Vicq d'Azyr). Others pass to e cerebral peduncle. A portion of the fibers cross to the opposite thalamus and cerebral peduncle.

The **posterior pillars** (Crura fornicis) are much larger bands which diverge widely from the posterior angles of the body. Each curves outward and backward over the thalamus (from which it is separated by the tela chorioidea) and is chiefly continued as the **fimbria** along the concave border of the hippocampus. The pillars give off fibers to form the alveus or white matter which covers the ventricular face of the hippocampi, and between them are transverse fibers which constitute the hippocampal commissure.

The **septum pellucidum** is the median partition between the two lateral ventricles. Its convex upper border blends with the corpus callosum and its concave lower border joins the fornix. Its anterior part is received into the genu of the corpus callosum. Traced backward it diminishes in height and the two edges meet at an acute angle at the splenium.

The septum consists of two layers (Laminæ septi pellucidi) which are in direct contact with each other. They consist of nerve-fibers and gray matter. The latter exists in considerable amount in the thicker part of the septum adjacent to the anterior pillars of the fornix. Many of the fibers of the septum pass up through the corpus callosum to the gyrus fornicatus. Others are connected with the subcallosal gyrus and the parolfactory area.

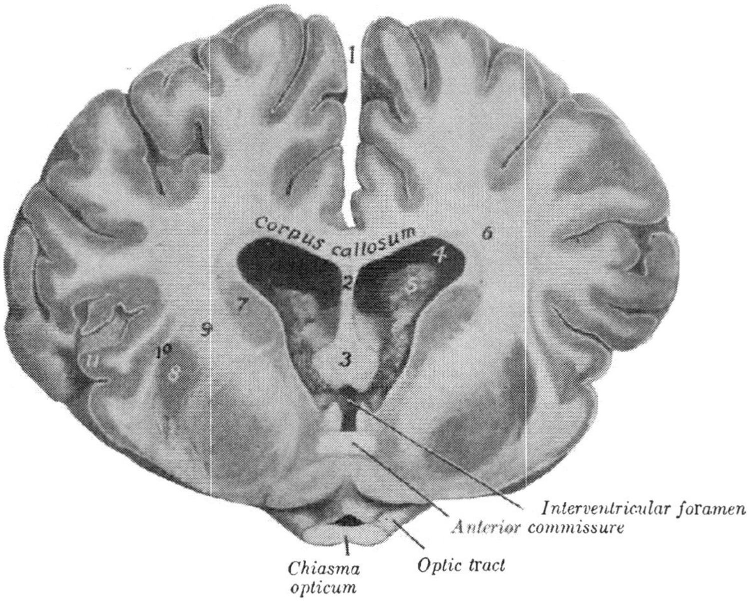

FIG. 512.—CROSS-SECTION OF BRAIN OF HORSE, ABOUT NATURAL SIZE.

Section passes through chiasma opticum, and is viewed from in front. *1*, Longitudinal fissure; *2*, septum pellucidum; *3*, columns (anterior pillars) of fornix; *4*, lateral ventricle; *5*, chorioid plexus; *6*, corpus medullare (central white matter) of hemisphere; *7*, caudate nucleus; *8*, lenticular nucleus; *9*, internal capsule; *10*, external capsule; *11*, insula.

The **lateral ventricle** (Ventriculus lateralis) is the irregular cavity in the interior of each cerebral hemisphere.[1] Each communicates with the third ventricle through the **interventricular foramen** (of Monro), and by a small canal with the cavity of the olfactory bulb. It is usual to describe the ventricle as consisting of three parts, viz., the central part or body, and anterior and inferior horns. The **anterior horn** (Cornu nasale) is the part in front of the interventricular foramen; it communicates ventrally with the olfactory cavity. The **central part** (Pars centralis) extends back to the splenium of the corpus callosum. It opens into the third ventricle through the interventricular foramen, which is situated between the fornix and the anterior part of the thalamus. The **inferior horn** (Cornu ventrale)

[1] It is hardly possible to get an accurate idea of the shape of the ventricle except by studying a cast of it. The size of the ventricles varies in different subjects, and it is not rare to find more or less disparity between the two ventricles of the same brain.

curves downward and forward into the pyriform lobe. The roof of the ventricle is formed by the corpus callosum and the inner wall is the septum pellucidum. After removal of the roof the floor is seen to be formed chiefly by two bodies. The anterior one is the caudate nucleus (Nucleus caudatus), a somewhat pear-shaped gray eminence, the long axis of which is directed obliquely upward, backward, and outward. Its anterior large end is termed the head, and the posterior long tapering end the tail. The posterior body, the **hippocampus,** is white on its ventricular surface, which is strongly convex. It curves outward and backward and then turns downward and forward to join the pyriform lobe. The two bodies are separated by an oblique groove which is occupied by the **chorioid plexus** of the lateral ventricle. This is the thickened edge of a fold of pia mater, the tela chorioidea (or velum interpositum), which lies between the hippocampus and the thalamus. It contains convolutions of small blood-vessels and in old subjects there may be calcareous concretions in it. The plexuses of the two sides are continuous through the interventricular foramen. On drawing the chorioid plexus backward a narrow

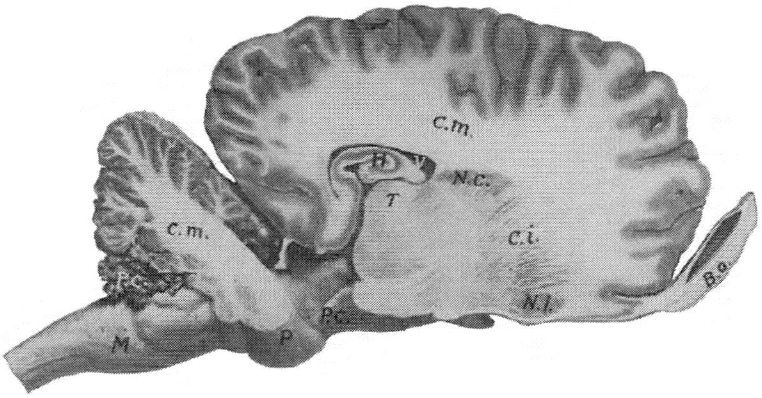

FIG. 513.—SAGITTAL SECTION OF BRAIN OF HORSE.

Section is cut about 1.5 cm. to the right of the median plane. *M*, Medulla oblongata; *P*, pons; *P.c.* (above *M*), chorioid plexus of fourth ventricle; *C.m.*, central white matter (corpus medullare) of cerebellum and of cerebrum; *P.c.* (in front of *P*), cerebral peduncle; *H*, hippocampus; *V*, lateral ventricle; *T*, thalamus; *N.c.*, caudate nucleus; *C.i.*, internal capsule; *N.l.*, lenticular nucleus; *B.o.*, olfactory bulb.

white band, the **stria terminalis** (or tænia semicircularis), is seen along the margin of the caudate nucleus, where it bounds the intermediate groove. The plexus partially covers a wider white band which is blended with the white substance of the hippocampus; this is the **posterior pillar of the fornix** and its continuation, the **fimbria.**

The **corpus striatum**[1] is the great basal ganglion of the hemisphere. It is situated in front of the thalamus and the cerebral peduncle, and its anterior rounded end appears on the base of the hemisphere at the trigonum olfactorium. It is composed of two masses of gray matter, the caudate and lenticular nuclei, separated incompletely by tracts of white matter which are known collectively as the internal capsule. The **caudate nucleus** (Nucleus caudatus) is the dorso-medial and larger of the two gray masses; it has been seen in the examination of the floor of the lateral ventricle. The **lenticular nucleus** (Nucleus lentiformis) lies ventro-laterally, over the trigonum olfactorium and the fossa transversa. It is related externally to a layer of white matter termed the **external capsule,** which separates it from a stratum of gray substance known as the **claustrum.** The two nuclei are fused in front, and

[1] The term arose from the striated appearance of the mass in sections cut in certain planes, the gray matter being cut up into strands by tracts of white fibers.

further back they are connected by strands of gray matter which intersect the internal capsule.

The amygdaloid nucleus (Nucleus amygdalæ) (Fig. 506) is an ovoid mass of gray matter situated external to the ventral horn of the lateral ventricle and below the posterior part of the lenticular nucleus. Some fibers of the stria terminalis are connected with it.

The internal capsule (Capsula interna) is a broad band of white matter situated between the thalamus and caudate nucleus internally and the lenticular nucleus externally. A sagittal section through the brain shows that it is in great part directly continuous with the basis or ventral part of the cerebral peduncle. It contains most of the so-called projection fibers of the hemisphere, which connect the cerebral cortex with nuclei of other and more posterior parts of the brain. When the fibers of the internal capsule are traced forward it is evident that they spread out in all directions to reach the cerebral cortex. This arrangement, in which the fibers of the corpus callosum participate, is termed the corona radiata.

The internal capsule also contains fibers which connect the corpus striatum with the thalamus. These are termed the thalamo-striate and strio-thalamic fibers respectively, according to the direction in which they conduct impulses.

The fibers of the stria terminalis connect the amygdaloid nucleus with the septum pellucidum and trigonum olfactorium. It is therefore probably part of the complex connections between the primary and secondary olfactory centers.

THE CRANIAL NERVES

The cranial or cerebral nerves (Nn. cerebrales) comprise twelve pairs which are designated from before backward numerically and by name. Their number, names, and functional characters are given in the subjoined table:

I.	Olfactory	Sensory (Smell)
II.	Optic	Sensory (Sight)
III.	Oculomotor	Motor
IV.	Trochlear	Motor
V.	Trigeminal	Mixed
VI.	Abducent	Motor
VII.	Facial	Mixed
VIII.	Auditory	Sensory (Hearing and Equilibration)
IX.	Glosso-pharyngeal	Mixed
X.	Vagus or Pneumogastric	Mixed
XI.	Spinal accessory	Motor
XII.	Hypoglossal	Motor

THE FIRST OR OLFACTORY NERVE

The olfactory nerve (N. olfactorius) is peculiar in that its fibers are not aggregated to form a trunk, but are connected in small bundles with the olfactory bulb. They are non-medullated, and are the central processes of the olfactory cells which are situated in the olfactory region of the mucous membrane of the nasal cavity. This region is distinguished by its brown color and comprises most of the lateral mass of the ethmoid, a small adjacent area of the superior turbinal, and the corresponding surface of the septum nasi. The nerve-bundles are inclosed in sheaths derived from the membranes of the brain and pass through the foramina of the cribriform plate to join the convex surface of the olfactory bulb. Some fibers come from the vomero-nasal organ of Jacobson.

THE SECOND OR OPTIC NERVE

The optic nerve (N. opticus) is composed of fibers which are the central processes of the ganglion cells of the retina. The fibers converge within the eyeball to the optic papilla, where they are collected into a round trunk, the optic nerve. The nerve thus formed pierces the chorioid and sclera, emerges from the posterior part of the eyeball, and passes backward and inward to the optic foramen. After traversing the latter it decussates with its fellow of the opposite side to form the optic chiasma or commissure. In the orbit the nerve is slightly flexuous and is embedded in the fat behind the eyeball and surrounded by the retractor oculi muscle. Its intraosseous part is an inch or more (ca. 3 cm.) long. The sheath of the nerve is formed by prolongations of the membranes of the brain, and includes continuations of the subdural and subarachnoid spaces.

The greater part of the fibers of the optic nerve cross in the chiasma to the tract of the opposite side. In the tract the fibers proceed to (1) the internal geniculate body, (2) the posterior part of the thalamus, and (3) the anterior quadrigeminal body (indirectly). The fibers which go to the internal geniculate body appear to belong to Gudden's commissure and to be non-visual in function. The visual fibers, which come from the outer part of the retina of the same side and the inner part of the retina of the opposite side, terminate about cells in the anterior quadrigeminal body and the part of the thalamus which corresponds to the pulvinar and external geniculate body of man. From the cells of the former fibers pass to the nuclei of the motor nerves of the eyeball, and complete the reflex arc. Fibers proceed from the cells of the thalamus to the visual area of the cortex in the occipital part of the hemisphere.

THE THIRD OR OCULOMOTOR NERVE

The oculomotor nerve (N. oculomotorius) arises by several radicles from the basal surface of the cerebral peduncle, a little lateral to the interpeduncular furrow. It turns sharply outward and forward, crosses over the cavernous sinus, and continnes above the maxillary nerve and in company with the ophthalmic nerve to the foramen lacerum orbitale. It emerges through the foramen with the latter nerve and the abducens and divides into two branches. The superior branch is short and divides into twigs which supply the rectus superior, retractor, and levator palpebræ superioris. The inferior branch (Figs. 438, 439) is larger and much longer. It supplies the motor fibers to the ciliary ganglion (which lies directly on this branch in the horse) and short branches to the rectus internus and rectus inferior, and continues forward on the latter to end in the inferior oblique muscle.

The deep origin of the fibers of the oculomotor nerve is in the oculomotor nucleus situated in the gray matter of the floor of the cerebral aqueduct in the region of the anterior corpora quadrigemina.

THE FOURTH OR TROCHLEAR NERVE

The trochlear or pathetic (N. trochlearis) is the smallest of the cranial nerves. It arises from the anterior cerebellar peduncle just behind the corpora quadrigemina, curves outward and forward, pierces the tentorium cerebelli, and passes forward along the outer border of the maxillary nerve (Figs. 504, 505). It emerges from the cranium through a small foramen immediately above the foramen lacerum orbitale or through the latter and passes forward along the inner wall of the orbit to end in the posterior part of the superior oblique muscle of the eyeball (Fig. 439).

The fibers of the fourth nerve spring from a nucleus in the gray matter of the floor of the cerebral aqueduct behind the oculomotor nucleus. The fibers run backward in the tegmentum, then turn upward and inward and undergo total decussation with those of the opposite nerve in the anterior part of the anterior medullary velum. In addition to this peculiarity it is the only nerve which is connected with the dorsal aspect of the brain.

THE FIFTH, TRIGEMINAL, OR TRIFACIAL NERVE

The trigeminal nerve (N. trigeminus) is the largest of the cranial series. It is connected with the lateral part of the pons by a large sensory root and a smaller motor root (Fig. 499).

The sensory root (Portio major) extends forward through a notch on the lower part of the petrosal crest and widens out to join the semilunar ganglion.

The **semilunar** (or Gasserian) **ganglion** (Ganglion semilunare) is a crescent-shaped mass of nerve-fibers and cells which overlies the antero-external part of the foramen lacerum basis cranii, and is partly embedded in the dense fibrous tissue which occupies the foramen except where vessels and nerves pass through. Its long axis, which is about an inch (2.5 cm.) in length, is directed forward and inward and its convex anterior face gives rise to the ophthalmic, the maxillary, and the sensory part of the mandibular division of the nerve. The surface of the ganglion is irregularly striated. It is connected by filaments with the adjacent carotid plexus of the sympathetic, and sends delicate twigs to the dura mater.

The fibers of the sensory root arise from the ganglion as axones of the ganglion cells, and the fibers of the nerves which extend peripherally from the ganglion are dendrites of the cells. The sensory root-fibers enter the tegmentum of the pons and divide into anterior and posterior branches, which terminate about the cells of the sensory nucleus of termination of the trigeminus. This nucleus extends from the pons to the sixth cervical segment of the spinal cord (Dexler). The posterior branches of the fibers are collected into a compact bundle, the spinal tract or root of the trigeminus, which lies lateral to the substantia gelatinosa in the medulla. The central connections of the sensory part of the trigeminus are very extensive. The most important paths are: (1) Axones of cells of the sensory nucleus and the substantia gelatinosa pass chiefly as arcuate fibers across the raphe to the thalamus, whence impulses are transmitted by thalamo-cortical fibers to the cerebral cortex. In ungulates a distinct tract extends from the anterior part of the sensory nucleus to the thalamus of the same side (Wallenberg). It is probable that collaterals of the arcuate fibers go to the motor nuclei of the fifth, seventh, ninth, and tenth cranial nerves. (2) Axones of cells of the sensory nucleus enter the posterior cerebellar peduncle of the same side and reach the cerebellar cortex. (3) Collaterals are distributed to the nuclei of origin of the hypoglossal and of the motor part of the trigeminal and facial nerves.

The motor root (Portio minor) extends forward beneath the sensory root and the semilunar ganglion and is incorporated with the mandibular division of the nerve. Its fibers arise chiefly from the so-called masticatory nucleus, which is situated in the pons near the inner face of the sensory nucleus; a few of these fibers come from the nucleus of the opposite side and cross in the raphe. Other fibers, which constitute the mesencephalic root, arise from cells in the outer part of the central gray matter of the mid-brain.

It is evident from the foregoing statements that the trigeminus has essentially the same arrangement as a typical spinal nerve. It divides into three branches.

I. The ophthalmic nerve (N. ophthalmicus) (Figs. 438, 439, 440) is purely sensory and is the smallest of the three branches of the trigeminus. It arises from the inner part of the front of the semilunar ganglion, passes forward along the outer side of the cavernous sinus, and is blended with the maxillary nerve for some distance. It enters the foramen lacerum orbitale with the third and sixth nerves and divides into three branches.

1. The lacrimal nerve (N. lacrimalis) runs forward on the rectus superior and the levator palpebræ superioris and ramifies chiefly in the lacrimal gland and the upper eyelid. A branch (Ramus zygomatico-temporalis) exchanges twigs with the zygomatic branch of the maxillary nerve, perforates the periorbita, and emerges from the orbital fossa behind the supraorbital process; it forms a plexus with branches of the auriculo-palpebral and frontal nerves, and ramifies in the skin of the temporal region.

2. The frontal nerve (N. frontalis), also termed the supraorbital, runs forward almost parallel with the superior oblique muscle, at first within, then outside of, the periorbita. It passes through the supraorbital foramen with the artery of like name and ramifies in the skin of the forehead and upper eyelid, forming a plexus with the lacrimal and auriculo-palpebral nerves. It divides into three branches.

3. The naso-ciliary nerve (N. naso-ciliaris), also termed the palpebro-nasal, runs forward along the inner side of the optic nerve between parts of the retractor muscle and divides into two branches. Of these the ethmoidal nerve (N. ethmoi-

dalis) is the continuation of the parent trunk. It accompanies the ethmoidal artery through the foramen of like name into the cranial cavity and crosses the lower part of the ethmoidal fossa. Leaving the cranium through an opening in the cribriform plate close to the crista galli, it enters the nasal cavity and ramifies in the mucous membrane of the septum nasi and the superior turbinal. The **infratrochlear** nerve (N. infratrochlearis) runs forward to the inner canthus and ramifies in the skin in this region; it detaches twigs to the conjunctiva and caruncula lacrimalis, and a long branch which supplies the third eyelid and the lacrimal ducts and sac. The naso-ciliary nerve furnishes the sensory or long root (Radix longa) of the ciliary ganglion.

The ciliary ganglion is placed on the inferior branch of the oculomotor nerve. It is usually not larger than a millet-seed, and is best found by following the nerve to the inferior oblique muscle back to its origin. The ganglion receives (*a*) sensory fibers from the naso-ciliary nerve; (*b*) motor fibers from the oculomotor nerve; and (c) sympathetic fibers from the sphenopalatine plexus. It detaches filaments which unite with twigs from the ophthalmic and maxillary nerves and from the sphenopalatine ganglion to form the ciliary plexus. From the latter emanate five to eight delicate short ciliary nerves (Nn. ciliares breves), which pursue a somewhat flexuous course along the optic nerve, pierce the sclera near the entrance of that nerve, and run forward between the sclera and chorioidea to the circumference of the iris. Here the branches of adjacent nerves anastomose to form a circular plexus (Plexus gangliosus ciliaris), from which filaments go to the ciliary body, iris, and cornea.

The circular fibers of the iris and the ciliary muscle are innervated by fibers derived from the oculomotor nerve, the radial fibers of the iris by the sympathetic.

II. The maxillary nerve (N. maxillaris), also termed the superior maxillary, is purely sensory and is much larger than the ophthalmic. It extends forward from the semilunar ganglion in the middle cranial fossa in the large groove on the root of the temporal wing of the sphenoid. It is related internally to the cavernous sinus and superiorly to the ophthalmic nerve, with which it is blended for some distance. It emerges through the foramen rotundum, passes forward in the pterygo-palatine fossa above the internal maxillary artery and embedded in fat, and is continued in the infraorbital canal as the infraorbital nerve (Fig. 439). Its branches are as follows:

1. The zygomatic nerve (N. zygomaticus s. subcutaneus malæ), also termed the orbital branch, arises before the maxillary nerve reaches the pterygo-palatine fossa (Figs. 438, 439, 514). It pierces the periorbita and divides into two or three delicate branches which pass along the surface of the external straight muscle to the external canthus and ramify chiefly in the lower lid and the adjacent skin. Anastomoses are formed with branches of the lacrimal nerve.

2. The sphenopalatine nerve (N. sphenopalatinus) is given off in the pterygopalatine fossa from the lower border of the maxillary nerve (Fig. 439). It is broad and flat and forms a plexus in which several small sphenopalatine ganglia are interposed. It divides into posterior nasal, and greater and lesser palatine nerves. (1) The posterior nasal nerve (N. nasalis aboralis) passes through the sphenopalatine foramen, in which it bears one or more minute ganglia, enters the nasal cavity, and divides into internal and external branches (Figs. 440, 464). The internal branch (N. septi narium) runs forward in the submucous tissue of the lower part of the septum nasi, gives twigs to the mucous membrane here and to the vomero-nasal organ (of Jacobson), passes through the palatine cleft and ramifies in the anterior part of the hard palate. The external branch (Ramus lateralis) ramifies in the mucous membrane of the inferior turbinal and the middle and inferior meatus nasi. (2) The greater or anterior palatine nerve (N. palatinus major s. anterior) (Figs.

438, 439) is the largest of the three branches. It runs forward in the palatine canal and groove and ramifies in the hard palate and gums. It also supplies twigs to the soft palate, and gives off branches which pass through the accessory palatine foramina to supply the mucous membrane of the inferior meatus.

The branches of the two nerves anastomose in the hard palate and form a plexus about the branches of the palatine arteries.

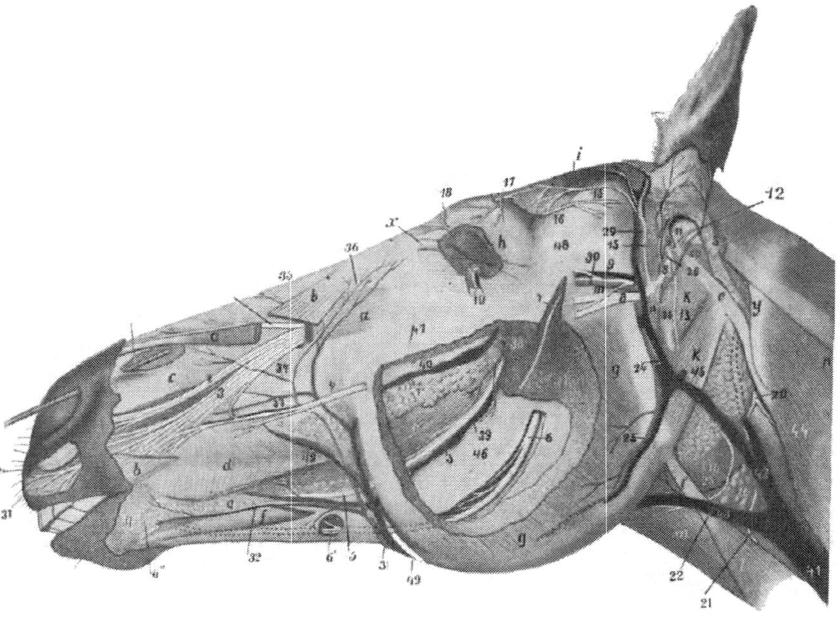

FIG. 514.—DISSECTION OF HEAD OF HORSE.

The masseter and superficial muscles and the parotid gland are in great part removed. *a, a*, Levator labii superioris proprius; *b, b*, levator nasolabialis; *c*, dilatator naris inferior; *d*, buccinator; *e*, common mass of buccinator and depressor labii inferioris; *f*, depressor labii inferioris; *g*, masseter; *h*, orbicularis oculi; *i*, temporalis; *k*, occipito-hyoideus; *k'*, stylo-maxillaris; *l*, sterno-cephalicus; *l'*, tendon of same; *m*, omo-hyoideus; *n*, crico-pharyngeus; *o*, mastoid tendon of mastoido-humeralis; *p*, splenius; *q*, inferior buccal and labial glands; *r*, superior buccal glands; *s*, remnant of parotid gland; *t*, submaxillary gland; *u*, anterior cervical (subparotid) lymph glands; *v*, probe passed into diverticulum nasi; *w*, cornu of alar cartilage; *x*, internal palpebral ligament; *y*, wing of atlas; *z*, scutiform cartilage of ear; *1*, external nasal nerve; *2*, anterior nasal nerve; *3*, superior labial nerve; *4*, anterior part of superior buccal nerve; *5*, buccinator nerve; *6, 6'*, inferior alveolar nerve; *6''*, mental nerve-continuation of *6*; *7*, masseteric nerve; *8*, facial nerve (cut); *9*, superficial temporal nerve; *10*, anastomosis between *9* and *8*; *11*, internal auricular nerve; *12*, posterior auricular nerve; *13*, digastric nerve; *14*, cervical branch of facial nerve (cut); *15*, auriculo-palpebral nerve; *16*, lacrimal nerve; *17*, frontal nerve; *18*, infratrochlear nerve; *19*, n. zygomaticus s. subcutaneus malæ; *20*, spinal accessory nerve; *21*, ventral branch of spinal accessory nerve (to sterno-cephalicus); *22*, ventral end branch of first cervical nerve; *23*, thyro-laryngeal artery; *24*, internal maxillary artery; *25*, masseteric artery; *26*, great (posterior) auricular artery; *27*, external branch of *26*; *28*, deep auricular artery; *29*, superficial temporal artery; *30*, transverse facial artery; *31*, facial artery; *32*, inferior labial artery; *33*, superior labial artery; *34*, lateral nasal artery; *35*, dorsal nasal artery; *36*, angular artery of eye; *37*, labial twigs of palato-labial artery—left uncolored by oversight; *38*, branch of buccinator artery; *39*, buccinator vein; *40*, vena reflexa; *41, 42*, jugular vein; *43*, external maxillary vein; *44*, inferior cerebral vein; *45*, stump of great auricular vein; *46*, ramus of mandible; *47*, facial crest; *48*, zygomatic arch; *49*, parotid duct. (After Ellenberger-Baum, Top. Anat. d. Pferdes.)

(3) The lesser or posterior palatine nerve (N. palatinus minor s. posterior), also termed the staphyline, is much the smallest of the three branches (Figs. 438, 439). It passes downward and forward with the palatine vein in the groove at the inner side of the tuber maxillare and ramifies in the soft palate.

The sphenopalatine ganglia and plexus (Fig. 515) lie on the perpendicular part of the palate bone and the pterygoid process under cover of the maxillary nerve. The afferent fibers of the plexus and ganglia come chiefly from the branches of the sphenopalatine nerve and the nerve of the pterygoid canal. Interspersed in these are several minute ganglia and one or more larger ones. The **nerve of the pterygoid canal** or **Vidian nerve** (N. canalis pterygoidei) is formed by the union of sympathetic fibers with the superficial petrosal branch of the facial nerve. It passes forward at first between the Eustachian tube and the sphenoid bone, enters the canal between the pterygoid bone and process, and joins the posterior part of the plexus. It is probable that it furnishes the motor fibers to the levator palati and palatinus muscles. Efferent filaments go to the periorbita and the ophthalmic vessels, and others accompany the branches of the maxillary nerve, around which they have a plexiform arrangement.

3. The **infraorbital nerve** (N. infraorbitalis) is the continuation of the maxillary trunk. It traverses the infraorbital canal, emerges through the infraorbital foramen, and divides into nasal and superior labial branches. Along its course it gives off **superior alveolar** or **dental** branches (Rami alveolares maxillæ), which supply the teeth, alveolar periosteum, and gums.

The delicate posterior alveolar branches are given off in the pterygo-palatine fossa, pass through small foramina in the tuber maxillare, and supply the posterior molar teeth and the maxillary sinus. The middle alveolar branches are given off in the infraorbital canal, and constitute the chief nerve-supply to the cheek teeth and the maxillary sinus. The anterior or incisor branch runs forward in the anterior alveolar or incisor canal and supplies branches to the canine and incisor teeth. The foregoing unite with each other to form the superior dental plexus, from which the dental and gingival branches are given off.

The **external nasal branches** (Rami nasales externi), two or three in number, accompany the levator labii superioris proprius and ramify in the dorsum nasi and the nasal diverticulum.

The large **anterior nasal branch** (Ramus nasalis anterior) passes over the nasal process of the premaxilla under cover of the dilatator naris inferior, gives branches to the nasal mucous membrane, and terminates in the skin of the upper lip.

The **superior labial branch** (Ramus labialis dorsalis) is the largest of the terminals of the infraorbital nerve. It passes downward and forward under the levator nasolabialis and, after supplying the skin of the anterior part of the cheek, forms a rich terminal ramification in the skin and mucous membrane of the upper lip. It anastomoses with the superior buccal branch of the facial nerve.

III. The **mandibular nerve** (N. mandibularis), also termed the inferior maxillary branch, is formed by the union of two roots; of these the large sensory root comes from the semilunar ganglion, and the small motor root is the pars minor of the trigeminus. It emerges from the cranium through the oval notch of the foramen lacerum, between the temporal wing of the sphenoid bone and the muscular process of the petrous temporal, and gives off the following branches:

1. The **masseteric nerve** (N. massetericus) (Figs. 437, 515) passes outward through the sigmoid notch of the mandible and enters the deep face of the masseter muscle, in which it ramifies.

2. The **deep temporal nerves** (Nn. temporales profundi) (Fig. 437), two or three in number, arise by a common trunk with the masseteric. They supply the temporal muscle.

3. The **buccinator nerve** (N. buccinatorius) passes obliquely forward through the anterior part of the external pterygoid muscle, then between the internal pterygoid and the tuber maxillare (Fig. 514). It continues forward in the submucous tissue of the cheek along the lower border of the buccinator and divides into branches which ramify in the mucous membrane and glands of the lips in the vicinity of the commissure. It supplies small branches to the external pterygoid and temporal muscles and detaches numerous collateral twigs to the mucous membrane of the cheek and to the buccal glands. It also communicates with the inferior buccal branch of the facial nerve.

4. The **pterygoid nerve** (N. pterygoideus) arises in common with the preceding, passes forward on the guttural pouch, and divides into branches for the pterygoid muscles (Fig. 515).

The **otic ganglion** (G. oticum) is situated near the origin of the pterygoid and buccinator nerves, and is related internally to the tensor palati and the Eustachian tube. It receives motor fibers from the pterygoid nerve and sensory fibers by the small superficial petrosal nerve from the tympanic plexus, through which communications are made with the facial and glosso-pharyngeal nerves. Sympathetic fibers are derived from the plexus on the internal maxillary artery. Efferent filaments go to the tensor palati, tensor tympani, and pterygoid muscles, and to the Eustachian tube.

The ganglion is small and somewhat difficult to demonstrate. In many cases it is replaced by a number of minute ganglia interspersed in a fine plexus.

5. The superficial temporal nerve (N. temporalis superficialis) (Figs. 437, 514, 515) runs outward across the pterygoideus externus, passes between the parotid gland and the neck of the ramus of the mandible, turns around the latter, and di vides into two branches. The upper branch (Ramus transversus faciei) accom-

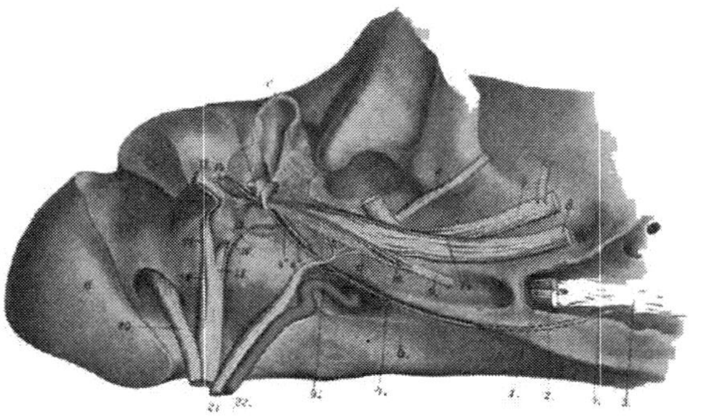

FIG. 515.—DEEP DISSECTION OF BASE OF CRANIUM, VIEWED FROM THE RIGHT AND BELOW.

The tympanic cavity is opened and the paramastoid process is sawn off. *a*, Occipital condyle; *b*, body of sphenoid; c, external auditory meatus (part removed); d, malleus; *e*, incus; *1*, stump of ophthalmic nerve; *2*, maxillary nerve (cut off); *3*, sphenopalatine plexus; *4*, Vidian nerve; *4*, deep petrosal nerve; *4″*, branch to tympanic plexus; *4‴*, superficial petrosal nerve; *5*, superficial temporal nerve (cut off); *6*, masseteric nerve (cut off); *7*, mandibular nerve (raised); *8*, lingual nerve (cut off); *9*, pterygoid nerve (cut); *10*, nerve to tensor tympani; *11*, otic ganglion; *12*, facial nerve; *13*, stapedial nerve; *14*, chorda tympani; *15*, glosso-pharyngeal nerve (cut); *16*, tympanic nerve; *17*, vagus (cut off); *18*, auricular branch of vagus; *19*, spinal accessory nerve (cut off); *20*, hypoglossal nerve (cut off); *21*, sympathetic nerve (cut off); *22*, internal carotid artery. (After Ellenberger, in Leisering's Atlas.)

panies the transverse facial vessels and ramifies in the skin of the cheek. The larger inferior branch unites with the inferior buccal division of the facial nerve.

Before its division the nerve gives off twigs to the guttural pouch, the parotid gland, the external ear, and the skin of the external auditory meatus and the membrana tympani. Branches from it concur with filaments from the cervical branch of the facial nerve in the formation of the auricular plexus.

6. The inferior alveolar or dental nerve (N. alveolaris mandibulæ) (Figs. 436, 437, 514) arises with the lingual by a common trunk which passes forward at first on the external pterygoid muscle, then inclines ventrally between the internal pterygoid and the ramus of the mandible. The lingual and alveolar separate at an acute angle, and the latter enters the mandibular foramen and courses in the canal within the ramus (Fig. 516). Emerging at the mental foramen, it terminates by dividing into six to eight inferior labial and mental branches, which ramify in the lower lip and chin. Before entering the bone, the nerve detaches the mylo-hyoid nerve (N. mylohyoideus), which runs downward and forward between the ramus and the mylo-hyoid muscle; it supplies that muscle, the anterior belly of the digastricus, and the skin of the anterior part of the submaxillary space. The dental

and gingival branches detached from the nerve within the mandible are arranged like the corresponding nerves of the upper jaw.

7. The **lingual** nerve (N. lingualis) arises by a common trunk with the inferior alveolar or dental nerve (Figs. 436, 437). After separating from the latter it runs downward and forward, lying at first between the ramus of the mandible and the internal pterygoid muscle, then on the inner face of the mylo-hyoid. On reaching the root of the tongue it divides into superficial and deep branches. The **superficial branch** (Ramus superficialis) runs forward on the stylo-glossus and accompanies the submaxillary duct on the deep face of the sublingual gland. It supplies the mucous membrane of the tongue and the floor of the mouth. At the root of the tongue it gives off a recurrent branch to the isthmus faucium, which communicates with the lingual branch of the glosso-pharyngeal nerve. The larger **deep branch** (Ramus profundus) turns around the lower edge of the hyo-glossus, passes upward and forward between that muscle and the genio-glossus, and continues forward on the latter to the tip of the tongue. It gives branches to the mucous membrane and the fungiform papillæ of the tongue, and anastomoses with branches of the hypo-

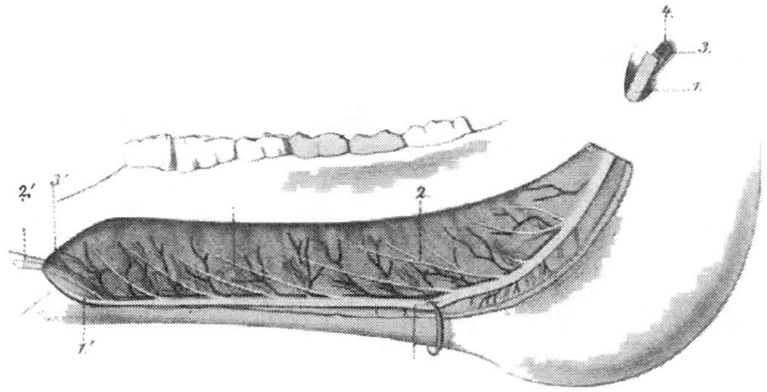

Fig. 516.—Part of Branch of Lower Jaw of Horse, Internal View.

The bone has been removed to show the vessels and nerves. *1, 1'*, inferior alveolar or dental nerve; *2, 2*, branches to cheek teeth and gums; *2'*, branch to canine and incisor teeth; *3, 3'*, inferior alveolar or dental artery; *4*, satellite vein. (After Leisering's Atlas.)

glossal nerve and with the superficial branch. Minute ganglia occur on the finer branches of the lingual nerve. The **chorda tympani** branch of the facial joins the lingual nerve at the origin of the latter and is incorporated with it in its distribution to the tongue.

THE SIXTH OR ABDUCENT NERVE

The **abducent nerve** (N. abducens) emerges from the brain behind the pons and just external to the pyramid (Fig. 499). It passes forward across the pons, pierces the dura mater, and accompanies the third and ophthalmic nerves, below which it emerges through the foramen lacerum orbitale. In the orbit it divides into two branches; the larger of these enters the external rectus, the smaller supplies the superior and external parts of the retractor muscle of the eyeball. Within the cranium it receives filaments from the carotid plexus of the sympathetic.

The fibers of the abducent nerve are axones of the large multipolar cells of the abducent nucleus which is situated beneath the eminentia teres of the floor of the fourth ventricle. The nucleus lies within the loop formed by the fibers of origin of the facial nerve. It is connected with (*a*) the anterior olive; (*b*) the oculomotor nucleus of the opposite side; (*c*) the motor area of the cerebral cortex by means of the pyramidal tract of the opposite side.

THE SEVENTH OR FACIAL NERVE

The facial nerve (N. facialis) has its superficial origin at the lateral part of the corpus trapezoideum, immediately behind the pons (Fig. 499). It passes outward in front of the eighth nerve and enters the internal auditory meatus. At the bottom of the meatus the two nerves part company, the facial coursing in the facial canal of the petrous temporal bone. The canal and nerve are at first directed outward between the vestibule and the cochlea, then curve backward and downward in the posterior wall of the tympanum to end at the stylo-mastoid foramen. The bend formed by the nerve is called the **knee** (Geniculum n. facialis) and bears at its highest point the round **geniculate ganglion** (G. geniculi).

The nerve consists of two parts, motor and sensory. The **motor part** constitutes the bulk of the nerve. Its deep origin is from the cells of the **facial nucleus,** which is situated in the medulla above the facial tubercle. On leaving the nucleus the root-fibers pass upward and inward, incline forward close to the median plane, and then bend sharply downward to the point of emergence. The highest point of the bend is subjacent to the gray matter of the eminentia teres in the floor of the fourth ventricle, and the abducent nucleus lies in the concavity of the curve. The small **sensory part** (N. intermedius) consists of axones of cells of the geniculate ganglion, which is interposed on the facial nerve as it bends downward in the facial canal. The fibers of this part after entering the medulla, pass to the nucleus of termination which it shares with the ninth and tenth nerves. The peripheral fibers from the geniculate ganglion constitute the chorda tympani.

After its emergence through the stylo-mastoid foramen (Fig. 514) the nerve passes downward, forward, and outward on the guttural pouch under cover of the parotid gland, and crosses between the origin of the superficial temporal and internal maxillary arteries internally and the superficial temporal vein externally. It then crosses the posterior border of the ramus of the mandible ventral to the transverse facial artery and about an inch and a half (ca. 3.5 to 4 cm.) below the articulation of the jaw. Emerging from beneath the parotid gland upon the masseter muscle, it receives the lower branch of the superficial temporal nerve, and divides into superior and inferior buccal branches. The following collateral branches are given off, the first five being detached within the facial canal, and the others between the stylo-mastoid foramen and the border of the jaw.

1. The **great superficial petrosal nerve** (N. petrosus superficialis major) arises from the geniculate ganglion.[1] It passes through the petrosal canal, contributes a filament to the tympanic plexus, receives the great deep petrosal nerve from the carotid plexus of the sympathetic, emerges through the foramen lacerum, and is continued as the Vidian nerve to the sphenopalatine plexus and ganglia (Fig. 515).

2. A delicate branch (R. anastomoticus cum plexu tympanico) emerges from the geniculate ganglion and unites with a filament issuing from the tympanic plexus to form the **small superficial petrosal nerve** (N. petrosus superficialis minor); this ends in the otic ganglion.

3. The **stapedial** nerve (N. stapedius) (Fig. 515) is a short filament detached from the facial nerve as it turns down in the facial canal. It innervates the stapedins muscle.

4. The **chorda tympani** (Fig. 515) is a small nerve which arises a little below the preceding and pursues a recurrent course in a small canal in the mastoid part of the temporal bone to reach the tympanic cavity. It traverses the latter, passing between the handle of the malleus and the long branch of the incus. Emerging through the petrotympanic fissure, the nerve passes downward and forward, crosses beneath the internal maxillary artery, and joins the lingual nerve. It sends twigs to the submaxillary and sublingual glands, and through its incorporation with the lingual nerve furnishes fibers to the mucous membrane of the anterior two-thirds of the tongue which are believed to mediate the sense of taste.

[1] Although this nerve springs directly from the ganglion, it contains motor as well as sensory fibers.

5. Anastomotic filaments unite with the auricular branch of the vagus near the stylomastoid foramen.

6. The **posterior auricular nerve** (N. auricularis posterior) arises from the facial at its emergence from the facial canal (Fig. 514). It runs upward and backward with the posterior auricular artery under cover of the parotid gland and supplies the posterior auricular muscles and the skin of the convex surface of the external ear. It anastomoses with branches of the first and second cervical nerves.

7. The **internal auricular nerve** (N. auricularis internus) springs from the facial close to or in common with the preceding (Fig. 514). It ascends in the parotid gland just behind the styloid process of the conchal cartilage, passes through an opening in the cartilage, and ramifies in the skin of the concave surface of the ear.

8. The **digastric branch** (R. digastricus) (Fig. 514) arises from the facial below the auricular nerves. Its branches innervate the posterior belly of the digastricus, the stylo-hyoideus, and the occipito-hyoideus. At its origin it gives off a small branch which forms a loop around the great auricular artery or its posterior branch and rejoins the trunk.

9. The **auriculo-palpebral nerve** (N. auriculo-palpebralis) (Fig. 514) arises from the upper edge of the facial near the posterior border of the ramus. It ascends in the parotid gland behind the superficial temporal artery, and terminates in anterior auricular and temporal branches. The **anterior auricular branches** form with branches of the trigeminus the **anterior auricular plexus**. They innervate the anterior auricular and parotido-auricularis muscles. The **temporal branch** runs forward and inward over the temporal muscle to the inner canthus of the eye, forms a plexus with the terminal branches of the ophthalmic nerve, and is distributed to the orbicularis oculi, corrugator supercilii, and levator nasolabialis.

10. The **cervical branch** (R. colli) (Fig. 435) arises from the ventral border of the facial opposite to the preceding nerve. It emerges obliquely through the parotid gland, passes downward and backward on or near the jugular vein, and anastomoses with the cutaneous branches of the cervical nerves. It gives branches to the parotido-auricularis and the cervical panniculus. In its course along the neck the nerve is reinforced by twigs from the cutaneous branches of the second to the sixth cervical nerves.

11. Small branches are detached to the guttural pouch and the parotid gland. The latter (Rami parotidei) concur with branches of the superficial temporal nerve in forming the **parotid plexus.**

The facial nerve usually terminates after a short course on the surface of the masseter by dividing into two buccal branches (Figs. 435, 461).

1. The **superior buccal nerve** (N. buccalis dorsalis) passes forward on the upper part of the masseter, dips under the zygomaticus, and continues along the lower border of the dilatator naris lateralis. It then runs under the last-named muscle and anastomoses with branches of the infraorbital nerve, and is distributed to the muscles of the cheek, upper lip, and nostril.

2. The **inferior buccal nerve** (N. buccalis ventralis) crosses the masseter obliquely and continues forward along the depressor labii inferioris. It is connected by variable anastomotic branches with the superior nerve. It gives collateral branches to the panniculus, buccinator, and depressor labii inferioris, and ramifies with the terminal branches of the inferior alveolar nerve in the lower lip.

The buccal nerves are subject to much variation in regard to their course, anastomoses, and relations to the sensory components derived from the superficial temporal nerve. Their distribution is constant. The point at which the branch of the superficial temporal nerve joins the facial is variable.

THE EIGHTH OR AUDITORY NERVE

The auditory **nerve** (N. acusticus) is connected with the lateral aspect of the medulla just behind and external to the facial (Fig. 499). It has two roots, vestibular and cochlear (Radix vestibularis et cochlearis)

The auditory nerve consists of two distinct parts which might well be regarded as separate nerves. The cochlear part mediates the sense of hearing, while the vestibular part is not auditory in function, but is concerned in the sense of the position of the body and the mechanism of equilibration.

The nerve passes outward to the internal auditory meatus, which it enters behind the facial nerve. In the meatus it divides into two nerves, of which the upper is the vestibular and the lower is the cochlear nerve.

1. The **vestibular nerve** (N. vestibuli) is distributed to the utriculus, the sacculus, and to the ampullæ of the semicircular canals, of the internal ear. In the internal auditory meatus the nerve is connected by filaments with the geniculate ganglion of the facial nerve. At the bottom of the meatus it bears the **vestibular ganglion** (G. vestibulare), from the cells of which the fibers of the nerve arise.

2. The **cochlear nerve** (N. cochleæ) detaches a filament to the sacculus, passes through the lamina cribrosa to the labyrinth, and is distributed to the organ of Corti in the cochlea.

The fibers of the vestibular nerve arise from the vestibular ganglion as central processes (axones) of the bipolar cells of the ganglion. The peripheral processes (dendrites) of the cells form arborizations about the deep ends of the hair-cells of the maculæ and cristæ acusticæ of the utriculus, sacculus, and semicircular canals. The fibers enter the medulla, pass between the restiform body and the spinal tract of the trigeminus, and spread out to end in the vestibular nucleus in the floor of the fourth ventricle. Among the central connections of the vestibular nerve are: (1) fibers which connect its nucleus with centers in the cerebellum (chiefly of the opposite side); (2) the vestibulo-spinal tract, which conveys impulses to the motor cells of the ventral columns of the spinal cord; (3) fibers which connect the nucleus with those of the abducent nerve of the same side, the third and fourth nerves, and the motor part of the trigeminus of both sides.

The fibers of the cochlear nerve are the central processes of the bipolar cells of the spiral ganglion of the cochlea. The peripheral processes of these cells end in relation to the hair-cells of the organ of Corti. Some of the nerve-fibers enter the ventral cochlear nucleus in the medulla close to the superficial origin of the nerve; others end in the dorsal nucleus of the tuberculum acusticum at the lateral angle of the floor of the fourth ventricle. From the ventral nucleus fibers pass in the corpus trapezoideum to the anterior olivary nucleus of the same and of the opposite side. Thence tracts pass to the nuclei of the motor nerves of the eye, and through the lateral fillet to the posterior quadrigeminal body and the internal geniculate body. The axones of the cells of the dorsal nucleus pass largely (as the striæ acusticæ) over the restiform body and across the floor of the fourth ventricle toward the median plane. They then turn ventrally, cross to the opposite side, and are continued by the lateral fillet. From the mid-brain a tract proceeds to the cortex of the temporal lobe of the hemisphere.

THE NINTH OR GLOSSO-PHARYNGEAL NERVE

The **glosso-pharyngeal nerve** (N. glossopharyngeus) is attached to the anterior part of the lateral aspect of the medulla by several filaments (Fig. 499). The root-bundles enter the furrow ventral to the restiform body; they are separated by a short interval from the origin of the facial nerve, but are not marked off behind from the roots of the vagus. The bundles converge laterally to form a nerve which perforates the dura mater and emerges through the foramen lacerum posterius just in front of the tenth nerve (Fig. 515). As it issues from the cranium the nerve bears a considerable ovoid gray enlargement, the **petrous ganglion** (G. petrosum).[1] It then curves downward and forward over the guttural pouch and behind the great cornu of the hyoid bone, crosses the deep face of the external carotid artery, and divides into pharyngeal and lingual branches (Fig. 437). The collateral branches are as follows:

1. The **tympanic nerve** (N. tympanicus) (Fig. 515) arises from the petrous

[1] This ganglion appears to be equivalent to the jugular or superior and petrous ganglia of man.

ganglion and passes upward between the petrous and tympanic parts of the temporal bone to reach the cavity of the tympanum. Here it breaks up into branches to form, along with branches from the carotid plexus of the sympathetic, the **tympanic plexus.** From the plexus branches pass to the mucous membrane of the tympanum and the Eustachian tube. The continuation of the nerve issues from the plexus and unites with a filament from the geniculate ganglion of the facial to form the small superficial petrosal nerve; this runs forward and ends in the otic ganglion.

Filaments also connect the petrous ganglion with the jugular ganglion of the vagus nerve and with the superior cervical ganglion of the sympathetic.

2. A considerable branch runs backward on the guttural pouch, contributes filaments to the pharyngeal plexus, and concurs with twigs from the vagus and the sympathetic in forming the carotid plexus on the terminal part of the carotid artery and on its chief branches. In this plexus is the small ganglion intercaroticum.

The **pharyngeal branch** (R. pharyngeus) (Fig. 437) is the smaller of the two terminal branches. It runs forward across the deep face of the great cornu of the hyoid bone and concurs with the pharyngeal branches of the vagus and with sympathetic filaments in forming the pharyngeal plexus; from this branches pass to the muscles and mucous membrane of the pharynx.

The **lingual branch** (R. lingualis) is the continuation of the trunk (Fig. 437). It runs along the posterior border of the great cornu of the hyoid bone in front of the external maxillary artery and dips under the hyo-glossus muscle. It gives collateral branches to the soft palate, isthmus faucium, and tonsil, and ends in the mucous membrane of the posterior part of the tongue, where it supplies gustatory fibers to the vallate papillæ. A considerable branch unites with a twig from the lingual nerve.

The glosso-pharyngeal is a mixed nerve, containing both motor and sensory fibers. The latter constitute the bulk of the nerve and include those which mediate the special sense of taste. They are processes of the cells of the petrous ganglion. The central processes of the ganglion cells enter the medulla, pass upward and inward through the formatio reticularis, and end in the nucleus of termination in the floor of the fourth ventricle. The motor fibers arise from dorsal and ventral efferent nuclei in the medulla. The glosso-pharyngeal shares these nuclei with the vagus and has practically the same central connections as that nerve (*q. v.*).

THE TENTH, VAGUS, OR PNEUMOGASTRIC NERVE

The **vagus** or **pneumogastric** (N. vagus) is the longest and most widely distributed of the cranial nerves; it is also remarkable for the connections which it forms with adjacent nerves and with the sympathetic. It is attached to the lateral aspect of the medulla by several filaments which are in series with those of the ninth nerve in front and the eleventh nerve behind (Fig. 499). The bundles converge to form a trunk which passes outward, pierces the dura mater, and emerges from the cranium through the foramen lacerum posterius (Fig. 515). In the foramen the nerve bears on its lateral aspect the elongated flattened **jugular ganglion** (G. jugulare).

The ganglion communicates with (*a*) the tympanic nerve, (*b*) the petrous ganglion of the ninth nerve, (*c*) the spinal accessory, and (*d*) the hypoglossal. It also gives off the **auricular branch** (R. auricularis), which runs forward below the petrous ganglion and passes through a small canal in the petrous temporal bone to gain the facial canal. Here it gives filaments to the facial and emerges with that nerve through the stylo-mastoid foramen. It ascends behind the external auditory meatus, dips under the rotator longus muscle, and passes through a foramen in the conchal cartilage to ramify in the integument which lines the meatus and the adjacent part of the ear.

Beyond the ganglion the vagus runs backward and downward with the spinal accessory in a fold of the guttural pouch (Fig. 437). Then the two nerves separate, allowing the hypoglossal to pass between them, and the vagus descends with the internal carotid artery and crosses the inner face of the origin of the occipital artery. Here it is joined by the cervical trunk of the sympathetic, and the two nerves continue along the dorsal aspect of the common carotid artery in a common sheath (Fig. 433). At the root of the neck the vagus separates from the sym-

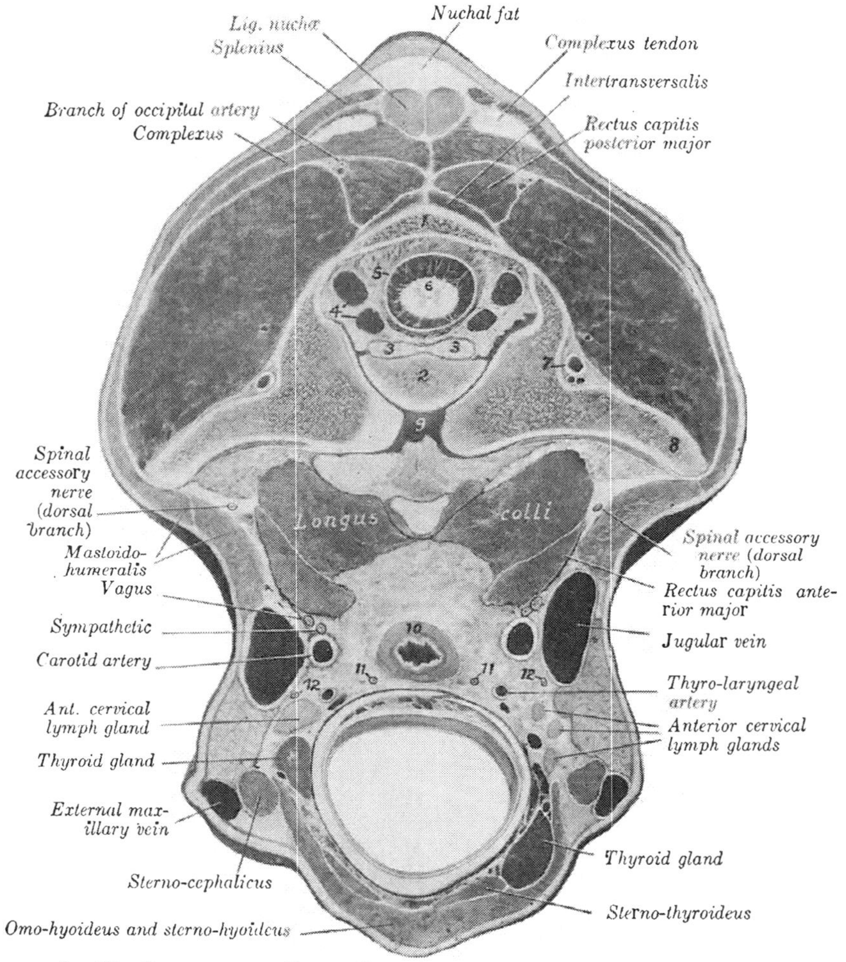

FIG. 517.—CROSS-SECTION OF NECK OF HORSE, PASSING THROUGH POSTERIOR PART OF ATLAS.

The head and neck were extended. *1*, Dorsal arch of atlas; *2*, odontoid process; *3*, odontoid ligament; *4*, vertebral sinuses; *5*, dura mater; *6*, spinal cord; *7*, vertebral artery; *8*, wing of atlas; *9*, atlanto-axial joint cavity; *10*, œsophagus; *11*, *11*, recurrent nerves; *12*, *12*, ventral branches of spinal accessory nerves. By an oversight the obliquus cap. post. (above wing of atlas) is unmarked.

pathetic, and from this point backward the relations of the right and left vagi differ somewhat and must be described separately.

The right vagus (Fig. 429) enters the thorax in the angle of divergence of the right brachial artery and the truncus bicaroticus. It then passes backward and slightly upward, crossing obliquely the outer surface of the brachiocephalic artery and the right face of the trachea. Reaching the dorsal surface of the latter near the bifurcation, it divides into dorsal and ventral branches.

The **left vagus** (Fig. 428) enters the thorax on the ventral face of the œsophagus, crosses obliquely under the left brachial artery, and passes back on the external surface of that vessel in company with a large cardiac nerve.[1] Separating from the latter, the vagus continues backward on the left face of the aorta, inclines to the upper surface of the left bronchus, and divides into dorsal and ventral branches.

The dorsal and ventral branches unite with the corresponding branches of the opposite nerve, thus forming **dorsal** and **ventral œsophageal trunks** (Truncus œsophageus dorsalis, ventralis). These run backward in the posterior mediastinum, above and below the œsophagus respectively, and enter the abdominal cavity through the hiatus œsophageus; they supply branches to the œsophagus and anastomose with each other. The dorsal trunk receives the major part of its fibers from the right vagus. After entering the abdomen it passes to the left of the cardia, gives branches to the visceral surface of the stomach, and ends in the cœliac and subsidiary plexuses. The ventral trunk passes to the lesser curvature of the stomach and ramifies on the parietal surface of the stomach; it forms here the anterior gastric plexus, from which branches are supplied also to the first part of the duodenum and to the liver.

The collateral branches of the vagus are as follows

1. The **pharyngeal branch** (R. pharyngeus) is given off in relation to the superior cervical ganglion, turns around the internal carotid artery, and runs downward and forward on the guttural pouch to the dorsal wall of the pharynx (Fig. 437). Here its branches concur with the pharyngeal branch of the ninth nerve and with filaments from the spinal accessory and the sympathetic in forming the **pharyngeal plexus.** This supplies numerous twigs to the pharynx, and a larger branch which passes along the side of the œsophagus and ramifies in its cervical part.

According to Ellenberger and Baum the pharyngeal plexus receives filaments also from the digastric, superior laryngeal, hypoglossal, and first cervical nerves. The branches of the plexus form secondary intermuscular and submucous plexuses, in which there are numerous minute ganglia.

2. The **superior** or **anterior laryngeal nerve** (N. laryngeus cranialis) is larger than the preceding and arises a little behind it (Fig. 437). It crosses the deep face of the origin of the external carotid artery, runs downward and forward over the lateral wall of the pharynx behind the hypoglossal nerve, and passes through the foramen below the anterior cornu of the thyroid cartilage. Its terminal branches ramify in the mucous membrane of the larynx, the floor of the pharynx, and the entrance to the œsophagus; they anastomose with those of the recurrent. At its origin the nerve gives off its small **external branch** (R. externus); this descends to the crico-thyroid muscle, which it supplies, and sends filaments to the crico-pharyngeus also. It may arise from the trunk of the vagus or from the pharyngeal branch.

At the point of origin of the superior laryngeal nerve there is a plexiform widening which is regarded by some authors as the homologue of the ganglion nodosum of man. From it a filament arises which, after a short course, rejoins the vagus or enters the sympathetic trunk. Stimulation of its central end causes a reduction of the blood-pressure, and it is therefore termed the depressor nerve (N. depressor).

3. The **recurrent nerve** (N. recurrens), also termed the inferior or posterior laryngeal nerve, differs on the two sides in its point of origin and in the first part of its course. The **right nerve** (Fig. 429) is given off opposite the second rib, turns around the dorso-cervical artery from without inward, runs forward on the lower part of the lateral surface of the trachea, and ascends in the neck on the ventral face of the common carotid artery. The **left nerve** (Fig. 428) arises from the vagus where the latter begins to cross the aortic arch. It passes back over the ligamentum

[1] In some cases the left vagus passes back below the junction of the jugular veins and the termination of the left brachial vein. It then runs backward and somewhat dorsally across the left face of the anterior vena cava to reach its usual position.

arteriosum, winds around the concavity of the aortic arch from without inward, runs forward on the lower part of the left face of the trachea, and continues in the neck in a similar position to the right nerve.

It is worthy of note that the left nerve passes beneath the bronchial lymph glands as it winds around the aorta; also that in the next part of its course it lies between the left surface of the trachea and the deep face of the aorta, and is then related to lymph glands which lie along the ventral aspect of the trachea. The left recurrent is often incorporated in part of its course in the anterior mediastinum with a deep cardiac nerve. Further, the left nerve lies at first ventral to, and then upon, the œsophagus in the neck. The right recurrent is given off from or in common with a considerable trunk which connects the vagus with the first thoracic ganglion of the sympathetic. The arrangement here is commonly more or less plexiform, and from it one or two cardiac nerves arise.

The terminal part of each nerve (Fig. 517) lies on the dorsal surface of the trachea, in relation to the œsophagus internally and the carotid artery above.[1] It passes between the crico-arytenoideus posterior and the crico-pharyngeus; the **terminal branches** supply all the muscles of the larynx except the crico-thyroid, and communicate with branches of the superior laryngeal nerve. **Collateral branches** are given off to the cardiac plexus (Rr. cardiaci), to the trachea (Rr. tracheales), to the œsophagus (Rr. œsophagei), and to the inferior cervical ganglion of the sympathetic.

4. **Cardiac branches** (Rr. cardiaci), usually two or three in number, are given off from each vagus within the thorax (Figs. 428, 429). These concur with the cardiac branches of the sympathetic and recurrent nerves to form the cardiac plexus, which innervates the heart and great vessels.

5. Small **tracheal and œsophageal branches** (Rr. tracheales et œsophagei) are given off from both vagi in the thorax. These concur with branches from the recurrent nerves and the inferior cervical and anterior thoracic ganglia of the sympathetic in forming the **posterior tracheal** and **œsophageal plexuses,** from which twigs go to the trachea, œsophagus, heart, and large vessels.

6. **Bronchial branches** (Rr. bronchiales) are detached at the roots of the lungs and unite with sympathetic filaments in forming the **pulmonary plexuses.** From the latter numerous branches proceed in a plexiform manner along the bronchi and vessels into the substance of the lungs.

The vagus and glosso-pharyngeal nerves are so closely associated in origin and central connections that they may be described together in this respect.

The **sensory fibers** arise from the petrous and jugular ganglia, and their central parts enter the lateral aspect of the medulla and divide into anterior and posterior branches like the fibers of the dorsal roots of the spinal nerves. Most of the fibers end in arborizations about the cells of the vago-glosso-pharyngeal nucleus of termination, which consists of two parts. Of these the **dorsal sensory nucleus** (Nucleus alæ cinereæ) is situated in the posterior part of the floor of the fourth ventricle and in the adjacent part of the closed portion of the medulla near the median plane. The other part is termed the **nucleus of the solitary tract,** and is so named because its cells are grouped about the bundle (Tractus solitarius) formed by the posterior divisions of the afferent nerve-fibers. It ends about the level of the pyramidal decussation. The secondary central connections are similar to those of the sensory part of the trigeminus.

The **motor fibers** (and those of the medullary part of the accessory) arise from the **dorsal motor nucleus** and the **ventral motor nucleus.** The cells of the former lie in groups along the ventro-medial side of the dorsal sensory nucleus. The latter, also termed the nucleus ambiguus, is situated more deeply in the lateral part of the formatio reticularis.

THE ELEVENTH OR SPINAL ACCESSORY NERVE

The **spinal accessory nerve** (N. accessorius) is purely motor. It consists of two parts which differ in origin and function.

The **medullary part** arises from the lateral aspect of the medulla by several rootlets which are behind and in series with those of the vagus (Fig. 499). The **spinal part** arises from the cervical part of the spinal cord by a series of fasciculi

[1] The nerve lies here about a finger's breadth above the thyroid gland. If, however, the gland is enlarged it may come in contact with the nerve. The same is true in regard to the relation to the anterior cervical lymph glands.

which emerge between the dorsal and ventral roots. The bundles unite to form a trunk which is very small at its origin at the fifth segment of the cord, but increases in size when traced toward the brain, since it continually receives accessions of fibers. It passes through the foramen magnum and joins the medullary part. The trunk thus formed sends its medullary fibers to the tenth and ninth nerves and emerges through the foramen lacerum posterius. It then runs backward and down-

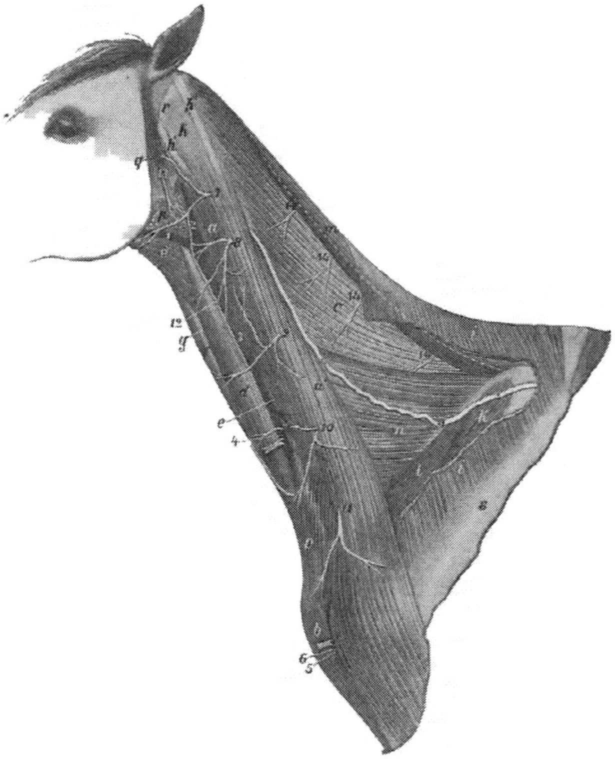

FIG. 518.—NECK OF HORSE, AFTER REMOVAL OF PART OF PANNICULUS AND TRAPEZIUS.

a, a', Mastoido-humeralis; *b*, anterior superficial pectoral muscle; *c*, cervical panniculus; *d*, sterno-cephalicus; *e*, omo-hyoideus; *f*, sterno-thyro-hyoideus; *g*, trachea; *h, h', h''*, tendons of splenius, mastoido-humeralis, and trachelo-mastoideus; *i*, trapezius cervicalis; *k*, supraspinatus; *l*, anterior deep pectoral muscle; *m*, rhomboideus cervicalis; *n*, serratus cervicis; *o*, splenius, upper and lower borders of which are indicated by dotted lines; *p*, parotid gland; q, parotido-auricularis muscle; *r*, wing of atlas; *s*, spine of scapula; *1*, external maxillary vein; *2, 3*, jugular vein; *4*, carotid artery; *5*, descending branch of inferior cervical artery; *6*, cephalic vein; *7–11*, ventral branches of second to seventh cervical nerves; *12*, cutaneous branch of second cervical nerve; *13*, cervical branch of facial nerve; *14*, terminal branches of dorsal divisions of cervical nerves; *15*, dorsal branch of spinal accessory nerve. (After Ellenberger-Baum, Top. Anat. d. Pferdes.)

ward with the vagus in a fold of the guttural pouch, separates from that nerve, crosses the deep face of the submaxillary gland and the occipital artery, and divides in the recessus atlantis into dorsal and ventral branches.

It is connected by anastomotic branches with the vagus and hypoglossal nerves and the superior cervical ganglion of the sympathetic, and contributes a branch to the pharyngeal plexus.

The **dorsal branch** (R. dorsalis) (Figs. 433, 517, 518) receives a twig from the second and third cervical nerves and turns around the atlantal tendon of the splenius under cover of the mastoido-humeralis. It then passes obliquely through the latter muscle and continues backward on the splenius and the cervical part of the serratus, inclines upward across the anterior deep pectoral and the supraspinatus, and enters the deep face of the trapezius, in which it ramifies.

The **ventral branch** (R. ventralis) (Fig. 436) is smaller. It enters the sterno-cephalicus muscle behind the cervical angle of the parotid gland.

The fibers of the spinal part of the accessory arise from the ventro-lateral cells of the ventral gray column of the cord as far back as the fifth cervical segment. The fibers of the medullary part come chiefly from the nucleus ambiguus in common with the motor fibers of the vagus.

THE TWELFTH OR HYPOGLOSSAL NERVE

The **hypoglossal nerve** (N. hypoglossus) is purely motor and innervates the muscles of the tongue (Fig. 437). Its root-fibers arise from the ventral face of the medulla in linear series about 3 to 4 mm. lateral to the posterior half of the pyramid (Fig. 499). The filaments converge to three or four bundles which perforate the dura mater and unite to form the trunk. The latter emerges through the hypoglossal foramen (Fig. 515) and runs downward and backward between the guttural pouch and the capsule of the atlanto-occipital articulation for a distance of a little less than an inch (ca. 2 cm.). It then passes between the tenth and eleventh nerves, turns downward and forward, crosses the external face of the external carotid artery, and continues over the pharynx parallel with the great cornu of the hyoid bone and behind the external maxillary artery. It then crosses beneath the artery, runs forward on the external face of the hyo-glossus muscle, and divides into its terminal branches (Rami linguales). The smaller branch supplies the stylo-glossus, hyo-glossus, and lingualis. The larger branch ramifies on the genio-glossus and supplies the remaining muscles. Anastomoses occur with branches of the lingual nerve.

In the first part of its course the nerve communicates with the superior cervical ganglion and with the ventral branch of the first cervical nerve, and gives filaments to the pharyngeal branch of the vagus and the pharyngeal plexus.

The fibers of the nerve arise from the hypoglossal nucleus, an elongated group of large multipolar cells situated chiefly under the posterior part of the floor of the fourth ventricle close to the median plane. The two nuclei are connected by commissural fibers. The other central connections include: (*a*) communications by the medial longitudinal fasciculus with the nuclei of termination of other cranial nerves; (*b*) cortico-nuclear fibers which come from the cortex by way of the internal capsule and the pyramids and go largely to the nucleus of the opposite side; (*c*) fibers which join the dorsal longitudinal bundle of Schütz, a tract which underlies the floor of the fourth ventricle and is traceable forward below the cerebral aqueduct.

THE SPINAL NERVES

The **spinal nerves** (Nervi spinales) are arranged in pairs, of which there are usually forty-two in the horse. They are designated according to their relations to the vertebral column as **cervical** (8), **thoracic** (18), **lumbar** (6), **sacral** (5), and **coccygeal** (5). Each nerve is connected with the spinal cord by two roots, dorsal and ventral (Fig. 497).

The **dorsal** (or superior) **root** (Radix dorsalis) is the larger of the two. Its fibers (Fila radicularia) spread out in fan shape and join the cord in a linear series along the dorso-lateral groove. Laterally the fibers converge to form a compact bundle, on which is a gray nodular enlargement, the **spinal ganglion** (Ganglion spinale). Beyond the ganglion the dorsal root joins the ventral root to constitute the nerve. The ganglia are external to the dura mater, and are situated in the intervertebral foramina, except in the case of the sacral and coccygeal nerves, the ganglia of which lie within the vertebral canal. Those of the coccygeal nerves are intradural.

The ganglia vary greatly in size; that of the first cervical nerve is scarcely as large as a hemp-seed, while that of the eighth cervical is about 2 cm. long and 1 cm. wide. On the large roots connected with the cervical and lumbar enlargement of the cord there are multiple ganglia of varying sizes interposed in the course of the root-bundles. The fibers of the dorsal roots arise from the cells of the spinal ganglia; each cell gives off a fiber which enters the spinal cord and another which passes into the nerve.

The **ventral** (or inferior) **root** (Radix ventralis) contains fewer fibers than the dorsal root, except in the case of the first cervical nerve. It arises from the ventral surface of the spinal cord (Fig. 495) by means of numerous small bundles of fibers which do not form a linear series but emerge from the cord over an area three to five millimeters in width (ventral root zone). The fibers are processes of the large cells of the ventral gray columns of the spinal cord. There is no ganglion on the ventral root.

In the cervical, thoracic, and anterior lumbar regions the bundles of both roots pass through separate openings in linear series in the dura mater before uniting into a root proper. Further back the bundles of each root unite within the dura. In the anterior part of the cervical region and in the thoracic part of the cord there are intervals of varying length between adjacent roots, but in some places the fibers of adjacent roots overlap and an exchange of fibers may be observed.

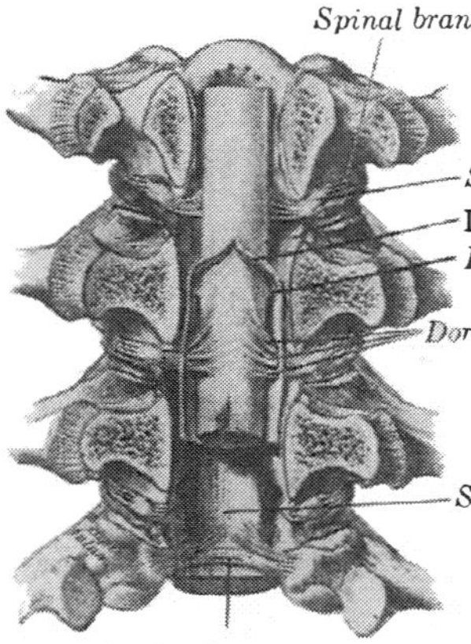

FIG. 519.—VERTEBRAL CANAL OPENED BY SAWING OFF THE ARCHES. (After Schmaltz, Atlas d. Anat. d. Pferdes.)

Many of the roots are directed almost straight outward or incline slightly backward, but the posterior lumbar, sacral, and coccygeal roots and nerves run backward to reach the foramina through which they emerge. The distance thus to be traversed increases from before backward, so that these nerves form a tapering sheaf around the conus medullaris and filum terminale in the last lumbar vertebra and the sacrum which is known as the cauda equina.

The **size** of the spinal nerves varies greatly. The largest are connected with the cervical and lumbar enlargements.

In or immediately after its emergence from the intervertebral foramen each spinal nerve gives off a small **meningeal or recurrent branch** (Ramus meningeus). This is joined by a bundle of fibers from the ramus communicans and enters the vertebral canal, in which it is distributed. Each nerve then divides into two primary branches, **dorsal** and **ventral** (Ramus dorsalis, ventralis). The **dorsal branches** are smaller than the ventral, except in the cervical region. They are distributed chiefly to the muscles and skin of the dorsal part of the body. The **ventral branches** supply in general the muscles and skin of the ventral parts of the body, including the limbs. Each nerve or its ventral branch is connected with an adjacent ganglion of the sympathetic system by at least one small short branch known as a **ramus communicans.** Many nerves have two and some have three such rami. A nerve may be connected with two ganglia, and a ganglion may be connected with two nerves.

The dorsal root is sensory or afferent, *i. e.*, it conveys impulses to the central system. Its fibers are axones of the cells of the spinal ganglion. The ventral root is motor or efferent, and conveys impulses toward the periphery. Its fibers are axones of the large cells in the ventral gray columns of the spinal cord. The common trunk or nerve formed by the union of the two roots contains both kinds of fibers, as do also their primary divisions. In addition to these fibers, which are distributed to the skeletal muscles and the skin, the spinal nerves contain fibers derived from the sympathetic system through the rami communicantes; these go to the glands and unstriped muscle and are designated secretory and vasomotor fibers.

THE CERVICAL NERVES

The **cervical nerves** (Nervi cervicales) (Figs. 431, 433, 518, 523) number eight pairs. Of these the first emerges through the intervertebral foramen of the atlas, the second through that of the axis, and the eighth between the last cervical and the first thoracic vertebræ.

The **dorsal branches** are distributed to the dorso-lateral muscles and skin of the neck. They divide usually into inner and outer branches. The internal branches (Rami mediales) run in general across the multifidus and the lamellar part of the ligamentum nuchæ to the skin of the upper border of the neck; they supply the deep lateral muscles and the skin. The external branches (Rami laterales) are chiefly muscular in their distribution. The dorsal branches of the third to the sixth nerves are connected by anastomotic branches to form the **dorsal cervical plexus.**

The **ventral branches** are smaller than the dorsal ones—an exception to the general rule. They increase in size from first to last. They supply in general the muscles and skin over the lateral and ventral aspect of the vertebræ, but the last three enter into the formation of the brachial plexus, and the three preceding the last give off the roots of the phrenic nerve. An irregular **ventral cervical plexus** is formed by anastomoses established between the ventral branches. The following special features may be noted:

The **first cervical nerve** emerges through the intervertebral (antero-internal) foramen of the atlas. Its **dorsal branch** (N. occipitalis) passes upward and outward between the obliqui capitis and the recti capitis dorsales and supplies branches to these muscles, the scutularis and posterior auricular muscles, and the skin of the poll. The **ventral branch** descends through the alar (antero-external) foramen of the atlas, crosses over the ventral straight muscles and the carotid artery under cover of the parotid gland, and divides into two branches. The anterior branch enters the omo-hyoideus muscle. The posterior branch passes downward and backward under cover of that muscle, unites with a branch of the ventral division of the second cervical nerve, and continues its course on the ventro-lateral surface of the trachea to enter the sterno-thyro-hyoideus behind the intermediate tendon. In the recessus atlantis the ventral branch is connected by one or more twigs with the superior cervical ganglion of the sympathetic, and a little lower with the hypoglossal nerve. It also sends branches to the ventral straight muscles of the head and the thyro-hyoideus. Below the atlas the ventral branch is crossed superficially by the spinal accessory nerve, the occipital artery, and the inferior cerebral vein.

The **second cervical nerve** is larger than the first. It emerges from the vertebral canal through the intervertebral foramen of the anterior part of the arch of the axis. Its **dorsal branch** ascends between the complexus and the ligamentum nuchæ and ramifies in the skin of the poll. The **ventral branch** gives off **muscular branches** to the rectus capitis anterior major, and **anastomotic branches** to the spinal accessory and the ventral divisions of the first and third cervical nerves;

one of these crosses over the carotid artery and concurs in the formation of the nerve to the sterno-thyro-hyoideus mentioned above. The ventral branch then becomes superficial by passing between the two parts of the mastoido-humeralis, and divides into posterior auricular and cutaneous branches. The **posterior auricular nerve** passes upward and forward on the parotid gland parallel with the posterior border of the parotido-auricularis to ramify on the convex face of the external ear. The **cutaneous nerve** of the neck (N. cutaneus colli) crosses the mastoido-humeralis muscle and turns backward along the course of the jugular vein. On the lower part of the parotid gland it is connected by a twig with the cervical cutaneous branch of the facial nerve. It gives off twigs to the subcutaneous muscles and the skin of the parotid and laryngeal regions and a long branch which passes forward in the submaxillary space.

The **third cervical nerve** leaves the vertebral canal through the foramen between the second and third cervical vertebræ. Its **dorsal branch** emerges between two bundles of the intertransversalis muscle accompanied by a branch of the vertebral artery, turns upward on the multifidus, and divides into several branches which radiate on the deep face of the complexus. It gives branches to these muscles and to the skin, and a twig which joins the corresponding branch of the fourth nerve. The **ventral branch** emerges through the intertransversalis below the bundle above which the dorsal branch appears. It gives branches to the trachelo-mastoideus, rectus capitis anterior major, longus colli, splenius, and mastoido-humeralis. It also gives off a large cutaneous nerve which passes out between the two parts of the mastoido-humeralis and divides into several divergent branches.

The **fourth** and **fifth cervical nerves** are distributed in general like the third. Their **dorsal branches** are united by anastomotic twigs with each other and with those of the third and sixth nerves to form the dorsal cervical plexus. The **ventral branch** of the fifth nerve often contributes a small twig to the phrenic nerve.

The **sixth cervical nerve** has a smaller **dorsal branch** than the fifth. Its **ventral branch** is larger and goes in part to the brachial plexus; it supplies twigs to the intertransversales, the longus colli, the mastoido-humeralis, and the cervical parts of the serratus and rhomboideus, furnishes a root of the phrenic nerve, and gives off several considerable subcutaneous branches. One of the latter ramifies on the thick part of the cervical panniculus, to which it gives branches; another and larger branch (N. supraclavicularis) sends twigs to the skin over the shoulder joint, and descends to the skin over the superficial pectoral muscles (Fig. 466).

The **seventh** and **eighth cervical nerves** have small **dorsal branches,** which ascend between the longissimus and multifidus, giving twigs to these muscles, the spinalis and semispinalis, the rhomboideus, and the skin. Their **ventral branches** are very large and concur in the formation of the brachial plexus; that of the seventh nerve contributes the posterior root of the phrenic nerve.

Phrenic Nerve

The **phrenic nerve** (N. phrenicus) (Figs. 428, 429, 433), the motor nerve to the diaphragm, is formed by the union of two or three roots which cross the superficial face of the scalenus muscle obliquely downward and backward. The chief roots come from the ventral branches of the sixth and seventh cervical nerves. The root derived from the fifth nerve is small and inconstant. The root from the seventh cervical comes by way of the brachial plexus. The course of the nerve is not the same on both sides. On the **right side** the nerve enters the thorax by passing between the brachial artery and the anterior vena cava. It then courses backward and somewhat downward over the right face of the anterior vena cava, crosses the pericardium, and continues along the posterior vena cava to the diaphragm. In the latter part of its course it is inclosed in a special fold of the right pleura and inclines gradually to the ventral face of the vein. On the left side the nerve enters the thorax between the left brachial and inferior cervical arteries, and then runs its entire course in the mediastinum. In the anterior mediastinum it lies along the brachiocephalic artery ventral to the left vagus and cardiac nerves, and crosses over the dorso-cervical vein. It then passes over the upper part of the pericardium and runs backward in the posterior mediastinum to reach the tendinous center of the diaphragm considerably to the left of the median plane. Each nerve is usually connected near its origin with the first thoracic ganglion of the sympathetic by a ramus communicans, and each terminates by dividing into several branches which are distributed to the corresponding part of the diaphragm.

The Brachial Plexus

The **brachial plexus** (Plexus brachialis) (Fig. 433) results from anastomoses established between the ventral branches of the last three cervical and first two thoracic nerves. It appears as a thick, wide band between the two parts of the scalenus muscle, and is covered by the anterior deep pectoral and subscapularis muscles. The largest root of the plexus is derived from the first thoracic nerve, while the root supplied by the sixth cervical nerve is quite small. Each of the three chief roots, *i. e.*, those from the last two cervical and the first thoracic nerve, is connected with the sympathetic by a ramus communicans.

The **branches** emanating from the plexus go for the most part to the thoracic limb, but some are distributed on the chest-wall. The names of the branches, and their arrangement so far as they can be conveniently examined before removal of the fore limb, are as follows:[1]

1. The large **suprascapular nerve** (N. suprascapularis) turns outward and forward and disappears between the supraspinatus and subscapularis.
2. The much smaller **subscapular nerves** (Nn. subscapulares), usually two primary trunks, arise close behind the suprascapular, run backward a short distance, and divide into several branches which enter the lower third of the subscapularis.
3. The **anterior thoracic** or **pectoral nerves** (N. pectorales craniales), three or four in number, arise from the anterior part of the plexus and from the loop formed by the musculo-cutaneous and median nerves. One enters the anterior deep pectoral muscle. Another passes out between the divisions of the deep pectoral to supply the superficial pectoral, giving a twig usually to the posterior deep muscle. The latter receives one or two other nerves.
4. The **musculo-cutaneous nerve** (N. musculocutaneus) arises from the anterior part of the plexus and passes over the outer face of the brachial artery, below which it is connected by a large but short branch with the median nerve, thus forming a loop in which the artery lies. One or two branches to the pectoral muscles are given off from the nerve or the loop.
5. The **median nerve** (N. medianus) is usually the largest branch of the brachial plexus. It lies at first above the brachial artery, then passes between the artery and vein to reach the anterior border of the former. It is easily recognized by its large size and the loop which it forms with the musculo-cutaneous nerve.
6. The **ulnar nerve** (N. ulnaris) arises with the median by a short common trunk. It descends behind the brachial artery and is accompanied a short distance by the radial nerve.
7. The **radial nerve** (N. radialis) arises from the posterior part of the plexus and is sometimes the largest branch. It descends behind the ulnar nerve over the origin of the subscapular artery and the lower part of the teres major, and

[1] In order to examine the plexus and the origins of its chief branches conveniently and with as little disturbance of relation as possible, the subject should be suspended in imitation of the natural position and the fore limb abducted as much as is necessary.

dips into the interstice between that muscle and the long and internal heads of the triceps.

8. The **axillary** or **circumflex nerve** (N. axillaris) arises behind the musculo cutaneous. It passes downward and backward on the inner face of the subscapu laris and disappears between that muscle and the subscapular artery.

9. The **long thoracic nerve** (N. thoracalis longus) is wide and thin. It passes backward across the surface of the serratus magnus, to which it is distributed. The branches which enter the muscle are given off both upward and downward in fairly regular fashion.

10. The **thoraco-dorsal nerve** (N. thoracodorsalis) passes upward and backward across the subscapularis muscle to ramify in the teres major and the latissimus dorsi.

11. The **external** (or subcutaneous) **thoracic nerve** arises by a common trunk with the ulnar. It runs backward and downward across the inner face of the tensor fasciæ antibrachii, communicates with the anterior pectoral branches, and gives twigs to the deep pectoral muscle. It then runs backward in company with the external thoracic or "spur" vein, gives branches to the latissimus dorsi and the deep pectoral, and ramifies in the panniculus and the skin of the abdominal wall. It communicates with perforating branches of the intercostal nerves. A branch from it, accompanied by a large perforating intercostal branch, winds around the lower border of the latissimus dorsi and ramifies in the panniculus on the outer surface of the arm.

The term posterior thoracic or pectoral nerves (Nn. pectorales caudales) may be used to include 8, 9, and 10.

Suprascapular Nerve

The **suprascapular** (Fig. 441) is a large nerve derived chiefly, if not exclusively, from the sixth and seventh cervical components of the brachial plexus. It passes between the supraspinatus and subscapularis muscles and turns around the distal fourth of the anterior border of the scapula to reach the supraspinous fossa. It gives branches to the supraspinatus and continues backward and upward into the infraspinous fossa, where it supplies the infraspinatus, deltoid, and teres minor muscles.

The direct relation of this nerve to the scapula renders it liable to injury, the result of which may be paralysis and atrophy of the muscles supplied by it.

Musculo-cutaneous Nerve

The **musculo-cutaneous nerve** (Fig. 441) arises close behind the suprascapular, and is derived chiefly from the part of the brachial plexus which is supplied by the seventh and eighth cervical nerves. It descends across the outer surface of the brachial artery, below which a great part of the nerve unites with the median to form the loop previously mentioned. It gives off a branch which enters the upper part of the belly of the coraco-brachialis, passes downward and forward between the two parts of that muscle or between the muscle and the bone, and divides into branches which enter the biceps brachii. It contributes one of the nerves to the pectoral muscles. In some cases this nerve sends a branch to join the cutaneous branch of the median.

Axillary Nerve

The **axillary nerve** (Figs. 441, 520), also termed the circumflex, derives its fibers from the eighth cervical and first thoracic roots of the brachial plexus. It runs downward and backward across the lower part of the subscapularis and dips in between that muscle and the subscapular artery at the level of the shoulder joint. Continuing outward in the interval between the teres minor and the long and external heads of the triceps, it reaches the deep face of the deltoid and divides into several divergent branches. The **muscular branches** supply the teres major, capsularis, teres minor, infraspinatus, deltoid, and mastoido-humeralis. The **cutaneous branch** (N. cutaneus brachii lateralis) runs downward and a little forward across the external head of the triceps and ramifies on the fascia on the front of the forearm and on the superficial pectoral muscle.

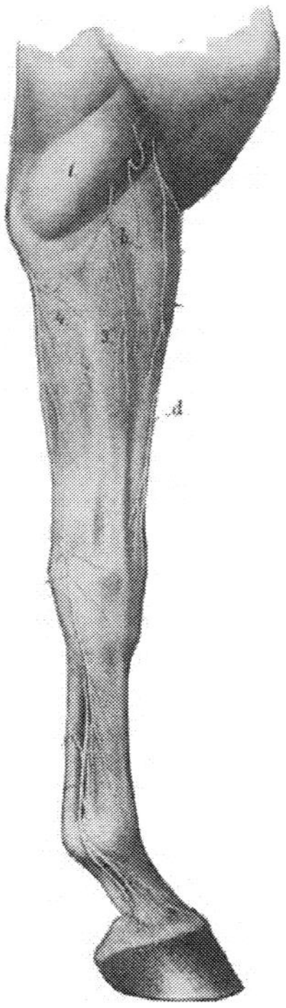

Fig. 520. — Cutaneous Nerves of Right Fore Limb of Horse, External Face.

a, Cutaneous branch of axillary nerve; *b*, cutaneous branches of radial nerve; *c*, posterior cutaneous branch of ulnar nerve; *d*, cutaneous branch of median nerve; *e*, superficial branch of ulnar nerve; *f*, external metacarpal nerve; *g*, anastomotic branch connecting internal and external metacarpal nerves; *1*, external head of triceps; *2*, extensor carpi radialis; *3*, anterior extensor; *4*, flexor carpi externus. (After Ellenberger, in Leisering's Atlas.)

Radial Nerve

The radial nerve (Figs. 441, 443, 520), also called the musculo-spiral, is sometimes the largest branch of the brachial plexus. Its fibers are derived from the seventh and eighth cervical and first thoracic roots of the plexus. It passes downward and backward over the inner surface of the subscapular artery and the teres major. In this part of its course it is related in front to the ulnar nerve, which separates it from the brachial vein. It detaches a branch to the tensor fasciæ antibrachii, passes outward in the interval between the teres major and the long and internal heads of the triceps, and gains the musculo-spiral groove of the humerus. Accompanied by a branch of the deep brachial artery, it runs obliquely downward and outward in the groove, covered externally by the external head of the triceps and the extensor carpi radialis, and reaches the flexion surface of the elbow joint. In this part of its course it gives off a muscular branch which ramifies in the long and external heads of the triceps and in the anconeus, and a **cutaneous nerve** (N. cutaneus antibrachii dorsalis); branches of the latter emerge below or through the external head of the triceps and ramify on the dorso-lateral surface of the forearm. At the elbow the nerve descends with the anterior radial vessels on the joint capsule between the brachialis and extensor carpi radialis, and supplies branches to the extensor carpi and the common or anterior extensor of the digit and (inconstantly) to the brachialis. Below the elbow joint the nerve detaches a large branch which passes back to the flexor carpi externus, and terminates by small branches which descend on the radius to enter the radial and ulnar heads of the common extensor, the lateral extensor, and the oblique extensor of the carpus. Thus the radial nerve innervates the extensors of the elbow, carpal and digital joints, and supplies also the flexor carpi externus.[1]

Ulnar Nerve

The **ulnar nerve** (Figs. 441, 442, 443, 520) arises with the median from the thoracic components of the brachial plexus. It descends between the brachial artery and vein, accompanied for a short distance by the radial nerve. It then crosses the vein and continues behind the latter along the anterior border of the tensor fasciæ antibrachii and dips under that muscle near the elbow. Here it is joined by the ulnar vessels and passes downward and backward over the internal

[1] Morphologically the last-named muscle belongs to the extensor group. In man and in the dog and many other animals it is an extensor in function.

epicondyle of the humerus. In the forearm it crosses obliquely the deep face of the ulnar head of the flexor carpi medius and descends under the deep fascia with the vessels, at first on the ulnar head of the perforans, and then between the middle and external flexors of the carpus. Near the level of the accessory carpal bone it divides into two terminal branches, superficial and deep. It gives off two principal collateral branches. The **cutaneous branch** (Ramus cutaneus palmaris) is detached just before the nerve passes under the tensor fasciæ antibrachii; it runs downward and backward on that muscle under cover of the posterior superficial pectoral, becomes superficial below the elbow and ramifies on the posterior surface and both sides of the forearm. The **muscular branch** is given off at the elbow joint and divides to supply the flexors of the digit and the middle flexor of the carpus. Of

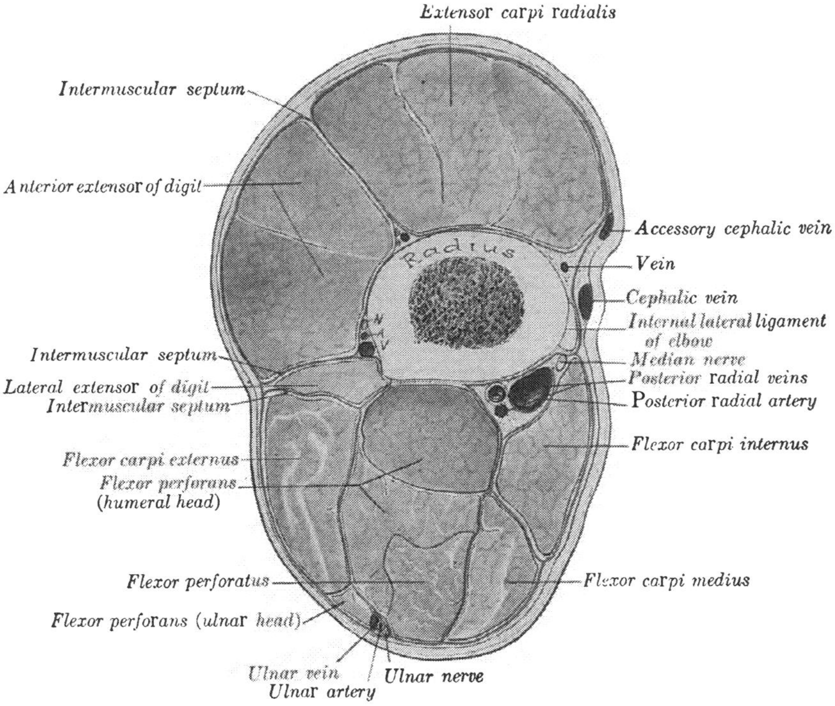

Fig. 521.—Cross-section of Forearm of Horse About Three inches (ca. 8 cm.) below the Elbow Joint. The deep fascia is designated by red line. *N, A. V*, interosseous vessels and nerve.

the two terminals, the **superficial branch** (Ramus superficialis) emerges between the tendons of insertion of the external and middle flexors of the carpus and ramifies on the dorso-lateral aspect of the carpus and metacarpus. The **deep branch** (Ramus profundus), after a very short course, unites under cover of the tendon of the flexor carpi medius with the outer branch of the median nerve to form the external metacarpal or volar nerve.

Median Nerve

The **median nerve** (Figs. 441, 442, 447, 520, 521) derives its fibers chiefly from the first thoracic root of the brachial plexus. It is usually the largest branch and it accompanies the chief arterial trunks to the distal part of the limb. It descends over the inner face of the brachial artery, which it crosses obliquely, and continues down the arm in front of the artery. Near its origin it is joined by a large branch with the musculo-cutaneous nerve, thus forming a loop in which the artery appears to be suspended. Near the elbow it crosses obliquely over the artery (posterior radial) and lies behind it on the internal lateral ligament. Below the joint it again crosses the artery and lies behind the radius and the lower part of the long internal lateral ligament.

At the elbow the nerve is covered by the posterior superficial pectoral muscle and is crossed by the large oblique connection between the cephalic and brachial veins. The variable and often plexiform venous arrangement renders approach to the nerve here undesirable. It can be reached

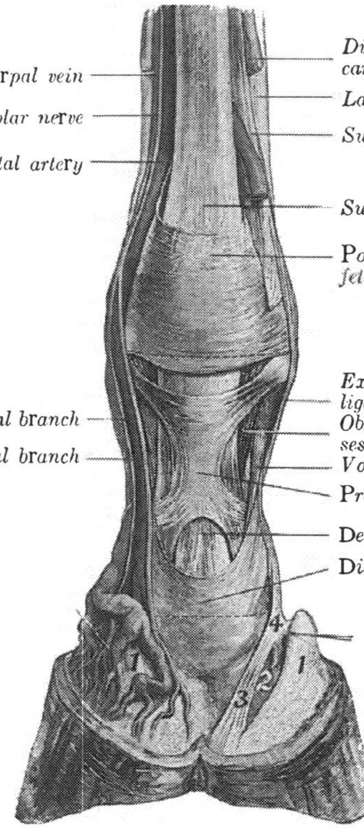

Fig. 522.—Dissection of Distal Part of Right Fore Limb of Horse, Viewed from Behind. *1* Lateral cartilage; *2, 3, 4*, ligaments from first phalanx to third sesamoid, bulb of heel, and lateral cartilage. (After Schmaltz, Atlas d. Anat. d. Pferdes.)

best by an incision just behind the lower part of the long internal lateral ligament; here the nerve lies under the deep fascia in the furrow between the radius and the anterior border of the flexor carpi internus, overlapped by the latter. In some cases the nerve retains its position in front of the artery at the elbow, and in others it crosses the deep face of the artery.

Passing beneath the internal flexor of the carpus, the nerve continues downward in the forearm with the posterior radial vessels, and divides at a variable distance above the carpus into two branches; these are the internal volar or metacarpal nerve and the branch which unites with the ulnar to form the corresponding external nerve.

At the proximal part of the forearm the nerve runs almost straight downward along the posterior border of the long internal lateral ligament, while the artery here inclines somewhat backward. Thus the nerve is superficial to the artery for a short distance, then lies in front of the latter to about the middle of the region, where it inclines a little backward and arrives at the interval between the internal and middle flexors of the carpus. The division may occur about the middle of the region, but commonly takes place in the distal third or fourth.

The collateral branches are as follows:

1. The **musculo-cutaneous branch** is in reality the continuation of the nerve of that name. It is given off about the middle of the arm, passes beneath the lower part of the biceps, and divides into muscular and cutaneous branches. The **muscular branch** enters the brachialis. The **cutaneous branch** emerges between the mastoido-humeralis and the biceps and divides into two branches; these descend on the fascia of the forearm with the cephalic vein and its accessory, and ramify on the front and inner face of the forearm, carpus, and metacarpus.

2. **Muscular branches** to the internal flexor of the carpus and the flexors of the digit are given off just as the nerve passes under the first named muscle.

3. The very small **interosseous nerve** passes through the interosseous space and is distributed chiefly to the periosteum, but in some cases twigs may go to the extensor muscles.

The **metacarpal** or volar **nerves**,[1] internal and external, are the continuations of the median and ulnar nerves in the distal part of the limb.

The **internal metacarpal** or volar **nerve** (N. volaris medialis) arises as the inner terminal branch of the median nerve at a variable distance above the carpus (Fig. 442). It descends through the carpal canal along the inner border of the superficial flexor tendon, and lies at first in front of the large metacarpal or common digital artery. It then passes behind the artery to the distal third of the metacarpus, where it lies behind the vein, the artery here becoming deeper in position. In addition to cutaneous twigs, the nerve gives off about the middle of the metacarpus a considerable **anastomotic branch** which winds obliquely downward and outward over the flexor tendons and joins the external nerve at the lower third of the metacarpus (Fig. 447). Near the fetlock the nerve divides into two digital branches.

1. The **dorsal** or **anterior digital branch** (Ramus dorsalis) descends at first between the digital artery and vein, then crosses over the vein and ramifies in the skin and the matrix of the hoof on the dorsal (anterior) face of the digit.

2. The volar or **posterior digital branch** (Ramus volaris) is the direct continuation of the trunk. It descends behind the digital artery, which it accompanies in its ramification. A **middle digital branch** is sometimes described as descending behind the vein. In some cases this branch is distinct, but usually there are instead several small twigs derived from the posterior branch, which cress very obliquely over the artery and anastomose in a variable manner with each other and with the anterior branch.

The **external metacarpal** or volar **nerve** (N. volaris lateralis) is formed by the union of the external terminal branch of the median with the deep branch of the ulnar nerve (Fig. 442). It descends with the internal volar or small metacarpal artery in the texture of the posterior annular ligament of the carpus. In the metacarpus it descends along the outer border of the deep flexor tendon behind the external metacarpal vein, and is accompanied by a small artery from the volar subcarpal arch. Toward the distal end of the metacarpus it is joined by the oblique branch from the internal nerve, and beyond this is arranged like the latter. Below the carpus it detaches a deep branch to the suspensory ligament and the interossei, and also supplies twigs to the skin.

Anastomoses are established between the digital branches, and the areas innervated by them are not well defined, but really overlap each other. In certain diseased conditions, however, in which the lesions are confined to the volar structures, relief from pain may be afforded by section of the volar branches only.

[1] In veterinary works these are frequently termed plantar nerves, which is an unfortunate misnomer. The writer inclines to the use of the old term metacarpal or common digital to designate the nerves as far as their divisions, and the term digital beyond this.

THE THORACIC NERVES

The thoracic **nerves** (Nn. thoracales) number eighteen on either side in the horse. They are designated numerically according to the vertebræ behind which they emerge. Most of them are arranged in a very similar manner and therefore do not require separate description. Each divides into a dorsal and a ventral branch, the latter being the larger.

The **dorsal branches** (Rami dorsales) emerge behind the levatores costarum and divide into internal and external branches. The internal branches ascend on the multifidus and supply the dorsal spinal muscles. The external branches run outward under the longissimus and emerge between that muscle and the transversalis costarum; after giving twigs to these muscles they pass through the latissimus dorsi and the lumbo-dorsal fascia and ramify as dorsal cutaneous nerves under the skin of the back (Fig. 523). In the region of the withers they give branches to the serratus anticus and rhomboideus, and their cutaneous terminals pass through these muscles and the dorso-scapular ligament to supply the skin over the ligamentum nuchæ and the scapular cartilage.

The **ventral branches** or **intercostal nerves** (Nn. intercostales) are much larger than the preceding, and are connected with the sympathetic by rami communicantes. The first goes almost entirely to the brachial plexus, but sends a fine branch downward in the first intercostal space which is expended in the muscle there without reaching the lower end of the space. The second ventral branch furnishes a considerable root to the brachial plexus, but its intercostal continuation is typical. The intercostal nerves (Fig. 184) descend in the intercostal spaces with the vessels of like name, at first between the intercostal muscles, and lower down chiefly between the pleura and the internal intercostal muscle. In the anterior spaces the artery lies along the posterior border of the rib, with the nerve in front of it; further back the nerve lies behind the border of the rib, with the artery in front of it. They supply the intercostal muscles, give off lateral perforating branches, and terminate in the following manner: The second to the sixth inclusive emerge through the spaces between the costal cartilages and concur in supplying the pectoral muscles. The second to the eighth give branches to the transversus thoracis. The succeeding ones give branches to the diaphragm, pass between the transverse and internal oblique muscles, give twigs to these, and end in the rectus abdominis. There are three series of cutaneous nerves given off by the intercostal nerves. The upper nerves emerge through the serratus magnus and the external intercostals about parallel with the digitations of the external oblique. The middle set perforate the origin of the latter muscle. The lower ones appear through the abdominal tunic. They supply branches to the abdominal muscles, the panniculus, and the skin. Some of the anterior ones anastomose with the posterior thoracic branches of the brachial plexus. The posterior three supply in part the skin of the flank. The ventral branch of the last thoracic nerve runs outward behind the last rib across the dorsal surface of the psoas major and divides into superficial and deep branches. The superficial branch passes between the obliquus internus and transversus abdominis, perforates the obliquus externus, and ramifies under the skin of the flank (Fig. 525). The deep branch descends on the inner face of the internal oblique to the rectus abdominis, in which it ends.

THE LUMBAR NERVES

There are six pairs of **lumbar nerves** (Nn. lumbales) in the horse, the last of which emerge between the last lumbar vertebra and the sacrum. The anterior two or three are about the same size as the thoracic nerves, but the others are much larger.

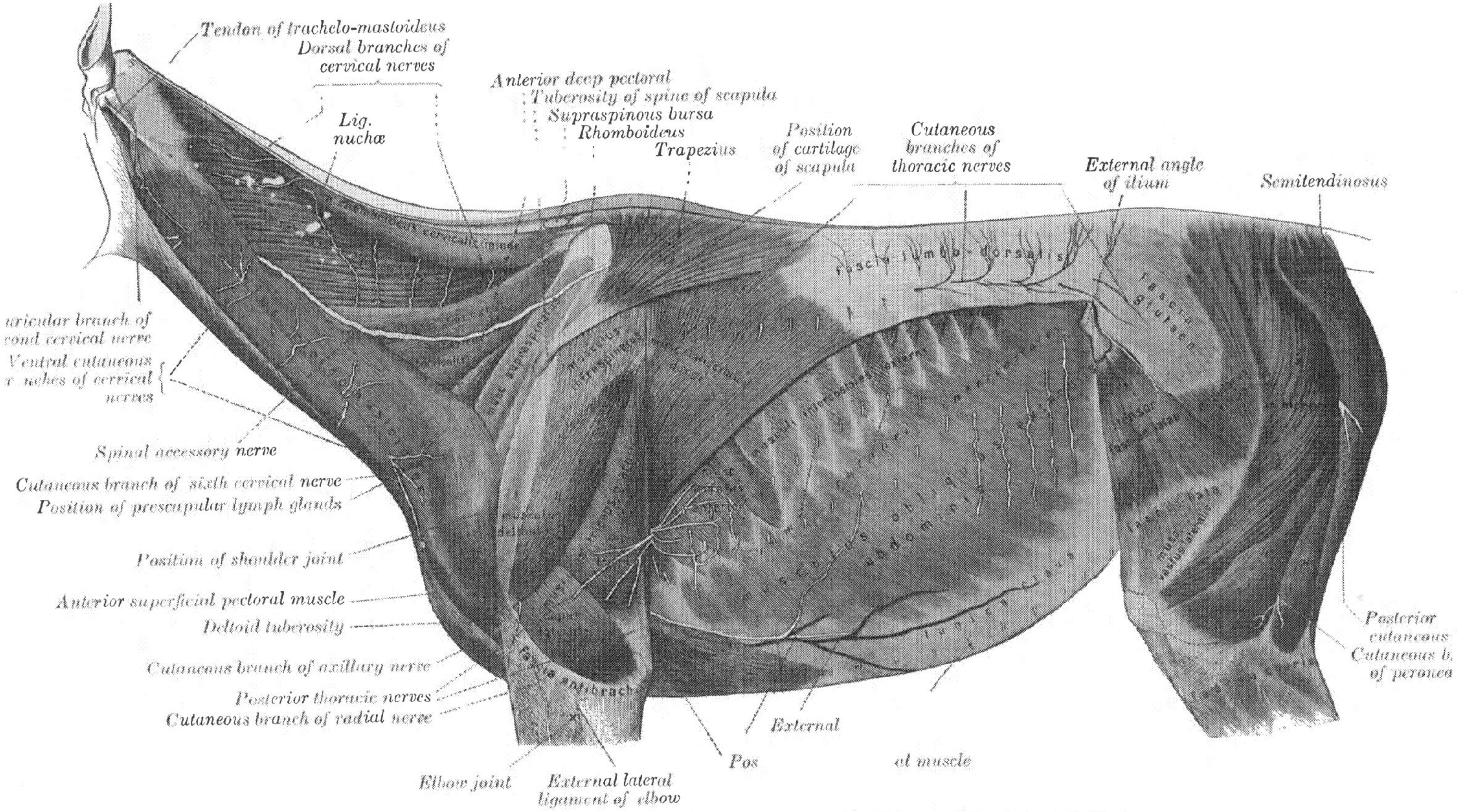

FIG. 523. —SUPERFICIAL NERVES OF NECK AND TRUNK OF HORS . (After Schmaltz, Atlas d. Anat. d. Pferdes.

Their dorsal branches are small in comparison with the ventral ones. They are distributed to the muscles and skin of the loins and croup in a fashion similar to those of the thoracic nerves.

The ventral branches are connected with the sympathetic by small rami communicantes, and give branches to the sublumbar muscles. Those of the first two nerves are arranged in a manner analogous to the corresponding branch of the last thoracic nerve.

The ventral branch of the first **lumbar nerve** is termed the **ilio-hypogastric nerve** (N. iliohypogastricus). It passes outward between the quadratus lumborum and the psoas major, and divides at the outer border of the latter into an anterior or superficial and a posterior or deep branch. The **anterior or superficial branch** passes over the upper edge of the internal oblique, descends between that muscle and the external oblique, perforates the latter, and runs downward and backward and ramifies under the skin of the posterior part of the flank and the outer surface of the thigh. It gives branches to the transversus and obliquus externus abdominis. The **posterior or deep branch** is smaller; it runs downward and back

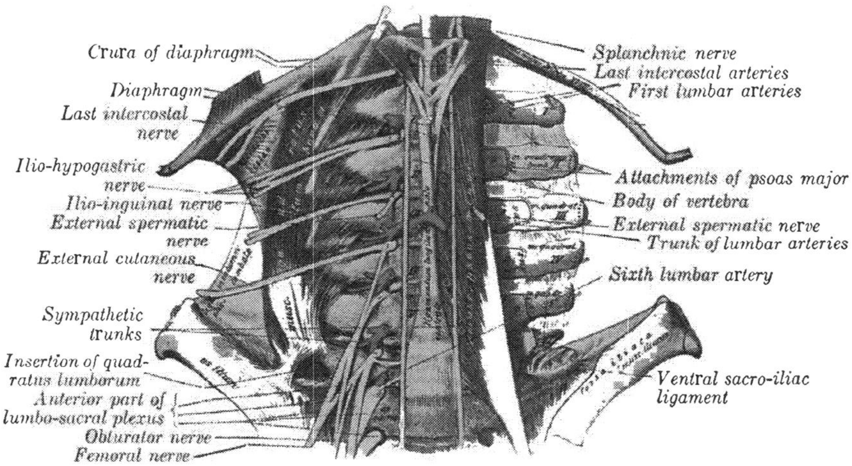

FIG. 524.—LUMBAR NERVES OF HORSE, VENTRAL VIEW. (After Schmaltz, Atlas d. Anat. d. Pferdes.)

ward beneath the peritoneum to the outer border of the rectus abdominis, gives branches to the internal oblique, and terminates in the rectus abdominis.

The ventral branch of the **second lumbar nerve** is connected by an anastomotic branch with that of the third nerve. It gives off a large branch to the psoas muscle and an inguinal branch, and is continued as the ilio-inguinal nerve. The **inguinal branch** (N. spermaticus externus) runs backward in the substance of the psoas minor, emerges a short distance in front of the circumflex iliac vessels, and runs backward and downward under the peritoneum to the internal inguinal ring. It gives branches to the internal oblique muscle and descends in the inguinal canal along the outer border of the cremaster (to which it detaches filaments) and ends subcutaneously in the scrotum and prepuce in the male, the mammary gland in the female. The **ilio-inguinal nerve** (N. ilioinguinalis) may be regarded as the continuation of the ventral branch. It runs parallel with the ilio-hypogastric nerve and has a similar arrangement. Its **anterior or superficial branch** perforates the external oblique muscle a little in front of the point of the hip, runs downward on the front of the thigh and the outer surface of the stifle, and gives off cutaneous branches. The **posterior or deep branch** runs behind and parallel with that of the ilio-hypogastricus, detaches branches to the internal oblique muscle, and descends the inguinal canal with the inguinal branch, to be distributed to the external genital organs and the surrounding skin in the inguinal region.

The ventral branch of the **third lumbar nerve** is connected by a small anastomotic branch with the second nerve and furnishes a root of the lumbo-sacral plexus. It gives off a branch to the psoas muscles, an inguinal branch, and is continued as the external cutaneous nerve. The **inguinal branch** (N. spermaticus externus) passes backward in the substance of the psoas minor, from which it emerges under cover of or near the circumflex iliac vessels. It then runs external to and parallel with the external iliac artery and descends in the inner part of the inguinal canal. It emerges at the external ring with the external pudic artery and ramifies in the external genital organs and the skin of the inguinal region. The **external cutaneous nerve** of the thigh (N. cutaneus femoris lateralis) runs backward in the substance of the psoas muscles and emerges at the outer border of the psoas minor. It then passes outward and backward on the iliac fascia and accompanies the posterior branch of the circumflex iliac artery. With this vessel it perforates the abdominal wall by passing between the external oblique and the iliacus a short distance below the point of the hip, and descends on the inner face of the tensor fasciæ latæ (near its anterior border) and ramifies subcutaneously in the region of the stifle.

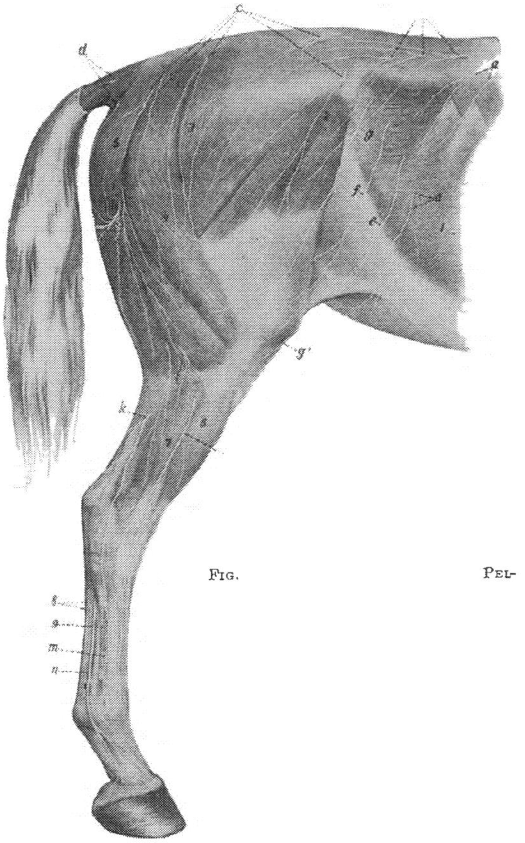

FIG. PEL-

The origin and disposition of some of the foregoing nerves are variable. In some cases the ilio-inguinal nerve ends in the psoas major, and appears then to be absent. The mode of formation of the inguinal nerves is very inconstant. The inner nerve may arise with one of the outer ones from a common trunk, or they may anastomose. The inguinal branch of the ilio-inguinal nerve often receives a twig from the ilio-hypogastric nerve.

The ventral branches of the **fourth, fifth,** and **sixth lumbar** nerves concur in the formation of the lumbo-sacral plexus.

LUMBO-SACRAL PLEXUS

This plexus (Fig. 451) results substantially from the union of the ventral branches of the last three lumbar and the first two sacral nerves, but it derives a small root from the third lumbar nerve also. The anterior part of the plexus lies in front of the internal iliac artery between the lumbar transverse processes and the psoas minor. The posterior part lies partly upon and partly in the texture of the sacro-sciatic ligament. From the plexus are derived the nerves of the pelvic limb, which are now to be described.

Femoral Nerve

The **femoral** (or anterior crural) nerve (N. femoralis) is derived chiefly from the fourth and fifth lumbar nerves, but commonly receives a fasciculus from the third nerve also (Fig. 524). It is the larger of the two nerves which are given off from the anterior part of the lumbo-sacral plexus. It runs backward at first between the psoas major and minor, then crosses the deep face of the tendon of insertion of the latter, and descends under cover of the sartorius in the furrow between the two heads of the iliacus. It gives off the saphenous nerve, crosses the lower part of the outer head of the iliacus, and divides into several branches which dip into the interstice between the rectus femoris and the vastus internus (Fig. 450). These branches are accompanied by the anterior femoral vessels and innervate the quadriceps femoris. Collateral muscular branches are supplied to the ilio-psoas and sartorius.

The **saphenous nerve** (N. saphenus) (Figs. 450, 451, 457) is given off as the parent trunk crosses the furrow between the psoas major and the outer head of the iliacus. It descends with the femoral vessels in the femoral canal, and gives branches to the sartorius, gracilis, and pectineus. About the middle of the thigh it divides into several branches which emerge from between the sartorius and gracilis, perforate the deep fascia and ramify on the inner surface and the front of the limb as far downward as the hock. The longer posterior branches accompany the saphenous vessels, while the anterior branches deviate forward toward the stifle and the anterior surface of the leg.

Obturator Nerve

This nerve (N. obturatorius) is derived from the ventral branches of the last three lumbar nerves (Fig. 524). It runs downward and backward, at first above and then upon the external iliac vein, inclines inward across the obturator vein, and passes through the anterior part of the obturator foramen in front of that vessel (Fig. 451). It continues downward through the obturator externus, and divides into several branches which innervate the obturator externus, pectineus, adductor, and gracilis muscles (Fig. 456).

Anterior Gluteal Nerve

This nerve (N. glutæus cranialis) is derived chiefly from the last lumbar and first sacral nerves. It divides into four or five branches which emerge through the great sacro-sciatic foramen with the divisions of the anterior gluteal artery and supply the gluteal and tensor fasciæ latæ muscles. The nerve to the latter and the anterior part of the superficial gluteus passes between the deep part of the gluteus medius and the deep gluteal muscle, and is accompanied on the iliacus by branches of the external circumflex vessels.

Posterior Gluteal Nerve

The **posterior gluteal nerve** (N. glutæus caudalis) is derived mainly from the sacral roots of the lumbo-sacral plexus (Figs. 451, 526). It divides into two trunks which emerge above the great sciatic nerve. The upper nerve passes backward on the sacro-sciatic ligament and divides into branches which enter the two heads of the biceps femoris; it supplies a branch to the posterior part of the middle gluteus, and a nerve which turns around the posterior border of the latter and enters the posterior head of the superficial gluteus. The inferior nerve runs downward and backward on the sacro-sciatic ligament and divides into the **posterior cutaneous nerve** and muscular branches which supply the semitendinosus. The former (N. cutaneus femoris caudalis) passes through the biceps femoris, emerges between that muscle and the semitendinosus a little below the level of the tuber ischii, and ramifies subcutaneously on the outer and posterior surfaces of the hip and thigh (Fig. 525).

Great Sciatic Nerve

The **great sciatic nerve** (N. ischiadicus) (Figs. 451, 455, 526), the largest in the body, is derived chiefly from the last lumbar and the sacral roots of the lumbo-sacral plexus, but may receive a fasciculus from the third sacral nerve also. It

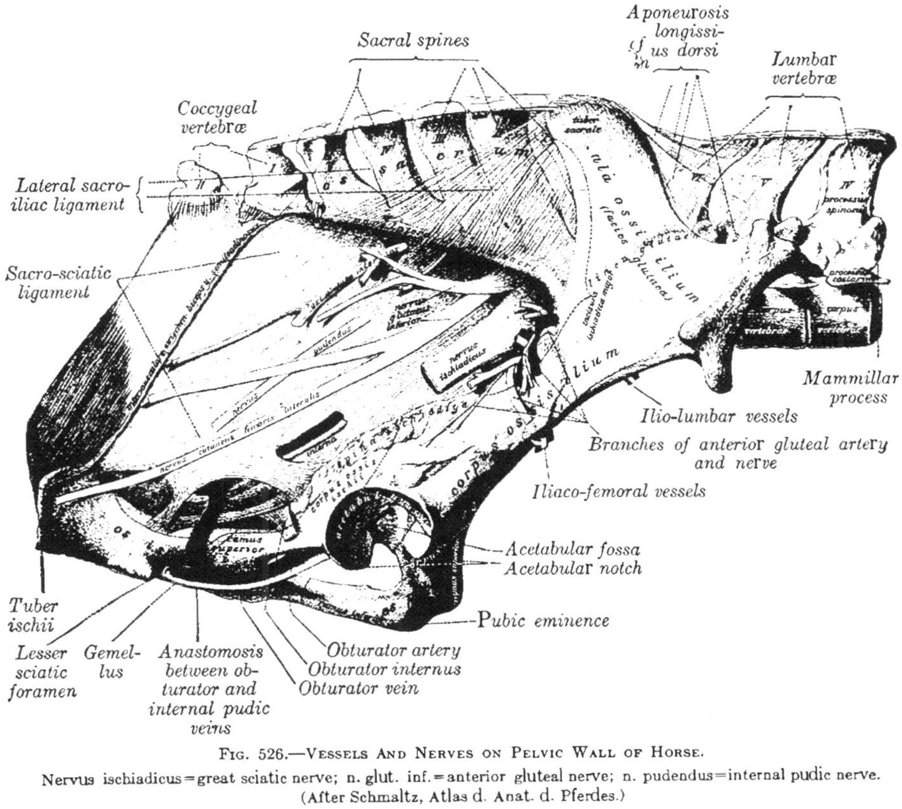

Fig. 526.—Vessels and Nerves on Pelvic Wall of Horse.
Nervus ischiadicus=great sciatic nerve; n. glut. inf.=anterior gluteal nerve; n. pudendus=internal pudic nerve. (After Schmaltz, Atlas d. Anat. d. Pferdes.)

emerges through the great sacro-sciatic foramen as a broad flat band—blended at first with the posterior gluteal nerve—which passes downward and backward on the lower part of the sacro-sciatic ligament and on the origin of the deep gluteus muscle. It turns downward in the hollow between the trochanter major and the tuber ischii over the gemellus, the tendon of the obturator internus, and the quadratus femoris. In its descent in the thigh it lies between the biceps femoris externally and the adductor, semimembranosus, and semitendinosus internally, and it is continued between the two heads of the gastrocnemius as the tibial nerve. Its chief branches are as follows:

1. In the pelvic part of its course the sciatic nerve supplies small branches to the obturator internus, gemellus, and quadratus femoris; the branch to the obturator internus reaches the muscle by passing through the anterior end of the lesser sacro-sciatic foramen.

2. As the sciatic nerve turns down behind the hip joint it gives off a large branch (Ramus muscularis proximalis) which divides to supply the semimembranosus and the short heads of the biceps femoris and semitendinosus.

3. The **posterior cutaneous nerve** of the leg or **external saphenous nerve** (N. cutaneus suræ posterior) is detached from the sciatic about the middle of the thigh. It receives a fasciculus from the peroneal nerve and descends with the recurrent tarsal vein on the outer face of the gastrocnemius to the distal third of the leg. Here it perforates the deep fascia and ramifies under the skin on the outer surface of the tarsus and metatarsus (Fig. 525).

4. The **peroneal** or **external popliteal nerve** (N. peronæus) (Figs. 455, 460, 527) is a large trunk which arises from the great sciatic nerve very shortly after the latter emerges from the pelvic cavity. It descends with the parent trunk to the origin of the gastrocnemius; here the peroneal nerve deviates outward and forward across the external face of the gastrocnemius under cover of the biceps femoris, and divides at the origin of the lateral extensor muscle into superficial and deep branches. The collateral branches include a twig to the biceps femoris, the reinforcing fasciculus detached about the middle of the thigh to the posterior cutaneous nerve, and, lower down, the **external cutaneous nerve** of the leg (Ramus cutaneus suræ lateralis). The latter, also known as the peroneal cutaneous nerve, emerges between the middle and posterior divisions of the biceps femoris at the level of the stifle joint and ramifies under the skin. The **superficial peroneal** or **musculo-cutaneous nerve** (N. peronæus superficialis) furnishes branches to the lateral extensor, and descends in the furrow between that muscle and the anterior extensor, perforates the deep fascia of the leg, and ramifies under the skin on the front and the outer face of the tarsus and metatarsus. The **deep peroneal** or **anterior tibial nerve** (N. peronæus profundus) is the direct continuation in point of size of the peroneal trunk. It dips in between the lateral and anterior extensors of the digit, gives branches to these muscles and the tibialis anterior, and descends in front of the intermuscular septum which separates the former. It continues downward behind the tendon of the anterior extensor and divides on the front of the hock into internal and external branches. The **internal branch** (Ramus medialis) passes down under the skin on the anterior face of the metatarsus and supplies the cutaneous fibers of this region. The **external branch** (Ramus lateralis) furnishes a twig to the extensor brevis muscle and descends with the great metatarsal artery. It supplies the skin on the outer face of the metatarsus and the fetlock.

In the greater part of its course in the leg the deep peroneal nerve is separated from the anterior tibial vessels by the tibialis anterior (muscular part of the flexor metatarsi). It should be noted that the outer of the two veins which almost always accompany the artery here is frequently very large, and the layer of muscle which intervenes between it and the nerve is often exceedingly thin. In the distal part of the leg the nerve is in direct contact with the vein, and on the front of the hock it lies behind the vessels.

Tibial Nerve

The **tibial nerve** (N. tibialis), also termed the posterior tibial, is the direct continuation of the great sciatic nerve (Figs. 451, 455, 458, 459, 527). It passes down between the two heads of the gastrocnemius, and accompanies the recurrent tibial vessels to the distal third of the leg, where it divides into internal and external plantar nerves. In the upper third of the leg it lies along the inner side of the superficial flexor under cover of the internal head of the gastrocnemius; lower down it is covered by the common deep fascia and is situated in the space between the deep flexor and the inner border of the tendo Achillis.

At the usual point of election for tibial neurectomy, *i. e.*, about a handbreadth above the level of the tuber calcis, the nerve lies in areolar tissue and fat in a fascial compartment formed by the special fascia of the deep flexor in front and by the common fascia and the accessory or tarsal tendon of the semitendinosus and biceps femoris behind and internally.

At its origin the tibial nerve gives off a **muscular branch** (Ramus muscularis distalis), the divisions of which pass between the two heads of the gastrocnemius and radiate to supply that muscle, the popliteus, the soleus, and the flexors of the digit. Small cutaneous twigs are also detached along the course of the nerve.

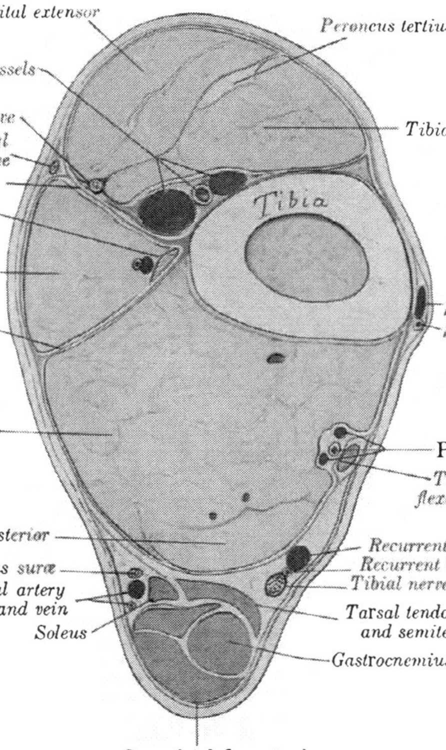

Fig. 527.—Cross-section of Distal Third of Left Leg of Horse.
The deep fascia is shown by red line.

Plantar Nerves

The **plantar nerves,** internal and external (N. plantaris medialis, lateralis), result from the bifurcation of the tibial nerve in the lower part of the leg (Figs. 458, 459). They continue at first in the same direction and relations as the parent trunk, in direct apposition and inclosed in a common sheath. At the hock they diverge at a very acute angle and descend in the tarsal canal behind the deep flexor tendon in company with the plantar arteries. The internal plantar nerve supplies cutaneous nerves to the inner aspect of the tarsus and metatarsus, descends along the inner border of the flexor tendons behind the superficial plantar metatarsal vessels, and is otherwise arranged like the corresponding volar nerve of the fore limb. The external plantar nerve deviates outward between the two flexor tendons to reach their outer border. It supplies a branch to the suspensory ligament, and in its further course resembles the corresponding nerve of the fore limb.

In so-called "tibial" neurectomy the operator really cuts the two plantar nerves which have not yet separated. The anastomotic branch between the two plantar nerves is smaller than that which connects the corresponding nerves of the fore limb, and is absent in 30 per cent. of the cases, according to Rudert.

Sacral Nerves

Five pairs of sacral nerves (Nn. sacrales) are present in the horse.

The small dorsal branches emerge through the dorsal sacral foramina and the space between the sacrum and the first coccygeal vertebra, and ramify in the muscles and skin of the sacral region and the adjacent part of the tail (Fig. 525). The fifth anastomoses with the dorsal branch of the first coccygeal nerve.

The ventral branches leave the vertebral canal through the ventral sacral foramina and the interval between the sacrum and first coccygeal vertebra. They are connected with the sympathetic by rami communicantes, and contribute branches to the pelvic plexus. The first and second are the largest, and unite with each other and with those of the last three lumbar nerves to form the lumbo-sacral plexus. The third and fourth are connected with each other, and the majority of their fibers go to form the pudic and posterior hæmorrhoidal nerves.

The pudic nerve (N. pudendus) (Figs. 451, 455, 526) accompanies the internal pudic artery to the ischial arch, turns around the latter, parting company with the artery, and pursues a flexuous course along the dorsum penis as the nervus dorsalis penis and ramifies in the glans and the penile layer of the prepuce. Within the pelvis it anastomoses with the posterior hæmorrhoidal nerve, and gives branches to the bladder and urethra, the terminal part of the rectum, and the skin and muscles of the anus (Fig. 452). It also supplies the nerve to the ischio-cavernosus muscle and numerous branches to the corpus cavernosum and corpus spongiosum. In the female it terminates in the clitoris and vulva (Fig. 453).

The posterior hæmorrhoidal nerve (N. hæmorrhoidalis caudalis) passes downward and backward above the pudic nerve, with which it anastomoses. It gives twigs to the terminal part of the rectum, the sphincter ani externus, and the surrounding skin (Fig. 452). In the female it supplies twigs to the vulva also (Fig. 453).

The ventral branch of the fifth nerve is small. It gives twigs to the sacrococcygeus ventralis lateralis and the skin of the root of the tail and joins the first coccygeal nerve.

Coccygeal Nerves

The coccygeal nerves (Nn. coccygei) commonly number five pairs. Their dorsal and ventral branches anastomose to form respectively two trunks on either side, which extend to the tip of the tail and supply its muscular and cutaneous nerves. The dorsal trunk runs with the dorso-lateral artery between the sacrococcygeus dorsalis and intertransversales muscles (Fig. 454). The ventral trunk accompanies the ventro-lateral artery below the intertransversales.

The Sympathetic Nervous System[1]

The sympathetic nervous system (Systema nervorum sympathicum) is that part of the nervous system which serves (1) to transmit stimuli to the heart-muscle, unstriped muscle, and glands; (2) to conduct impulses from the viscera to the cerebrospinal system.

Many of the fibers are derived from the cerebrospinal system and are rearranged and distributed in the sympathetic system. Numerous sympathetic fibers are contributed to the cerebro-

[1] The special statements of this description refer to the system of the horse. A few important differential features will be mentioned in the account of the nervous system of the other animals.

spinal nerves, through which they are distributed to the unstriped muscular tissue and glands, as vasomotor, pilomotor, and secretory nerves. The sympathetic, like the cerebrospinal system, consists of **neurones**, each of which comprises the cell-body, an axone, and numerous branched dendrites. The cell-bodies are aggregated into **ganglia**, some of which are large and more or less constant in position and form, while others are microscopic and are scattered in an irregular manner through the peripheral part of the system. It is probable that simple visceral reflexes may be mediated by sympathetic neurones alone.

In descriptive anatomy the sympathetic system is regarded as consisting of (1) a chain of **ganglia** extending along either side of the vertebral column and connected by association fibers to form the sympathetic **trunk**; (2) **central branches** to and from the cerebrospinal nerves; (3) **peripheral branches**, which form plexuses with each other and the cerebrospinal nerves; (4) the **peripheral ganglia** which are interposed in the plexuses.

The **sympathetic trunk** (Truncus sympathicus) extends on either side from the base of the cranium to the tail. In it are interposed, at intervals of varying regularity, the **ganglia of the sympathetic trunk** (Ganglia trunci sympathici). These are connected with the cerebrospinal nerves by central branches, the **rami communicantes.**

Two kinds of rami communicantes occur. Of these, one type consists largely of medullated fibers derived from the spinal nerves and ganglia; they have therefore a white appearance, and are termed **white rami.** They contain both efferent and afferent fibers. The **efferent splanchnic fibers** are derived from the ventral roots of the spinal nerves and terminate in great part about the cells of the nearest sympathetic ganglion; others end in more distant or in peripheral ganglia. The **afferent splanchnic fibers** are chiefly peripheral processes of the cells of the spinal ganglia, but some are sympathetic fibers which enter the spinal nerve-trunk and terminate about cells of the spinal ganglion. The **gray rami** consist mainly of non-medullated fibers derived from the sympathetic ganglia directly or through the trunk, which proceed centrally to the spinal nerves and are distributed along the somatic divisions of the latter to unstriped muscle and glands as **vasomotor, pilomotor,** and **secretory fibers.** Some go to the membranes of the spinal cord, and a few terminate about cells of the spinal ganglia as sensory sympathetic fibers.

Similar but more complex and irregular communications which exist between the sympathetic system and the cranial nerves—with the exception of the first and second—have been referred to in the accounts of the latter.

It is convenient for descriptive purposes to divide the sympathetic system into cephalic, cervical, thoracic, abdominal, and pelvic parts.

1. The **cephalic part** (Pars cephalica systematis sympathici) comprises the **otic, sphenopalatine,** and **ciliary ganglia,** which may be regarded as homologues of the ganglia of the trunk of other regions. It also includes three plexuses formed by branches derived from the superior cervical ganglion. The ganglion gives off two or three filaments which subdivide to form the **internal carotid plexus** around the artery of like name. The cavernous plexus surrounds the artery within the cavernous sinus and communicates with that of the opposite side. The **external carotid plexus** is formed around the homonymous artery, and filaments from it go to the vessel and its branches and to the salivary glands.

2. The **cervical part** (Pars cervicalis s. sympathici) includes two ganglia and the trunk which connects them.

The **superior** or **anterior cervical ganglion** (G. cervicale craniale) lies on the guttural pouch below the occipito-atlantal articulation (Fig. 437). It is reddish-gray in color, fusiform, and about an inch (ca. 2 to 3 cm.) in length. It is connected by rami communicantes with the last four cranial and first cervical nerves, sends branches to form the plexuses mentioned above, and contributes to the pharyngeal plexus.

The **cervical trunk** of the sympathetic connects the superior and inferior cervical ganglia. On leaving the former it is associated in a common sheath with the vagus along the dorsal face of the common carotid artery. At the root of the neck it separates from the vagus and joins the inferior ganglion.

The **inferior** or **posterior cervical ganglion** (G. cervicale caudale) is situated under the first rib and the insertion of the scalenus (Figs. 428, 429). On the right side it lies upon the longus colli and the trachea, on the left side upon the same muscle and the œsophagus. It is flattened, very irregular and variable in outline, and is blended more or less with the first thoracic ganglion. It is connected by large gray rami with the ventral branches of the last two cervical nerves, and by small filaments with the recurrent nerve. It receives a nerve—termed by Schmaltz the nervus transversarius—which accompanies the vertebral artery; through it rami come from the second to the sixth cervical nerves inclusive.

A middle cervical ganglion may be present, and occurs oftenest on the right side. It lies on the carotid artery an inch or two in front of the first rib and is intercalated in the vago-sympathetic trunk.

The cardiac nerves (Nn. cardiaci) are formed by branches from the inferior cervical and first thoracic ganglia, together with twigs from the sympathetic trunks and the vagi. They form a plexus (P. cardiacus) on the ventral face of the trachea with each other and with branches of the vagus and recurrent nerves. They are subject to considerable variation, but their general arrangement may be stated as follows:

(*a*) On the right side there are usually two cardiac nerves. Of these one passes back with the vagus in the angle between the right brachial artery and the common carotid trunk, pierces the pericardium, crosses the aortic arch, and divides into branches which are mingled with those of the left nerves. The second crosses obliquely over the right face of the trachea and joins the vagus, where the latter gives off the right recurrent nerve; a small plexus is formed here, from which two or three cardiac branches are detached. These pass back beneath the trachea and ramify on the atria and ventricles.

(*b*) On the left side there are commonly three cardiac nerves. One of these is distributed to the great vessels in the anterior mediastinum. The largest passes back at first with the vagus beneath the arch of the left brachial artery, inclines downward, perforates the pericardium, and divides into two branches. One branch passes beneath the bifurcation of the pulmonary artery and is distributed to the left atrium. The larger branch dips in between the aorta and the pulmonary artery, gives twigs to these vessels, and ramifies on the ventricles, especially along the course of the right coronary artery. The third nerve crosses the deep face of the left brachial artery, passes back below the trachea, and unites with filaments of a right cardiac nerve. It passes around the aorta and ramifies chiefly along the course of the left coronary artery on the left face of the ventricles.

3. The thoracic part (Pars thoracalis systematis sympathici) extends below the costo-vertebral joints from the inferior cervical ganglion to the upper border of the diaphragm, and passes between the latter and the psoas minor to be continued by the abdominal part.

The trunk is concealed in the first part of its course by the outer border of the longus colli, but further back it is visible under the pleura.

The ganglia are arranged segmentally at each intercostal space and partly on the heads of the ribs. They are flattened and are small and fusiform, with the exception of the first. This (G. thoracale primum) is extensive, irregularly quadrilateral in outline, and is united with the inferior cervical ganglion. The ganglia are connected with the thoracic nerves by white and gray rami communicantes.

The visceral branches comprise aortic, cardiac, pulmonary, and œsophageal branches, and the splanchnic nerves. The aortic branches ramify on the thoracic artery, forming around that vessel the thoracic aortic plexus (P. aorticus thoracalis). The cardiac branches concur with those of the vagus in forming the cardiac plexus (P. cardiacus). From this branches go to form the coronary plexuses (P. coronarii) along the course of the vessels of like name. The pulmonary branches join with corresponding branches of the vagus and filaments from the cardiac plexus in forming the pulmonary plexus (P. pulmonalis) at the root of the lung. Branches of the plexus, on which are minute ganglia, ramify with the bronchi in the substance of the lung.[1] The **œsophageal branches** join with those of the vagus in the formation of the **œsophageal plexus** (P. œsophageus).

The **great splanchnic nerve** (N. splanchnicus major) arises by a series of roots derived from the sixth or seventh to the fifteenth or sixteenth thoracic ganglia inclusive. It extends at first along the inner side of the thoracic trunk, then crosses the latter ventrally, passes back between the crus of the diaphragm and the outer border of the psoas minor, and joins the cœliac ganglion. It is small at its origin, but becomes considerably larger than the sympathetic trunk. Near its termination it bears the small **splanchnic ganglion**, from which and from the nerve, filaments go to the aorta, the œsophagus, and the vertebræ.

The **small splanchnic nerve** (N. splanchnicus minor) is formed by roots derived from the last two or three thoracic ganglia. It runs back with the great splanchnic nerve, but ends in the cœliac or in the renal and adrenal plexuses.

This nerve is not always present and is variable in arrangement. The roots communicate by filaments with the great splanchnic.

4. The **abdominal part** of the sympathetic trunk (Pars abdominalis systematis sympathici) lies along the inner border of the psoas minor, above the aorta on the left side and the posterior vena cava on the right (Fig. 524). The trunk is smaller than the thoracic part, and presents usually six small fusiform **lumbar ganglia** (G. lumbalia), which are connected by rami communicantes with the ventral divisions of the lumbar nerves. Visceral branches go to the aortic and hypogastric plexuses, and to the cœliac and mesenteric ganglia.

5. The **pelvic part** of the sympathetic trunk (Pars pelvina systematis sympathici) begins at the last lumbar ganglion and extends along the pelvic surface of the sacrum internal to the emergence of the ventral branches of the sacral nerves (Fig. 451). At the third segment of the sacrum the trunk divides into internal and external branches. The internal branch inclines to the median plane and unites with the opposite branch. At the junction there is often found the small **coccygeal ganglion** (G. impar), which lies on the coccygeal artery at the joint between the first and second coccygeal vertebræ. A filament from the ganglion accompanies the artery. The external branch communicates with the last two sacral nerves and joins the ventral coccygeal nerves. Ganglia occur near each of the first three sacral foramina, and are connected by gray rami communicantes with the adjacent spinal nerves. The visceral branches are distributed through the hypogastric plexus. They supply motor fibers to the longitudinal and inhibitory fibers to the circular muscular coat of the rectum, motor fibers to the bladder and uterus, and the vaso-dilator fibers (Nn. erigentes) to the penis.

THE ABDOMINAL AND PELVIC PLEXUSES

The chief plexuses which distribute nerves to the viscera and vessels of the abdominal and pelvic cavities are two in number, the solar and the pelvic. From them fibers proceed to form numerous subsidiary plexuses which are named according to the organs which they supply or the vessels which they enlace.

The Solar Plexus

The **solar plexus** (Fig. 450) is situated on the dorsal wall of the abdominal cavity in relation to the aorta and the origin of its chief visceral branches. It comprises the cœliaco-mesenteric ganglia and the cœliac and anterior mesenteric plexuses.

[1] The right and left plexuses communicate with each other, so that both lungs receive fibers from both vagi.

The **cœliaco-mesenteric ganglia**[1] are two in number, right and left. They are situated on each side of the aorta, in relation to the origin of the cœliac and anterior mesenteric arteries. The right ganglion is concealed by the posterior vena cava; it is irregularly quadrilateral and is about two inches (4 to 6 cm.) in length. The left ganglion is largely covered by the left adrenal; it is narrower than the right one and is three or four inches (ca. 8 to 10 cm.) long. The two ganglia are united by irregular connecting branches in front of and behind the anterior mesenteric artery.[2] Each receives the splanchnic nerve of its own side and branches from the dorsal œsophageal continuation of the vagus nerves. Branches from the ganglia and the cords which connect them pass back to the small stellate **posterior mesenteric ganglia**, which are situated at the origin of the posterior mesenteric artery.

The **cœliac plexus** (P. cœliacus) consists of a felt-work of nerve-fibers in which are small ganglia. It surrounds the cœliac artery and from it proceed the following unpaired secondary plexuses which accompany the arterial branches:

1. The **gastric plexus** (P. gastricus) enlaces the gastric artery and divides like the artery into two parts, forming the anterior and posterior gastric plexuses. These receive branches of the vagus nerves.

2. The **hepatic plexus** (P. hepaticus) is formed by several nerves of considerable size which accompany the hepatic artery and the portal vein. It receives fibers from the left vagus, ramifies in the liver, and gives off branches which accompany the collateral branches of the hepatic artery and supply the areas in which these vessels are distributed.

3. The **splenic plexus** (P. lienalis) resembles the preceding in its arrangement. In addition to its terminal branches to the spleen, it gives collateral twigs to the pancreas and the left part of the greater curvature of the stomach.

The **anterior mesenteric plexus** (P. mesentericus cranialis) is formed mainly by branches from the posterior part of the cœliaco-mesenteric ganglia; it is continuous with the cœliac plexus in front and the posterior mesenteric behind. It surrounds the anterior mesenteric trunk and its branches, and supplies the viscera to which these vessels are distributed.

The **posterior mesenteric plexus** (P. mesentericus caudalis) accompanies the artery of like name in its distribution.

The secondary plexuses which accompany the branches of the mesenteric arteries give off branches which form two fine peripheral plexuses in the wall of the intestine. One of these, the **myenteric plexus** (P. myentericus) or plexus of Auerbach, lies between the layers of the muscular coat, and is provided with microscopic ganglia. The other is in the submucous tissue, and is therefore termed the **submucous plexus** (P. submucosus) or plexus of Meissner.

The following paired plexuses are derived mainly from branches of the cœliac and aortic plexuses:

1. The **renal plexuses** (P. renales) proceed largely from the cœliaco-mesenteric ganglia, but receive fibers also from the small splanchnic nerves. They enlace the renal arteries and supply the kidneys. Minute renal ganglia occur on the course of the nerves along the renal vessels.

2. The **adrenal plexuses** (P. suprarenales) are formed by a relatively very large number of fine fibers derived in great part directly from the cœliaco-mesenteric ganglia. Numerous minute ganglia occur in their meshes.

3 *a*. The **spermatic plexuses** (P. spermatici) proceed largely from the aortic and renal plexuses. Each accompanies the corresponding (internal) spermatic artery to the testicle.

3 *b*. The **utero-ovarian plexuses** (P. ovarici) are the homologues in the female

[1] It has been customary to designate these in veterinary works as the semilunar or cœliac ganglia, but in the horse they evidently include the anterior mesenteric ganglia as well.

[2] A good preparation of the ganglia in the horse is often difficult to obtain on account of aneurysm of the artery and the formation of a quantity of connective tissue about it.

of the preceding. They accompany the utero-ovarian arteries to the ovary and the cornua of the uterus.

The **hypogastric** or **pelvic plexus** (P. hypogastricus) is the pelvic continuation of the aortic and posterior mesenteric plexuses. The chief nerves which form it enter the pelvic cavity ventral to the large vessels, anastomose with each other and with branches from the third and fourth sacral nerves, and ramify on the pelvic viscera. The peripheral plexuses derived therefrom are named according to the organs which they supply; the chief of these are the **hæmorrhoidal, vesical, utero-vaginal, prostatic, cavernous** (of the penis or clitoris).

THE NERVOUS SYSTEM OF THE OX[1]

The **spinal cord** resembles that of the horse in conformation and structure. In cattle of medium size its length is about 165 to 170 cm. (ca. 65 to 67 inches) and its weight about 240 to 250 grams (ca. 8 ounces).

In a cow 140 cm. in height Dexler found the weight of the cord (including the intradural nerve-roots) to be 260 g. and the length 162 cm. The lengths of the regions were: cervical 41 cm., thoracic 72 cm., lumbar 32 cm., sacral 7 cm.

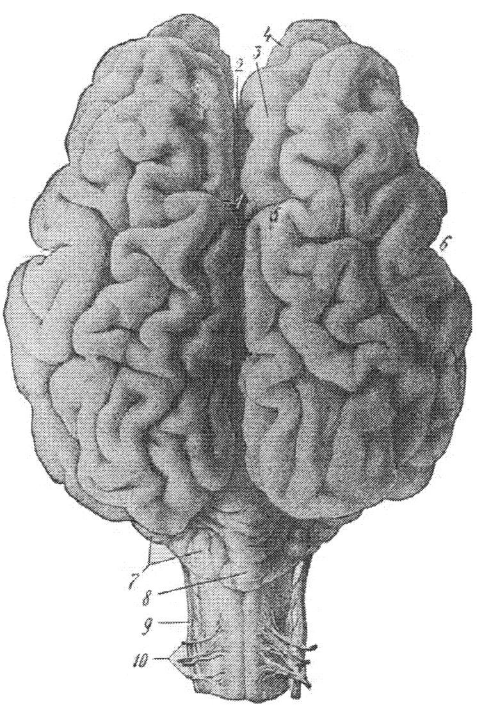

Fig. 528.—Brain of Cow, Dorsal View.

1, Sulcus transversus; *2*, longitudinal fissure; *3*, antero-internal frontal gyrus; *4*, olfactory bulb; *5*, marginal or sagittal pole of hemisphere; *6*, lateral fissure (of Sylvius); *7*, hemisphere of cerebellum; *8*, vermis of same; *9*, accessory nerve; *10*, dorsal root of first cervical nerve. (Ellenberger-Baum, Anat. d. Haustiere.)

The **brain** has an average weight of about 500 grams (ca. 16 to 17 ounces). Its differences in general form are correlated with those noted in the consideration of the cranial cavity.

The **medulla** is short, wide, and thick. Its ventral face is strongly convex. The pyramids are narrow, short, and close together in front. Near the decussation there is a well-defined oval prominence on either side which indicates the position of the posterior olive. The corpus trapezoideum is large; it has no central part between the pyramids. The external arcuate fibers are distinct. The restiform bodies are short and thick and diverge more strongly than in the horse. The floor of the fourth ventricle is only about two-thirds as long as in the horse. The area acustica is a well-marked oval prominence lateral to the middle part of the limiting sulcus. The tuberculum acusticum at the origin of the auditory nerve is very large. The anterior fovea is distinct. The posterior recess of the fourth ventricle communicates through the foramen of Magendie (Apertura mediana) with the subarachnoid space.

[1] Only the most salient differences as compared with the horse will be mentioned.

The pons is smaller, both transversely and longitudinally, than that of the horse. It is strongly convex and has a distinct central depression.

The cerebellum is smaller and more angular in form than in the horse. The vermis is large and has a distinct depression on its anterior face for the posterior corpora quadrigemina. The hemispheres are relatively small and are not clearly divided into tabulations. The anterior peduncles are very short.

The cerebral peduncles are short. A small eminence in the locus perforatus posticus is caused by the presence of the interpeduncular ganglion. The internal geniculate body is prominent. The pineal body is long and fusiform, and is often pigmented in spots. The third ventricle forms two considerable recesses in relation to the pineal body: one (R. pinealis) extends up into the body; the other (R. suprapinealis) is a long tubular prolongation in front of it.

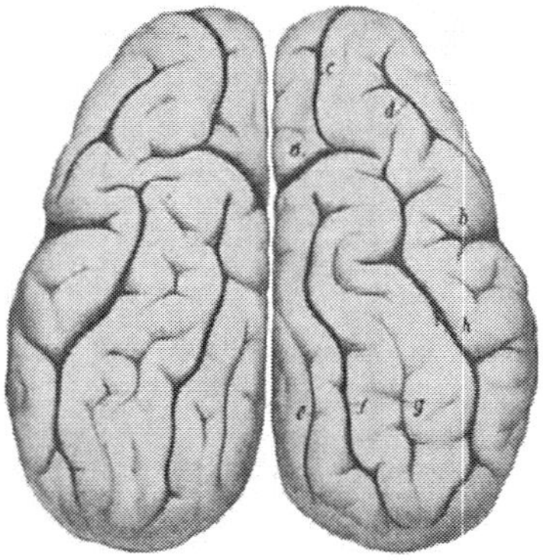

FIG. 529.—CEREBRAL HEMISPHERES OF OX, DORSAL VIEW.

a, Transverse fissure; b, lateral fissure (of Sylvius); c, coronal fissure; d, diagonal fissure; e, entomarginal fissure; f, marginal fissure; g, ectomarginal fissure; h, suprasylvian fissure. (After Ellenberger, in Leisering's Atlas.)

The optic tracts cross the cerebral peduncles almost at a right angle.

The pituitary body is situated in a deep fossa and is surrounded by a plexus of vessels.

The cerebral hemispheres are shorter, higher, and relatively wider than in the horse. The frontal poles are small, the occipital large. Viewed from the side, the dorsal surface is strongly convex. The highest point of the dorso-medial border is a little in front of its middle and forms a marked prominence termed the sagittal or marginal pole (Polus sagittalis s. prominentia marginalis dorsalis). Anterior to this the border drops abruptly, being cut into by the deep transverse fissure. The arachnoid on the basal and anterior parts of the hemispheres is usually pigmented. The corpus callosum extends through a little more than a third of the length of the hemisphere. The pattern of the fissures and gyri of the pallium is somewhat simpler than in the horse.

1. The lateral fissure (of Sylvius) is very deep. Its middle branch extends almost vertically upward on the middle of the lateral surface of the hemisphere, and is separated by a gyrus of variable width from the suprasylvian fissure. The anterior branch runs forward about parallel with the sulcus rhinalis anterior, from which it is separated by the short gyri of the insula. The latter are covered to a small extent only by the overhanging gyri (operculum). The posterior branch may run back a distance of only about 1.5 cm. and end in T-shaped manner, or it may join the sulcus rhinalis posterior.

2. The suprasylvian fissure is deep and very distinct. It extends in an undulating manner from the lateral surface of the occipital pole to the outer side of the sagittal pole. Here it may be interrupted or may be continued by the coronal fissure, which descends to the frontal pole and divides into two short branches.

3. The diagonal fissure (S. diagonalis) begins in front of the stem of the lateral fissure and runs upward and forward. Its form is very variable.

4. The transverse fissure cuts obliquely into the dorsal border in front of the sagittal pole. It is short and deep and commonly communicates with the suprasylvian and coronal fissures.

5. The marginal fissure is distinct. It extends from the sagittal pole to the occipital pole. It is flexuous and deviates outward somewhat in its posterior two-thirds.

6. The entomarginal fissure lies medial and parallel to the posterior part of the preceding.

7. The ectomarginal fissure is lateral and parallel to the marginal fissure. It does not extend so far in either direction as the latter and is often more or less broken up by annectent gyri.

8. The sulcus rhinalis is more open than in the horse, since it is not overlapped by the gyri above it.

9. The calloso-marginal fissure is flexuous and not so regular as in the horse. It is often

interrupted at or near the level of the genu of the corpus callosum, in which case the **genual fissure** continues it downward.

10. The **crucial fissure** is faint and is confined to the medial surface. It lies about one centimeter in front of the transverse fissure and commonly joins the calloso-marginal fissure below.

11. Short and variable fissures occur in front of and behind the middle branch of the lateral fissure (F. ectosylvia anterior, posterior).

The **olfactory bulb** is much smaller than in the horse. The external olfactory tract is large, the inner one small and not distinct.

The **cranial nerves** have in general the same superficial origin as in the horse. The more important differences in other respects are as follows:

The **oculomotor nerve** is larger than in the horse. It emerges with the fourth, sixth, ophthalmic, and maxillary nerves through the large foramen, which is equivalent to the foramen lacerum orbitale and foramen rotundum of the horse.

The internal branch of the **lacrimal nerve** supplies twigs to the mucous membrane of the frontal sinus; the large outer branch runs backward and supplies the matrix of the horn. The **frontal nerve** emerges from the orbit below the supraorbital process. The **naso-ciliary nerve** is large and sends filaments to the ocular muscles. The **ciliary ganglion** is somewhat larger than in the horse and is connected with the lower division of the oculomotor nerve by several short filaments. In consequence of the absence of the canine and upper incisor teeth the corresponding branch of the infraorbital nerve is naturally wanting. The **mandibular nerve** emerges through the foramen ovale. The **superficial temporal nerve** gives off a large branch which joins the superior buccal division of the facial on the masseter, about half-way between the zygomatic arch and the angle of the jaw. The **otic ganglion** is larger than in the horse. According to Moussu the buccinator nerve furnishes excito-secretory twigs to the parotid and inferior buccal glands.

The **facial nerve** divides into its two terminal branches before reaching the border of the jaw. The **superior buccal nerve** is the larger of the two; it crosses the masseter much lower than in the horse. The relatively small **inferior buccal nerve** runs beneath the parotid or in the gland substance parallel with the border of the lower jaw, crosses under the insertion of the sterno-cephalicus, and runs forward along the depressor labii inferioris. At the point where it crosses the facial vein and parotid duct it gives off an anastomotic branch to the superior nerve. The **auriculo-palpebral** nerve is large.

The **vagus** bears—in addition to the relatively large **jugular ganglion**—a **ganglion nodosum** at the point of origin of the superior laryngeal nerve. The trunk is large. The **pharyngeal branch** is large and anastomoses with the superior and external laryngeal nerves. The latter commonly arises directly from the trunk. The **superior œsophageal trunk** communicates with the splanchnic nerve, contributes twigs to the hepatic plexus, and ramifies chiefly on the right surface of the rumen and the adjacent surface of the abomasum. The **inferior œsophageal trunk** supplies branches to the hepatic plexus and to all the divisions of the stomach.

The **spinal accessory nerve** presents two special features. The part which joins the jugular ganglion bears a small ganglion. The ventral branch supplies both parts of the sterno-cephalicus.

The **hypoglossal nerve** is large. It is connected with the ventral division of the first cervical nerve by a branch of considerable size, and detaches a long branch which runs backward along the carotid artery

The **spinal nerves** resemble those of the horse in origin and general arrangement. The thoracic nerves number thirteen pairs. The more important differences in the limb-plexuses and their branches are as follows:

The **brachial plexus** is formed by the ventral branches of the last three cervical and first thoracic nerves; the second thoracic nerve furnishes no root, but the ventral branch of the sixth cervical goes almost entirely to the plexus after giving off the nerve to the rhomboideus and the cervical part of the serratus magnus.

The differences in the nerves above the elbow are not of sufficient moment to receive notice in this brief account, but below this point there are naturally important special features correlated chiefly with the arrangement of the digits.

The **radial nerve** is continued below the elbow by a large **cutaneous branch** (N. cutaneus antibrachii dorsalis) which emerges at the lower border of the exter

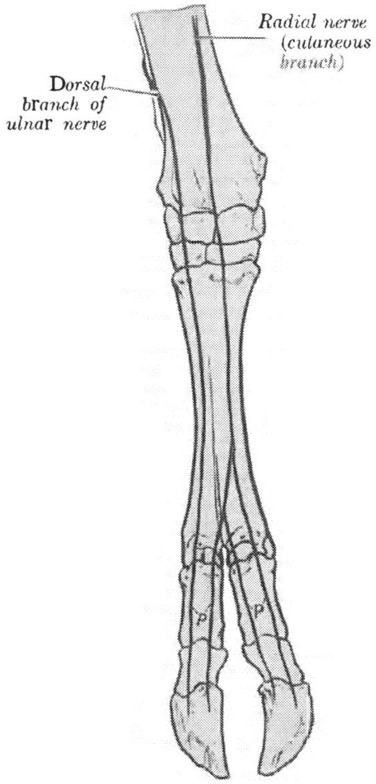

Fig. 530.—Nerves of Distal Part of Right Fore Limb of Ox, Anterior View (Schematic).
p, Dorsal digital nerves.

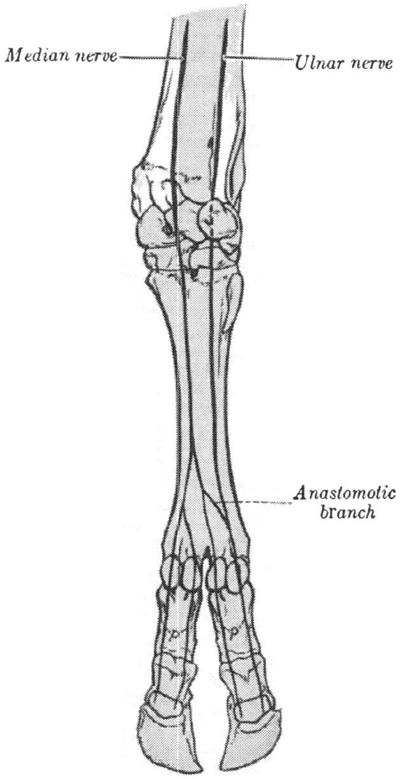

Fig. 531.—Nerves of Distal Part of Right Fore Limb of Ox, Posterior View (Schematic).
p, Volar digital nerves.

nal head of the triceps and descends on the dorsal aspect of the limb. It communicates above the carpus with the cutaneous branch of the median nerve and terminates in three **dorsal digital nerves**; two of these descend along the axial or interdigital side of the dorsal surface of the chief digits, and the third along the inner (abaxial) side of the inner chief digit.

The **ulnar nerve** divides at a variable distance down the forearm into two branches. The dorsal or **superficial branch** emerges between the tendons of the external and middle flexors of the carpus, and is continued as the **external dorsal digital nerve** on the outer chief digit. The volar or **deep branch** descends along the superficial digital flexor, gives a branch to the suspensory ligament below the carpus, and unites with the external branch of the median nerve to form the **external volar digital nerve.**

The **median nerve** is much larger than the ulnar. It passes beneath the pronator teres, descends the forearm as in the horse, and divides in the distal part of the metacarpus into two branches. The **internal branch** gives twigs to the inner small digit and is continued on the inner side of the volar surface of the inner chief digit as the **internal volar digital nerve** (N. digitalis medialis digiti III); it also concurs with the outer branch in forming the two digital nerves which descend along the interdigital aspect of the chief digits. The **external branch** is larger. It bifurcates,

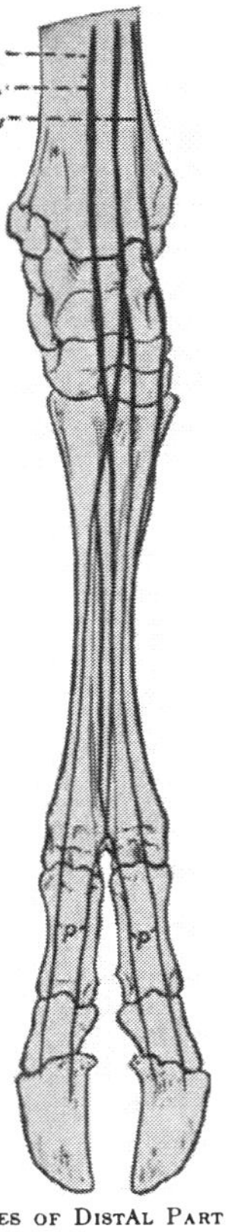

FIG. 532.—NERVES OF DISTAL PART OF RIGHT HIND LIMB OF OX, ANTERIOR VIEW (SCHEMATIC). *p*, Dorsal digital nerves.

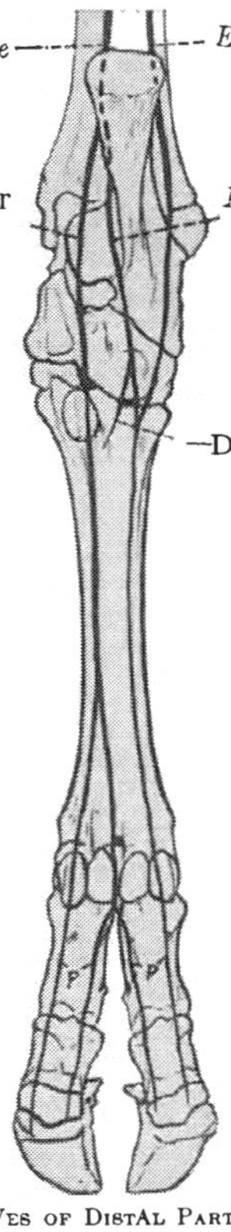

FIG. 533.—NERVES OF DISTAL PART OF RIGHT HIND LIMB OF OX, POSTERIOR VIEW (SCHEMATIC). *p*, Plantar digital nerves.

and one division unites with the twig from the internal branch to form a common digital trunk. From the latter two digital nerves proceed as mentioned above; these are the **external** and **internal** volar **digital nerves** of the internal and external chief digits respectively (N. digitalis volaris lateralis digiti III, medialis digiti IV). The other division unites with the volar branch of the ulnar nerve to form the **external** volar **digital nerve** of the external chief digit (N. digitalis lateralis digiti IV).

The **lumbo-sacral plexus** and its branches to the pelvis and thigh present no very striking special features.

The **superficial peroneal nerve** is much larger than in the horse. After crossing beneath the peroneus longus it passes down on the front of the tarsus and metatarsus and divides into three branches. The internal and external branches descend as the **internal** and **external dorsal digital nerves** on the chief digits. The larger middle branch joins a branch of the deep peroneal nerve in the interdigital space, and from this union proceed the dorsal digital nerves which descend on the opposed surfaces of the chief digits.

The **deep peroneal nerve** descends in the leg as in the horse and continues down the anterior groove of the metatarsus with the dorsal metatarsal artery. Its terminal branches concur with branches from the superficial peroneal nerve in the formation of the two axial dorsal digital **nerves** (N. dig. dors. lat. dig. III et dig. dors. med. dig. IV pedis), and with a branch of the internal plantar nerve in the formation of corresponding plantar digital nerves.

The tibial **nerve** divides at the back of the hock into internal and external plantar nerves. The **internal plantar nerve** descends between the superficial flexor tendon and the suspensory ligament and divides into two branches; the inner branch descends as the **internal plantar digital nerve** (N. dig. plant. med. dig. III) along the inner side of the flexor tendons of the inner chief digit; the outer branch turns around the flexor tendons to reach the interdigital space, where it concurs with a branch of the deep peroneal nerve in the formation of two **axial plantar digital nerves** (N. dig. plant. lat. dig. III et dig. plant. med. dig. IV) which descend on the opposed surfaces of the chief digits. The **external plantar nerve** descends along the outer border of the flexor tendons, gives a branch to the suspensory ligament and to the external small digit, and continues along the outer face of the external digit as the **external plantar digital nerve** (N. dig. plant. lat. dig. IV).

The **sympathetic system** closely resembles that of the horse in its general arrangement, and only a few differential features will receive attention. The **superior cervical ganglion** is closer to the cranial base and is thicker than in the horse; its branches to the carotid and cavernous plexuses are large, and no connection is formed with the spinal accessory nerve. The **cervical trunk** is smaller than in the horse, and arises by two or three bundles from the superior cervical ganglion behind its middle. The **inferior cervical ganglion** is distinctly separable from the first thoracic; the latter is large. There are thirteen pairs of thoracic **ganglia.** The **cœliaco-mesenteric ganglia** are plexiform, not compact. There are five pairs of **sacral ganglia,** and the right and left trunks are connected here by transverse anastomoses.

THE NERVOUS SYSTEM OF THE PIG

The **spinal cord** weighs about 42 grams (Ellenberger-Baum). It is almost circular in cross-section, except at the enlargements, where it is somewhat flattened dorsoventrally. The conus medullaris extends to the anterior part of the third sacral segment. The epidural space is occupied by a large quantity of fat.

The **brain** in adults of medium size weighs about 125 grams (ca. 4 to 4½ ounces). When viewed from above, it is seen to have an elongated oval form. The occipital poles overlie the cerebellum to a small extent only; the frontal poles are rounded and relatively large, but do not conceal the ends of the olfactory bulbs. The **medulla** is relatively broad. The cuneate tubercle is very large and is limited externally by a groove. The corpus trapezoideum is very wide laterally. The **pons** is less prominent than in the ox. The **cerebellum** is very wide and short. Its anterior face is flattened and presents a depression for the corpora quadrigemina. The vermis is large. The hemispheres consist of an inner large and an outer small part. The cerebral **peduncles** are very short. The posterior corpora quadrigemina are wide apart, rounded, and relatively large. The internal geniculate body is prominent. The **cerebral hemispheres** are somewhat bean-shaped in lateral profile, the convex border being dorsal. The arrangement of the gyri and sulci is simpler than in the horse or ox. The principal fissures are as follows:

1. The **lateral fissure** (of Sylvius) begins at the sulcus rhinalis and runs upward and somewhat backward on the depressed part of the lateral surface of the hemisphere; it appears unbranched on superficial examination, but when the gyrus which almost completely conceals the insula is raised, an anterior branch is exposed which forms the dorsal boundary of the insula.

2. The **suprasylvian fissure** pursues a curved course approximately parallel with the dorso-medial border of the hemisphere. Its posterior end is separated by a short interval from the sulcus rhinalis posterior. From its highest point a branch proceeds obliquely upward and forward, crosses the dorso-medial border, and joins the splenial fissure.

3. The **diagonal fissure** crosses the anterior part of the lateral surface. It is directed obliquely downward and backward.

4. The **coronal fissure** is constant and deep. It is directed upward and inward over the frontal pole, continues backward near the dorso-medial border, and usually ends by passing obliquely over the border to the inner surface of the hemisphere.

5. The **presylvian fissure** begins—apparently as a branch of the sulcus rhinalis anterior—about 2 cm. in front of the lateral fissure, and curves over the lateral aspect of the frontal pole.

6. The **marginal fissure** begins behind the cruciate fissure close to the dorsomedial border and extends in a gentle curve backward almost to the occipital pole.

7. The **ectomarginal fissure** lies above and nearly parallel to the posterior part of the suprasylvian fissure.

8. The **entomarginal fissure** lies along the posterior part of the dorso-medial border.

9. The **calloso-marginal fissure** consists of two separate parts. The more extensive posterior part is termed the **splenial fissure.** It extends from the tentorial aspect of the hemisphere in a direction parallel with the corpus callosum nearly to the middle of the medial surface; it is continued by the cruciate fissure and is also connected with the suprasylvian and coronal fissures by branches which pass obliquely upward and forward. The anterior part, the **genual fissure,** lies about midway between the anterior part of the corpus callosum and the dorsomedial border.

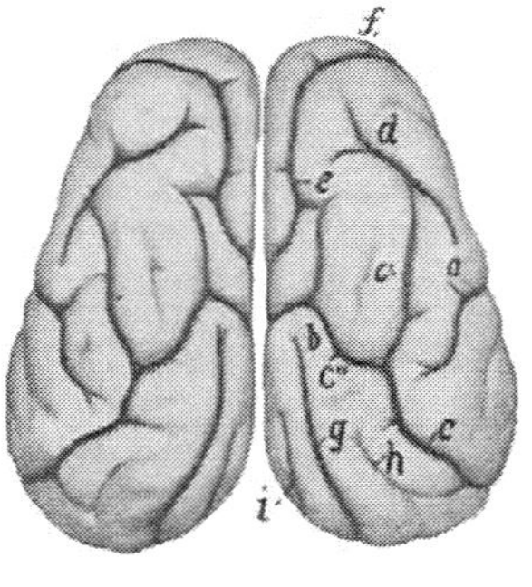

FIG. 534.—CEREBRAL HEMISPHERES OF PIG, DORSAL VIEW.

a, Upper part of lateral fissure (of Sylvius); *b*, cruciate fissure; *c*, suprasylvian fissure, with its anterior branch (*c'*) and upper branch (*c''*); *d*, diagonal fissure; *e*, coronal fissure; *f*, presylvian fissure; *g*, marginal fissure; *h*, ectomarginal fissure; *i*, entomarginal fissure. (After Ellenberger, in Leisering's Atlas.)

10. The **cruciate fissure** is short and shallow. It runs obliquely upward and forward from the anterior end of the splenial fissure on the inner surface of the hemisphere.

11. The **sulcus rhinalis** extends in an undulating manner along the entire lower part of the lateral surface of the hemisphere and forms the upper limit of the rhinencephalon.

The **olfactory bulbs** are very large and the **tracts** extremely broad and short. The trigonum olfactorium is so prominent as to be termed the **tuberculum olfactorium.**

The **cranial nerves** present the following special features:

The **third, fourth, sixth,** and the **ophthalmic** and **maxillary divisions** of the fifth **nerve,** emerge together as in the ox.

The **lacrimal nerve** resembles that of the horse, the **frontal** that of the ox. The **naso-ciliary nerve** is relatively large and sends numerous filaments to the ocular muscles. The **maxillary nerve** has a very short course in the pterygo-palatine fossa. The **infraorbital nerve** is large in correlation with the development of the snout which receives numerous branches. The **mandibular nerve** emerges through the foramen lacerum anterius. The **superficial temporal nerve** is small; according to Moussu it furnishes the excito-secretory fibers to the upper part of the parotid gland, while those going to the lower part are derived from the mylo-hyoid nerve.

The **inferior buccal nerve** passes downward and forward under cover of the parotid gland and accompanies the parotid duct, with which it turns around the lower border of the jaw in front of the masseter.

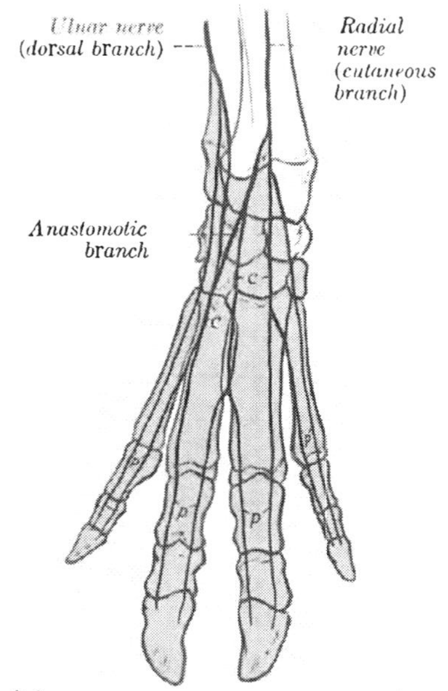

FIG. 535.—NERVES OF DISTAL PART OF RIGHT FORE LIMB OF PIG, ANTERIOR VIEW (SCHEMATIC).
c, Dorsal common digital nerves; *p*, dorsal proper digital nerves.

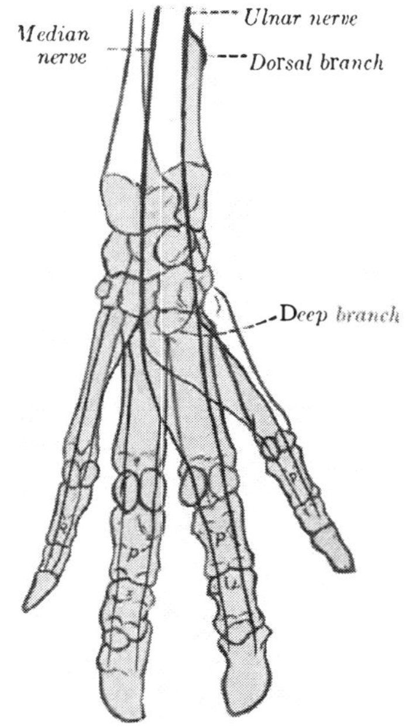

FIG. 536.—NERVES OF DISTAL PART OF RIGHT FORE LIMB OF PIG, POSTERIOR VIEW (SCHEMATIC).
p, Volar proper digital nerves.

The vagus bears a **jugular ganglion** and a **ganglion nodosum;** the latter occurs at the point of origin of the superior laryngeal nerve, and may be as large as a small pea. Proximal to this the vagus is easily divided into two strands, one of which is the accessory component. The œsophageal trunks form a posterior œsophageal plexus, as in man, from which two nerves issue. The inferior nerve is small and ramifies on the parietal surface of the stomach. The superior trunk is much larger; it gives branches to the stomach, crosses the lesser curvature of that organ, and joins the solar plexus.

The **hypoglossal nerve** may present a small dorsal root, on which there is a minute hypoglossal ganglion (of Froriep).

The **spinal nerves** number on each side eight in the cervical region, fourteen (commonly) in the thoracic, seven in the lumbar, and four in the sacral. Some of the special features of the nerves of the limbs are as follows:

The **brachial plexus** is derived from the same nerves as in the ox, but the root furnished by the sixth cervical is relatively smaller. The plexus consists of two parts, the upper of which emerges above the scalenus, the lower between the two parts of that muscle. The more important differences in the nerves emanating from the plexus from the arrangement in the ox occur in the lower part of the limb. The cutaneous branch of the **radial nerve** divides at the carpus into branches which concur with the dorsal branch of the ulnar nerve in supplying the **dorsal digital nerves,** two for each digit. The **volar digital nerves,** also two for each digit, are formed by the terminal branches of the **median nerve** and the volar or deep branch

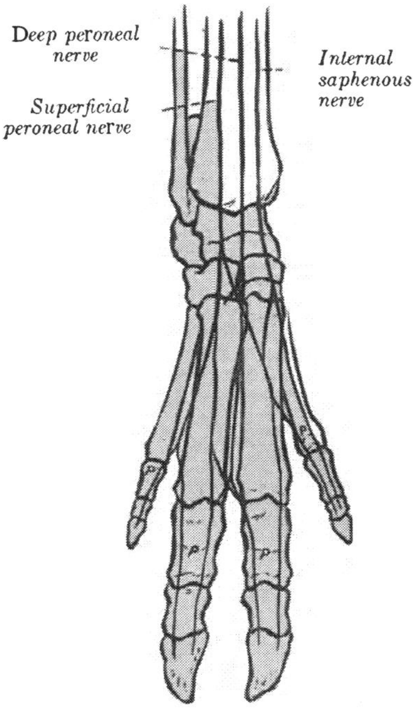

FIG. 537.—NERVES OF DISTAL PART OF RIGHT HIND LIMB OF PIG, ANTERIOR VIEW (SCHEMATIC).
p, Dorsal proper digital nerves.

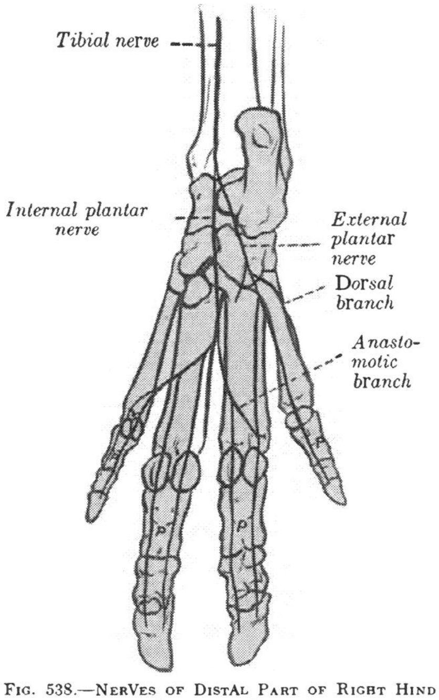

FIG. 538.—NERVES OF DISTAL PART OF RIGHT HIND LIMB OF PIG, POSTERIOR VIEW (SCHEMATIC).
p, Plantar proper digital nerves.

of the **ulnar nerve.** The formation and arrangement of the digital nerves are indicated in the annexed schematic figures.

The **lumbo-sacral plexus** is derived from the ventral branches of the last three lumbar and first sacral nerves. The distribution of the branches of the plexus differs chiefly in the distal part of the limb. The **superficial peroneal nerve** is large and terminates by forming the greater part of the **dorsal digital nerves.** The latter, two for each digit, are also in part formed by the terminal branches of the **deep peroneal nerve.**

The **tibial nerve** divides at the tarsus into **internal** and **external plantar nerves.** The latter divide to form the **plantar digital nerves,** two for each digit. In addition, the external plantar nerve supplies a branch to the dorsal aspect of the outer (fifth) digit. The arrangement of the digital nerves is indicated by the annexed schematic figures.

The **sympathetic system** of the pig has received very little attention from anatomists. The **superior cervical ganglion** is long and fusiform. It gives off filaments which join the vagus near the ganglion nodosum. The **cervical trunk** is short and relatively larger than in the ox; it is inclosed in a common sheath with the vagus in the neck and separates from that nerve to join the **middle cervical ganglion** at the thoracic inlet.

THE NERVOUS SYSTEM OF THE DOG

The **spinal cord** is almost circular in cross-section except at the well-marked cervical and lumbar enlargements, where it is compressed dorso-ventrally. The conus medullaris lies over the junction of the sixth and seventh lumbar vertebræ.

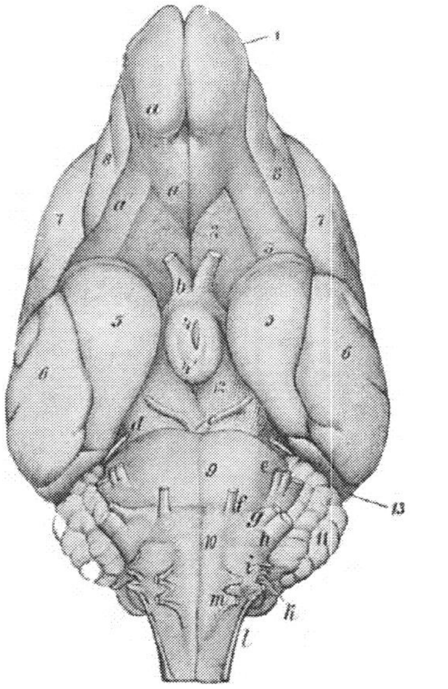

FIG. 539.—BASE OF BRAIN OF DOG.

a, Olfactory bulb; *a*,′ *a*″, external and internal olfactory tracts; *b*, optic nerve; *c*, oculomotor nerve; *d*, trochlear nerve; *e*, trigeminus; *f*, abducens; *g*, facial; *h*, auditory; *i*, glosso-pharyngeal; k, vagus; *l*, spinal accessory; *m*, hypoglossal; *2*, trigonum olfactorium; *3*, anterior perforated substance; *4*, tuber cinereum and infundibulum; *4′*, mammillary body; *5*, pyriform lobe; *6*, temporal lobe; *7*, parietal lobe; *8*, frontal lobe; *9*, pons; *10*, medulla oblongata; *11*, cerebellum; *12*, cerebral peduncle; *13*, occipital lobe. (Ellenberger-Baum, Anat. d. Hundes.)

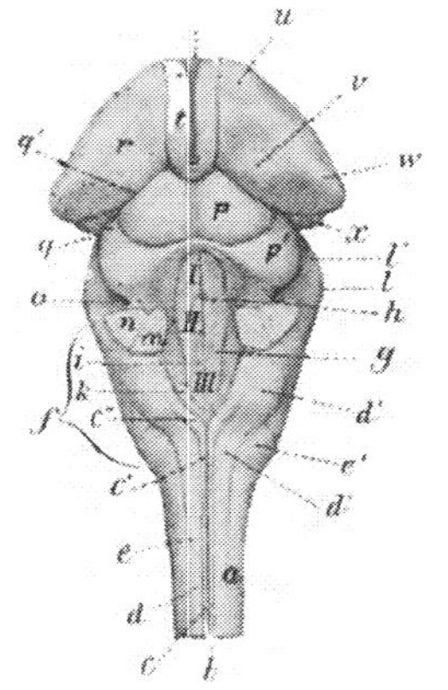

FIG. 540.—BRAIN STEM OF DOG, DORSAL VIEW.

a, Spinal cord; *b*, dorsal median groove; *c*, *c*′, funiculus gracilis; *c*″, clava; *d*, *d*′, funiculus cuneatus; *d*″, tuberculum cuneatum; *e*, funiculus lateralis; *e*′, tuberculum Rolandi; *f*, medulla oblongata; *I*, *II*, *III*, floor of fourth ventricle (fossa rhomboidea); *g*, limiting groove; *h*, median fissure; *i*, eminentia medialis; k, ala cinerea; *l*, *l*′, pons; *m*, posterior peduncle, and *n*, middle peduncle of cerebellum (cut); *o*, anterior peduncle of cerebellum; *p*, *p*′, corpora quadrigemina, anterior and posterior; *q*, *q*′, peduncles (brachia) of corpora quadrigemina; *r*, thalamus; *s*, massa intermedia; *t*, stria medullaris; *u*, anterior tubercle of thalamus; *v*, pulvinar; *w*, corpus geniculatum laterale; *x*, corpus geniculatum mediale. (After Ellenberger, in Leisering's Atlas.)

The length of the cord of a rather large dog was found to be about 38 cm.; of this, the cervical part was 11 cm., the thoracic 17.4 cm., the lumbar about 7 cm., and the sacro-coccygeal about 2.6 cm. (Flatau-Jacobson).

The **brain** weighs about 60 to 70 g. in dogs of medium size, but there is, of course, a wide range of weight in the different breeds. Thus in small terriers the weight is 30 g. or even less, while in very large dogs it may exceed 150 g. It corresponds much more closely with the cranium in size and general form than in the animals previously described; this is specially true of the small breeds, in which the bony crests and frontal sinuses are little developed.

The medulla is broad and thick. Its ventral surface is strongly convex from side to side. The pyramids are large and prominent and are limited by distinct median and lateral grooves. The olivary eminence is a well-defined oval elevation situated between the pyramid and the superficial origin of the hypoglossal nerve. The external arcuate fibers form a wide band which crosses the lateral surface obliquely upward and forward, and obscures the groove which limits the restiform

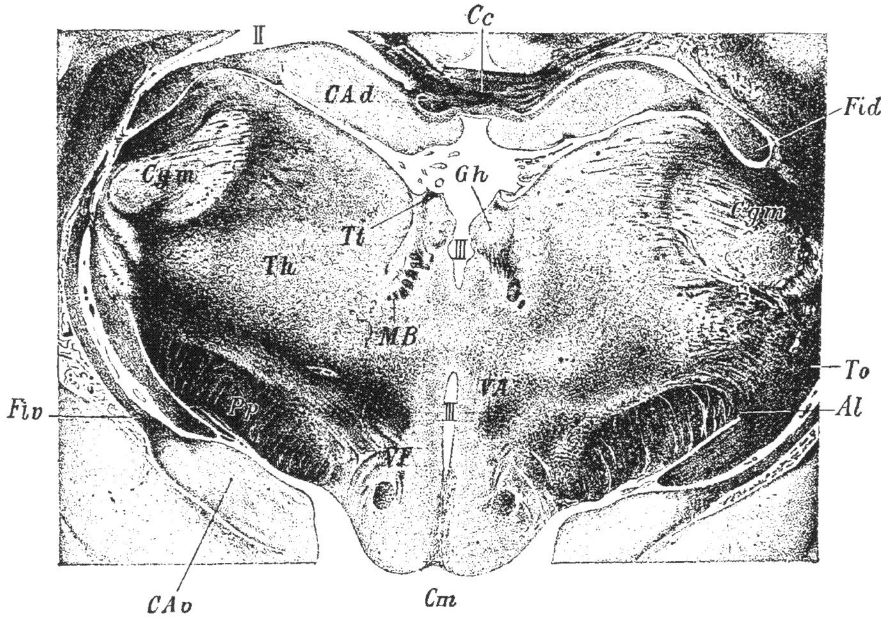

FIG. 541.—PART OF CROSS-SECTION OF BRAIN OF DOG, PASSING THROUGH GANGLION HABENULÆ.

Al, Ansa lenticularis of thalamic radiation; *C a d*, dorsal end of hippocampus; *C a v*, ventral end of same; C c, corpus callosum; *C g m*, corpus geniculatum mediale; *C m*, corpus mammillare; *F i* d, fimbria; *F i v*, ventral part of fimbria; *G h*, ganglion habenulæ; *M B*, fasciculus retroflexus; *P* p, pes pedunculi; *T h*, thalamus; *T o*, tractus opticus; *T t*, habenula; *V A*, fasciculus thalamo-mammillaris; *V F*, fornix ventralis; *II*, lateral ventricle; *III*, third ventricle. (After Probst.)

body externally. The cuneate tubercle is distinct. The rhomboid fossa is deep and narrow.

The pons is relatively small. The corpus trapezoideum is very wide and is divided by the pyramids into two lateral parts. The cerebellum is very broad, but is low and also compressed from before backward. Rather more than half of it is overlapped by the cerebral hemispheres. The anterior surface is accurately adapted to the concave tentorial surfaces of the hemispheres and to the posterior corpora quadrigemina and their commissure. The posterior surface is almost vertical and is convex centrally and flattened laterally. The vermis is prominent and in general well defined, although it is connected in its middle part with the hemispheres. The latter are three-sided and consist of four lobules. The anterior peduncles are very short.

The posterior corpora quadrigemina are large, very wide apart, and prominent, and are connected by a curved commissure. The internal geniculate body is large.

In the deep interpeduncular fossa are two small bands which indicate the course of the fasciculi retroflexi, tracts which connect the habenular and interpeduncular ganglia. The mammillary body is double. The tuber cinereum is relatively large. The pituitary body is circular and rather small.

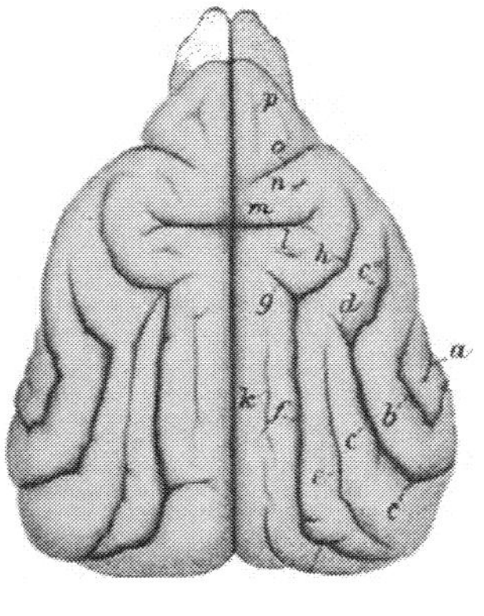

FIG. 542.—CEREBRUM OF DOG, DORSAL VIEW.

a, End of lateral fissure (of Sylvius); *b*, ectosylvian fissure; *c*, *c'*, *c''*, suprasylvian fissure; d, fissura ansata minor; *e*, ectolateral fissure; *f*, ectomarginal or collateral fissure; *g*, fissura ansata; *h*, coronal fissure; *i*, medilateral fissure; *k*, entomarginal fissure; *l*, postcruciate fissure; *m*, cruciate fissure; *o*, presylvian fissure; p, fissura prorea. (After Ellenberger, in Leisering's Atlas.)

The cerebral hemispheres are very broad behind and diminish in width anteriorly; there is a sudden narrowing at the frontal poles, which are flattened laterally. The tentorial surfaces are concave and form a deep cavity which receives the anterior part of the cerebellum. The arrangement of the fissures and gyri is simpler than in the animals previously examined. The chief fissures are as follows:

1. The lateral fissure (of Sylvius) extends upward and backward from the sulcus rhinalis a little behind the middle of the lateral surface of the hemisphere.

2. The ectosylvian fissure has approximately the shape of an inverted U, and curves over the lateral fissure. It is regarded as consisting of three parts—anterior, middle, and posterior (F. ectosylvia anterior, media, posterior).

3. The suprasylvian fissure lies above and approximately concentric with the preceding. It also consists of three parts—anterior, middle, and posterior.

4. The ectomarginal or collateral fissure runs forward on the dorsal aspect of the hemisphere almost parallel with the dorso-medial border. A little in front of the middle of the surface it gives off a short ansate fissure (F. ansata) which runs obliquely inward and forward, and is continued by the coronal fissure.

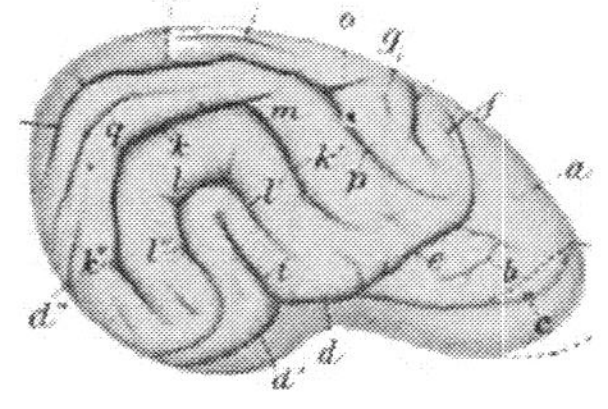

FIG. 543.—FISSURES OF LATERAL SURFACE OF CEREBRUM OF DOG, RIGHT SIDE.

a, Fissura prorea; *b*, frontal fissure; *c*, olfactory fissure; *d*, d', sulcus rhinalis; *e*, presylvian fissure; *f*, precruciate fissure; *g*, postcruciate fissure; *h*, cruciate fissure; *i*, lateral fissure (of Sylvius); *k*, *k'*, *k''*, suprasylvian fissure; *l*, *l'*, *l''*, ectosylvian fissure; *m*, fissura ansata minor; *n*, ectomarginal or collateral fissure; *o*, fissura ansata; *p*, coronal fissure; *q*, ectolateral fissure; r, medilateral fissure; *s*, entomarginal fissure. (After Ellenberger, in Leisering's Atlas.)

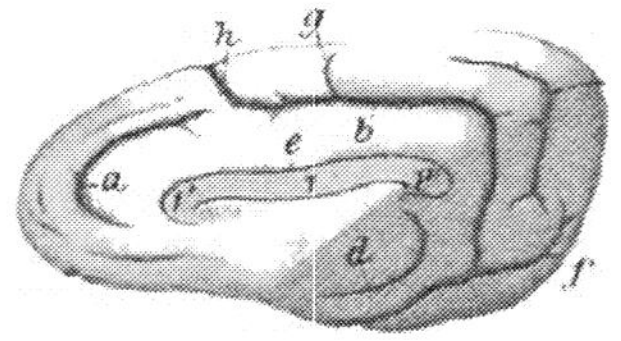

FIG. 544.—RIGHT CEREBRAL HEMISPHERE OF DOG, INNER SIDE.

1, Corpus callosum; *1'*, genu, *1''*, splenium of corpus callosum; *a*, genual fissure; *b*, splenial fissure; c, suprasplenial fissure; d, hippocampal fissure; *e*, sulcus corporis callosi; *f*, postsplenial fissure; *g*, lesser cruciate fissure; *h*, cruciate fissure. (After Ellenberger, in Leisering's Atlas.)

5. The coronal fissure is the continuation of the ectomarginal. It runs forward and downward, curving around the cruciate fissure, and ends behind the middle of the presylvian fissure.

6. The **ectolateral fissure** lies between the posterior part of the ectomarginal fissure and the suprasylvian fissure.

7. The **entomarginal fissure** lies between the anterior part of the ectomarginal fissure and the dorso-medial border. It is often indistinct and not rarely absent.

8. The **presylvian fissure** begins at the sulcus rhinalis, a little in front of its middle, and curves over the anterior third of the lateral surface of the hemisphere in front of the coronal fissure.

9. The **cruciate fissure** is the deepest and most characteristic. It cuts deeply into the anterior third of the dorso-medial border and runs almost straight outward. It is continuous on the inner surface of the hemisphere with the calloso-marginal or splenial fissure.

10. The sulcus **rhinalis** is continued on the tentorial surface of the hemisphere

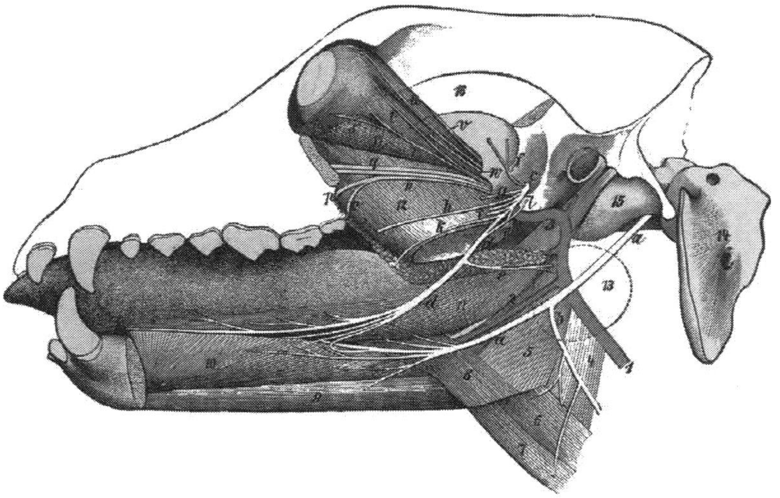

FIG. 545.—DEEP DISSECTION OF HEAD OF DOG, SHOWING ESPECIALLY TRIGEMINAL AND HYPOGLOSSAL NERVES.

a, Hypoglossal nerve; *b*, cervical branch of *a*; c, mandibular division of trigeminus; d, lingual nerve; *e*, nerve to submaxillary gland; *f*, deep temporal nerve; *g*, pterygoid nerve; *h*, buccinator nerve (cut); *i*, inferior alveolar or dental nerve; *k*, staphyline branch of lingual nerve; *l*, chorda tympani; *m*, mylo-hyoid nerve; *n*, sphenopalatine nerve; *o*, lesser palatine nerve; p, great palatine nerve; q, infraorbital nerves; *r*, subcutaneus malæ; *s*, branch of oculomotor nerve to inferior oblique muscle; *t*, lacrimal nerve; *u*, frontal nerve; *v*, trochlear nerve; *w*, abducens; *1*, carotid artery; *2*, lingual artery; *3*, internal maxillary artery; *4*, thyro-pharyngeus muscle; *5*, hyo-pharyngeus muscle; *6*, thyro-hyoideus; *7*, sterno-hyoideus; *8*, baseo-glossus, *9*, genio-hyoideus; *10*, genio-glossus; *11*, stylo-glossus; *12*, pterygoideus internus; *13*, outline of submaxillary gland (dotted); *14*, atlas; *15*, bulba ossea; *16*, zygomatic arch (dotted); *17*, rectus oculi inferior; *18*, obliquus oculi inferior. (Ellenberger-Baum, Anat. d. Hundes.)

by the occipito-temporal fissure. Anteriorly it is prolonged as the olfactory fissure, which is concealed by the olfactory bulb and tract.

11. The **calloso-marginal** or **splenial fissure** is parallel with the splenium and middle part of the corpus callosum on the inner surface of the hemisphere. It is continuous in front with the cruciate fissure and runs downward and outward across the tentorial surface to join the occipito-temporal fissure and sulcus rhinalis. It gives off from its highest part the short lesser or accessory cruciate fissure.

12. The **suprasplenial fissure** runs almost parallel with the posterior part of the calloso-marginal fissure on the inner and tentorial surfaces of the hemisphere.

The **olfactory bulb** is large and is strongly compressed laterally; its anterior end projects beyond the frontal pole of the hemisphere. The tract is short and is also flattened laterally. Both contain a narrow cavity which communicates with the lateral ventricle. The pyriform lobe is large and rounded.

The cranial nerves present the following special features which are worthy of notice:

The ophthalmic nerve gives off lacrimal, frontal, long ciliary, ethmoidal, and infratrochlear branches. The lacrimal nerve arises from the ophthalmic at its origin;[1] its recurrent branch emerges at the orbital ligament and concurs with the zygomatic and frontal nerves in the formation of the anterior auricular plexus. The frontal nerve emerges from the orbit in front of the upper end of the orbital ligament, ramifies in the upper lid and the adjacent skin of the forehead, and sends branches backward to the anterior auricular plexus. The long ciliary nerve accompanies the optic nerve and divides into several branches which pierce the posterior part of the sclera. The ethmoidal nerve gives off internal nasal branches and ends in the muzzle. The infratrochlear nerve runs forward between the internal

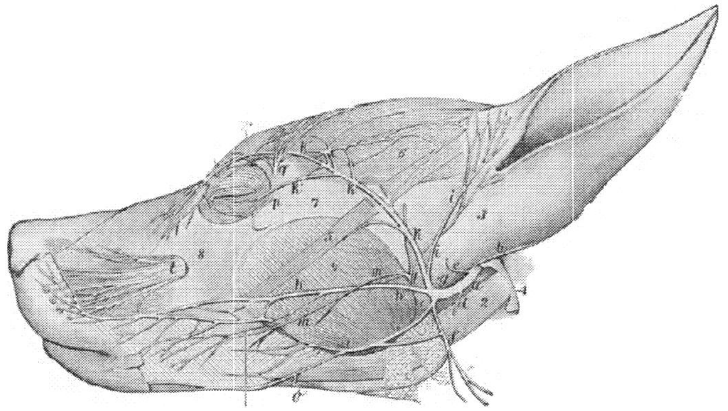

FIG. 546.—NERVES OF FACE OF DOG. PAROTID GLAND IS REMOVED.

a, Facial nerve; *b*, posterior auricular nerve; c, internal auricular nerve; d, digastric nerve; c, inferior buccal nerve; *f*, cervical branch of facial; *g*, auriculo-palpebral; *h*, superior buccal nerve; *i*, temporal branch; *k*, *k'*, *k''*, zygomatic branch; *l*, auriculo-temporal; *m*, malar branch of *l*; *n*, buccinator nerve; *o*, mylo-hyoid branch; *p*, subcutaneus malæ; *q*, lacrimal nerve; r, frontal nerve; *s*, infratrochlear nerve; *t*, infraorbital nerve; *1*, paramastoid process; *2*, digastricus muscle; *3*, base of concha; *4*, masseter; *5*, zygomaticus; *6*, scutularis; *7*, zygomatic arch; *8*, maxilla. (Ellenberger-Baum, Anat. d. Hundes.)

straight and the superior oblique muscles of the eye and ramifies on the face in the vicinity of the inner canthus.

The maxillary nerve, after giving off the zygomatic, divides into infraorbital and sphenopalatine branches. The zygomatic nerve emerges through an opening in the upper part of the orbital ligament and ramifies in the lower lid and on the adjacent surface of the face. The infraorbital nerves, two in number, divide within the infraorbital canal and after their emergence upon the face, thus forming seven or eight external nasal and superior labial branches. The sphenopalatine nerve gives off lesser and greater palatine and posterior nasal nerves.

The mandibular nerve passes out through the foramen ovale. The superficial temporal nerve divides into auricular, temporal, and malar branches; the last-named crosses the masseter and ramifies with the buccal nerves. The mylo-hyoid nerve is given off from the mandibular nerve almost immediately after the latter emerges from the cranium; it innervates the mylo-hyoideus and digastricus and gives off a branch which turns around the lower jaw, joins the inferior buccal nerve,

[1] The origin of the lacrimal nerve is such that Ellenberger-Baum and Martin describe it as a branch of the maxillary nerve.

and ramifies on the lateral surface of the face. The **inferior alveolar nerve** arises by a common trunk with the mylo-hyoid; it gives off dental branches and terminates in mental and inferior labial branches. The **lingual nerve** supplies vaso-dilator and excito-secretory filaments to the submaxillary and sublingual salivary glands; these fibers are derived from the chorda tympani.

The **facial nerve** divides near the posterior border of the jaw into four branches. The upper branch is the **auriculo-palpebral nerve,** which divides after a very short course into anterior auricular and zygomatic branches. The latter curves upward and forward across the zygomatic arch toward the eye, and divides into branches which supply the eyelids and nasal region and concur with the frontal and lacrimal nerves in forming the anterior auricular plexus. The **superior buccal nerve** accompanies the parotid duct across the masseter. The **inferior buccal nerve** runs forward along the lower border of the masseter and the mandible. The two nerves ramify on the cheek and anastomose with each other and the infraorbital nerves to form a plexus from which branches go to the muscles of the lips and nostrils. The **cervical branch** runs downward and backward over the submaxillary gland and ramifies in the cervical panniculus; it communicates with the inferior buccal nerve and sends twigs to the parotido-auricularis muscle and the submaxillary space.

The **vagus** bears a **jugular ganglion** and a **ganglion nodosum.** The latter is situated near the superior cervical ganglion on the rectus capitis anterior major and dorsal to the carotid artery; it is fusiform and may be about half an inch (ca. 1 to 1.5 cm.) long in a large dog. In its course in the neck the nerve is inclosed with the sympathetic trunk in a common sheath and is related ventrally to the common carotid artery. The formation of dorsal and ventral **œsophageal trunks** by the union of the dorsal and ventral divisions of the two nerves takes place at the hiatus œsophageus. The **dorsal trunk** concurs with branches of the solar plexus in forming the **posterior gastric plexus** on the visceral surface of the stomach. The **ventral trunk** ramifies on the parietal surface of the stomach, forming the **anterior gastric plexus,** from which a considerable branch passes along the lesser curvature to the pylorus. Some special features of the collateral branches are: Two pharyngeal branches are present. The **superior pharyngeal branch** arises from the vagus above the ganglion nodosum. It passes under the deep face of the carotid artery and descends on the lateral surface of the pharynx to end in the crico-thyroid muscle. It furnishes a root of the inferior pharyngeal branch, and communicates with the pharyngeal branch of the ninth and with the superior laryngeal and hypoglossal nerves. The **inferior pharyngeal branch** is formed by the union of roots derived from the superior pharyngeal nerve and the ganglion nodosum, together with filaments from the superior cervical ganglion. It crosses the side of the pharynx behind the superior pharyngeal and ramifies on the posterior constrictor of the pharynx and the origin of the œsophagus. It contributes filaments to the pharyngeal plexus, communicates with the recurrent nerve, and supplies twigs to the thyroid gland. The **pharyngeal plexus** is formed on the lateral surface of the pharynx by branches of the pharyngeal nerves and the communications above described; branches from it innervate the muscles and mucous membrane of the pharynx. The **superior laryngeal nerve** arises from the ganglion nodosum and descends over the side of the pharynx, crossing beneath the carotid artery and the superior laryngeal nerve. It passes through the thyroid notch and ramifies in the mucous membrane of the larynx. It communicates with the superior cervical ganglion and the superior pharyngeal branch of the vagus, and gives twigs to the hyo-pharyngeus muscle. Immediately after its entrance into the larynx it gives off a large branch which, instead of uniting with the recurrent as in the other animals, has a peculiar arrangement. It runs back near the dorsal border of the thyroid cartilage, gives a branch to the crico-arytenoideus posterior as it passes over that muscle, and continues along the trachea internal to the recurrent nerve. At the thoracic inlet it communicates with the inferior cervical ganglion and continues backward to unite with the vagus at or near the point of origin of the recurrent nerve. Its collateral filaments supply the trachea and concur with the inferior pharyngeal branch in forming a plexus on the cervical part of the œsophagus which innervates that tube.[1] The **depressor nerve** is a very delicate filament which arises usually from the superior laryngeal nerve and accompanies the vago-sympathetic trunk to the thorax; its fibers reach the heart through the cardiac nerves. The **pulmonary** and **posterior œsophageal plexuses** are highly developed.

The **hypoglossal nerve** gives off a long branch (R. descendens) which runs downward and backward across the pharynx and larynx, communicates with the ventral branch of the first cervical nerve, and supplies the thyro-hyoid, sterno hyoid, and sterno-thyroid muscles.

The **spinal nerves** number thirty-six or thirty-seven on either side, and comprise eight cervical, thirteen thoracic, seven lumbar, and five or six coccygeal.

The **brachial plexus** (Fig. 487) is derived from the ventral branches of the last four cervical and first thoracic nerves; the root supplied by the fifth cervical nerve is very small. The roots unite at the lower border of the scalenus. The more important special features in the arrangement of the nerves which emanate from the plexus are as follows:

The **musculo-cutaneous nerve** passes between the coraco-brachialis and the brachial artery and descends in the arm in front of the artery. At the shoulder joint it gives off branches to the biceps and coraco-brachialis, and in the lower third of the arm is connected with the median nerve by an oblique branch. It terminates near the elbow by dividing into a branch for the brachialis and a small cutaneous nerve which passes down over the inner face of the elbow and, inclining a little forward, descends over the deep fascia of the forearm to the carpus.

The **radial nerve** descends behind the ulnar nerve, gives branches to the extensors of the elbow, dips in between the internal head of the triceps and the accessory head of the anconeus, winds around the arm, and divides between the brachialis and the external head of the triceps into two branches. The **deep branch** (R. profundus) supplies the extensor and supinator muscles on the forearm. The **superficial branch** (R. superficialis) emerges upon the flexor surface of the elbow and divides into two branches which terminate by supplying two **dorsal digital nerves** to each digit, except the fifth, which receives its outer dorsal nerve from the ulnar. The inner branch descends along the inner side of the cephalic vein to the carpus, where it divides into dorsal digital nerves for the first digit and the inner side of the second. The outer branch is much larger. It runs downward on the middle of the front of the forearm and supplies the remaining dorsal digital nerves except that to the outer side of the fifth digit.

The **ulnar nerve** is as large as or larger than the median, with which it is united for some distance. At the distal third of the arm it separates from the median and passes over the internal epicondyle of the humerus. At the proximal part of the forearm it gives off the dorsal **branch** (R. dorsalis), which supplies cutaneous twigs to the dorso-lateral surface of the lower part of the forearm and carpus and terminates as the **external dorsal digital nerve** of the fifth digit. Descending under cover of the flexor carpi ulnaris, the ulnar nerve inclines inward under the tendon of insertion of that muscle and divides into superficial and deep branches. The **superficial branch** (R. superficialis) runs downward along the outer border of the flexor tendons, gives off the **external volar digital nerve of the fifth digit** (N. dig. vol. lat. dig. V), and a branch (N. met. vol. IV) which descends in the space between the fourth and fifth metacarpal bones and unites with the deep branch. The **deep**

[1] Lesbre terms this the tracheo-œsophageal branch, and considers that it must be regarded as an accessory or internal recurrent nerve.

branch (R. profundus) descends in the carpal canal and divides under the deep flexor tendon into its terminal branches. The smaller of these supply the volar metacarpal muscles. The larger terminals are the three volar **common** digital **nerves** (Nn. dig. vol. comm. II, III, IV), which descend along the second, third, and fourth intermetacarpal spaces, subdivide, and concur with the volar metacarpal branches of the median nerve in forming the **volar proper** digital **nerves** (Nn. dig. vol. proprii).

The **median nerve** descends behind the brachial artery, passes over the internal epicondyle of the humerus, then under the pronator teres, and continues in the forearm under cover of the flexor carpi radialis. It gives branches below the elbow

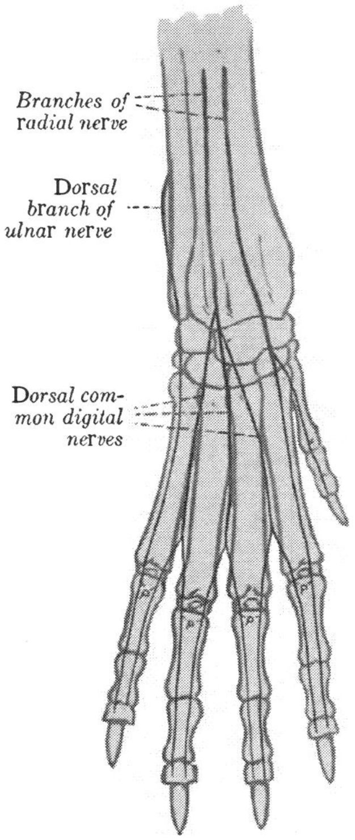

FIG. 547.—NERVES OF DISTAL PART OF RIGHT FORE LIMB OF DOG, ANTERIOR VIEW (SCHEMATIC).
p, Dorsal proper digital nerves.

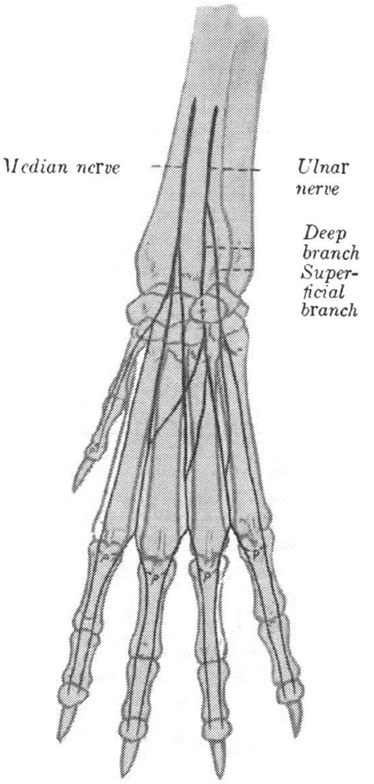

FIG. 548.—NERVES OF DISTAL PART OF RIGHT FORE LIMB OF DOG, POSTERIOR VIEW (SCHEMATIC).
p, Volar proper digital nerves.

to the flexor and pronator muscles, and lower down a palmar branch to the skin on the inner and posterior aspect of the carpus, and terminates between the superficial and deep flexor tendons by dividing into three volar **metacarpal nerves** (N. met. vol. I, II, III). These descend in the first, second, and third intermetacarpal spaces and unite with the volar common digital nerves in forming volar proper digital nerves. The arrangement of the digital nerves is indicated in the annexed schematic figures.

The **lumbo-sacral plexus** is formed from the ventral branches of the last five lumbar and first sacral nerves. The more important special facts in regard to the nerves of the pelvic limb are as follows:

The **saphenous nerve** (Fig. 492) is relatively large, and, in fact, might be considered as the continuation of the femoral nerve. It descends at first in front of the femoral artery, then passes over the lower part of the inner surface of the thigh with the saphenous artery, continues down the leg with the dorsal branch of that vessel, and anastomoses with branches of the superficial peroneal nerve. It supplies cutaneous twigs from the stifle to the metatarsus.

The **peroneal nerve** separates from the tibial above the origin of the gastrocnemius, runs downward and forward across the outer head of that muscle, passes between the deep flexor of the digit and the peroneus longus, and divides into superficial and deep branches. The **superficial peroneal nerve** descends the leg along the peroneus tertius and longus, gives off a **dorsal branch** to the first digit (N. cutaneus dorsalis medialis), and divides at the proximal part of the metatarsus into three

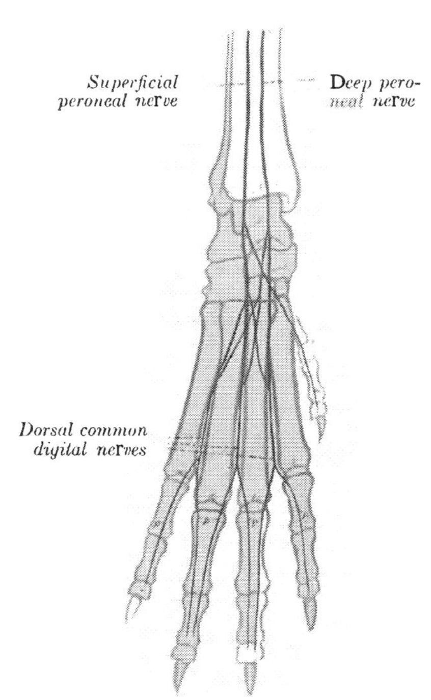

Fig. 549.—Nerves of Distal Part of Right Hind Limb of Dog, Anterior View (Schematic).
p, Dorsal proper digital nerves.

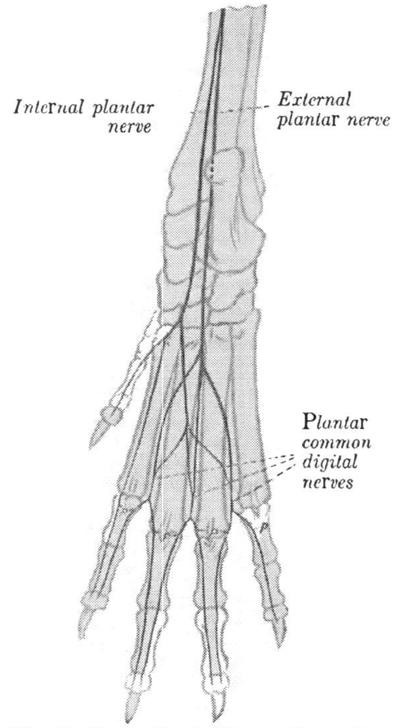

Fig. 550.—Nerves of Distal Part of Right Hind Limb of Dog. Posterior View (Schematic).
p, Plantar proper digital nerves.

dorsal common digital nerves (Nn. dig pedis dors. comm. II, III, IV). These descend with the superficial dorsal metatarsal arteries and concur with branches of the deep peroneal nerve in forming **dorsal proper digital nerves** (Nn. dig. ped. prop. dorsales). The **deep peroneal nerve** passes down the leg with the anterior tibial vessels. It gives twigs to the hock joint and the extensor brevis muscle, and divides into three dorsal **metatarsal nerves** (Nn. met. dors. II, III, IV); these descend with the corresponding arteries along the intermetatarsal spaces and unite with the dorsal common digital nerves in supplying the dorsal proper digital nerves.

The tibial **nerve** divides at the tarsus into two plantar branches. The **internal plantar nerve** descends along the inner border of the superficial flexor tendon and divides near the middle of the metatarsus into two branches. Of these, the internal branch constitutes the first **plantar common digital nerve** (N dig. comm. plant. I). The outer branch descends on the superficial flexor tendon and divides into three **plantar metatarsal nerves** (Nn. met. plant. II, III, IV), which unite with the plantar common digital nerves. The **external plantar nerve** passes down between the flexor tendons, sends twigs to the muscles on the plantar surface of the metatarsus, and divides into three **plantar common digital nerves** (Nn. dig. comm. plant. II, III, IV). These descend with the deep plantar metatarsal arteries in the second, third, and fourth intermetatarsal spaces, receive the plantar metatarsal nerves, and divide into **plantar proper digital nerves,** which pass down the opposed surfaces of the second to the fifth digits.

The **sympathetic system** presents few special features worthy of mention. The **superior cervical ganglion** lies above the ganglion nodosum close to the cranial base and internal to the origin of the internal carotid and occipital arteries. It forms connections directly or through the carotid plexus with the last seven cranial and first cervical nerves. The **cervical trunk** unites with the vagus so intimately as to form a vago-sympathetic trunk. There may be a small **middle cervical ganglion** in front of the inferior cervical ganglion. The latter is usually distinct from the first thoracic ganglion, which is stellate and lies on the longus colli opposite the second rib and intercostal space.

ÆSTHESIOLOGY

THE SENSE ORGANS AND COMMON INTEGUMENT

The **organs of the senses** (Organa sensuum) receive external stimuli and conduct impulses to the brain which result in sensations of sight, hearing, taste, smell, and touch. They consist essentially of specially differentiated cells, the neuro-epithelium, and a conduction path which is simple in the more generalized sense organs, elaborate in those which are highly specialized—the eye and the ear.

THE SENSE ORGANS AND SKIN OF THE HORSE

THE EYE

The **eye or organ** of vision (Organon visus) in the broader sense of the term comprises the eyeball or globe of the eye, the optic nerve, and certain accessory

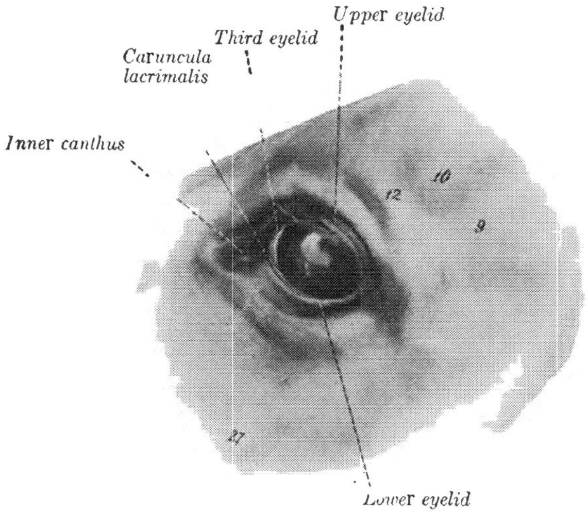

FIG. 551.—LEFT EYE OF HORSE.

9 Zygomatic arch; *10*, supraorbital depression; *12*, supraorbital process; *27*, facial crest. (After Ellenberger-Baum, Anat. für Künstler.)

organs associated therewith. The accessory organs (Organa oculi accessoria) are the orbital fasciæ and muscles, the eyelids and conjunctiva, and the lacrimal apparatus. These structures will be considered in the order in which they may be most conveniently examined, taking the horse as a type. The bony walls of the orbit have been described in connection with the skull; the periorbita, a fibrous membrane which incloses the eyeball together with its muscles, vessels, and nerves, may be appropriately included in the account of the fasciæ.

THE EYELIDS AND CONJUNCTIVA

The **eyelids,** upper and lower (Palpebra superior et inferior), are movable folds of integument situated in front of the eveball. When closed, they cover the entrance to the orbit and the anterior surface of the eyeball. The upper lid is much more extensive and more movable than the lower one, and its free edge is more concave. The interval between the lids is termed the **palpebral fissure** (Rima palpebrarum). When the eye is closed, it is an oblique slit about two inches (ca. 5 cm.) in length; when open, it is biconvex in outline. The ends of the fissure are the **angles** or **canthi,** and are distinguished as **internal** or **nasal,** and **external** or **temporal** (Angulus oculi medialis, lateralis). The external angle is rounded when the eye is open, but the internal angle is narrowed to form a ⊃-shaped bay or recess, termed the **lacrimal lake** (Lacus lacrimalis). In this there is a rounded, pigmented prominence known as the **lacrimal caruncle** (Caruncula lacrimalis); it is about the size of a small pea and is covered with modified skin, connected with that of the inner commissure, from which project a number of hairs provided with sebaceous glands. The lids unite on either side and form the **commissures,** internal and external (Commissura palpebrarum medialis, lateralis). The **anterior surface** of the lids (Facies anterior palpebrarum) is convex and presents a variable number of long tactile hairs in addition to the ordinary but very short hairs. A considerable number of tactile hairs are scattered over the lower part of the lower lid, but on the upper lid they are very scanty. The infrapalpebral depression (Sulcus infrapalpebralis) indicates somewhat indistinctly the limit of the lower lid. The upper lid is marked by two furrows when raised. The **posterior surface** (Facies posterior palpebrarum) is adapted to the free surface of the eyeball and is covered by the palpebral conjunctiva. The free border of the lid is smooth and usually black. It has a well-defined posterior margin (Limbus palpebralis posterior), along which the ducts of the tarsal glands open. The anterior margin (Limbus palpebralis anterior) bears stiff hairs termed the **cilia** or eyelashes. On the upper lid the cilia are long and numerous except at its inner third, where they are very small or absent. On the lower lid the cilia are often scarcely distinguishable from the ordinary hairs; in other cases they may be clearly seen except near the external canthus, and are much finer and shorter than those of the upper lid. The edge of each lid is pierced near the internal angle by a

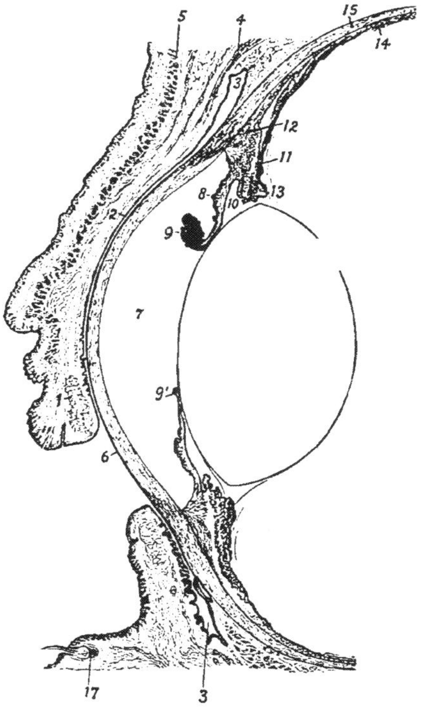

FIG. 552.—VERTICAL SECTION OF ANTERIOR PART OF EYE OF HORSE, WITH LIDS HALF CLOSED.

1, Tarsal gland of upper lid; *2*, palpebral conjunctiva; *3*, fornix conjunctivæ; *4*, levator palpebræ superioris; *5*, orbicularis oculi; *6*, cornea; *7*, anterior chamber; *8*, iris; *9*, *9'*, granula iridis; *10*, posterior chamber; *11*, ciliary process; *12*, ciliary muscle; *13*, ciliary zone or suspensory lig. of lens; *14*, chorioid; *15*, sclera; *16*, lens; *17*, root of tactile hair. (After Bayer, Augenheilkunde.)

minute, slit-like opening, the **punctum lacrimalis,** which is the entrance to the lacrimal duct or canaliculus.

Structure of the Eyelids.—The skin of the eyelids is thin and freely movable, except near the free edge, where it is more firmly attached. The underlying subcutaneous tissue is destitute of fat. The **muscular layer** consists chiefly of the elliptical bundles of the orbicularis oculi, with which are associated fibers of the corrugator supercilii in the upper lid and the malaris in the lower lid. At the inner side there is a fibrous band, the **palpebral ligament,** which is attached to the lacrimal tubercle and furnishes origin to some fibers of the orbicularis. At the inner commissure a bundle detached from the orbicularis passes inward behind the lacrimal sac, and is known as the pars lacrimalis or Horner's muscle. At the outer side an indistinct palpebral raphe occurs where fibers of the orbicularis decussate. The **fibrous layer** is thicker and denser along the free edge of the lid, forming here the **tarsus.** The tarsus furnishes insertion to a layer of unstriped muscle known as the tarsal muscle (of Müller). The **tarsal glands** (Glandulæ tarsales) are partly embedded in the deep face of the tarsus, and are visible when the lid is everted if the conjunctiva is not too strongly pigmented. They are arranged in a linear series, close together, and with their long axes perpendicular to the free edge of each lid. In the upper lid they number forty-five to fifty; in the lower, thirty to thirty-five. Each consists of a tubular duct beset with numerous alveoli, in which a

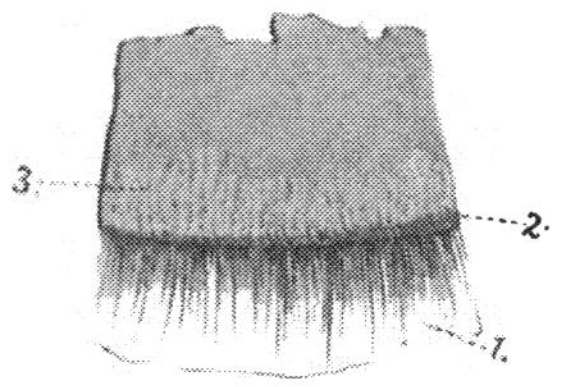

Fig. 553.—Piece of Upper Eyelid, Inner Surface.
1, Cilia; 2, limbus palp. posterior; 3, tarsal glands. (After Ellenberger, in Leisering's Atlas.)

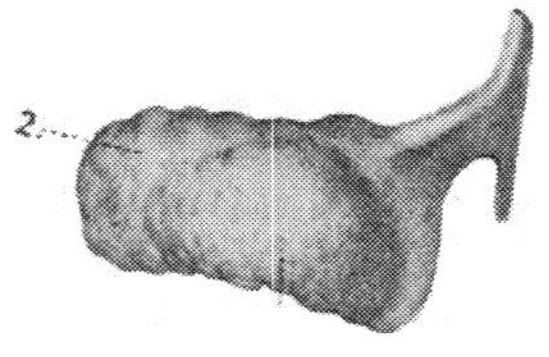

Fig. 554.—Cartilage of Third Eyelid of Horse, Convex Surface.
1, Gland; 2, fat surrounding deep part of cartilage. (After Ellenberger, in Leisering's Atlas.)

fatty substance, the **palpebral sebum,** is secreted. The **palpebral conjunctiva** lines the posterior surface of the eyelids.

The **conjunctiva** is the mucous membrane which lines the lids as **palpebral conjunctiva** (C. palpebrarum) and is reflected upon the anterior part of the eyeball as bulbar **conjunctiva** (C. bulbi); the line of reflection is termed the **fornix conjunctivæ.** The palpebral part is closely adherent to the tarsus, but is loosely attached further back. It is papillated and is covered with stratified cylindrical epithelium in which many goblet-cells are present. In the fornix and its vicinity there are tubular glands (of Henle). Near the inner angle there are numerous lymph nodules. The conjunctiva of the outer part of the upper lid is pierced near the fornix by the orifices of the excretory ducts of the lacrimal gland. The bulbar conjunctiva is loosely attached to the anterior part of the sclera and is pigmented in the vicinity of the corneo-scleral junction. On the cornea it is represented by a stratified epithelium.

When the lids are in apposition, the conjunctiva (including the epithelium of the cornea) forms a complete **conjunctival sac,** as the capillary space between the lids and the eyeball is termed.

The **third eyelid** (Palpebra tertia) is situated at the inner angle of the eye (Figs. 551, 556). It consists of a semilunar fold of the conjunctiva, known as the **membrana nictitans,** which covers and partly incloses a curved plate of hyaline cartilage. Its marginal part is thin and usually more or less pigmented. The cartilage has an elongated quadrilateral outline. The part of it which lies in the membrana is wide and thin. The deep part is narrower and thicker and is embedded in fat at the inner side of the eyeball. Numerous minute lymph nodules occur in the membrana nictitans, and the deep part of the cartilage is surrounded by a gland which resembles the lacrimal gland in structure (Glandula superficialis palpebræ tertiæ).

Ordinarily the third eyelid extends very little over the inner end of the cornea, but when the eyeball is strongly retracted (as in tetanus) the membrana is protruded over it so as to measure about an inch (ca. 2 to 3 cm.) in its middle. This effect results from the pressure of the eyeball and its muscles on the fat which surrounds the deep part of the cartilage.

Vessels and Nerves.—The **arteries** which chiefly supply the eyelids and conjunctiva are branches of the ophthalmic and facial arteries, and the blood is drained away by corresponding veins. The **sensory nerves** are branches of the ophthalmic and maxillary divisions of the trigeminus. The **motor nerves** to the orbicularis oculi, corrugator supercilii, and malaris come from the facial nerve, the levator palpebræ superioris is innervated by the oculomotor, and the unstriped muscle of the lids by the sympathetic.

THE LACRIMAL APPARATUS

The **lacrimal apparatus** (Apparatus lacrimalis) comprises: (1) the lacrimal gland, which secretes the clear lacrimal fluid; (2) the excretory ducts of the gland; (3) the two lacrimal ducts or canaliculi, lacrimal sac, and naso-lacrimal duct, which receive the fluid and convey it to the nostril.

The **lacrimal gland** (Glandula lacrimalis) is situated between the supraorbital process and the dorso-lateral surface of the eyeball (Fig. 438). It is flattened, oval in outline, and measures about two inches (ca. 5 cm.) transversely and an inch or more (2.5 to 3 cm.) in the sagittal direction. Its upper face is convex and is related to the concave lower surface of the supraorbital process. The lower face is concave in adaptation to the eyeball, from which it is separated by the periorbita. The **excretory ducts** (Ductuli excretorii) are very small and are twelve to sixteen in number; they open into the outer part of the conjunctival sac along a line a little in front of the fornix conjunctivæ superior. In appearance and structure the gland resembles the parotid. It receives its blood-supply chiefly from the lacrimal artery. The sensory nerve is the lacrimal, and the secretory fibers are derived from the sympathetic.

The **puncta lacrimalia** are the entrances to the two lacrimal ducts. Each is a fine slit-like opening (about 2 mm. long), situated close behind the free edge of the lid and about a third of an inch (ca. 8 mm.) from the internal canthus. The **lacrimal ducts** (Ductus lacrimales), upper and lower, begin at the puncta and converge at the inner commissure to open into the **lacrimal sac.** The latter (Saccus lacrimalis) may be regarded as the dilated origin of the naso-lacrimal duct. It occupies the funnel-like origin of the bony lacrimal canal, and leads to the **naso-lacrimal duct** (Ductus naso-lacrimalis), which passes forward and a little downward along the outer wall of the frontal sinus and the nasal cavity and opens near the lower commissure of the nostril. Its length is about ten to twelve inches (ca. 25 to 30 cm.). In the first part of its course it is inclosed in the osseous lacrimal canal; further forward it lies in the lacrimal groove of the maxilla, covered at first by a plate of cartilage and then by the mucous membrane of the middle meatus. The terminal part lies in the inferior turbinal fold and opens on the skin of the floor of the nostril near the transition to mucous membrane. Accessory openings may occur a little further back.

The first part of the duct, about 6 to 7 mm. in diameter, extends in a gentle curve, convex dorsally, from the internal commissure toward a point just above the level of the infraorbital foramen. The second part (isthmus) is narrower (ca. 3 to 4 mm.); it extends forward and a little ventrally about to a transverse plane through the first cheek tooth and lies in the groove above the inferior turbinal crest. Beyond this the duct inclines upward and widens very considerably, crosses the nasal process of the premaxilla obliquely, and contracts at its termination. The mucous membrane may present valvular folds, the most distinct of which is situated at the origin.

THE PERIORBITA

The **periorbita** or ocular sheath is a conical fibrous membrane which incloses the eyeball with its muscles, vessels, nerves, etc. Its apex is attached around the optic and lacerated foramina, and its base is in part attached to the bony rim of the orbit, in part continuous with the fibrous layer of the lids. Its inner part, which is in contact with the orbital wall, is thin; incorporated with it beneath the root of the supraorbital process is the bar of cartilage around which the superior oblique muscle is reflected. The outer part is thicker, and is strengthened by an elastic band which is attached to the pterygoid crest and furnishes origin to the thin unstriped orbital muscle. A quantity of fat (Corpus adiposum extraorbitale) lies about the periorbita, and within it is the intraorbital adipose tissue (Corpus adiposum intraorbitale) which fills the interstices between the eyeball, muscles, etc.

THE ORBITAL FASCIÆ AND OCULAR MUSCLES (Figs. 438, 439, 555)

The straight muscles of the eyeball and the oblique muscles in part are inclosed in fibrous sheaths (Fasciæ musculares), formed by superficial and deep layers of fascia, which are united by intermuscular septa in the interstices between the muscles. The **superficial fascia** is thin; it blends in front with the fibrous layer of the eyelids and is attached behind around the optic foramen. The **deep fascia** consists anteriorly of two layers, one of which is continuous with the fibrous tissue of the lids, while the other is attached at the corneo-scleral junction.

The posterior part of the eyeball is covered by the **bulbar fascia** or capsule of Tenon (Fascia bulbi), so that between them a lymph space (Spatium interfasciale) is inclosed which communicates with the subdural space along the course of the optic nerve.

The levator **palpebræ superioris** muscle[1] is a thin band about half an inch in width which lies above the rectus superior. It is narrow at its origin above and behind the ethmoidal foramen and ends by an expanded tendon in the upper lid. Its action is to raise the upper lid.

The **recti oculi** (Mm. recti bulbi) are four in number and are designated according to their positions as **superior, inferior, internal,** and **external.** They are all band-like, arise close together around the optic foramen, and diverge as they pass forward to the eyeball. On reaching the latter they end in thin tendons which are inserted into the sclera in front of the equator of the eyeball.

The **retractor** oculi (M. retractor bulbi) surrounds the optic nerve, and is incompletely divided into four parts which alternate with the recti. They arise around the optic nerve and are inserted into the sclera behind the recti.

The **obliquus oculi superior** (M. obliquus bulbi dorsalis s. superior) is the longest and narrowest of the ocular muscles. It arises near the ethmoidal foramen and passes forward internal to the rectus internus. Under the root of the supraorbital process it is reflected almost at a right angle around a cartilaginous pulley (trochlea), which is attached to the anterior part of the inner wall of the orbit, a bursa being interposed here. The muscle is then directed outward and somewhat forward, and ends in a thin tendon which passes between the rectus superior and the eyeball, and is inserted into the sclera between the superior and external recti, about half an inch behind the margin of the cornea.

The **obliquus** oculi **inferior** (M. obliquus bulbi ventralis s. inferior) is wide and

[1] This belongs to the upper eyelid, but is described here on account of its position.

much shorter than the recti. It arises from the inner wall of the orbit in the small depression (Fossa muscularis) behind the lacrimal fossa. It curves around the rectus inferior and is inserted into the sclera near and partly beneath the rectus externus.

Actions.—The superior and inferior recti rotate the eyeball about a transverse axis, moving the vertex of the cornea upward and downward respectively. Similarly the internal and external recti rotate the eyeball about a vertical axis, turning the vertex of the cornea inward and outward respectively. The oblique muscles rotate the eyeball about a longitudinal axis; the superior oblique raises the outer end of the pupil, while the inferior oblique lowers it. The retractor as a whole draws the eyeball backward, and its parts may separately reinforce the corresponding recti. Also the four recti acting together will retract the eyeball.

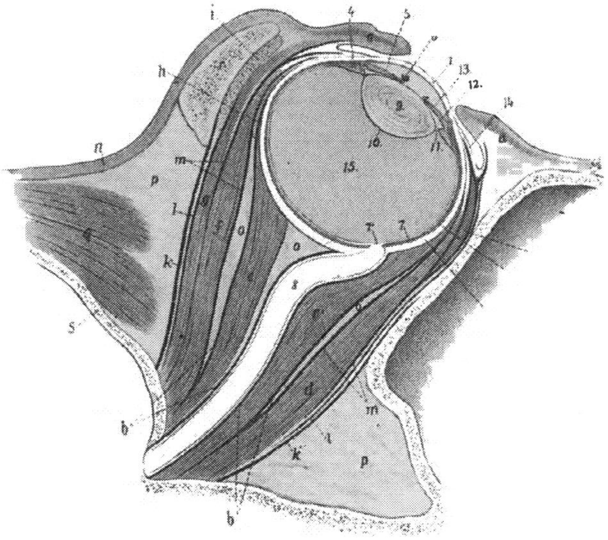

FIG. 555.—VERTICAL AXIAL SECTION OF ORBIT OF HORSE.

a, Eyelids; *b*, bulbar fascia (Tenon's capsule); *c*, *c'*, retractor bulbi; *d*, rectus oculi inferior; *e*, obliquus oculi inferior (in cross-section); *f*, rectus oculi superior; *g*, levator palpebræ superioris; *h*, obliquus oculi superior (in cross-section); *i*, lacrimal gland; k, *k'*, periorbita; *l*, superficial fascia; *m*, deep fascia; *n*. skin; *o*, retrobulbar fat; *p*, extraorbital fat; *q*, temporalis muscle; *r*, supraorbital process; *s*, cranial wall; *1*, cornea; *2*, sclera; *3*, chorioidea; *4*, ciliary muscle; *5*, iris; *6*, granula iridis; *7*, retina; *7'*, optic papilla; *8*, optic nerve; *9*, crystalline lens; *10*, capsule of lens; *11*, ciliary zone; *12*, posterior chamber; *13* anterior chamber; *14*, conjunctiva bulbi; *15*, vitreous body. (After Ellenberger, in Leisering's Atlas.)

The actual movements of the eyeball are by no means so simple as might be inferred from the foregoing general statements. Practically all movements are produced by the coördinated actions of several muscles, involving combinations which are quite complex and difficult to analyze accurately. Further complication is caused by the fact that the recti are not inserted at equal distances from the equator and the axes of rotation of the oblique muscles do not correspond to the longitudinal axis of the eyeball.

Nerve-supply.—The oculomotor nerve supplies the foregoing muscles, with the exception of the rectus externus and obliquus superior, which are innervated by the abducens and trochlearis respectively.

THE EYEBALL

The **eyeball** (Bulbus oculi) is situated in the anterior part of the orbital cavity, protected in front by the eyelids and conjunctiva, in its middle by the complete orbital ring, and related behind to the bulbar fascia, fat, and ocular muscles.

It has the form approximately of an oblate spheroid, but is composed of the segments of two spheres of different sizes. The anterior, transparent, corneal segment has a radius of curvature of about 17 mm., and the posterior, opaque, scleral segment a radius of about 25 mm. The anterior segment therefore projects more strongly, and the junction of the two segments is marked externally by a broad, shallow groove, the sulcus scleræ. The central points of the anterior and posterior curvatures of the eyeball are termed respectively the **anterior** and **posterior poles** (Polus anterior, posterior), and the line connecting the poles is the **optic axis** (Axis oculi externa). The angle of divergence of the optic axes is about 137 degrees. The **equator** (Æquator) is an imaginary line drawn around the eyeball midway between its poles, and **meridians** (Meridiani) are lines drawn around it through the poles.

The average transverse diameter of the eyeball is about 5 cm., the vertical about 4.5 cm., and the axial about 4.25 cm. The distance from the anterior pole to the point of entrance of the optic nerve is about 3 cm.

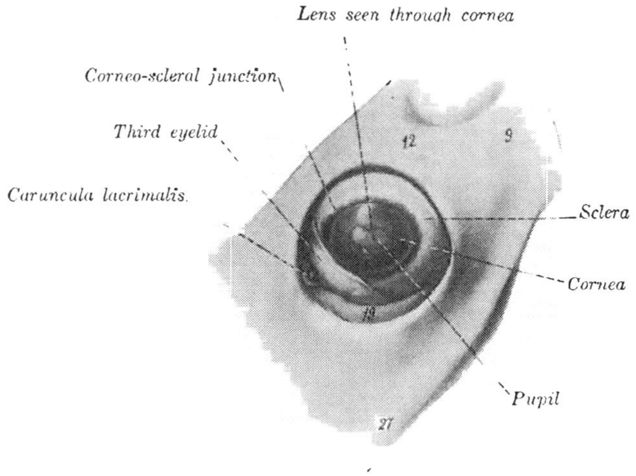

FIG. 556.—LEFT EYEBALL OF HORSE, *in situ*, AFTER REMOVAL OF UPPER AND LOWER LIDS.
9 Zygomatic arch; *12*, supraorbital process; *19*, orbital fat; *27*, facial crest. (After Ellenberger-Baum Anat. für Künstler.)

The eyeball consists of three concentric tunics or coats, within which three refractive media are inclosed.

THE FIBROUS TUNIC

The **fibrous tunic** (Tunica fibrosa oculi) is the external coat and is composed of a posterior opaque part, the sclera, and a transparent anterior part, the cornea.

The **sclera,** popularly termed the "white of the eye," is a dense fibrous membrane which forms about four-fifths of the fibrous tunic. Thickest in the vicinity of the posterior pole (ca. 2 mm.), it thins at the equator (ca. 0.4 mm.), and increases in thickness toward the junction with the cornea (ca. 1.3 mm.). It is in general white, but may have a bluish tinge in its thinnest parts. Its external surface furnishes insertion to the ocular muscles and is covered by the conjunctiva scleræ in its anterior part. The episcleral tissue, which is richly supplied with vessels and nerves, attaches the conjunctiva to the sclera; it is abundant and loosely meshed except at the junction with the cornea. The inner surface is attached to the chorioid coat by a layer of delicate, pigmented, connective tissue, the **lamina**

fusca. The anterior border is oval, the long axis being transverse, and is continuous with the cornea. The transition from the opaque scleral tissue to the transparent corneal substance occurs in such manner that the sclera appears to form a groove (Rima cornealis), into which the cornea fits somewhat as a watch-glass in the case. Near the corneo-scleral junction there is a circular venous plexus, the **plexus s. sinus venosus scleræ,** formerly called the canal of Schlemm. The optic nerve passes through the posterior part of the sclera a little below and external to the posterior pole. The opening for the nerve is crossed by interlacing fibrous strands, forming the **lamina cribrosa scleræ.**

The sclera consists of interlacing bundles of white fibrous tissue, associated with which there are a few elastic fibers. The bundles are arranged chiefly in meridional and equatorial layers. The very limited blood-supply is derived from the ciliary arteries, and the veins open into the venæ vorticosæ and ciliary veins.

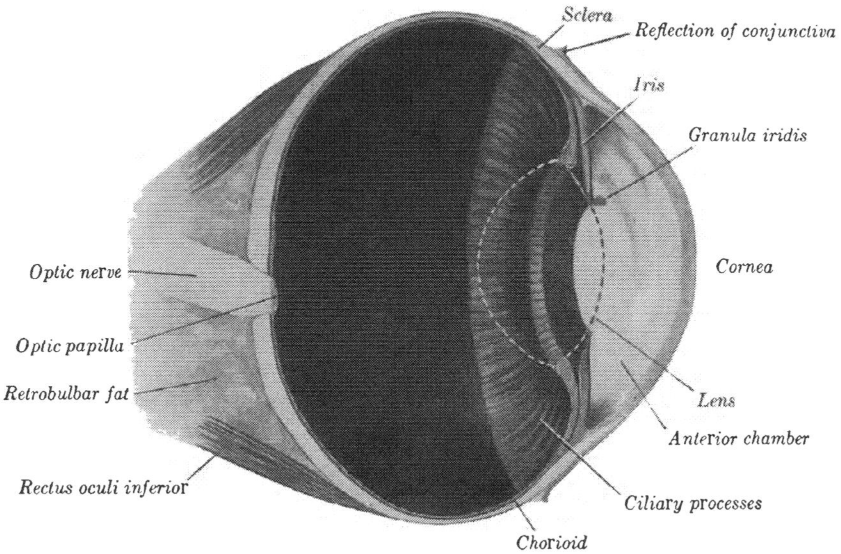

FIG. 557.—VERTICAL SECTION OF EYEBALL OF HORSE, ABOUT $\frac{3}{2}$.
The contour of the crystalline lens is dotted.

The lymphatics are represented by intercommunicating cell spaces. The nerves are derived from the ciliary nerves.

The **cornea** forms the anterior fifth of the fibrous tunic. It is transparent, colorless, and non-vascular. Viewed from in front it is oval in outline, the long axis being transverse and the broad end internal; it appears more nearly circular when viewed from behind. Its **anterior surface** (Facies anterior) is convex and is more strongly curved than the sclera; its central part is termed the **vertex corneæ.** The **posterior surface** (Facies posterior) is concave; it forms the anterior boundary of the anterior chamber, and is in contact with the aqueous humor. The margin (limbus corneæ) joins the sclera; the latter overlaps the cornea more in front than behind, and more above and below than at the sides, thus explaining the difference in outline of the two surfaces. The cornea is thinnest at the vertex.

The cornea consists, from before backward, of the following layers: (1) The **epithelium corneæ** is continuous with that of the conjunctiva scleræ, and is of the stratified squamous type. (2) The **lamina limitans anterior** is merely a condensation of the next layer. (3) The **substantia propria** forms the bulk of the cornea and is composed of interlacing bundles of connective tissue, arranged in part in lamellæ disposed parallel with the surface. In the amorphous cement substance between the lamellæ are flattened connective-tissue cells, the corneal corpuscles. These have branching processes which unite with those of other cells, thus forming a protoplasmic network.[1] (4) The **lamina elastica posterior,** also termed the membrane of Descemet or Demours, is a thin and practically homogeneous membrane which is less intimately attached to the substantia propria than the anterior lamina. It is clear, glistening, and elastic. At the periphery the lamina divides into three sets of fibers. The anterior fibers join the sclera, the middle give attachment to the ciliary muscle, while the posterior pass into the iris and form the **ligamentum pectinatum** iridis. (5) The **endothelium** (cameræ anterioris) consists of a layer of flattened polygonal cells, and is reflected on to the anterior surface of the iris.

The cornea is without blood-vessels except at its periphery, where the terminal twigs of the vessels of the sclera and conjunctiva terminate in loops. The **nerves** are derived from the ciliary nerves. They form a plexus around the periphery (Plexus annularis), from which fibers pass into the substantia propria, become non-medullated, and form the fundamental or stroma plexus. From this perforating branches pass through the anterior limiting layer and form a subepithelial plexus, from which filaments ascend between the epithelial cells. Other branches from the plexuses in the substantia propria end as fibrils which are in close relation with the corneal corpuscles.

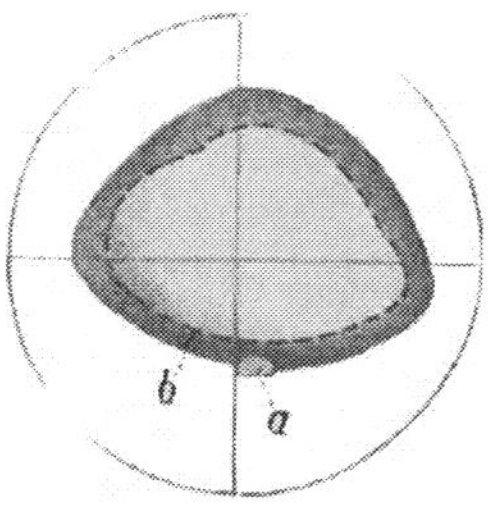

FIG. 558.—TAPETUM OF HORSE. *a*, Optic papilla; *b*, lower border of tapetum. (After Ellenberger, in Leisering's Atlas.)

THE VASCULAR TUNIC

The **vascular tunic** (Tunica vasculosa oculi) lies internal to the fibrous coat; it comprises three parts—the chorioid, the ciliary body, and the iris.

1. The **chorioid** (Chorioidea) is a thin membrane which lies between the sclera and retina. It is in general rather loosely attached to the sclera by the lamina fusca, but is intimately adherent at the point of entrance of the optic nerve and less closely in places where the ciliary vessels and nerves pass through. The inner surface is in contact with the layer of pigmented cells of the retina, which adhere so closely to the chorioid that they were formerly regarded as a part of the latter. The general color of the chorioid is dark brown, but an extensive semilunar area a little above the level of the optic papilla has a remarkable metallic luster, and is termed the **tapetum** of the chorioid (Tapetum chorioideæ). The appearance here varies in different individuals, but the prevailing colors in most cases are iridescent blue and green in various nuances shading into yellow. Posteriorly the chorioid is perforated by the optic nerve, and anteriorly it is continuous with the ciliary body.

The chorioid consists of four layers, which from without inward are as follows: (1) The **lamina suprachorioidea** consists of interlacing fine lamellæ of fibrous tissue, each containing a network of elastic tissue. Among these are large-branched, pigmented, connective-tissue cells. The spaces between the lamellæ are lined with endothelium, and form a system of lymph-clefts which together form the perichorioid space (Spatium perichorioideale). (2) The **lamina vasculosa** is the outer part

[1] According to Piersol the system of spaces and canaliculi in the substantia propria is completely filled by the cells and their processes, upon which the nutrition of the cornea largely depends. The lamina elastica anterior, formerly described as a distinct layer between the corneal epithelium and the substantia propria, does not exist as such, but there is a condensation of the superficial part of the latter, which Rollett termed the anterior limiting layer; it is not elastic.

of the proper tissue of the chorioid. It contains the larger blood-vessels, which are supported by connective-tissue and elastic fibers. (3) The **lamina chorio-capillaris** consists of an extremely rich network of capillaries embedded in an almost homogeneous matrix. Between it and the lamina vasculosa is a laver of fibro-elastic tissue, the **tapetum fibrosum,** which causes the metallic luster mentioned above. (4) The **lamina basalis** is very thin and transparent. It is composed of an inner homogeneous part and an outer elastic part.

2. The **ciliary body** (Corpus ciliare), the middle part of the vascular coat, connects the chorioid with the periphery of the iris. In meridional section it has the form of a narrow triangle, the base of which is next to the iris. On its inner side are the ciliary processes and on its outer side the ciliary muscle. It consists of three parts—the ciliary ring, ciliary processes, and ciliary muscle. The **ciliary ring** (Orbicularis ciliaris) is the posterior zone, which is distinguished from the chorioid mainly by its greater thickness and the absence of the chorio-capillaris. Its inner face presents numerous fine meridional ridges, by the union of which the ciliary processes are formed. The **ciliary processes** (Processus ciliares), more than a hundred in number, form a circle of radial folds which surround the lens and furnish attachment to the zonula ciliaris or suspensory ligament of the latter. They are small at their origin on the ciliary ring and become much thicker and higher toward their inner ends. The width of the circle formed by them is narrower at the inner side than elsewhere. Their bases extend forward to the periphery of the iris, and their inner ends are close to the margin of the lens. They bear numerous secondary folds. Their inner surface is covered by a continuation of the lamina basalis of the chorioid, on which there are two layers of epithelial cells which constitute the pars ciliaris retinæ. They consist of a rich network of tortuous vessels supported in pigmented connective tissue. The **ciliary muscle** (M. ciliaris) (Figs. 552, 555, 559) constitutes the outer part of the ciliary body, and lies between the sclera and the ciliary processes. It forms a circular band of unstriped muscle, the fibers of which are for the most part directed meridionally. They arise from the inner surface of the sclera and from the ligamentum pectinatum iridis close to the corneo-scleral junction, and run backward along the sclera to be inserted into the ciliary processes and ring. When the muscle contracts, it pulls the processes and ring forward, thus slackening the ciliary zone or suspensory ligament of the lens, and allowing the latter to become more convex. This is the mechanism of accommodation for near objects.

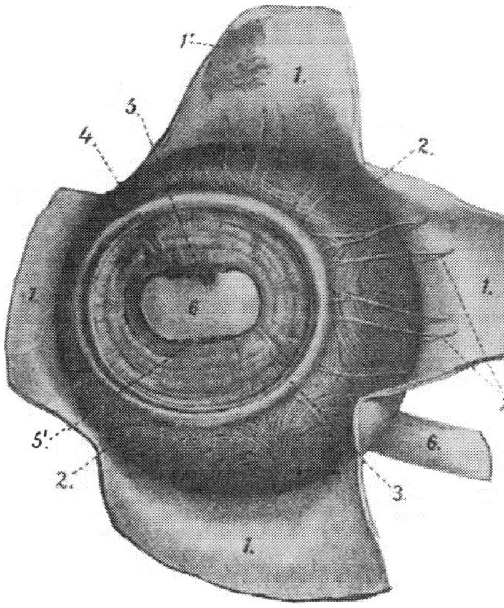

FIG. 559.—VASCULAR TUNIC OF EYEBALL OF HORSE, FRONT VIEW.

The cornea is removed and the sclera is reflected in flaps. *1*, Sclera; *1'*, lamina fusca; *2*, chorioidea; *2'*, ciliary veins; *3*, ciliary muscle; *4*, iris; *5*, *5'*, granula iridis; *6*, pupil, through which the lens is visible. (After Ellenberger, in Leisering's Atlas.)

In man the muscle has the form of a prismatic ring which is triangular in meridional section, the base being directed toward the periphery of the iris. It consists chiefly of meridional fibers, but a ring of circular fibers forms the inner angle of its base. In the horse the muscle is much less developed, and has the form of a flat band; it does not contain circular fibers, but the arrangement is rendered more or less plexiform by the existence of oblique and equatorial fibers.

3. The **iris** (Figs. 552, 557, 559) is a muscular diaphragm placed in front of the lens, and is visible through the cornea. It is pierced centrally by an elliptical opening, the **pupil** (Pupilla), which varies in size during life and determines the amount of light admitted to act on the retina. In strong light the vertical diameter of the pupil is very short, but the opening is almost circular when the pupil is fully dilated. The **ciliary** border (Margo ciliaris) or periphery of the iris is continuous with the ciliary body and is connected with the corneo-scleral junction by the ligamentum pectinatum iridis. The ligament consists of strands of connective tissue which are attached externally to the corneo-scleral junction. Its bundles interlace and inclose spaces (Spatia anguli iridis) which are lined with endothelium and communicate with the anterior chamber. The **pupillary border** (Margo pupillaris) surrounds the pupil. Its upper part bears in its middle several black masses of variable size, termed the **granula iridis** or corpora nigra; similar, but much smaller, projections may be seen on the lower margin of the pupil. The **anterior surface** (Facies anterior) determines the color of the eye, which is dark brown usually. It is marked by delicate concentric lines (Plicæ iridis), which fade out near the pupil. The smooth, narrow, central part is termed the pupillary zone or annulus iridis minor, while the much broader plicated part is the ciliary zone or annulus iridis major. The **posterior surface** (Facies posterior) is usually black. It bears numerous fine radial lines except at the pupillary margin. Its central part is in contact with the anterior surface of the lens, but peripherally the two are separated by a narrow space termed the posterior chamber. The iris consists chiefly of the **stroma iridis,** a delicate framework of connective tissue, which supports numerous blood-vessels, and contains branched pigmented cells. The muscular tissue (unstriped) consists of a sphincter and a dilator of the pupil. The **sphincter pupillæ** lies in the posterior part around the pupil, with which the fibers are largely concentric. The **dilatator pupillæ** consists of fibers which radiate outward from the sphincter to the ciliary border. The anterior surface of the iris is covered by a continuation of the endothelium of the cornea. Beneath this is a condensation of the stroma, in which the cells are close together and are full of pigmented granules.[1] There appear to be minute clefts here by which the lymph-spaces of the stroma communicate with the anterior chamber. The posterior surface is covered by a pigmented epithelium, the stratum pigmenti iridis, which is a continuation of that of the ciliary body.

The **arteries** of the vascular tunic come from the ciliary branches of the ophthalmic artery. The arteries of the chorioidea are derived chiefly from the short posterior ciliary arteries. These perforate the sclera around the posterior pole, run forward in the lamina vasculosa, and form the rich capillary network of the choriocapillaris. The two long ciliary arteries perforate the sclera obliquely near the optic nerve; they run forward in the lamina suprachorioidea in the horizontal meridian, one on the inner, the other on the outer, side of the eyeball. On reaching the ciliary body each divides into diverging branches; the subdivisions of these unite with each other and with twigs of the anterior ciliary arteries to form a circular anastomosis, the **circulus arteriosus major.** From this branches go to the ciliary muscle and processes and to the iris. The two anterior ciliary arteries, dorsal and ventral, form an episcleral plexus around the corneo-scleral junction, and give off branches which perforate the sclera. These supply twigs to the ciliary muscle and recurrent branches to the chorioid, and assist in forming the circulus arteriosus major.

The blood is carried away from the vascular tunic chiefly by four or five venous

[1] In albinos the pigment is absent here, as elsewhere, and the iris is pinkish in color.

trunks, the **venæ vorticosæ,** which are formed by the convergence in whorls of numerous veins, coming not only from the chorioid, but also from the ciliary body and iris. The venæ vorticosæ perforate the sclera about at the equator and join the veins of the ocular muscles.

The **nerves** come from the long and short ciliary nerves. They form a plexus in the lamina suprachorioidea, which contains ganglion cells, and sends numerous non-medullated fibers chiefly to the blood-vessels of the chorioid. At the ciliary muscle a second plexus (P. gangliosus ciliaris) is formed, which supplies the muscle and sends fibers to the iris. The sphincter pupillæ is supplied by fibers derived from the oculomotor nerve, while the dilatator pupillæ is innervated by the sympathetic.

THE RETINA

The **retina** or nervous tunic of the eyeball is a delicate membrane which extends from the entrance of the optic nerve to the margin of the pupil. It consists of

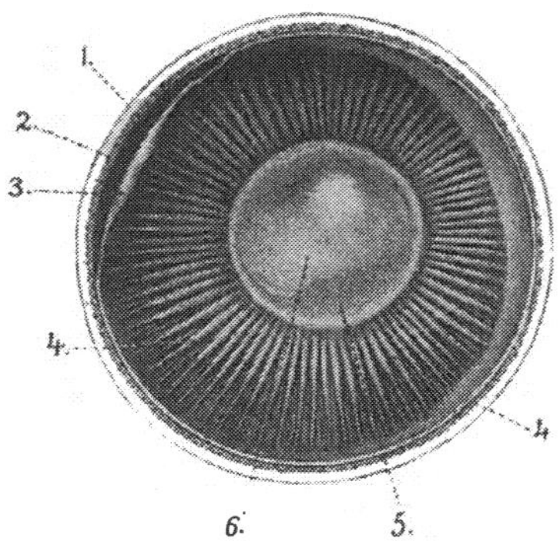

FIG. 560.—INNER SURFACE OF ANTERIOR PART OF EYEBALL OF HORSE (EQUATORIAL SECTION).

1, Sclera; *2*, chorioidea; *3*, retina (drawn away from chorioidea); *4*, ciliary processes; *5*, crystalline lens, through which the pupil (*6*) is seen. (After Ellenberger, in Leisering's Atlas.)

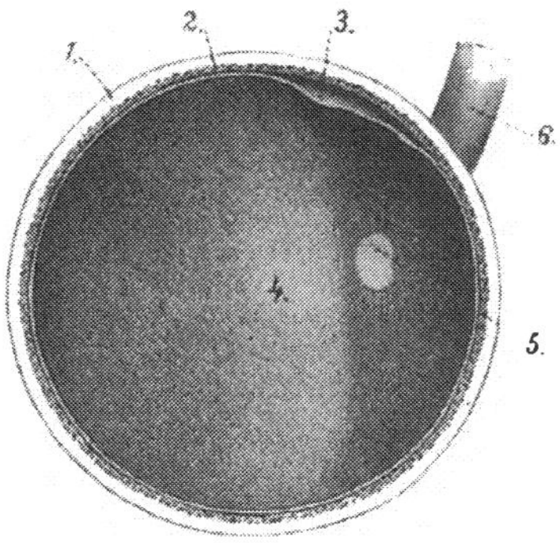

FIG. 561.—FUNDUS OCULI, SEEN ON EQUATORIAL SECTION OF EYEBALL OF HORSE.

1, Sclera; *2*, chorioidea; *3*, retina (loosened); *4*, tapetum; *5*, optic papilla; *6*, optic nerve. (After Ellenberger, in Leisering's Atlas.)

three parts. The large posterior part, which alone contains the nervous elements, including the special neuro-epithelium and the optic nerve-fibers, is termed the **pars optica retinæ.** It extends forward to the ciliary body, where it terminates at an irregular line called the **ora serrata.** Here the retina rapidly loses its nervous elements, becomes much thinner, and is continued over the ciliary body and the posterior surface of the iris by two layers of epithelial cells. In the **pars ciliaris retinæ** the inner stratum is non-pigmented, while the outer layer is a direct continuation of the stratum pigmenti of the pars optica. In the **pars iridica retinæ** both are pigmented. In the dead subject the pars optica is an opaque, gray, soft membrane which can be stripped of the chorioid, leaving most of its outer pigmented layer on the latter. During life it is transparent, except as to its pigmented epithelium, and the reddish appearance of the fundus as viewed by the ophthalmoscope is caused by the blood in the network of the choriocapillaris. The entrance of the optic nerve forms a sharply defined, oval, light area, the **optic papilla** (Papilla nervi optici), situated about 15 mm. below the horizontal meridian and 3 to 4 mm. external to the vertical meridian. The central part of the papilla is slightly depressed (Excavatio papillæ n. optici).

The transverse diameter of the papilla is about 6 to 7 mm., and the vertical about 4 to 5 mm. It is commonly situated a little below the margin of the tapetum, but the latter may extend down somewhat on either side of the papilla. The lower margin is often indented a little. In inspection of the fundus with the ophthalmoscope numerous fine branches of the arteria centralis retinæ are seen radiating from the periphery of the papilla.

The optic nerve fibers converge from all parts of the pars optica to the papilla, where they collect into bundles which traverse the lamina cribrosa of the chorioidea and sclera, and constitute the optic nerve. The **area centralis retinæ** is a round spot, 2 to 3 mm. in diameter, situated above and external to the optic papilla; it corresponds to the macula lutea of man, which is histologically more highly differentiated than the rest of the retina and is the area of most acute vision.

The **structure** of the retina is very complex. It consists of nervous elements which are supported in a peculiar sustentacular tissue, and are covered externally by a layer of pigmented epithelium (Stratum pigmenti retinæ). The nervous elements comprise a highly specialized neuro-epithelium, the rods and cones; ganglion-cells, the axones of which form the optic nerve; and intermediate neurones. Ten layers may be recognized in sections microscopically.[1]

The **arteries** of the retina are derived from the arteria centralis retinæ and anastomotic branches from the short ciliary arteries. The arteria centralis enters the optic nerve a short distance behind the eyeball and runs in the axis of the nerve. The artery divides 2 to 3 mm. before reaching the papilla, and gives off thirty to forty branches which radiate in the posterior part of the retina and divide dichotomously into end-arteries. The anterior part of the retina is non-vascular. The veins accompany the arteries except in the capillary plexuses; their walls consist merely of a layer of endothelial cells, around which are a lymph-channel and sheath.

CHAMBERS OF THE EYE AND AQUEOUS HUMOR

The **anterior chamber** of the eye (Camera oculi anterior) is inclosed in front by the cornea and behind by the iris and lens (Figs. 552, 555, 557). It communicates through the pupil with the **posterior chamber** (Camera oculi posterior); this is a small annular space, triangular in cross-section, which is bounded in front by the iris, behind by the peripheral part of the lens and its ligament, and externally by the ciliary processes. The chambers are filled by the **aqueous humor** (Humor aqueus), a clear fluid which consists of about 98 per cent. of water, with a little sodium chlorid and traces of albumin and extractives. It is carried off chiefly through the spaces (of Fontana) in the zonula ciliaris or suspensory ligament of the lens into the plexus venosus scleræ.

REFRACTIVE MEDIA OF THE EYEBALL

The **vitreous body** (Corpus vitreum) is a semifluid transparent substance situated between the crystalline lens and the retina. In front it presents a deep cavity, the **fossa hyaloidea,** which receives the posterior surface of the lens. It consists of a framework of delicate fibrils, the **stroma vitreum,** the meshes of which are filled by the fluid **humor vitreus.** The surface is covered by a condensation of the stroma known as the membrana hyaloidea.

The **crystalline lens** (Lens crystallina) is a biconvex, transparent body, situated in front of the vitreous body and in partial contact with the posterior surface of the iris. Its periphery, the **æquator lentis,** is almost circular and is closely surrounded by the ciliary processes. The **anterior surface** (Facies anterior) is convex; it is bathed by the aqueous humor and is in contact with the iris to an extent which varies with the state of the pupil. The **posterior surface** (Facies posterior) is much

[1] For the minute structure of the retina reference must be made to histological works.

more strongly curved than the anterior. It rests in the fossa of the vitreous body. The central points of the surfaces are the **anterior** and **posterior poles** (Polus anterior et posterior lentis), and the line which connects them is the axis of the lens (Axis lentis).

The transverse diameter of the lens is about 2 cm., the vertical diameter is slightly smaller, and the axis measures about 13 mm. The radius of curvature of the anterior surface is 13.5 mm., and of the posterior surface 9.5 to 10 mm. But the curvatures of its surfaces—especially that of the anterior—vary during life according as the eye is accommodated for near or far vision.

The **zonula ciliaris** (of Zinn) or suspensory ligament of the lens (Fig. 552) consists of delicate fibers (Fibræ zonulares) which pass in a meridional direction from the ciliary processes to the capsule of the equator of the lens. Many fibers cross each other, and the spaces between the fibers (Spatia zonularia) are filled with aqueous humor; they communicate with each other and with the posterior chamber.

The **substance** of the lens (Substantia lentis) is inclosed by a structureless, highly elastic membrane, the **capsule** of the lens (Capsula lentis), and consists of a softer **substantia corticalis,** and a dense central part, the **nucleus lentis.** The capsule is thickest on the anterior surface, and here it is lined by a layer of flat polygonal cells, the epithelium of the lens capsule. The lens substance, when hardened, is seen to consist of concentric laminæ arranged somewhat like the layers of an onion, and united by an amorphous cement substance. The laminæ consist of lens fibers, hexagonal in section, and of very different lengths. Faint lines radiate from the poles and indicate the edges of layers of cement substance which unite the groups of lens fibers. These lines, the **radii lentis,** are three in number in the fœtus and new-born, and form with each other angles of 120 degrees. On the anterior surface one is directed upward from the pole and the other two diverge downward; on the posterior surface one is directed downward and the others diverge upward. The developed lens has neither vessels nor nerves.

In the fœtus the lens is nearly globular, and is soft and pinkish in color. During part of fœtal life it is surrounded by a vascular network, the tunica vasculosa lentis. This is derived chiefly from a temporary vessel, the hyaloid artery, which is a continuation forward of the arteria centralis retinæ through the hyaloid canal that traverses the vitreous body. In old age the lens tends to lose its elasticity and transparency; it also becomes flatter and the nucleus especially grows denser.

THE EAR

The ear or organ of hearing (Organon auditus) consists of three natural divisions—external, middle, and internal.

THE EXTERNAL EAR

The **external ear** (Auris externa) comprises (1) the **auricula,** a funnel-like organ which collects the sound waves, together with its muscles, and (2) the **external auditory canal,** which conveys these waves to the tympanic membrane, the partition which separates the canal from the cavity of the middle ear.

The **auricula** or pinna is attached by its base around the external auditory canal in such a manner as to be freely movable. In the following description it will be assumed that the opening is directed outward and that the long axis is practically vertical. It has two surfaces, two borders, a base, and an apex. The convex surface or dorsum (Dorsum auriculæ) faces inward and is widest in its middle part; its lower part is almost circular in curvature, while above it narrows and flattens. The concave surface (Scapha) is the reverse of the dorsum; it presents several ridges which subside toward the apex. The anterior border is sinuous; it is largely convex, but becomes concave near the apex. It divides below into two diverging parts (crura helicis). The posterior border is convex. The apex is flattened, pointed, and curved a little forward. The base is strongly convex. It is attached to the external auditory process of the petrous temporal bone, and around this there is a quantity of fat. The parotid gland overlaps it below and externally. The structure of the external ear comprises a framework of cartilages (which are chiefly elastic), the integument, and a complicated arrangement of muscles.

The **conchal** or **auricular cartilage** (Cartilago auriculæ) determines the shape of the ear; its form can be made out without dissection, except below, where it is concealed by the muscles and the parotid gland. The basal part is coiled to form a tube, which incloses the cavity of the concha (Cavum conchæ). This part is funnel-shaped and curves outward and a little backward. Its internal (medial) surface is strongly convex, forming a prominence termed the **eminentia conchæ.** The lowest part of the internal margin bears a narrow, pointed prolongation, the **styloid process.** This process is about an inch long and projects downward externally over the annular cartilage; the guttural pouch is attached to its free end. Behind its base there is a foramen through which the auricular branch of the vagus passes.

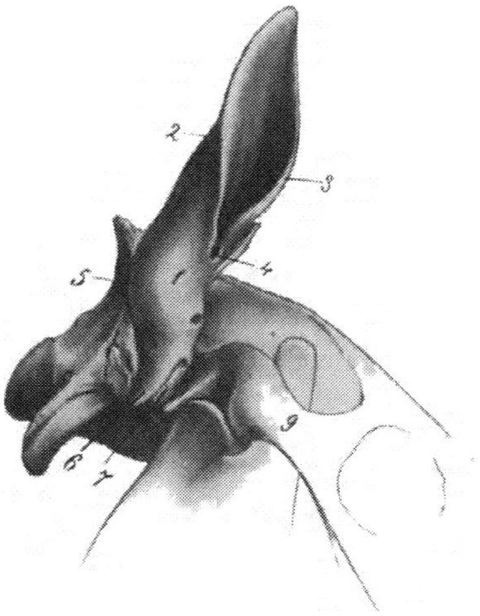

FIG. 562.—CONCHAL AND ANNULAR CARTILAGES OF EAR OF HORSE, EXTERNAL VIEW.

1, Base of concha; *2*, posterior border, *3*, anterior border of concha; *4*, intertragic notch; *5*, eminentia conchæ; *6*, styloid process; *7*, annular cartilage; *9*, zygomatic arch. (After Ellenberger-Baum, Anat. für Künstler.)

The **annular cartilage** (Cartilago annularis) is a quadrilateral plate, curved to form about three-fourths of a ring; its ends are a little less than half an inch (ca. 1 cm.) apart internally and are united by elastic tissue. It embraces the external auditory process and forms with the lower part of the conchal cartilage the cartilaginous part of the external auditory canal.

The **scutiform cartilage** (Cartilago scutiformis s. scutulum) is an irregular quadrilateral plate which lies on the temporal muscle in front of the base of the conchal cartilage. Its superficial face is slightly convex from side to side and its deep face is correspondingly concave. The anterior end is thin and rounded; the posterior part or base is wider and thicker, and its inner angle is prolonged by a pointed process half an inch or more in length. The cartilage moves very freely over the underlying parts.

The **external auditory canal** or **meatus** leads from the cavum conchæ to the tympanic membrane. It does not continue the general direction of the cavity of the concha, but extends inward, downward, and slightly forward. It consists of a cartilaginous part formed by the lower part of the conchal cartilage and the annular cartilage, and an osseous part formed by the external auditory process of the temporal bone. These are united by elastic membranes to form a complete tube. Its caliber diminishes from without inward, so that the lumen of the inner end is about half of that of the outer end.

The **skin** on the convex surface of the concha presents no special features; it is attached to the cartilage by a considerable amount of subcutaneous tissue except at the apex. The integument which lines the concave surface is intimately adherent to the cartilage and is relatively dark in color. There are three or four cutaneous ridges which run about parallel with the borders of the conchal cartilage, but do not extend to the apex or the cavum conchæ. The upper and marginal parts and the ridges are covered with long hairs, but between the ridges and below it is thin, covered sparsely with very fine hairs, and supplied with numerous sebaceous glands. In the external auditory canal the skin becomes thinner; in the cartilaginous part it is supplied with numerous large, coiled, **ceruminous glands** (Glandulæ ceruminosæ) and is sparsely covered with very fine hairs; in the osseous part the glands are small and few or absent and there are no hairs.

THE AURICULAR MUSCLES

The **auricular muscles** may be subdivided into two sets, viz., (*a*) extrinsic muscles, which arise on the head and adjacent part of the neck, and move the external ear as a whole, and (*b*) intrinsic muscles, which are confined to the auricula. In this connection the scutiform cartilage may be regarded as a sesamoid cartilage intercalated in the course of some of the muscles.

The **extrinsic** muscles are as follows:

1. The **scutularis** is a thin muscular sheet situated subcutaneously over the temporalis muscle. Its fibers arise from the zygomatic arch and the frontal and sagittal crests, and converge to the scutiform cartilage. It consists of three parts.

(*a*) The **fronto-scutularis** comprises temporal and frontal parts, which arise from the zygomatic arch and the frontal crest, and are inserted into the outer and anterior borders of the scutiform cartilage respectively.

(*b*) The **interscutularis** arises from the sagittal crest, over which it is in part continuous with the muscle of the opposite side. Its fibers converge to the inner border of the scutiform cartilage.

(*c*) The **cervico-scutularis** is not well defined from the preceding muscle. It arises from the occipital crest and is inserted into the inner border of the scutiform cartilage.

2. The **anterior auricular** muscles (Mm. auriculares nasales) are four in number.

(*a*) The **zygomatico-auricularis** arises from the zygomatic arch and the parotid fascia, and is inserted into the outer face of the base of the conchal cartilage under cover of the parotido-auricularis.

(*b*) The **scutulo-auricularis superficialis inferior** arises on the outer part of the superficial face of the scutiform cartilage and ends on the base of the conchal cartilage with the preceding muscle.

(*c*) The **scutulo-auricularis superficialis** medius arises from the posterior part of the deep surface of the scutiform cartilage and is inserted into the dorsum of the conchal cartilage, close to the lower part of its anterior border and above and behind the preceding muscle. It receives a slip from the cervico-scutularis.

(*d*) The **scutulo-auricularis superficialis** superior is a thin slip which is detached from the interscutularis over the inner border of the scutiform cartilage. It ends on the anterior aspect of the lower part of the dorsum of the conchal cartilage.

3. The **superior** auricular muscles (Mm. auriculares dorsales) are two in number.

(*a*) The **scutulo-auricularis superficialis** accessorius is a narrow band which is largely covered by the preceding muscle. It arises from the posterior prolongation and the adjacent part of the superficial face of the scutiform cartilage, and is inserted into the convex surface of the conchal cartilage internal to the preceding muscle, the two crossing each other at an acute angle.

(*b*) The **parieto-auricularis** is flat and triangular; it arises from the sagittal crest under cover of the cervico-scutularis, runs outward and a little backward, and is inserted by a flat tendon into the lower part of the convex surface of the concha under cover of the cervico-auricularis superficialis.

4. The **posterior auricular** muscles (Mm. auriculares caudales) are three in number.

(*a*) The **cervico-auricularis superficialis** is a thin triangular sheet. It is wide at its origin from the occipital crest and the adjacent part of the ligamentum nuchæ,

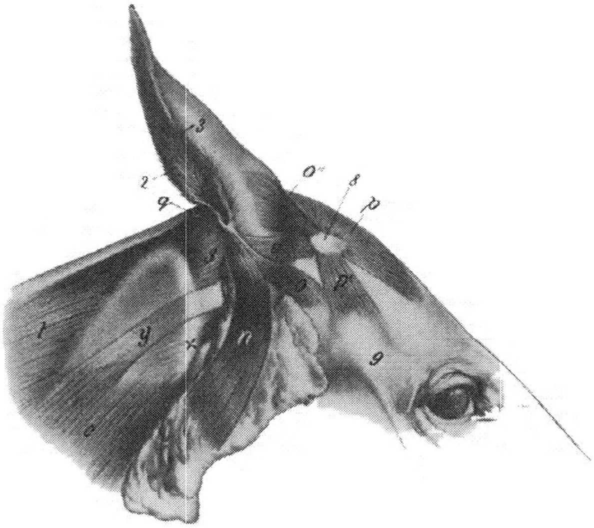

FIG. 563.—EXTERNAL EAR OF HORSE AND ITS MUSCLES, LATERAL VIEW.

2, Posterior border, *3*, anterior border of auricula; *8*, scutiform cartilage; *9*, zygomatic arch; *n*, parotido-auricularis; *o*, zygomatico-auricularis; *o'*, scutulo-auricularis superficialis inferior; *o''*, scutulo-auricularis superficialis medius et superior; *p*, interscutularis; p', fronto-scutularis (pars temporalis); q, cervico-auricularis profundus major; *s*, small (or anterior) oblique muscle of head; *t*, splenius; *y*, tendon of mastoido-humeralis; c, mastoido-humeralis; *x*, wing of atlas. (After Ellenberger-Baum, Anat. für Künstler.)

and becomes narrower as it passes outward to be inserted into the inner side of the convex surface of the concha.

(*b*) The **cervico-auricularis profundus** major arises from the ligamentum nuchæ, partly beneath and partly behind the preceding muscle. It is directed outward and is inserted into the postero-external aspect of the base of the ear, partly under cover of the parotido-auricularis.

(*c*) The **cervico-auricularis profundus minor** arises under the preceding muscle and passes downward and outward to be inserted into the lowest part of the convex surface of the concha, partly under cover of the parotid gland.

5. The **parotido-auricularis** (s. M. auricularis inferior) is a ribbon-like muscle which lies on the parotid gland. It is thin and wide at its origin from the fascia on the lower part of the parotid gland and becomes somewhat narrower and thicker as it passes upward. It is inserted into the conchal cartilage just below the angle of junction of its borders.

6. The **deep auricular** or rotator **muscles** (M. auriculares profundi s. rotatores auriculæ), two in number, are situated under the scutiform cartilage and the base of the concha and cross each other.

(*a*) The **scutulo-auricularis profundus** major is the strongest of the auricular muscles. It is flat and is about an inch wide. It arises from the deep face of the scutiform cartilage and passes backward to end on and below the most prominent part of the base of the concha (eminentia conchæ).

(*b*) The **scutulo-auricularis profundus minor** lies between the base of the concha and the preceding muscle, and is best seen when the latter is cut and reflected.

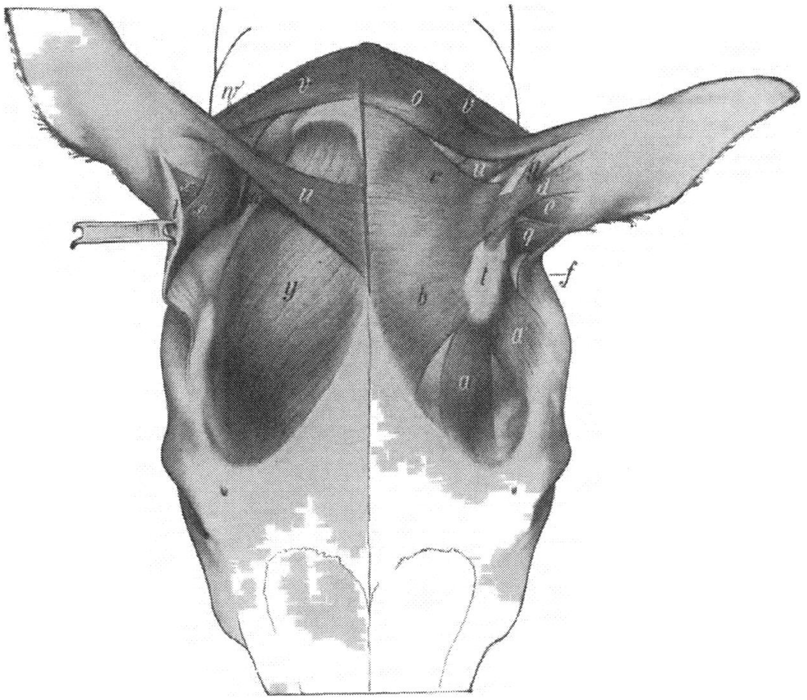

FIG. 564.—MUSCLES OF EXTERNAL EAR OF HORSE, VIEWED FROM ABOVE.

On the right side parts of the superficial muscles have been removed and the scutiform cartilage turned back to display the deeper muscles. *a*, Frontal part, *a'*, temporal part of fronto-scutularis; *b*, interscutularis; *c*, cervico-scutularis; d, *e*, scutulo-auricularis superficialis superior and medius; *f*, zygomatico-auricularis; *g*, scutulo-auricularis superficialis accessorius; *o*, cervico-auricularis superficialis; q, scutulo-auricularis superficialis inferior; *t*, scutiform cartilage; *u*, parieto-auricularis; *v*, cervico-auricularis profundus major; *w*, cervico-auricularis prof. minor; *x*, *x'*, scutulo-auricularis prof. major et minor; *y*, temporalis. (Ellenberger-Baum, Anat. d. Haustiere.)

It is flat and about an inch in length. It arises from the posterior part of the deep face of the scutiform cartilage and from the cervico-scutularis, and passes downward, backward, and outward to be inserted into the base of the concha under cover of the preceding muscle.

7. The **tragicus** or mastoido-auricularis is a small muscle which arises from the temporal bone just behind the external auditory process and from the annular cartilage; it passes upward to be inserted into the lower part of the anterior border of the conchal cartilage.

The **intrinsic muscles** are very small and of little importance. They are as follows:

1. The **antitragicus** consists of a few bundles which are attached to the conchal

cartilage behind the junction of its two borders, and are partially blended with the insertion of the parotido-auricularis.

2. The **helicis** is a small muscle attached in a position opposite to the preceding on the anterior border of the conchal cartilage; it extends also into the depression between the two divisions of the border. It is in part continuous with the insertion of the parotido-auricularis.

3. The **verticalis auriculæ**[1] is a thin stratum of muscular and tendinous fibers which extends upward on the posterior surface of the concha from the eminentia conchæ.

Actions.—The base of the concha is rounded and rests in a pad of fat (Corpus adiposum auriculæ), so that the movements of the external ear resemble those of a ball-and-socket joint. It is noticeable that movements about the longitudinal and transverse axes are accompanied by rotation. When the ear is vertical or drawn forward ("pricked up"), the opening is usually directed forward; conversely, when the ears are "laid back," the opening faces backward. These movements evidently result from the coördinated actions of several muscles which are very complex and cannot be discussed in detail here. The scutularis acting as a whole fixes the scutiform cartilage, so that the muscles which arise on the latter act efficiently on the concha. The anterior auricular muscles in general erect the ear and turn the opening forward. The interscutularis concurs in this action, causing adduction and a symmetrical position of the ears; it also acts directly on the conchal cartilage, since the scutulo-auricularis superficialis superior is in reality a conchal insertion of the interscutularis. The scutulo-auricularis superficialis accessorius draws the concha forward and turns the opening outward. The parieto-auricularis adducts the concha and inclines it forward. The cervico-auricularis superficialis is chiefly an adductor of the conchal cartilage, and directs the opening outward. The cervico-auricularis profundus major turns the opening outward and, acting with the parotido-auricularis, inclines the ear toward the poll. The cervico-auricularis profundus minor tends to direct the opening downward and outward. The parotido-auricularis draws the ear downward and backward, and acts with the cervico-auricularis profundus major in "laying back the ears"; the deep auricular muscles concur in these actions. The tragicus shortens the external auditory canal. The actions of the intrinsic muscles are inappreciable.

The **arteries** of the external ear are derived from the anterior auricular branch of the superficial temporal, the posterior or great auricular branch of the internal maxillary, and the anterior branch of the occipital artery.

The motor **nerves** to the muscles come from the auricular and auriculo-palpebral branches of the facial nerve and from the first and second cervical nerves. The sensory nerves are supplied by the superficial temporal branch of the mandibular nerve and the auricular branch of the vagus.

THE MIDDLE EAR

The **middle ear** (Auris media) or **tympanic cavity** (Cavum tympani) is a space in the tympanic and petrous parts of the temporal bone situated between the membrana tympani and the internal ear. It is a pneumatic cavity, which is lined by mucous membrane, and communicates with the pharynx and the guttural pouch by the Eustachian tube. It contains a chain of auditory ossicles by which the vibrations of the membrana tympani are transmitted to the internal ear.

The cavity consists of: (1) A main part or atrium, which lies immediately to the inner side of the membrana tympani; (2) the recessus epitympanicus, situated above the level of the membrane and containing the upper part of the malleus

[1] Ellenberger and Baum regard this as the homologue of the transversus and obliquus auriculæ of man.

and the greater part of the incus; (3) a relatively large ventral recess in the bulla ossea.

The **external wall** (Paries membranacea) is formed largely by the thin **membrana tympani,** which closes the inner end of the external auditory canal, and thus forms the septum between the external and middle parts of the ear. The membrane is an oval disc, which slopes obliquely downward and inward at an angle of about 30 degrees with the lower wall of the external auditory canal. The circumference is attached in a groove (Sulcus tympanicus) in the thin ring of bone (Annulus tympanicus) which almost completely surrounds it. The handle of the malleus (the outermost of the auditory ossicles) is attached to the inner surface of the membrane and draws the central part inward, producing a slight concavity of the outer surface. The periphery is thickened, forming the annulus fibrosus. The membrana tympani consists of three layers. The external cutaneous layer (Stratum cutaneum) is a prolongation of the lining of the external auditory meatus. The middle fibrous layer or membrana propria includes two chief sets

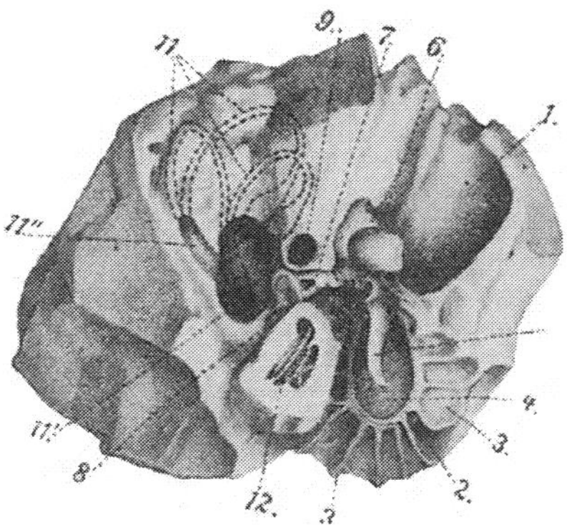

Fig. 565.—Right Petrous Temporal Bone of Horse, Antero-internal View.

1, External auditory meatus; *2,* annulus tympanicus; *3,* laminæ radiating from *2;* *4,* membrana tympani; *5,* malleus; *6,* incus; *7,* stapes; *8,* fenestra cochleæ (s. rotundum); *9,* facial canal; *11, 11'',* semicircular canals; *11',* vestibule; *12* cochlea. (After Ellenberger, in Leisering's Atlas.)

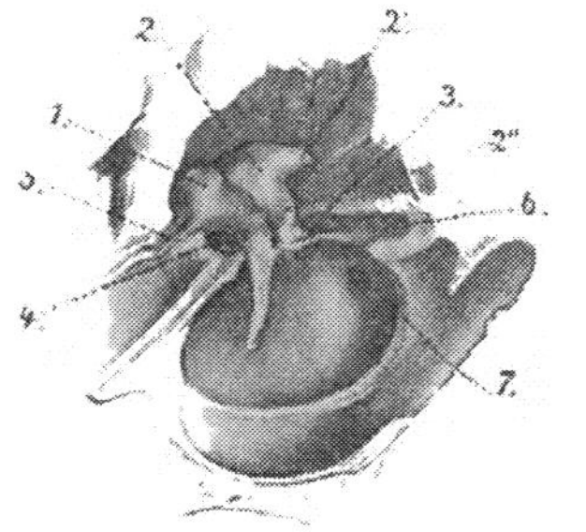

Fig. 566.—Right Auditory Ossicles and Membrana Tympani, Enlarged and Viewed from Inner Side and Below.

1, Malleus; *2,* incus; *2', 2'',* short and long processes of *2;* *3,* stapes; *4,* tensor tympani; *5,* ligament attaching long process of malleus; *6,* stapedius muscle; *7,* fenestra cochleæ (s. rotundum). (After Ellenberger, in Leisering's Atlas.)

of fibers; the outer stratum (Stratum radiatum) consists of fibers which radiate from the handle of the malleus, while the inner stratum (Stratum circulare) is composed of circular fibers which are best developed peripherally. There are also branched or dendritic fibers in part of the membrane. The internal mucous layer (Stratum mucosum) is a part of the general mucous membrane which lines the tympanic cavity

The **internal wall** of the tympanic cavity (Paries labyrinthica) separates it from the internal ear; it presents a number of special features. The **promontory** (Promontorium) is a distinct eminence near the center which corresponds to the first coil of the cochlea, and is marked by a faint groove for the superficial petrosal nerve. Above this is the **fenestra vestibuli** (s. ovalis), a reniform opening which is closed by the foot-plate of the stapes and its annular ligament. The **fenestra cochleæ** (s. rotundum) is situated below and behind the preceding; it is an irregularly oval opening and is closed by a thin membrane (Membrana tympani secundaria), which separates the tympanic cavity from the scala tympani of the cochlea.

The **anterior wall** (Paries tubaria) is narrow, and is pierced by the slit-like tympanic opening of the Eustachian tube. Above this and incompletely separated from it by a thin plate of bone is the semicanal for the tensor tympani muscle.

The superior wall or roof (Paries tegmentalis) is crossed in its inner part by the facial nerve; here the facial canal is more or less deficient ventrally, and the nerve is covered by the mucous membrane of the tympanum.

The posterior wall (Paries mastoidea) presents nothing of importance; a tympanic antrum and mastoid cells, such as are found behind the tympanic cavity proper in man and many animals, are not present in the horse.

The inferior wall or floor (Paries tympanica) is concave and thin. It is crossed by delicate curved ridges, which radiate from the greater part of the annulus tympanicus.

The auditory ossicles (Ossicula auditus) form a chain which extends from the outer to the inner wall of the cavity. They are named, from without inward, the **malleus**, the **incus**, the **os lenticulare**, and the **stapes**. The first is attached to the inner surface of the tympanic membrane and the last is fixed in the fenestra vestibuli.

The **malleus** or hammer, the largest of the ossicles, consists of a head, neck, handle, and two processes. The **head** (Capitulum mallei) is situated in the epitympanic recess. It is smooth and convex above and in front, and presents

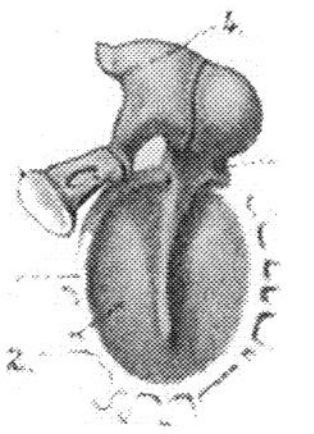

FIG. 567.—AUDITORY OSSICLES AND MEMBRANI TYMPANI, INNER VIEW, ENLARGED.

1, Annulus tympanicus; *2*, membrana tympani; *3*, malleus; *4*, incus; *5*, stapes. (After Ellenberger, in Leisering's Atlas.)

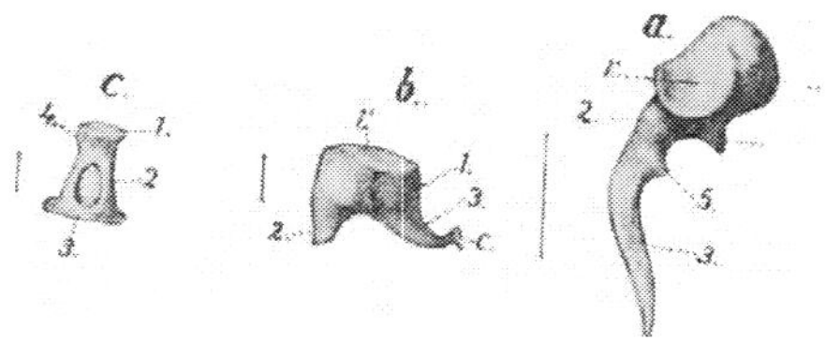

FIG. 568.—RIGHT AUDITORY OSSICLES, ENLARGED AS INDICATED BY LINES GIVING THEIR ACTUAL LENGTH.

a, Malleus; *1*, head; *2*, neck; *3*, handle; *4*, long process; *5*, muscular process. **b**, Incus; *1*, body; *2*, short branch; *3*, long branch; *c*, os lenticulare. **c**, Stapes; *1*, head; *2*, crus; *3*, base; *4*, attachment of stapedius. (After Ellenberger, in Leisering's Atlas.)

on its postero-internal aspect a concave facet for articulation with the body of the incus. The **neck** (Collum mallei) is the constricted part below the head; its inner surface is crossed by the chorda tympani. The **handle** (Manubrium mallei) is directed downward, inward, and a little forward from the neck, and is attached along its entire length to the membrana tympani. On its inner surface, near the upper end, there is a slight projection to which the tendon of the tensor tympani muscle is attached. The long process (Processus longus) is a pointed spicule which projects forward from the neck toward the petro-tympanic fissure. The short process (Processus brevis) is a slight projection of the outer side of the neck, and is attached to the upper part of the membrana tympani.

The **incus** or anvil is situated chiefly in the epitympanic recess. It may be said to resemble a bicuspid tooth with two divergent roots, and consists of a body and two processes. The **body** (Corpus incudis) articulates with the head of the hammer. The long process (Crus longum) projects downward from the body and then curves inward; its extremity has attached to it a small nodule of bone, the **os lenticulare**, which articulates with the head of the stapes. The short process (Crus breve) projects chiefly backward, and is attached to the wall of the recess by a small ligament.

The **stapes** or stirrup consists of a head, two crura, and a base. The **head**

(Capitulum stapedis) is directed outward and articulates with the os lenticulare. The crura, anterior and posterior (Crus anterius, posterius), are directed inward from the head, and join the ends of the base. The base or foot-plate (Basis stapedis) occupies the fenestra vestibuli, to which it is attached. The space between the crura and the base is closed by a membrane.

The **articulations** and **ligaments** of the auditory ossicles comprise: (1) A diarthrodial joint between the head of the malleus and the body of the incus (Articulatio incudomalleolaris), inclosed by a capsule. (2) An enarthrosis between the os lenticulare and the head of the stapes (Articulatio incudostapedia), also surrounded by a capsule. (3) The base of the stapes is attached to the margin of the fenestra vestibuli by a ring of elastic fibers (Lig. annulare bascos stapedis). (4) Small ligaments attach the head of the malleus and the short crus of the incus to the roof of the epitympanic recess. (5) The axial ligament (of Helmholtz) attaches the neck of the malleus to a small projection (Spina tympanica anterior) above and in front of the annulus tympanicus.

The **muscles** of the auditory ossicles are two in number, viz., the tensor tympani and the stapedius. The **tensor tympani** arises from the upper wall of the osseous Eustachian tube, and ends in a delicate tendon which bends outward and is inserted into the handle of the malleus near its upper end. When it contracts, it draws the handle of the malleus inward and tenses the membrana tympani; it probably also rotates the malleus around its long axis. It is innervated by the motor part of the trigeminus through the otic ganglion. The **stapedius** arises from a small prominence (Eminentia pyramidalis) of the posterior wall of the tympanum, runs forward on the facial nerve, and is inserted into the neck of the stapes. Its action is to draw the head of the stapes backward and rotate the anterior end of the base outward, thus tensing the annular ligament. It is innervated by the facial nerve.

The **tympanic mucous membrane** (Tunica mucosa tympanica) is continuous with that of the pharynx and the guttural pouch through the Eustachian tube. It is thin, closely united with the underlying periosteum, and is reflected over the ossicles, ligaments, and muscles, the chorda tympani, and the facial nerve in the open part of the facial canal. It contains minute lymph nodules and small mucous glands (Glandulæ tympanicæ). The epithelium is in general columnar ciliated, but over the membrana tympani, ossicles, and promontory it is flattened.

The **artery** of the tympanum is the stylo-mastoid, a small vessel which arises from the posterior auricular branch of the internal maxillary artery. It enters the tympanum through the stylomastoid foramen, and forms a circle around the tympanic membrane. The **nerves** of the mucous membrane come from the tympanic plexus.

The Eustachian Tube

The **Eustachian** or **auditory** tube (Tuba auditiva [Eustachii]) extends from the tympanic cavity to the pharynx; it transmits air to the former and equalizes the pressure on the two surfaces of the membrana tympani. It is directed forward, downward, and slightly inward, and is four to five inches (ca. 10 to 12 cm.) in length. Its posterior extremity lies at the inner side of the root of the muscular process of the petrous temporal, and communicates with the anterior part of the tympanic cavity by the small slit-like **tympanic opening** (Ostium tympanicum tubæ auditivæ). For a distance of about a quarter of an inch (ca. 6 to 7 mm.) in front of this opening it is a complete tube, with a curved lumen which is little more than a capillary space. Further forward it has the form of a plate which widens anteriorly and is curved to inclose a narrow groove, that opens ventrally into an extensive diverticulum termed the guttural pouch. The **pharyngeal opening** (Ostium pharyngeum tubæ auditivæ) is situated on the postero-superior part of the lateral wall of the pharynx just below the level of the posterior nares. It is a slit, an inch or more (ca. 3 cm.) in length, which slopes downward and backward. It is bounded internally by the thin free edge of the tube, from the lower part of which a fold of mucous membrane (Plica salpingo-pharyngea) extends in the same direction on the lateral wall of the pharynx for a distance of a little more than an inch usually. The outer boundary of the opening is the lateral wall of the pharynx. The basis of the tube is a plate of fibro-cartilage (Cartilago tubæ auditivæ) which is firmly attached dorsally to the fibrous tissue which closes the foramen lacerum basis cranii, the temporal wing of the sphenoid, and the pterygoid bone.[1] On cross-section the cartilage (except at its tympanic end) is seen to consist of two laminæ which are continuous with each other above. The internal lamina (Lamina medialis) gradually widens toward the pharyngeal end, where it forms a broad valvular flap. This is convex internally, and its thin anterior edge forms the inner margin of the pharyngeal opening. Behind this the lamina has a thick free edge which projects ventrally from the roof of the guttural pouch. The external lamina (Lamina lateralis) is narrow and thin, and is related externally to the levator and tensor palati muscles, which are in part attached to it; it does not exist at the pharyngeal end of the tube. The mucous membrane of the tube is continuous behind with that of the tympanum and in front with that of the pharynx. On either side it is reflected to form a large diverticulum, the guttural pouch. It is covered with ciliated epithelium, and contains mucous glands and lymph nodules.

The pharyngeal opening appears to be closed ordinarily, but the tube opens during deglutition. This action is apparently produced by the part of the palato-pharyngeus muscle which is attached to the tube.

The Guttural Pouches

The guttural pouches, right and left (Figs. 255, 256, 569), are large mucous sacs, each of which is a ventral diverticulum of the Eustachian tube (Diverticulum tubæ auditivæ); they are not present in the domesticated animals other than the equidæ. They are situated between the base of the cranium and the atlas above and the pharynx below. Medially they are in apposition in great part, but are to some extent separated by the intervening ventral straight muscles of the head. The anterior end is a small cul-de-sac which lies below the body of the presphenoid between the Eustachian tube and the median recess of the pharynx. The posterior extremity lies near or below the atlantal attachment of the longus colli. The pouch is related dorsally to the base of the cranium, the atlanto-occipital joint capsule, and the ventral straight muscles. Ventrally it lies on the pharynx and the origin of the œsophagus. Laterally the relations are numerous and complex. They comprise the pterygoid, levator palati, tensor palati, stylo-hyoideus, and digastricus muscles; the parotid and submaxillary glands; the external carotid, internal maxillary, and external maxillary arteries; the internal maxillary and jugular veins; the pharyngeal or guttural lymph glands; the glosso-pharyngeal, hypoglossal, and superior laryngeal nerves. The vagus, accessory, and sympathetic nerves, the superior cervical ganglion, the internal carotid artery, and the inferior cerebral vein are situated in a fold of the upper wall of the pouch. The pouch is reflected around the anterior border of the great cornu of the hyoid bone so as to clothe both surfaces of the upper part of the latter. It thus forms an outer compartment, which extends backward external to the great cornu and the occipito-hyoideus muscle; it is related externally to the parotid gland, the articulation of the jaw, the ascending part of the internal maxillary artery, the superficial temporal artery, and the facial nerve; dorsally it covers the mandibular nerve and its chief branches, and is attached to the styloid process of the conchal cartilage.

[1] There is, strictly speaking, no osseous part of the tube such as occurs in man. In the horse the cartilage extends to the tympanic orifice.

Each pouch communicates with the pharynx through the pharyngeal orifice of the Eustachian tube, and is in direct continuity with the mucous membrane of the latter.

The wall of the pouch is a delicate mucous membrane which is in general rather loosely attached to the surrounding structures. It is covered with ciliated epithelium and is supplied with mucous glands.

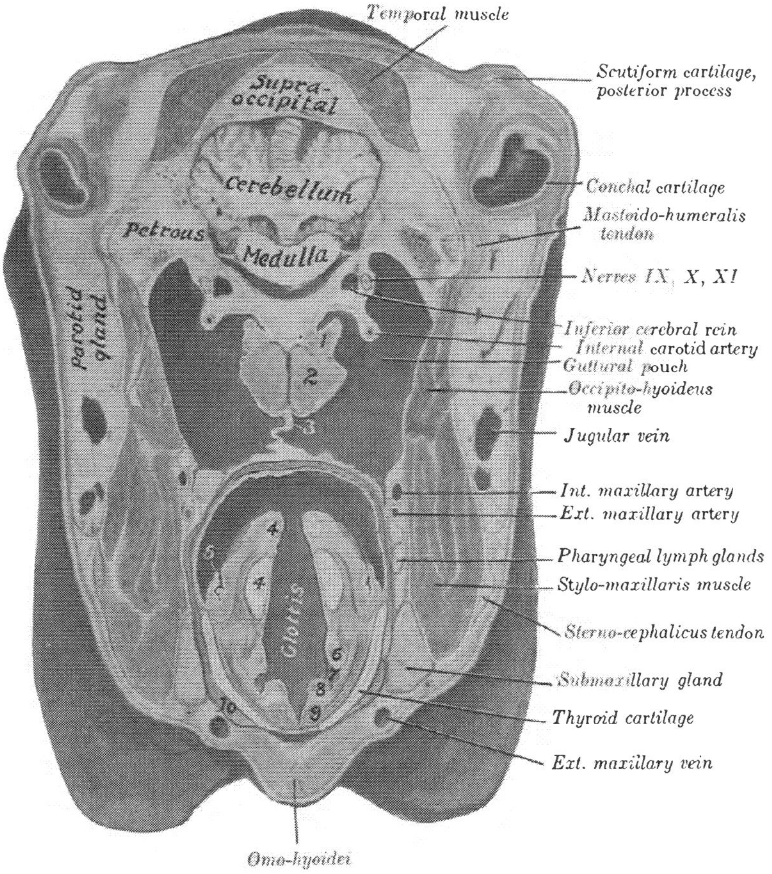

FIG. 569.—CROSS-SECTION OF HEAD OF HORSE.

The section passes through the base of the external ear and just behind the posterior border of the lower jaw. *1*, Rectus capitis anterior minor; *2*, rectus capitis anterior major; *3*, inner walls of guttural pouches in apposition; *4*, *4*, arytenoid cartilage, upper piece apex; *5*, posterior pillar of soft palate; *6*, false vocal cord; *7*, lateral ventricle of larynx; *8*, true vocal cord; *9*, vocal muscle; *10*, thyro-hyoideus muscle.

It is worthy of note that the pharyngeal orifice of the Eustachian tube is at such a level as to provide (in the ordinary position of the head) only an overflow outlet for the escape of fluid which may accumulate in the pouch. The two pouches are often unequal in size, and variations in regard to the distance which they extend backward are not uncommon. In one case, a small aged horse, the right pouch extended along the œsophagus about five inches (ca. 12 cm.) behind the ventral tubercle of the atlas, and the left one a little more than two inches (ca. 6 cm.). No pathological changes were apparent, and the condition was not recognizable externally. Cases of extreme size—so-called tympanites—of the pouches occur, and are apparently congenital defects. In a case in a yearling colt, the head of which was 24 inches long, the left pouch extended about 12 inches (ca. 30 cm.) behind the tubercle of the atlas, and had a capacity of six quarts.

The anterior end formed a cul-de-sac about two inches (ca. 5 cm.) long between the Eustachian tube and levator palati internally and the internal pterygoid muscle externally.

THE INTERNAL EAR

The **internal ear** or labyrinth (Auris interna s. Labyrinthus) consists of two parts, viz.: (1) a complex membranous sac, which supports the auditory cells and the peripheral ramifications of the auditory nerve; (2) a series of cavities in the petrous temporal bone, which inclose the membranous part. The first is called the **membranous labyrinth,** and contains a fluid, the **endolymph.** The second is the **osseous labyrinth.** The two are separated by the **perilymphatic space,** which is occupied by a fluid termed the **perilymph.**

THE OSSEOUS LABYRINTH

The **osseous labyrinth** (Labyrinthus osseus) (Fig. 565) is excavated in the petrous temporal bone to the inner side of the tympanic cavity. It consists of three divisions: (1) a middle part, the **vestibule;** (2) an anterior one, the **cochlea;** and (3) a posterior one, the **semicircular canals.**

1. The **vestibule** (Vestibulum) is the central part of the osseous labyrinth, and communicates in front with the cochlea, behind with the semicircular canals. It is a small, irregularly ovoid cavity, which is about 5 to 6 mm. in length. Its outer wall separates it from the tympanic cavity, and in it is the **fenestra vestibuli,** which is occupied by the base of the stapes. The inner wall corresponds to the fundus of the internal auditory meatus. It is crossed by an oblique ridge, the **crista vestibuli,** which separates two recesses. The anterior and smaller of these is the **recessus sphæricus,** which lodges the saccule of the membranous labyrinth. In its lower part there are about a dozen minute foramina which transmit filaments of the vestibular nerve to the saccule. The posterior and larger depression is the **recessus ellipticus,** which lodges the utricle of the membranous labyrinth. The crista vestibuli divides below into two divergent branches, which include between them the small **recessus cochlearis;** this is perforated by small foramina, through which nerve-bundles reach the ductus cochlearis. Similar foramina in the recessus ellipticus and the crista vestibuli transmit nerve filaments to the utricle and the ampullæ of the superior and external semicircular ducts. The anterior wall is pierced by an opening which leads into the scala vestibuli of the cochlea. The posterior part of the vestibule presents the four openings of the semicircular canals. The inner opening of the **aquæductus vestibuli** is a small slit behind the lower part of the crista vestibuli. The aquæductus passes backward in the petrous temporal bone, and opens on the inner surface of the latter near the middle of its posterior border; it contains the ductus endolymphaticus.

2. The osseous **semicircular canals** (Canales semicirculares ossei), three in number, are situated behind and above the vestibule. They are at right angles to each other, and are designated according to their positions as superior, posterior, and external. They communicate with the vestibule by four openings only, since the inner end of the superior and the upper end of the posterior canal unite to form a common canal (Crus commune), and the ampullate ends of the superior and external canals have a common orifice. Each canal forms about two-thirds of a circle, one end of which is enlarged and termed the **ampulla.** The **superior canal** (Canalis semicircularis superior) is nearly vertical and is placed obliquely with regard to a sagittal plane, so that its outer limb is further forward than the inner one. The antero-external end is the ampulla and opens into the vestibule with that of the external canal. The opposite non-dilated end joins the adjacent end of the posterior canal to form the crus commune, which opens into the supero-internal part of the vestibule. The **posterior canal** (Canalis semicircularis posterior) is

also nearly vertical. Its ampulla is below, and opens into the vestibule directly, while the non-dilated end joins that of the superior canal. The **external canal** (Canalis semicircularis lateralis) is nearly horizontal. Its ampulla is external and opens into the vestibule with that of the superior canal.

3. The **cochlea** is the anterior part of the bony labyrinth. It has the form of a short blunt cone, the **base** of which (Basis cochleæ) corresponds to the anterior part of the fundus of the internal auditory meatus, while the **apex** or **cupola** (Cupula) is directed outward, forward, and downward. It measures about 7 mm. across the base and about 4 mm. from base to apex. It consists of a **spiral canal** (Canalis spiralis cochleæ), which forms two and a half turns around a central column termed the **modiolus.** The modiolus diminishes rapidly in diameter from base to apex. Its base (Basis modioli) corresponds to the area cochleæ of the fundus of the internal auditory meatus, and its apex extends nearly to the cupola. Projecting from the modiolus like the thread of a screw is a thin plate of bone, the **lamina spiralis ossea.** This begins between the two fenestræ and ends near the cupola as a hook-like process (Hamulus laminæ spiralis). The lamina extends about half-way to the periphery of the cochlea and partially divides the cavity into two passages; of these, the upper one is termed the **scala vestibuli,** and the lower the **scala tympani.** The membrana basilaris extends from the free margin of the lamina to the outer wall of the cochlea and completes the septum between the two scalæ, but they communicate through the opening (Helicotrema) at the cupola. The modiolus is traversed by an axial canal which transmits the nerves to the apical coil, and by a spiral canal (canalis spiralis modioli), which follows the attached border of the lamina spiralis, and contains the spiral ganglion and vein. Close to the beginning of the scala tympani is the inner orifice of the **aquæductus cochleæ,** a small canal which opens behind the internal auditory meatus, and establishes a communication between the scala tympani and the subarachnoid space.

The **internal** auditory **meatus** has been described in part (*vide* Osteology). The fundus of the meatus is divided by a ridge (Crista transversa) into upper and lower parts. The anterior part of the upper depression (Area n. facialis) presents the cranial opening of the facial canal; and the posterior part (Area vestibularis superior) is perforated by foramina for the passage of nerves to the utricle and the ampullæ of the superior and external membranous semicircular canals. The anterior part of the inferior depression (Area cochleæ) presents a central foramen and a spiral tract of minute foramina (Tractus spiralis foraminosus) for the passage of nerves to the cochlea. Behind these is an area of small openings which transmit nerves to the saccule (Area vestibularis inferior), and a single foramen (F. singulare) for the passage of a nerve to the ampulla of the posterior semicircular canal.

The Membranous Labyrinth

The **membranous labyrinth** (Labyrinthus membranaceus) lies within, but does not fill, the osseous labyrinth. It is attached to the latter by delicate trabeculæ which traverse the perilymphatic space. It conforms more or less closely to the bony labyrinth, but consists of four divisions, since the vestibule contains two membranous sacs—the utricle and saccule.

1. The **utricle** (Utriculus), the larger of the two sacs, lies in the posterosuperior part of the vestibule, largely in the recessus ellipticus. It receives the openings of the membranous semicircular canals, and the small **ductus utriculo-saccularis** leads from its lower part to the ductus endolymphaticus.

2. The **saccule** (Sacculus) is situated in the recessus sphæricus of the vestibule. From its lower part the ductus **reuniens** proceeds to open into the ductus cochlearis, a little in front of the blind end of the latter. A second narrow tube, the **ductus endolymphaticus,** passes from the posterior part of the saccule, and is joined by the ductus utriculo-saccularis; it then traverses the aquæductus vestibuli, and term-

inates under the dura mater on the posterior part of the internal surface of the petrous temporal bone in a dilated blind end, the saccus endolymphaticus.

3. The **membranous semicircular canals** (Ductus semicirculares) correspond in general to the osseous canals already described, but it may be noted that while the ampullæ of the membranous canals nearly fill those of the osseous canals, the other parts of the membranous canals only occupy about one-fourth of the bony cavities.

4. The **cochlear duct** (Ductus cochlearis) is a spiral tube situated within the cochlea. It begins by a blind end (Cæcum vestibulare) in the cochlear recess of the vestibule, and ends by a second blind end (Cæcum cupulare), which is attached to the cupola of the cochlea. The vestibular part is connected with the saccule by the ductus reuniens. The duct is triangular in cross-section, and it is usual to regard it as having three walls. The vestibular wall or roof, which separates the cochlear duct from the scala vestibuli, is formed by the very delicate **membrana vestibularis** (of Reissner), which extends obliquely from the lamina spiralis ossea to the outer wall of the cochlea. The tympanic wall or floor intervenes between the cochlear duct and the scala tympani; it is formed by the periosteum of the marginal part of the lamina spiralis and the **membrana basilaris,** which stretches between the free edge of the lamina and the outer wall of the cochlea. The outer wall consists of the fibrous lining of the cochlea, which is greatly thickened to form the **ligamentum spirale cochleæ.**

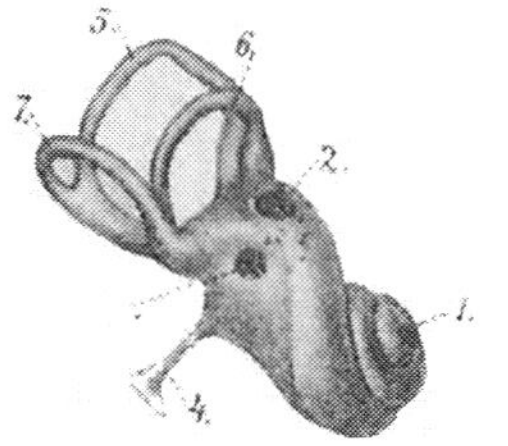

FIG. 570.—LEFT MEMBRANOUS LABYRINTH (ENLARGED).

1, Cochlea; *2*, fenestra vestibuli; *3*, fenestra cochleæ; *4*, ductus endolymphaticus; *5*, superior, *6*, external, *7*, inferior semicircular canal. (After Ellenberger, in Leisering's Atlas.)

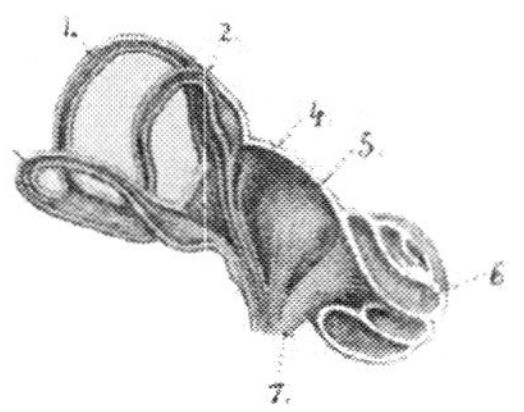

FIG. 571.—SCHEMATIC SECTIONAL VIEW OF LABYRINTH (ENLARGED).

1, *2*, *3*, Superior, external, and inferior semicircular canals; *4*, utricle; *5*, saccule; *6*, cochlea; *7*, auditory nerve. (After Ellenberger, in Leisering's Atlas.)

Structure.[1]—The membranous labyrinth consists in general of an outer thin fibrous layer, a middle transparent tunic, and an internal epithelium, composed of flattened cells. But in certain situations special and remarkable structures occur, among which are the following: (1) The **maculæ acusticæ** appear as small whitish thickenings of the inner walls of the saccule and utricle. The epithelium here consists of two kinds of cells, viz., supporting cells and hair cells. The latter are flask-shaped and are surrounded by the fusiform supporting cells. The free end of each hair cell bears a stiff, hair-like process composed of a bundle of cilia. Fibers of the saccular and utricular branches of the vestibular nerve form arborizations about the basal parts of the hair cells. Adherent to the surface of the maculæ are fine crystals of lime salts, embedded in a mucoid substance, and termed otoconia. (2) The **cristæ acusticæ** are linear thickenings of the wall of each ampulla of the membranous semicircular canals. Their structure is similar to that of the maculæ. (3) The **spiral organ** of Corti (Organon spirale) is an epithelial elevation which is situated upon the inner part of the membrana basilaris, and extends the entire length of the ductus cochlearis. It is very complicated in structure, but consists

[1] For the finer structure reference is to be made to the histological literature.

essentially of remarkable supporting cells and hair cells. Fibers of the cochlear nerve ramify about the basal parts of the hair cells.

Vessels and Nerves.—The **artery** of the internal ear is the internal auditory artery, a very small vessel which usually arises from the posterior cerebellar artery, and enters the internal auditory meatus. The **veins** go to the inferior petrosal sinus. The **vestibular nerve** is distributed to the utricle, saccule, and membranous semicircular canals, and mediates equilibration. The **cochlear nerve** gives a branch to the saccule and enters the central canal of the modiolus. Along its course it gives off fibers which radiate outward between the two plates of the lamina spiralis ossea, and ramify about the hair cells of the organ of Corti. The **ganglion spirale** or ganglion of Corti is situated in the spiral canal of the modiolus near the fixed border of the lamina spiralis. The cochlear nerve mediates the sense of hearing.

THE SKIN

The **skin** or **common integument** (Integumentum commune) is the protective covering of the body, and is continuous at the natural openings with the mucous membranes of the digestive, respiratory, and urogenital tracts. It contains peripheral ramifications of the sensory nerves, and is thus an important sense organ. It is the principal factor in the regulation of the temperature of the body, and by means of its glands it plays an important part in secretion and excretion. Some of its special horny modifications or appendages are used as organs of prehension or as weapons.

The **thickness** of the skin varies in the different species, on different parts of the body of the same animal, and also with the breed, sex, and age. The **color** also varies greatly, but this is masked in most places by the covering of hair or wool. The skin is in general highly elastic and resistant.

Permanent **folds** of the skin (Plicæ cutis) occur in certain situations, and in some places there are cutaneous **pouches** or **diverticula** (Sinus cutis).

The skin is attached to the underlying parts by the **subcutis** or **superficial fascia** (Tela subcutanea). This consists of connective tissue containing elastic fibers and fat. When the fat forms a layer of considerable thickness, it is termed the **panniculus adiposus.** Over a considerable part of the body the subcutis contains striped muscle, the **panniculus carnosus** (M. cutaneus); in some regions the fibers of the muscle are inserted into the skin, and their contraction twitches the skin or produces temporary folds.[1] The amount of subcutaneous tissue varies widely; in some places it is abundant, so that the skin can be raised considerably; in other situations it is practically absent and the skin is closely adherent to the subjacent structures. **Subcutaneous bursæ** often develop over prominent parts of the skeleton where there is much pressure or friction.

Structure.—The integument consists of the cutis or skin proper and its epidermal appendages, *e. g.*, hairs, hoofs, claws, horns, etc. The **cutis** consists of two distinct strata, viz., a superficial epithelial layer, the **epidermis,** and a deep connective-tissue layer, the **corium.**

The **epidermis** is a non-vascular, stratified epithelium of varying thickness. It presents the openings of the cutaneous glands and the hair-follicles, and its deep surface is adapted to the corium.[2] It is divisible into a superficial, harder, drier part, the **stratum corneum,** and a deeper, softer, moister part, the **stratum germinativum.** The cells of the latter contain pigment, and by their proliferation compensate the loss by desquamation of the superficial part of the stratum corneum.

[1] This muscle has been described in the Myology.

[2] To prevent a possible misapprehension, it may be stated that the epidermis primarily molds the corium, and that the glands and hair-follicles are invaginations of the epidermis.

In many places further subdivision into strata is evident on properly prepared cross-sections.

The **corium** consists essentially of a feltwork of connective-tissue and elastic fibers. It is well supplied with vessels and nerves, and contains the cutaneous glands, the hair-follicles, and unstriped muscle. The deeper part of the corium, the **tunica propria,** consists of a relatively loose network of coarse bundles of fibers, and in most places there is no clear line of demarcation between it and the subcutis. The superficial part, the **corpus papillare,** is of finer texture and is free from fat. Its superficial face is thickly beset with blunt conical prominences, the **papillæ,** which are received into corresponding depressions of the epidermis. They contain vascular loops and nerves, or, in certain situations, special nerve-endings.

The papillæ are best developed where the epidermis is thick and hairs are small or absent. On thickly-haired regions they are small or even absent. On certain parts of the body (anus, vulva, prepuce, scrotum, eyelids, etc.) the corium contains pigment in its connective-tissue cells.

The **glands** of the skin (Glandulæ cutis) are chiefly of two kinds, sudoriferous and sebaceous.

The **sudoriferous** or **sweat glands** (Glandulæ sudoriferæ) consist of a tube, the lower, secretory part of which is coiled in the deep part of the corium or in the subcutis to form a round or oval ball (Corpus glandulæ sudoriferæ). The excretory duct (Ductus sudoriferus) passes almost straight up through the corium, but pursues a more or less flexuous course through the epidermis, and opens into a hair-follicle or by a funnel-shaped pore (Porus sudoriferus) on the surface of the skin.

The **sebaceous glands** (Glandulæ sebaceæ) are in great part associated with the hairs, into the follicles of which they open. Their size varies widely, and is in general in inverse ratio to that of the hair. The larger ones are easily seen with the naked eye, and appear as small, pale yellow or brownish bodies. In certain situations (*e. g.*, the labia vulvæ, anus, prepuce) they are independent of the hairs and are well developed. In form they may be branched alveolar, simple alveolar, or even tubular in type. They secrete a fatty substance, the **sebum cutaneum,** which serves as a protective against moisture, and may also (by its aromatic constituents) play an important part in the sexual life of animals.

The two kinds of glands described above are those which are most widely distributed, but many special types occur. Some of these are to be regarded as modified sweat glands, *e. g.*, the naso-labial glands of the ox, the glands of the snout of the pig, and the glands of the plantar cushion of the horse. Others, *e. g.*, the tarsal (or Meibomian) glands of the eyelids, are modified sebaceous. Still others are not yet classified satisfactorily. Some of these special types have been referred to in previous chapters, and others will receive attention in the special descriptions which follow. The mammary glands are highly modified cutaneous glands, which are intimately associated in function with the genital organs, and have been described with the latter.

Vessels and Nerves.—The **arteries** of the skin enter from the subcutis, where they communicate freely. In the deeper part of the corium they form a plexus, and another network is formed under the papillæ. Small vessels from the deep plexus go to the fat and sweat glands, and the subpapillary plexus sends fine branches to the papillæ, hair-follicles, and sebaceous glands. The **veins** form two plexuses, one beneath the papillæ, and another at the junction of the corium and subcutis. The **lymph vessels** form subpapillary and subcutaneous plexuses.

The **nerves** vary widely in number in different parts of the skin. The terminal fibers either end free in the epidermis and in certain parts of the corium, or form special microscopic corpuscles of several kinds.

THE APPENDAGES OF THE SKIN

The appendages of the skin are modifications of the epidermis, and comprise the hairs, hoofs, claws, horns, etc.

The **hairs** (Pili) cover almost the entire surface of the body in the domesticated mammals, and some parts which appear at first sight to be bare are found on close inspection to be provided with sparse and very fine hair. The hairs are constantly being shed and replaced, but at certain periods in the horse, for example, they fall out in great numbers, constituting the shedding of the coat. It is customary to distinguish the ordinary hairs (the coat), which determine the color of the animal, from the special varieties found in certain places. Among the latter are the long **tactile hairs** about the lips, nostrils, and eyes; the **eyelashes** or **cilia**; the **tragi** of the external ear; and the **vibrissæ** of the nostrils. Other special features will be noted in the discussion of the skin of the various species. The hairs are directed in such a way as to form more or less definite **hair-streams** (Flumina pilorum), and at certain points these converge to form **vortices** (Vortices pilorum).

The part of the hair above the surface of the skin is the **shaft** (Scapus pili), while the root (Radix pili) is embedded in a depression termed the **hair-follicle**

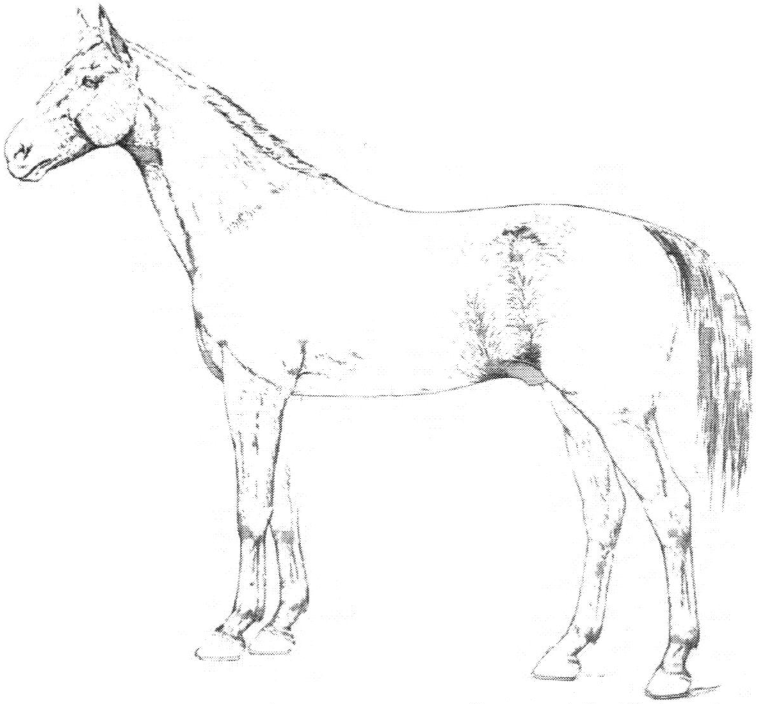

Fig. 572.—Lateral View of Horse to Show Hair-streams and Vortices. (After Ellenberger-Baum, Anat. für Künstler.)

(Folliculus pili). A vascular **papilla** (Papilla pili) projects up in the fundus of the follicle and is capped by the expanded end of the root, the **bulb** of the hair (Bulbus pili). The hair-follicles extend obliquely into the corium to a varying depth; in the case of the long tactile hairs they reach to the underlying muscle. Most of the follicles have attached to them small unstriped muscles known as the **arrectores pilorum**; these are attached at an acute angle to the under side of the deep part of the follicle, and their contraction causes erection of the hair and compression of the sebaceous glands, one or more of which open into the follicle.

The hairs are composed of epidermal cells, and consist from without inward of three parts. The **cuticle** is composed of horny, scale-like cells which overlap like slates on a roof. The **cortex** consists of horny fusiform cells which are packed close together and contain pigment. The **medulla** is the central core of softer, cubical or polyhedral cells; it contains some pigment and air-spaces.

The hair-follicles, being invaginations of the skin, are composed of a central epidermal part, and a peripheral layer which corresponds in structure to the corium. The follicles of the tactile hairs have remarkably thick walls which contain blood-sinuses between their outer and inner layers; in ungulates the sinuses are crossed by trabeculæ and assume the character of cavernous or erectile tissue.

The **hoofs, claws, horns,** and other horny structures consist of closely packed epidermal cells which have undergone cornification. In structure they might be compared to hairs matted together by intervening epidermal cells. They cover a specialized corium known as their **matrix,** from which the stratum germinativum derives its nutrition.

THE SKIN OF THE HORSE

The **thickness** of the skin of the horse varies from 1 to 5 mm. in different regions, and is greatest at the attachment of the mane and the ventral surface of the tail.

The **glands** are numerous and are larger than those of the other domesticated animals. The sebaceous glands are specially developed on the lips, the prepuce, mammary glands, perineum, and labia of the vulva. The sweat glands are yellow or brown in color. They occur in almost all parts of the skin, but are largest and most numerous on the outer wing of the nostril, the flank, mammary glands, and free part of the penis.

In addition to the ordinary and tactile **hairs** certain regions present coarse hairs of great length. The mane (Juba) springs from the dorsal border of the neck and the adjacent part of the withers; its anterior part, which covers the forehead to a variable extent, is termed the foretop (Cirrus capitis). The tail, with the exception of its ventral surface, bears very large and long hairs (Cirrus caudæ). The tuft of long hairs on the flexion surface of the fetlock (Cirrus pedis) gave rise to the popular name of this region.

The development of these special hairs varies widely, and is in general much greater in the draft breeds than in others. In Shire and Clydesdale horses, for instance, the hair on the volar aspect of the metacarpus and metatarsus and fetlock is often so long and abundant as to account for the term "feather," which is commonly applied to it by horsemen.

THE HOOF

The hoof[1] (Unguis) is the horny covering of the distal end of the digit. It is convenient to divide it for description into three parts, termed the wall, sole, and frog.

1. The **wall** is defined as the part of the hoof which is visible when the foot is placed on the ground.[2] It covers the front and sides of the foot, and is reflected posteriorly at an acute angle to form the **bars.** The latter (Pars inflexa medialis, lateralis) appear on the ground surface of the hoof as convergent ridges, which subside in front and are fused with the sole; they are united with each other by the frog. For topographic purposes the wall may be divided into an anterior part or "toe" (Pars ungulæ dorsalis), lateral parts or "quarters" (Pars ungulæ medialis, lateralis), and the angles or "heels" (Pars ungularis medialis, laterales). It presents two surfaces and two borders.

The outer surface is convex from side to side and slopes obliquely from edge to edge. In front the angle of inclination on the ground plane is about 50° for the fore limb, 55° for the hind limb; on the sides the angle gradually increases and is 100° at the angles. The curve of the wall is wider on the external than on the

[1] The hoof may be loosened and removed intact by allowing the foot to macerate or by boiling it.

[2] The term foot is used here in the popular sense, *i. e.*, to designate the hoof and the structures inclosed within it.

internal side, and the external quarter is more oblique than the internal one. The surface is smooth and is crossed by more or less distinct ridges, which are parallel with the coronary border and indicate variations in the activity of the growth of the hoof. It is also marked by fine parallel striæ, which extend from border to border in an almost rectilinear manner.

The slope of the wall varies considerably in apparently normal hoofs. Lungwitz found by careful measurements of 56 fore and 36 hind feet the following average angles:

	Fore Foot	Hind Foot
Toe	47.26°	54.1°
Inner angle	101.57°	96.50°
Outer angle	101.37°	96.1°

The wall of the fore foot may even be more upright than that of the hind, and may have an angle of 60°. The length of the wall at the toe, quarters, and heels is in the ratio of about 3 : 2 : 1 in the fore foot and about 2 : 1½ : 1 in the hind hoof.

The inner surface is concave from side to side, and bears about six hundred thin **primary laminæ** (Cristæ ungulæ), which extend from the coronary groove to the junction of wall and sole. Each bears a hundred or more **secondary laminæ** on its surfaces, so that the arrangement is pennate on cross-section. These horny laminæ are continued on the inner surface of the bars, and alternate with corresponding laminæ of the matrix.

The **proximal** or **coronary border** (Margo occultus) is thin. Its outer aspect is covered by a layer of soft horn known as the **periople**; this appears as a ring-like prominence above and gradually fades out below; at the angle it forms a wide cap or bulb and blends centrally with the frog. The inner aspect of the border is excavated to form the **coronary groove** (Sulcus coronalis ungulæ), which contains the thick coronary matrix. The groove is deepest in front, narrows on the sides, and is wide and shallow at the heels.[1] It is perforated by innumerable small, funnel-like openings which are occupied by the papillæ of the coronary matrix in the natural state.

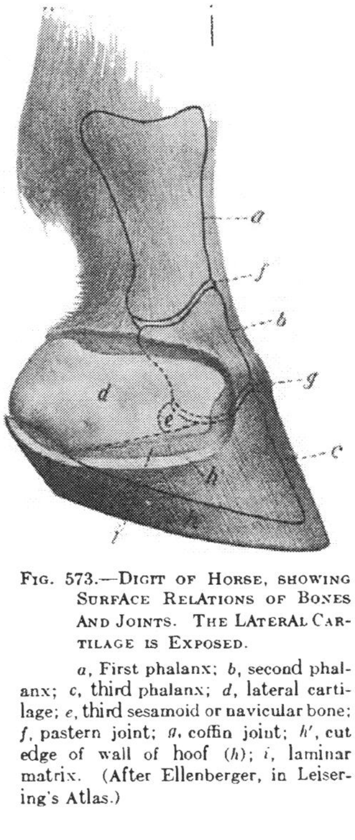

Fig. 573.—Digit of Horse, showing Surface Relations of Bones and Joints. The Lateral Cartilage is Exposed.

a, First phalanx; *b*, second phalanx; *c*, third phalanx; *d*, lateral cartilage; *e*, third sesamoid or navicular bone; *f*, pastern joint; *g*, coffin joint; *h'*, cut edge of wall of hoof (*h*); *i*, laminar matrix. (After Ellenberger, in Leisering's Atlas.)

The **distal** or **ground border** (Margo liber) of the unshod hoof comes in contact with the ground. Its thickness is greatest in front and decreases considerably from before backward on the sides, but there is a slight increase at the angles. Its inner face is united with the periphery of the sole by horn of lighter color and softer texture, which appears on the ground surface of the hoof as the **white line**.

In the case of horses at liberty the wall is usually worn off to the level of the adjacent sole, but if the ground is too soft the wall is likely to become unduly long and split or break or undergo deformation. On very hard or rough ground, on the other hand, the wear may be in excess of the growth. In the case of shod horses it is necessary to remove the excess of growth of the wall at each shoeing. The **thickness** of the wall at the toe, quarters, and heels is about in the ratio of 4 : 3 : 2 for the fore foot and about 3 : 2½ : 2 for the hind foot.

2. The **sole** (Solea ungulæ) forms the greater part of the ground surface of the hoof. It is somewhat crescentic in outline, and presents two surfaces and two borders.

[1] The wide groove at the heels, however, contains chiefly the matrix of the periople.

The **superior** or **inner surface** is convex, and slopes with a varying degree of obliquity downward to the convex border. It presents numerous small funnel-like openings which contain the papillæ of the sole matrix in the natural state

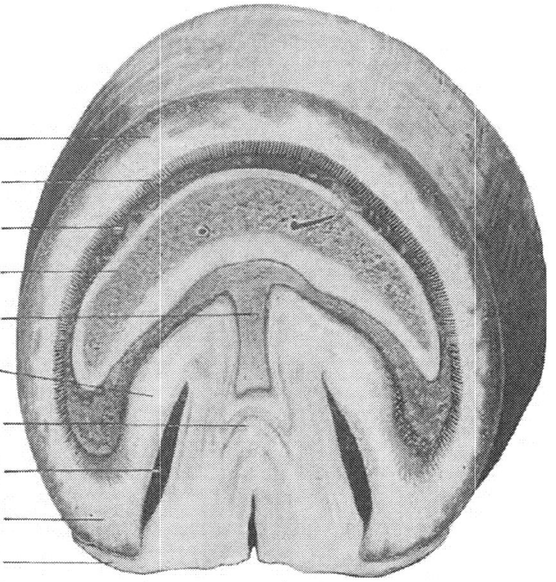

FIG. 574.—CROSS-SECTION OF FOOT OF HORSE, CUT PARALLEL WITH THE CORONARY BORDER

The **inferior** or **ground surface** is the converse of the preceding. It is normally arched—and more strongly in the hind than in the fore foot—but the curvature is subject to wide variation; in heavy draft horses the sole is commonly less curved

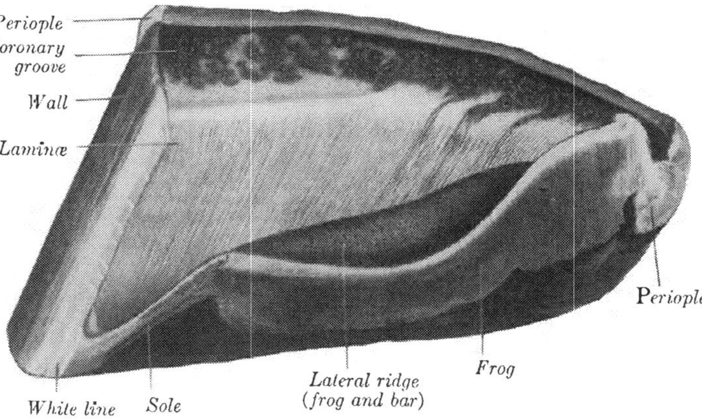

FIG. 575.—HALF OF HOOF OF HORSE, INTERNAL SURFACE

than in the lighter breeds and may even be flat. The surface is usually rough, since the horn exfoliates here in irregular flakes.

The **convex border** is joined to the wall by relatively soft horn, previously referred to as forming the white line on the ground surface of the hoof. The angle of junction is rounded internally and presents a number of low ridges and specially large openings for the papillæ of the matrix. There is frequently a ridge of larger size at the toe.

The **concave border** has the form of a deep angle which is occupied by the bars and frog. By its junction with these it forms two pronounced ridges in the interior of the foot. The parts of the sole between the wall and bars may be termed its angles.

3. The frog (Furea ungulæ) is a wedge-shaped mass which occupies the angle between the bars and sole, and extends considerably below these on the ground surface of the foot. It may be described as having four surfaces, a base, and an apex.

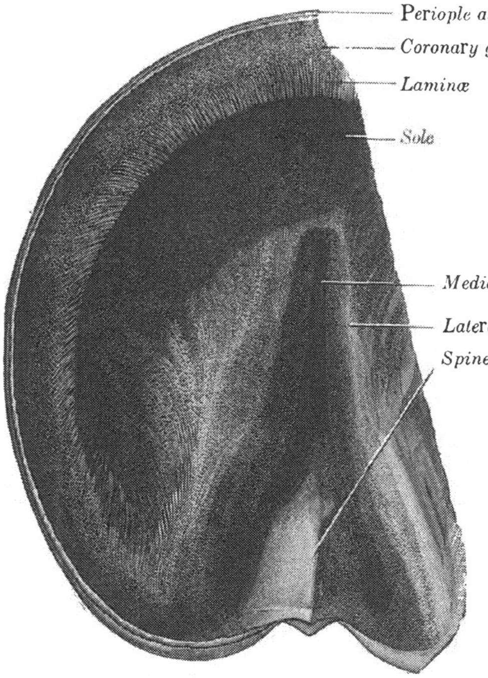

FIG. 576.—INTERNAL SURFACE OF PART OF HOOF OF HORSE. (After Schmaltz, Atlas d. Anat. d. Pferdes.)

The **superior** or **internal surface** is deeply concave from side to side. It bears a central ridge, the **spine** or **"frog-stay"** (Spina furcæ ungulæ), which is high posteriorly and subsides abruptly in front. On either side of this is a deep depression, bounded outwardly by the rounded ridge formed by the junction of the frog with the bar and sole. This surface presents fine striæ and openings for the papillæ of the frog matrix.

The **inferior** or **ground surface** presents a **central** furrow (Sulcus intercruralis), which is bounded by two ridges or crura (Crura furcæ ungulæ); these converge and form the apex.

The **sides** (Facies medialis et lateralis) are united at the upper part with the bars and sole, but are free below and form the central wall of the deep **lateral furrows** (Sulci cruroparietales), which are bounded outwardly by the bars.

The **base** is wide and high. It is depressed centrally and prominent at the sides, where it unites with the angles of the walls; the junction here is covered by the expanded periople and constitutes the bulb of the hoof.

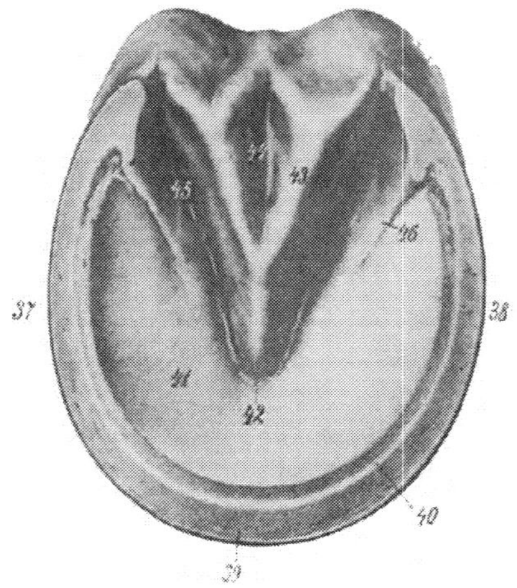

FIG. 577.—HOOF OF HORSE, RIGHT FORE FOOT GROUND SURFACE.

37, inner quarter; *38*, outer quarter; *39*, ground border of wall (toe); *40*, white line; *41*, sole; *42*, apex of frog; *43*, lateral ridge of frog; *44*, central furrow of frog; *45*, lateral furrow between frog and bar; *46*, bar. (After Ellenberger-Baum, Anat. für Künstler.)

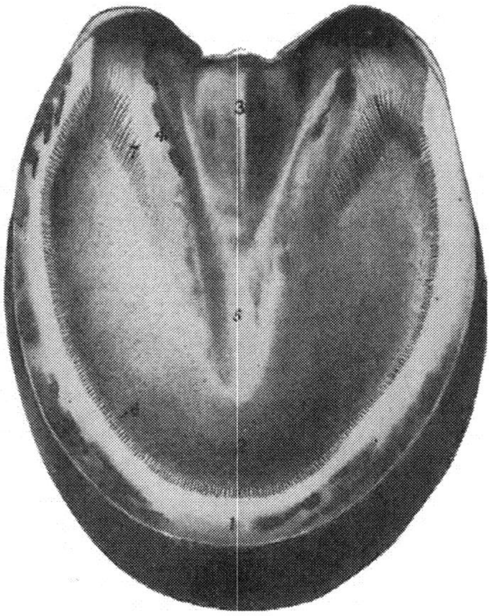

FIG. 578.—HORIZONTAL SECTION OF HOOF OF HORSE.

The section is cut just above the ridges of the frog and bars and parallel with the ground surface. *1*, Wall; *2*, sole; *3*, median ridge of frog; *4*, lateral ridge formed by junction of frog and bar; *5*, median furrow over apex of frog; *6*, laminæ of wall; *7*, laminæ of bar.

The **apex** occupies the central angle of the concave border of the sole, and forms a blunt, round prominence a little in front of the middle of the ground surface of the hoof.

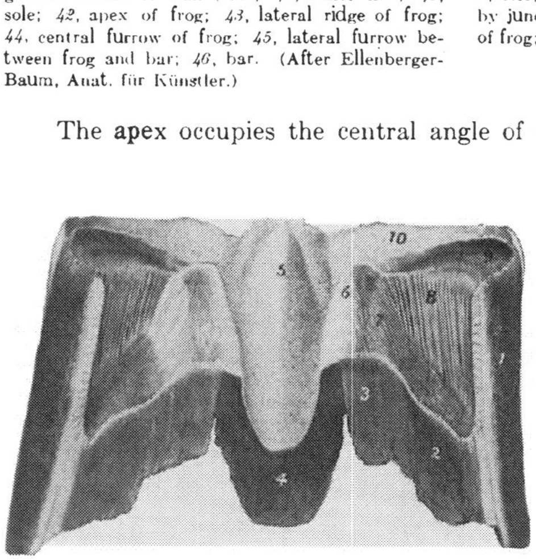

FIG. 579.—FRONTAL SECTION OF HOOF OF HORSE, POSTERIOR PART VIEWED FROM IN FRONT.

1, Wall; *2*, sole; *3*, bar; *4*, frog; *5*, median ridge of frog; *6*, lateral ridge formed by junction of frog and bar; *7*, laminæ of bar; *8*, laminæ of wall; *9*, coronary groove; *10*, periople of heel.

Structure of the Hoof.—The hoof is composed of epithelial cells which are more or less completely keratinized except in its deepest part, the **stratum germinativum;** here the cells have not undergone cornification, and by their proliferation maintain the growth of the hoof. The cells are in part arranged to form tubes which are united by intertubular epithelium, and inclose medullary cells and air-spaces.

The **wall** may be regarded as consisting of three layers. The external layer consists of the periople and the stratum vitreum. The **periople** is composed of soft, non-pigmented tubular horn. It is continuous with the epidermis above, and extends downward a variable distance.

Usually it forms a distinct band somewhat less than an inch wide, except at the heels, where it is much wider, and caps the angle of inflection of the wall proper. The **stratum vitreum** is a thin layer of horny scales which gives the wall below the periople its smooth, glossy appearance. The **middle** or **tubular layer** forms the bulk of the wall, and is the densest part of the hoof. Its horn tubes run in a straight direction from the coronary to the ground border. In dark hoofs it is pigmented except in its deep part. The internal or laminar layer consists of the **primary** and **secondary laminæ** and is non-pigmented. The laminæ are narrow and thin at their origin at the lower margin of the coronary groove, but become wider and thicker below. At the junction of the wall and sole they are united by interlaminar horn to form the white line. Only the central part of the laminæ becomes fully keratinized. They are composed of non-tubular horn in the normal state.

The **sole** consists of tubular and intertubular horn. The tubes run parallel with those of the wall and vary much in size.

The **frog** is composed of relatively soft horn, which is much more elastic than that of the wall or sole, and is not fully keratinized. The horn tubes in it are slightly flexuous.

The hoof is non-vascular and receives its nutrition from the matrix. It is also destitute of nerves.

The Matrix of the Hoof

The **matrix** of the hoof (Matrix ungulæ) is the specially modified and highly vascular part of the corium of the common integument which furnishes nutrition to the hoof. It is convenient to divide it into five parts which nourish corresponding parts of the hoof.

1. The **perioplic matrix** or **ring** (Margo matricis ungulæ) is a band 5 to 6 mm. in width which lies in a groove between the periople and the coronary border of the wall. It is continuous above with the corium of the skin, and is marked off by a groove from the coronary matrix. At the heels it widens and blends with the matrix of the frog. It bears very fine, short papillæ which curve downward and are received in depressions of the periople, to which it supplies nutrition.

2. The **coronary matrix** or **cushion** (Corona matricis ungulæ) is the thick part of the corium which occupies the coronary groove, and furnishes nutrition to the bulk of the wall. It diminishes in width and thickness posteriorly, and along the upper border of the bar it is not very clearly defined from the matrix of the frog. The convex superficial surface is thickly covered with papillæ 4 to 6 mm. in length, which are received into the funnel-like openings of the coronary groove. At the heels and along the bars the papillæ are arranged in rows, separated by fine furrows. The deep surface is attached to the extensor tendon and the lateral cartilages by an abundant subcutis which contains many elastic fibers and a rich venous plexus.

3. The **laminar matrix** (Latus matricis ungulæ)—also termed the sensitive laminæ—bears primary and secondary laminæ which are interleaved with the hornv laminæ of the wall and bars in the natural state. It is attached to the wall surface of the third phalanx by a modified periosteum (Stratum periosteale) which contains a close-meshed network of vessels, and to the lower part of the lateral cartilages by a subcutis which contains a rich venous plexus. The laminæ are small at their origin above, become wider below, and end in several papillæ 4 to 5 mm. in length. The sensitive laminæ supply nutrition to the horny laminæ and to the interlaminar horn of the white line.

4. The **sole matrix** (Latus volare matricis ungulæ)—also termed the sensitive sole—corresponds to the horny sole, to which it supplies nutrition. It is often more or less pigmented and bears long papillæ, which are specially large along the

convex border and at the angles. Centrally it is continuous with the matrix of the frog and bars. The deep surface is attached to the sole surface of the third phalanx by a modified and highly vascular periosteum.

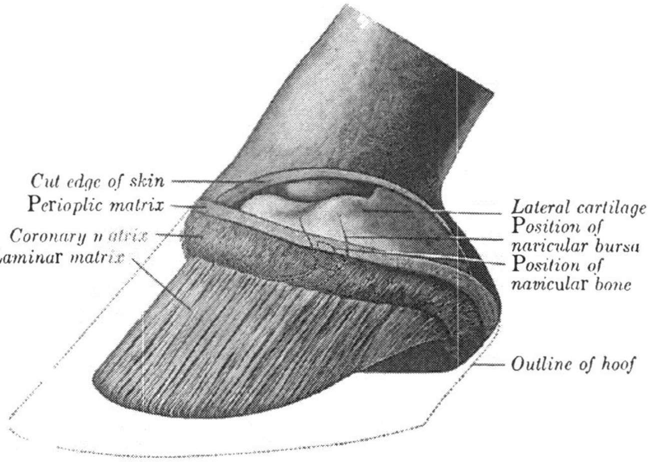

FIG. 580.—LATERAL VIEW OF FOOT OF HORSE AFTER REMOVAL OF HOOF AND PART OF SKIN. (After Schmaltz, Atlas d. Anat. d. Pferdes.)

5. The **frog matrix** (Furca matricis ungulæ)—also called the sensitive frog—is moulded on the deep surface of the frog and bears small papillæ. Its deep face is

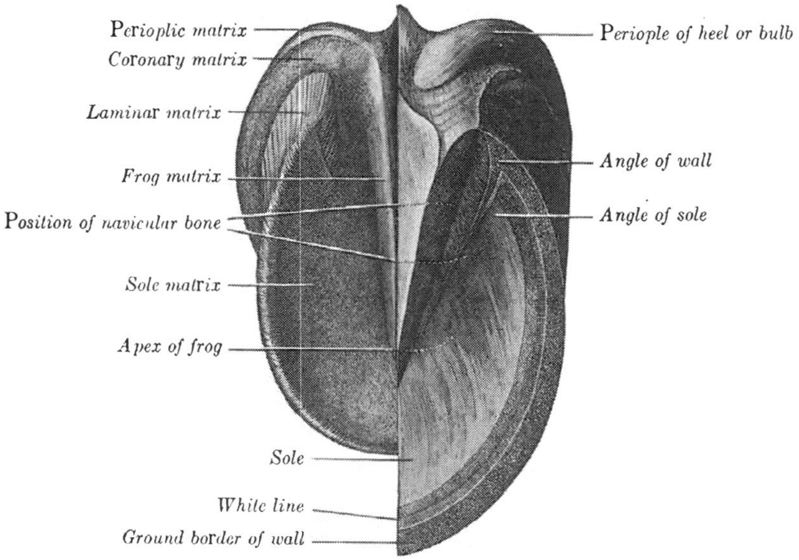

FIG. 581.—GROUND SURFACE OF FOOT OF HORSE AFTER REMOVAL OF HALF OF HOOF. (After Schmaltz, Atlas d. Anat. d. Pferdes.)

blended with the plantar cushion. The germinal cells of the frog derive their nutrition from this part of the matrix.

The **digital** or **plantar cushion** (Torus digitalis) is an important part of the elastic apparatus of the foot. It is a wedge-shaped mass which overlies the frog. It presents for description four surfaces, a base, and an apex. The **superior surface** faces upward and forward and is connected with the distal fibrous sheath of the deep flexor tendon. The **inferior surface**, covered by the matrix of the frog, is moulded on the upper face of the frog. The **lateral surfaces** are related chiefly to the lateral cartilages; inferiorly the cushion is closely attached to the cartilages, but higher up a rich venous plexus intervenes. The **base**, situated posteriorly, is partly subcutaneous, and is divided by a central depression into two rounded prominences termed the bulbs of the plantar cushion. The **apex** lies under the terminal part of the deep flexor tendon. The cushion is poorly supplied with vessels. It consists of a feltwork of fibrous trabeculæ and elastic fibers, in the meshes of which are masses of fat. The bulbs are soft and loose in texture and contain a relatively large amount of fat, but toward the apex the cushion becomes denser and more purely white fibrous in structure. Branched **coil glands** occur chiefly in the part of the cushion which overlies the central ridge of the frog. Their ducts pursue a slightly flexuous course through the matrix and pass in a spiral manner through the frog. Their secretion contains fat.

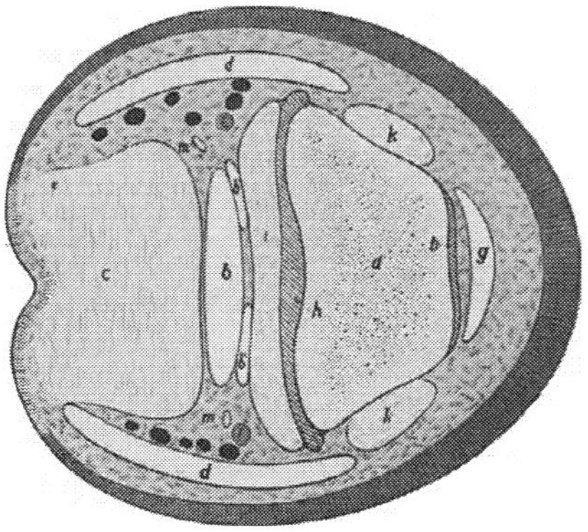

FIG. 582.—CROSS-SECTION OF DIGIT OF HORSE, THROUGH DISTAL END OF SECOND PHALANX.

a, Second phalanx; *b*, deep flexor tendon; *b'*, digital synovial sheath; *c*, plantar cushion; *d*, lateral cartilage; *e*, skin; *f*, hoof; *g*, anterior extensor tendon; *h*, cavity of coffin joint; *i*, suspensory ligament of navicular bone; k, lateral ligament of coffin joint; *l*, digital artery; *m*, digital nerve. (After Ellenberger, in Leisering's Atlas.)

Vessels and Nerves.—The matrix is richly supplied with blood by the **digital arteries.** The **veins** are valveless, and form remarkable plexuses which communicate freely with each other and are drained by the digital veins. The **lymph vessels** form subpapillary plexuses in the matrix of the sole and frog, and a wider-meshed plexus at the base of the plantar cushion. A considerable lymph vessel lies in the attached edge of each of the laminæ. The **nerves** are branches of the digital nerves; some fibers end in lamellar corpuscles and end-bulbs.

The **ergot** is a small mass of horn which is situated in the tuft of hair at the flexion surface of the fetlock. It is the vestige of the second and fourth digits of extinct equidæ, and hence is absent in cases in which these digits are developed. A small tendinous band, 3 to 5 mm. in width, extends downward and slightly forward from the fibrous basis of the ergot on each side, crosses over the digital vessels and nerves very obliquely, and blends below with the digital fascia and the plantar cushion. It is known as the ligament or tendon of the ergot.

The term **chestnut** is applied to the masses of horn which occur on the inner surface of the forearm about a handbreadth above the carpus, and on the lower part of the inner face of the tarsus. They have an elongated oval form and are flattened. They are regarded usually as vestiges of the first digit. That of the hind limb is absent in the donkey and very small in the mule.

These horny vestiges are quite variable in form and size and are correlated with the fineness or coarseness of the integument in general. The supracarpal chestnut is about 1½ to 2½ inches long, oval in outline, the proximal end being pointed; it overlies the flexor carpi internus at a quite variable distance above the carpus, and hence should not be used as a surgical landmark. The tarsal chestnut lies at a point behind the lower part of the internal lateral ligament of the hock. When well developed it is about 2 to 2½ inches long, broad below and produced above to form a long pointed end, with a short blunt anterior process. They are composed of horn somewhat like that of the frog.

ORGAN OF SMELL

The peripheral part of the olfactory apparatus or organ of smell (Organon olfactus) is that part of the nasal mucous membrane which was referred to in the description of the nasal cavity as the olfactory region; this (Regio olfactoria) is limited to the ethmo-turbinals and the adjacent part of the superior turbinal and the septum nasi, in which the fibers of the olfactory nerve ramify. It is distinguished by its yellow-brown color, thickness, and softness. It contains characteristic tubular **olfactory glands** (of Bowman), which are lined by a single layer of pigmented cells, and a neuro-epithelium, the **olfactory cells**, the central processes of which extend as non-medullated fibers to the olfactory bulb.

The epithelium is non-ciliated and is covered by a structureless limiting layer. It consists essentially of three kinds of cells, supporting, basal, and olfactory. The supporting cells are of long columnar form above and contain pigment granules; below they taper and often branch, and their central processes unite with those of adjacent cells to form a protoplasmic network. The basal cells are branched and lie on a basement membrane. The olfactory cells are situated between the supporting cells; they have the form of long narrow rods, with an enlarged lower part which is occupied by the nucleus. The peripheral end pierces the limiting membrane and bears a tuft of fine hair-like cilia (olfactory hairs). A central process extends from the nucleated pole of the cell to the olfactory bulb as a non-medullated olfactory nerve-fiber.

The **vomero-nasal organ** (of Jacobson) lies along each side of the anterior part of the lower border of the septum nasi. It communicates with the nasal cavity through the naso-palatine canal. It consists of a tube of hyaline cartilage lined with mucous membrane; a small part of the latter along the inner side is olfactory in character.

THE ORGAN OF TASTE

The peripheral part of the gustatory apparatus (Organon gustus) is formed by the microscopic **taste buds** (Calyculi gustatorii), which occur especially in the foliate, fungiform, and vallate papillæ, in the free edge and anterior pillars of the soft palate, and the oral surface of the epiglottis. The taste buds are ovoid masses, which occupy corresponding recesses in the ordinary epithelium; each presents a minute opening, the gustatory pore. The buds consist of fusiform supporting cells grouped around central gustatory **cells**. The latter are long and narrow; the peripheral end of each bears a small filament, the gustatory hair, which projects at the gustatory pore; the central end is produced to form a fine process which is often branched. The taste buds are innervated by fibers of the glosso-pharyngeal nerve and the lingual branch of the trigeminus.

SENSE ORGANS AND SKIN OF THE OX

THE EYE

The **eyelids** are thick, prominent, and less pliable than those of the horse. The lower lid bears a considerable number of cilia, which are, however, finer than those of the upper lid. The tarsal glands are more deeply embedded and therefore not so evident. The **conjunctiva** of the lower lid presents folds or ridges, and one or two prominences which contain numerous leukocytes; the conjunctival epithelium is transitional in type. The superficial part of the cartilage of the **third eyelid** is leaf or shovel-shaped and thicker than in the horse; the edge bears a narrower process, on which there is a transverse bar, giving the arrangement some resemblance to an anchor. The **gland** of the third eyelid is very large—an inch or more in length—and may be divided into two parts. The deep part is pink and consists of loose lobules, but the much larger superficial part is more compact. There are two large and several smaller excretory ducts. The subconjunctival tissue of the third eyelid contains lymph nodules, which are specially numerous on the bulbar side.

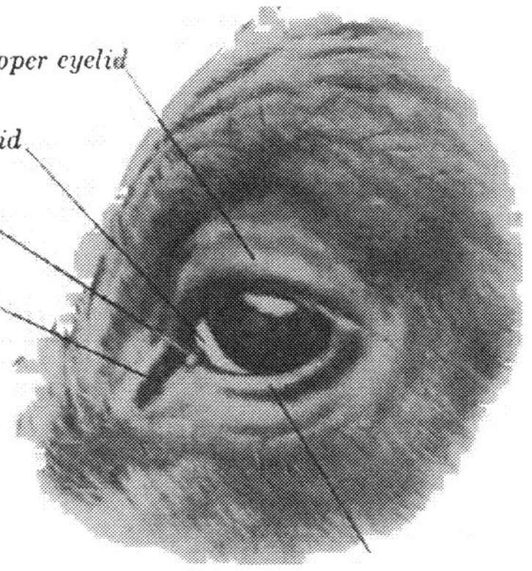

FIG. 583.—EYE OF OX. (After Ellenberger-Baum, Anat. für Künstler.)

The **lacrimal gland** is thick and distinctly lobulated. It is more or less clearly divided into a thick upper and a thinner lower part (Glandula lacrimalis superior, inferior). There are six to eight larger excretory ducts and several smaller ones. The **naso-lacrimal** duct is shorter than in the horse, and is almost straight. Its terminal part is inclosed between two plates of cartilage, and it opens near the nostril on the outer wall; the orifice is placed on the inner side of the alar fold of the inferior turbinal, and is therefore not easily found.

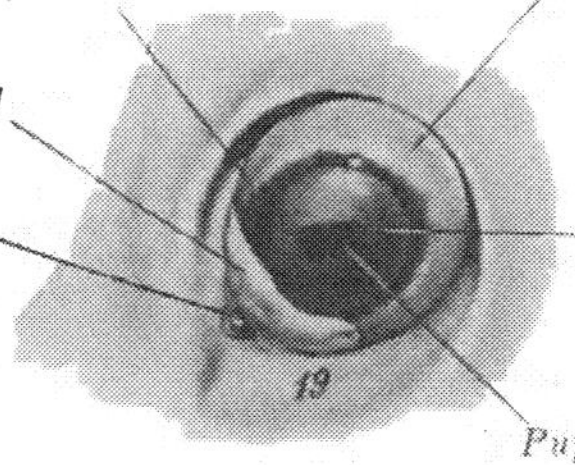

FIG. 584.—LEFT EYEBALL OF OX *in situ*, EXTERNAL VIEW.
19, Orbital fat. (After Ellenberger-Baum, Anat. für Künstler.)

The **eyeball** resembles that of the horse in shape, but is considerably smaller.

The average transverse diameter is about 42 mm., the vertical diameter 41 mm., and the axis 36 mm. The angle between the axes is about 119°.

The **sclera** is often more or less pigmented; where non-pigmented it may have a bluish tinge. The point of entrance of the optic nerve is about 2 mm. external to the vertical meridian, and about 7 mm. below the horizontal meridian.

The thickness of the sclera is about 2 mm. at the posterior pole, 1 mm. at the equator, and 1.2 to 1.5 mm. near the cornea.

The **cornea** is thicker than that of the horse.

The **tapetum** of the chorioidea is extensive at the outer side, but is a narrow strip internally. It has a metallic luster, shading from a brilliant green to a deep blue; centrally it has a reddish sheen.

The **iris** is usually very dark colored. The granula form a continuous series of small nodules along the upper margin of the pupil and are most prominent centrally; they are very small on the lower margin.

The **optic papilla** is much smaller and is not so sharply defined on ophthalmoscopic examination as that of the horse. Several relatively large retinal arteries radiate from the center of the papilla to the periphery of the retina. They may be seen to wind spirally around the veins, which are very large.

The arteria centralis retinæ arises from a posterior ciliary artery and divides close to the optic papilla into three branches usually; of these the upper is larger than the two lateral branches. The retina is more vascular than that of the horse; it has a round area centralis at the inner side, which is continued outward by a narrow strip of a similar histological structure.

The **vitreous body** is less fluid than that of the horse.

THE EAR

The **external ear** is inclined outward. The middle part is much wider and less curved than in the horse. The apex is also wide and does not curve forward. The lower part of the anterior border is bent backward and bears long hairs. The posterior border is thin and is regularly convex, except below, where it is indented. The opening is wide and the concave surface presents four ridges; the convex surface presents corresponding depressions. The styloid process of the conchal cartilage is short and blunt. The edges of the annular cartilage are in contact at the inner side and the upper border is notched externally. The scutiform cartilage is a very irregular quadrilateral plate; it is situated on the lateral aspect of the cranium with its concave surface in contact with the fat and temporalis muscle. The osseous external auditory meatus is directed practically straight inward; it is about twice as long as that of the horse, and tapers very gradually from without inward. The chief special characters of the **auricular muscles** are as follows: (1) The scutularis blends with the frontalis muscle. The interscutularis arises from the base of the processus cornu (or the corresponding area in polled cattle) and from the frontal crest. (2) The cervico-scutularis arises from the posterior surface of the cranium below the frontal eminence, and receives slips from the parieto-auricularis and cervico-auricularis superficialis. (3) The zygomatico-auricularis and scutulo-auricularis superficialis inferior are fused. (4) The scutulo-auricularis superficialis superior is distinct from the interscutularis; it arises from the superficial face of the scutiform cartilage. (5) The cervico-auricularis superficialis arises from the ligamentum nuchæ and ends on the convex surface of the conchal cartilage. (6) The parieto-auricularis arises from the nuchal surface of the frontal bone, the adjacent part of the parietal bone, and the ligamentum nuchæ; it is inserted below the preceding muscle. (7) The scutulo-auricularis superficialis accessorius arises from the superficial face of the scutiform cartilage and is inserted by a round tendon into the anterior part of the convex surface of the conchal cartilage. (8) The cervico-auricularis profundus minor consists of two fasciculi; the inner, narrow part is deep red in color, and arises from the fascia of the cervical muscles external to the occipital attachment of the ligamentum nuchæ; the outer, wider part is pale, and arises beneath the cervico-auricularis superficialis, indirectly from the scutiform cartilage. The two unite and are inserted into the lower aspect of the base of the conchal cartilage. (9) The scutulo-auricularis profundus minor arises from the temporal crest above the external auditory meatus and is inserted into the anterior part of the deep face of the scutiform cartilage.

The **cavum tympani** is small; it communicates ventrally with the air-cells of the bulla ossea. The tympanic membrane is nearly circular and is not so oblique as in the horse. The auditory ossicles are smaller than those of the horse; the malleus is more curved, the body of the incus is longer, and there is a small prominence on the front of the head of the stapes for the attachment of the stapedius muscle.

The **Eustachian tube** is small and is only about two inches long. The pharyngeal opening is small and is situated on the side of the fornix of the pharynx close to the base of the cranium. There is no flap-like expansion of the cartilage, but the inner border of the orifice is formed by a fold of mucous membrane.

The **internal ear** has essentially the same arrangement as in the horse.

COMMON INTEGUMENT

The thickness of the **skin** of the ox is greater than that of any of the other domesticated animals; in general it is about 3 to 4 mm., but at the root of the tail and the point of the hock it is about 5 mm. and on the brisket 6 to 7 mm. The variably developed prominence at the anterior part of the pectoral region known as the brisket consists of a fold of skin (Plica colli ventralis longitudinalis), which contains posteriorly a mass composed of coarse fibrous trabeculæ and fat.

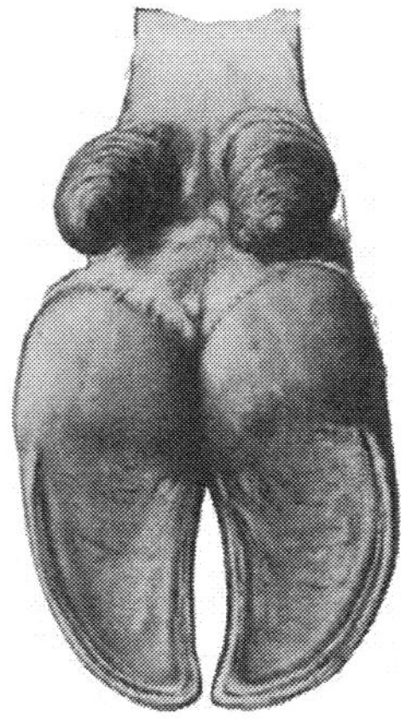

Fig. 585.—Claws of Ox, Volar Aspect. (After Ellenberger-Baum, Anat. für Künstler.)

The **cutaneous glands** are fewer and less developed than in the horse. Except about the natural openings, at the point of the hock, and the flexion surface of the fetlock, the **sweat glands** do not form a coil, but are enlarged at the deep end and are variably flexuous. The **sebaceous glands** are best developed about the natural openings and on the udder, but there are none on the teats. The **naso-labial glands** form a thick layer under the bare skin of the muzzle. They are compound tubular glands and are lined with cubical epithelium. The openings of their excretory ducts are easily seen.

The **hairs** are extremely variable in color and size in the different breeds and in different individuals. The hair of the frontal region is often curly, especially in the bull. There is no mane, and the long hairs of the tail occur only at the end, where they form the "brush" (Cirrus caudæ).

The **claws,** four in number on each limb, cover the ends of the digits. Those of the chief digits conform in a general way to the shape of the third phalanges, and each may be regarded as having three surfaces. The abaxial or outer surface is convex from side to side, and is marked by ridges parallel with the coronary border. Its anterior part is concave from edge to edge, and the angle which it forms with the ground is about 30°. The interdigital or inner surface is concave and grooved; it touches the opposite claw only at its ends. The inferior or ground surface consists of two parts, viz., a slightly concave sole, which is pointed in front and widens behind, and a prominent bulb of soft thin horn, which is continuous above with the skin. The claw may be regarded as consisting of three parts—periople, wall, and sole. The periople surrounds the coronary border in the form of a flat band, which is about half an inch wide, except at the heels, where it widens to cover the entire surface. The wall forms most of the abaxial or outer part of the claw and is reflected in front upon the interdigital surface. It thins out toward the bulb or heel, which appears, as stated above, to consist of the thin expansion of the periople. The sole occupies the angle of inflection of the wall;

it is continuous without demarcation with the periople of the bulb. The perioplic matrix bears relatively long papillæ. The coronary matrix is much less developed than in the horse and its papillæ are short. The sensitive laminæ are much narrower and are more numerous than in the horse; secondary laminæ are not present. The matrix of the sole is not marked off behind from that of the periople; its papillæ are very small and close together. The matrix of the bulbs is separated from the flexor tendon by a mass of elastic, fatty tissue, which is analogous with the plantar cushion of the horse. The papillæ here are long and often compound.

The accessory digits bear short conical horn capsules which resemble in a general way those of the chief digits, and have a similar matrix, which covers one or two nodular vestigial phalanges. From these a fibrous band descends obliquely

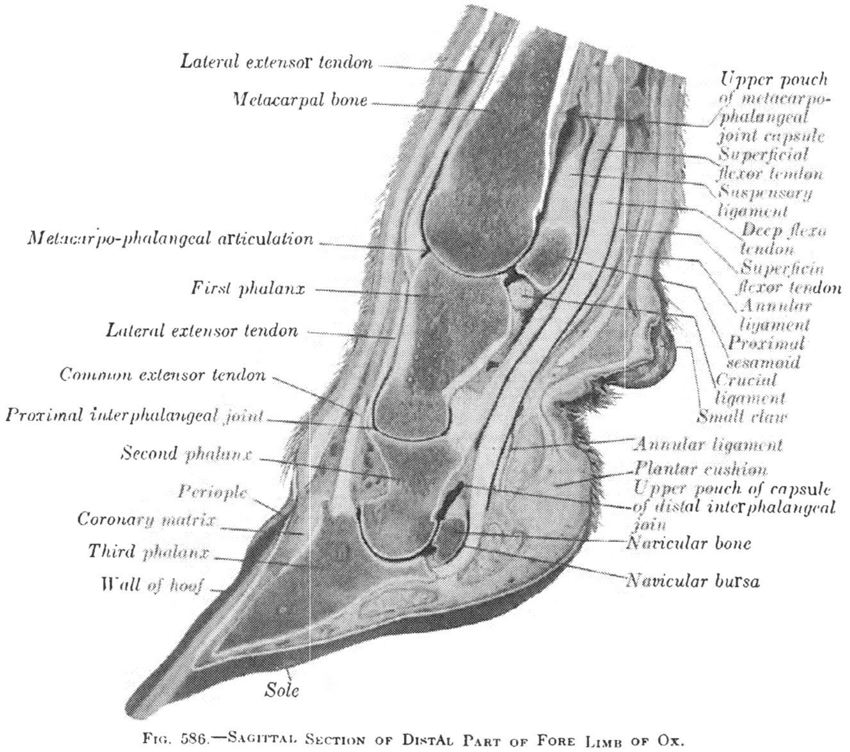

FIG. 586.—SAGITTAL SECTION OF DISTAL PART OF FORE LIMB OF OX.

on the volar aspect of each chief digit and is attached below to the distal phalanx and sesamoid bones, sending fibers also to the elastic pad of the heel.

The **horns** (Cornua) inclose the horn processes of the frontal bones (except in the polled breeds). They vary very greatly in size, form, and curvature. The root or base of the horn (Radix cornus) has a thin edge which is continuous with the epidermis. It is covered by a thin layer of soft horn similar to the periople of the hoof of the horse. Near the root the horn is encircled by variable rings. Toward the apex (Apex cornus) the thickness of the horn increases till it becomes practically a solid mass. The horn consists mainly of tubes which are very close together, except at the rings, where there is more intertubular horn. The **matrix** of the horn (Matrix cornus) is united to the horn process by periosteum which is traversed by numerous blood-vessels. The matrix at the root of the horn is thick and bears long, slender papillæ; in the body of the horn it becomes thin and the papillæ are smaller, but increase in size apically. Rudimentary papillated laminæ also occur.

The **skin** of the **sheep** varies in thickness from 0.5 to 3 mm., but differs greatly in fineness and in other respects in various breeds. In Merinos considerable folds occur on the neck. Cutaneous pouches (Sinus cutis) are constantly present in certain situations. The **infraorbital** or **lacrimal pouch** (Sinus cutaneus infraorbitalis) is an invagination about half an inch in depth, which is situated in front of the inner angle of the eye. It bears scattered fine hairs, into the follicles of which large compound sebaceous glands open; coil glands are also present. The secretion of the glands is fatty and forms a yellow sticky covering on the skin when dry. The **inguinal** (or mammary) **pouch** (Sinus cutaneus inguinalis) is much more extensive, and is situated in the inguinal region in both sexes. The skin of the pouch bears scattered fine hairs and contains well-developed sebaceous glands and exceedingly large coil glands. The **interdigital pouch** (Sinus cutaneus interdigitalis) is a peculiar tubular invagination of the integument which opens at the anterior part of the interdigital cleft. On sagittal section it appears as a bent tube, an inch or more (ca. 2.5 to 3 cm.) in length, and about a fourth of an inch (ca. 6 to 7 mm.) in diameter. The pouch extends downward and backward, and then curves sharply upward between the distal ends of the proximal phalanges. Its deep blind end is somewhat ampullate. The subcutis forms a capsule around it. The skin of the pouch is thin and pale; it bears fine colorless hairs, the follicles of which receive the secretion of several sebaceous gands. The coil glands here are compound and very large; they open into the hair-follicles or directly into the pouch. The secretion of the glands is a colorless fatty substance. The skin is covered in great part by wool, which is similar in structure to hair, but is finer, curly, and usually contains no medullary cells. The follicles of the wool are curved, and are arranged more or less distinctly in groups of ten or a dozen, several of which open in common on the surface. A considerable part of the face and the limbs is covered with short, stiff hair, and long hairs occur more or less interspersed among the wool. The claws resemble those of the ox. The horns, when present, are more or less prismatic, distinctly ringed, and vary in length and curvature in different breeds. Their structure is similar to those of the ox.

The olfactory and gustatory organs resemble in general those of the horse.

SENSE ORGANS AND INTEGUMENT OF THE PIG

THE EYE

The posterior part of the orbital margin is formed chiefly by the orbital ligament, which extends from the extremely short supraorbital process to the small eminence at the junction of the malar and the zygomatic process of the temporal.

Cilia occur only on the upper eyelid. The inner canthus is prolonged by a groove on the infraorbital region. The tarsal glands are very short and curved. The conjunctival epithelium is of the transitional type with many goblet cells.

The deep part of the cartilage of the third eyelid is broad and spoon-like, the superficial part somewhat anchor-shaped. In addition to the gland which surrounds the deep part of the cartilage, there is a deeper gland of Harder (Glandula palpebræ tertiæ profunda), which is surrounded by a distinct capsule and a blood-sinus. This gland is brownish or yellowish-gray in color, elliptical in outline, and about an inch (2 to 3 cm.) in length. It is situated deeply below the attachment of the inferior oblique muscle.

The caruncula lacrimalis has the form of a ridge; it divides into two branches which join the skin at the inner commissure. It is red in color and contains numerous large coil glands.

The lacrimal gland is mucous in type. There is no lacrimal sac, and the two lacrimal ducts pass through separate openings at the infraorbital margin. The naso-lacrimal duct is usually short and opens into the inferior meatus at the posterior end of the inferior turbinal.[1]

The eyeball appears small, partly on account of the narrowness of the palpebral opening; it closely approaches the spherical form. The cornea, although in reality almost circular, appears oval when viewed from the front, the inner end being much the broader. The chorioid has no tapetum. The iris is usually dark grayish-brown or yellowish-brown, but sometimes has a blue tinge. The pupil is a transverse oval in ordinary light, but almost circular when dilated; granula are not present. The optic papilla is nearer the posterior pole than in the horse and ox, and has a distinct central artery and vein.

THE EAR

The external ear differs considerably in size, thickness, and position. It may be carried vertically, inclined inward, or hang downward. It is relatively wide and is little curved except at the base. The concave surface presents several cutaneous ridges which correspond approximately with the long axis of the ear. The anterior border of the concha is strongly recurved in its lower part, and divides into two branches, one of which passes almost horizontally backward in the cavum conchæ, while the other continues the general direction of the border. The posterior border is slightly concave above, strongly convex below, forming a prominence somewhat analogous to the lobule of the human ear. The osseous external auditory meatus is very long and is directed downward and inward. The tympanic membrane is almost circular.

The tympanic cavity proper is small, but it is continuous with the numerous cells of the large bulla ossea. The Eustachian tube is short; its pharyngeal opening is situated in the upper part of the wall of the pharynx immediately behind the posterior nares. It is somewhat infundibular, and is bounded internally by a thick fold of mucous membrane (Torus tubarius).

THE SKIN AND APPENDAGES

The thickness of the skin in improved breeds is 1 to 2 mm. Fat usually accumulates in the subcutis and forms a distinct and often extremely thick panniculus adiposus over the greater part of the body.

The sebaceous glands are in general small and much fewer than in the other animals. The sweat glands, on the other hand, are large, yellow or brownish in color, and are in many places visible to the naked eye. At the inner side of the carpus there are small cutaneous diverticula, the so-called carpal glands, into which numerous compound coil glands open. Large glands also occur in the skin of the digits and interdigital space. Compound tubular glands are present in the skin of the snout. Large sebaceous and sweat glands are found at the entrance to the preputial diverticulum.

The hairs are sparsely scattered in improved breeds—indeed, in some cases the skin is almost bare. The long hairs or bristles are arranged usually in groups

[1] The lower punctum lacrimale is frequently absent and the corresponding duct therefore blind. There is often a duct or its remnant which opens below the inferior turbinal fold, but is not connected behind with the functional duct.

of three. They are most developed on the neck and back. The bristles about the snout and the chin are sinus hairs.

The **claws** and their matrix resemble those of the ox, but the bulbs are more prominent and form a greater part of the ground surface; they are also better defined from the sole, which is small. The claws of the accessory digits are more developed and their parts better differentiated than those of the ox.

The olfactory region is extensive in correlation with the large size of the olfactory bulbs; the mucous membrane here is brown in color.

SENSE ORGANS AND INTEGUMENT OF THE DOG

THE EYE

The posterior margin of the orbit is formed by the orbital ligament, as in the pig. The orbital axes if produced backward would include an angle of about 79°, the optic axes an angle of about 92.5° (Koschel).

The lower eyelid has no distinct cilia. The inner angle is wide, the lacus lacrimalis shallow, and the caruncula lacrimalis small and yellowish-brown. The conjunctival epithelium is cylindrical, with many goblet cells. The gland which surrounds the deep end of the cartilage of the third eyelid is large and pink; it is a mixed gland.

The lacrimal gland is flat and lies chiefly under the orbital ligament. It is pink in color and mixed in structure. The naso-lacrimal duct is variable in arrangement and may differ on the two sides. It may open into the inferior meatus immediately after its emergence from the osseous lacrimal canal; thence it continues forward and opens on the lateral wall of the nostril below the inferior turbinal fold.

The eyeball is almost spherical and is relatively large, especially in the small breeds. The sclera is thick in the ciliary region, where it contains a well-developed venous plexus; in the vicinity of the equator it is thin, and the chorioid shows through it. The cornea is almost circular. The chorioid is richly pigmented, and presents a well-defined **tapetum cellulosum;** this is somewhat triangular in outline and has a metallic luster. Its color is often golden green, shading to blue peripherally, but the blue tone may predominate, and in other cases it is mainly golden yellow or reddish-yellow. The appearance is due to several layers of peculiar flattened polygonal cells. The ciliary muscle is more developed than in the other species. The iris is commonly light or yellow brown, but not rarely has a blue tinge; the color often differs in the two eyes. The pupil is round; its edge is either smooth or bears minute round prominences. The retina presents a round area centralis external to the optic papilla. The latter is variable in outline; commonly it has the form of a triangle with the angles rounded off, but is often round or oval. Branches of the central vessels of the retina radiate from the middle of the papilla. The surfaces of the lens are not so strongly curved as in the other domestic animals, and there is little difference in the radius of curvature of the two surfaces.

THE EAR

The external ear differs greatly in size and form in the various breeds; in most it is relatively wide and thin and the greater part of it hangs down over the opening. The anterior border has a prominence (Spina helicis) at its lower part, and below this it divides into two branches (Crura helicis). One of these continues down to a blunt point, while the other turns in to the cavity of the concha. The posterior border forms a pouch below its middle, and is thick and rounded in its basal part. Here the conchal cartilage bears a pointed process (Processus uncinatus), which projects upward and backward. The outer wall of the cavum conchæ is supported by a quadrilateral plate (Tragus) above and a semiannular cartilage below. The concave surface presents several cutaneous folds, and in the cavum conchæ there are ridges and irregular prominences. There are long hairs on the borders, apex, and the folds of the concave surface, but the skin of the cavum conchæ is bare. The annular cartilage is a complete ring. The osseous external auditory meatus is wide and extremely short.

The auricular muscles are thin. The scutularis is extensive and is divisible into interscutularis and fronto-scutularis. It partly covers the occipitalis muscle, which is oval and unpaired and ends in the fascia of the frontal region. The scutulo-auriculares superficiales, inferior et accessorius, and the cervico-scutularis are not differentiated as separate muscles. The cervico-auricularis superficialis and the parieto-auricularis both bifurcate and are inserted into the base of the concha and the scutiform cartilage. The parotido-auricularis is narrow and almost long enough to meet the opposite muscle. The tragicus consists of two parts; of these the lateral one is long and arises from the border of the mandible above the angular process. The helicis and the verticalis auriculæ are well developed.

The tympanic cavity is very roomy, extending ventrally into the large but simple cavity of the bulla ossea. The tympanic membrane is extensive and oval. The promontory is very pronounced. The auditory ossicles are large. The Eustachian tube is short, and has a fibrous outer wall. Its pharyngeal opening is an oblique slit situated on the lateral wall of the naso-pharyngeal meatus, and is margined internally by a thick mucous fold.

The cochlea has three and a half turns and is more sharply pointed than in the ungulates.

THE SKIN AND APPENDAGES

The skin varies greatly in thickness in different breeds. It is remarkably loose on the dorsal aspect of the neck and trunk, where it can be raised in extensive folds. The coat is also subject to extreme variation in length, thickness, color, etc. The hairs are arranged in groups of three to a large extent. The sebaceous glands are best developed in the short and rough haired breeds. They are largest and most numerous at the lips, anus, dorsal surface of the trunk, and sternal region. The sweat glands are relatively better developed in the long and fine haired breeds. The largest are found in the digital pads. Coil glands occur in the skin of the muzzle, the perineum, and the paranal pouches.

On the flexion surface of the carpus and digit there are hairless, cushion-like pads. The carpal pad (Torus carpalis) is situated medial and distal to the accessory carpal bone. The metacarpal and metatarsal pads (Torus metacarpalis, metatarsalis) are the largest and are situated behind the distal ends of the metacarpal or metatarsal bones and the greater part of the first phalanges. They are somewhat heart-shaped, with two unequal lateral lobes, and the apex distal. The metapodio-phalangeal joints rest on them when the paw supports the weight. The digital pads (Tori digitales) are oval and are much smaller; they similarly support the second digital joints. That of the first digit is small on the fore limb, and usually absent from the hind limb. Each receives two suspensory bands from the tubercles at the distal end of the corresponding second phalanx. The pads have a basis of fibro-elastic tissue and fat, which is intimately adherent to the skin and is connected by trabeculæ with the bones and tendons. The epidermis is thick and largely keratinized, and is studded with numerous rounded papillæ which are readily seen with the naked eye. The corium has large papillæ, and contains sweat glands and lamellar corpuscles.

The **claws** (Ungues) correspond in form to the ungual part of the distal phalanges which they inclose. The horn of the claw consists of a body or wall and a sole. The former is strongly curved in both directions, and is compressed laterally. Its root or coronary border fits into the depression under the bony collar or ungual crest of the third phalanx and is covered by skin. The lateral borders converge and inclose the sole anteriorly. The matrix presents a coronary part which bears papillæ only near the coronary border. On the dorsal surface it is thickened to form a ridge, and the corresponding part of the horny covering is thick and maintains the pointed character of the claw. The matrix of the sides of the wall bears small laminæ which converge to the matrix of the sole. The latter is papillated. When the flexor muscles are inactive, the distal phalanges and the claws are maintained in dorsal flexion by two elastic ligaments. These arise from the tubercles at the proximal end of the second phalanx and converge to the dorsal aspect of the ungual crest of the third phalanx.

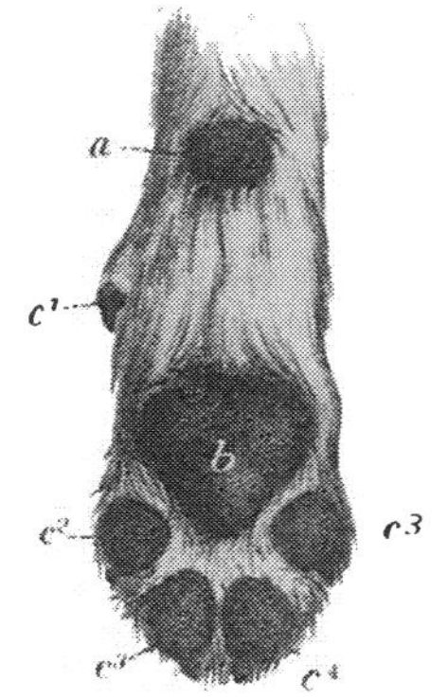

Fig. 587.—Pads of Paw of Dog.
a Carpal pad; b, metacarpal pad; c^1–c^5, digital pads. (From Leisering's Atlas.)

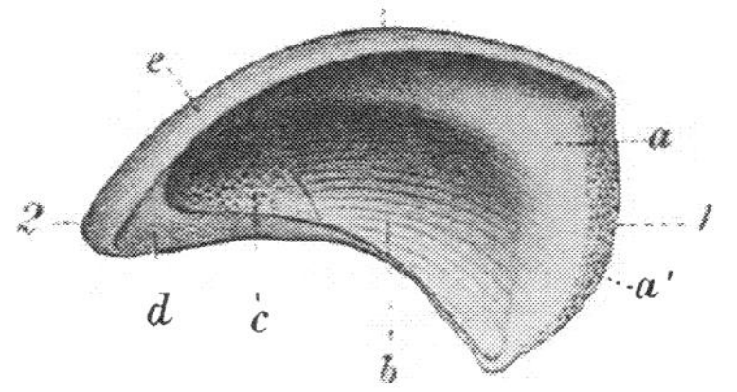

Fig. 588.—Half of Claw of Dog, inner Surface.
a, a', Coronary part, b, volar part of wall· c, sole; d, section of c; e, section of wall; 1, coronary border; 2, apex; 3, dorsal surface. (From Leisering's Atlas.)

OLFACTORY AND GUSTATORY ORGANS

The **olfactory region** lies above the lamina transversa, which separates it from the naso-pharyngeal meatus. The mucous membrane is distinguished by its thickness and yellow color, and is very extensive. It covers about half of the large ethmoturbinals, and one-third to one-half of the septum nasi. The ethmoturbinal which projects into the frontal sinus and the adjacent inner wall of the sinus is olfactory in character. Olfactory nerve-fibers ramify in the vomero-nasal organ (of Jacobson).

The gustatory apparatus presents no special features of importance.

INDEX

muscle,

of

This book has been produced in line with the EU GPSR guidelines about the safety of products.

The General Product Safety Regulation is the European Union's updated framework for ensuring that all consumer products, including books, are safe for consumers.

This book has been printed by CPI books GmbH. The printer has issued safety certificates for the materials - like ink, paper and glue - being used.

The product identifier is: 9786256629363

The author is responsible for the content of the book, is the publisher of the works and bears full responsibility for it.

The book has been published via Bookmundo. Bookmundo enables any author to share their stories with the rest of the world via printed books and ebooks and a broad distribution network.

Bookmundo will act as an intermediary in regard to questions about safety and will address them to the printer / author. Should there be any question in regard to the safety of the product, please contact us.

Bookmundo
Delftsestraat 33
3013AE Rotterdam
The Netherlands
info@bookmundo.com

FSC
www.fsc.org
MIX
Papier | Fördert gute Waldnutzung
FSC® C083411

Kolibri 360 GmbH
Ferdinand-Jühlke-Straße 7
99095 Erfurt, Deutschland
produktsicherheit@kolibri360.de